Dacie and Lewis
PRACTICAL
HAEMATOLOGY

Dacie and Lewis
PRACTICAL HAEMATOLOGY

Tenth Edition

S. Mitchell Lewis, BSc, MD, FRCPath, DCP, FIBMS

Emeritus Reader in Haematology,
University of London;
Senior Research Fellow in Haematology, Imperial College School of Medicine,
Hammersmith Hospital, London, UK

Barbara J. Bain, FRACP, FRCPath

Professor of Diagnostic Haematology,
St. Mary's Hospital Campus of Imperial College
Faculty of Medicine, London, UK

Imelda Bates, MD, FRCP, FRCPath

Senior Lecturer in Tropical Haematology,
Liverpool School of Tropical Medicine,
University of Liverpool, Liverpool, UK

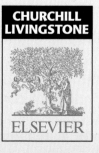

CHURCHILL
LIVINGSTONE

ELSEVIER

CHURCHILL
LIVINGSTONE
ELSEVIER

1600 John F. Kennedy Blvd.
Ste 1800
Philadelphia, PA 19103-2899

PRACTICAL HAEMATOLOGY

ISBN-13: 978-0-443-06660-3
ISBN-10: 0-443-06660-4

Notice

Knowledge and best practice in this field are constantly changing. As new research and experience broaden our knowledge, changes in practice, treatment, and drug therapy may become necessary or appropriate. Readers are advised to check the most current information provided (i) on procedures featured or (ii) by the manufacturer of each product to be administered, to verify the recommended dose or formula, the method and duration of administration, and contraindications. It is the responsibility of the practitioner, relying on their own experience and knowledge of the patient, to make diagnoses, to determine dosages and the best treatment for each individual patient, and to take all appropriate safety precautions. To the fullest extent of the law, neither the Publisher nor the Authors assume any liability for any injury and/or damage to persons or property arising out or related to any use of the material contained in this book.

The Publisher

Previous editions copyrighted 1950, 1956, 1963, 1968, 1975, 1984, 1991, 1995, 2001.

Library of Congress Cataloging-in-Publication Data
Dacie and Lewis practical haematology/[edited by] S. Mitchell Lewis, Barbara J. Bain, Imelda Bates.–10th ed.
    p.; cm.
Rev. ed. of: Practical haematology/Sir John V. Dacie, S.M. Lewis. 8th ed. 1995.
Includes bibliographical references and index.
ISBN 0-443-06660-4
1. Blood–Examination. 2. Hematology–Technique.
[DNLM: 1. Hematologic Diseases–diagnosis. 2. Hematologic Tests. 3. Blood. 4. Laboratory Techniques and Procedures. QY 400 D1177 2006] I. Title: Practical haematology. II. Lewis, S.M. (Shirley Mitchell) III. Bain, Barbara J. IV. Bates, Imelda. V. Dacie, John V. (John Vivian), Sir. VI. Dacie, John V. (John Vivian), Sir. Practical haematology.
RB45.D24 2006
616.07'561–dc22

2005053767

Acquisitions Editor: Dolores Meloni
Developmental Editor: Kristina Oberle
Project Manager: David Saltzberg
Printed in Germany
Last digit is the print number: 9 8 7 6 5 4 3 2 1

Contents

Contributors

Barbara J. Bain, FRACP, FRCPath
Imperial College Faculty of Medicine
St. Mary's Hospital
London, UK

Imelda Bates, MD, FRCP, FRCPath
Liverpool School of Tropical Medicine
University of Liverpool
Liverpool, UK

Sheena Blackmore CSci, FIBMS
Department of Haematology
Good Hope Hospital NHS Trust
Birmingham, UK

Anne Bradshaw, BSc, FIBMS, DMLM
Department of Haematology
Hammersmith Hospital
London, UK

Daniel Catovsky, FRCP, FRCPath, DSc, FMedSci
Royal Marsden Hospital
The Institute of Cancer Research
London, UK

Barbara De la Salle, MSc, CSci, FIBMS
UK NEQAS (H)
Watford General Hospital
Watford, UK

Inderjeet Dokal, MD, FRCP, FRCPath
Department of Haematology
Imperial College Faculty of Medicine
Hammersmith Hospital
London, UK

Malcolm Hamilton, MRCP, FRCPath
Haematology Department
Good Hope Hospital
Sutton Coldfield, UK

Jaspal Kaeda, PhD, FIBMS, GiBiol
Department of Haematology
Hammersmith Hospital
London, UK

Sue Knowles, BSc, MB, FRCP, FRCPath
Department of Haematology
St. Helier's Hospital
Carshalton, Surrey, UK

Mike Laffan, DM, FRCP, FRCPath
Department of Haematology
Imperial College Faculty of Medicine
Hammersmith Hospital
London, UK

Mark D. Layton, FRCP, FRCPCH
Department of Haematology
Imperial College Faculty of Medicine
Hammersmith Hospital
London, UK

S. Mitchell Lewis, BSc, MD, FRCPath, DCP, FIBMS
Department of Haematology
Imperial College School of Medicine
Hammersmith Hospital
London, UK

Richard Manning, BSc, FIBMS
Department of Haematology
Hammersmith Hospital
London, UK

Estella Matutes, MD, PhD, FRCPath
Royal Marsden Hospital
The Institute of Cancer Research
London, UK

Barry Mendelow, MD
Department of Haematology
University of Witwatersrand
Johannesburg, South Africa

Clare Milkins, BSc, CSci, FIBMS
UK NEQAS (BGS)
Watford General Hospital
Watford, UK

Ricardo Morilla, MSc
Royal Marsden Hospital
Department of Academic Haematology
London, UK

Fiona Regan, MRCP, MRCPath
Department of Haematology
Hammersmith Hospital
London, UK

David Roper, FIBMS, MSc
Department of Haematology
Hammersmith Hospital
London, UK

Megan Rowley, FRCP, FRCPath
Department of Haematology
Kingston Hospital
Kingston, UK

David Swirsky, FRCP, MRCPath
Department of Haematology
Leeds General Infirmary
Leeds, UK

Noriyuki Tatsumi, MD, PhD
International Buddhist University
Osaka, Japan

Tom Vulliamy, BA, PhD
Department of Haematology
Hammersmith Hospital
London, UK

Barbara Wild, PhD, FIBMS
Department of Haematology
King's College Hospital
London, UK

Nay Win, FRCP, FRCPath
Red Cell Immunohaematology
National Blood Service: Tooting Centre
London, UK

Mark Worwood, BSc, PhD, FRCPath, FMed Sci
Department of Haematology
Cardiff University School of Medicine
Heath Park, Cardiff, UK

Preface

This 10th edition celebrates the 55th year of *Practical Haematology*. The first edition by J.V. Dacie was published in 1950. This work, and subsequent editions with Mitchell Lewis as co-author, were based on the haematology course for the London University Diploma of Clinical Pathology (DCP) and subsequently the MSc in Haematology at the then Royal Postgraduate Medical School.

Medical science has expanded exponentially in the last half century, but no discipline has expanded more than haematology in both its clinical and laboratory aspects. Originally laboratory haematology was virtually restricted to the "blood count" with a counting chamber and a microscope. The blood count remains an essential test as it provides an important component for diagnosis and patient management, but today automated instruments analyse the physico-chemical properties of individual blood cells and provide precise metrological data on the red cells, leucocytes, and platelets at a speed that would have been beyond imagination in those early days. Sophisticated technology enables complex analyses to be performed routinely in many laboratories; these include DNA studies, immunophenotyping for leukaemia classification, diagnosis of megaloblastic anaemias, and radio isotope measurements. However, we recognize that many of the more sophisticated tests are not readily available in all laboratories, and a chapter is devoted to the essential tests in under-resourced laboratories and health centres. We also take account of the increasing use of commercially available ready-to-use kits for many laboratory tests and the trend for some tests to be performed at point-of-care; advice is given on the supporting role of the laboratory in order to ensure the reliability of this latter practice.

Another advance with enormous impact is the internet. Virtually every topic is to be found, often with an overwhelming amount of information, from a single key word. We have indicated a few important Websites that are relevant to haematology, including those of manufacturers of specialized devices and reagents.

Biomedical scientists are increasingly responsible for laboratory practice as medically qualified haematologists become more concerned with clinical care of patients. But both groups should be aware of the importance of effective laboratory organization and management, the need to maintain a high technical standard in the laboratory, with well-established quality control, and an understanding of the clinical relevance of haematological investigations. The principles for good laboratory practice were established by Dacie in his first edition, when he wrote that "all those concerned with laboratory work should understand what is the significance of the tests that they carry out, the relative value of haematological investigations and the order in which they should be undertaken." We have attempted to maintain his approach in context and style, albeit appropriately updated to meet present-day practices.

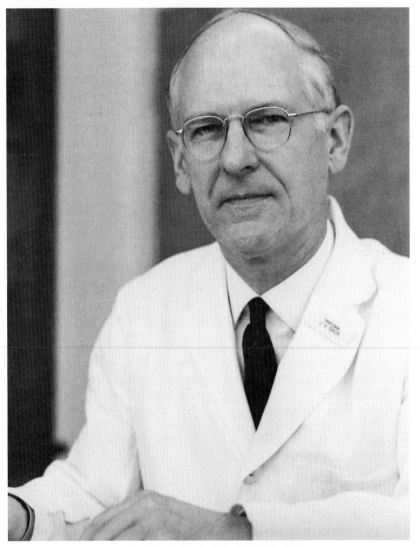

Sir John V Dacie, MD, FRCPath, FRS
1912–2005

We are grateful to all our contributors whose names are listed on pages vii–viii, and also to other colleagues who gave us learned advice on specific topics. These include, especially, Michel Deenmamode (Radioisotopes), Mark Griffin (Health & Safety), Julia Howard (Cytogenetics), John Meek (Clinical Chemistry), Andrew Osei-Bimpong (General Haematology).

As a fifty-five-year tribute, this edition is dedicated to Sir John Dacie, to his students from many countries whose subsequent distinguished careers were inspired by him, and to the centre of excellence that he created in the former Royal Postgraduate Medical School, University of London, now Faculty of Medicine of Imperial College at Hammersmith Hospital.

S. Mitchell Lewis
Barbara J. Bain
Imelda Bates

Abbreviations

2,3 DPG	2,3-diphosphoglycerate	CHAD	cold haemagglutinin disease
2-ME	2-mercaptoethanol	CLL	chronic lymphocytic leukaemia
ABC	antibody binding capacity	CLL/PL	chronic lymphocytic leukaemia with increased prolymphocytes
ACD	acid-citrate dextrose		
ACRES	amplification created restriction enzyme site	CML	chronic myeloid leukaemia
		CPD	cirtate–phosphate–dextrose
ADA	adenosine deaminase	CTP	cytosine triphosphate
ADP	adenosine-diphosphate	CV	coefficient of variation
AET	2-aminoethyl-*iso*-thiouronium	Cy	cytoplasmic
AIHA	autoimmune haemolytic anaemia	DAB	diaminobenzidine
ALL	acute lymphoblastic leukaemia	DAT	direct antiglobulin test
AML	acute myeloid leukaemia	DMSO	dimethylsulphoxide
ANAE	alpha-naphthyl acetate esterase	DNA	deoxyribonucleic acid
ANB	alpha-naphthyl butyrate	DTT	dithiothreitol
APAAP	alkaline phosphatase anti-alkaline phosphatase	EDTA	ethylenediaminetetraacetic acid
		EGIL	European Group for the Immunological Classification of Leukaemias
APTT	activated partial thromboplastin time		
ARMS	amplification refractory mutation system	ELISA	enzyme-linked immunosorbent assay
ASOH	allele-specific oligonucleotide hybridization	FAB	French-American-British (classification)
		FDPs	fibrin/fibrinogen degratation products
AT	antithrombin	FVL	factor V Leiden
ATLL	adult T-cell leukaemia/lymphoma	FITC	fluorescein isothiocyanate
ATP	adenosine triphosphate	FSc	forward light scatter
BCSH	British Committee for Standards in Haematology	g	either gram or relative centrifugal force, as appropriate
bp	base pair	G6PD	glucose-6-phosphate dehydrogenase
B-PLL	B-cell prolymphocytic leukaemia	GPI	glycosylphosphatidylinositol
BM	bone marrow	Hb	haemoglobin or haemoglobin concentration
BSA	bovine serum albumin		
C	complement	HbCO	carboxyhaemoglobin
C3, C3d, C3sg	complement components	HCL	hairy cell leukaemia
		HCT	haematocrit
CAE	naphthol AS-D chloroacetate esterase	HDW	haemoglobin distribution width
CD	cluster of differentiation		

HEMPAS	hereditary erythroblastic multinuclearity with positive acidified-serum test	PCH	paroxysmal cold haemoglobinuria
Hi	methaemoglobin	PCR	polymerase chain reaction
HiCN	cyanmethaemoglobin	PCV	packed cell volume
HIV	human immunodeficiency virus	PDW	platelet distribution width
HPFH	hereditary persistence of fetal haemoglobin	PE	phycoerythrin
		pI	isoelectric point
HPLC	high performance liquid chromatography	PK	pyruvate kinase
HVR	hypervariable region	PML	protein encoded by *PML* gene
IAT	indirect antiglobulin test	PNH	paroxysmal nocturnal haemoglobinuria
ICSH	International Council (formerly Committee) for Standardization in Haematology	PT	prothrombin time
		PVP	polyvinyl pyrrolidine
		QSC	quantum simply cellular
IEF	isoelectric focusing	RID	radial immunodiffusion
Ig	immunoglobulin	RE	restriction enzyme
IgA	immunoglobulin A	RBC	red blood cell count
IgD	immunoglobulin D	RDW	red cell distribution width
IgE	immunoglobulin E	RFLP	restriction fragment-length polymorphism
IgG	immunoglobulin G	RNA	ribonucleic acid
IgM	immunoglobulin M	RT	reverse transcriptase
IP	immunoperoxidase	RT-PCR	reverse transcriptase-polymerase chain reaction
iu	international units		
kb	kilobase	SD	standard deviation
LISS	low ionic strength saline	SDS	sodium dodecyl sulphate
McAb	monoclonal antibody	SHb	sulphhaemoglobin
MCH	mean cell haemoglobin	SLVL	splenic lymphoma with villous lymphocytes
MCHC	mean cell haemoglobin concentration		
MCV	mean cell volume	SmIg	surface immunoglobulin
MDS	myelodysplastic syndrome or syndromes	SOP	standard operating procedure
MESF	molecules equivalent soluble fluorochrome	SSc	sideways light scatter
		SSCP	single-strand conformation polymorphism
MGG	May-Grünwald-Giemsa	TAE	Tris acetate EDTA (buffer)
MoAb	monoclonal antibody	TBE	Tris borate EDTA (buffer)
MPO	myeloperoxidase	TBS	Tris-buffered saline
MPV	mean platelet volume	TCR	T-cell receptor
NAP	neutrophil alkaline phosphatase	TE	Tris-EDTA (buffer)
NEQAS	national external quality assessment	TEB	Tris-EDTA-borate (buffer)
NISS	normal ionic strength saline	TNCC	total nucleated cell count
NRBC	nucleated red blood cell	t-PA	tissue plasminogen activator
NSE	non-specific esterase	TT	thrombin time
PA	plasminogen activator	UIBC	unsaturated iron-binding capacity
PAS	periodic acid-Schiff	UV	ultraviolet
PB	peripheral blood	vol	volume
PBS	phosphate-buffered saline	v/v	volume/volume
PBS-azide-BSA	phosphate-buffered saline containing sodium azide and bovine serum albumin	WBC	white cell count
		WHO	World Health Organization
		w/v	weight/volume

EDITORIAL NOTE

In keeping with recommendations from the International Organization for Standardardization (ISO), the World Health Organization (WHO), and other international authorities, we have used the Système International (SI) for expressing quantities and units (see p. 696). Concentration of solutions is expressed either in mol/l (for substance concentration) or g/l (for mass concentration), whichever is more appropriate. While we are aware that in some countries g/dl is still in common use for expressing haemoglobin concentration, in keeping with the internationally agreed convention we have expressed Hb in g/l. To convert this to g/dl divide the quantity by 10.

We have indicated the source of a reagent, kit, or device if there is a single manufacturer or if a specific make is recommended. If no source is indicated, suitable material or equipment will generally be available from different suppliers. Catalogues from these manufacturers and detailed information on the use of their unique devices can be found on their Websites.

1 Collection and handling of blood

S. Mitchell Lewis and Noriyuki Tatsumi

In investigating physiological function and malfunction of blood, accurate and precise methodology is essential to ensure, as far as possible, that tests do not give misleading information because of technical errors. Obtaining the specimen is the first step toward analytic procedures. It is important to use appropriate blood containers and to avoid faults in specimen collection, storage, and transport to the laboratory. Venous blood generally is used for most haematological examinations and for chemistry tests; capillary skin puncture samples can be almost as satisfactory for some purposes if a free flow of blood is obtained (see p. 4), but in general this procedure should be restricted to children and to some "point-of-care" screening tests that require only a drop or two of blood. Bone marrow aspirates are described in Chapter 6.

BIOHAZARD PRECAUTIONS

Special care must be taken to avoid risk of infection from various pathogens during all aspects of laboratory practice, and the safety procedures described in Chapter 25 must be followed as far as

possible when collecting blood. The operator should wear disposable plastic or thin rubber gloves. It is also desirable to wear a protective apron or gown and, if necessary, glasses or goggles. Care must be taken to prevent injuries, especially when handling syringes, needles, and lancets.

Disposable sterilized syringes, needles, and lancets should be used if at all possible, and they should never be reused. Reusable items must, after use, always be sterilized in an autoclave or hot-air oven at 160°C for 1 hour (see p. 652).

STANDARDIZED PROCEDURE

The constituents of the blood may be altered by a number of factors, which are listed in Table 1.1. It is important to have a standard procedure for the collecting and handling of blood specimens. Recommendations for standardizing the procedure have been published.[1-3]

VENOUS BLOOD

It is now common practice for specimen collection to be undertaken by specially trained phlebotomists,

---

*Some individuals may have an allergic reaction to either plastic or rubber gloves (see p. 650).

Table 1.1   Causes of Misleading Results from Discrepancies in Specimen Collection
Precollection
Toilet within 30 min; food or water intake within 2 hours
Smoking
Physical activity (including fast walking) within 20 min
Stress
Drugs or dietary supplement administration within 8 hours
During Collection
Different times (diurnal variance)
Posture: lying, standing, or sitting
Haemoconcentration from prolonged tourniquet pressure
Excessive negative pressure when drawing blood into syringe
Incorrect type of tube
Capillary vs. venous blood
Handling of Specimen
Insufficient or excess anticoagulant
Inadequate mixing of blood with anticoagulant
Error in patient and/or specimen identification
Inadequate specimen storage conditions
Delay in transit to laboratory

Table 1.2   Phlebotomy Tray
Syringes and needles
Tourniquet
Specimen containers (or evacuated tube system)—plain and with various anticoagulants
Request form
70% isopropyl alcohol swabs or 0.5% chlorhexidine
Sterile gauze swabs or cellulose pads
Adhesive dressings
Self-sealing plastic bags
Rack to hold specimens upright during process of filling
(A puncture-resistant disposal container should also be available.)

and there are published guidelines that set out an appropriate training programme.[1,4]

Phlebotomy Tray

It is convenient to have a tray that contains all the requirements for blood collection (Table 1.2).

Disposable Plastic Syringes and Disposable Needles

The needles should not be too fine, too large, or too long; those of 19 or 21G* are suitable for most adults, and 23G (especially with a short shaft of about 15 mm) is suitable for children. It may be

*The International Organization for Standardization has established a standard (ISO 7864) that relates the following diameters for the different gauges: 19G = 1.1 mm, 21G = 0.8 mm, 23G = 0.6 mm.

helpful to collect the blood by means of a winged ("butterfly") needle connected to a length of plastic tubing, which can be attached to the nozzle of the syringe or to a needle for entering the cap of an evacuated container (see later discussion).

Specimen Containers

The common containers for haematology tests are available commercially with dipotassium, tripotassium, or disodium ethylenediaminetetra-acetic acid (EDTA) as anticoagulant, and they are marked at a level to indicate the correct amount of blood to be added. Containers are also available containing trisodium citrate, heparin, or acid citrate dextrose, and there are containers with no additive, which are used when serum is required. Design requirements and other specifications for specimen collection containers have been described in a number of national and international standards (e.g., that of the International Council for Standardization in Haematology[5]), and there is also a European standard (EN 14820). Unfortunately, there is not yet universal agreement regarding the colours for identifying containers with different additives; phlebotomists should familiarize themselves with the colours used by their own suppliers.

Evacuated tube systems, which are now in common use, consist of a glass or plastic tube/container (with or without anticoagulant) under defined vacuum, a needle, and a needle holder that secures the needle to the tube. The main advantage is that the cap can be pierced, so that it is not necessary to remove it either to fill the tube, or subsequently to withdraw samples for analysis, thus minimizing the risk of aerosol discharge of the contents.[6,7] An evacuated system is useful when multiple samples in different anticoagulants are required. The vacuum controls the amount of blood that enters the tube, ensuring an adequate specimen for the subsequent tests and the correct proportion of anticoagulant when this is present. Silicone-coated evacuated tubes can be used for routine coagulation screening tests.

Phlebotomy Procedure

The phlebotomist should first check the patient's identity, making sure that it corresponds to the details on the request form, and also ensure that the phlebotomy tray contains all the required specimen containers.

Blood is best withdrawn from an antecubital vein or other visible veins in the forearm by means of either an evacuated tube or a syringe. It is usually recommended that the skin be cleaned with 70% alcohol (e.g., isopropanol) or 0.5% chlorhexidine and allowed to dry spontaneously before being punctured; however, some doubts have been expressed on the utility of this practice for preventing infection at the venepuncture site.[8] Care must also be taken when using a tourniquet to avoid contaminating it with blood, because infection risks have been reported during blood collection.[9] The tourniquet should be applied just above the venepuncture site and released as soon as the blood begins to flow into the syringe or evacuated tube—delay in releasing it leads to fluid shift and haemoconcentration as a result of venous blood stagnation.[4] It should be possible with practice to obtain venous blood even from patients with difficult veins (except for very young children). A butterfly needle is especially useful when a series of samples is required.

Successful venepuncture may be facilitated by keeping the subject's arm warm, applying to the upper arm a sphygmomanometer cuff kept at approximately diastolic pressure, and tapping the skin over the site of the vein a few times. After cleaning and drying the site and applying a tourniquet, ask the patient to make a fist a few times. Veins suitable for puncture will usually become apparent. If the veins are very small, a butterfly needle or 23G needle should enable at least 2 ml of blood to be obtained satisfactorily. In patients who are obese, it may be easier to use a vein on the dorsum of the hand, after warming it by immersion in warm water; however,

this site is not generally recommended because vein punctures here tend to bleed into surrounding tissues more readily than at other sites. Venepuncture should not be attempted over a site of scarring or haematoma.

If a syringe is used for blood collection, the piston of the syringe should be withdrawn slowly and no attempt should be made to withdraw blood faster than the vein is filling. Anticoagulated specimens must be mixed by inverting the containers several times. Haemolysis can be avoided or minimized by using clean apparatus, withdrawing the blood slowly, not using too fine a needle, delivering the blood gently into the receiver, and avoiding frothing during the withdrawal of the blood and subsequent mixing with the anticoagulant. If the blood is drawn too slowly or inadequately mixed with the anticoagulant, some coagulation may occur. After collection, the containers must be firmly capped to minimize the risk of leakage.

If blood collection fails, it is important to remain calm and consider the possible cause of the failure. This includes poor technique, especially stabbing rather than holding the needle parallel to the surface of the skin as it enters; this may result in the needle passing through the vein. After two or three unsuccessful attempts, it may be wise to refer the patient to another operator after a short rest.

After obtaining the blood and releasing the tourniquet, remove the needle and then press a sterile swab over the puncture site, applying pressure on the swab. The arm should be elevated after withdrawal of the needle, and pressure should continue to be applied to the swab with the arm elevated for a few minutes before checking that bleeding has completely ceased. Then cover the puncture site with a small adhesive dressing.

Obtaining blood from an indwelling line or catheter is a potential source of error. Because it is common practice to flush lines with heparin, they must be flushed free from heparin before any blood is collected for laboratory tests. If intravenous fluids are being transfused into an arm, the blood sample should not be collected from that arm.

Postphlebotomy Procedure

The phlebotomist should again check the patient's identity and ensure that it corresponds to the details on the request form. In addition to the request form being labelled, it is essential that every specimen is labelled with adequate patient identification immediately after the samples have been obtained. On the labels this should include at least surname and forename or initials, hospital number, date of birth, and date and time of specimen collection. The same information must be given on the request form, together with ward or department, name of requesting clinician, and test(s) requested. When relevant, a biohazard warning also must be affixed to the container and to the request form. If automated patient identification is available, both the label and the request form should be bar-coded with the relevant data.

Specimens should be sent in individual plastic bags separated from the request forms to prevent contamination of the forms in the event of leakage. Alternatively, the specimen tubes must be set upright in a holder or rack and placed in a carrier together with the request forms for transport to the laboratory.

Waste Disposal

Without separating the needle from the syringe, place both, together with the used swab and any other dressings, in a puncture-resistant container for disposal (see p. 653). If it is essential to dispose of the needle separately, it should be detached from the syringe only with forceps or a similar tool. Alternatively, the needle can be destroyed *in situ* with a special device (e.g., Sharp-X, Biomedical Disposal Inc., www.biodisposal.com).

CAPILLARY BLOOD

Skin puncture can be used for obtaining a small amount of blood either for direct use in an analytic process or for collecting into capillary tubes coated with heparin for packed cell volume or into a special anticoagulated microcollection device (p. 5). These methods are mostly used when it is not possible to obtain venous blood (e.g., in infants younger than 1 year, in cases of gross obesity, or for point-of-care blood tests).

Collection of Capillary Blood

Skin puncture is carried out with a needle or lancet. In adults and older children blood can be obtained from a finger; the recommended site is the distal digit of the third or fourth finger on its palmar surface, about 3–5 mm lateral from the nail bed. Formerly the ear lobe was commonly used, but it is no longer recommended because reduced blood flow renders it unrepresentative of the circulating blood.[1] In infants, satisfactory samples can be obtained by a deep puncture of the plantar surface of the heel in the area shown in Figure 1.1. Because the heel should be very warm, it may be necessary to bathe it in hot water. The central plantar area and the posterior curvature should not be punctured in small infants to avoid the risk of injury and possible infection to the underlying tarsal bones, especially in newborns.

Clean the area with 70% alcohol (e.g., isopropanol) and allow to dry. Puncture the skin to a depth of 2–3 mm with a sterile disposable lancet. Wipe away the first drop of blood with dry sterile gauze. If necessary, squeeze very gently to encourage a free flow of blood. Collect the second and following drops

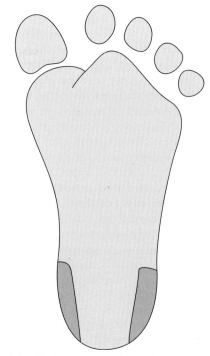

Figure 1.1   Skin puncture in infants. Puncture must be restricted to the outer medial and lateral portions of the plantar surface of the foot where indicated by the shaded area.

directly onto a reagent strip or by a 10 ml or 20 ml micropipette for immediate dispensing into diluent. A free flow of blood is essential, and only the very gentlest squeezing is permissible; ideally, large drops of blood should exude slowly but spontaneously. If it is necessary to squeeze firmly to obtain blood, the results are unreliable. If the poor flow is the result of the sampling site being cold and cyanosed, then the figures obtained for haemoglobin, red blood cell count (RBC), and leucocyte count are usually too high.

There are methods for collecting the blood into a capillary tube fixed into the cap of a microcontainer to allow the blood to pass by capillary action into the container (e.g., Microtainer*).[10] In another system (Unopette*), a calibrated capillary is completely filled with blood and linked to a premeasured volume of diluent.[11] An adequate puncture with a free flow of blood can also enable a larger volume to be collected, drop by drop, into a plastic or glass container.[12]

After use, lancets (and needles) should be placed in a puncture-resistant container for subsequent waste disposal. They must never be reused on another individual.

Blood Film Preparation

Ideally, blood films should be made immediately after the blood has been collected. Because blood samples are usually sent to the laboratory after a variable delay, there are advantages in preparing blood films when the phlebotomy is carried out. The phlebotomy tray might include some clean glass slides and spreaders, and phlebotomists should be given appropriate training for film preparation, as described in Chapter 4. An automated device for making smears is also available.[13] When films are not made on site, they should be made in the laboratory without delay as soon as the specimens have been received.

DIFFERENCES BETWEEN CAPILLARY AND VENOUS BLOOD

Venous blood and "capillary" blood are not quite the same. Blood from a skin puncture is a mixture of blood from arterioles, veins, and capillaries, and it

contains some interstitial and intracellular fluid.[1,4,14] Although some studies have suggested that there are negligible differences when a free flow of blood has been obtained,[15] others have shown definite differences in composition between skin puncture and venous blood samples in neonates,[16] children,[17] and adults.[18] The differences may be exaggerated by cold with resulting slow capillary blood flow.[4]

The packed cell volume (PCV), RBC, and haemoglobin concentration (Hb) of capillary blood are slightly greater than in venous blood. The total leucocyte and neutrophil counts are higher by about 8%; the monocyte count is higher by about 12%, and in some cases by as much as 100%, especially in children. Conversely, the platelet count appears to be higher in venous than in capillary blood; this is on average by about 9% and in some cases by as much as 32%.[16-18] This may be the result of adhesion of platelets to the site of the skin puncture.

SERUM

The difference between plasma and serum is that the latter lacks fibrinogen and some of the coagulation factors. Blood collected to obtain serum should be delivered into sterile tubes with caps or commercially available, plain (nonanticoagulant), evacuated collection tubes and allowed to clot undisturbed for about 1 hour at room temperature.[†] Then the clot should be loosened gently from the container wall by means of a wooden stick or a thin plastic or glass rod. Rough handling will cause lysis. The tube should be closed with a cap/stopper. Some products contain a clot activator combined with a gel for accelerated separation of serum (e.g., serum separator tubes*).

The tubes, with or without a serum separator, are centrifuged for 10 min at about 1200 g. The supernatant serum then is pipetted into another tube and centrifuged again for 10 min at about 1200 g. The supernatant serum is transferred to tubes for tests or for storage. For most tests, serum should be kept at 4°C until used, but if testing is delayed, serum can be stored at –20°C for up to 3 months and at –40°C or less for long-term storage. Frozen specimens should be thawed on the bench or in a

---

*BD Ltd.

†Room temperature is usually taken as 18–25°C.

waterbath at room temperature, then inverted several times to ensure homogeneity before use for a test. Do not refreeze thawed specimens.

Defibrinating Whole Blood

The procedure described in Chapter 28 (p. 708) can be used to obtain plasma-free red cells, e.g., when investigating certain types of haemolytic anaemia. Cell morphology is well preserved in this process.

Cold Agglutinins

If cold agglutinins are to be titrated, the blood must be kept at 37°C until the serum has separated. If cold agglutinins are known to be present in high concentration, it is best to bring the patient to the laboratory and collect blood into a previously warmed syringe and then to deliver the blood into containers that have been kept warm at 37°C. When filled, the containers should be promptly replaced in the 37°C waterbath. In this way, it is possible to obtain serum free from haemoglobin even when cold antibodies capable of causing agglutination at temperatures as high as 30°C are present. A practical way of warming the syringe is to place it in its container for 10 min in an oven at approximately 50°C or for about 30 min in a 37°C incubator. When the clot has retracted in the sample and clear serum has been expressed, the serum is removed by a Pasteur pipette and transferred to a tube that has been warmed by being allowed to stand in a waterbath. It is then rapidly centrifuged so as to rid it of any suspended red cells.

ANTICOAGULANTS

EDTA and sodium citrate remove calcium, which is essential for coagulation. Calcium is either precipitated as insoluble oxalate (crystals of which may be seen in oxalated blood) or bound in a nonionized form. Heparin binds to antithrombin, thus inhibiting the interaction of several clotting factors.

EDTA is used for blood counts; sodium citrate is used for coagulation testing and erythrocyte sedimentation rate (ESR). For better long-term preservation of red cells for certain tests and for transfusion purposes, citrate is used in combination with dextrose in the form of acid–citrate–dextrose (ACD), citrate–phosphate–dextrose (CPD), or Alsever's

solution (p. 689). Anticoagulant mixtures are also used to compensate for disadvantages in each and to meet the needs of the analytic process[19,20]; these include ACD, CPD, or heparin combined with EDTA and EDTA, citrate, or heparin combined with sodium fluoride. Any anticoagulant can be used for collecting blood for flow cytometry.[19,21]

Ethylenediaminetetra-Acetic Acid

The sodium and potassium salts of EDTA are powerful anticoagulants, and they are especially suitable for routine haematological work. EDTA acts by its chelating effect on the calcium molecules in blood. To achieve this requires a concentration of 1.2 mg of the anhydrous salt per ml of blood (c 4 mmol). The dipotassium salt is very soluble (1650 g/l) and is to be preferred on this account to the disodium salt, which is considerably less soluble (108 g/l).[22] Coating the inside surface of the blood collection tube with a thin layer of EDTA improves the speed of its uptake by the blood.

The dilithium salt of EDTA is equally effective as an anticoagulant,[23] and its use has the advantage that the same sample of blood can be used for chemical investigation. However, it is less soluble than the dipotassium salt (160 g/l).

The tripotassium salt dispensed in liquid form has been recommended in the United States by the Clinical and Laboratory Standards Institute (formerly the National Committee for Clinical Laboratory Standards, or NCCLS).[3] However, blood delivered into this solution will be slightly diluted, and the tripotassium salt produces some shrinkage of red cells, which results in a 2–3% decrease in PCV within 4 hours of collection, followed by a gradual increase in mean cell volume (MCV). By contrast, there are negligible changes when the dipotassium salt is used.[1,4] Accordingly, the International Council for Standardization in Haematology recommends the dipotassium salt at a concentration of 1.50 ± 0.25 mg/ml of blood.[24] Na$_3$-EDTA is not recommended because of its high pH.

Excess of EDTA, irrespective of which salt, affects both red cells and leucocytes, causing shrinkage and degenerative changes. EDTA in excess of 2 mg/ml of blood may result in a significant decrease in PCV by centrifugation and increase in mean cell haemoglobin concentration (MCHC).[4] The platelets are also affected; excess of EDTA causes them to swell and then disintegrate, leading to an artificially high platelet count because the fragments are large enough to be counted as normal platelets. Care must therefore be taken to ensure that the correct amount of blood is added and that by repeated inversions of the container the anticoagulant is thoroughly mixed in the blood added to it. Blood films made from EDTA blood may fail to demonstrate basophilic stippling of the red cells in lead poisoning. EDTA has also been shown to cause leucoagglutination affecting both neutrophils and lymphocytes,[25] and it is responsible for the activity of a naturally occurring antiplatelet autoantibody, which may sometimes cause platelet adherence to neutrophils in blood films (see p. 111). Monocyte activation measured by release of tissue factor and tumor necrosis factor activity has been reported as being lower with EDTA than with citrate and heparin. Similarly, neutrophil activation measured by lipopolysaccharide-induced release of lactoferrin is low with EDTA. EDTA also appears to suppress platelet degranulation.[26]

Trisodium Citrate

For coagulation studies 9 volumes of blood are added to 1 volume of 109 mmol/l sodium citrate solution (32 g/l of $Na_3C_6H_5O_7.2H_2O$*).[27] This ratio of anticoagulant to blood is critical as osmotic effects and changes in free calcium ion concentration affect coagulation test results.

For the ESR, 4 volumes of blood are added to 1 volume of the sodium citrate solution (109 mmol/l) and immediately well mixed with it. The mixture is taken up in a Westergren tube.[28]

Heparin

Lithium or sodium salt of heparin at a concentration of 10–20 iu per ml of blood is a commonly used anticoagulant for chemistry, gas analysis, and emergency tests. It does not alter the size of the red cells, and it is recommended when it is important to reduce to a minimum the chance of lysis occurring after blood has been withdrawn. It is thus the best anticoagulant for osmotic fragility tests and is suitable for immunophenotyping.

However, heparin is not suitable for blood counts because it often induces platelet and leucocyte

---

*Or 38 g/l of $2Na_3C_6H_5O_7.11H_2O$

clumping.[4,29,30] It also should not be used for making blood films because it gives a faint blue colouration to the background when the films are stained by Romanowsky dyes, especially in the presence of abnormal proteins. It inhibits enzyme activity,[19] and it should not be used in the study of polymerase chain reaction with restriction enzymes.[31]

EFFECTS OF STORAGE ON THE BLOOD COUNT

Various changes take place in anticoagulated blood when it is stored at room temperature, and these changes occur more rapidly at higher ambient temperatures. These occur regardless of the anticoagulant, although they are less marked in blood in ACD, CPD, or Alsever's solution than in EDTA blood and greater in the tripotassium salt than in the dipotassium salt of EDTA. The RBC, white blood cell count (WBC), platelet count, and red cell indices are usually stable for 8 hours after blood collection, although as the red cells start to swell the PCV and MCV start to increase, osmotic fragility increases, and the ESR decreases. When the blood is kept at 4°C, the effects on the blood count are usually insignificant for up to 24 hours. Thus, for many purposes blood may safely be allowed to stand overnight in the refrigerator if precautions against freezing are taken. Nevertheless, it is best to count leucocytes and especially platelets within 2 hours, and it should be noted that the decrease in leucocyte count and a progressive decrease in the absolute lymphocyte count may become marked within a few hours, especially if there is an excessive amount of EDTA (>4.5 mg/ml).[21] Storage beyond 24 hours at 4°C results in erroneous data for automated white cell differential counts, although the extent depends on instrument performance and the manufacturer's recommendation, which should be followed when an automated counting method is used. One study using an aperture impedance analyzer on blood left at room temperature showed WBC and neutrophils to be stable for 2–3 days, but other leucocytes were stable for only a few hours.[32]

Reticulocyte counts are unchanged when the blood is kept in either EDTA or ACD anticoagulant for 24 hours at 4°C, but at room temperature the count begins to decrease within 6 hours. Nucleated red cells disappear in the blood specimen within 1–2 days at room temperature.

Haemoglobin concentration remains unchanged for days, provided that the blood does not become infected, as shown by turbidity or discoloration of the specimen. However, within 2–3 days, and especially at high ambient temperatures, the blood begins to lyse, resulting in a decrease in the RBC and PCV, with an increase in the calculated MCH and MCHC.

Coagulation test stability is critical for diagnosis and treatment of coagulopathies. NCCLS has recommended that tests be carried out within 2 hours when the blood or plasma is stored at 22–24°C, 4 hours at 4°C, 2 weeks at –20°C, and 6 months at –70°C.[2]

For a serum or plasma test, blood should be centrifuged within 5 hours of collection. For vitamin B_{12} and folate assays, the serum or plasma should be kept at 4°C or at –20°C if storage for more than 2–3 weeks is required. For long-term storage, specimens should be divided into several aliquots to avoid repeated freezing and thawing.

Inappropriate handling of blood specimens during transfer to the laboratory (e.g., excess shaking) may causes haemolysis, partial coagulation, and cell disintegration. Shipping of specimens requires special packaging.

EFFECTS OF STORAGE ON BLOOD CELL MORPHOLOGY

Changes in blood cell morphology occur easily even in short-time storage. The changes are not solely a result of the presence of an anticoagulant because they also occur in defibrinated blood. Irrespective of anticoagulant, films made from blood that has been standing for not more than 1 hour at room temperature are not easily distinguished from films made immediately after collection of the blood. By 3 hours, changes may be discernible, and by 12–18 hours these become striking. Some but not all neutrophils are affected; their nuclei may stain more homogeneously than in fresh blood, the nuclear lobes may become separated, and the cytoplasmic margin may appear ragged or less well defined; small vacuoles appear in the cytoplasm (Fig. 1.2A, B). Some or many of the large monocytes develop marked changes; small vacuoles appear in the cytoplasm and the nucleus undergoes irregular lobulation, which may almost amount to disintegration (Fig. 1.2C). Lymphocytes undergo similar changes: a few vacuoles may be seen in the cytoplasm, nuclei stain more homogeneously than usual, and in some the nucleus undergoes budding (giving rise to nuclei with two or three lobes) (Fig. 1.2D–F). Normal red cells are little affected by standing

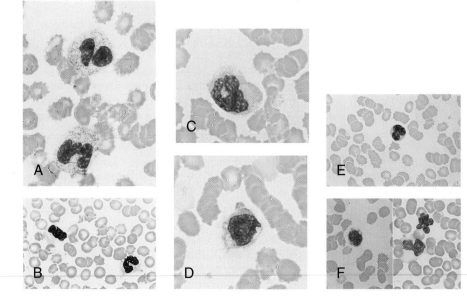

Figure 1.2   Effect of storage on blood cell morphology. Photomicrographs from films made from ethylenediaminetetra-acetic acid (EDTA) blood after 24 hours at 20°C. A and B: Polymorphnuclear neutrophil; C: Monocytes; D, E, and F: Lymphocytes. Red cell crenation is prominent in B and E.

for up to 6 hours at room temperature. Longer periods lead to progressive crenation and sphering (Fig. 1.2B, E, and F). With an excess of EDTA, a marked degree of crenation occurs within a few hours. All the previously mentioned changes are retarded but not abolished in blood kept at 4°C. Their occurrence underlines the importance of making films as soon as possible after the blood has been collected. However, as a rule, delay of up to 3 hours is permissible.

These artefactual changes must be distinguished from apoptosis, which is a controlled process of programmed cell death that occurs when the cytokines and growth factors regulating cell survival are depleted or inhibited, with mitochondrial dysfunction as a key event.[33,34] Apoptosis is characterized morphologically (Fig. 1.3) by cell shrinkage with cytoplasmic condensation around the nuclear membrane and indentations in the nucleus, followed by its fragmentation; finally the cell remnants form dense basophilic masses (the apoptotic bodies). Apoptotic neutrophils with a single apoptotic body may be confused with nucleated red cells if the cytoplasmic features are not appreciated. The remnants are removed from the circulation by phagocytosis, and usually in a film only an occasional apoptotic cell is seen, surrounded by viable cells.[35] More frequent apoptotic cells can be seen in leukaemia.

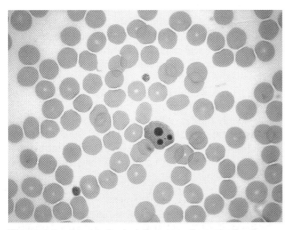

Figure 1.3   Morphological features of apoptosis. See text.

SAMPLE HOMOGENEITY

To ensure even dispersal of the blood cells, it is essential that specimens are mixed effectively immediately prior to taking a sample for testing. Place the specimen tube on a mechanical rotating mixer for at least 2 min or invert the tube 8–10 times by hand. If the specimen has been stored at 4°C, it will be viscid and the blood should be allowed to warm up to room temperature before mixing.

REFERENCES

1. Tatsumi N, Miwa S, Lewis SM, International Council for Standardization in Haematology/International Society of Hematology 2002 Specimen collection, storage, and transportation to the laboratory for hematological tests. International Journal of Hematology 75:261–268.
2. NCCLS 2003 Procedures for the collection of diagnostic blood specimens by venipuncture. Approved standard, 5th edition. H3-A5. NCCLS, Wayne PA.
3. NCCLS 2003 Tubes and additives for venous blood specimen collection. Approved standard, 5th edition. NCCLS, Wayne PA.
4. Van Assendelft OW, Simmons A 1995 Specimen collection, handling, storage and variability. In: Lewis SM, Koepke JA (eds) Hematology Laboratory Management and Practice, p. 109–127. Butterworth Heinemann, Oxford.
5 Tatsumi N, van Assendelft OW, Naka K 2002 ICSH recommendation for blood specimen collection for hematological analysis. Laboratory Hematology 8:1–6.
6. Katz L 1975 Evacuated blood-collection tubes—the backflow hazard. Canadian Medical Association Journal 113:208–213.
7. Katsuda I 2003. Safety of evacuated-blood collection tubes. Japanese Journal of Clinical Pathology 23 (suppl 2):168.
8. Sutton CD, White SA, Edwards R 1999 A prospective controlled trial of the efficacy of isopropyl alcohol wipes before venesection in surgical patients. Annals of the Royal College of Surgeons 81:183–186.
9. Golder M, Chen CLH, O'Shea S et al 2000 Potential risk of cross-infection during peripheral-venous access by contaminated tourniquets. Lancet 355:44.

10. Meitis S 1988 Skin puncture and blood collection techniques for infants: updates and problems. Clinical Chemistry 34:1890–1894.

11. Hicks JR, Rowland GL, Buffone GJ 1976 Evaluation of a new blood collection device ("Microtainer") that is suitable for pediatric use. Clinical Chemistry 22:2034–2036.

12. Freudlich MH, Gerarde HW 1963 A new, automatic disposable system for blood count and hemoglobin. Blood 21:648–655.

13. Tatsumi N, Pierre R 2002 Automated image processing; past, present, and future of blood cell morphology identification. Clinics in Laboratory Medicine 22:299–316.

14. Conway AM, Hinchliffe RF, Earland J et al 1998 Measurement of hemoglobin using single drops of skin puncture blood: is precision acceptable? Journal of Clinical Pathology 51:248–250.

15. Yang Z-W, Yang S-H, Chen L, et al 2001 Comparison of blood counts in venous, finger tip and arterial blood and their measurement variation. Clinical and Laboratory Haematology 23:155–159.

16. Kayiran SM, Özbek N, Turan M, et al 2003 Significant differences between capillary and venous complete blood counts in the neonatal period. Clinical and Laboratory Haematology 25:9–16.

17. Daae LNW, Hallerud M, Halvorsen S 1988 A comparison between haematological parameters in "capillary" and venous blood samples from hospitalized children aged 3 months to 14 years. Scandinavian Journal of Clinical and Laboratory Investigation 51:651–654.

18. Daae LNW, Halvorsen S, Mathison PM, et al 1988 A comparison between haematological parameters in "capillary" and venous blood from healthy adults. Scandinavian Journal of Clinical and Laboratory Investigation 48:723–726.

19. Narayanan S 2000 The pre-analytic phase: an important component of laboratory medicine. American Journal of Clinical Pathology 113:429–457.

20. Tatsumi N 2003 Universal anticoagulants. Japanese Society of Thrombosis and Haemostasis 13:158–168.

21. NCCLS 1997 Clinical application of flow cytometry: quality assurance and immunophenotyping of peripheral blood lymphocytes. Document H43-A, NCCLS, Wayne PA.

22. Hadley GG, Weiss SP 1955 Further notes on use of salts of ethylene diaminetetraacetic acid (EDTA) as anticoagulants. American Journal of Clinical Pathology 25:1090–1093.

23. Sacker LS, Sanders KE, Page B et al 1959 Dilithium sequestrene as an anticoagulant. Journal of Clinical Pathology 12:254–257.

24. International Council for Standardization in Haematology 1993. Recommendations for ethylenediaminetetraacetic acid anticoagulation of blood for blood cell counting and sizing. American Journal of Clinical Pathology 100:371–372.

25. Deal I, Hernandez AM, Pierre RV 1995 Ethylenediamine tetraacetic acid-associated leukoaggulutination. American Journal of Clinical Pathology 103:338–340.

26. Engstad CS, Gutteberg TJ, Osterud B 1997 Modulation of cell activation by four commonly used anticoagulants. Thrombosis and Haemostasis 77:690–696.

27. Ingram GIC, Hills M 1976 The prothrombin time test; effect of varying citrate concentration. Thrombosis and Haemostasis 36:230–236.

28. International Committee for Standardization in Haematology 1977 Recommendation for measurement of erythrocyte sedimentation rate of human blood. American Journal of Clinical Pathology 66:505–507.

29. Salzman EW, Rosenberg RD 1980 Effect of heparin and heparin fractions on platelet aggregation. Journal of Clinical Investigation 65:64–73.

30. Hirsh J, Levine NM 1992 Low molecular weight heparin. Blood 79:1–9.

31. Yokota M, Tatsumi N, Nathalang O et al 1999 Effects of heparin on polymerase chain reaction for blood white cells. Journal of Clinical and Laboratory Analysis 13:133–140.

32. Gulati GL, Hyland LJ, Kocher W, et al 2002 Changes in automated complete blood cell count and differential leucocyte count results induced by storage of blood at room temperature. Archives of Pathology and Laboratory Medicine 126:336–342.

33. Kerr JF, Wylie AH, Curie AR 1972 Apoptosis: a basic biological phenomenon with wide-ranging implications in tissue kinetics. British Journal of Cancer 26:239–257.

34. Wylie AH, Kerr JFR, Currie AR 1980 Cell death: the significance of apoptosis. International Review of Cytology 68:251–306.

35. Lach-Szyrma V, Brito-Babapulle F 1999 The clinical significance of apoptotic cells in peripheral blood smears. Clinical and Laboratory Haematology 21:277–280.

2 Reference ranges and normal values

S. Mitchell Lewis

A number of factors affect haematological values in apparently healthy individuals. As described in Chapter 1, these include the technique and timing of blood collection, transport and storage of specimens, differences in the subject's posture when the sample is taken, prior physical activity, or whether the subject is confined to bed. Variation in the analytic methods used may also affect the measurements. These can all be standardized.

More problematic are the inherent variables as a result of sex, age, occupation, body build, genetic background, and adaptation to diet and to environment (especially altitude). These factors must be recognized when establishing physiologically normal values. Furthermore, it is difficult to be certain in any survey of a population for the purposes of obtaining data from which normal ranges may be constructed that the "normal" subjects are completely healthy and do not have nutritional deficiencies (especially iron deficiency, which is prevalent in many countries), mild chronic infections, parasitic infestations, or the effects of smoking.

Haematological values for the normal and abnormal will overlap, and a value within the recognized normal range may be definitely pathological in a particular subject. For these reasons the concept of "normal values" and "normal ranges" has been replaced by *reference values* and the *reference range,* which is defined by *reference limits* and obtained from measurements on the *reference population* for a particular test. The reference range is also termed the *reference interval.*[1,2] Ideally, each laboratory should establish a databank of reference values that take account of the variables mentioned earlier, so that an individual's result can be expressed and interpreted relative to a comparable apparently normal population, insofar as normal can be defined.

REFERENCE RANGES

A reference range for a specified population can be established from measurements on a relatively small number of subjects (discussed later) if they are assumed to be representative of the population as a whole.[2] The conditions for obtaining samples from the individuals and the analytic procedures must be standardized, whereas data should be analyzed separately for different variables such as individuals who are in bed or ambulant, smokers or nonsmokers, and so on. The samples should be collected at about the same time of day, preferably in the morning before breakfast; the last meal should have been eaten not later than 9 p.m. on the previous evening and at that time alcohol should have been restricted to one bottle of beer or an equivalent amount of other alcoholic drink.[3]

STATISTICAL PROCEDURES

In biological measurements it is usually assumed that the data will fit a specified type of pattern, either symmetric (Gaussian) or asymmetric with a skewed distribution (non-Gaussian). With a Gaussian distribution, the *arithmetic mean* ($\bar{x}$) can be obtained by dividing the sum of all measurements by the number of observations. The *mode* is the value that occurs most frequently, and the *median* (m) is the point at which there are an equal number of observations above and below it. In a true Gaussian distribution they should all be the same. The standard deviation (SD) can be calculated as described on p. 698.

If the data fit a Gaussian distribution, when plotted as a frequency histogram the pattern shown in Figure 2.1 is obtained. Taking the mode and the calculated SD as reference points, a Gaussian curve is superimposed on the histogram. From this curve, practical reference limits can be determined even if the original histogram included outlying results from some subjects not belonging to the normal population. Limits representing the 95% reference range are calculated from arithmetic mean ±2SD (or more accurately ± 1.96SD).

When there is a log normal (skew) distribution of measurements, the range to –2SD may even extend to zero (Fig. 2.2A). To avoid this anomaly, the data should be plotted on semilogarithmic graph paper to obtain a normal distribution histogram (Fig. 2.2B). To calculate the mean and SD the data should be converted to their logarithms by means of a calculator with the appropriate facility. The log-mean value is obtained by adding the logs of all the measurements and dividing by the number of observations. The log SD is calculated by the formula on p. 698, and the results are then converted to their antilogs to express the data in the arithmetic scale. This process can also be carried out on a computer with an appropriate statistical program.

When it is not possible to make an assumption about the type of distribution, a nonparametric procedure may be used instead to obtain the median and SD. For this, the data are sorted out and ranked according to increasing quantitative values, and the median is calculated as illustrated in Table 2.1. To obtain an approximation of the SD, the range that comprises the middle 50% spread (i.e., between 25% and 75% of results) is read and divided by 1.35. This represents 1SD.[4]

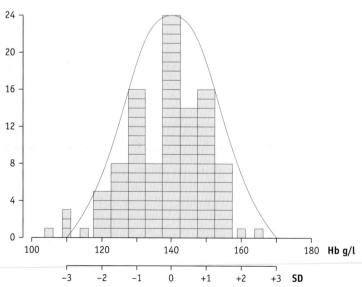

Figure 2.1   Example of establishing a reference range. Histogram of data of haemoglobin measurements in a population, with Gaussian curve superimposed. The ordinate shows the number that occurred at each reference point. The mean was 140 g/l; the reference ranges at 1SD, 2SD, and 3SD are indicated.

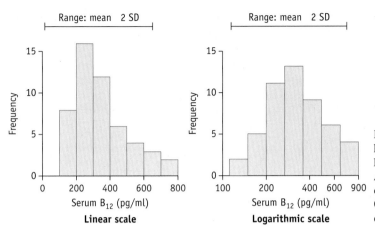

Figure 2.2   Example of conversion to a log normal distribution. Data of vitamin B_{12} measurements in a population. A: Arithmetic scale: Mean 340; 2SD range calculated as 10–665 pg/ml. B: Geometric scale: Mean 308; 2SD range calculated as 120–780 pg/ml.

Table 2.1   Illustration of calculation of median*

Rank no.	1	2	3	4	5	6	7	8	9	10	11
Haemoglobin g/l	110	112	113	115	115	118	120	122	124	126	127

If the total (n) is an odd number, the rank position for the median is calculated from $\frac{(n+1)}{2}$; (i.e., position 6 = 118 g/l).

Rank no.	1	2	3	4	5	6	7	8	9	10
Haemoglobin g/l	110	112	113	115	115	118	120	122	124	126

If the total (n) is an even number, the rank position for the median lies between $\frac{n}{2}$ and $\frac{(n+2)}{2}$; (i.e., between

rank positions 5 and 6 = $\frac{(115+118)}{2}$ = 116.5 g/l).

*In practice a larger number would be required for meaningful statistics (see text).

Confidence Limits

In any of the methods of analysis, a reasonably reliable estimate can be obtained with 40 values, although a larger number (120 or more) is preferable (Fig. 2.3).[5] When a large set of reference values is unattainable and precise estimation is impossible, a smaller number of values may still serve as a useful clinical guide. Confidence limits define the reliability (e.g., 95% or 99%) of the established reference values when assessing the significance of a test result, especially when it is on the borderline between normal and abnormal. Calculation of confidence limits is described on p. 698. Another

important measurement is the coefficient of variance (CV) of the test because a wide CV is likely to influence its clinical utility (see p. 629).

NORMAL REFERENCE VALUES

The data given in Tables 2.2, 2.3, and 2.4 provide general guidance to normal reference values that are applicable to most healthy adults and children, respectively, in industrialized countries. The data have been derived from personal observations as well as various published reports.[6-11] However, slightly different ranges may be found in individual laboratories where different analyzers and methods

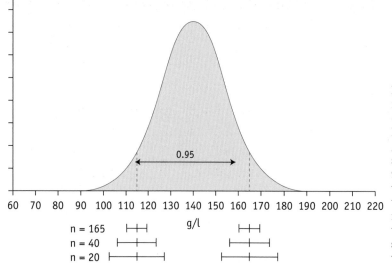

60 70 80 90 100 110 120 130 140 150 160 170 180 190 200 210 220

g/l

n = 165

n = 40

n = 20

Figure 2.3 Effect of sample size on reference values. A smoothed distribution graph was obtained for haemoglobin measurement from a group of normal women; the ordinate shows the frequency distribution. The 95% reference interval is defined by the lower and higher reference limits, which are 115 and 165 g/l, respectively. The confidence levels for these values are shown for three sample sizes of 20, 40, and 165 values, respectively.

Table 2.2   Haematological values for normal adults expressed as a mean ±2SD (95% range)

Red blood cell count		Differential white cell count	
Men	$5.0 \pm 0.5 \times 10^{12}$/l	Neutrophils	$2.0–7.0 \times 10^9$/l (40–80%)
Women	$4.3 \pm 0.5 \times 10^{12}$/l	Lymphocytes	$1.0–3.0 \times 10^9$/l (20–40%)
		Monocytes	$0.2–1.0 \times 10^9$/l (2–10%)
Haemoglobin		Eosinophils	$0.02–0.5 \times 10^9$/l (1–6%)
Men	150 ± 20 g/l	Basophils	$0.02–0.1 \times 10^9$/l (<1–2%)
Women	135 ± 15 g/l		
		Lymphocyte subsets (approximations from ranges in published data)	
Packed cell volume (PCV) or Haematocrit (Hct)			
Men	0.45 ± 0.05 (l/l)	CD3	$0.6–2.5 \times 10^9$/l (60–85%)
Women	0.41 ± 0.05 (l/l)	CD4	$0.4–1.5 \times 10^9$/l (30–50%)
		CD8	$0.2–1.1 \times 10^9$/l (10–35%)
Mean cell volume (MCV)		CD4/CD8 ratio	0.7–3.5
Men and women	92 ± 9 fl		
		Platelet count	$280 \pm 130 \times 10^9$/l
Mean cell haemoglobin (MCH)			
Men and women	29.5 ± 2.5 pg	**Bleeding time**	
		Ivy's method	2–7 min
Mean cell haemoglobin concentration (MCHC)		Template method	2.5–9.5 min
Men and women	330 ± 15 g/l		
		Prothrombin time	
Red cell distribution width (RDW)		Recombinant	11–16 s
As coefficient of variation (CV)	12.8 ± 1.2%	thromboplastin	10–12 s
As standard deviation (SD)	42.5 ± 3.5 fl		
		Activated partial thombo-plastin time (APTT)	30–40 s
Red cell diameter (mean values)			
Dry films	6.7–7.7 mm	**Thrombin time**	15–19 s
Red cell density	1092–1100 g/l	**Plasma fibrinogen**	
		Clauss	2.0–4.0 g/l
Reticulocyte count	$50–100 \times 10^9$/l (0.5–2.5%)	Dry clot	1.5–4.0 g/l
White blood cell count	$4.0–10.0 \times 10^9$/l		

Table 2.2 Haematological values for normal adults expressed as a mean ±2SD (95% range)—cont'd

Fibrinogen titre	≥128		Transferrin saturation	16–50%
Plasminogen	0.75–1.60 u/ml		Ferritin	
Euglobulin lysis time	90–240 min		Men	15–300 µgl/l (median 100 µg/l)
Antithrombin	0.75–1.25 u/ml		Women	15–200 µgl/l (median 40 µgl/l)
β-Thromboglobulin	<50 ng/ml		Serum vitamin B_{12}	180–640 ng/l
Platelet factor 4	<10 ng/ml		Serum folate	3–20 µg/l (6.8–45 nmol/l)
Protein C			Red Cell folate	160–640 µg/l (0.36–1.45 µmol/l)
Function	0.70–1.40 u/ml			
Antigen	0.61–1.32 u/ml		Plasma haemoglobin	10–40 mg/l
Protein S			Serum haptoglobin	
Total	0.78–1.37 u/ml		Radial immunodiffusion	0.8–2.7 g/l
Free	0.68–1.52 u/ml		Haemoglobin binding	
Activity			capacity	0.3–2.0 g/l
Men	0.60–1.35 u/ml		Hb A_2	2.2–3.5%
Women	0.55–1.35 u/ml		Hb F	<1.0%
Heparin cofactor II	0.55–1.45 u/ml		Methaemoglobin	<2.0%
Median red cell fragility (MCF) (g/l NaCl)			Sedimentation rate (mm in 1 hour at 20 ± 3°C)	
Fresh blood	4.0–4.45 g/l NaCl		Men	
24h at 37°C	4.65–5.9 g/l NaCl		17–50 yr	10 or <
Cold agglutinin titre (4°C)<64			51–60 yr	12 or <
			61–70 yr	14 or <
Blood volume (normalized to "ideal weight")			>70 yr	30 or <
Red cell volume			Women 17–50 yr	12 or <
Men	30 ± 5 ml/kg		51–60 yr	19 or <
Women	25 ± 5 ml/kg		61–70 yr	20 or <
Plasma volume	45 ± 5 ml/kg		>70 yr	35 or <
Total blood volume	70 ± 10 ml/kg		Plasma viscosity	
Red cell lifespan	120 ± 30 days		25°C	1.50–1.72 mPa/s
Serum iron			37°C	1.16–1.33 mPa/s
Men and Women	10–30 µmol/(c 0.6–1.7 mg/l)			
Total iron-binding	47–70 µmol/l			
capacity	(c 2.5–4.0 mg/l)			

are used. The reference interval, which comprises a range of ±2SD from the mean, indicates the limits that should cover 95% of normal subjects; 99% of normal subjects will be included in a range of ±3SD. Age and sex differences have been taken into account for some values. Even so, the wide ranges that are shown for some tests reflect the influence of various factors, as described below. Narrower ranges would be expected under standardized conditions. Because modern analyzers provide a high level of technical precision, even small differences in successive measurements may be significant. It is thus important to establish and understand the limits of physiological variation for various tests. The

Table 2.3   Haematological values for normal infants (amalgamation of data derived from various sources; expressed as mean ±2SD or 95% Range)*

	Birth	Day 3	Day 7	Day 14	1 Month	2 Months	3–6 Months
Red blood cell count (RBC) × 10^{12}/l	6.0 ± 1.0	5.3 ± 1.3	5.1±1.2	4.9±1.3	4.2 ± 1.2	3.7 ± 0.6	4.7 ± 0.6
Haemoglobin g/l	180 ± 40	80 ± 30	175±4	165±4	140 ± 25	112 ± 18	126 ± 15
Packed cell volume (PCV) l/l	0.60 ± 0.15	0.56 ± 0.11	0.54 ± 0.12	0.51 ± 0.2	0.43 ± 0.10	0.35 ± 0.07	0.35 ± 0.05
Mean cell volume (MCV) fl	110 ± 10	105 ± 13	107 ± 19	105 ± 19	104 ± 12	95 ± 8	76 ± 8
Mean cell Hb (MCH) pg	34 ± 3	34 ± 3	34 ± 3	34 ± 3	33 ± 3	30 ± 3	27 ± 3
Mean cell Hb conc (MCHC) g/l	330 ± 30	330 ± 40	330 ± 50	330 ± 50	330 ± 40	320 ± 35	330 ± 30
Reticulocytes × 10^{9}/l	120–400	50–350	50–100	50–100	20–60	30–50	40–100
White blood cell count (WBC) × 10^{9}/l	18 ± 8	15 ± 8	14 ± 8	14 ± 8	12 ± 7	10 ± 5	12 ± 6
Neutrophils × 10^{9}/l	4–14	3–5	3–6	3–7	3–9	1–5	1–6
Lymphocytes × 10^{9}/l	3–8	2–8	3–9	3–9	3–16	4–10	4–12
Monocytes × 10^{9}/l	0.5–2.0	0.5–1.0	0.1–1.7	0.1–1.7	0.3–1.0	0.4–1.2	0.2–1.2
Eosinophils × 10^{9}/l	0.1–1.0	0.1–2.0	0.1–0.8	0.1–0.9	0.2–1.0	0.1–1.0	0.1–1.0
Lymphocyte subsets (× 10^{9}/l)**							
CD3		3.1–5.6				2.4–6.5	2.0–5.3
CD4		2.2–4.3				1.4–5.6	1.5–3.2
CD8		0.9–1.8				0.7–2.5	0.5–1.6
CD4/CD8 ratio		1.1–4.5				1.1–4.4	1.1–4.2
Platelets × 10^{9}/l	100–450	210–500	160–500	170–500	200–500	210–650	200–550

*There have been some reports of WBC and platelet counts being lower in venous blood than in capillary blood samples, although still within these reference ranges. In one study venous blood from a newborn gave lower values for haemoglobin, RBC, and WBC than capillary blood but gave higher values for platelets and lymphocytes.[60]
**Approximations because wide variations have been reported in different studies.

blood count data and other test results can then provide sensitive indications of minor abnormalities that may be important in clinical interpretation and health screening.

It should be noted that in Table 2.2 the differential white cell count is shown as percentages and in absolute numbers. Automated analysers provide absolute counts for each type of leucocyte, and because proportional (percentage) counting is less likely to interpret correctly their absolute increase or decrease, the International Council for Standardization in Haematology has recommended that the differential leucocyte count should always be given as the absolute number of each cell type

Table 2.4　Haematological values for normal children (amalgamation of data derived from various sources; expressed as mean $\pm$2SD or 95% Range)

	1 Year	2–6 Years	6–12 Years
Red cell count $\times 10^{12}$/l	4.5 $\pm$ 0.6	4.6 $\pm$ 0.6	4.6 $\pm$ 0.6
Haemoglobin g/l	126 $\pm$ 15	125 $\pm$ 15	135 $\pm$ 20
Packed cell volume (PCV) l/l	0.34 $\pm$ 0.04	0.37 $\pm$ 0.03	0.40 $\pm$ 0.05
Mean cell volume (MCV) fl	78 $\pm$ 6	81 $\pm$ 6	86 $\pm$ 9
Mean cell Hb (MCH) pg	27 $\pm$ 2	27 $\pm$ 3	29 $\pm$ 4
Mean cell Hb conc (MCHC) g/l	340 $\pm$ 20	340 $\pm$ 30	340 $\pm$ 30
Reticulocytes $\times 10^9$/l	30–100	30–100	30–100
White cell count $\times 10^9$/l	11 $\pm$ 5	10 $\pm$ 5	9 $\pm$ 4
Neutrophils $\times 10^9$/l	1–7	1.5–8	2–8
Lymphocytes $\times 10^9$/l	3.5–11	6–9	1–5
Monocytes $\times 10^9$/l	0.2–1.0	0.2–1.0	0.2–1.0
Eosinophils $\times 10^9$/l	0.1–1.0	0.1–1.0	0.1–1.0
Lymphocyte subsets ($\times 10^9$/l)*			
CD3	1.5–5.4	1.6–4.2	0.9–2.5
CD4	1.0–3.6	0.9–2.9	0.5–1.5
CD8	0.6–2.2	0.6–2.0	0.4–1.2
CD4/CD8 ratio	1.0–3.0	0.9–2.7	1.0–3.0
Platelets $\times 10^9$/l	200–550	200–490	170–450

*Approximations because wide variations have been reported in different studies.

per unit volume of blood.[12] The neutrophil:lymphocyte ratio obtained from a differential leucocyte count should be regarded only as an approximation.

PHYSIOLOGICAL VARIATIONS IN THE BLOOD COUNT

Red Cell Components

There is considerable variation in the red blood cell count (RBC) and haemoglobin concentration (Hb) at different periods of life. At birth the haemoglobin is higher than at any period subsequently (Table 2.3). The RBC is high immediately after birth,[6,13] and values for haemoglobin greater than 200 g/l, RBC higher than 6.0 $\times 10^{12}$/l, and a packed cell volume (PCV) of 0.65 are encountered frequently when the cord is tied late after delivery. Probably it is the cessation of pulsation of the umbilical artery in the cord as well as the uterine contractions that result in much of the blood contained in the placenta reentering the infant's circulation. After the immediate postnatal period, the Hb falls fairly steeply to a minimum by about the second month (Fig. 2.4). The RBC and PCV also fall, although less steeply, and the cells may become microcytic with the development of iron deficiency. The changes in the mean cell haemoglobin (MCH), mean cell haemoglobin concentration, and mean cell volume (MCV) from the neonate through infancy to early childhood are shown in Tables 2.3 and 2.4.

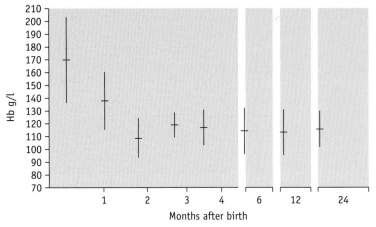

Figure 2.4   Changes in haemoglobin values in the first 2 years after birth. The perpendicular lines show means and 2SD ranges.

The Hb and RBC normally increase gradually to almost adult levels by puberty.[7] However, in a health survey of apparently normal men and women in Britain, mean haemoglobin values of 145 g/l for men and 128 g/l for women have been reported[9]; the lower normal limits for haemoglobin (i.e., 2SD below the mean) are usually taken as 130 and 120 g/l, respectively, but in some apparently normal men and women lower limits of 120 and 110 g/l, respectively, were noted. Statistically, at least 1% of a normal population have levels at 3SD below the mean, but in some studies there have been considerably larger numbers.[9] It is possible that some have nutritional deficiencies, especially iron deficiency, without clinical effects. The levels in women tend to be significantly lower than those of men.[9,14] Apart from a hormonal influence on haemopoiesis, iron deficiency is likely to be a factor influencing the difference; the extent to which menstrual blood loss is a significant factor is not clear because a loss of up to 100 ml of blood with each period may lead to iron depletion although without anaemia.[15,16] Moreover, arrest of menstruation by oral contraceptives causes an increase in serum iron without affecting the haemoglobin level.[17] There may be ethnic differences. A major national health survey in the United States over a 6-year period has shown that in socially comparable populations the haemoglobin in Black Americans is 5–10 g/l lower than their White counterparts at all ages and as much as 20 g/l lower in the first 2 years of life.[18]

Table 2.5 Haemoglobin values in pregnancy	
1st trimester	124–135 g/l
2nd trimester	110–117 g/l
3rd trimester	106–109 g/l*
Mean values postpartum	
Day 2	104 g/l
Week 1	107 g/l
Week 3	116 g/l
Month 2	119 g/l

*Normal values (120 g/l or higher) may be found when supplementary iron is being given.

Pregnancy

In normal pregnancy, there is an increase in erythropoietic activity.[19] However, at the same time, an increase in plasma volume occurs,[20,21] and this results in a progressive decrease in haemoglobin, PCV, and RBC (Table 2.5). The level returns to normal about a week after delivery. There is a slight increase in MCV during the second trimester.[22] Serum ferritin decreases in early pregnancy and usually remains low throughout pregnancy, even when supplementary iron is given,[23] although the decrease in haemoglobin is less marked.

Old Age

In healthy men and women, haemoglobin, RBC, PCV and related parameters remain remarkably constant until the sixth decade. Aging is, however, a gradual process, the start of which is arbitrary. In many studies it is assumed to be 65 years, but anaemia becomes more common in those older than 70–75 years.[24–26] This is less marked in women than in men, so that a difference of 20 g/l in younger age groups is reduced to 10 g/l or less in old age. There is a concomitant increase in serum iron, although serum ferritin levels remain higher in men than in women. The factors to be considered for the lower haemoglobin in the elderly include diminished erythropoietic reserves with decrease in erythroid progenitors in the bone marrow, cobalamin deficiency, and chronic inflammatory disease or chronic blood loss (which is often overlooked).[24,25] Moderate or severe anaemia should never be attributed to aging *per se* until underlying disease has been excluded; however, a significant number of elderly subjects with anaemia have no identifiable clinical or nutritional causes.

Transient Changes

In addition to the permanent effects of age and sex, there seem to be transient fluctuations, the significance of which is often difficult to assess.

Exercise

It is not clear whether light exercise increases the RBC or haemoglobin significantly above the baseline observed with the subject at rest; the effects may be small enough to be submerged in the technical errors of estimation. More significant changes occur in endurance athletes—for example, long-distance runners who may develop so-called "sports anaemia" with a slightly lower haemoglobin and RBC, thought to be the result of increased plasma volume).[27,28] Conversely, in sprinters who require a short burst of very strenuous muscular activity, the RBC increases by 0.5×10^{12}/l and haemoglobin by 15 g/l, largely because of reduction in plasma volume and to a lesser extent to the re-entry into the circulation of cells previously sequestered in the spleen.[29] This is a transient event that occurs in athletes immediately after a race, whereas at all other times there are no significant differences in haemoglobin and PCV between these athletes and nonathletic controls—a point to be aware of when checking athletes for "dope"-related effects.[30,31]

Decreased levels of serum iron and ferritin occur during endurance training, possibly associated with loss of iron in sweat.[32] These effects of exercise must be distinguished from a form of haemolysis known as "runner's anaemia" or "march haemoglobinuria," which occurs as a result of pounding of the feet on the ground.[33]

Posture

There is a small but significant alteration in the plasma volume with an increase in haemoglobin and PCV as the posture changes from lying to sitting, especially in women[34]; conversely, change from walking about to lying down results in a 5–10% decrease in the Hb and PCV. Thus, subjects should rest for 5–10 min before their blood is collected. The difference in position of the arm during venous sampling, whether dependent or held at atrial level, can also affect the PCV.

These aspects highlight the importance of using a standardized method for blood collection. This is discussed in Chapter 1 and differences between venous and capillary blood are described on p. 5.

Diurnal and Seasonal Variation

Changes in Hb and RBC during the course of the day are usually slight, about 3%, with negligible changes in the MCV and MCH. However, variation of 20% occurs with reticulocytes.[8] Serum erythropoietin has a marked diurnal variation, being lowest at 8 a.m., with increases by 40% at 4 p.m. and 60% at 8 p.m.[35] Pronounced, but variable, diurnal variations are also seen in serum iron and ferritin.[36,37] Because fluctuations will also occur in patients taking iron-containing supplements, the timing of specimen collection must also take this into account.[37] It has been suggested that minor seasonal variations also occur, but the evidence for this is conflicting.[38–40]

Altitude

The effect of altitude is to increase the Hb and PCV and increase the number of circulating red cells with a lower MCV. The magnitude of the poly-cythaemia depends on the degree of hypoxaemia.[41] At an altitude of 2000 metres (c 6500 ft), haemoglobin is c 8–10 g/l and PCV is 0.025 higher than at sea level; at 3000 metres (c 10,000 ft), haemoglobin is c 20 g/l and PCV is 0.060 higher, and at 4000 metres (c 13,000 feet) haemoglobin is

35 g/l and PCV is 0.110 higher. Corresponding increases occur at intermediate and at higher altitudes.[42] These increases appear to be the result of both increased erythropoiesis as a result of the hypoxic stimulus and the decrease in plasma volume that occurs at high altitudes.

Smoking

Cigarette smoking affects Hb, RBC, PCV, and MCV (see p. 21).

Leucocyte Count

The effect of age is indicated in Tables 2.2, 2.3, and 2.4; at birth, the total leucocyte count is high; neutrophils predominate, reaching a peak of c 13.0 $\times 10^9$/l at 12 hours, then falling to c 4.0 $\times 10^9$/l over the next few weeks, and then to a level at which the count remains steady. The lymphocytes decrease during the first 3 days of life often to a low level of c 2.0–2.5 $\times 10^9$/l and then rise up to the 10th day; after this time, they are the predominant cell (up to about 60%) until the 5th to 7th year when they give way to the neutrophils. From that age onward, the levels are the same as for adults.[7] There are also slight sex differences; the total leucocyte count and the neutrophil count may be slightly higher in girls than in boys,[7] and in women than in men.[43] After menopause, the counts fall in women so that they tend to become lower than in men of similar age.[15,43]

People differ considerably in their leucocyte counts. Some tend to maintain a relatively constant level over long periods; others have counts that may vary by as much as 100% at different times. In some subjects, there appears to be a rhythm, occurring in cycles of 14 to 23 days, and in women this may be related to some extent to the menstrual cycle. Some forms of oral contraception have been reported to raise the leucocyte count.[43] There is no clearcut diurnal variation, but minimum counts are found in the morning with the subject at rest, and during the course of a day there may be differences of 14% for the total leucocyte count, 10% for neutrophils, 14% for lymphocytes, and 20% for eosinophils[8]; in some cases this may result in a reversed neutrophil:lymphocyte ratio. Random activity may raise the count slightly; strenuous exercise causes increases of up to 30 $\times 10^9$/l, chiefly because of decreased splenic blood flow resulting in reduced pooling of neutrophils in the spleen and to some extent because of liberation into the bloodstream of neutrophils formerly sequestered in shutdown capillaries and in the spleen.[44] Large numbers of lymphocytes and monocytes also enter the bloodstream during strenuous exercise. However, there have also been reports of neutropenia and lymphopenia in athletes undergoing daily training sessions.[45,46]

Adrenaline (epinephrine) injection causes an increase in the leucocyte count; here, too, increases in the numbers of all major types of leucocytes (and platelets) occur, possibly reflecting the extent of the reservoir of mature blood cells present not only in the bone marrow and spleen but also in other tissues and organs of the body. Emotion may possibly cause an increase in the leucocyte count in a similar way. A transient lymphocytosis with a reversed neutrophil:lymphocyte ratio occurs in adults with physical stress or trauma.[47] This may also occur in patients when visiting their doctors. The effect of ingestion of food is uncertain. Cigarette smoking has an effect on the leucocyte count (see p. 21).

A moderate leucocytosis of up to 15 $\times 10^9$/l is common during pregnancy, owing to a neutrophilia, with the peak in the second trimester.[22] The count returns to normal levels a week or so after delivery.[48]

The environment may influence the leucocyte count. Thus, in tropical Africa, there is a tendency for a reversal of the neutrophil:lymphocyte ratio in individuals with a low total leucocyte count.[49] This may partly result from endemic parasitic and protozoal disease; however, genetics are also likely to play a part because significantly lower leucocyte counts, especially neutrophil counts, have also been observed in Africans living in Britain.[50] In some tropical areas, reactive eosinophilia or monocytosis is sufficiently common to be regarded as a (normal?) reference value for that population. Elderly people receiving influenza vaccination show a lower total leucocyte count owing to a decrease in lymphocytes.[51]

Platelet Count

There is a slight diurnal variation of about 5%[8]; this occurs during the course of a day as well as from day to day. Within the wide normal reference range, there are some ethnic differences, and in healthy West Indians and Africans platelet counts may on average be 10–20% lower than those in Europeans living in the same environment.[52] There may be a sex difference; thus, in women, the platelet count has been reported to be about 20% higher than in men.[53] A decrease in the platelet count may occur in women at about the time of menstruation. There are no obvious age differences; however, in the first year after birth the platelet count tends to be at the higher level of the adult normal reference range. Strenuous exercise causes a 30–40% increase in platelet count[44]; the mechanism is similar to that which occurs with leucocytes.

Other Blood Constituents

As with the blood count, variations from normal reference values occur in respect of sex, age, stress, diurnal fluctuation, and so on. These are described in the relevant chapters.

Effects of Smoking

Cigarette smoking has a significant effect on many haematological normal reference values.[54] Some effects may be transient, and their severity varies between individuals as well as by the number of cigarettes smoked. Smoking 10 or more cigarettes a day results in slightly higher Hb, PCV, and MCV.[40,55] This is probably a consequence of the accumulation of carboxyhaemoglobin in the blood together with a decrease in plasma volume. After a single cigarette, the carboxyhaemoglobin level increases by about 1%,[56] and in heavy smokers the carboxyhaemoglobin may constitute c 4–5% of the total Hb. There may be polycythaemia.[57]

The leucocyte count increases, largely as a result of an increase in the neutrophils, and neutrophil function may be affected.[14,54,58] Lymphocytes are also affected with an increase in CD4-positive and total lymphocyte count.[54,58,59]

Smokers tend to have higher platelet counts than nonsmokers, but the counts decrease rapidly on cessation of smoking.[54] Studies of platelet aggregation and adhesiveness have given equivocal results, but there appears to be a consistent increase in platelet turnover with decreased platelet survival and increased plasma β-thromboglobulin. Elevated fibrinogen concentration (with increased plasma viscosity) and reduced protein S have been reported, but smoking does not seem to have any consistent effects on the fibrinolytic system.[54]

The influence of smoking on the blood is summarized in Table 2.6.

Table 2.6   Effects of cigarette smoking*[54–59]

Increased	Decreased
Haemoglobin (Hb)	Plasma volume
Red cell count (RBC)	Protein S
Packed cell volume (PCV)	
Mean cell volume (MCV)	
Mean cell haemoglobin (MCH)	
White cell count (WBC)	
Neutrophil count	
Lymphocyte count	
T cells (CD4-positive)	
Monocyte count	
Carboxyhaemoglobin (>2 %)	
Platelet count (transient)	
Mean platelet volume	
Fibrinogen	
β-thromboglobulin	
von Willebrand factor	
Red cell mass	
Haptoglobins	
Plasma viscosity	
Whole blood viscosity	
Erythrocyte sedimentation rate (ESR)	

*Extent of change from normal reference values varies with individuals and amount smoked; some effects may occur only during and immediately after smoking. Some effects may be transient, and their severity varies between individuals as well as by the number of cigarettes smoked.

REFERENCES

1. International Committee for Standardization in Haematology 1981 The theory of reference values. Clinical and Laboratory Haematology 3:369–373.
2. International Federation of Clinical Chemistry and International Council for Standardization in Haematology 1987 The theory of reference values Part 6: Presentation of observed values related to reference values. Journal of Clinical Biochemistry 25:657–662.

3. International Committee for Standardization in Haematology 1982 Standardization of blood specimen collection procedures for reference values. Clinical and Laboratory Haematology 4:83–86.

4. Tukey JW 1977 Exploratory data analysis. Addison-Wesley, Reading MA.

5. International Federation of Clinical Chemistry and International Council for Standardization in Haematology 1987 The theory of reference values Part 5: Statistical treatment of collected reference values. Determination of reference limits. Journal of Clinical Chemistry and Clinical Biochemistry 25:645–656.

6. Lilleyman JS, Hann IM, Blanchette VS 1999 Pediatric hematology, 2nd ed., Churchill Livingstone, London.

7. Taylor MRH, Holland CV, Spencer R, et al 1997 Haematological reference ranges for school children. Clinical and Laboratory Haematology 19:1–15.

8. Richardson Jones A, Twedt D, Swaim W, et al 1996 Diurnal change of blood count analytes in normal subjects. American Journal of Clinical Pathology 106:723–727.

9. White A, Nicolaas G, Foster K, et al 1991 Health Survey for England: Office of population census and surveys—Social Survey Division. HMSO, London.

10. Bellamy GJ, Hinchliffe RF, Crawshaw KC 2000 Total and differential leucocyte counts in infants at 2, 5 and 13 months of age. Clinical and Laboratory Haematology 22:81–87.

11. Handin RI, Lux SE, Stossel TP 2003 Blood—Principles and Practice of Hematology, 2nd ed., p. 2219. Lippincott Williams and Wilkins, Philadelphia.

12. International Council for Standardization in Haematology: Expert Panel on Cytometry 1995 Recommendation of the International Council for Standardization in Haematology on reporting differential leucocyte counts. Clinical and Laboratory Haematology 17:113.

13. Özbek N, Gürakan B, Kayiran SM 2000 Complete blood cell counts in capillary and venous blood of healthy term newborns. Acta Haematologica 103:226–228.

14. Helman N, Rubenstein LS 1975 The effects of age, sex and smoking on erythrocytes and leukocytes. American Journal of Clinical Pathology 63:35–44.

15. Cruickshank JM, Alexander MK 1970 The effect of age, parity, haemoglobin level and oral contraceptive preparations on the normal leucocyte count. British Journal of Haematology 18:541.

16. Hallberg L, Hogdahl AM, Nilsson L, et al 1966 Menstrual blood loss and iron deficiency. Acta Medica Scandinavica 180:639–650.

17. Burton JL 1967 Effect of oral contraceptives on haemoglobin, packed cell volume, serum-iron and total iron-binding capacity in healthy women. Lancet 1:978–980.

18. Houwen B, van Assendelft OW 2002 Haemoglobinometry: screening and routine practice. In: Rowan RM, van Assendelft OW, Preston FE (eds) Advanced Laboratory Methods in Haematology, pp 182–190, Arnold, London.

19. McMullin MF, White R, Lappin T, et al 2003 Haemoglobin during pregnancy: relationship to erythropoietin and haematinic status. European Journal of Haematology 71:44–50.

20. Chesley LC 1972 Plasma and red cell volumes during pregnancy. American Journal of Obstetrics and Gynecology 112:440–450.

21. Large RD, Dynesius R 1973 Blood volume changes during normal pregnancy. Clinics in Haematology 2:433–451.

22. Balloch AJ, Cauchi MN 1993 Reference ranges for haematology parameters in pregnancy derived from patient populations. Clinical and Laboratory Haematology 15:7–14.

23. Howells MR, Jones SE, Napier JAF, et al 1986 Erythropoiesis in pregnancy. British Journal of Haematology 64:595–599.

24. Carmel R 2001 Anemia and aging: an overview of clinical, diagnostic and biological issues. Blood Reviews 15:9–18.

25. Nilsson-Ehle H, Jagenburg R, Landahl S, et al 2000 Blood haemoglobin declines in the elderly: implications for reference intervals from age 70 to 85. European Journal of Haematology 65:297–305.

26. Mattila KS, Kuusela V, Pelliniemi TT, et al 1986 Haematological laboratory findings in the elderly; influence of age and sex. Scandinavian Journal of Clinical and Laboratory Investigation 46:411–415.

27. Smith JA 1995 Exercise, training and red blood cell turnover. Sports Medicine 19:9–31.

28. Green HJ, Sutton JR, Coates G, et al 1991 Response of red cell and plasma volume to prolonged training in humans. Journal of Applied Physiology 70:1810–1815.

29. Allsop P, Peters AM, Arnot RN, et al 1992 Intrasplenic blood cell kinetics in man before and after brief maximal exercise. Clinical Science 83:47–54.

30. Marx JJM, Vergouwen PCJ 1998 Packed-cell volume in elite athletes. Lancet 352:451–452.

31. Lippi G, Franchini M, Guidi G 2002 Haematocrit measurement and antidoping policies. Clinical and Laboratory Haematology 24:65–66.
32. Cook JD 1994 The effect of endurance training on iron metabolism. Seminars in Hematology 31:146–154.
33. Davidson RJL 1964 March or exertional haemoglobinuria. Seminars in Haematology 6:150–161.
34. Felding P, Tryding N, Hyltoft Petersen P, et al 1980 Effects of posture on concentration of blood constituents in healthy adults: practical application of blood specimen collection procedures recommended by the Scandinavian Committee on Reference Values. Scandinavian Journal of Clinical and Laboratory Investigation 40:615–621.
35. Wide L, Bengtsson C, Birgegård G 1989 Circadian rhythm of erythropoietin in human serum. British Journal of Haematology 72:85–90.
36. Romslo I, Talstad I 1988 Day-to-day variations in serum iron, serum iron binding capacity, serum ferritin and erythrocyte protoporphyrin concentration in anaemic subjects. European Journal of Haematology 40:79.
37. Dale JC, Burritt MF, Zinsmeister AR 2002 Diurnal variation of serum iron, iron-binding capacity, transferrin saturation and ferritin levels. American Journal of Clinical Pathology 117:802–808.
38. Costongs GMPJ, Janson PCW, Bas BM, et al 1985 Short-term and long-term intra-individual variations and critical differences of haematological laboratory parameters. Journal of Clinical Chemistry and Biochemistry 23:69–76.
39. Ross DW, Ayscue LH, Watson J, et al 1988 Stability of hematologic parameters in healthy subjects: intraindividual versus interindividual variation. American Journal of Clinical Pathology 90:262–267.
40. Kristal-Boneh E, Froom P, Harari G, et al 1997 Seasonal differences in blood cell parameters and the association with cigarette smoking. Clinical and Laboratory Haematology 19:177–181
41. Ruiz-Arguelles GJ, Sanchez-Medal L, Loria A, et al 1980 Red cell indices in normal adults residing at altitudes from sea level to 2670 meters. American Journal of Hematology 8:265–271.
42. Myhre LD, Dill DB, Hall FG, et al 1970 Blood volume changes during three week residence at high altitude. Clinical Chemistry 16:7–14.
43. England JM, Bain BJ 1976 Total and differential leucocyte count. British Journal of Haematology 33:1–7.
44. Allsop P, Arnot R, Gwilliam M et al 1988 Does splenic autotransfusion occur during high intensity cycle exercise in man. Journal of Physiology (London) 407:24P
45. Watson HG, Meiklejohn DJ 2001 Leucopenia in professional football players. British Journal of Haematology 112:824–827.
46. Bain BJ, Philllips D, Thomson K, et al 2000 Investigation of the effect of marathon running on leucocyte counts of subjects of different ethnic origins: relevance to the aetiology of ethnic neutropenia. British Journal of Haematology 108:483–487.
47. Karandikar NJ, Hotchkiss EC, McKenna RW 2002 Transient stress lymphocytosis: an immunophenotypic characterization of the most common cause of newly identified adult lymphocytosis in a tertiary hospital. American Journal of Clinical Pathology 117:819–825.
48. Cruickshank JM 1970 The effects of parity on the leucocyte count in pregnant and non-pregnant women. British Journal of Haematology 18:531–540.
49. Woodliff HJ, Kataaha PK, Tibaleka AK, et al 1972 Total leucocyte count in Africans. Lancet 2:875.
50. Bain BJ, Seed M, Godsland I 1984 Normal values for peripheral blood white cell counts in women of four different ethnic origins. Journal of Clinical Pathology 37:188–193.
51. Cummins D, Wilson ME, Foulger KJ, et al 1998 Haematological changes associated with influenza vaccination in people aged over 65: case report and prospective study. Clinical and Laboratory Haematology 20:285–287.
52. Bain BJ, Seed M 1986 Platelet count and platelet size in healthy Africans and West Indians. Clinical and Laboratory Haematology 8:43–48.
53. Stevens RF, Alexander MK 1977 A sex difference in the platelet count. British Journal of Haematology 37:295–300.
54. Bain BJ 1992 The haematological effects of smoking. Journal of Smoking-related Diseases 3:99–108.
55. Whitehead TP, Robinson D, Allaway SL, et al 1995 The effects of cigarette smoking and alcohol consumption on blood haemoglobin, erythrocytes and leucocytes: a dose related study on male subjects. Clinical and Laboratory Haematology 17:131–138.
56. Russell MA, Wilson C, Cole PV, et al 1973 Comparison of increases in carboxyhaemoglobin after smoking "extramild" and "non mild" cigarettes. Lancet 2:687–690.
57. Smith JR, Landaw SA 1978 Smoker's polycythemia. New England Journal of Medicine 298:6–10.

58. Parry H, Cohen S, Schlarb J 1997 Smoking, alcohol consumption and leukocyte counts. American Journal of Clinical Pathology 107:64–67.

59. Bain BJ, Rothwell M, Feher MD et al 1992 Acute changes in haematological parameters on cessation of smoking. Journal of the Royal Society of Medicine 85:80–82.

60. Kayiran SM, Özbek N, Turan M, et al 2003 Significant differences between capillary and venous complete blood counts in the neonatal period. Clinical and Laboratory Haematology 25:9–16.

3 Basic haematological techniques

Barbara J Bain, S. Mitchell Lewis, and Imelda Bates

It is possible to use manual, semiautomated, or automated techniques to determine the various components of the full blood count (FBC). Manual techniques are generally low cost with regard to equipment and reagents but are labour intensive; automated techniques entail high capital costs but permit rapid performance of a large number of blood counts by a smaller number of laboratory workers. Automated techniques are more precise, but their accuracy depends on correct calibration and the use of reagents that are usually specific for the particular analyzer. Many laboratories now use automated techniques almost exclusively, but certain manual techniques are necessary as reference for standardization of the methods. Manual methods may also be needed to deal with samples that have unusual characteristics that may give discrepant results with automated analyzers.

All the tests discussed in this chapter can be performed on venous or free-flowing capillary blood that has been anticoagulated with ethylenedi-aminetetra-acetic acid (EDTA) (p. 6). Thorough mixing of the blood specimen before sampling is essential for accurate test results. Ideally, tests should be performed within 6 hours of obtaining the blood specimen because some test results are altered by longer periods of storage. However, results that are sufficiently reliable for clinical purposes can usually be obtained on blood stored for up to 24 hours at 4°C (see p. 7).

HAEMOGLOBINOMETRY

The haemoglobin concentration (Hb) of a solution may be estimated by measurement of its colour, by its power of combining with oxygen or carbon monoxide, or by its iron content. The methods to be described are all colour or light-intensity matching techniques, which also measure, to a varying extent, any methaemoglobin (Hi) or sulphaemoglobin (SHb) that may be present. The oxygen-combining capacity of blood is 1.34 ml O_2 per g haemoglobin. Ideally, for assessing *clinical* anaemia, a functional estimation of Hb should be carried out by measurement of oxygen capacity, but this is hardly practical in the routine haematology laboratory. It gives results that are at least 2% lower than those given by the other methods, probably because a small proportion of inert pigment is always present. The iron content of haemoglobin can be estimated accurately,[1] but again the method is impractical for routine purposes. Estimations based on iron content are generally taken as authentic, but iron bound to inactive pigment is included. Iron content is converted into haemoglobin by assuming the following relationship: 0.347 g iron = 100 g haemoglobin.[2]

MEASUREMENT OF HAEMOGLOBIN CONCENTRATION USING A SPECTROMETER (SPECTROPHOTOMETER) OR PHOTOELECTRIC COLORIMETER

Two methods are in common use: (a) haemiglobincyanide (HiCN; cyanmethaemoglobin) method, and (b) oxyhaemoglobin (HbO_2) method. There is little to choose in accuracy between these methods, although a major advantage of the HiCN method is the availability of a stable and reliable reference preparation.

Although the HiCN reagent contains cyanide, there is only 50 mg of potassium cyanide per litre and 600–1000 ml would have to be swallowed to produce serious effects. However, the use of potassium cyanide has been viewed as a potential hazard; alternative nonhazardous reagents that have been proposed are sodium azide[3] and sodium lauryl sulphate,[4,5] which convert haemoglobin to haemiglobinazide and haemiglobinsulphate, respectively. They are used in some automated systems, but no stable standards are available, and they, too, are toxic substances that must be handled with care.

Other methods that have been used include Sahli's acid-haematin method, which is less accurate because the colour develops slowly, is unstable, and begins to fade almost immediately after it reaches its peak. The alkaline-haematin method gives a true estimate of total Hb even if carboxyhaemoglobin (HbCO), Hi, or SHb is present; plasma proteins and lipids have little effect on the development of colour, although they cause turbidity. The original method was more cumbersome and less accurate than the HiCN or HbO_2 methods, but a modified method has been developed in which blood is diluted in an alkaline solution with nonionic detergent and read in a spectrometer at an absorbance of 575 nm against a standard solution of chlorohaemin.[6,7] One evaluation has given encouraging results,[8] although another study has shown a bias of 2.6% when compared with the reference method, with non-linearity in the relationship between haemoglobin concentration and absorbance at high and low haemoglobins.[9]

HAEMIGLOBINCYANIDE (CYANMETHAEMOGLOBIN) METHOD

The haemiglobincyanide (cyanmethaemoglobin) method is the internationally recommended method for determining the haemoglobin[2] concentration of blood.* The basis of the method is dilution of blood in a solution containing potassium cyanide and potassium ferricyanide. Haemoglobin, Hi, and HbCO, but not SHb, are converted to HiCN. The absorbance of the solution is then measured in a spectrometer at a wavelength of 540 nm or a photoelectric colorimeter with a yellow–green filter (e.g., Ilford 625, Wratten 74, Chance 0 Gr1).

Diluent

The original (Drabkin's) reagent had a pH of 8.6. The following modified solution, Drabkin-type reagent, as recommended by the International Committee for Standardization in Haematology,[2] has a pH of 7.0–7.4. It is less likely to cause turbidity from precipitation of plasma proteins and requires a shorter conversion time (3–5 min) than the original Drabkin's solution, but it has the disadvantage that the detergent causes some frothing:

Potassium ferricyanide (0.607 mmol/l)	200 mg
Potassium cyanide (0.768 mmol/l)	50 mg
Potassium dihydrogen phosphate	
(1.029 mmol/l)	140 mg
Nonionic detergent	1 ml
Distilled or deionized water	To 1 litre

Suitable nonionic detergents include Nonidet P40 (VWR International, Merck, Eurolab) and Triton X-100 (Aldrich).

The pH should be 7.0–7.4 and must be checked with a pH meter at least once a month. The diluent should be clear and pale yellow in colour. When measured against water as a blank in a spectrometer at a wavelength of 540 nm, absorbance must be zero. If stored at room temperature in a brown borosilicate glass bottle, the solution keeps for several months. If the ambient temperature is higher than 30°C, the solution should be stored in the refrigerator but brought to room temperature before use. It must not be allowed to freeze. The reagent must be discarded if it becomes turbid, if the pH is found to be outside the 7.0–7.4 range, or if it has an absorbance other than zero at 540 nm against a water blank.

Haemiglobincyanide Reference Standard

With the advent of HiCN solution, which is stable for many years, other standards have become outmoded.[10] The International Committee for Standardization in Haematology[2] has defined specifications on the basis of a relative molecular mass (molecular weight) of human haemoglobin of 64458 (i.e., 16114 as the monomer) and a millimolar area absorbance (coefficient extinction) of 11.0.*

Some standards are prepared from ox blood, which has the same coefficient extinction but a molecular weight of 64532 (16133 as the monomer). These specifications have been widely adopted; a World Health Organization (WHO) International Standard has been established, and a comparable reference material is also available from the European Community Bureau of Reference (BCR) (see p. 694). Preparations that conform to these international specifications are available commercially. They contain 550–850 mg of haemoglobin per litre, and the exact concentration is indicated on the label.

The HiCN solution is dispensed in 10 ml sealed ampoules and is regarded as a dilution of whole blood. The original Hb that it represents is obtained by multiplying the figure stated on the label by the dilution to be applied to the blood sample. Thus, if the standard solution contains 800 mg (0.8 g) of haemoglobin per litre, it will have the same optical density as a blood sample containing 160 g/l of

---

*In some countries cyanide reagents are no longer available.

*That is, the absorbance of a solution containing 55.8 mg of haemoglobin iron per litre at 540 nm.

haemoglobin if diluted 1 to 200, or as one containing 200 g/l of haemoglobin if diluted 1 to 250.[†]

The HiCN reference preparation is intended primarily for direct comparison with blood that is converted to HiCN. It can also be used for the standardization of a whole-blood standard in the HbO_2 method (discussed later).

Method

Make a 1 in 201 dilution of blood by adding 20 µl of blood to 4 ml of diluent. Stopper the tube containing the solution and invert it several times. Let the test sample stand at room temperature for at least 5 min (to ensure the complete conversion of haemoglobin to haemiglobinocyanide), and then pour it into a cuvette and read the absorbance in a spectrometer at 540 nm or in a photoelectric colorimeter with a suitable filter (e.g., Ilford 625, Wratten 74, Chance 0 Gr1) against a reagent blank. The absorbance of the test sample must be measured within 6 hours of its initial dilution. The absorbance of a commercially available HiCN standard (brought to room temperature if previously stored in a refrigerator) should also be compared to a reagent blank in the same spectrometer or photoelectric colorimeter as the patient sample. The standard should be kept in the dark, and, to ensure that contamination is avoided, any unused solution should be discarded at the end of the day on which the ampoule is opened.

Calculation of Haemoglobin Concentration

$$Hb\ (g/l) = \frac{*A^{540}\ of\ test\ sample}{A^{540}\ of\ standard} \times Conc.\ of\ standard \times \frac{Dilution\ factor\ (201)^{\ddagger}}{1000}$$

Preparation of Standard Graph and Standard Table

When many blood samples are to be tested, it is convenient to read the results from a standard graph or table relating absorbance readings to haemoglobin in g/l for the individual instrument. This graph should be prepared each time a new photometer is put into use or when a bulb or other components are replaced. It can be prepared as follows.

Prepare five dilutions of the HiCN reference standard (or equivalent preparation) (brought to room temperature) with the cyanide–ferricyanide reagent according to Table 3.1. Because the graph will be used to determine the haemoglobin measurements, it is essential that the dilutions are performed accurately.

The haemoglobin concentration of the reference preparation in each tube should be plotted against the absorbance measurement. For example, if the label on the reference preparation states that it contains 800 mg/l, (i.e. 0.8 g/l) and the method for haemoglobin measurement uses a dilution of 1:201, the respective haemoglobin concentrations of tubes 1–5 would be 160 g/l, 120 g/l, 80 g/l, 40 g/l, and zero.

Using linear graph paper, plot the absorbance values on the vertical axis and the haemoglobin values[‡] on the horizontal axis. (If the readings are in percentage transmittance, use semilogarithmic paper with the transmittance recorded on the vertical, or log, scale.) The points should fit a straight line that passes through the origin. Providing that the standard has been correctly diluted, this provides a check that the calibration of the photometer is linear. From the graph, it is possible to construct a table of readings and corresponding haemoglobin values. This is more convenient than reading values from a graph when large numbers of measurements are made. It is important that the performance of the instrument does not vary and that its calibration remains constant in relation to haemoglobin measurements. To ensure this, the reference preparation should be measured at frequent intervals, preferably with each batch of blood samples.

The main advantages of the HiCN method for haemoglobin determination are that it allows direct comparison with the reference standard and that the readings need not be made immediately after

---

[†]Within the SI system, haemoglobin may be expressed in terms of substance concentration as µmol/l or in mass concentration as g/l (or g/dl) or µmol/l = g/l × 0.062. For clinical purposes, there are practical advantages in expressing haemoglobin in mass concentration per litre or per decilitre (dl).

[‡]Absorbance; formerly called optical density. In some instruments, measurements are read as percentage transmittance.

[†]Or 251 if initial dilution is 1 in 250 (i.e., 20 µl blood to 5 ml reagent).

Table 3.1   Dilutions of haemiglobincyanide (HiCN) reference solution for preparation of standard graph

Tube	Haemoglobin* (%)	HiCN volume (ml)	Reagent volume (ml)
1	100 (full strength)	4.0 (neat)	None
2	75	3.0	1.0
3	50	2.0	2.0
4	25	1.0	3.0
5	0	None	4.0 (neat)

*As percent of haemoglobin in reference solution.

dilution so batching of samples is possible. It also has the advantage that all forms of haemoglobin, except SHb, are readily converted to HiCN.

The rate of conversion of blood containing HbCO is markedly slow. This difficulty can be overcome by prolonging the reaction time to 30 min before reading.[1] The difference between the 5 and 30 min readings can be used as a semiquantitative method for estimating the percentage of HbCO in the blood.

As referred to earlier, lauryl sulphate[5] or sodium azide[3] can be used as nonhazardous substitutes for potassium cyanide. However, no stable standards are available for these methods so a sample of blood that has first had a haemoglobin value assigned by the HiCN method needs to be used as a secondary standard.

Abnormal plasma proteins or a high leucocyte count may result in turbidity when the blood is diluted in the Drabkin-type reagent. The turbidity can be avoided by centrifuging the diluted sample or by increasing the concentration of potassium dihydrogen phosphate to 33 mmol/l (4.0 g/l).[12]

OXYHAEMOGLOBIN METHOD

The HbO_2 method is the simplest and quickest method for general use with a photometer. Its disadvantage is that it is not possible to prepare a stable HbO_2 standard, so the calibration of these instruments should be checked regularly using HiCN reference solutions or a secondary standard of preserved blood or lysate (p. 27). The reliability of the method is not affected by a moderate increase in plasma bilirubin, but it is not satisfactory in the presence of carboxy, met, or SHb.

Method

Wash 20 ml of blood into a tube containing 4 ml of 0.4 ml/l ammonia (specific gravity 0.88) to give a ×201 dilution. Use a tightly fitting stopper and mix by inverting the tube several times. The solution of HbO_2 is then ready for matching against a standard in a spectrometer at 540 nm or a photometer with a yellow–green filter (e.g., Ilford 625) against a water blank. If the absorbance of the haemoglobin solution exceeds 0.7, dilute the blood further with an equal volume of water, and read again. Fresh ammonia solution must be made up each week. Once diluted, the blood sample is stable at 20°C for about 2 days.

Standard

A standard should be prepared from a specimen of normal anticoagulated whole blood. Its haemoglobin is first determined by the HiCN method (p. 27). The blood is then diluted 1:201 by pipetting 20 ml of the well-mixed blood into 4 ml of ammonia; sequential dilutions are made in ammonia, and absorbance is read in a spectrometer at 540 nm or photometer using a yellow–green filter (Ilford 625, Wratten 74, or Chance 0 Gr 1). The readings are plotted on arithmetic graph paper. Linearity of response is checked, and absorbance is related to haemoglobin from the measurement obtained in the original sample by the HiCN method.

Colorimeters and light filters unfortunately differ sufficiently one from the other to make it essential to check the chosen standard at frequent intervals against a HiCN reference preparation in the photometer in which it is going to be used. It is probably preferable to use a new fresh whole-blood sample each day as a secondary standard after measuring its haemoglobin by the HiCN method. Preserved blood (p. 660) or lysate (p. 661) can be used instead.

Direct calculation from a standard:

$$Hb \ (g/l) = \frac{A^{540} \ \text{test sample}}{A^{540} \ \text{standard}} \times \frac{\text{Conc. of}}{\text{standard}} \times \frac{\text{Dilution factor}}{1000}$$

If the HiCN method is not available, a neutral grey filter of 0.475 density (Ilford or Chance) can be used as a calibration standard. This corresponds to a 1:201 dilution of blood with 146 g/l haemoglobin in a 1-cm cuvette at a wavelength of 540 nm.

DIRECT SPECTROMETRY

The haemoglobin of a diluted blood sample can be determined by spectrometry without the need for a standard, provided that the spectrometer has been correctly calibrated. The blood is diluted 1:201 (or 1:251) with cyanide–ferricyanide reagent (p. 27), and the absorbance is measured at 540 nm. Haemoglobin is calculated as follows:

$$Hb \ (g/l) = \frac{A^{540} \ \text{HiCN} \times 16114 \times \text{Dilution factor}}{11.0 \times d \times 1000}$$

$$\text{or } Hb \ (\mu mol/l) = \frac{A^{540} \ \text{HiCN} \times \text{Dilution factor}}{11.0 \times d \times 1000}$$

where A^{540} = absorbance of solution at 540 nm; 16114 = monomeric molecular weight of haemoglobin; dilution = 201 when 20 ml of blood are diluted in 4 ml of reagent; 11.0 = millimolar coefficient extinction; d = layer thickness in cm; and 1000 = conversion of mg to g.

When assigning a value to a haemoglobin solution that may be used as a reference preparation, it is necessary first to calibrate the spectrometer. This requires checking wavelength with a holmium oxide filter, absorbance with a set of calibrated neutral density filters, and stray light with a neutral density filter at 220 nm.* Matched optical or quartz glass cuvettes with a transmission difference of <1% at 200 nm should be used. Subsequently, the calibration of the spectrophotometer can be checked by verifying that it gives an accurate reading of the HiCN standard. Slight deviations from the expected A^{540} HiCN value for the standard may be used to

correct the results of test samples for a bias in measurement.[2]

DIRECT READING PORTABLE HAEMOGLOBINOMETERS

Colour Comparators

These are simple clinical devices that compare the colour of blood against a range of colours representing haemoglobin concentrations. They are intended for anaemia screening in the absence of laboratory facilities and are described in Chapter 27.

Portable Haemoglobinometers

Portable haemoglobinometers have a built-in filter and a scale calibrated for direct reading of haemoglobin in g/dl or g/l. They are generally based on the HbO_2 method. A number of instruments are now available that use a light-emitting diode of appropriate wavelength and are standardized to give the same results as with the HiCN method.

The HemoCue system (HemoCue AB, Ängelsholm, SE-262 23, Sweden) is a well-established method for haemoglobinometry. It consists of a precalibrated, portable, battery-operated spectrometer; no dilution is necessary because blood is run by capillary action directly into a cuvette containing sodium nitrite and sodium azide, which convert the haemoglobin to azidemethaemoglobin. The absorbance is measured at wavelengths of 565 and 880 nm. Measurements are not affected by high levels of bilirubin, lipids, or white cells, and it is sufficiently reliable for use as a laboratory instrument; it is easy for nontechnical personnel to operate and is thus also suitable for use at point-of-care. The cuvettes must be stored in a container with a drying agent and kept within the temperature range of 15–30°C.

The DHT Haemoglobinometer (Gordon-Keeble, Barton Mills, IP28 7DX, UK) is a direct reading precalibrated spectrometer that measures haemoglobin in blood diluted 1:100 in 0.4 g/l ammoniated water. It functions at a set wavelength of 523 nm, which has been chosen as the crossover of absorption curves of the common forms of haemoglobin, all of which are included in the measurement. A

---

*For example, from National Physical Laboratory, Teddington, TW11 0LW, UK.

validation study on a batch of blood samples showed some results within 2–3% of the reference method, but there are generally differences of 8–10%, with the DHT instrument tending to read higher than the reference method (data at www.gordon-keeble.co.uk/haemoglobin).

Noninvasive Screening Tests

Methods are being developed for using near infrared spectroscopy at body sites, mainly a finger, to identify the spectral pattern of haemoglobin in an underlying blood vessel and derive a measurement of haemoglobin concentration. Early studies have shown an approximate correlation with blood haemoglobinometry.[13,14]

Range of Haemoglobin in Health

See Chapter 2, Tables 2.2, 2.3, and 2.4. It should be noted that there are sex differences, diurnal variations, and environmental and physiological factors that must also be taken into account.

PACKED CELL VOLUME OR HAEMATOCRIT

The packed cell volume (PCV) can be used as a simple screening test for anaemia, as a reference method for calibrating automated blood count systems, and as a rough guide to the accuracy of haemoglobin measurements. The haematocrit ×1000 is about three times the haemoglobin expressed in g/l. In conjunction with estimations of haemoglobin and red blood cell count (RBC), it can be used in the calculation of red cell indices. However, its use in under-resourced laboratories may be limited by the need for a specialized centrifuge and a reliable supply of capillary tubes.

MICROHAEMATOCRIT METHOD[15]

The microhaematocrit method[15] is carried out on blood contained in capillary tubes 75 mm in length and having an internal diameter of about 1 mm. The tubes may be plain for use with anticoagulated blood samples or coated inside with 1 iu of heparin for the direct collection of capillary blood. The centrifuge used for the capillary tubes provides a centrifugal force of c 12000 g, and 5 min centrifugation results in a constant PCV. When the PCV is greater than 0.5, it may be necessary to centrifuge for a further 5 min.

Allow blood from a well-mixed specimen, or from a free flow of blood by skin puncture, to enter the tube by capillarity, leaving at least 15 mm unfilled. Then seal the tube by a plastic seal (e.g. Cristaseal, Hawksley, Lancing, Sussex). Sealing the tube by heating is not recommended because the seals tend to be tapered and there is the likelihood of lysis. After centrifugation for 5 min, measure the proportion of cells to the whole column (i.e., the PCV) using a reading device.

Accuracy of Microhaematocrit

The microhaematocrit method has an adequate level of accuracy and precision for clinical utility.[16] However, attention must be paid to a number of factors that may produce an inaccurate result.

Anticoagulant

K_2-EDTA is recommended, because K_3-EDTA causes shrinking of the red cells, reducing the PCV by about 2%. Anticoagulant concentration in excess of 2.2 mg/ml may also cause a falsely low PCV as a result of cell shrinkage.

Blood Sample

Because the PCV gradually increases with storage, the test should be performed within 6 hours of collecting the blood sample, but a delay of up to 24 hours is acceptable if the blood is kept at 4°C.

Failure to mix the blood sample adequately will produce an inaccurate result. The degree of oxygenation of the blood also affects the result because the PCV of venous blood is ~2% higher than that of fully aerated blood (which has lost CO_2 and taken up O_2).[17] To ensure adequate oxygenation and sample mixing, the free air space above the sample should be >20% of the container volume.

Capillary Tubes

Variation of the bore of the tubes may cause serious errors if they are not within the narrow limits of defined specifications that should be met by manu-facturers: length 75 $\pm$ 0.5 mm; internal diameter 1.07–1.25 mm, wall thickness 0.18–0.23 mm; and bore taper not exceeding 2% of the internal diameter over the entire length of the tube.[16]

Centrifuge

Centrifuges should be checked at intervals (at least annually) by a tachometer for speed and by a stopwatch for timer accuracy. Efficiency of packing should also be tested by centrifuging samples of normal and polycythaemic blood for varying times from 5 to 10 min to determine the minimum time for complete packing of the red cells.

Reading

The test should be read as soon as possible after centrifugation because the red cells begin to swell and the interface becomes progressively more indistinct. To avoid errors in reading with the special reading device, a magnifying glass should be used. White cells and platelets (the buffy coat) must be excluded as far as possible from the reading of the packed red cells. If a special reading device is not available, the ratio of red cell column to whole column can be calculated from measurements obtained by placing the tube against arithmetic graph paper or against a ruler.

Plasma Trapping

The amount of plasma trapped between red cells, especially in the lower end of the red cell column, and red cell dehydration during centrifugation generally counterbalance each other, and the error caused by trapped plasma is usually not more than 0.01 PCV units. Thus, in routine practice, it is unnecessary to correct for trapped plasma, but if the PCV is required for calibrating a blood cell analyser or for calculating blood volume, the observed PCV should be reduced by a 2% correction factor after it has been centrifuged for 5 min or for 10 min with polycythaemic blood.[18] It is, however, prefer-able to use the surrogate reference method. Plasma trapping is increased in macrocytic anaemias,[19] spherocytosis, thalassaemia, hypochromic anaemias, and sickle cell anaemia[20]; it may be as high as 20% in sickle cell anaemia if all the cells are sickled.[19]

Haemoglobin is measured by routine method on blood specimens in a range of haemoglobin con-centrations. Samples of the same specimens are then taken into special borosilicate glass capillary tubes, which are centrifuged for 5 min or longer to achieve full red cell packing. The tubes are then broken at the midpoint of the packed red cells, blood is extracted with a micropipette, and its haemoglobin is measured. PCV is calculated as the ratio of the Hb of whole blood to that of the packed cells. This method is appropriate for instrument and reagent manufacturers, but it is time-consuming and requires significant expertise, which makes it impractical for occasional use in routine laboratories. Accordingly, the International Council for Standardization in Haematology (ICSH) has developed a "surrogate reference method."[22]

Surrogate Reference Method

Equipment

Standard microhaematocrit centrifuge

Borosilicate glass capillary tubes with the following specifications: length 75 $\pm$ 0.5 mm; inner diameter 1.55 $\pm$ 0.085 mm; outer diameter 1.9 $\pm$ 0.085 mm*

Capillary tube holder consisting of a 75- $\times$ 25-mm glass slide mounted on a 75- $\times$ 50-mm slide.

Microscope fitted with a vernier scale and ocular crossbar.

Method

1. Take up duplicate samples of well-mixed blood into the specified capillary tubes and centrifuge as described on p. 31.
2. Promptly remove the tubes from the centrifuge, position each in turn against the edge of the 25-mm slide, and place this on the stage of the microscope.
3. Ensure that the capillary tube is aligned in a true horizontal position relative to the field of view

---

*For example, Drummond Scientific, Broomall, PA 19008: Catalogue # 1-000-7510.

and, using low power, note on the vernier scale the lengths of the tube at the interfaces of (a) red cells and seal, (b) red cells and leucocytes, and (c) plasma and air.

4. Calculate the spun PCV = (B–A)/(C–A). Determine the acceptability of paired measurements— duplicates must agree within 0.007 units; if they do not, the paired tests must be repeated.
5. Calculate the surrogate reference PCV from the formula[†]:

$$\frac{\text{Spun PCV} - 0.0119}{0.9736}$$

If the surrogate reference measurements are to be used to validate equipment or methods, a minimum of six different blood samples are required, at least two in each of the ranges of PCV 0.20–0.25, 0.40–0.45, and 0.60–0.65. If necessary, the PCV of normal samples may be adjusted by the appropriate addition or removal of autologous plasma.

Range of Packed Cell Volume in Health

See Chapter 2.

MANUAL CELL COUNTS AND RED CELL INDICES

The principles of manual cell counts, the use of the haemocytometer counting chamber for manually counting white cells and platelets, and the limitations of these measurements are described in Chapter 27.

An accurate RBC enables the mean cell volume (MCV) and mean cell haemoglobin (MCH) to be calculated. In well-equipped laboratories, where these indices are provided by an automated system (p. 46), they are of considerable clinical importance and are widely used in the classification of anaemia. Where automated analysers are not used, manual RBCs (and consequently, calculations of these red cell indices) are so inaccurate and time-consuming that they have become obsolete.

The only measurement that can be obtained with reasonable accuracy by manual methods is mean cell haemoglobin concentration (MCHC) because this is derived from Hb and PCV from the following formula:

$$\text{MCHC (g/l)} = \text{Hb (g/l)} \div \text{PCV (l/l)}.$$

Range of MCHC in Health

See Chapter 2.

BASOPHIL AND EOSINOPHIL COUNTS

Count the percentage of eosinophils or basophils in a differential count of all the leucocytes on a stained blood film. If fewer than 500 cells are seen in the film, continue the count on a second film. Then calculate the eosinophil or basophil count per litre from the total leucocyte count. It is essential to have thin, preferably short, films with the leucocytes evenly distributed throughout the film and readily identified (p. 34).

Range of Eosinophil Count in Health

See Chapter 2.

There is normally considerable diurnal variation in the eosinophil count, and differences amounting to as much as 100% have been recorded. The lowest counts are found in the morning (10 a.m. to noon) and the highest at night (midnight to 4 a.m.).[23–24] For a review of the causes of eosinophilia, see reference 25.

Range of Basophil Count in Health

See Chapter 2.

Gilbert and Ornstein[26] reported a 95% distribution in normal subjects of $0.01–0.08 \times 10^9$/l. There are no age or sex differences, although serial counts have shown lower levels during ovulation.[27]

MANUAL DIFFERENTIAL LEUCOCYTE COUNT

Differential leucocyte counts are usually performed by visual examination of blood films that are pre-

---

[†]This formula applies only to the specified capillary tubes; other tubes require specific validation by the ICSH Reference method[21] so that an appropriate formula can be derived.

pared on slides by the spread or "wedge" technique. Unfortunately, even in well-spread films, the distribution of the various cell types is not totally random (see below).

For a reliable differential count on films spread on slides, the film must not be too thin and the tail of the film should be smooth. To achieve this, the film should be made with a rapid movement using a smooth glass spreader. This should result in a film in which there is some overlap of the red cells, diminishing to separation near the tail, and in which the white cells in the body of the film are not too badly shrunken. If the film is too thin, or if a rough-edged spreader is used, many of the white cells, perhaps even 50% of them, accumulate at the edges and in the tail (Fig. 3.1). Moreover, a gross qualitative irregularity in distribution is the rule: polymorphonuclear neutrophils and monocytes predominate at the margins and the tail; lymphocytes predominate in the middle of the film (Fig. 3.2). This separation probably depends on differences in stickiness, size, and specific gravity of the different types of cells.

Differences in distribution of the various types of cells are probably always present to a small extent even in well-made films. Various systems for performing the differential count have been advocated, but none can compensate for the gross irregularities in distribution in a badly made film. On well-made films, the following technique of counting is recommended.

Method

Count the cells using a ×40 objective in a strip running the whole length of the film. Avoid the lateral edges of the film. Inspect the film from the head to the tail, and if fewer than 100 cells are encountered in a single narrow strip, examine one or more additional strips until at least 100 cells have been counted. Each longitudinal strip represents the blood drawn out from a small part of the original drop of blood when it has spread out between the slide and spreader (Fig. 3.3). If all the cells are counted in such a strip, the differential totals will closely approximate the true differential count. This technique is liable to error if cells in the thick part of the film cannot be identified; also, it does not allow for any excess of neutrophils and monocytes

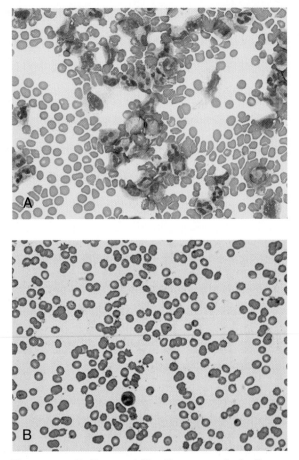

Figure 3.1 Badly spread film. Two areas of a badly spread film from a patient with a white blood cell count of 20×10^9/l showing (A) many leucocytes in the tail; and (B) very few leucocytes in body of film.

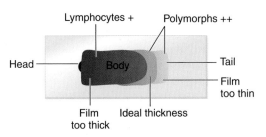

Figure 3.2 Schematic drawing of a blood film made on a slide. The film has been spread from left to right. An indication is given of the way the white blood cells are distributed (see text).

at the edges of the film, but this preponderance is slight in a well-made film and in practice makes little difference to the result.

This technique is easy to carry out; with high counts ($10-30 \times 10^9$ cells per litre) a short, 2–3 cm, film is desirable. In patients with very high counts (as in leukaemia), the method has to be abandoned and the cells should be counted in any well-spread area where the cell types are easy to identify. Other systems of counting, such as the "battlement" count, are more elaborate but may minimize error owing to variation of distribution of cells between the centre and the edge of the film. The results of the differential count can be recorded using a multiple manual register or they can directly entered onto a computer.

The variance of the differential count depends not only on artefactual differences in distribution owing to the process of spreading, but also on "random" distribution; together they are by far the most important cause of unreliable differential counts. The random distribution means that, if a total of 100 cells are counted, with a true neutrophil proportion of 50%, the range (±2SD) within which 95% of the counts will fall is of the order of ±14% (i.e., 36–64%) neutrophils. A 200-cell count can provide a more accurate estimate; in the previous example, the ±2SD range will be about 40–60%. In a 500-cell count, the range would be reduced to 44–56% neutrophils. In practice, a 100- or 200-cell count is recommended as a routine procedure. However, if abnormal cells are present in small numbers, they

are more likely to be detected when 200–500 cell counts are performed than with a 100-cell count.

Reporting the Differential Leucocyte Count

The differential count, expressed as the percentage of each type of cell, should be related to the total leucocyte count and the results should be reported in absolute numbers ($\times 10^9$/l). Myelocytes and metamyelocytes, if present, are recorded separately from neutrophils. Band (stab) cells are generally counted as neutrophils, but it may be useful to record them separately. They normally constitute less than 6% of the neutrophils; an increase may point to an inflammatory process even in the absence of an absolute leucocytosis.[28] However, the band cell count is imprecise, and, although it is sometimes recommended in infants, it has been found to be unhelpful in predicting occult bacteraemia in this group.[29]

Correcting the Count for Nucleated Red Blood Cells

When nucleated red blood cells (NRBC) are present, they will be included in the total WBC, which is really a "total nucleated cell count" (TNCC). They should also be included in the differential count, as a percentage of the TNCC, and reported in absolute numbers ($\times 10^9$/l) in the same way as the different types of leucocytes. If they are present in significant numbers, the TNCC should be corrected to obtain the true total WBC. Thus, for example, if total WBC is 8.0×10^9/l and the percentage of NRBCs on the differential count is 25%, then

$$\text{Corrected WBC} = 8 - (8 \times 25/100) = 6 \times 10^9/\text{l}.$$

Care should be taken to differentiate small lymphocytes from nucleated red blood cells (e.g., Chapter 5, Figure 5.64).

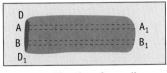

→ Direction of spreading

Figure 3.3   Schematic drawing illustrating the longitudinal method of performing differential leucocyte counts. The original drop of blood spreads out between spreader and slide (D–D_1). The film is made in such a way that representative strips of films, such as A–A_1 and B–B_1, are formed from blood originally at A and B, respectively. To perform an accurate differential count, all the leucocytes in one or more strips, such as A–A_1 and B–B_1, should be inspected and classified.

Reference Differential White Cell Count

A reference method is required to validate the accuracy of automated systems (to be described later). The method that has been used widely for this purpose is essentially similar to the routine manual procedure on stained blood films, but to ensure adequate precision a 200-cell count is carried out by two independent observers, each on two films prepared from the same sample.[30] However, this is still too imprecise for cells with a low frequency, and attempts have been made to establish a reference method using flow cytometry with specific monoclonal-antibody labeling of the specific cell types, including immature leucocytes.[31,32]

Range of Differential White Cells in Health

See Chapter 2.

PLATELET COUNT

The method for manual counting of platelets using a counting chamber is described on page 677. If an RBC by a semiautomated counter is available, it is possible to obtain an approximation of the platelet count by counting the proportion of platelets to red cells in a thin part of a film made from an EDTA blood sample, using the ×100 oil-immersion objective and, if possible, eyepieces provided with an adjustable diaphragm, as for a reticulocyte count.

RETICULOCYTE COUNT

Reticulocytes are juvenile red cells; they contain remnants of the ribosomal ribonucleic acid (RNA) that was present in larger amounts in the cytoplasm of the nucleated precursors from which they were derived. Ribosomes have the property of reacting with certain basic dyes such as azure B, brilliant cresyl blue, or New methylene blue (see below) to form a blue or purple precipitate of granules or filaments.

This reaction takes place only in vitally stained unfixed preparations. Stages of maturation can be identified by their morphological features. The most immature reticulocytes are those with the largest amount of precipitable material; in the least immature, only a few dots or short strands are seen. Reticulocytes can be classified into four groups, ranging from the most immature reticulocytes, with a large clump of reticulin (group I), to the most mature, with a few granules of reticulin (group IV) (Fig. 3.4).

If a blood film is allowed to dry and is afterwards fixed with methanol, reticulocytes appear as poly-chromatic red cells staining diffusely basophilic if the film is stained with one of the basic dyes.

Complete loss of basophilic material probably occurs in the bloodstream and, particularly, in the spleen after the cells have left the bone marrow.[33] This maturation is thought to take 2–3 days, of which about 24 hours are spent in the circulation.

The number of reticulocytes in the peripheral blood is a fairly accurate reflection of erythropoietic activity, assuming that the reticulocytes are released normally from the bone marrow and that they remain in circulation for the normal time period. These assumptions are not always valid because an increased erythropoietic stimulus leads to premature release into the circulation. The average maturation time of these so-called "stress" or stimulated reticulocytes may be as long as 3 days. In such cases, a higher than normal proportion of immature reticulocytes will be found in circulation. A more precise assessment of reticulocyte maturation is possible by quantitative flow cytometry of their RNA content. Nevertheless, adequate information is usually obtained from a simple reticulocyte count recorded either as a percentage of the red cells or, preferably, when the RBC is known, as an absolute number per l. When there is severe anaemia, the reticulocyte count should be corrected for the anaemia and expressed as a reticulocyte index.[34]

$$\text{Reticulocyte index} = \text{Observed reticulocyte\%} \times \frac{\text{Measured Hb or PCV}}{\text{Appropriate normal Hb or PCV}}$$

Reticulocyte Stains

Better and more reliable results are obtained with New methylene blue* than with brilliant cresyl blue. New methylene blue stains the reticulofilamentous material in reticulocytes more deeply and more uniformly than does brilliant cresyl blue, which varies from sample to sample in its staining ability. Azure B is a satisfactory substitute for New methylene blue; it has the advantage that the dye does not precipitate, and it is available in pure form.[38] It is used in the same concentration, and the staining procedure is the same as with New methylene blue.

---

*New methylene blue is chemically different from methylene blue, which is a poor reticulocyte stain.

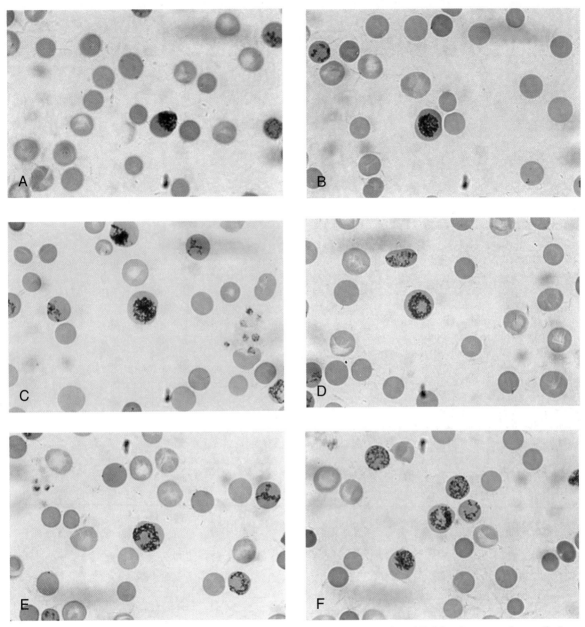

Figure 3.4   Photomicrographs of reticulocytes showing stages of maturation. A and B: Most immature (group I); C and D: Intermediate (group II); E and F: Later stage intermediate (group III).

Staining Solution

Dissolve 1.0 g of New methylene blue (CI 52030) or azure B (CI 52010) in 100 ml of iso-osmotic phosphate buffer pH 6.5.

Method

Deliver 2 or 3 drops of the dye solution into a 75- × 10-mm plastic tube by means of a plastic Pasteur pipette. Add 2–4 volumes of the patient's EDTA-

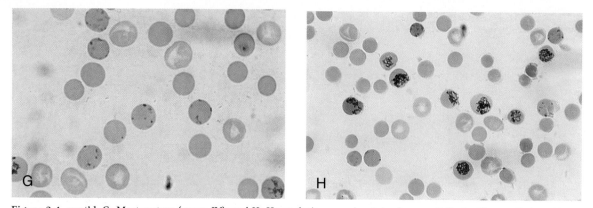

Figure 3.4, cont'd G: Most mature (group IV); and H: Haemolytic anaemia, stained supravitally by New methylene blue.

anticoagulated blood to the dye solution and mix. Keep the mixture at 37°C for 15–20 min. Resuspend the red cells by gentle mixing, and make films on glass slides in the usual way. When dry, examine the films without fixing or counterstaining.

The exact volume of blood to be added to the dye solution for optimal staining depends on the RBC. A larger proportion of anaemic blood, and a smaller proportion of polycythaemic blood, should be added than of normal blood. In a successful preparation, the reticulofilamentous material should be stained deep blue and the nonreticulated cells should be stained diffuse shades of pale greenish blue. Films should not be counterstained. The reticulofilamentous material is not better defined after counterstaining, and precipitated stain overlying cells may cause confusion. Moreover, Heinz bodies will not be visible in fixed and counterstained preparations. If the stained preparation is examined under phase contrast, both the mature red cells and reticulocytes are well defined. By this technique, late reticulocytes characterized by the presence of remnants of filaments or threads are readily distinguished from cells containing inclusion bodies. Satisfactory counts may be made on blood that has been allowed to stand (unstained) for as long as 24 hours, although the count will tend to decrease after 6–8 hours unless the blood is kept at 4°C.

Counting Reticulocytes

An area of film should be chosen for the count where the cells are undistorted and where the staining is good. A common fault is to make the film too thin; however, the cells should not overlap. To count the cells, use the ×100 oil-immersion objective and, if possible, eyepieces provided with an adjustable diaphragm. If eyepieces with an adjustable diaphragm are not available, a paper or cardboard diaphragm, in the centre of which has been cut a small square with sides about 4 mm in length, can be inserted into an eyepiece and used as a less convenient substitute.

The counting procedure should be appropriate to the number of reticulocytes present. Very large numbers of cells have to be surveyed if a reasonably accurate count is to be obtained when only small numbers of reticulocytes are present. When the count is less than 10%, a convenient method is to survey successive fields until at least 100 reticulocytes have been counted and to count the total red cells in at least 10 fields to determine the average number of red cells per field.

Calculation

Number of reticulocytes in n fields = x
Average number of red cells per field = y
Total number of red cells in n fields = n × y
Reticulocyte percentage = [x ÷ (n × y)] × 100%
Absolute reticulocyte count = % × RBC

Thus, when the reticulocyte percentage is 3.3 and the RBC is 5×10^{12}/l, the absolute reticulocyte count per litre is as follows: $[3.3/100] \times 5 \times 10^{12} = 165 \times 10^{9}$

It is essential that the reticulocyte preparation be well spread to ensure an even distribution of cells in successive fields.

When the reticulocyte count exceeds 10%, only a relatively small number of cells will have to be surveyed to obtain a standard error of 10%.

An alternative method is based on the principle of balanced sampling, using a Miller ocular.* This is an eyepiece giving a square field, in the corner of which is a smaller ruled square, one-ninth the area of the total square (Fig. 3.5). Reticulocytes are counted in the large square, and the total number of red cells are counted in the small square.

The number of fields that should be surveyed to obtain a desired degree of precision depends on the proportion of reticulocytes (Table 3.2).

It is essential that the reticulocyte preparation be well spread and well stained. Other important factors that affect the accuracy of the count are the visual acuity and patience of the observer and the quality and resolving power of the microscope. The most accurate counts are carried out by a conscientious observer who has no knowledge of the supposed reticulocyte level, thus eliminating the effect of conscious or unconscious bias.

Differentiating between Reticulocytes and Other Red Cell Inclusions

The decision as to what is and what is not a reticulocyte may be difficult because the most mature reticulocytes contain only a few dots or threads of reticulofilamentous material. Fortunately, in well-stained preparations viewed under the light microscope, the Pappenheimer (iron-containing) type of granular material—usually present as a single small dot, less commonly as multiple dots—stains a darker shade of blue than does the reticulofilamentous material of the reticulocyte. As described earlier, phase contrast will help to distinguish them. If there is any doubt, Pappenheimer bodies can be identified by overstaining the film for iron by Perls' reaction.

HbH undergoes denaturation in the presence of brilliant cresyl blue or New methylene blue, resulting in round inclusion bodies that stain greenish-blue (see Chapter 13, Figs. 13.6 and 13.7). These can be easily differentiated from reticulofilamentous material (Fig. 13.8).

Heinz bodies are also stained by New methylene blue, but they stain a lighter shade of blue than the

---

*For example, Graticules Ltd., Morley Road, Tonbridge, UK.

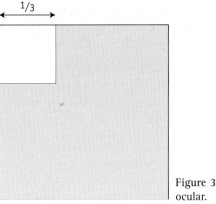

1/3

Figure 3.5   Miller ocular.

Table 3.2   Accuracy of reticulocyte counts with Miller ocular

	Reticulocytes	Standard error (σ)		
Percent	Proportion (p)	2%	5%	10%
1	0.01	27,500	4,400	1,100
2	0.02	13,600	2,180	550
5	0.05	5,280	845	210
10	0.10	2,500	400	100
25	0.25	835	135	35

Columns 3–5 indicate the total number of red cells to be counted *in the small squares* so as to give the required standard error at different reticulocyte levels. It is derived from the following:

$$\sigma = \sqrt{p(1 - p)/\lambda}$$

where p = Number of reticulocytes in n large squares ÷ (number of red cells in n small squares × f); f = ratio of large to small squares (i.e., 9); and λ = approximate total number of cells in n large squares.

reticulofilamentous material of reticulocytes and stain well with methyl violet (Figs. 13.5 and 13.6).

Fluorescence Methods for Performing a Reticulocyte Count

Reticulocytes can be counted manually by fluorescence microscopy on appropriately stained films.[36] Add 1 volume of acridine orange solution (50 mg/100 ml of 9 g/l NaCl) to 1 volume of blood.

Mix gently for 2 min; make films on glass slides, dry rapidly, and examine by a fluorescent microscope. RNA gives an orange–red fluorescence, whereas nuclear material (DNA) fluoresces yellow. Although the amount of fluorescence is proportional to the amount of RNA, the brightness and colour of the fluorescence fluctuates and the preparation quickly fades when exposed to light; also, it requires a special fluorescence microscope. It is thus not suitable for routine use for reticulocyte counting.

Fluorescent staining combined with flow cytometry has been developed as a method for automated reticulocyte counting (see p. 52).

Manual Reference Method

The manual reference method[37,38] is essentially the same procedure as for the routine method, the supravitally stained films slides being examined by bright field or phase contrast. Reticulocytes are identified as non-nucleated red cells that contain at least two blue staining particles or one particle linked to a filamentous thread; every non-nucleated cell in each field must be classified as a red cell or a reticulocyte. Three suitable blood films must be selected for each sample, and counting is performed by moving from field to field in a battlement pattern until sufficient red cells have been counted to satisfy precision requirement (Table 3.2). An objective is a variance of 2%, but this is impractical when the reticulocyte proportion is in the range 0.01–0.02.

Range of Reticulocyte Count in Health

The range of reticulocyte in adults and children is $50–100 \times 10^9/l$ (0.5–2.5%). In infants (full term, cord blood) it is 2–5% (see p. 16).

AUTOMATED BLOOD COUNT TECHNIQUES

A variety of automated instruments for performing blood counts are in widespread use. Semiautomated instruments require some steps (e.g., dilution of a blood sample) to be carried out by the operator. Fully automated instruments require only that an appropriate blood sample is presented to the instrument. Semiautomated instruments often measure a small number of components (e.g., WBC and Hb). Fully automated multichannel instruments usually measure from 8 to 20 components, including some variables that have no equivalent in manual techniques. Automated instruments usually have a high level of precision, which, for cell counting and cell-sizing techniques, is greatly superior to that achievable with manual techniques. If instruments are carefully calibrated and their correct operation is ensured by quality control procedures, they produce test results that are generally accurate. When blood has abnormal characteristics, the results for one or more parameters may be aberrant; instruments are designed so that such inconsistent results are "flagged" for subsequent review. The abnormal characteristics that lead to inaccurate counts vary between instruments, so it is important for instrument operators to be familiar with the types of factitious results to which their instruments are prone.

Blood cell counters may have automated procedures for sample recognition (e.g., by bar-coding), for ensuring that adequate sample mixing occurs, for taking up the test sample automatically, and for detection of clots or inadequately sized samples. Ideally, blood sampling is carried out by piercing the cap of a closed tube so that samples that carry an infection hazard can be handled with maximum safety.

Laboratories performing large numbers of blood counts each day require fully automated blood counters capable of the rapid production of accurate and precise blood counts, including platelet counts and differential counts, either three-part or five- to seven-part. The sample throughput required varies with the workload and the timing of arrival of blood specimens in the laboratory, but for most large laboratories a throughput of 100 or more samples per hour is required. Sample size and the availability of a "predilute" mode are particularly relevant if the laboratory receives many paediatric specimens.

Choice of an instrument for an individual laboratory, as well as for point-of-care sites outside the laboratory (see p. 638), should take account of capital expenditure and running costs, including maintenance and reagents; size of instrument; requirements of services such as water, compressed air, drainage, and an electricity supply with stable voltage; environmental disturbance by generation of heat, vibration, and noise; any influence on performance by the ambient temperature and humidity; storage requirements for the often bulky reagents; ease of operation; and the likely level of support that can be expected from the manufacturer.

A practical guide on the principles of the various systems has been published,[39] and there are guidelines to help in the choice of an instrument suitable for the needs of an individual laboratory and also to assess its performance, as compared with the claims of the manufacturer, when it has been installed and is being used in routine practice.[40] Choice of instrument may be aided by reference to published reports of instrument evaluations, of which there are many, including reports from the U.K. Medicines and Healthcare products Regulatory Agency (formerly Medical Devices Agency) and related monographs.[39,41–43] Some semiautomated instruments aspirate a sample of accurately determined volume and so can perform absolute cell counts and accurate estimations of Hb. Most automated instruments, however, count for a specified period of time rather than on an exact volume of blood; they therefore require calibration by means of the direct counts derived from instruments counting cells in a defined volume of diluted blood. For some variables, instruments are calibrated by the manufacturer, but others require calibration in the laboratory. Performance characteristics of an instrument vary over time, so periodic recalibration is needed, both when quality control procedures indicate the necessity and when certain components are replaced.

HAEMOGLOBIN CONCENTRATION

Most automated counters measure haemoglobin by a modification of the manual HiCN method with cyanide reagent or with a nonhazardous chemical such as sodium lauryl sulphate, which avoids possible environmental hazards from disposal of large volumes of cyanide-containing waste. Modifications include alterations in the concentration of reagents and in the temperature and pH of the reaction. A nonionic detergent is included to ensure rapid cell lysis and to reduce turbidity caused by cell membranes and plasma lipids. Measurements of absorbance are made at a set time interval after mixing of blood and the active reagents but before the reaction is completed.

RED BLOOD CELL COUNT

Red cells and other blood cells can be counted in systems based on either aperture impedance or light-scattering technology. Because large numbers of cells can be counted rapidly, there is a high level of precision. Consequently, electronic counts have rendered the RBC and the red cell indices derived from it (the MCV and the MCH) of much greater clinical relevance than was possible when only a slow and imprecise manual RBC was available.

COUNTING SYSTEMS

Impedance Counting

Impedance counting, first described by Wallace Coulter in 1956,[44] depends on the fact that red cells are poor conductors of electricity, whereas certain diluents are good conductors; this difference forms the basis of the counting systems used in Beckman–Coulter, Sysmex, Abbott, Roche, and a number of other instruments.

For a cell count, blood is highly diluted in a buffered electrolyte solution. The flow rate of this diluted sample is controlled by a mercury siphon (as in the original Coulter system) or by displacement of a tightly fitting piston. This result is a measured volume of the sample passing through an aperture tube of specific dimensions (e.g., 100 mm in diameter and 70 mm in length). By means of a constant source of electricity, a direct current is maintained between two electrodes, one in the sample beaker or the chamber surrounding the aperture tube and another inside the aperture tube. As a blood cell is carried through the aperture, it displaces some of the conducting fluid and increases the electrical resistance. This produces a corresponding change in potential between the electrodes, which lasts as long as the red cell takes to pass though the aperture; the height of the pulses produced indicates the volume of the cells passing through. The pulses can be displayed on an oscillograph screen. The pulses are led to a threshold circuit provided with an amplitude discriminator for selecting the minimal pulse height, which will be counted (Fig. 3.6). The height of the pulses is used to determine the volume of the red cells.

Light Scattering

Red cells and other blood cells may be counted by means of electro-optical detectors.[45] A diluted cell suspension flows through an aperture so that the cells pass, in single file, in front of a light source; light is scattered by the cells passing through the light beam. The scattered light is detected by a photomultiplier or photodiode, which converts it into electrical impulses that are accumulated and counted. The amount of light scattered is proportional to the surface area and therefore the volume of the cell so that the height of the electrical pulses can be used to estimate the cell volume. The high-intensity coherent laser beams used in current instruments have superior optical qualities to the noncoherent tungsten light of earlier instruments. Sheathed flow allows cells to flow in an axial stream with a diameter not much greater than that of a red cell; light can be precisely focused on this stream of cells. Electro-optical detectors are used for red cell sizing and counting in Bayer-Technicon systems and for white cell differential counting in a number of other instruments.

RELIABILITY OF ELECTRONIC COUNTERS

Electronic counts are precise, but care needs to be taken so that they are also accurate. The recorded count on the same sample may vary from instrument to instrument and even between different models of the same instrument. Inaccuracy may be introduced by coincidence (i.e., by two cells passing through an orifice simultaneously and being counted as one cell, or by a pulse being generated during the electronic dead time of the circuit); by recirculation of cells that have already been counted; by red cell agglutination (which causes a clump of cells to be counted as one cell); and by the counting of bubbles, lipid droplets, microorganisms, or extraneous particles as cells. Faulty maintenance may lead to variation in the volume aspirated or the flow rate. Single-channel instruments may have their thresholds set incorrectly, and multichannel instruments may be incorrectly calibrated.

A statistical correction may be applied for coincidence (coincidence correction); in some instruments, this is done automatically by electronic editing. Errors of coincidence can be detected by carrying out a series of measurements at various dilutions of the same specimen, plotting the data on graph paper, and then extrapolating the graph to

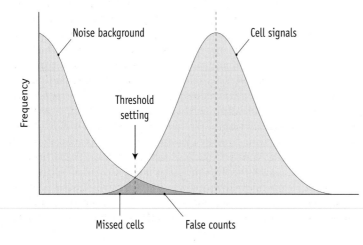

Figure 3.6   Effect of threshold discrimination (horizontal axis) in separating cell signals from background noise.

the baseline for the true value. Alternatively, the need for coincidence correction can be avoided by having the dimensions and flow characteristics of the aperture through which the cells pass such that cells can only pass in single file; this may be achieved by sheath flow or hydrodynamic focusing in which diluted blood is injected into a sheath of fluid as it flows into the sensing zone. This induces the cells to pass through the centre of the sensing zone in single file and free of distortion. Coincidence can be more effectively reduced with sheathed flow and precisely focused light in an electro-optical detector than in an impedance counter so that less dilution of the blood sample is needed.[45] Electrical impulses generated by recirculation of cells can be eliminated by electronic editing; alternatively, recirculation of cells in the region of the aperture can be prevented by "sweep flow" in which a directed stream of diluent sweeps cells and debris away from the aperture, thus preventing cells from being recounted and debris from being counted as cells.

Inaccurate counts consequent on red cell agglutination are usually the result of cold agglutinins. They are recognized as erroneous because of an associated marked factitious elevation of the MCV. A correct count can be achieved by prewarming the blood sample and, if necessary, also prewarming the diluent.

A correct RBC and, particularly, a correct measurement of the MCV is dependent on the use of an appropriate diluent. For impedance counters, pH, temperature, and rate of ionization have to be standardized and remain constant because changes alter the electrical field and may lead to artefactual alterations in the size, shape, and stability of the blood cells in the diluent. Diluents must be free of particles and give a background count of less than 50 particles in the measured volume. The correct diluent for each individual instrument must be used; other diluents, even those made by the same manufacturer, may not be interchangeable. Any laboratories using diluents other than those recommended by the manufacturer of the instrument must satisfy themselves that no error is being introduced.

For red cell counting in simple single-channel counters a suitable diluent requires a pH of 7.0–7.5 and osmolality of 340 ± 10 mmol. Physiological saline (9 g/l NaCl) or phosphate-buffered saline, which have the advantages of simplicity and ready availability, can be used as a red cell diluent, provided that the counts are performed immediately after dilution to avoid errors owing to sphering. Commercial solutions of saline (for intravenous use) are usually particle-free. Other solutions may require filtration through a 0.22- or 0.45-mm micropore filter to remove dust.

Setting Discrimination Thresholds

An accurate RBC requires that thresholds be set so that all red cells, but a minimum of other cells, are included in the count. Some counters have a lower threshold but no upper threshold so that white cells are included in the "RBC." Because the WBC is usually very low in relation to the RBC, this is not usually of practical importance; however, an appreciable error can be introduced if the WBC is greatly elevated, particularly if the patient is also anaemic. The setting of the lower threshold is of considerable importance because it is necessary to ensure that microcytic red cells are included in the count without also counting large platelets.

Current multichannel instruments, both impedance counters and counters using light-scattering technology, have thresholds that are either precalibrated by the manufacturer or are automatically adjusted, depending on the characteristics of individual blood samples. Single-channel impedance instruments capable of performing a direct RBC require setting of thresholds so as to separate pulses generated by red cells from background noise and from pulses generated by platelets. This is done by adjusting the aperture current and the pulse amplification. A simple method is to dilute a fresh blood sample and carry out successive counts on the suspension, while the lower threshold control is moved incrementally from its maximum to its minimum position. At the maximum position, the count should be zero or close to zero, and the counts will increase as the amplitude is reduced. The counts at each setting are plotted on arithmetic graph paper (Fig. 3.7). The correct threshold setting is at the left of the horizontal part of the graph before the line begins to slope. It is important to check that the setting selected is valid for microcytic cells. The threshold can be defined more precisely for an individual sample by means of a pulse height analyser linked to the counting system. The lower threshold is correctly set if beyond this point there are less than

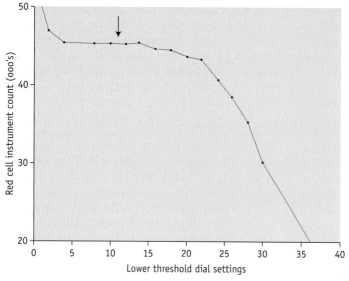

Figure 3.7   Method to establish working conditions of cell counters. The correct setting of the threshold (at arrow) is intended to exclude noise pulses without loss of the signal pulses produced by the blood cells.

0.5% of the counts at the peak (mode) of the pulse size distribution curve (Fig. 3.6).

PACKED CELL VOLUME AND MEAN CELL VOLUME

Modern automated blood cell counters estimate PCV by technology that has little connection with packing red cells by centrifugation. It is sometimes convenient to use different terms to distinguish the manual and automated tests, and for this reason the International Council for Standardization in Haematology has suggested that the term "haematocrit" (Hct) rather than PCV should be used for the automated measurement. However, it should be noted that, in the past, the terms "packed cell volume" and "haematocrit" have been used interchangeably for the manual procedure.

With automated instruments, the derivation of the RBC, PCV, and MCV are closely interrelated. The passage of a cell through the aperture of an impedance counter or through the beam of light of a light-scattering instrument leads to the generation of an electrical pulse the height of which is proportional to cell volume. The number of pulses generated allows the RBC to be determined, as discussed earlier. Pulse height analysis allows either the MCV or the PCV to be determined. If the average pulse height is computed, this is indicative of the MCV, and the PCV can be derived by multiplying the estimated MCV by the RBC. Similarly, if the pulse heights are summated, this figure is indicative of the PCV, and the MCV can, in turn, be derived by dividing the PCV by the RBC.

Automated instruments require calibration before the PCV or MCV can be determined. Calibration of the PCV can be based on manual PCV determinations. Alternatively, the MCV can be calibrated by means of the pulse heights generated by latex beads,* stabilized cells, or some other calibrant containing particles of known size; however, unfixed human red cells that are biconcave and flexible will not necessarily show the same characteristics in a cell counter as latex particles or some other artificial calibrant. Aperture-impedance systems measure an apparent volume that is greater than the true volume, being influenced by a "shape factor"[46]; this factor is less than 1.1 for young, flexible red cells; is between 1.1 and 1.2 for fixed biconcave cells; and is about 1.5 for spheres, whether they be fixed cells or latex spheres.[45,46]

The MCV, and therefore the PCV, as determined by an automated counter, will vary with certain cell

---

*BCR Certified preparations available from Institute for Reference Materials and Measurements (IRMM) (see p. 695).

characteristics other than volume. As indicated earlier, such characteristics include shape, which in turn is partly determined by flexibility. With impedance counters, the normal disc-shaped red cell becomes elongated into a cigar shape as it passes through the aperture; this is caused by deformation in response to shear force, which occurs in cells of normal flexibility. Cells with a reduced haemoglobin concentration undergo more elongation than normal cells; this leads to a reduced "shape factor," a reduced pulse height in relation to the true size of the cell, and underestimation of the MCV. Conversely, cells with abnormally rigid membranes and cells such as spherocytes with a high haemoglobin concentration will undergo less deformation than normal and the MCV will be overestimated. Earlier light-scattering instruments also underestimated the volume of red cells with a reduced haemoglobin concentration because light scattering was affected by the haemoglobin concentration.[47] These artefacts are seen even with normal red cells of varying haemoglobin concentration but are more apparent with red cells from patients with defects in haemoglobin synthesis such as those from patients with iron deficiency. Light-scattering instruments have been developed to avoid artefacts of this type. Cells are isovolumetrically sphered so that their light-scattering characteristics are uniform and should follow the laws of physics. Light scattering by each individual cell is measured at two angles: forward scatter (FSC or FSc) and side scatter (SSC or SSc) at an angle of 90°, which permits computation of both its volume and its haemoglobin concentration[47]; the latter measurement is designated the cellular haemoglobin concentration mean (CHCM) to distinguish it from the traditional MCHC derived from the Hb and the PCV. If all measurements are accurate, the CHCM and the MCHC should give the same results, thus providing an internal quality control mechanism.

The automated MCV and PCV are prone to certain errors that do not occur or are less of a problem with manual methods. These include those resulting from microclots or partial clotting of the specimen, extreme microcytosis, and the presence of cryoglobulins or cold agglutinins; the last is a relatively common cause of factitious elevation of the MCV because clumps of cells are sized as if they were single cells. Because the RBC is under-estimated, the PCV is less affected, although it is also inaccurate. It is rare for warm agglutinins to cause a similar problem. Sickling may cause a factitious increase in MCV and PCV, whereas alterations in plasma osmolarity occurring, for example, in severe hyperglycaemia also cause factitious elevation of the MCV and PCV.[43,48,49]

RED CELL INDICES

Red cell indices traditionally have been the derived parameters of MCV, MCH, and MCHC; more recently, red cell distribution width (RDW) has also been included and, for some instruments, haemoglobin distribution width (HDW). These indices are the basis for classifying anaemias, and in various combinations they have been used to aid in the distinction between iron deficiency and thalassaemias.[50-52] It is important to note, however, that these formulae may not be consistent between different instruments, and their use provides only a guide to the most likely diagnosis. When diagnosis is important, as in preconceptual or antenatal screening for thalassaemia, definitive tests are required, even in patients whose red cell indices are more suggestive of iron deficiency.

Mean Cell Volume

As described earlier, in automated systems, MCV is measured directly, but in semiautomated counters MCV is calculated by dividing the PCV by RBC.

Thus, for example, if the PCV is 0.45 (i.e., 0.45 litres of red cells per litre of blood) and the RBC is 5×10^{12} per litre,

$$\text{Volume of 1 cell} = 0.45 \div 5 \times 10^{12}$$
$$= 90 \text{ femtolitres (fl)}$$

Mean Cell Haemoglobin and Mean Cell Haemoglobin Concentration

MCH is derived from the Hb divided by RBC.

Thus, for example, if there are 150 g of Hb and 5×10^{12} red cells per litre,

$$\text{MCH} = 150 \div 5 \times 10^{12} = 3 \div 10^{11}\text{g}$$
$$= 30 \text{ picograms (pg)}.$$

The MCHC is derived in the traditional manner (p. 33) from the Hb and the PCV with instruments that measure the PCV and calculate the MCV, whereas when the MCV is measured directly and the PCV is calculated, the MCHC is derived from the Hb, MCV, and RBC according to the following formula:

$$\text{MCHC (g/l)} = \frac{\text{Hb (g/l)} \times 1000}{\text{MCV (fl)} \times \text{RBC} \times 10^{-12}/\text{l}}$$

For example, if Hb is 150 g/l, MCV is 90 fl, and RBC is $5 \times 10^{12}/\text{l}$,

$$\text{MCHC} = 150 \times \frac{1000}{90 \times 5}$$

$$= 333 \text{ g/l}$$

As automated counters were developed and introduced, it was noted that the lowered MCHC that, with manual methods, had been a useful indicator of hypochromia in early iron deficiency was a less sensitive indicator of developing iron deficiency. The explanation of this is complex. In iron deficiency, there is not only true hypochromia but also increased plasma trapping within the column of red cells in a microhaematocrit tube that increases the PCV and exaggerates the decrease in the MCHC. The lowered MCHC is thus partly a true reflection of hypochromia and partly an artefact. When the MCHC is derived by automated counters, the artefact of increased plasma trapping is no longer present, but the instruments are also less sensitive to a true reduction of the MCHC because of the underestimation of the size of hypochromic red cells described earlier. Because the MCHC is calculated from the formula given earlier, the underestimation of the MCV leads to an over-estimation of the MCHC. The MCHC thus shows little alteration as cells become hypochromic. Where CHCM is available, it is a more directly measured equivalent of the MCHC. This provides improved sensitivity to iron deficiency because MCHC and the CHCM decrease as hypochromia develops.[53]

VARIATIONS IN RED CELL VOLUMES: RED CELL DISTRIBUTION WIDTH

Automated instruments produce volume distribution histograms that allow the presence of more than one population of cells to be appreciated. Instruments may also assess the percentage of cells falling above and below given MCV thresholds and "flag" the presence of an increased number of microcytes or macrocytes. Such measurements may indicate the presence of a small but significant increase in the percentage of either microcytes or macrocytes before there has been any change in the MCV.

Most instruments also produce a quantitative measurement of the variation in cell volume, an equivalent of the microscopic assessment of the degree of anisocytosis. This new parameter has been named the "red cell distribution width." The RDW is derived from pulse height analysis and can be expressed either as the standard deviation (in fl) or as the coefficient of variation (CV) (%) of the measurements of the red cell volume. Current Beckman-Coulter and Bayer-Technicon instruments express the RDW as the SD, and Sysmex instruments express it as either the SD or the CV. The normal reference range is in the order of $12.8 \pm 1.2\%$ as CV and 42.5 ± 3.5 fl as SD. However, widely different ranges have been reported; therefore it is important for laboratories to determine their own reference ranges. The RDW expressed as the CV has been found of some value in distinguishing between iron deficiency (RDW usually increased) and thalassaemia trait (RDW usually normal) and between megaloblastic anaemia (RDW often increased) and other causes of macrocytosis (RDW more often normal).

VARIATION IN RED CELL HAEMOGLOBINIZATION: HAEMOGLOBIN DISTRIBUTION WIDTH

Instruments that determine the haemoglobin concentration of individual red cells provide distribution curves of the haemoglobin concentration and are able to "flag" the presence of increased numbers of hypochromic cells and hyperchromic cells. The degree of variation in red cell haemoglobinization is quantified as the haemoglobin distribution width or HDW; this is the CV of the measurements of haemoglobin concentration of individual cells. The normal 95% range is 1.82–2.64. Because the volume of individual red cells is determined, it is possible to distinguish between hypochromic microcytes, which are indicative of a defect in haemoglobin synthesis, and hypochromic macrocytes, which often represent reticulocytes.[54] The identification of an increased percentage of hyperchromic cells may be caused by the presence of spherocytes, irregularly contracted cells, or sickled cells.

TOTAL WHITE BLOOD CELL COUNT

The total WBC is determined in whole blood in which red cells have been lysed. The lytic agent is required to destroy the red cells and reduce the red cell stroma to a residue that causes no detectable response in the counting system without affecting leucocytes in such a manner that the ability of the system to count them is altered. Various manufacturers recommend specific reagents, and for multichannel instruments that also perform an automated differential count use of the recommended reagent is essential. For a simple single-channel impedance counter, the following fluid is satisfactory:

Cetrimide 20 g
10% formaldehyde (in 9 g/l NaCl) 2 ml
Glacial acetic acid 16 ml
NaCl 6 g
Water to 1 litre

Relatively simple instruments are also available that determine the Hb and the WBC by consecutive measurements on the one blood sample. The diluent contains a reagent to lyse the red cells and another to convert haemoglobin to haemoglobin cyanide. Hb is measured by a modified HiCN method, and white cells are counted by impedance technology. Apart from the reagents specified by the manufacturers, a diluent containing potassium cyanide and potassium ferricyanide together with ethylhexadecyldimethyl-ammonium bromide can be used.[55,56]

Fully automated multichannel instruments perform WBCs by impedance or light-scattering technology or both. Residual particles in a diluted blood sample are counted after red cell lysis or, in the case of some light-scattering instruments, after the red cells have been rendered transparent. Thresholds are set to exclude normal platelets from the count, although giant platelets are included. Some or all of any nucleated red cells present are usually included, so that when nucleated red cells are present the count approximates more to the TNCC than to the WBC.

Factitiously low automated WBCs occasionally occur as a consequence of leucocyte agglutination, prolonged sample storage, or abnormally fragile cells (e.g., in leukaemia). Factitiously high counts are more common and usually result from failure of lysis of red cells. With certain instruments this may occur with the cells of neonates or be consequent on uraemia or on the presence of an abnormal hae-moglobin such as haemoglobin S or haemoglobin C; high counts may also be the result of microclots, platelet clumping, or the presence of a cryoglobulin.

AUTOMATED DIFFERENTIAL COUNT

Most automated differential counters that are now available use flow cytometry incorporated into a full blood counter rather than being stand-alone differential counters. Increasingly, automated blood cell counters have a differential counting capacity, providing either a three-part or a five- to seven-part differential count. Counts are performed on diluted whole blood in which red cells are either lysed or are rendered transparent. A three-part differential count assigns cells to categories usually designated: (a) "granulocytes" or "large cells"; (b) "lymphocytes" or "small cells"; and (c) "monocytes," "mononuclear cells," or "middle cells." In theory, the granulocyte category includes eosinophils and basophils, but in practice it is common for an appreciable proportion of cells of these types to be excluded from the granulocyte category and to be counted instead in the monocyte category.[57]

Five- to seven-part differential counts classify cells as neutrophils, eosinophils, basophils, lymphocytes, and monocytes and in an extended differential count may also include large immature cells (com-posed of blasts and immature granulocytes) and atypical lymphocytes (including small blasts). Automated instruments performing three-part or five-to seven-part differential counts are able to "flag" or reject counts from the majority of samples with nucleated red cells, myelocytes, promyelocytes, blasts, and atypical lymphocytes. To a lesser extent, instruments incorporating a three-part differential count, although not capable of enumerating eosinophils or basophils, are able to flag a significant proportion of samples that have an increased number of one of these cell types.

Both impedance counters and light-scattering instruments are capable of producing three-part differential counts from a single channel; the categorization is based on the different volume of various types of cell following partial lysis and cytoplasmic shrinkage. Most five- to seven-part differential counts require two or more channels in which cell volume and other characteristics are analysed by various modalities (Table 3.3). Analysis may be dependent only on volume and other physical characteristics of the cell or also on binding of certain dyes to granules or activity of cellular enzymes such as peroxidase. Technologies used to study cell characteristics include light scattering and absorbance and impedance measurements with low- and high-frequency electromagnetic current or radiofrequency current. Cells may have been exposed to lytic agents, or a cytochemical reaction may have occurred before cell characteristics are studied. Two-parameter analysis or more complex discriminant functions divide cells into clusters that can be matched with the position of the various white cell clusters in normal blood. Thresholds, some fixed and some variable, divide clusters from one another, permitting cells in each cluster to be counted.

Automated differential counters using flow cytometry classify far more cells than is possible with a manual differential count. Automated counts are consequently much more precise than manual counts; however, with certain cell categories—specifically monocytes and basophils—the degree of precision is sometimes less than would be expected for the number of cells counted, indicating that such cells are not always classified in a consistent manner. The accuracy of automated counters is less impressive than their precision. With all types of counters, unusual cell characteristics or ageing of a blood specimen can lead to misclassification of cells. Although the majority of samples containing abnormal cells are "flagged," this is not invariably so; the presence of nucleated red cells, immature granulocytes, atypical lymphocytes, and blasts (even occasionally quite large numbers of blasts) may not give rise to a "flag." However, human observers performing a 100-cell manual differential count also miss significant abnormalities. In general, automated counts have compared favourably with routine manual counts, especially if the instruments are assigned only two functions—performing dif-

Table 3.3 Automated full blood counters with a five-part or more differential counting capacity*	
Instrument and manufacturer	Technology used for differential count
Coulter STKS, GEN-S, LH 700 series	Impedance with low-frequency electromagnetic current Impedance with high-frequency electromagnetic current Laser light scattering
Sysmex SE series, XE2100	Impedance with low-frequency direct current Impedance with radiofrequency current
Bayer H series, Advia	Light scattering and absorbance following peroxidase reaction Two-angle light scatter following differential cytoplasmic stripping
Abbott Cell-Dyn 3500	Four light-scattering parameters: forward light scatter, orthogonal light scatter, narrow-angle light scatter, and depolarized orthogonal light scatter
Cobas Argos 5	Electrical impedance with intact cells and following differential cytoplasmic stripping Light absorbance

*In addition to the blood counters listed here, there are an increasing number of instruments on the market that are capable of providing full differential counts using various technologies.

ferential counts on normal samples and "flagging" abnormal samples. If morphological abnormalities are flagged, microscopic examination of a stained blood film should always be undertaken.

The instrument–reagent systems that have been developed to permit automated differential counts often include some, but not all, NRBC in the total "WBC." Thus, in the presence of a significant number of NRBC, the total count is neither a true "WBC" nor a true "TNCC" and the absolute WBC counts calculated from the total will necessarily be somewhat erroneous. This differs from the situation with earlier instruments that included any nucleated red cells in the "WBC." It may be possible to make some assessment of the proportion of the NRBCs included in the total count by studying the graphic output of the instrument, and some instruments also specifically identify and count these cells; otherwise, if accurate absolute counts of different leucocyte types are needed, it is necessary to revert to earlier instruments to provide the TNCC and to correct it to a WBC by means of a differential count.

Instruments currently in use that count NRBC and correct the WBC for NRBC interference include the Abbott CellDyn 4000, the Sysmex XE2100, and the Beckman-Coulter LH750.

Differential counters based on pattern recognition in stained blood films were initially preferred by many haematologists, but they were relatively slow, and because they could count only a small number of cells in a reasonable time, the precision of the automated count was no better than that of a manual count. However, with improved computing technology and with the use of artificial neural networks, such instruments (e.g., DiffMaster, CellVision AB, SE-223 70, Lund, Sweden) are now capable of providing a useful differential count on blood samples containing abnormal cells. Up to 30 films an hour can be processed and reviewed, and abnormal cells can be reclassified if required.

New White Cell Parameters

Many instruments are able to "flag" the presence of atypical or "variant" lymphocytes by features such as alteration in size and in impedance or light-scattering characteristics. Automated white cell counters can also analyse cell characteristics by novel technologies and identify cell types by features that differ greatly from those used when a blood film is examined visually. It is possible, for example, to identify eosinophils by the ability of their granules to polarize light[58] or to detect a left shift or the presence of blasts by the reduced light scattering of the nuclei of more immature granulocytes. There is also the potential to produce information that is not directly analogous with that available from a manual differential count. Instruments that incorporate a cytochemical reaction give information on enzyme activity expressed as the mean peroxidase activity index (MPXI). An increased MPXI has been observed in infections, in some myelodysplasias and leukaemias, in the acquired immune deficiency syndrome (AIDS), and in megaloblastic anaemia, whereas a reduced MPXI occurs in inherited and acquired neutrophil peroxidase deficiency.[53,59,60] Such measurements have the potential for clinical usefulness. The percentage of immature granulocytes as measured by the Sysmex XE2100 has, for example, been found to be predictive of infection, although it should be noted that it was no more predictive than the absolute neutrophil count.[61] It has been suggested that the parameters used for defining leucocyte types might also allow detection of the presence of malaria pigment as a screening test in areas where malaria is prevalent.[62,63]

AUTOMATED INSTRUMENT GRAPHICS

Fully automated instruments produce a graphic display of much of the data produced. This is displayed on a colour monitor and can be printed, either in black and white or in colour. Inspection of the graphic display can give further information beyond that which is available from assessment of the numeric data. Displays usually include histograms of red cell, white cell, and platelet size and sometimes histograms of red cell haemoglobin concentration and scatter plots of size versus haemoglobin concentration. Differential counts are graphically represented as scatter plots of two variables or scatterplots of discriminant functions derived from more than two variables.

Typical printouts of histograms or scatter-plots of current automated instruments are shown in Fig. 3.8.

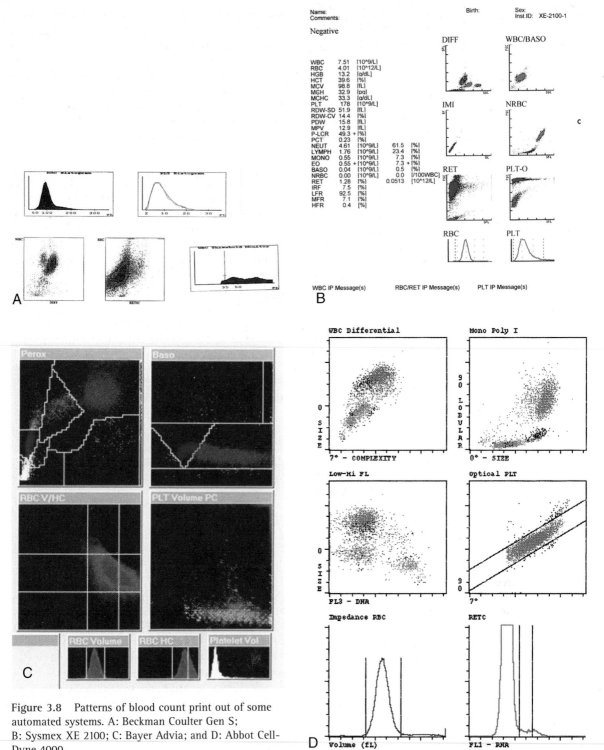

Figure 3.8 Patterns of blood count print out of some automated systems. A: Beckman Coulter Gen S; B: Sysmex XE 2100; C: Bayer Advia; and D: Abbot Cell-Dyne 4000.

PLATELET COUNT

Platelets can be counted in whole blood using the same techniques of electrical or electro-optical detection as are used for counting red cells. An upper threshold is needed to separate platelets from red cells, and a lower threshold is needed to separate platelets from debris and electronic noise. Recirculation of red cells near the aperture should be prevented, as pulses produced may simulate those generated by platelets. Three techniques for setting thresholds have been used: (a) platelets can be counted between two fixed thresholds (e.g., between 2 and 20 fl); (b) pulses between fixed thresholds can be counted with subsequent fitting of a curve and extrapolation so that platelets falling outside the fixed thresholds are included in the computed count; and (c) thresholds can vary automatically, depending on the characteristics of individual blood samples, to make allowance for microcytic or fragmented red cells or for giant platelets.

A new method for platelet counting by flow cytometry has been developed.[64] Platelets in a blood sample are labelled fluorescently with a specific monoclonal antibody or combination of antibodies, and by measuring the RBC:platelet ratio the platelet count can be calculated. Suitable antibodies to platelet antigens are CD41, CD42, and CD61. This method using CD41 and CD61 has been adopted by the International Council for Standardization in Haematology as the reference method.[65] Some instruments now provide an automated immunological platelet count for diagnostic use. Although these instruments can count platelets down to levels of 10×10^9/l or less, it should be noted that precision at these levels is often poor with CVs of 22–66% being observed and with mean counts differing appreciably between instruments.[66]

Factitiously low automated platelet counts may be the result of giant platelets being identified as red cells, EDTA-induced platelet clumping, and satellitism (p. 112). Misleadingly high platelet counts may be due to markedly microcytic or fragmented red cells, to cell fragments in leukaemia,[67] or to bacteria or fungi.

After labelling with specific immunological markers, it is possible to identify young platelets with a higher RNA content.[64,68-70] By analogy with the reticulocyte count, these have been called "reticulated platelets," and it has been suggested that an increased number in the circulation is a sensitive and early indication of regeneration of thromboboiesis in aplastic anaemia. However, because there is a constant exchange of platelets between the circulation and the spleen, it is not clear whether their presence in the blood has the same significance as reticulocytes.

Platelet Count in Health

In health, there are approximately $150–400 \times 10^9$ platelets per litre of blood. The counts are somewhat higher in women than in men,[71] and there is a cycling, with slightly lower count at about the time of menstruation.[72] Lower platelet counts have been observed in apparently healthy West Indians and Africans than in Caucasians.[73]

Mean Platelet Volume

The same techniques that are used to size red cells can be applied to platelets. The calculated mean platelet volume (MPV) is very dependent on the technique of measurement and on length and conditions of storage prior to testing the blood. When MPV is measured by impedance technology, it has been found to vary inversely with the platelet count in normal subjects. If this curve is extrapolated, it has been found that data fit the extrapolated curve when thrombocytopenia is caused by peripheral platelet destruction; however, the MPV is lower than predicted when thrombocytopenia is caused by megaloblastic anaemia or bone marrow failure.[74] The MPV is generally greater than predicted in myeloproliferative disorders, but differentiating essential thrombocythaemia from reactive thrombocytosis on this basis has not been very successful.

Other platelet parameters that can be computed by automated counters include the platelet distribution width (PDW), which is a measure of platelet anisocytosis, and the "plateletcrit," which is the product of the MPV and platelet count and, by analogy with the haematocrit, may be seen as indicative of the volume of circulating platelets in a unit volume of blood. The PDW has been found to be of some use in distinguishing essential thrombocythaemia (PDW increased) from reactive thrombocytosis (PDW normal). The plateletcrit does not appear to provide any information of clinical value.

RETICULOCYTE COUNT

Automated reticulocyte counts have been developed by using the fact that various dyes and fluorochromes combine with the RNA of reticulocytes.[34,75] Following binding of the dye, fluorescent cells can be enumerated using a flow cytometer. Most fully automated blood counters now incorporate a reticulocyte counting capacity so that use of a stand-alone reticulocyte counter is no longer necessary and use of a general purpose flow cytometer is no longer appropriate. An international standard for this method has been published by NCCLS in collaboration with ICSH.[38] The dyes used in the different systems include auramine O (Sysmex), thiazole orange (ABX), CD4K 530 (Abbott), as well as nonfluorescent dyes such as oxazine 750 (Bayer-Technicon) and the traditional New methylene blue (Beckman-Coulter, Abbott).

After staining, it is necessary to separate the reticulocytes from unstained red cells, and, because the dyes also combine with DNA of nucleated cells, these cells must also be excluded. The threshold for this exclusion is determined by the intensity of fluorescence and particle sizing. Although the separation of reticulocytes from mature red cells is not always clearcut, automated reticulocyte counts correlate well with manual reticulocyte counts, although absolute counts may differ because automated counts are dependent on the conditions of incubation and the method of calibrating the instrument.[75] Precision is much superior to that of the manual count because many more cells are counted and the subjective element inherent in recognizing late reticulocytes is eliminated. Potential sources of inaccuracy are the inclusion of some leucocytes and platelets and, less often, Howell–Jolly bodies or malarial parasites in the "reticulocyte" count.

Automated reticulocyte counts are fairly stable in blood that has been stored for 1–2 days at room temperature or up to 3–5 days at 4°C.

Immature Reticulocyte Fraction

Fully automated instruments provide a measure of the various degrees of reticulocyte maturation because the most immature reticulocytes, produced when erythropoietin levels are high, have more RNA and fluoresce more strongly than the mature reticulocytes normally present in the peripheral blood. Parameters indicating reticulocyte immaturity have potential clinical relevance. For example, an increase in mean fluorescence intensity indicative of the presence of immature reticulocytes has been noted as an early sign of engraftment following bone marrow transplantation.

The characteristics of reticulocyte output in different types of anaemias can be especially appreciated from an output bivariate graph relating fluorescent intensity to reticulocyte count.[34] As described earlier, low total count with a relatively high immature reticulocyte fraction (IRF) is indicative of a repopulating marrow, whereas a reticulocytopenia with low IRF is typical of severe aplastic anaemia or renal failure A high total count with high IRF occurs in acute haemolysis and blood loss, whereas a low to normal total count with a high IRF occurs in dyserythropiesis and in early response to haematinics.[76–78] The appearance of reticulocytes with high fluorescence also heralds response when severe aplastic anaemia is being treated with immunosuppressive therapy,[76] and is a reliable indication of haemopoietic regeneration after marrow ablative chemotherapy. A high IRF has also been found to be useful in predicting the optimal time for stem cell harvests in some but not all studies.[79] A normal total count with an unexpectedly high IRF in athletes has been suggested as a method to detect "doping" with erythropoietin.[80] It may also be useful in deciding whether a macrocytic anaemia is megaloblastic or nonmegaloblastic.[81]

Reticulocyte Counts in Health

The normal reticulocyte count in men or women is: $50–100 \times 10^9/l$ (0.5–2.5%).

However, reference ranges reported for automated reticulocyte counts have varied considerably between methods, and it is important for laboratories to establish their own values.

CALIBRATION OF AUTOMATED BLOOD CELL COUNTERS

The following methods are recommended for calibrating an automated blood cell counter[82,83]:

1. By using fresh normal blood specimens to which values have been assigned for Hb, PCV, RBC, WBC, and platelet count by standardized reference methods
2. By use of a stable calibrant (either preserved blood or a substitute) to which values appropriate for the instrument in question have been assigned by comparison with fresh normal blood
3. By use of a commercial calibrant with assigned values suitable for the instrument in question

For reasons of convenience and economy, control materials are commonly used as calibrants; but this practice is not recommended. Such materials are not sufficiently stable to serve as calibrants and their stated values are often approximations that are not assigned by reference methods. They are designed to give test results within a stated range over a stated period rather than a specific result.

The procedure for assigning values to fresh blood samples and indirectly to a stable calibrant is as follows:

1. 4 ml blood specimens are obtained from three haematologically normal volunteers and are anticoagulated with K_2 EDTA.
2. The Hb value is assigned by using the haemiglobincyanide method and the mean of two measurements.
3. The PCV is assigned by the microhaematocrit method, taking the mean of measurements in four microhaematocrit tubes.
4. The RBC is assigned by performing counts on a single-channel aperture-impedance counter capable of performing a direct cell count; the mean of two dilutions, each counted twice, is used.
5. The MCV is assigned by calculation from the RBC and PCV.
6. The WBC is assigned by performing counts on a single-channel aperture-impedance instrument capable of performing direct cell counts; the mean of two dilutions, each counted twice, is used.
7. The platelet count is assigned by using a flow

cytometer capable of measuring the ratio of platelets to red cells; the platelet count is calculated from the ratio and an independently measured RBC. Where fluorescent monoclonal antibody labelling is available, the ICSH/ISLH reference method[65] should be used. In preparations intended as a differential leucocyte count or a reticulocyte count calibrant, assign the values by the reference manual methods,[30,37] as described on p. 33 and p. 40, respectively

To calibrate the automated counter directly from the three fresh blood samples, perform two counts with each sample and take the means. If the measured counts differ from those assigned, recalibrate the counter appropriately.

To calibrate a stable calibrant, perform two counts on the calibrant and on each fresh sample using the automated instrument, A, and take the means. From the ratio of the test results on fresh blood to those on the calibrator, assign corrected values to the calibrator by using the following calculations.

Corrected calibrator value =

$$A_c \times \sqrt[3]{\frac{D_{F1}}{A_{FI}} \times \frac{D_{F2}}{A_{F2}} \times \frac{D_{F3}}{A_{F3}}}$$

where:

A_C = measurement of calibrator by automated counter

A_F = measurement of the fresh bloods (1, 2, and 3) by automated counter

D_F = direct measurement of the fresh bloods (1, 2, and 3).

Considerable care is required to ensure that the initial measurements on the fresh blood are as accurate as possible. Dilutions should be made with individually calibrated pipettes and grade A volumetric flasks. The cell counter should be calibrated as described on p. 43, with a signal-to-noise ratio of greater than 100:1 and the count corrected for coincidence. Details of procedures to be used are described by the International Committee for Standardization in Haematology.[84] Procedures for verification of the performance of multichannel analysers by the users have also been published by ICSH[40] and in the United States by the National Committee for Clinical Laboratory Standards.[85]

FLAGGING OF AUTOMATED BLOOD COUNTS[86-87]

"Flagging" refers to a signal that the specimen being analysed may have a significant abnormality because one or more of the blood count variables are outside specified limits (usually 2SD) or there is a qualitative abnormality that requires a quality control check and/or additional investigation. This usually includes a blood film review. Although it is theoretically desirable for every blood count to include examination of a stained film, this is being challenged by increasing workloads requiring time- and cost-effective rationalization, as well as by the use of automated analyzers that report differential leucocyte counts on every specimen. Consequently, fewer blood films are being examined micro-scopically. Thus, a decision of when a blood film should be made, stained, and examined should take account of flagging and the need to ensure analytic reliability. This includes a check of any significant changes from a recent previous count (delta-check), as well as any specific clinical circumstances. The following is a guide to this selection.

Blood count request: Is it a first time count or repeat count?

First time count: Is it a routine screening test or special category?

If Routine: Analyzer report for blood count alone
Film required if any flags are signalled

If Special category: **Film required:**
1. Diagnosed blood disease patients
2. Patients receiving radiotherapy and/or chemotherapy
3. Renal disease
4. Neonates
5. Intensive care unit
6. If special tests have also been requested for: infectious mononucleosis, haemolytic anaemia, enzymopathy, abnormal haemoglobins
7. If the clinical details on the request form indicate lymphadenopathy, splenomegaly, jaundice or suggest the possibility of leukaemia or lymphoma
8. Specific requests by clinician

Repeat count: **Film required:**

1. Delta check positive when compared with previous record
2. Any flag occurs in present count
3. On each occasion for patients with known blood diseases, for neonates, and when specifically requested by clinicians

REFERENCES

1. Zijlstra WG, van Kampen EJ 1960 Standardization of hemoglobinometry. I. The extinction coefficient of hemiglobincyanide at l = 540mm: $e^{540}HiCN$. Clinica Chimica Acta 91:719–726.
2. International Committee for Standardization in Haematology 1996 Recommendations for Reference Method for Haemoglobinometry in Human Blood (ICSH Standard 1995) and Specifications for International Haemiglobincyanide Standard, 4th ed., Journal of Clinical Pathology 49, 271–274.
3. Vanzetti G 1966 An azide-methemoglobin method for hemoglobin determination in blood. Journal of Laboratory and Clinical Medicine 67:116–126.
4. Oshiro I, Takenaka T, Maeda J 1982 New method for hemoglobin determination by using sodium lauryl sulfate (SLS). Clinical Biochemistry 15:83–88.
5. Lewis SM, Garvey B, Manning R, et al 1991 Lauryl sulphate haemoglobin: a non-hazardous substitute for HiCN in haemoglobinometry. Clinical and Laboratory Haematology 13:279–290.
6. Zander R, Land W, Wolf HU 1984 Alkaline haematin D-575, a new tool for the determination of haemoglobin as an alternative to the cyanhaemiglobin method. I. Description of the method. Clinical Chimica Acta 136:83–93
7. Wolff HU, Land W, Zander R 1984 Alkaline haematin D-575, a new tool for the determination of haemoglobin as an alternative to the cyanhaemiglobin method. 11. Standardization of the method using pure chlorohaemin. Clinical Chimica Acta 136:95–104.
8. Lema OE, Carter JY, Arube PA et al 1994 Evaluation of the alkaline haematin D-575 method for hamoglobin estimation in east Africa. Bulletin of World Health Organization 72:937–941.
9. van Assendelft OW, Zijlstra WG 1989 Observations on the alkaline haematin/detergent complex proposed for measuring haemoglobin concentration. Journal of Clinical Chemistry and Clinical Biochemistry 27:191–195.
10. Van Assendelft OW, Buursma A, Zijlstra WG 1996 Stability of haemiglobincyanide standards. Journal of Clinical Pathology 49:275–277

11. Van Kampen EJ, Zijlstra WG 1983 Spectrophotometry of hemoglobin and hemoglobin derivatives. Advances in Clinical Chemistry 23:199–257.

12. Matsubara T, Okuzono H, Senba U 1979 Modification of Van Kampen–Zijlstra's reagent for the hemiglobincyanide method. Clinica Chimica Acta 93:163–164.

13. Kinoshita Y, Yamane T, Takubo T et al 2002 Measurement of hemoglobin concentrations using the Astrim noninvasive blood vessel monitoring apparatus. Acta Haematologica 108:109–110.

14. Rendell M, Anderson E, Schlueter W et al 2003 Determination of hemoglobin levels in the finger using near infra-red spectroscopy. Clinical and Laboratory Haematology 25:93–97.

15. International Council for Standardization in Haematology 1980 Recommendations for reference method for determination by centrifugation of packed cell volume of blood. Journal of Clinical Pathology 33:1–2.

16. World Health Organization 2000 Recommended method for the determination of packed cell volume by centrifugation (Prepared by Expert Panel on Cytometry of the International Council for Standardization in Haematology) Document WHO/DIL/00.2:1–9, WHO, Geneva.

17. Bryner MA, Houwen B, Westengard J, et al 1997 The spun haematocrit and mean red cell volume are affected by changes in the oxygenation state of red blood cells. Clinical and Laboratory Haematology 19:99–103.

18. International Committee for Standardization in Haematology 1980 Recommended methods for measurement of red-cell and plasma volume. Journal of Nuclear Medicine 21:793–800.

19. England JM, Walford DM, Waters DAW 1972 Reassessment of the reliability of the haematocrit. British Journal of Haematology 23:247–256.

20. Pearson TC, Guthrie DL 1982 Trapped plasma in microhematocrit. American Journal of Clinical Pathology 78:770–772.

21. Expert Panel on Cytometry of the International Council for Standardization in Haematology 2001 Recommendations for reference method for the packed cell volume (ICSH Standard). Laboratory Hematology 7:148–170.

22. Bull BS, Fujimoto K, Houwen B et al 2003 International Council for Standardization in Haematology (ICSH) Recommendations for "surrogate reference" method for the packed cell volume. Laboratory Hematology 9:1–9.

23. Rothenberg ME 1998 Eosinophilia. New England Journal of Medicine 338:1592–1699.

24. Uhrbrand H 1958 The number of circulating eosinophils: normal figures and spontaneous variations. Acta Medica Scandinavica 160:99–104.

25. Brito-Babapulle F 2003 The eosinophilias, including the idiopathic hypereosinophilic syndrome. British Journal of Haematology 121:203–223.

26. Gilbert HS, Ornstein L 1975 Basophil counting with a new staining method using Alcian blue. Blood 46:279–286.

27. Mettler L, Shirwani D 1974 Direct basophil count for timing ovulation. Fertility and Sterility 25:718–723.

28. Mathy KA, Koepke JA 1974 The clinical usefulness of segmented vs stab neutrophil criteria for differential leucocyte counts. American Journal of Clinical Pathology 61:947–958.

29. Gombos M, Bienkowski R, Gochman R, et al 1998 The absolute neutrophil count: Is it the best indicator for occult bacteraemia in infants? American Journal of Clinical Pathology 109:221–225.

30. National Committee for Clinical Laboratory Standards 1992 Reference leukocyte differential count (proportional) and evaluation of instrument methods. Approved standard. NCCLS document H20-A. NCCLS, Wayne, PA.

31. Hubl W, Wolfbauer G, Andert S et al 1997 Towards a new reference method for the leukocyte five-part differential. Cytometry 30:72–84.

32. Fujimoto H. Sakata T, Hamaguchi Y et al 2000 Flow cytometric method for enumeration and classification of reactive immature granulocyte populations. Cytometry 42:371–378.

33. Groom AC, Schmidt EE 1990 Microcirculatory blood flow through the spleen. In AJ Bowdler (ed) The spleen: structure, function and clinical significance, p 45–102. Chapman and Hall, London.

34. D'Onofrio G, Zini G, Rowan RM 2002 Reticulocyte counting: methods and clinical applications. In: RM Rowan, OW van Assendelft, FE Preston (eds) Advanced laboratory methods in haematology, pp. 78–126. Arnold, London.

35. Wittekind D, Schulte E 1987 Standardized azure B as a reticulocyte stain. Clinical and Laboratory Haematology 9:395–398.

36. Jahanmehr SAH, Hyde K, Geary CG, et al 1987 Simple technique for fluorescence staining of blood cells with acridine orange. Journal of Clinical Pathology 40:926–929

37. International Council for Standardization in Haematology 1998 Proposed reference method for reticulocyte counting based on the determination of the reticulocyte to red cell ratio. Clinical and Laboratory Haematology 20:77–79.

38. National Committee for Clinical Laboratory Standards and International Council for Standardization in Haematology 2004 Methods for reticulocyte counting (automated blood cell counters, flow cytometry, and supravital dyes); approved guideline, 2nd ed., Document H44-A2. Vol 24 (8). NCCLS, Wayne PA.

39. Groner W, Simson E 1995 Practical guide to modern haematology analyzers. Wiley, Chichester.

40. International Council for Standardization in Haematology 1994 Guidelines for the evaluation of blood cell analysers including those used for differential leucocyte and reticulocyte counting and cell marker applications. Clinical and Laboratory Haematology 16:157–174.

41. Bain BJ 2000 Blood cells: a practical guide, 3rd ed., Blackwell Science Oxford.

42. Simson E, Ross DW, Kocher WD 1988 Atlas of automated cytochemical hematology. Technicon, Tarrytown, NY.

43. Houwen B 2002 The blood count. In: RM Rowan, OW van Assendelft, FE Preston (Eds) Advanced laboratory methods in haematology, pp. 19–44. Arnold, London.

44. Coulter WH 1956 High speed automatic blood cell counter and cell size analyser. Proceedings of National Electronics Conference 12:1034–1040.

45. Thom R 1990 Automated red cell analysis. Bailliere's Clinical Haematology 3:837–850.

46. England JM, van Assendelft OW 1986 Automated blood counters and their evaluation. In: Rowan RM, England JM (eds) Automation and quality assurance in haematology. Blackwell Scientific, Oxford.

47. Mohandas N, Kim YR, Tycko DH, et al 1986 Accurate and independent measurement of volume and hemoglobin concentration of individual red cells by laser scattering. Blood 68:506–513.

48. Evan-Wong L, Davidson RJ 1983 Raised Coulter mean corpuscular volume in diabetic ketoacidosis, and its underlying association with marked plasma hyperosmolarity. Journal of Clinical Pathology 36:334–336.

49. Holt JT, DeWandler MJ, Arvan DA 1982 Spurious elevation of the electronically determined mean corpuscular volume and hematocrit caused by hyperglycemia. American Journal of Clinical Pathology 77:561–567

50. Bentley SA, Ayscue LH, Watson JM, et al 1989 The clinical utility of discriminant functions in the differential diagnosis of microcytic anemias. Blood Cells 15:575–582.

51. Lafferty JD, Crowther MA, Ali MA, et al 1996 The evaluation of various mathematical RBC indices and their efficacy in discriminating between thalassemic and non-thalassemic microcytosis. American Journal of Clinical Pathology 106:201–295.

52. Green R, King R, 1989 A new red cell discriminant incorporating volume dispersion for differentiating iron deficiency anemia from thalassemia minor. Blood Cells 15:481–491.

53. Ross DW, Bentley SA 1986 Evaluation of an automated hematology system (Technicon H-1). Archives of Pathology and Laboratory Medicine 110:803–808.

54. Bain BJ, Cavill I 1993 Hypochromic macrocytes— are they reticulocytes? Journal of Clinical Pathology 46:963–964.

55. Ballard BCD 1972 Lysing agent for the Coulter S. Journal of Clinical Pathology 25:460.

56. Skinnider LF, Musglow E 1972 A stromatolysing and cyanide reagent for use with the Coulter Counter Model S. American Journal of Clinical Pathology 57:537–538.

57. Bain BJ 1986 An assessment of the three population differential count on the Coulter Model S Plus IV. Clinical and Laboratory Haematology 8:347–359.

58. Cornbleet PJ, Myrick D, Judkins S, et al 1992 Evaluation of the CELL-DYN 3000 differential. American Journal of Clinical Pathology 98:603–614.

59. D'Onofrio G, Zini G, Tommasi M, et al 1992 Anomalie ultramorpholigiche dei granulociti neutrofili nelle infezioni da virus HIV. Atti del V Incontro del Club Utilizzatori Sistemi Ematologici Bayer-Technicon, Montecatini Terme, 1991.

60. Taylor C, Bain BJ 1991 Technicon H1 automated white cell parameters in the diagnosis of megaloblastic erythropoiesis. European Journal of Haematology 46:248–249.

61. Ansari-Lari MA, Kickler TS and Borowitz MJ 2003 Immature granulocyte measurement using the Sysmex XE-2100. American Journal of Clinical Pathology 120:795–799

62. Fourcade C, Casbas MJ, Belaouni H et al 2004 Automated detection of malaria by means of the haematology analyser Coulter GEN.S. Clinical and Laboratory Haematology 26:367–372.

63. Hänscheid T, Pinto BG, Cristino JM, et al 2000 Malaria diagnosis with the haematology analyser Cell-Dyne 3500: what does the instrument detect? Clinical and Laboratory Haematology 22:259–261.

64. Ault KA 2001 The clinical utility of flow cytometry in the study of platelets. Seminars in Hematology 38:160–168.

65. ICSH (Expert Panel on Cytometry) and International Society of Laboratory Hematology (ISLH) 2001

Platelet counting by the PLT/RBC ratio—a reference method. American Journal of Clinical Pathology. 115:460–464.

66. Parker-Williams J 2003 Immunoplatelet counting: platelet transfusions. British Journal of Haematology 123:750–751.

67. van der Meer W, MacKenzie MA, Dinnisson JWB, et al 2003 Pseudoplatelets: a retrospective study of their incidence and interference with platelet counting. Journal of Clinical Pathology 56:772–774.

68. Takubo T, Yamane T, Hino M, et al 1998 Usefulness of determining reticulated and large platelets in idiopathic thrombocytopenic purpura. Acta Haematologica 99:109–110.

69. Macchi I, Chamlian V, Sadoun A et al 2002 Comparison of reticulated platelet count and mean platelet volume determination in the evaluation of bone marrow recovery after aplastic chemotherapy. European Journal of Haematology 69:152–157.

70. Robinson MSC, Mackie IJ, Machin SJ, Harrison P 2000 Two colour analysis of reticulated platelets. Clinical and Laboratory Haematology 22:211–213.

71. Bain BJ 1985 Platelet count and platelet size in males and females. Scandinavian Journal of Haematology 35:77–79.

72. Morley A 1969 A platelet cycle in normal individuals. Australasian Annals of Medicine 18:127–129.

73. Bain BJ, Seed M 1986 Platelet count and platelet size in Africans and West Indians. Clinical and Laboratory Haematology 8:43–48.

74. Bessman JD, Williams LJ, Gilmer PR 1982 Platelet size in health and hematologic disease. American Journal of Clinical Pathology 78:150–153.

75. Riley RS, Ben-Ezra JM, Tidwell A, et al 2002 Reticulocyte analysis by flow cytometry and other techniques. Haematology/Oncology Clinics of North America 16:378–420.

76. Sica S, Sora F, Laurenti L, et al 1999 Highly fluorescent reticulocyte count predicts haemopoietic recovery after immunosuppression for severe aplastic anaemia. Clinical and Laboratory Haematology 21:387–389.

77. Davies SV, Cavill I, Bentley N, et al 1992 Evaluation of erythropoiesis after bone marrow transplantation: quantitative reticulocyte counting. British Journal of Haematology 81:12–17.

78. Davis BH, Bigelow N, Ball ED et al 1989 Utility of flow cytometric reticulocyte quantification as a predictor of engraftment in autologous bone marrow transplantation. American Journal of Hematology 32:81–87.

79. Gowans ID, Hepburn MD, Clark DM, et al 1999 The role of the Sysmex SE9000 immature myeloid index and Sysmex R2000 reticulocyte parameters in optimizing the timing of peripheral blood cell harvesting in patients with lymphoma and myeloma. Clinical and Laboratory Haematology 21:331–336.

80. Parisotto R, Gore CJ, Emslie KR et al 2000 A novel method utilizing markers of altered erythropoiesis for the detection on recombinant human erythropoietin abuse in athletes. Haematologica 85:564–572.

81. Torres Gomez A, Casaño J, Sanchez J et al 2003 Utility of reticulocyte maturation parameters in the differential diagnosis of macrocytic anaemias. Clinical and Laboratory Haematology 25:283–288.

82. International Committee for Standardization in Haematology; Expert Panel on Cytometry 1988 The assignment of values to fresh blood used for calibrating automated blood cell counters. Clinical and Laboratory Haematology 10:203–212.

83. Lewis SM, England JM, Rowan RM 1991 Current concerns in haematology 3: Blood count calibration. Journal of Clinical Pathology 44:881–884.

84. International Council for Standardization in Haematology 1994 Reference method for the enumeration of erythrocytes and leucocytes. Clinical and Laboratory Haematology 16:131–138

85. National Committee for Clinical Laboratory Standards 1996 Performance goals for the internal quality control of multichannel hematology analyzers; approved standard. NCCLS, Wayne, PA.

86. British Committee for Standards in Haematology 1991 Assessment of the need for blood film examination with blood counts by aperture-impedance systems. In: Roberts B (ed) Standard Haematology Practice, pp. 34–42 Blackwell Scientific, Oxford.

87. Koepke JA 2002 Instrument flagging and blood film review. In: Rowan RM, van Assendelft OW, Preston FE (eds) Advanced laboratory methods in haematology pp. 64–77. Arnold, London.

4

Preparation and staining methods for blood and bone marrow films

Barbara J. Bain and S. Mitchell Lewis

PREPARATION OF BLOOD FILMS ON SLIDES

Blood films should be made on clean glass slides. Films made on coverglasses have negligible advantages and are unsuitable for modern laboratory practice. Films may be spread by hand or by means of an automated slide spreader, the latter being either a stand-alone instrument or a component of an automated blood cell counter.

Manual Method

Blood films can be prepared from fresh blood with no anticoagulant added or from ethylenedi-aminetetra-acetic acid (EDTA)-anticoagulated blood. Heparinized blood should not generally be used because its staining characteristics differ from those of EDTA-anticoagulated blood. Good films can be made in the following manner, using clean slides, if necessary wiped free from dust immediately before use. Slides should measure 75 × 25 mm and approximately 1 mm thick; ideally, they should be frosted at one end to facilitate labelling, but these are more expensive.

First, make a spreader from a glass slide that has a smooth end. Using a glass cutter, break off one corner of the slide, leaving a width of about 18 mm as the spreader. A spreader can be used repeatedly unless the edge becomes chipped, but it must be thoroughly washed and dried between films.

Place a small drop of blood in the centre line of a slide about 1 cm from one end. Then, without delay, place a spreader in front of the drop at an angle of about 30 degrees to the slide and move it back to make contact with the drop. The drop should spread out quickly along the line of contact. With a steady movement of the hand, spread the drop of blood along the slide. The spreader must not be lifted off until the last trace of blood has been spread out; with a correctly sized drop, the film should be about 3 cm in length. It is important that the film of blood finishes at least 1 cm before the end of the slide (Figure 4.1).

The thickness of the film can be regulated by varying the pressure and speed of spreading and by changing the angle at which the spreader is held. With anaemic blood, the correct thickness is achieved by using a wider angle, and, conversely, with polycythaemic blood, the angle should be narrower.

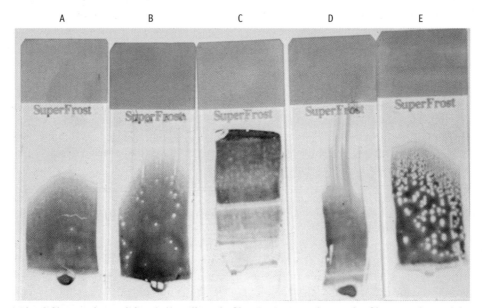

Figure 4.1 Blood films made on slides. A: A well-made film. B: An irregular patchy film on a dusty slide. C: A film that is too thick. D: A film that has been spread with inconsistent pressure and using an irregularly edged spreader, resulting in long tails. E: A film made on a very greasy slide.

The ideal thickness is such that on microscopy there is some overlap of red cells throughout much of the film's length (see p. 33). The leucocytes should be easily recognizable throughout most of the film. With poorly made films the leucocytes will be unevenly distributed, with monocytes and other large leucocytes being pushed to the end and the sides of the spread. An irregular streaky film will occur if the slide is greasy, and dust on the surface will cause patchy spots (Figure 4.1).

The films should be allowed to dry in the air. In humid conditions the films may be exposed to a current of warm air (e.g., from a hairdryer), but this should be in a microbiological safety hood.

Automated Methods

The manufacturer's instructions should be followed unless local experience has demonstrated that variation of the recommended technique achieves better results.

Labelling Blood Films

The film should be labelled immediately after spreading. Write either a laboratory reference number or the name of the patient and the date in pencil on the frosted end of the slide or on the film itself (writing on the thickest part, which is least suitable for microscopic examination). A label written in pencil will not be removed by staining. A paper label should be affixed to the slide later. If blood films are to be stored for future reference, apply the paper label in such a manner that it is easily read when the slides are filed.

In a computerized laboratory, bar-coded specimen identification labels are convenient and preferable.

Fixing Blood Films

To preserve the morphology of the cells, films must be fixed as described on page 63. This must be done without delay, and the films should never be left unfixed for more than a few hours. If films are sent to the laboratory by post, it is preferable that, when possible, they are thoroughly dried and fixed before dispatch.

Bone Marrow Films

The method for preparation of films from aspirated bone marrow is described on page 119. They should be made without delay. At least one film should be fixed for a Perls' stain, and, if necessary, films should be fixed in the appropriate fixatives for special staining (Chapter 13); others should be fixed and stained with a Romanowsky stain as described later. Crushed bone marrow particles and touch preparations from trephine biopsy specimens can be stained in the same manner.

STAINING BLOOD AND BONE MARROW FILMS

Romanowsky stains are used universally for routine staining of blood films, and satisfactory results can be obtained. The remarkable property of the Romanowsky dyes of making subtle distinctions in shades of staining, and of staining granules differentially, depends on two components—azure B (trimethylthionin) and eosin Y (tetrabromofluorescein).[1,2]

The original Romanowsky combination was polychrome methylene blue and eosin. Several of the stains now used routinely that are based on azure B also include methylene blue, but the need for this is debatable. Its presence in the stain is thought by some to enhance the staining of nucleoli and polychromatic red cells; in its absence, normal neutrophil granules tend to stain heavily and may resemble "toxic granules" in conventionally stained films.[3]

There are a number of causes of variation in staining. One of the main factors is the presence of contaminants in the commercial dyes and a simple combination of pure azure B and eosin Y might be considered preferable to the more complex stains because this ensures consistent results from batch to batch.[1,4,5] However, in practice, absolutely pure dyes are expensive, and it is sufficient to ensure that the stains contain at least 80% of the appropriate dye.[6] Among the Romanowsky stains now in use, Jenner is the simplest and Giemsa is the most complex. Leishman's stain, which occupies an intermediate position, is still widely used in the routine staining of blood films, although the results are inferior to those obtained by the combined May-Grünwald-Giemsa, Jenner-Giemsa, and azure B-eosin Y methods. Wright's stain, which is widely used in North America, gives results that are similar to those obtained with Leishman's stain, whereas Wright-Giemsa is similar to May-Grünwald-Giemsa.

A pH to the alkaline side of neutrality accentuates the azure component at the expense of the eosin and vice versa. A pH of 6.8 is usually recommended for general use, but to some extent this depends on personal preference. (When looking for malaria parasites, a pH of 7.2 is recommended to see Schüffner's dots.) To achieve a uniform pH, 50 ml of 66 mmol/l Sörensen's phosphate buffer (p. 692) may be added to each 1 litre of the water used in diluting the stains and washing the films.

The mechanism by which certain components of a cell's structure stain with particular dyes and other components fail to do so depends on complex differences in binding of the dyes to chemical structures and interactions between the dye molecules.[7] Azure B is bound to anionic molecules, and eosin Y is bound to cationic sites on proteins.

Thus, the acidic groupings of the nucleic acids and proteins of the cell nuclei and primitive cytoplasm determine their uptake of the basic dye azure B, and, conversely, the presence of basic groupings on the haemoglobin molecule results in its affinity for acidic dyes and its staining by eosin. The granules in the cytoplasm of neutrophil leucocytes are weakly stained by the azure complexes. Eosinophilic granules contain a spermine derivative with an alkaline grouping that stains strongly with the acidic component of the dye, whereas basophilic granules contain heparin, which has an affinity for the basic component of the dye. These effects depend on molar equilibrium between the two dyes in time-dependent reactions.[2] DNA binds rapidly, RNA more slowly, and haemoglobin more slowly still; hence the need to have the correct azure B to eosin ratio to avoid contamination of the dyes and to stain for the right time. Standardized stains and staining method have been proposed (p. 64).

The colour reactions of the Romanowsky effect are shown in Table 4.1; causes of variation in staining are given in Table 4.2.

Table 4.1   Colour responses of blood cells to Romanowsky staining

Cellular component	Colour
Nuclei	
Chromatin	Purple
Nucleoli	Light blue
Cytoplasm	
Erythroblast	Dark blue
Erythrocyte	Dark pink
Reticulocyte	Grey–blue
Lymphocyte	Blue
Metamyelocyte	Pink
Monocyte	Grey–blue
Myelocyte	Pink
Neutrophil	Pink/orange
Promyelocyte	Blue
Basophil	Blue
Granules	
Promyelocyte (primary granules)	Red or purple
Basophil	Purple black
Eosinophil	Red–orange
Neutrophil	Purple
Toxic granules	Dark blue
Platelet	Purple
Other inclusions	
Auer body	Purple
Cabot ring	Purple
Howell-Jolly body	Purple
Döhle body	Light blue

Preparation of Solutions of Romanowsky Dyes

May-Grünwald Stain

Weigh out 0.3 g of the powdered dye and transfer to a conical flask of 200–250 ml capacity. Add 100 ml of methanol and warm the mixture to 50°C. Allow the flask to cool to c 20°C and shake several times during the day. After letting it stand for 24 hours, filter the solution. It is then ready for use, no "ripening" being required.

Jenner's Stain

Prepare a 5 g/l solution in methanol in exactly the same way as described earlier for the May-Grünwald stain.

Table 4.2 Factors giving rise to faulty staining

Appearances	Causes
Too blue, nuclei	Eosin concentration too low
Blue to black	Incorrect preparation of stock Stock stain exposed to bright daylight Batch of stain solution overused Impure dyes Staining time too short Staining solution too acid Smear too thick Inadequate time in buffer solution
Too pink	Incorrect proportion of azure B-eosin Y Impure dyes Buffer pH too low Excessive washing in buffer solution
Pale staining	Old staining solution Overused staining solution Incorrect preparation of stock Impure dyes, especially azure A and/or C High ambient temperature
Neutrophil granules not stained	Insufficient azure B
Neutrophil granules Dark blue/black (pseudo-toxic)	Excess azure B
Other stain anomalies	Various contaminating dyes and metal salts
Stain deposit on film	Stain solution left in uncovered jar Stain solution not filtered
Blue background	Inadequate fixation or prolonged storage before fixation Blood collected into heparin as anticoagulant

Giemsa's Stain

Weigh 1 g of the powdered dye and transfer to a conical flask of 200–250 ml capacity. Add 100 ml of methanol and warm the mixture to 50°C; keep at this temperature for 15 min with occasional shaking, then filter the solution. It is then ready for use, but it will improve on standing for a few hours.

Azure B-Eosin Y Stock Solution

The stock solution includes azure B, tetrafluoroborate, or thiocyanate (Colour index 52010), >80% pure, and Eosin Y (Colour index 45380), >80% pure.

Dissolve 0.6 g of azure B in 60 ml dimethyl sulphoxide (DMSO) and 0.2 g of eosin Y in 50 ml DMSO; preheat the DMSO at 37°C before adding the dyes. Stand at 37°C, shaking vigorously for 30 sec at 5-min intervals until both dyes are completely dissolved. Add the eosin Y solution to the azure B solution and stir well. This stock solution should remain stable for several months if kept at room temperature in the dark. DMSO will crystallize below 18°C; if necessary, allow it to redissolve before use.

Leishman's Stain

Weigh out 0.2 g of the powdered dye, and transfer it to a conical flask of 200–250 ml capacity. Add 100 ml of methanol and warm the mixture to 50°C for 15 min, occasionally shaking it. Allow the flask to cool and filter. It is then ready for use, but it will improve on standing.

Buffered Water

Make up 50 ml of 66 mmol/l Sörensen's phosphate buffer of the required pH to 1 litre with water at a pH of 6.8 (see p. 692). An alternative buffer may be prepared from buffer tablets, which are available commercially. Solutions of the required pH are obtained by dissolving the tablets in water.

STAINING METHODS

May-Grünwald-Giemsa Stain

Dry the films in the air, then fix by immersing in a jar of methanol for 5–10 min. For bone marrow films, allow a longer time to ensure thorough drying and then leave for it 15–20 min in the methanol. Films should be fixed as soon as possible after they are made. If they are left unfixed at room temperature for several days, it may be found that the background of dried plasma stains a pale blue that is impossible to remove without spoiling the staining of the blood cells. It is important to prevent any contact with water before fixation is complete. Methyl alcohol (methanol) is the fixative of choice, although ethyl alcohol ("absolute alcohol") can also be used. To prevent the alcohol from becoming contaminated with absorbed water, it must be stored in a bottle with a tightly fitting stopper and not left exposed to the atmosphere, especially in humid climates. Methylated spirits must not be used because it contains water.

Transfer the fixed films to a staining jar containing May-Grünwald stain freshly diluted with an equal volume of buffered water. After the films have been allowed to stain for about 15 min, transfer them without washing to a jar containing Giemsa's stain freshly diluted with 9 volumes of buffered water, pH 6.8.

After staining for 10–15 min, transfer the slides to a jar containing buffered water, pH 6.8, rapidly wash in three or four changes of water, and finally allow to stand undisturbed in water for a short time (usually 2–5 min) for differentiation to take place. This may be controlled by inspection of the wet slide under the low power of the microscope; with experience, the naked-eye colour of the film is often a good guide. The slides should be transferred from one staining solution to the other without being allowed to dry. Because the intensity of the staining is affected by any variation in the thickness of a film, it is not easy to obtain uniform staining throughout a film's length.

When differentiation is complete, stand the slides upright to dry. This method is designed for staining a number of films at the same time. Single slides may be stained by flooding the slide with a combined fixative and staining solution (e.g., Leishman's stain, discussed later), but it is important to ensure that the methanol used as fixative is completely water-free. As little as 1% water may affect the appearance of the films, and a higher water content causes gross changes (Fig. 4.2). The red cells will also be affected by traces of detergent on inadequately washed slides (see Fig. 27.5, p. 684).

The diluted stains usually retain their staining powers sufficiently well for several batches of slides to be stained in them. They must be made up freshly each day, and it is probably best to stain the day's films in two batches, morning and afternoon. There is no need to filter the stains before use unless a deposit is present.

Standardized Romanowsky Stain

The standardized Romanowsky stain[2,5] is based on a method with pure dyes proposed by the International Committee for Standardization in Haematology. Its advantage is that it ensures consistent results from batch to batch so that it can be used for checking the performance of other stains and for automated pattern recognition methods. Its disadvantage in a routine laboratory is that it requires the use of DMSO, which is a potentially toxic solvent with an unpleasant smell. Furthermore, the stained films tend to fade after a few months, so this stain should not be used for staining bone marrow films that are to be stored for future reference.

Fixative

Mix 1 volume of stock solution of azure B-eosin Y with 14 volumes of methanol.

Staining Solution

Immediately before use, dilute 1 volume of the stock solution (discussed previously) with 14 volumes of HEPES (N-2-hydroxyethylpiperazine-N'-2-ethane-sulfonic acid) buffer, pH 6.6 (p. 691). This solution is stable for about 8 hours.[8]

Method

Dry the films in the air. Leave for 3 min in the fixative. Leave the slides in the diluted staining solution for 15 min. Rinse in phosphate buffer solution, pH 6.8, for 1 min. Then rinse with water, air dry, and mount.

When several batches of films are being stained in succession, the staining solution should be renewed at intervals (e.g., after each 50 slides). Loss of staining power is usually the result of precipitation of the eosin Y, and this will result in the nuclei staining blue instead of purple (see Table 4.2).

Jenner-Giemsa Stain

Jenner's stain may be substituted for May-Grünwald stain in the technique described on the previous page. The results are a little less satisfactory. The stain is used with 4 volumes of buffered water,

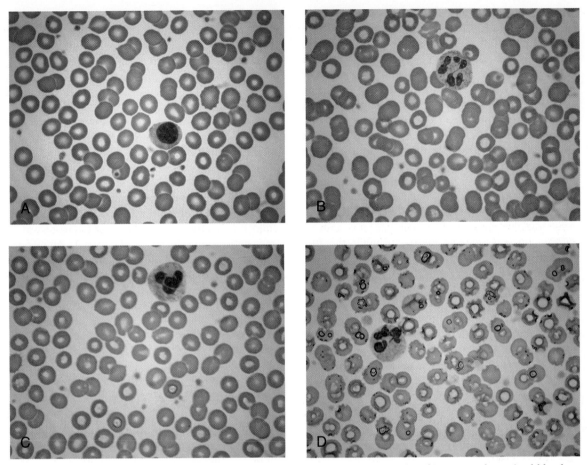

Figure 4.2   Blood film appearances following methanol fixation. Photomicrographs of Romanowsky-stained blood films that have been fixed in methanol containing: A: 1% water; B: 3% water; C: 4% water; and D: 10% water. The red cells and leucocytes are well fixed in A and B but badly fixed in C and D.

and the films, after being fixed in methanol, are immersed in it for approximately 4 min before being transferred to the Giemsa's stain. They should be allowed to stain in the latter solution for 7–10 min. Differentiation is carried out as described earlier.

Leishman's Stain

Air dry the film and flood the slide with the stain. After 2 min, add double the volume of water and stain the film for 5–7 min. Then wash it in a stream of buffered water until it has acquired a pinkish tinge (up to 2 min). After the back of the slide has been wiped clean, set it upright to dry.

Automated Staining

Automatic staining machines are available that enable large batches of slides to be handled. They may be either stand-alone staining machines or a part of a large automated blood counting instrument. In many instances, the instrument spreads, fixes, and stains blood films. Some automated instruments incorporating staining can only be programmed to prepare and stain a single film per sample. Others can prepare and stain multiple films from a single blood sample; this is useful in a teaching programme with a large number of students. Some systems apply staining solutions to slides lying horizontally (flat-bed staining), whereas others either immerse a slide or slides in a bath of staining solution ("dip-and-dunk" technique) or spray stain onto slides in a cytocentrifuge. Problems include increased background staining, inadequate staining of neutrophil granules, degranulation of basophils, and blue or green rather than pink staining of erythrocytes. These problems are usually related to the specific stains and staining protocols used rather than to the type of instrument, although flat-bed stainers are more likely to cause problems with stain deposit. However, as a rule, staining is satisfactory provided that reliable stains are used and there is careful control of the cycle time and other variables.[9] Flat-bed stainers may not stain an entire film (e.g., a bone marrow film) if the film exceeds the standard length.

Rapid Staining Method

Field's method[10,11] was introduced to provide a quick method for staining thick films for malaria parasites (see below). With some modifications, it can be used fairly satisfactorily for the rapid staining of thin films. The stains are available commercially ready for use, or they can be prepared as follows.

Stains

Stain A (Polychromed Methylene Blue)

Methylene blue	1.3 g
Disodium hydrogen phosphate (Na$_2$ HPO$_4$ 12H$_2$O)	12.6 g
Potassium dihydrogen phosphate (KH$_2$ PO$_4$)	6.25 g
Water	500 ml

Dissolve the methylene blue and the disodium hydrogen phosphate in 50 ml of water. Then boil the solution in a waterbath almost to dryness to "polychrome" the dye. Add the potassium dihydrogen phosphate and 500 ml of freshly boiled water. After stirring to dissolve the stain, set aside the solution for 24 hours before filtering. Filter again before use. The pH is 6.6–6.8.

Alternatively, azure B may be added to the methylene blue in the proportion of 0.5 g of azure B to 0.8 g of methylene blue, and the combined dyes are then dissolved directly in the phosphate buffer solution.

Stain B (Eosin)

Eosin	1.3 g
Disodium hydrogen phosphate (NaHPO$_4$ 12H$_2$O)	12.6 g
Potassium dihydrogen phosphate (KH$_2$PO$_4$)	6.25 g
Water	500 ml

Dissolve the phosphates in warm freshly boiled water, and then add the dye. Filter the solution after letting it stand for 24 hours.

Method

Fix the film for 10–15 sec in methanol. Pour off the methanol and drop on the slide 12 drops of diluted Stain B (1 volume of stain to 4 volumes of water). Immediately, add 12 drops of Stain A. Agitate the slide to mix the stains. After 1 min, rinse the slide in water, then differentiate the film for 5 sec in phosphate buffer at pH 6.6, wash the slide in water, and then place it on end to drain and dry. Two-stage stains of this type are also available commercially.

Mounting of Coverglass

When thoroughly dry, cover the blood film with a rectangular No. 1 coverglass, using for this purpose a mountant, which is miscible with xylol (e.g., DPX Mountant, Merck). For a temporary mount, cedarwood oil may be used.

The coverglass should be large enough to overlie the whole film, so that the edges and the tail of the film can be examined. If a neutral mounting medium is used, the staining should be preserved for many years if kept in the dark. Although it is probable that stained films keep best unmounted, there are objections to this course: it is almost impossible to keep the slides free from dust and from being scratched, and in the absence of a coverglass the observer is tempted to examine the film solely with the oil-immersion objective, a practice that is to be deprecated because it is important to have a general overview of the film before studying specific cells.

EXAMINATION OF WET BLOOD FILM PREPARATIONS

The examination of a drop of blood sealed between a slide and coverglass is sometimes of considerable value. The preparation may be examined in several ways: by ordinary illumination, by dark-ground, or by Nomarski (interference) illumination. Chemically clean slides and coverglasses (p. 695) should be used,* and the blood should be allowed to spread out thinly between them. If the glass surfaces are free from dust, the blood will spread out spontaneously, and pressure, which is undesirable, should not be necessary. The edges of the preparation may be sealed with a melted mixture of equal parts of petroleum jelly and paraffin wax or with nail varnish.

Red Cells

Rouleaux Formation

Rouleaux formation is typically seen in varying degrees in wet preparations of whole blood and must be distinguished from autoagglutination. The distinction is sometimes a matter of considerable difficulty, particularly when, as not infrequently happens, rouleaux formation is superimposed on agglutination. The rouleaux, too, may be notably irregular in haemolytic anaemias characterized by spherocytosis, whereas the clumping caused by massive rouleaux formation of normal type may closely simulate true agglutination. This pseudoagglutination owing to massive rouleaux formation may be distinguished from true agglutination in two ways:

1. By noting that the red cells, although forming parts of larger clumps, are mostly arranged side by side as in typical rouleaux.
2. By adding 3–4 volumes of 9 g/l NaCl to the preparation. Pseudoagglutination owing to massive rouleaux formation should either disperse completely or transform itself into typical rouleaux. The addition of saline to blood that has undergone true agglutination may cause the agglutinates to break up somewhat, but a major degree of it is likely to persist and typical rouleaux will not be seen.

Anisocytosis and *poikilocytosis* can be recognized in "wet" preparations of blood, but the tendency to crenation and the formation of rouleaux tend to make observations on shape changes rather difficult. Such changes can best be studied in a wet

preparation after fixation. For this, dilute a sample of freshly collected heparinized or EDTA-blood in 10 volumes of iso-osmotic phosphate buffer, pH 7.4 (see p. 691) and immediately fix with an equal volume of 0.3% glutaraldehyde in iso-osmotic phosphate buffer, pH 7.4. After standing for 5 min, add 1 drop of this suspension to 4 drops of glycerol, and place 1–2 drops on a glass slide that is then sealed.[12]

Pitting occurs normally in less than 2% of the red cells; an increase of more than 4% is an indication of splenic dysfunction. The pits are readily identified by Nomarski illumination or electron microscopy when they have the appearance of small crater-like indentations on the cell surface.[13]

Sickling of red cells in "wet" preparations of blood is described in Chapter 12.

Crystals of Hb C can be demonstrated by incubating a sample of blood with an equal volume of 30 g/l sodium chloride for 4 hours at 37°C. In blood with Hb C disease this induces formation of intracellular Hb C crystals, large, clear deposits of amorphous material that are well shown when the preparation is then stained by any Romanowsky stain.[14] They can also be demonstrated in Hb SC red cells.

Cryoglobulinaemia

To identify cryoglobulinaemia, put a drop of blood from an EDTA sample that has been kept at room temperature onto a glass slide, cover it with a glass coverslip, and examine it by phase contrast microscopy. The cryoglobulin will be seen as large clear amorphous material or as refringent precipitates that disappear when the slide is warmed to 37°C.

This is a useful test when an automated blood count gives anomalous results with spuriously elevated white blood cell and platelet counts.[15]

Leucocytes

The motility of leucocytes can be readily studied in heparinized blood if the microscope stage can be warmed to about 37°C. Usually, only the granulocytes show significant progressive movements. However, the examination of living neutrophils in plasma is not useful in day-to-day routine haematological practice. Specialized microscopy techniques applicable to leucocytes are discussed in the 8th edition of this book.

*Precleaned slides and coverglasses are available commercially

SEPARATION AND CONCENTRATION OF BLOOD CELLS

A number of methods are available for the concentration of leucocytes or abnormal cells when they are present in only small numbers in the peripheral blood. Concentrates are most simply prepared from the buffy coat of centrifuged blood. However, most methods affect to some extent subsequent staining properties, chemical reactions, and viability of the separated cells.

Making a Buffy Coat Preparation

Centrifuge an EDTA blood sample in a plastic tube for 5–10 min at 1200–1500 g. Then remove the supernatant plasma carefully with a fine plastic pipette, and with the same pipette deposit the platelet and underlying leucocyte layers onto one or two slides. Mix the buffy coat in a drop of the patient's plasma and then spread the films. Allow them to dry in the air and then fix and stain in the usual way.

When leucocytes are scanty or if many slides are to be made, it is worthwhile centrifuging the blood twice; first, about 5 ml are centrifuged and a second tube is then filled from the upper cell layers of this sample.

As an alternative to centrifugation, the blood may be allowed to sediment by placing the tube vertically on the bench without disturbance, with or without the help of sedimentation-enhancing agents such as fibrinogen, dextran, gum acacia, Ficoll (Pharmacia), or methylcellulose.[16] Bøyum's reagent[17] (methylcellulose and sodium metrizoate) is particularly suitable for obtaining leucocyte preparations with minimal red cell contamination.

Utility of the Buffy Coat

It is well known that atypical or primitive blood cells circulate in small numbers in the peripheral blood in health. Thus, atypical mononuclear cells, metamyelocytes, and megakaryocytes may be found. Even promyelocytes, blasts, and nucleated red cells may occasionally be seen but only in very small numbers. Efrati and Rozenszajn[18] described a method for the quantitative assessment of the numbers of atypical cells in normal blood and gave figures for the incidence of megakaryocyte fragments (e.g., mean 21.8 per 1 ml of blood) and of atypical mononuclears and metamyelocytes and myelocytes. In cord blood, the incidence of all types of primitive cells is considerably greater.[19]

In disease, abnormal cells may be seen in buffy coat preparations in much larger numbers than in films of whole blood (Fig. 4.3). Another example, for instance, is megakaryocytes and immature cells of the granulocyte series found in relatively large numbers in disseminated carcinoma.[20] Megaloblasts, if present, may help in the diagnosis of a megaloblastic anaemia. Haemophagocytosis, which is more often observed in the bone marrow, may also sometimes be demonstrated in buffy coat preparations.[21] Erythrophagocytosis may be conspicuous in cases of autoimmune haemolytic anaemia (Figure 4.4). In systemic lupus erythematosus (SLE) a few LE cells may be found, but this is not the best way to demonstrate LE cells; moreover, the detection of LE cells for the diagnosis of SLE has been supplanted by immunological tests for the detection of antinuclear or anti-DNA antibodies.

Buffy coat films can be useful for the detection of bacteria, fungi, or parasites within neutrophils, monocytes, or circulating macrophages; they also can help find ringed sideroblasts in the myelodysplastic syndromes, or other cells that may be present

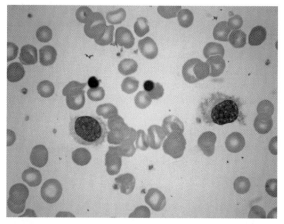

Figure 4.3   Buffy coat film. From blood of a patient with pancytopenia showing two hairy cells, an erythroblast, and a bare nucleus. Only rare cells resembling hairy cells were seen in the conventional film, whereas the buffy coat film showed many such cells.

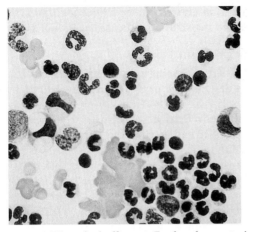

Figure 4.4   Film of a buffy coat. Erythrophagocytosis in autoimmune haemolytic anaemia.

in very small numbers (e.g., hairy cells in hairy cell leukaemia). With the availability of monoclonal antibodies reactive with epithelial and other tumour cells, immunocytochemical techniques can now be applied for the identification of infrequent neoplastic cells.

Separation of Specific Cell Populations

It is now possible to identify specific cell populations by flow cytometric immunophenotyping, and the need for separation of mononuclear cells from blood has diminished. However, differences in density of cells can also be used to separate individual cell types, using gradient solutions of selected specific gravity.[17,33] This is also a useful method for use in leucocyte imaging with radio-isotope-labelled neutrophils (see p. 374). A simple convenient technique has been described for layering the blood or bone marrow over the density preparations.[22] The median density values for the main haemopoietic cells are as follows:

Erythrocytes	1100
Eosinophils	1090
Neutrophils	1085
Myelocytes	1075
Lymphocytes	1070
Monocytes	1064
Myeloblasts	1062
Platelets	1035

PARASITES DETECTABLE IN BLOOD, BONE MARROW, OR SPLENIC ASPIRATES

There are now a number of screening tests for diagnosing malaria based on the detection of malarial antigens (see Chapter 22). However, the essential method for a definitive diagnosis remains the finding of parasites in a blood film and the identification of the species by morphology.[23,24] Only brief outlines of the microscopic diagnoses are given in this chapter. For more detailed accounts, readers are referred to a parasitology textbook. In addition to the *Plasmodia* that give rise to malaria, the other important parasites to be found in the blood are *leishmaniae, Babesiae,* trypanosomes, microfilaria, and ehrlichiosis.

In addition to standard thin films, thick films are extremely useful when parasites are scanty, and these should be prepared and examined as a routine, although identification of the species is less easy than in thin films and mixed infections may be missed. If 5 min are spent examining a thick film, this is equivalent to about 1 hour spent in traversing a thin film. Once the presence of parasites has been confirmed, a thin film should be used for determining the species and, in the case of *Plasmodium falciparum,* for assessing the severity of the infection by counting the percentage of positive cells.

Low levels of parasitaemia detected by immunological tests may be missed by microscopy, and proficiency testing studies have demonstrated the need for all laboratories, and especially those lacking expertise, to take part in external quality control programmes and to refer problematic cases to more experienced centres.[25,26]

Thick blood films are also useful for the detection of microfilaria. When they are used for this purpose, it is important to scan the entire film using a low-power objective, or parasites may be missed. Examination of wet preparations of blood can be used for diagnosis of microfilariae and has the advantage that the parasites are easily detected because they are moving. A stained film is necessary for confirmation of species. Wet preparations are also useful for the detection of trypanosomes and the spirochaetes of relapsing fever. The presence of small numbers of trypanosomes or spirochaetes is revealed by occasional slight agitation of groups of red cells. Examination of a stained film confirms their nature.

EXAMINATION OF BLOOD FILMS FOR PARASITES

Making Thick Films

Make a thick film by placing a small drop of blood in the centre of a slide and spreading it out with a corner of another slide to cover an area about four times its original area. The correct thickness for a satisfactory film will have been achieved if, with the slide placed on a piece of newspaper, small print is just visible.

Allow the film to dry thoroughly for at least 30 min at 37°C. If it is necessary to hurry the procedure, the slide can be left near a light bulb where the temperature is 50-60°C, but not touching it, for about 7 min; the quality of the film may deteriorate if it is overheated. Absolutely fresh films, although apparently dry, often wash off in the stain.

Staining Thick Films

Field's method of staining[10,11] is quick and usually satisfactory for thick films, but the method is not practical for staining large numbers of films; for this purpose the Giemsa, Leishman; or azure B-eosin Y methods are more suitable. Careful attention to pH is critical for satisfactory staining of parasites

Field's Stain

The preparation of the stains is described on page 66.

1. Dip the slide with the dried film on it into Stain A for 3 sec.
2. Dip into a jar of tap water for 3 sec with gentle agitation.
3. Dip into Stain B for 3 sec.
4. Wash gently in tap water for a few seconds until all excess stain is removed.
5. Drain the slide vertically and leave to dry. Do not blot.

Giemsa's stain

1. Dry the films thoroughly, as explained previously.
2. Immerse the slides for 20–30 min in a staining jar containing Giemsa's stain freshly diluted with 20 volumes of buffered water (pH 7.2).

3. Wash in buffered water pH 7.2 for 3 min.
4. Stand the slides upright to dry. Do not blot.

Azure B-Eosin Y Stain

1. Prepare a staining solution from the stock stain, as described on page 63, but using HEPES buffer at pH 7.2.
2. After the films have been dried and treated as described earlier, stain for 10 min in the staining solution.
3. Rinse for 1 min in buffered water, pH 7.2.
4. Stand the slides upright to dry. Do not blot.

Sometimes when thick films are stained, they become overlaid by a residue of stain or spoilt by the envelopes of the lysed red cells. These defects can be minimized by adding 0.1% Triton X-100 to the buffer before diluting the stock stain.[27] An alternative, but more laborious, method is to lyse 1 volume of blood with 3 volumes of 1% saponin in saline for 10 min, then centrifuge for 5 min, decant the supernatant, and make films from the residual pellet.[28]

STAINING THIN FILMS FOR PARASITES

Thin films should be stained with Giemsa's stain or Leishman's stain at pH 7.2, not with a standard May-Grünwald-Giemsa stain.

Leishman's Stain

Use commercially available stain or prepare stain as follows:

1. Add glass beads to 500 ml of methanol.
2. Add 1.5 g of Leishman's powder.
3. Shake well, leave on a rotary shaker during the day, then incubate at 37°C overnight.

There is no need to filter.

Method

1. Make a thin film and air dry rapidly.
2. Place the film on a staining rack, flood with Leishman's stain, and leave for 30 sec to 1 min to fix.

3. Add twice as much buffered distilled water (preferably from a plastic wash bottle because this permits better mixing of the solution), pH 7.2.
4. Leave to stain for 10 min.
5. Wash off stain with tap water.

Thick blood films are also useful for the detection of microfilariae. When they are used for this purpose, it is important to scan the entire film using a low-power objective or parasites may be missed. Examination of fresh liquid blood (see below) can also be used for the identification of microfilariae and has the advantage that, because the parasites are moving, they are easily detected. A stained film is necessary for confirmation of species.

MALARIA

Methods for staining and examination of thin and thick blood films for *Plasmodium* were described earlier. Films for malaria must be made no longer than 3–4 hours after blood collection. Morphological criteria for differentiation of malaria parasites are given in Table 4.3 and illustrated in Figure 4.5. Two other morphological-based screening methods are available.

Table 4.3   Morphological differentiation of malaria parasites

	P. falciparum	P. vivax	P. ovale	P. malariae
Infected red cells	Normal size*; Maurer's clefts[†]	Enlarged; Schüffner's dots[†]	Enlarged; oval and fimbriated; Schüffner's dots[†]	Normal or microcytic; stippling not usually seen
Ring forms (early trophozoites)	Delicate; frequently 2 or more; accolé forms[§]; small chromatin dot	Large, thick; usually single (occasionally 2) in cell; large chromatin dot	Thick, compact rings	Very small, compact rings
Later trophozoites	Compact, vacuolated; sometimes 2 chromatin dots	Amoeboid; central vacuole; light blue cytoplasm	Smaller than P. vivax; slightly amoeboid	Band across cell; deep blue cytoplasm
Schizonts	18–24 merozoites filling $^2/_3$ of cell	12–24 merozoites, irregularly arranged	8–12 merozoites filling $^3/_4$ of cell	6–12 merozoites in daisy-head around central mass of pigment
Pigment	Dark to black clumped mass	Fine granular; yellow–brown	Coarse light brown	Dark, prominent at all stages
Gametocytes	Crescent of sausage-shaped; diffuse chromatin; single nucleus	Spherical, compact, almost fills cell; single nucleus	Oval; fills $^3/_4$ of cell; similar to but smaller than P. vivax	Round; fills $^1/_2$ to $^2/_3$ of cell; similar to P. vivax but smaller, with no Schüffner's dots

*In *P. falciparum*, it is important to report the percentage of red cells that are infected.
[†]Large, irregularly shaped, red-staining dots.
[‡]Fine stippling.
[§]That is, marginalized to edge of cell ("appliqué").

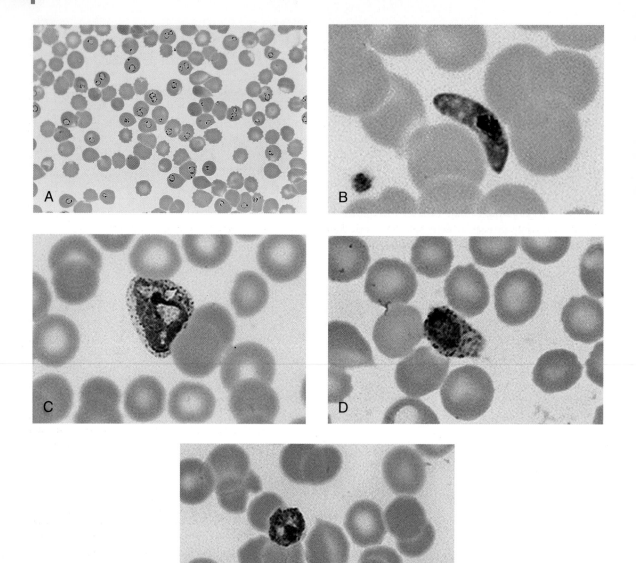

Figure 4.5   Malaria parasites. A: *P. falciparum*: trophozoites; B: *P. falciparum*: gametocyte. C: *P. vivax*: trophozoites; D: *P. ovale*: trophozoites; E: *P. malariae*: trophozoites.

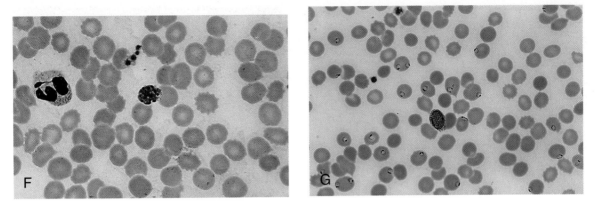

Figure 4.5, cont'd F: *P. malariae*: schizont; and G: *P. falciparum* and *P. vivax*: mixed infection.

Fluorescence Microscopy

Red cells containing malaria parasites fluoresce when examined by fluorescence microscopy after staining with acridine orange.[29,30] This has a sensitivity of about 90% in acute infections but only 50% at lower levels of parasitaemia, and false-positive readings may occur with Howell–Jolly bodies and reticulocytes.[23] When positive, it is necessary to examine a conventionally stained blood film to identify the species.

Quantitative Buffy Coat Method

The quantitative buffy coat (QBC) method (BD Diagnostic Systems) is another procedure for detection of parasites by fluorescent microscopy. The blood is centrifuged in capillary tubes that are coated with acridine orange. It is fairly sensitive but requires expensive equipment and has the disadvantage of false-positive results in the presence of Howell–Jolly bodies and reticulocytes. When positive, identification of species will require examination of a stained blood film, but it is useful as an initial screening test.[23,31]

LEISHMANIASIS

Leishmania species are transmitted by the bite of an infected female sandfly and are associated with a variety of clinical conditions including visceral, mucous, and cutaneous leishmaniasis. Visceral leishmaniasis may present to the haematologist as splenomegaly, hepatomegaly, fever, lymph-adenopathy, or pancytopenia, and it is being increasingly reported in patients with human immunodeficiency virus (HIV) infection. Serological studies are recommended as the initial diagnostic tests in suspected leishmaniasis. In advanced stages of the disease, parasites can be found in phagocytic cells in spleen, lymph nodes, bone marrow, and peripheral blood. Culture of aspirated bone marrow is, however, a more sensitive diagnostic technique than microscopy.

Diagnosis of Leishmaniasis in the Haematology Laboratory

Leishmaniasis is diagnosed in the haematology laboratory by direct visualization of the amastigotes (often referred to as Leishman-Donovan bodies). Buffy coat preparations of peripheral blood or aspirates (see p. 68 for preparation of buffy coats) from marrow, spleen, lymph nodes, or skin lesions should be spread on a slide to make a thin smear and stained with Leishman's or Giemsa's stain (pH 7.2) for 20 min (p. 63). Amastigotes are seen within monocytes or, less commonly, in neutrophils in peripheral blood and in macrophages in bone marrow aspirates. They are small, round bodies 2–4 mm in diameter with indistinct cytoplasm, a nucleus, and a small rod-shaped kinetoplast (Figure 4.6A). Occasionally amastigotes may be seen lying free between cells.

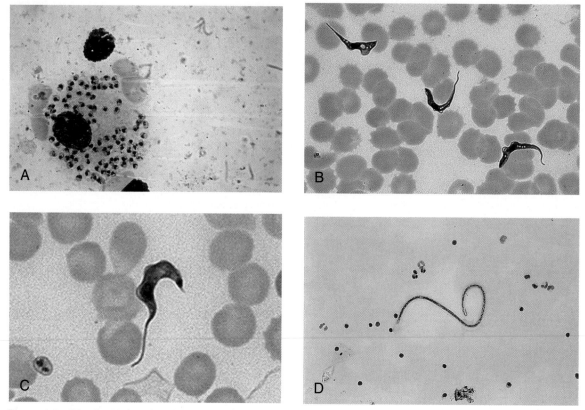

Figure 4.6   Blood parasites. A: Leishmaniasis (Leishman-Donovan bodies); B: African trypanosomiasis; C: Trypanosomiasis (*T. cruzi*); and D: microfilaria.

TRYPANOSOMIASIS

African Trypanosomiasis

African trypanosomiasis (sleeping sickness) is caused by *Trypanosoma brucei gambiense* (West Africa and western Central Africa) and *Trypanosoma brucei rhodesiense* (East, Central, and Southern Africa); it is transmitted by a few species of tsetse fly. The trypomastigotes can be found in blood, lymph node aspirates, and cerebrospinal fluid, but repeated examinations and concentration techniques may be needed before they are detected. Serological investigations may also be helpful in diagnosis.

American Trypanosomiasis

American trypanosomiasis (Chagas' disease) is caused by *Trypanosoma cruzi*, which is transmitted by the Reduviidae bug, subfamily *Triatominae*. Chagas' disease is only found in tropical and subtropical South and Central American countries. Trypomastigotes can only be found circulating in the blood in the acute form of Chagas' disease. Because the trypomastigotes are more fragile than those causing African trypanosomiasis, serology rather than morphology is recommended for initial screening. In the haematology laboratory, tests that detect motile organisms are more sensitive than those that require fixed, stained preparations.

Diagnosis of Trypanosomiasis in the Haematology Laboratory

Care should be taken when handling samples suspected of being infected with trypomastigotes because infection can occur if the organisms penetrate the skin. Several techniques are available for examining specimens for the presence of trypomastigotes.

Wet Preparations

If present in high concentrations, trypomastigotes can be seen thrashing among the cells on a fresh, unstained wet preparation of blood or lymph node fluid. Preparations should be examined within 4 hours of sampling (this time can be extended if a few milligrams of glucose are added to the specimen) using a ×40 objective and a partially closed condenser iris or dark-field or phase contrast microscopy.

Thick Blood Films or Chancre Aspirates

Examination of a thick film allows more of the sample to be examined rapidly, but *T. cruzi* are easily damaged by the spreading of specimens for thick films. Thick films are prepared by spreading a drop of blood on a slide to cover a 15–20-mm diameter area and staining with Giemsa staining technique or Field's rapid technique (p. 66) as for malaria smears. Microscopically, *T. b. gambiense* and *T. b. rhodesiense* cannot be distinguished from each other; they are 13–42 mm long with a single flagellum, a centrally placed nucleus, and a small dotlike kinetoplast. *T. cruzi* measures 12–30 mm and has a larger kinetoplast than *T. b. gambiense* and *T. b. rhodesiense* (Fig. 4.6B, C).

Concentration Techniques

Quantitative Buffy Coat Method

The QBC method[31,32] is referred to on p. 73. After centrifugation, the tube should be left to stand upright for 5 min, and the plasma interface area is then examined for motile trypomastigotes. This has been suggested as the "gold standard" for diagnosis.

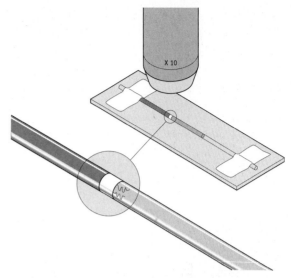

Figure 4.7   Capillary tube concentration method. Method used for detecting trypomastigotes or microfilariae in blood. See text.

Capillary Tube Method

Fill one or two micro-haematocrit capillary tubes with EDTA or citrated blood. Seal the ends and centrifuge for about 5 min as for microhaematocrit. Then lay the capillary tubes adjacent to each other on a microscope slide, and secure both ends onto the slide with adhesive tape (Figure 4.7). Examine the plasma just below the red cell and buffy layer immediately for motile trypomastigotes using a ×20 or ×10 objective with the condenser iris partially closed or by dark-field microscopy.

FILARIASIS AND LOIASIS

Filariasis involving the lymphatics is the cause of elephantiasis. It is caused by the filarial worms *Brugia malayi*, *Wuchereria bancrofti*, and *Brugia timori*, whereas filarial infection of the subcutaneous tissues is caused by *Loa loa*. The larvae of these worms, microfilariae, are transmitted by mosquito to humans, where they can be found in the blood and where they show periodicity with fluctuating levels at different times of the day (Figure 4.6D).

Diagnosis of Filariasis in the Haematology Laboratory

Blood concentrations of microfilariae are often higher in capillary blood than venous blood. However, even when blood has been collected at the appropriate time, microfilariae can be scanty, so that serological or rapid immunochromatographic tests and concentration techniques may be required.

Wet Preparation

A thick blood film is prepared from 20 µl blood and stained as for malaria smears (p. 71).

Concentration Techniques

Filtration Method

The filtration method is the most sensitive concentration method for microfilariae, but samples must be handled gently to preserve the organisms. Anticoagulated blood (10 ml), followed by 10 ml of methylene blue or azure B saline solution, are passed through a transparent polycarbonate membrane filter of 3-mm porosity attached to a syringe. The filter is placed face upward on a slide, a drop of saline is added, and a coverslip is placed on top. The entire membrane is examined microscopically for motile microfilariae using a ×10 objective and a partially closed condenser iris or dark-field microscopy.

Quantitative Buffy Coat and Microhaematocrit Methods

Microfilariae can be detected using the same methods as for detection of trypomastigotes (see above).

Lyzed Capillary Blood

Blood (1 ml) is mixed with 9 ml of 2% formalin and centrifuged at 1000 g for 5 min. All the deposit is placed on a slide and 1 drop of Field's stain A or 1% methylene blue is added to facilitate species identification. Motile microfilariae can be seen using a ×10 objective with a partially closed condenser iris or dark-field microscopy.

BABESIOSIS

Babesiosis results from a tickbourne intraerythrocytic protozoan, *Babesia*. Humans are infected by chance in the natural cycle of transmission between the tick and its domestic or wild animal host. It is especially prevalent in subtropical and tropical countries. The infection results in high fever accompanied by jaundice and severe haemolytic anaemia with haemoglobinuria; there is a leucocytosis with neutrophilia.

The parasites can be seen in the erythrocytes in Giemsa-stained blood films. Morphologically they are variable round or oval bodies that may be mistaken for the ring form of plasmodium, but it can be distinguished by characteristically dividing cells consisting of two daughter cells held together by a thin strand of cytoplasm; also, no pigment occurs in erythrocytes infected with older stages of *Babesia*.

EHRLICHOSIS

Ehrlichosis is a tickbourne fever in which clusters of small organisms may be seen in Giemsa-stained blood smears. The detection of organisms within neutrophils or monocytes is important for its diagnosis.

REFERENCES

1. Wittekind D 1979 On the nature of Romanowsky dyes and the Romanowsky Giemsa effect. Clinical and Laboratory Haematology 1:247–262.
2. Horobin RW, Walter KJ 1987 Understanding Romanowsky staining. I. the Romanowsky-Giemsa effect in blood smears. Azure B-eosin as a substitute for May-Grünwald-Giemsa and Jenner-Giemsa stains. Microscopica Acta 79:153–156.
3. Marshall PN 1978 Romanowsky-type stains in haematology. Histochemical Journal 10:1–29.
4. Wittekind DH, Kretschmer V, Sohmer I 1982 Azure B-eosin Y stain as the standard Romanowsky-Giemsa stain. British Journal of Haematology 5:391–393.
5. International Committee for Standardization in Haematology 1984 ICSH reference method for staining of blood and bone marrow films by azure B and eosin Y (Romanowsky stain). British Journal of Haematology 57:707–710.
6. Schenk EA, Willis CT 1989 Note from the Biological Stain Commission: certification of Wright stain solution. Stain Technology 64:152–153.

7. Wittekind DH 1983 On the nature of Romanowsky-Giemsa staining and its significance for cytochemistry and histochemistry: an overall view. Histochemical Journal 15:1029–1047.

8. Bind M, Huiges W, Halie MR 1985 Stability of azure B-eosin Y staining solutions. British Journal of Haematology 59:73–78.

9. Hayashi M, Gauthier S, Tatsumi N 1996 Evaluation of an automated slide preparation and staining unit. Sysmex Journal International 6:63–69.

10. Field JW 1940–41 The morphology of malarial parasites in thick blood films. IV. The identification of species and phase. Transactions of the Royal Society of Tropical Medicine and Hygiene 34:405–414.

11. Field JW 1941–42 Further notes on a method of staining malarial parasites in thick films. Transactions of the Royal Society of Tropical Medicine and Hygiene 35:35.

12. Zipursky A, Brown E, Palko J, et al 1983 The erythrocyte differential count in newborn infants. American Journal of Pediatric Hematology and Oncology 5:45–51.

13. Sills RH 1989 Hyposplenism. In: Pochedly C, Sills RH, Schwartz AD (Eds) Disorders of the spleen. Marcel Dekker, New York.

14. Nagel RL, Fabry ME, Steinberg MH 2003 The paradox of Hemoglobin SC disease. Blood Reviews 17:167–178

15. Fohlen-Walter A, Jacob C, Lacompte T, et al 2002 Laboratory identification of cryoglobulinema from automated blood cell counts, fresh blood samples, and blood films. American Journal of Clinical Pathology 117:606–614.

16. Bloemendal H (Ed) 1977 Cell separation methods. Elsevier-North Holland, Amsterdam.

17. Bøyum A 1984 Separation of lymphocytes, granulocytes and monocytes from human blood using iodinated density gradient media. Methods in Enzymology 108:88–102.

18. Efrati P, Rozenszajn L 1960 The morphology of buffy coat in normal human adults. Blood 16:1012–1019.

19. Efrati P, Rozenszajn L, Shapira E 1961 The morphology of buffy coat from cord blood of normal human newborns. Blood 17:497–503.

20. Romsdahl MM, McGrew EA, McGrath RG, et al 1964 Hematopoietic nucleated cells in the peripheral venous blood of patients with carcinoma. Cancer (Philadelphia) 17:1400–1404.

21. Linn YC, Tien SL, Lim LC, et al 1995 Haematophagocytosis in bone marrow aspirate: a review of the clinical course of 10 cases. Acta Haematologica 94:182–191.

22. Islam A 1995 A new, fast and convenient method for layering blood or bone marrow over density gradient medium. Journal of Clinical Pathology 48:686–688

23. Hänscheid T 1999. Diagnosis of malaria: a review of alternatives to conventional microscopy. Clinical and Laboratory Haematology 21:235–245.

24. Moody AH, Chiodini PL 2000 Methods for the detection of blood parasites. Clinical and Laboratory Haematology 22:189–202.

25. Thomson ST, Lohmann RC, Crawford L et al 2000 External quality assessment in the examination of blood films for malaria parasites within Ontario, Canada. Archives of Pathology and Laboratory Medicine 124:57–60.

26. Bell D, GO R, Miguel C et al 2001 Diagnosis of malaria in a remote area of the Philippines: comparison of techniques and their acceptance by health workers and the community. Bulletin of the World Health Organization 79:933–941.

27. Melvin DM, Brooke MM 1955 Triton X-100 in Giemsa staining of blood parasites. Stain Technology 30:269–275.

28. Gleeson RM 1997 An improved method for thick film preparation using saponin as a lysing agent. Clinical and Laboratory Haematology 19:249–251.

29. Lowe BS, Jeffa NF, New L 1996 Acridine orange fluorescence techniques as alternatives to traditional Giemsa staining for the diagnosis of malaria in developing countries. Transactions of the Royal Society of Tropical Medicine and Hygiene 90:30–34.

30. Gay T, Traore B. Zanoni J et al 1996 Direct acridine orange fluorescence examination of blood slides compared to current techniques for malaria diagnosis. Transactions of the Royal Society of Tropical Medicine and Hygiene 90:516–518.

31. Craig MH, Sharp BL 1997 Comparative evaluation of four techniques for the diagnosis of *Plasmodium falciparum* infections. Transactions of the Royal Society of Tropical Medicine and Hygiene 91:279–282.

32. Bailey W, Smith D 1994 The quantitative buffy coat for the diagnosis of trypanosomes. Tropical Doctor 24:54–56.

33. Ali FMK 1986 Separation of human blood and bone marrow cells. Wright, Bristol.

5 Blood cell morphology in health and disease

Barbara J. Bain

Examination of a fixed and stained blood film is an essential part of a haematological investigation, and it cannot be emphasized too strongly that, to obtain maximum information from the examination, the films must be well spread, well stained, and examined systematically. Details of the recommended procedure for examination are given later in this chapter.

The most important red cell abnormalities, as seen in fixed and stained films, are described and illustrated, and some notes on their significance and diagnostic importance are added. Leucocyte and platelet abnormalities are also described and, where appropriate, are illustrated. The slides were stained with May-Grünwald-Giemsa. Variations in the colours are the result of photographic processing and whether a daylight blue filter was used in the microscope.

EXAMINATION OF BLOOD FILMS

Blood films should be examined systematically, starting with macroscopic observation of the stained film and then progressing from low-power to high-power microscopic examination. It is useless to place a drop of immersion oil randomly on the film and then to examine it using the high-power ×100 objective.

First, the film should be examined macroscopically to assess whether the spreading technique was satisfactory and to judge its staining characteristics and whether there are any abnormal particles present that may represent large platelet aggregates, cryoglobulin deposits, or clumps of tumour cells. Either before or after macroscopic assessment, the film should be covered with a coverglass (coverslip) using a neutral medium as mountant. Next the film should be inspected under a low magnification (with a ×10 or ×20 objective) to: (a) get an idea of the quality of the preparation; (b) assess whether red cell agglutination, excessive rouleaux formation, or platelet aggregation is present; (c) assess the number, distribution, and staining of the leucocytes; and (d) find an area where the red cells are evenly distributed and are not distorted. A large part of the film should be scanned to detect scanty abnormal cells such as occasional granulocyte precursors or nucleated red blood cells.

Having selected a suitable area, a ×40 or ×50 objective or ×60 oil-immersion objective should then be used. A much better appreciation of variation in red cell size, shape, and staining can be obtained with one of these objectives than with the ×100 oil-immersion lens. It should be possible to detect features such as toxic granulation or the presence of Howell–Jolly bodies or Pappenheimer bodies. The major part of the assessment of a blood film is usually done at this power. The ×100 objective in combination with ×6 or ×10 eyepieces should be used only for the final examination of unusual cells

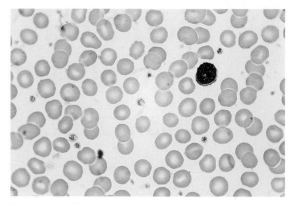

Figure 5.1   Photomicrograph of blood films. Film of a healthy adult.

and for looking at fine details such as punctate basophilia or Auer rods. Whether it is necessary to examine a film with a ×100 objective depends on the clinical features, the blood count, and the nature of any morphologic abnormality detected at lower power.

Because the diagnosis of the type of anaemia or other abnormality present usually depends on comprehension of the whole picture the film presents, the red cells, leucocytes, and platelets should all be systematically examined. The film examination also serves to validate the automated blood count, distinguishing, for example, between true macrocytosis and factitious macrocytosis caused by the presence of a cold agglutinin and, similarly, between true thrombocytopenia and factitious thrombocytopenia caused by platelet aggregation or satellitism.

RED CELL MORPHOLOGY

In health, the red blood cells vary relatively little in size and shape (Fig. 5.1). In well-spread, dried, and stained films the great majority of cells have round, smooth contours and diameters within the comparatively narrow range of 6.0–8.5 mm. As a rough guide, normal red cell size appears to be about the same as that of the nucleus of a small lymphocyte on the dried film (Fig. 5.1). The red cells stain quite deeply with the eosin component of Romanowsky dyes, particularly at the periphery of the cell in consequence of the cell's normal biconcavity. A small but variable proportion of cells in well-made films (usually less than 10%) are definitely oval rather than round, and a very small percentage may be contracted and have an irregular contour or appear to have lost part of their substance as the result of fragmentation (schistocytes). According to Marsh, the percentage of "pyknocytes" (irregularly contracted cells) and schistocytes in normal blood does not exceed 0.1% and the proportion is usually considerably less than this, whereas in normal, full-term infants the proportion is higher, 0.3–1.9%, and in premature infants it is still higher, up to 5.6%.[1]

Normal and pathological red cells are subject to considerable distortion in the spreading of a film, and, as already mentioned, it is imperative to scan films carefully to find an area where the red cells are least distorted before attempting to examine the cells in detail. Such an area can usually be found toward the tail of the film, although not actually at the tail. Rouleaux often form rapidly in blood after withdrawal from the body and may be conspicuous even in films made at a patient's bedside. They are particularly noticeable in the thicker parts of a film that have dried more slowly. Ideally, red cells should be examined in an area in which there are no rouleaux and the red cells are touching but with little overlap. The film in the chosen area must not be so thin as to cause red cell distortion; if the tail of the film is examined, a false impression of spherocytosis may be gained. The varying appearances of different areas of the same blood film are illustrated in Figures 5.2, 5.3, and 5.4. The area illustrated in Figure 5.2 would clearly be the best for looking at red cells critically.

The advantages and disadvantages of examining red cells suspended in plasma have been referred to briefly in Chapter 4 (p. 67). By this means, red cells can be seen in the absence of artefacts produced by drying, and abnormalities in size and shape can be better and more reliably appreciated than in films of blood dried on slides. However, the ease and rapidity with which dried films can be made, and

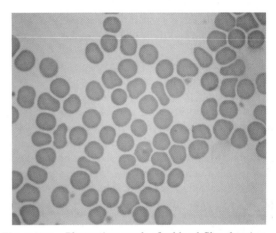

Figure 5.3 Photomicrograph of a blood film showing an area that is too thin for examination (same film as Figure 5.2).

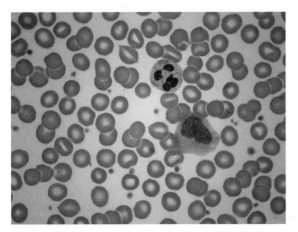

Figure 5.2 Photomicrograph of a blood film. Ideal thickness for examination.

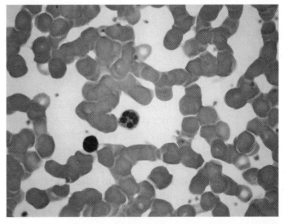

Figure 5.4 Photomicrograph of a blood film showing an area that is too thick for examination (same film as Figure 5.2).

their permanence, give them an overwhelming advantage in routine studies.

In disease, abnormality in the red cell picture stems from four main causes:

1. Abnormal erythropoiesis that may be effective or ineffective
2. Inadequate haemoglobin formation
3. Damage to, or changes affecting, the red cells after leaving the bone marrow, including the effects of reduced or absent splenic function
4. Attempts by the bone marrow to compensate for anaemia by increased erythropoiesis.

These processes result, respectively, in the following abnormalities of the red cells:

a. Increased variation in size (anisocytosis) and shape (poikilocytosis) and punctate basophilia
b. Reduced or unequal haemoglobin content (hypochromasia, anisochromasia, or dimorphism)
c. Spherocytosis, irregular contraction, elliptocytosis, or fragmentation (schistocytosis); the presence of Pappenheimer bodies, Howell–Jolly bodies, and a variable number of certain specific poikilocytes (target cells, acanthocytes, and spherocytes)
d. Signs of immaturity (polychromasia and erythroblastaemia).

ABNORMAL ERYTHROPOIESIS

Anisocytosis ($\alpha\nu\iota\sigma\sigma\zeta$, unequal) and Poikilocytosis ($\pi\sigma\iota\kappa\iota\lambda\sigma\zeta$, varied)

Anisocytosis and poikilocytosis are nonspecific features of almost any blood disorder. The terms imply more variation in size or shape than is normally present (Figs. 5.5 and 5.6). Anisocytosis may be a result of the presence of cells larger than normal (macrocytosis), cells smaller than normal (microcytosis), or both; frequently both macrocytes and microcytes are present (Fig. 5.5).

Poikilocytes are produced in many types of abnormal erythropoiesis—for example, megaloblastic anaemia (Fig. 5.7), iron deficiency anaemia, thalassaemia, myelofibrosis (both idiopathic and secondary) (Fig. 5.8), congenital dyserythropoietic anaemia (Fig. 5.9), and the myelodysplastic syndromes. Elliptocytes and ovalocytes are among the poikilocytes that may be present when there is dyserythropoiesis; they are often present in megaloblastic anaemia (macro-ovalocytes) and in iron deficiency anaemia ("pencil cells"), but they may also be seen in myelodysplastic syndromes and in idiopathic myelofibrosis (see Fig. 5.8). The number of elliptocytes and "tailed-poikilocytes"

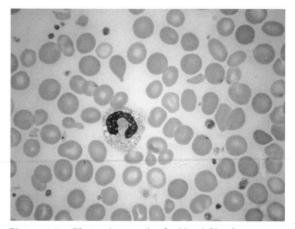

Figure 5.5   Photomicrograph of a blood film from a patient with a myelodysplastic/myeloproliferative condition, unclassified. Shows moderate anisocytosis, anisochromasia, and poikilocytosis. There is one neutrophil band form.

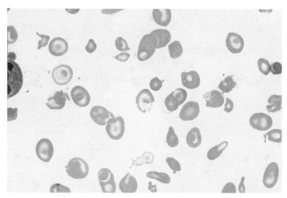

Figure 5.6   Photomicrograph of a blood film from a patient with compound heterozygosity for haemoglobin E and β° thalassaemia. Shows marked anisocytosis and poikilocytosis.

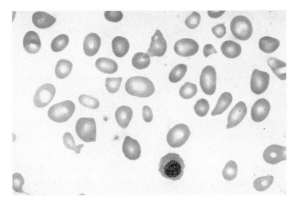

Figure 5.7 Photomicrograph of a blood film. Pernicious anaemia. Shows marked anisocytosis, moderate poikilocytosis (including oval macrocytes and teardrop cells), and a megaloblast.

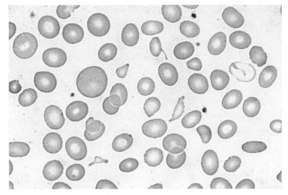

Figure 5.9 Photomicrograph of a blood film. Congenital dyserythropoietic anaemia type II. Shows marked anisocytosis, marked poikilocytosis, one unusually large macrocyte, and one severely hypochromic cell.

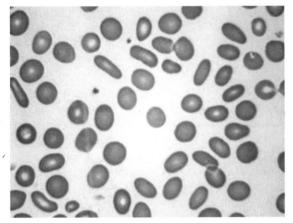

Figure 5.8 Photomicrograph of a blood film. Idiopathic myelofibrosis. Many of the erythrocytes are elliptical or oval.

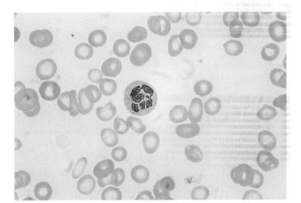

Figure 5.10 Photomicrograph of a blood film. Megaloblastic anaemia. Shows macrocytes, oval macrocytes, and a hypersegmented neutrophil.

(teardrop poikilocytes) has been observed to correlate with the severity of iron deficiency anaemia.[2] Poikilocytes are not only characteristic of disordered erythropoiesis but are also seen in various congenital haemolytic anaemias caused by membrane defects and in acquired conditions such as microangiopathic haemolytic anaemia and oxidant damage; in these disorders, the abnormality of shape results from damage to cells after formation and is described later in this chapter.

Macrocytes

Classically found in megaloblastic anaemias (Fig. 5.10), but macrocytes are also present in some cases of aplastic anaemia, myelodysplastic syndromes, and other dyserythropoietic states. In patients being treated with hydroxycarbamide (previously known as hydroxyurea) the red cells are often macrocytic. A common cause of macrocytosis is excess alcohol intake, and it occurs in alcoholic and other types of chronic liver disease. In these conditions, the red cells tend to be fairly uniform in size and shape and there may also be stomatocytes (Fig. 5.11). In the rare type III form of congenital dyserythropoietic anaemia, some of the macrocytes are exceptionally large. Another rare cause of macrocytosis is benign familial macrocytosis.[3] Macrocytosis also occurs whenever there is an increased rate of erythropoiesis, because of the presence of reticulocytes. Their presence is suspected in routinely stained films because of the slight basophilia, giving rise to polychromasia (p. 99) and is easily confirmed by special stains (e.g., New methylene blue, see p. 38). These polychromatic macrocytes should be distinguished from other macrocytes because the diagnostic significance is quite different.

Microcytes

The presence of microcytes usually results from a defect in haemoglobin formation. Microcytosis is characteristic of iron deficiency anaemia (Fig. 5.12), various types of thalassaemia (Fig. 5.13), and severe cases of anaemia of chronic disease. Causes that are more rare include congenital and acquired sideroblastic anaemias. Microcytosis related to a defect in haemoglobin synthesis should be distinguished from red cell fragmentation or schistocytosis (see p. 91). Both abnormalities can lead to a reduction of the mean cell volume (MCV). However, it should be noted that a low MCV is common in association with a defect in haemoglobin synthesis, whereas it is uncommon in fragmentation syndromes because the fragments usually comprise only a small percentage of erythrocytes.

Basophilic Stippling

Basophilic stippling (or punctate basophilia) means the presence of numerous basophilic granules distributed throughout the cell (Fig. 5.14); in contrast to Pappenheimer bodies (see below), they do not give a positive Perls' reaction for ionized iron. Basophilic stippling has quite a different significance from diffuse cytoplasmic basophilia. It is indicative of disturbed rather than increased erythropoiesis. It occurs in many blood diseases: thalassaemia,

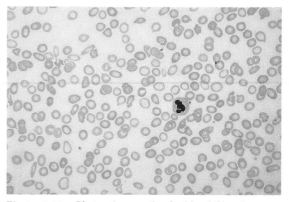

Figure 5.12   Photomicrograph of a blood film. Iron deficiency anaemia. Shows hypochromia, microcytosis, and poikilocytosis.

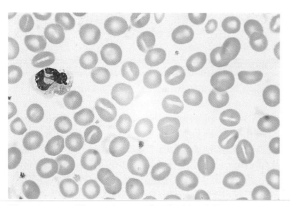

Figure 5.11   Photomicrograph of a blood film. Liver disease. Shows macrocytosis and stomatocytosis.

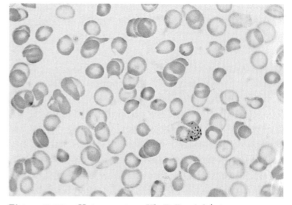

Figure 5.13   Heterozygous Hb D-Punjab/ β thalassaemia. Shows anisocytosis, poikilocytosis, hypochromia, microcytosis, and basophilic stippling.

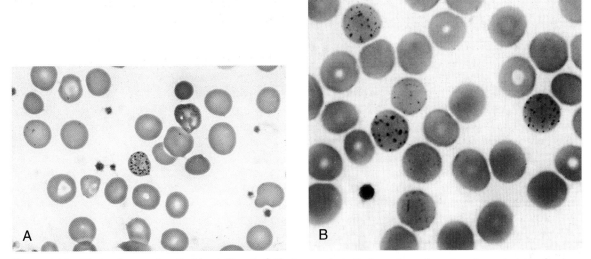

Figure 5.14   Photomicrographs of a blood film. A: β Thalassaemia trait shows hypochromia, microcytosis, and basophilic stippling. B: Erythropoietic porphyria. Shows prominent basophilic stippling.

megaloblastic anaemias, infections, liver disease, poisoning by lead and other heavy metals, unstable haemoglobins, and pyrimidine-5'-nucleotidase deficiency.[4]

INADEQUATE HAEMOGLOBIN FORMATION

Hypochromasia (Hypochromia) (υπορ, under)

The term *hypochromasia*, or now, more often, *hypochromia*, refers to the presence of red cells that stain unusually palely. (In doubtful cases, it is wise to compare the staining of the suspect film with that of a normal film stained at the same time.) There are two possible causes: a lowered haemoglobin concentration and abnormal thinness of the red cells. A lowered haemoglobin concentration results from impaired haemoglobin synthesis. This may stem from failure of haem synthesis—iron deficiency is a very common cause (Fig. 5.15) and sideroblastic anaemia (Fig. 5.16) is a rare cause—or failure of globin synthesis as in the thalassaemias (Fig. 5.17). Haemoglobin synthesis may also be impaired in chronic infections and other inflammatory conditions. It cannot be too strongly stressed that a

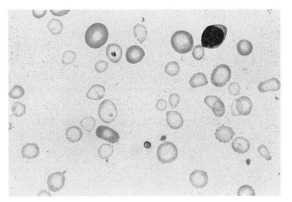

Figure 5.15   Photomicrograph of a blood film. Iron deficiency anaemia. Shows a marked degree of hypochromia, microcytosis, marked anisocytosis, and mild poikilocytosis; there are some normally haemoglobinized cells.

hypochromic blood picture does not necessarily mean iron deficiency, although this is the most common cause. In iron deficiency, the red cells are characteristically hypochromic and microcytic, but the extent of these abnormalities depends on the severity; hypochromia may be minor and may be overlooked if the haemoglobin concentration (Hb) exceeds 100 g/l. In heterozygous α+ or α°

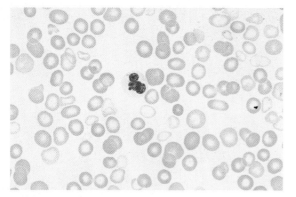

Figure 5.16   Photomicrograph of a blood film. Acquired sideroblastic anaemia (refractory anaemia with ring sideroblasts). Shows a dimorphic blood film with a mixture of normochromic normocytic cells and hypochromic microcytes; there are also several polychromatic macrocytes.

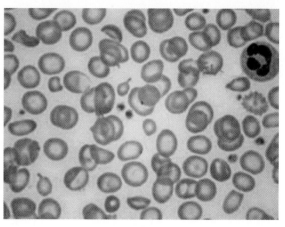

Figure 5.17   Photomicrograph of a blood film. Haemoglobin H disease. Shows microcytosis, moderate hypochromia, moderate anisocytosis, and some poikilocytes (including teardrop poikilocytes and red cell fragments).

thalassaemia, or heterozygous β thalassaemia, hypochromia is often less marked, in relation to the degree of microcytosis, than in iron deficiency. The presence of target cells or basophilic stippling also favours a diagnosis of thalassaemia trait rather than iron deficiency. In homozygous β thalassaemia, the abnormalities are greater than in iron deficiency at the same Hb and nucleated red cells are usually present, whereas they are not a feature of iron deficiency. If the patient is being transfused regularly, normal donor cells will also be present (Fig. 5.18).

Anisochromasia (ανισoζ, unequal) and Dimorphic Red Cell Population

A distinction should be made between anisochromasia, in which there is abnormal variability in staining of red cells, and a dimorphic picture, in which there are two distinct populations. Anisochromasia, in which some but not all of the red cells stain palely, is characteristic of a changing situation. It can occur during the development or resolution of iron deficiency anaemia (Fig. 5.19) or the anaemia of chronic disease. In thalassaemia trait, in contrast, anisochromasia is much less common. A dimorphic blood film can be seen in several circumstances. It can occur when an iron deficiency anaemia responds

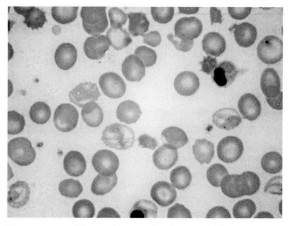

Figure 5.18   Photomicrograph of a blood film. β Thalassaemia major. Shows a dimorphic blood film. The normal cells are transfused cells. The patient's own cells show severe hypochromia. There are three nucleated red blood cells.

to iron therapy, after the transfusion of normal blood to a patient with a hypochromic anaemia (Fig. 5.19), and in sideroblastic anaemia (Fig. 5.20). In acquired sideroblastic anaemia as a feature of myelodysplasia, the two populations of cells are usually hypochromic microcytic and normochromic macrocytic, respectively.

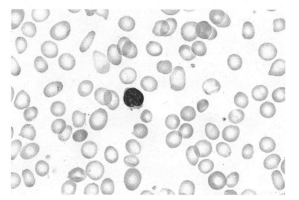

Figure 5.19 Photomicrograph of a blood film. Iron-deficiency anaemia. Shows a constant gradation of haemoglobinization of cells (i.e., anisochromasia). There is one elliptocyte.

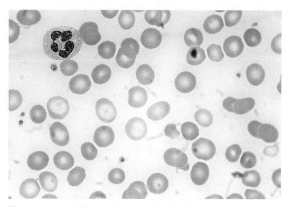

Figure 5.20 Photomicrograph of a blood film. Acquired sideroblastic anaemia. Shows two distinct populations of cells: hypochromic cells, which also tend to be microcytic, and normocytic normochromic cells.

DAMAGE TO RED CELLS AFTER FORMATION

Poikilocytosis can result not only from abnormal erythropoiesis but also from damage to red cells after their formation. The damage may be consequent on an intrinsic abnormality of the red cell such as a haemoglobinopathy, a membrane defect, or an enzyme defect that renders the cell prone to shape alteration. Poikilocytosis can also result from extrinsic causes, as when a red cell is damaged by drugs, chemicals, or toxins; by heat; or by abnormal mechanical forces. Poikilocytes of specific shapes suggest different aetiologic factors.

Hyperchromasia (Hyperchromia) (υπερ, over)

Unusually deep staining of the red cells with a lack of central pallor may be seen in two circumstances: first, in the presence of macrocytes and second, when cells are abnormally rounded. In macrocytosis, as in neonatal blood and megaloblastic anaemias, it is the increased red cell thickness that causes the hyperchromia, and the mean cell haemoglobin concentration is normal. When hyperchromia results from cells being of abnormal shape, the red cell thickness is greater than normal and the MCHC is increased. Abnormally rounded cells may be

either spherocytes or irregularly contracted cells. The distinction between these two cell types is of diagnostic importance.

Spherocytosis (σφαιρα, a sphere)

Spherocytes are cells that are more spheroidal (i.e., less disc-like) than normal red cells but maintain a regular outline. Their diameter is less and their thickness is greater than normal. Only in extreme instances are they almost spherical in shape. It is useful to draw a distinction between spherocytes of normal size and microspherocytes; the latter result from red cell fragmentation or from removal of a considerable proportion of the red cell membrane by splenic or other macrophages. Spherocytes may result from genetic defects of the red cell membrane as in hereditary spherocytosis (Fig. 5.21); from the interaction between immunoglobulin- or complement-coated red cells and phagocytic cells, as in ABO haemolytic disease of the newborn (Fig. 5.22) and autoimmune haemolytic anaemia (Fig. 5.23); and from the action of bacterial toxins (e.g., *Clostridium perfringens* lecithinase (Fig. 5.24).

Spherocytes usually appear perfectly round in contour in stained films; they have to be carefully distinguished from both irregularly contracted cells and "crenated spheres" or sphero-echinocytes (Fig. 5.25), which are the end result of crenation (see p. 93). Sphero-echinocytes develop as artefacts

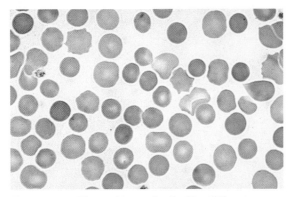

Figure 5.21   Photomicrograph of a blood film. Hereditary spherocytosis. Shows a moderate degree of spherocytosis and anisocytosis. Note the round contour of the spherocytes.

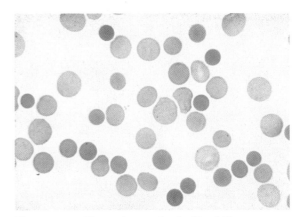

Figure 5.23   Photomicrograph of a blood film. Autoimmune haemolytic anaemia. Shows marked spherocytosis and anisocytosis. There are numerous polychromatic macrocytes.

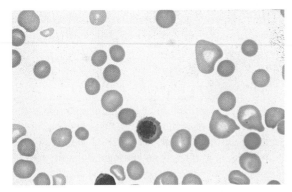

Figure 5.22   Photomicrograph of a blood film. ABO haemolytic disease of the newborn. Spherocytosis is intense, and there are several polychromatic macrocytes.

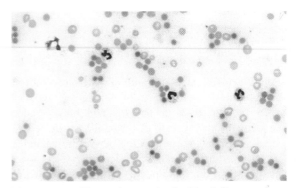

Figure 5.24   Photomicrograph of a blood film. *Clostridium perfringens* septicaemia. Shows an extreme degree of spherocytosis; note the round contour of the spherocytes. A markedly dimorphic picture.

especially in blood that has been allowed to stand before films are spread (Fig. 5.26). Sphero-echinocytes are also present in the blood of patients with hereditary spherocytosis who have been splenectomized. The blood film of a patient who has been transfused with stored blood may show a proportion of sphero-echinocytes (Fig. 5.27).

Irregularly Contracted Red Cells

There are a number of causes of irregularly contracted cells. In drug- or chemical-induced haemolytic anaemias, a proportion of the red cells are smaller than normal and unusually densely stained (i.e., they appear contracted) and their margins are slightly or moderately irregular and may be partly concave (Fig. 5.28). These may be cells from which Heinz bodies have been extracted by the spleen. Similar cells may be seen in films of some unstable haemoglobinopathies before splenectomy (e.g., that caused by the presence of Hb Köln or Hb St Mary's; Fig. 5.29) and in haemoglobin E homozygosity (Fig. 5.30) and, to a lesser extent, haemoglobin E heterozygosity. Heinz bodies are not normally visible in Romanowsky-stained blood films, but they may be seen in such films as pale pink–staining bodies at

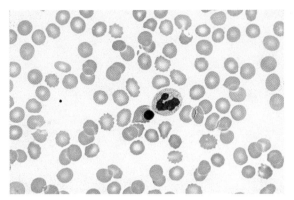

Figure 5.25   Photomicrograph of a blood film. Sodium chlorate poisoning. Shows sphero-echinocytes, one keratocyte, and one nucleated red cell.

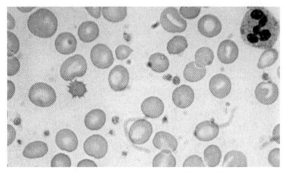

Figure 5.27   Photomicrograph of a blood film. Posttransfusion, showing one sphero-echinocyte.

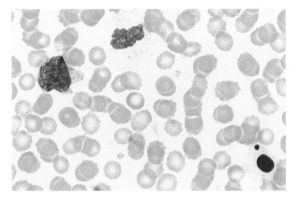

Figure 5.26   Photomicrograph of a blood film. Normal blood after 24 hours at c 20°C. Shows a marked degree of crenation; also degenerative changes in white cells.

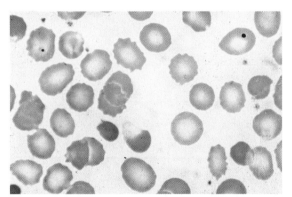

Figure 5.28   Photomicrograph of a blood film. Haemolytic anaemia caused by an overdose of phenacetin. Shows four irregularly contracted cells and crenation.

the cell margin or even protruding from the erythrocytes in severe unstable haemoglobin haemolytic anaemias after splenectomy and in acute oxidant-induced haemolytic aneamia. An extreme degree of irregular contraction is characteristic of severe favism or any other very acute haemolytic episode in individuals who are glucose-6-phosphate dehydrogenase deficient; it is typical to see cells in which the haemoglobin appears to have contracted away from the cell membrane, an appearance sometimes referred to as a hemi-ghost (Fig. 5.31). Irregularly contracted cells can be seen in small numbers in β thalassaemia trait, in heterozygosity for haemoglobin C. There may be a considerable number in haemoglobin C homozygosity, and in this condition haemoglobin C crystals may also be seen (Fig. 5.32).

A type of irregular contraction of unknown origin has been described by the term "pyknocytosis."[5] The pyknocytes closely resemble chemically damaged red cells. As already mentioned (p. 81), a small number of pyknocytes may be found in the blood of infants in the first few weeks of life, especially in premature infants. The term "infantile pyknocytosis" refers to a transient haemolytic anaemia, related to glutathione peroxidase and selenium deficiency, affecting infants in whom many pyknocytes are present (Fig. 5.33).[5,6]

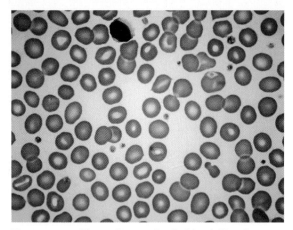

Figure 5.29   Photomicrograph of a blood film. An unstable haemoglobin haemolytic anaemia (haemoglobin St Mary's). Shows several irregularly contracted cells.

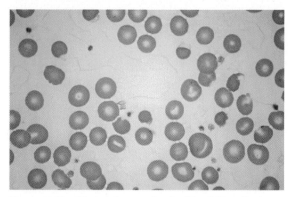

Figure 5.31   Photomicrograph of a blood film. Favism. Shows numerous markedly contracted cells. Note condensation and contraction of haemoglobin from the cell membrane.

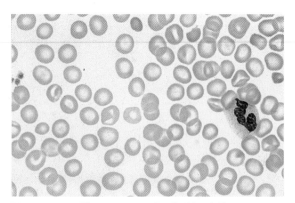

Figure 5.30   Photomicrograph of a blood film. Haemoglobin E homozygosity showing four irregularly contracted cells and target cells.

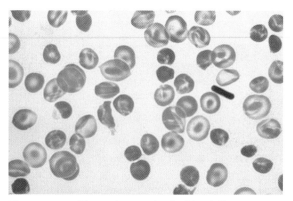

Figure 5.32   Photomicrograph of a blood film. Haemoglobin C disease (homozygosity for haemoglobin C). Shows many target cells, irregularly contracted cells, and a crystal of haemoglobin C. Sometimes it is apparent that haemoglobin C crystals are within otherwise empty red cell membranes.

Elliptocytosis and Ovalocytosis

Elliptocytes are often present in large numbers in hereditary elliptocytosis (Fig. 5.34). In hereditary pyropoikilocytosis, elliptocytes are only one of the many types of poikilocyte present (Fig. 5.35). Southeast Asian ovalocytosis is characterized by the presence of a variable number of elliptocytes, macro-ovalocytes, and stomatocytes (Fig. 5.36). In all these conditions, the reticulocytes are round in contour (i.e., the cell assumes an abnormal shape only in the late stages of maturation). They are therefore acquired defects of red cell shape, although the causative condition is inherited.

SPICULATED CELLS AND RED CELL FRAGMENTATION

The terminology applied to spiculated cells has been confusing because the same terms have been used to designate different types of cells. For this reason the term "burr cell" should be discarded and the terms recommended by Bessis[7] should be adopted. On the basis of scanning electron microscopy (discussed later), he distinguished four types of spiculated cell—

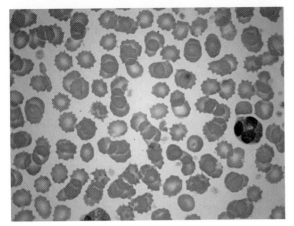

Figure 5.33   Photomicrograph of a blood film. Infantile pyknocytosis. Shows irregularly contracted cells similar to those seen in chemical- or drug-induced haemolytic anaemias.

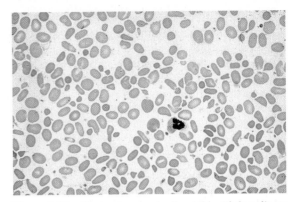

Figure 5.35   Photomicrograph of a child with hereditary pyropoikilocytosis. Shows spherocytes, elliptocytes, red cell fragments, and polychromatic macrocytes.

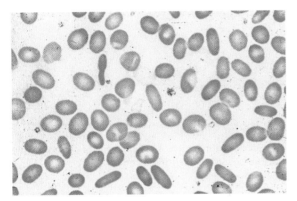

Figure 5.34   Photomicrograph of a blood film. Hereditary elliptocytosis. Many of the cells are elliptical, and others are oval.

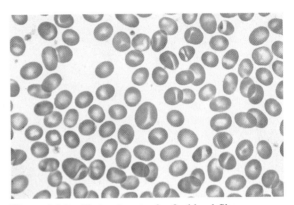

Figure 5.36   Photomicrograph of a blood film. Southeast Asian ovalocytosis. Shows stomatocytes, macrostomatocytes, and macro-ovalocytes.

schistocyte, keratocyte, acanthocyte, and echinocyte. The term *echinocyte* is used for the crenated cell. It is differentiated from the acanthocyte on the basis of the number, shape, and disposition of the spicules.

Schistocytosis (Fragmentation) (σχιστος, cleft)

Schistocytes or erythrocyte fragments are found in many blood diseases. They are smaller than normal red cells and of varying shape. Sometimes they have sharp angles or spines (spurs), and sometimes they

are round in contour, usually staining deeply but occasionally palely as the result of loss of haemoglobin at the time of fragmentation. If they are both round and densely staining, they may be referred to as microspherocytes. They occur in the following situations:

1. In certain genetically determined disorders (e.g., thalassaemias, congenital dyserythropoietic anaemia, and hereditary pyropoikilocytosis)
2. In acquired disorders of red cell formation when erythropoiesis is megaloblastic or dyserythropoietic

3. As the consequence of mechanical stresses (e.g., in the microangiopathic haemolytic anaemias; Figs. 5.37–5.39) and in cardiac haemolytic anaemias that are usually caused by a perivalvular leak accompanied by turbulence of left ventricular flow (Fig. 5.40)

4. As the result of direct thermal injury as in severe burns (Fig. 5.41).

In burns, schistocytes are often rounded, being either microspherocytes or very small disc-shaped fragments. In addition, erythrocytes may be seen to be budding off small rounded blebs of cytoplasm. Not infrequently, as, for instance in the haemolytic-uraemic syndrome in children, the blood picture is made more bizarre by the superimposition of varying degrees of echinocytic change. Schistocytes are also a feature of thrombotic thrombocytopenia purpura.[8]

Keratocytes ($\kappa\varepsilon\rho\alpha\zeta$, horn)

Keratocytes have pairs of spicules, usually either one pair or two pairs. They may be formed either by removal of a Heinz body by the pitting action of the spleen (Fig. 5.42) or by mechanical damage (Figs. 5.43–5.44). The terms "helmet cell" and "bite

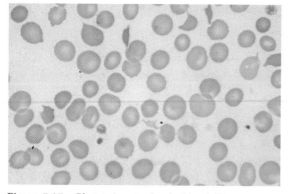

Figure 5.37 Photomicrograph of a blood film. Microangiopathic haemolytic anaemia. Shows angular red cell fragments.

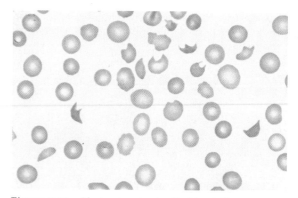

Figure 5.39 Photomicrograph of a blood film. Microangiopathic haemolytic anaemia. Shows numerous bizarre-shaped red cell fragments.

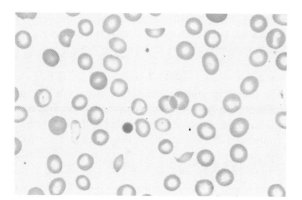

Figure 5.38 Photomicrograph of a blood film. Microangiopathic haemolytic anaemia in systemic lupus erythematosus. Shows one very dense microspherocyte and red cell fragments.

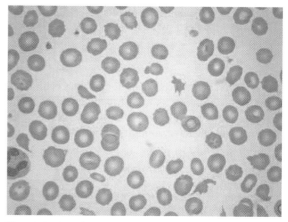

Figure 5.40 Photomicrograph of a blood film. Postcardiac surgery haemolytic anaemia. Shows numerous irregularly shaped cell fragments.

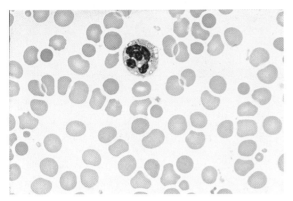

Figure 5.41   Photomicrograph of a blood film. Severe burns. Shows many very small, rounded red cell fragments (microspherocytes) and one crenated cell.

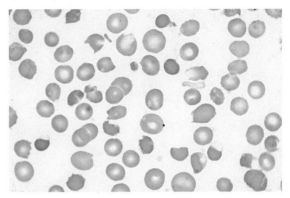

Figure 5.43   Photomicrograph of a blood film. Haemolytic anaemia caused by dapsone. Shows many irregularly contracted cells, three cells with haemoglobin retracted from the red cell membrane, and one keratocyte.

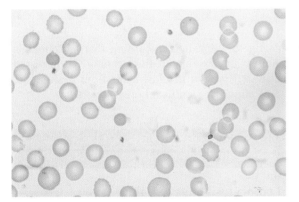

Figure 5.42   Photomicrograph of a blood film. Keratocytes and irregularly contracted cells in a patient with haemolysis caused by glucose-6-phosphate dehydrogenase deficiency.

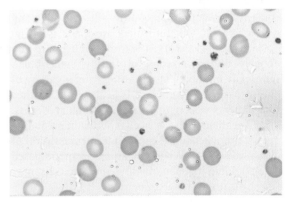

Figure 5.44   Photomicrograph of a blood film. Two keratocytes in a patient with microangiopathic haemolytic anaemia.

cell" have sometimes been used to describe keratocytes.

Acanthocytosis ($\alpha\kappa\alpha\nu\theta\alpha$, spine)

The term *acanthocytosis* was introduced to describe an abnormality of the red cell in which there are a small number of spicules of inconstant length, thickness, and shape, irregularly disposed over the surface of the cell (Fig. 5.45). They are often associated with abnormal phospholipid metabolism[9–11] or with inherited abnormalities of red cell membrane proteins as in the McLeod phenotype,

caused by lack of the Kell precursor (Kx).[12] They are present in varying numbers following splenectomy and in hyposplenism. A similar cell occurs in severe liver disease ("spur cell" anaemia).[13]

Echinocytosis ($\varepsilon\chi\iota\nu o\zeta$, sea-urchin or hedgehog)

Echinocytosis or crenation describes the process by which red cells develop many or numerous short, regular projections from their surface (see Figs. 5.25 and 5.26). First described by Ponder[14] as disc–sphere transformation, crenation has many causes. A few

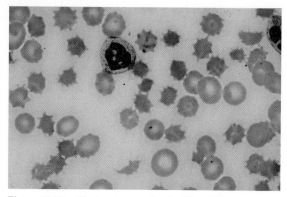

Figure 5.45 Photomicrograph of a blood film. Liver failure. Acanthocytes are conspicuous.

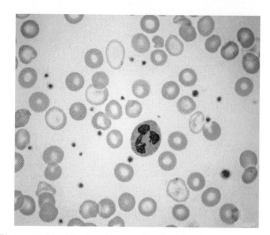

Figure 5.46 Photomicrograph of a blood film. β thalassaemia major, after splenectomy. Shows one target cell and cells grossly deficient in haemoglobin, which are leptocytes. There are some transfused cells.

crenated cells may be seen in many blood films, even in those from healthy subjects. Crenation regularly develops if blood is allowed to stand overnight at 20°C before films are made (see Fig. 5.26). It may be a marked feature, for obscure and probably diverse reasons, in freshly made blood films made from patients suffering from a variety of illnesses, especially uraemia. It is also seen in films from patients undergoing cardiopulmonary bypass. Marked echinocytosis has been reported in premature infants after exchange transfusion or transfusion of normal red cells.[15] When crenation is superimposed on an underlying abnormality, the red cells may appear bizarre in the extreme.

Crenation also occurs as an artefact if red cells are washed free from plasma and suspended in 9 g/l NaCl between glass surfaces, particularly at a raised pH; it also occurs in the presence of traces of fatty substances on the slides on which films are made and in the presence of traces of chemicals that at higher concentrations cause lysis.

The end stages of crenation are the "finely crenated sphere" and the "spherical form," which closely resemble spherocytes. The disc–sphere transformation may be reversible (e.g., that produced by washing cells free from plasma), and in this respect the contracted "spherical form" (which has not lost surface) is quite distinct from the "spherocyte" (which has lost surface), although they may closely resemble one another in stained films.

If echinocytosis is observed in a film, it usually represents a storage artefact caused by delay in making the film. It is a warning that morphologic features in the blood film cannot be assessed reliably. If present in films made from fresh blood, it is a clinically significant observation.

MISCELLANEOUS ERYTHROCYTE ABNORMALITIES

Leptocytosis (λεπτος, thin)

The term *leptocytosis* has been used to describe unusually thin red cells, as in severe iron deficiency or thalassaemia in which the cells may stain as rings of membrane with a little attached haemoglobin with large, almost unstained, central areas (Fig. 5.46).

Target Cells

The term *target cell* refers to a cell in which there is a central round stained area and a peripheral rim of haemoglobinized cytoplasm separated by non-staining or more lightly staining cytoplasm. Target cells result from cells having a surface that is disproportionately large compared with their volume. They may be normal in size, microcytic, or macrocytic. They are seen in films in chronic liver diseases in which the cell membrane may be loaded with cholesterol (Fig. 5.47), in hereditary hypo-betalipoproteinaemia,[16] and in varying numbers in iron deficiency anaemia and in thalassaemia (see Fig. 5.46). They are often conspicuous in certain haemoglobinopathies (e.g., haemoglobin C/β° tha-lassaemia; Fig. 5.48), haemoglobin C disease (Fig. 5.49), haemoglobin H disease (Fig. 5.50), sickle cell anaemia, sickle cell/haemoglobin C disease (Fig. 5.51), sickle cell/β thalassaemia, and haemoglobin E disease. Smaller numbers are usual in haemoglobin C trait, haemoglobin E trait, and postsplenectomy. Splenectomy in thalassaemia may result in an extreme degree of leptocytosis and target cell formation.

Stomatocytosis (στομα, mouth)

Stomatocytes are red cells in which the central biconcave area appears slitlike in dried films. In "wet" preparations, the stomatocyte is a cup-shaped red cell. The slitlike appearance of the cell's con-cavity, as seen in dried films, is thus to some extent an artefact. The term was first used to describe the appearance of some of the cells in a rare type of haemolytic anaemia, hereditary stomatocytosis.[17] They are also a feature of southeast Asian ovalocytosis. They have been described as being particularly frequent in films of Australians of

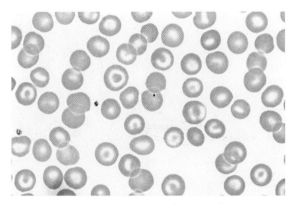

Figure 5.47   Photomicrograph of a blood film. Alcoholic liver disease. Shows many target cells.

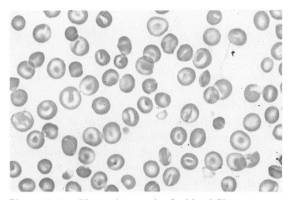

Figure 5.49   Photomicrograph of a blood film. Haemoglobin C homozygosity. Shows numerous target cells and irrregularly contracted cells.

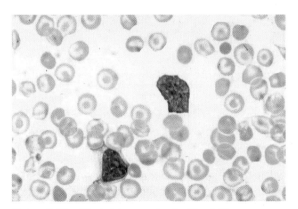

Figure 5.48   Photomicrograph of a blood film. Haemoglobin C/β° thalassaemia compound heteozygosity showing target cells, irregularly contracted cells, and one spherocyte.

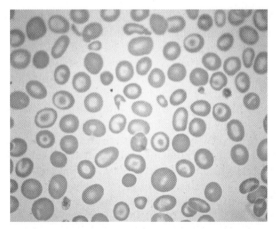

Figure 5.50   Photomicrograph of a blood film. Haemoglobin H disease. Shows target cells, hypochromic cells, and poikilocytes.

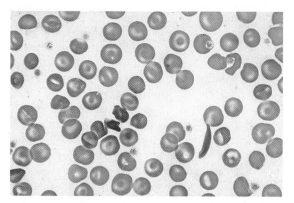

Figure 5.51 Photomicrograph of a blood film. Sickle cell/haemoglobin C disease. Shows a sickle cell, target cells, and two SC poikilocytes.

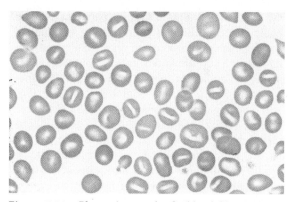

Figure 5.52 Photomicrograph of a blood film. Patient with chronic myeloid leukaemia taking hydroxycarbamide. Shows stomatocytosis. Many of the cells have a slit-like central unstained area.

Mediterranean origin.[18,19] Subsequently, stomatocytes were recognized in acquired conditions and occasionally they are prominent (Fig. 5.52). They are observed in liver disease, in alcoholism,[20] and occasionally in the myelodysplastic syndromes. There is a suspicion that in some films the occurrence of stomatocytosis is an *in vitro* artefact because it is known that the change can be produced by decreased pH and as the result of exposure to cationic detergent-like compounds and nonpenetrating anions.[21]

Sickle Cells

The varied film appearances in sickle cell anaemia are illustrated in Figures 5.53, 5.54, and 5.55. Sickle cells are almost always present in films of freshly withdrawn blood of adults with homozygosity for haemoglobin S. However, sickle cells are usually absent in neonates and are rare in adult patients with a high haemoglobin F percentage. Sometimes many irreversibly sickled cells are present, and in all cases massive sickling takes place when the blood is subjected to anoxia (see p. 292). In films of fresh blood, the sickled cells vary in shape between elliptical forms and sickles. Target cells are also often a feature of blood films from patients with sickle cell anaemia, and Howell–Jolly bodies are found when there is splenic atrophy.

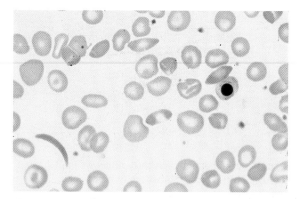

Figure 5.53 Photomicrograph of a blood film. Sickle cell anaemia (homozygosity for haemoglobin S). Shows a sickled cell, boat-shaped cells, and a nucleated red cell and target cells.

Haemoglobin C Crystals and SC Poikilocytes

In patients with homozygosity for haemoglobin C, target cells and irregularly contracted cells are usually numerous and there may be occasional straight-edged haemoglobin C crystals, either extracellularly (see Fig. 5.32) or within the ghost of a red cell. In patients who are compound heterozygotes for both haemoglobin S and haemoglobin C, the film may resemble that of haemoglobin C disease (see Fig. 5.32). In other patients, there are elliptical cells, rare sickle cells, and sometimes distinctive SC poikilocytes (Fig. 5.56).

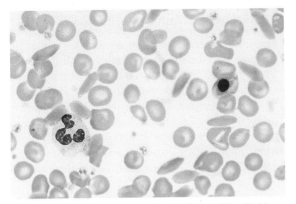

Figure 5.54   Photomicrograph of a blood film. Sickle cell anaemia (homozygosity for haemoglobin S). Shows boat-shaped cells and a nucleated red blood cell.

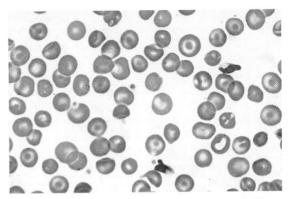

Figure 5.56   Photomicrograph of a blood film. Sickle cell/ haemoglobin C disease showing SC poikilocytes and target cells.

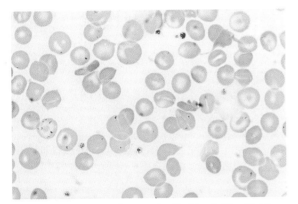

Figure 5.55   Photomicrograph of a blood film. Sickle cell anaemia (homozygosity for haemoglobin S). Shows elliptical sickle cells, target cells, and Pappenheimer bodies.

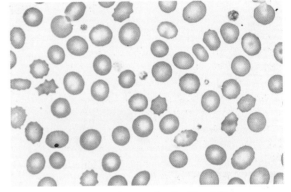

Figure 5.57   Photomicrograph of a blood film. Postsplenectomy. Shows acanthocytes, a target cell, and a Howell–Jolly body.

Erythrocyte Inclusions

The possibility of sometimes suspecting the presence of Heinz bodies on a routinely stained film and the detection of haemoglobin crystals within red cells has already been mentioned. Other red cell inclusions include Howell–Jolly bodies and Pappenheimer bodies.

Howell–Jolly Bodies

These are nuclear remnants and (usually singly) may be seen in a small percentage of red cells in pernicious anaemia. Cells containing them are regularly present after splenectomy and where there has been splenic atrophy (Fig. 5.57). Usually only a few such cells are present, but they may be numerous in cases of coeliac disease in which there is splenic atrophy and coexisting folate deficiency.

Pappenheimer Bodies

Pappenheimer bodies are small peripherally sited basophilic (almost black) erythrocyte inclusions. Usually only a small number are present in a cell.

They are composed of haemosiderin, and their presence is related to iron overload and hyposplenism (Figs. 5.58 and 5.59). Sometimes they are found in the majority of circulating red cells. Their nature can be confirmed by means of a Perls' stain. They correspond to the siderotic granules of siderocytes and are never distributed in large numbers throughout the cells as in classical punctate basophilia. However, a single cell may show both punctate basophilia and Pappenheimer bodies. With Perls' stain, the former granules are pink, whereas the latter are blue.

Rouleaux and Autoagglutination

The differences between rouleaux and autoagglutination are described on page 67, and there is usually no difficulty in determining which is which in stained films (Figs. 5.60 and 5.61). However, in myelomatosis and in other conditions in which there is intense rouleaux formation, the rouleaux may simulate autoagglutination. Even so, if the film, apparently showing autoagglutination, is carefully scanned, an area in which rouleaux can be

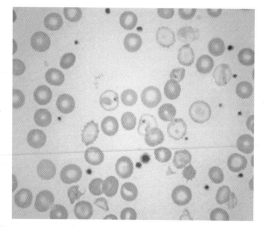

Figure 5.58   Photomicrograph of a blood film. β Thalassaemia major, patient of regular blood transfusions, showing Pappenheimer bodies in several poorly haemoglobinized cells.

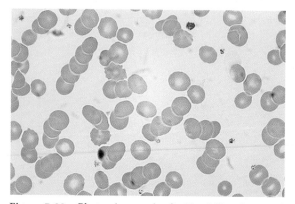

Figure 5.60   Photomicrograph of a blood film. Increased rouleaux formation in a patient with bacterial infection.

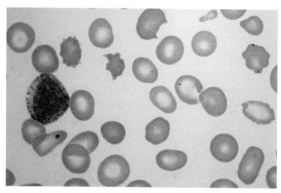

Figure 5.59   Photomicrograph of a blood film. Autoimmune thrombocytopenic purpura, postsplenectomy showing a Pappenheimer body and a Howell-Jolly body.

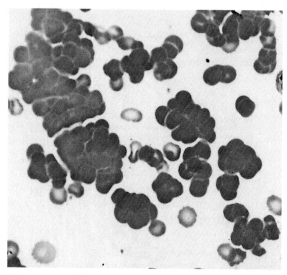

Figure 5.61   Photomicrograph of a blood film. Shows massive autoagglutination in a patient with chronic cold haemagglutinin disease (compare with Fig. 5.60).

clearly seen will almost certainly be found. Rouleaux occur to some extent in all films, and their presence adds point, as has been mentioned, to the importance of careful selection of the area of film to be examined.

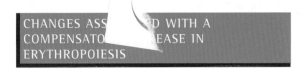

CHANGES ASSOCIATED WITH A COMPENSATORY INCREASE IN ERYTHROPOIESIS

Polychromasia (πολθζ, many)

The term *polychromasia* suggests that the red cells are being stained many colours. In practice, it means that some of the red cells stain shades of bluish grey (Fig. 5.62)—these are the reticulocytes. Cells staining shades of blue, "blue polychromasia," are unusually young reticulocytes. "Blue polychromasia" is most often seen when there is either an intense erythropoietic drive or when there is extramedullary erythropoiesis, as, for instance, in myelofibrosis or carcinomatosis.

Erythroblastaemia

Erythroblasts may be found in the blood films of almost any patient with a severe anaemia; they are, however, very unusual in aplastic anaemia, and their presence should lead to this diagnosis being doubted. They are more common in children than in adults, and large numbers are a very characteristic finding in haemolytic disease of the newborn. Small numbers can be found in the cord blood of normal infants, whereas quite large numbers are found in that of premature infants.

When large numbers of erythroblasts are present, many of them are probably derived from extramedullary foci of erythropoiesis (e.g., in the liver and spleen). This seems likely to be true, for instance, in haemolytic disease of the newborn, leucaemia, myelofibrosis, and carcinomatosis. In myelofibrosis and carcinomatosis, the number of erythroblasts is often disproportionately high for the degree of anaemia, and a few immature granulocytes are usually also present (so-called leucoerythroblastic anaemia) (Fig. 5.63).

Erythroblasts can usually be found in the peripheral blood after splenectomy, and many may be present in severe anaemia and in the presence of extramedullary erythropoiesis (Fig. 5.64). Large numbers are frequently seen in the blood films of patients with sickle cell anaemia in painful crises. Small numbers of erythroblasts are not uncommon in blood from patients suffering from cyanotic heart failure or septicaemia.

It should be noted that when the term *normoblast* is used, it implies that erythroid maturation is normoblastic. *Erythroblast* is a more general term that also includes megaloblasts.

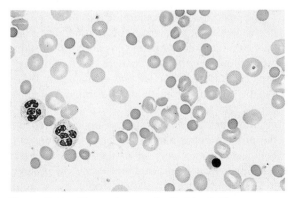

Figure 5.62 Photomicrograph of a blood film. Polychromasia. Some red cells stain shades of bluish grey.

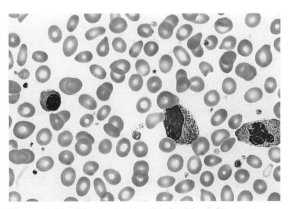

Figure 5.63 Photomicrograph of a blood film. Idiopathic myelofibrosis. Shows a leucoerythroblastic blood film, teardrop poikilocytes, and ovalocytes.

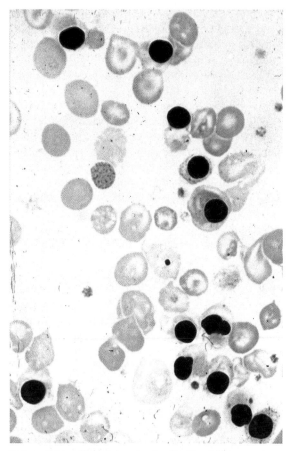

Figure 5.64   Photomicrograph of a blood film.
β Thalassaemia major with inadequate blood transfusion support. There are numerous erythroblasts; there are also hypochromic cells, target cells, and a cell containing a Howell–Jolly body.

EFFECTS OF SPLENECTOMY AND HYPOSPLENISM

Some of the effects of splenectomy and hyposplenism have already been mentioned—namely, the occurrence of target cells, acanthocytes, Howell–Jolly bodies, and Pappenheimer bodies (see Fig. 5.57). In addition, there may be neutrophilia (early after splenectomy), lymphocytosis, thrombocytosis, and giant platelets. In people who are haematologically normal, the blood film features of hyposplenism are variable—sometimes striking and sometimes very minor.

SCANNING ELECTRON MICROSCOPY

The morphology of red cells, as illustrated in this chapter, may be distorted by spreading and drying films in the traditional way. A more authentic portrayal of red cell shape *in vivo* can be seen by scanning electron microscopy. This provided the means for a critical reexamination of red cell morphology. Bessis and his co-workers published excellent photographs of pathologic red cells and, from their appearances, proposed a terminology[7,21,22] that we have generally adopted in this chapter. They also discussed the difficult question of the *in vivo* significance of crenation (echinocytic change) observed *in vitro*. It seems that neither echinocytosis nor acanthocytosis is necessarily associated with increased haemolysis. It cannot be concluded, either, that crenation is occurring *in vivo*, when the phenomenon is markedly evident in films made on glass slides. To ensure that cells are crenated in any blood sample as it is withdrawn, Brecher and Bessis recommended that the blood be examined immediately between plastic, instead of glass coverslips or slides, to avoid the known "echinocytogenic" effect of glass surfaces, probably caused by alkalinity.[22] Nevertheless, for practical purposes, if a blood film of a freshly drawn blood specimen shows echinocytosis and other films prepared using the same glass slides do not, the abnormality can be accepted as genuine.

The specialized procedure of scanning electron microscopy is not practical as a routine but helps in understanding the nature of cells observed in stained blood films. Morphologic changes in red cells may be very complex. Echinocytic and stomatocytic change can be superimposed on other pathological forms, giving rise to "sickle-stomatocytes" and "stomato-acanthocytes." Acanthocytes can undergo crenation, the product being termed an "acantho-echinocyte." Following splenectomy in patients with hereditary spherocytosis, sphero-acanthocytes may be observed.

The appearance of various cells by scanning electron microscopy is illustrated in Figures 5.65 to 5.72.

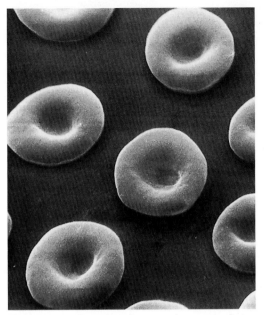

Figure 5.65   Scanning electron microscope photograph. Normal red cells.

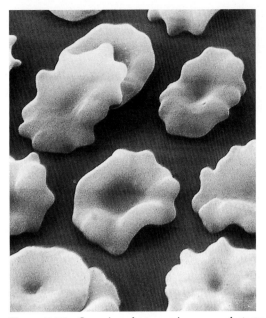

Figure 5.67   Scanning electron microscope photograph. Normal blood after standing overnight. Note crenation.

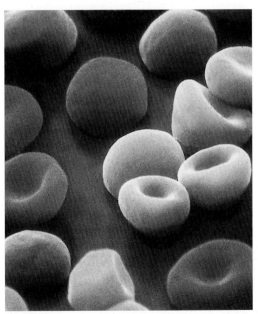

Figure 5.66   Scanning electron microscope photograph. Hereditary spherocytosis. Note the round shape of spherocytes. (Compare with Fig. 5.65; also see blood film appearances as shown in Fig. 5.21.)

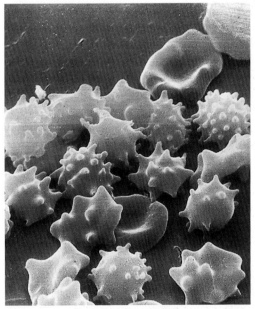

Figure 5.68   Scanning electron microscope photograph. Acanthocytosis. Some cells also show crenation and contraction. (Compare with Fig. 5.67; see also blood film appearances as shown in Fig. 5.45.)

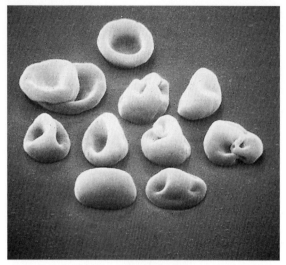

Figure 5.69 Scanning electron microscope photograph. Drug-induced haemolysis; see blood film appearances shown in Figure 5.43.

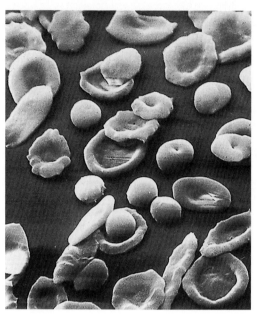

Figure 5.70 Scanning electron microscope photograph. Iron deficiency anaemia. (Compare with Fig. 5.71, and see also Fig. 5.12.)

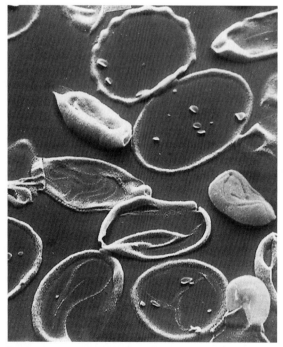

Figure 5.71 Scanning electron microscope photograph. Sickle cell anaemia (homozygosity for haemoglobin S). Shows sickled cells.

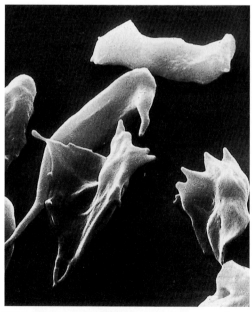

Figure 5.72 Scanning electron microscope photograph. β Thalassaemia major, postsplenectomy. Shows cells grossly deficient in haemoglobin; there are also contracted cells and poikilocytes. In the hypochromic cells, inclusions are seen, corresponding to Pappenheimer bodies.

MORPHOLOGY OF LEUCOCYTES

This section will include a description of the normal leucocytes, some congenital anomalies, and reactive changes that are commonly encountered. To describe adequately the various changes found in malignant conditions would require a lengthy text and many illustrations that are beyond the scope of this book. They will be referred to briefly here, but for detailed reference readers should consult an atlas on blood cells. For classification of the acute leukaemias, see the original description by the FAB (French–American–British) group[23] and the subsequent revision.[24] There is also a World Health Organization classification,[25] which supercedes the FAB classifications when facilities are available for fully characterizing leukaemia. However, the FAB classification remains useful as a widely accepted scheme for the morphologic description of leukaemias.

POLYMORPHONUCLEAR NEUTROPHILS

In normal adults, neutrophils account for more than half the circulating leucocytes. They are the main defence of the body against pyogenic bacterial infections. Normal neutrophils are uniform in size, with an apparent diameter of *about* 13 μm on a film. They have a segmented nucleus and, when stained, pink/orange cytoplasm with fine granulation (Fig. 5.73). The majority of neutrophils have three nuclear segments (lobes) connected by tapering chromatin strands. The chromatin shows clumping and is usually condensed at the nuclear periphery. A small percentage have four lobes, and occasionally five lobes may be seen. Up to 8% of circulating neutrophils are unsegmented or partly segmented ("band" forms) (discussed later).

In women, 2–3% of the neutrophils show an appendage at a terminal nuclear segment. This "drumstick" is about 1.5 μm in diameter and is connected to the nucleus by a short stalk. It represents the inactive X chromosome and corresponds to the Barr body of buccal cells.

Occasionally, red cells will adhere to neutrophils, forming rosettes. The mechanism is unknown, but it is likely to be immune; usually it appears to be of no clinical significance but occasionally it is seen in an immune haemolytic anaemia. Leucoagglutination also occurs as an *in vitro* artefact.[26] Occasionally neutrophils (and/or monocytes) have phagocytosed erythrocytes (Fig. 5.74). This is particularly common in paroxysmal cold haemoglobinuria

It is extremely important to ensure the consistency of staining of the blood films using a standardised Romanowsky method (see Chapter 4) because changes in the staining density, colour, and appearance of cytoplasmic granulation, if not artefact, may have diagnostic significance. Common neutrophil abnormalities are described later in this chapter.

Granules

Toxic granulation is the term used to describe an increase in staining density and possibly number of granules that occurs regularly with bacterial infection and often with other causes of inflammation (Fig. 5.75). It can also be a feature of administration of granulocyte colony-stimulating factor. Fractionally larger, coarser granules may be seen in aplastic anaemia and myelofibrosis. Conversely, poorly staining (hypogranular) and agranular neutrophils occur in the myelodysplastic syndromes (Fig. 5.76) and in some forms of myeloid leukaemia.

There are rare inherited disorders that are manifest by abnormal neutrophils. In the Alder–Reilly anomaly, the granules are very large, are discrete, stain deep red, and may obscure the nucleus (Fig. 5.77). Other leucocytes, including some lymphocytes, also show the abnormal granules. In the Chediak–Higashi syndrome there are giant but scanty azurophilic granules (Fig. 5.78), and the other leucocyte types may also be affected. Alder–Reilly neutrophils function normally, but in Chediak–Higashi syndrome there is a functional defect that is manifested by susceptibility to severe infection.

Vacuoles

In blood films spread without delay, the presence of vacuoles in the neutrophils is usually indicative of severe sepsis, when toxic granulation is usually also present. Vacuoles will develop as an artefact with prolonged standing of the blood before films are made (see Chapter 1, Fig. 1.2, p. 8).

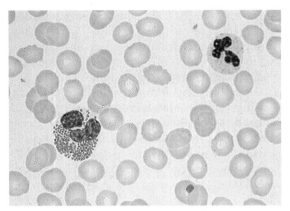

Figure 5.73   Photomicrograph of a blood film. Normal polymorphonuclear neutrophil and normal eosinophil.

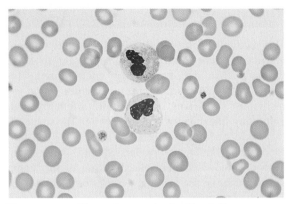

Figure 5.76   Photomicrograph of a blood film. Myelodysplastic syndrome. Shows a hypogranular neutrophil and a normally granulated neutrophil.

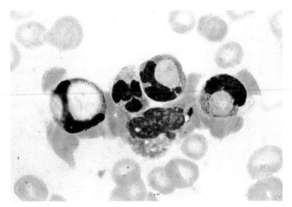

Figure 5.74   Photomicrograph of a blood film. Erythrophagocytosis in a patient with a positive direct antiglobulin test.

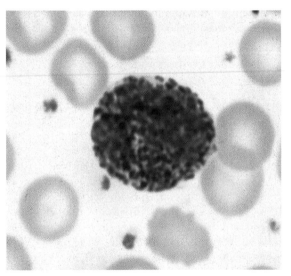

Figure 5.77   Photomicrograph of a blood film. Alder–Reilly anomaly. The nucleus is obscured by the cytoplasmic granules.

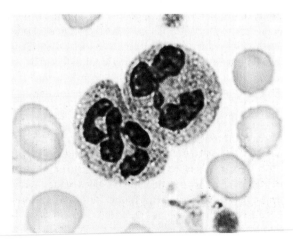

Figure 5.75   Photomicrograph of a blood film. Severe infection. Neutrophils show toxic granulation.

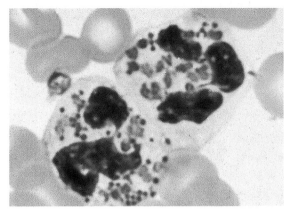

Figure 5.78   Photomicrograph of a blood film. Chediak–Higashi syndrome. Neutrophils show abnormal granules.

Bacteria

Very rarely, in the presence of overwhelming septicaemia (e.g., meningococcal or pneumococcal), bacteria may be seen within vacuoles or apparently lying free in the cytoplasm of neutrophils. When blood is taken from an infected central line, clumps of bacteria or fungi may be seen scattered in the film as well as in neutrophils in phagocytic vacuoles (Fig. 5.79). In premature infants with staphylococcal septicaemia, the detection of bacteria in neutrophils helps in early diagnosis.[27]

Döhle Bodies

Döhle bodies are small, round or oval, pale blue-grey structures usually found at the periphery of the neutrophil. They consist of ribosomes and endoplasmic reticulum. They are seen in bacterial infections. There is also a benign inherited condition known as *May–Hegglin anomaly* with a similar but not identical morphologic structure; in this condition, the inclusions occur in all types of leucocytes except lymphocytes.

Nuclei

Segmentation of the nucleus of the neutrophil is a normal event as the cell matures from the myelocyte. With the three-lobed neutrophil as a marker, a shift to the left (less mature) or to the right (hypermature) can be recognized (Table 5.1). A left shift with band forms, metamyelocytes, and perhaps

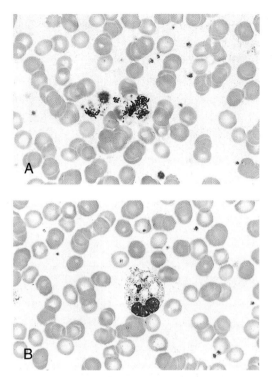

Figure 5.79   Photomicrograph of a blood film. Blood collected from infected site, showing bacteria (A) in scattered clumps and in a neutrophil (B).

occasional myelocytes is common in sepsis (Fig. 5.80), when it is usually accompanied by toxic granulation. If promyelocytes and myeloblasts are also present, it is likely to be a feature of a leuco-erythroblastic anaemia or leukaemia (Fig. 5.81); occasionally this extreme picture may be seen in very severe infections, when it is called "leukaemoid reaction." A left shift, with a significant number of band forms, occurs normally in pregnancy.

Hypersegmentation

The presence of hypersegmented neutrophils, with five or more nuclear segments, is an important diagnostic feature of megaloblastic anaemias. In florid megaloblastic states, neutrophils are often enlarged and their nuclei may have six or more segments connected by particularly fine chromatin bridges (see Fig. 5.10). A right shift with moderately hypersegmented neutrophils may also be seen in uraemia and not infrequently in iron deficiency.[28] Hypersegmentation can be seen after cytotoxic

Table 5.1 Stages of Granulocyte maturation

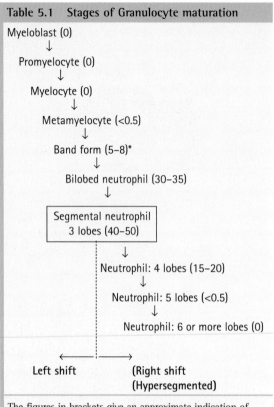

Myeloblast (0)
↓
Promyelocyte (0)
↓
Myelocyte (0)
↓
Metamyelocyte (<0.5)
↓
Band form (5–8)*
↓
Bilobed neutrophil (30–35)
↓

Segmental neutrophil
3 lobes (40–50)
↓
Neutrophil: 4 lobes (15–20)
↓
Neutrophil: 5 lobes (<0.5)
↓
Neutrophil: 6 or more lobes (0)

←————— ┊ —————→
Left shift **(Right shift**
(Hypersegmented)

The figures in brackets give an approximate indication of
the number per 100 neutrophils in a normal film. They are
intended only as a rough guide.
*However, according to the United States Health and
Nutrition Examination surveys, the normal band count is
lower—about 0.5% of the neutrophils.[37]

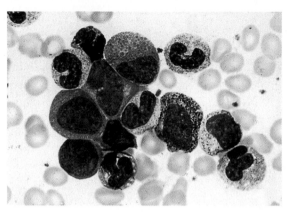

Figure 5.81 Photomicrograph of a blood film. Chronic granulocytic leukaemia. There is a left shift with band forms, metamyelocytes, myelocytes, and one myeloblast.

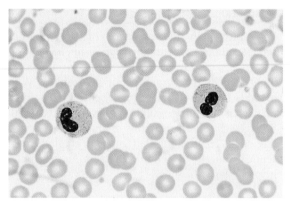

Figure 5.82 Photomicrograph of a blood film. Pelger–Huët anomaly. Shows hypolobated neutrophils.

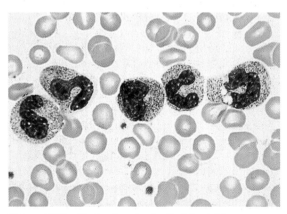

Figure 5.80 Photomicrograph of a blood film. Infection. Shows left shift of the neutrophils, with toxic granulation.

treatment, especially with methotrexate. Patients undergoing hydroxycarbamide treatment sometimes develop markedly hypersegmented neutrophils.

Pelger–Huët Cells

The Pelger–Huët anomaly is a benign inherited condition in which neutrophil nuclei fail to segment properly. The majority of circulating neutrophils have only two discrete equal-sized lobes connected by a thin chromatin bridge (Fig. 5.82). The chromatin is coarsely clumped, and granule content is normal.

A similar acquired morphologic anomaly, known as pseudo-Pelger cells or the acquired Pelger–Huët anomaly, may be seen in myelodysplastic syndromes, acute myeloid leukaemia with dysplastic maturation, and occasionally in chronic granulocytic leukaemia (during the accelerated phase) (Fig. 5.83). In these conditions, the neutrophils are often hypogranular and they tend to have a markedly irregular nuclear pattern.

Pyknotic Neutrophils (Apoptosis)

Small numbers of dead or dying cells may normally be found in the blood, especially when there is an infection. They may also develop in normal blood *in vitro* after standing for 12–18 hours, even if kept at 4°C. These cells have round, dense, featureless nuclei, and their cytoplasm tends to be dark pink (see p. 9 and Fig. 1.3). It is important not to confuse these cells with erythroblasts.

EOSINOPHILS

Eosinophils are a little larger than neutrophils, 12–17 μm in diameter. They usually have two nuclear lobes or segments, and the cytoplasm is packed with distinctive spherical gold/orange (eosinophilic) granules (see Figs. 5.73 and 5.84). The underlying cytoplasm, which is usually obscured by the granules, is pale blue. Prolonged steroid administration causes eosinopenia. Moderate eosinophilia occurs in allergic conditions; more severe eosinophilia (20–50 × 10⁹/l) may be seen in parasitic infections, and even greater numbers may be seen in other reactive eosinophilias, eosinophilic leukaemia, and the idiopathic hypereosinophilic syndrome. Reactive eosinophilia with very high counts may be seen in T-cell lymphoma, B-cell lymphoma, and acute lymphoblastic leukaemia. Eosinophils are part of the leukaemic population in chronic granulocytic leukaemia, and this is occasionally so in acute myeloid leukaemia.

BASOPHILS

Basophils are the rarest (<1%) of the circulating leucocytes. Their nuclear segments tend to fold up on each other, resulting in a compact irregular

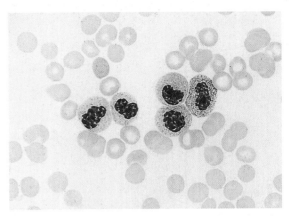

Figure 5.83   Photomicrograph of a blood film. Chronic granulocytic leukaemia. There are five "pseudo-Pelger" cells; this abnormality is not seen in the chronic phase of this disease.

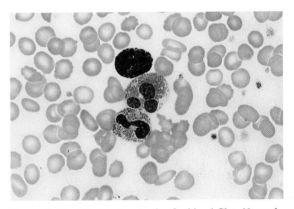

Figure 5.84   Photomicrograph of a blood film. Normal adult. Shows a basophil, an eosinophil, and a neutrophil.

dense nucleus resembling a closed lotus flower. The distinctive, large, variably sized, dark blue or purple granules of the cytoplasm (Fig. 5.84) often obscure the nucleus; they are rich in histamine, serotonin, and heparin substances. Basophils tend to degranulate, leaving cytoplasmic vacuoles.

Basophils are present in increased numbers in myeloproliferative disorders and are especially prominent in chronic granulocytic leukaemia; in the latter condition, when basophils are more than 10% of the differential leucocyte count, this is a sign of impending accelerated phase or blast crisis.

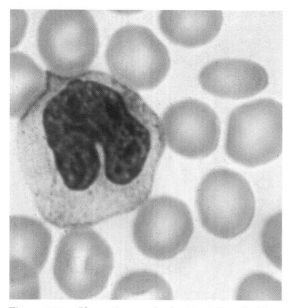

Figure 5.85   Photomicrograph of a blood film. Healthy adult. Monocyte.

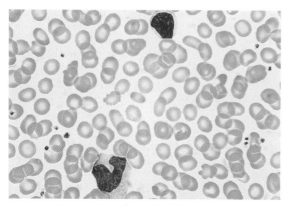

Figure 5.86   Photomicrograph of a blood film. Healthy adult. Shows a monocyte and a lymphocyte.

MONOCYTES

Monocytes are the largest of the circulating leucocytes, 15–18 μm in diameter. They have bluish-grey cytoplasm that contains variable numbers of fine reddish granules. The nucleus is large and curved, often in the shape of a horseshoe, but it may be folded or curled (Figs. 5.85 and 5.86). It never undergoes segmentation. The chromatin is finer and more evenly distributed in the nucleus than in neutrophil nuclei. An increased number of monocytes occur in some chronic infections and inflammatory conditions such as tuberculosis and Crohn's disease, in chronic myeloid leukaemias (particularly atypical chronic myeloid leukaemia and chronic myelomonocytic leukaemia), and in acute leukaemias with a monocytic component. In chronic myelomonocytic leukaemia, the mature monocyte count may reach as high as $100 \times 10^9/l$. It is occasionally difficult to distinguish monocytes from the large activated T lymphocytes produced in infectious mononucleosis or from circulating high-grade lymphoma cells.

LYMPHOCYTES

The majority of circulating lymphocytes are small cells with a thin rim of cytoplasm, occasionally containing scanty azurophilic granules (see Figs. 5.1 and 5.87). Nuclei are remarkably uniform in size (about 9 μm in diameter). This provides a useful guide for estimating red cell size (normally about 7–8 μm) on the blood film. Some 10% of circulating lymphocytes are larger, with more abundant pale blue cytoplasm containing azurophilic granules (Fig. 5.87). The nuclei of lymphocytes have homogeneous chromatin with some clumping at the nuclear periphery. About 85% of the circulating lymphocytes are T cells or natural killer (NK) cells.

In infections, both bacterial and viral, transforming lymphocytes may be present. These immunoblasts or "Türk" cells are 10–15 μm in diameter, with a round nucleus and abundant, deeply basophilic cytoplasm (Fig. 5.88). They may develop into plasmacytoid lymphocytes and plasma cells, and these are occasionally seen in the blood in severe infections. In the absence of infection, multiple myeloma must be excluded. In viral infection, "reactive lymphocytes" appear in the blood. These have slightly larger nuclei with more open chromatin and abundant cytoplasm that may be irregular. The most extreme examples of these cells are usually found in infectious mononucleosis (Fig. 5.89). These "glandular fever" cells have irregular nuclei and abundant cytoplasm that is basophilic at the periphery; they have a tendency to appear, on a blood film, to have flowed around adjacent erythrocytes.

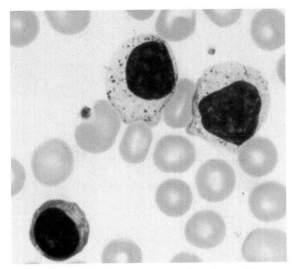

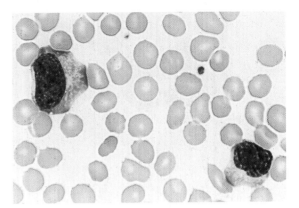

Figure 5.89   Photomicrograph of a blood film. Infectious mononucleosis. There are two activated lymphocytes ("atypical mononuclear cells").

Figure 5.87   Photomicrograph of a blood film. Shows a small lymphocyte and two large granular lymphocytes with azurophilic granules.

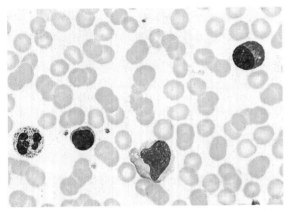

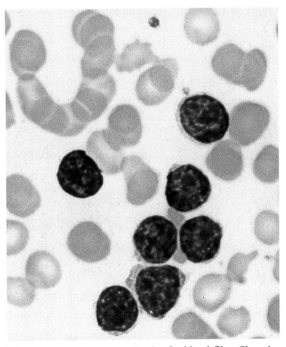

Figure 5.88   Photomicrograph of a blood film. Viral infection. Shows a Türk cell, another reactive lymphocyte, and a small lymphocyte.

Figure 5.90   Photomicrograph of a blood film. Chronic lymphocytic leukaemia. The cells are small lymphocytes; note that rouleaux formation is increased.

   Malignant lymphoid cells vary enormously in their morphology. The commonest malignancy is chronic lymphocytic leukaemia, the leukaemic population being composed almost exclusively of small lymphocytes (Fig. 5.90), sometimes with a few larger nucleolated cells. In prolymphocytic leukaemia, the majority of cells are a little larger than small lymphocytes with more cytoplasm and usually one distinct nucleolus (Fig. 5.91). Lym-phoblasts of acute lymphoblastic leukaemia (Figs. 5.92 and 5.93) vary in size from only slightly larger than lymphocytes to cells of 15–17 µm diameter. The nuclei generally have diffuse chromatin, but there may be some chromatin condensation in the

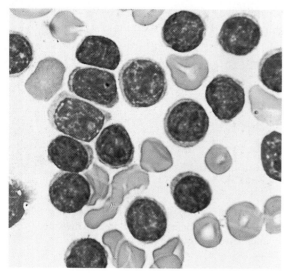

Figure 5.91   Photomicrograph of a blood film. Prolymphocytic leukaemia. There is a uniform population of prolymphocytes.

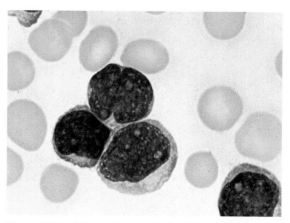

Figure 5.93   Photomicrograph of a blood film. Acute lymphoblastic leukaemia (FAB L1 type). Shows lymphoblasts.

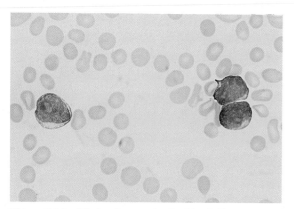

Figure 5.92   Photomicrograph of a blood film. Philadelphia-positive acute lymphoblastic leukaemia (FAB L1 category). Shows three lymphoblasts.

smaller blasts. The cytoplasm varies from weakly to strongly basophilic.

Circulating lymphoma cells vary markedly in size, depending on the type of lymphoma. When there is a lymphocytosis, the lymphocytes are usually far less uniform than in chronic lymphocytic leukaemia, and the lymphoma cells frequently have irregular lobed, indented, or cleaved nuclei and relatively scanty agranular cytoplasm that varies in its degree of basophilia. Lobulated lymphocytes are a feature of HTLV-I (human T-lymphotropic virus type I) infection and of adult T-cell leukaemia/ lymphoma. However, lymphocytes with definite lobulation are also a common storage artefact in blood kept for 18–24 hours at room temperature (see p. 7).

Lymphocytes predominate in the blood films of infants and young children. In this age range, large lymphocytes and reactive lymphocytes tend to be conspicuous, and a small number of lymphoblasts may also be present.

PLATELET MORPHOLOGY

Normal platelets are 1–3 μm in diameter. They are irregular in outline with fine red granules that may be scattered or centralized. A small number of larger platelets, up to 5 μm in diameter, may be seen in normal films. Larger platelets are seen in the blood when platelet production is increased (Fig. 5.94) and in hyposplenism (Fig. 5.95). Thus, for example, in severe immune thrombocytopenia, some large platelets will be seen on the film. Very high platelet counts as a feature of a myeloproliferative disorder may be associated with extreme platelet anisocytosis, with some platelets being as large as red cells and often with some agranular or hypogranular platelets (Fig. 5.96). The platelet count frequently

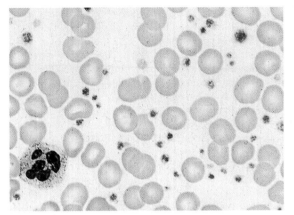

Figure 5.94   Photomicrograph of a blood film. Essential thrombocythaemia. Shows platelet anisocytosis and increased numbers of platelets

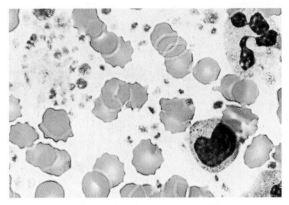

Figure 5.96   Photomicrograph of a blood film. Myeloproliferative disorder. Shows platelet anisocytosis with some giant platelets.

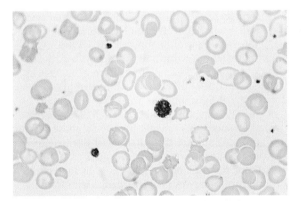

Figure 5.95   Photomicrograph of a blood film. Hyposplenism in coeliac disease. Shows giant platelet.

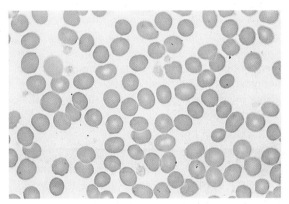

Figure 5.97   Photomicrograph of a blood film. Grey platelet syndrome. Shows agranular platelets.

increases with acute inflammatory stress or bleeding but seldom to more than $1000 \times 10^9/l$. More than this, unless the patient is critically ill, the cause is usually a myeloproliferative disorder.

Characteristic morphologic features are seen in two inherited platelet disorders associated with bleeding. These are the Bernard–Soulier syndrome, in which there are giant platelets with defective ristocetin response, and the grey platelet syndrome, in which the platelets lack granules and have a ghostlike appearance on the stained blood film (Fig. 5.97). Thrombocytopenia may also be present in the May–Hegglin anomaly (see p. 104).

In about 1% of individuals, ethylenediaminetetra-acetic acid (EDTA) anticoagulant causes platelet clumping, resulting in pseudothrombocytopenia.[29] It does not occur when the blood is collected into any other anticoagulant.[30] This phenomenon may be detected when it gives rise to a "flag" on an automated blood cell counter; it is identifiable on the blood film. It is not associated with any coagulation disturbance, and platelet function is normal. Occasionally, EDTA may also inhibit the staining of platelets.[31]

Occasionally, platelets may be seen adhering to neutrophils (Fig. 5.98).[32–35] This has been reported in

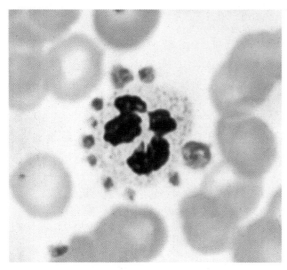

Figure 5.98   Photomicrograph of a blood film. Shows adhesion of platelets to a neutrophil (platelet satellism).

patients who have demonstrable antiplatelet autoantibodies,[36] but it is more commonly seen in apparently healthy individuals. It is not seen in films made directly from blood that has not been anticoagulated.

REFERENCES

1. Marsh GW 1966 Abnormal contraction, distortion and fragmentation in human red cells. London University MD thesis.
2. Rodgers MS, Chang C-C, Kass L 1999 Elliptocytosis and tailed poikilocytes correlate with severity of iron deficiency anemia. American Journal of Clinical Pathology 111:672–675.
3. Sechi LA, De Carll S, Catena C, et al 1996 Benign familial macrocytosis. Clinical and Laboratory Haematology 18:41–43.
4. Rees DC, Dudley JA, Marinaki A 2003 Review: pyrimidine 5'nucleotidase deficiency. British Journal of Haematology 120:375–383.
5. Tuffy P, Brown AK, Zuelzer WW 1959 Infantile pyknocytosis: a common erythrocyte abnormality of the first trimester. American Journal of Diseases of Children 98:227–241.
6. Keimowitz R, Desforges JF 1965 Infantile pyknocytosis. New England Journal of Medicine 273:1152–1154.
7. Bessis M 1972 Red cell shapes: an illustrated classification and its rationale. Nouvelle Revue Francaise d'Hematologie 12:721–745.
8. Burns ER, Lou Y, Pathak A 2004 Morphological diagnosis of thrombotic thrombocytopenic purpura. American Journal of Hematology 75, 18–21.
9. Estes JW, Morley TJ, Levine IM et al 1967 A new hereditary acanthocytosis syndrome. American Journal of Medicine 42:868–881.
10. Mier M, Schwartz SO, Boshes B 1960 Acanthrocytosis [sic], pigmented degeneration of the retina and ataxic neuropathy: a genetically determined syndrome with associated metabolic disorder. Blood 16:1586–1608.
11. Salt HB, Wolfe OH, Lloyd JK, et al 1960 On having no beta-lipoprotein: a syndrome comprising a-beta-lipoprotinaemia, acanthocytosis, and steatorrhoea. Lancet ii:325–329.
12. Wimer BM, Marsh WL, Taswel HF, et al 1977 Haematological changes associated with the McLeod phenotype of the Kell blood group system. British Journal of Haematology 36:219–224.
13. Silber R, Amorosi EL, Howe J, et al 1966 Spur-shaped erythrocytes in Laennec's cirrhosis. New England Journal of Medicine 275:639–643.
14. Ponder E 1948 Hemolysis and related phenomena. Grune & Stratton, New York.
15. Feo CJ, Tchernia G, Subtu E, et al 1978 Observation of echinocytosis in eight patients: a phase contrast and SEM study. British Journal of Haematology 40:519–526.
16. Crook M, Williams W, Schey S 1998 Target cells and stomatocytes in heterozygous familial hypobetalipoproteinaemia. European Journal of Haematology 60:68–69.
17. Lock SP, Sephton Smith R, Hardisty RM 1961 Stomatocytosis: a hereditary red cell anomaly associated with haemolytic anaemia. British Journal of Haematology 7:303–314.
18. Ducrou W, Kimber RJ 1969 Stomatocytes, haemolytic anaemia and abdominal pain in Mediterranean migrants: some examples of a new syndrome? Medical Journal of Australia ii:1087–1091.
19. Norman JG 1969 Stomatocytosis in migrants of Mediterranean origin. Medical Journal of Australia i:315.
20. Douglass C, Twomey J 1970 Transient stomatocytosis with hemolysis: a previously unrecognized complication of alcoholism. Annals of Internal Medicine 72:159–164.
21. Weed RI, Bessis M 1973 The discocyte-stomatocyte equilibrium of normal and pathologic red cells. Blood 41:471–475.

22. Brecher G, Bessis M 1972 Present status of spiculated red cells and their relationship to the discocyte–echinocyte transformation: a critical review. Blood 40:333–344.

23. Bennett JM, Catovsky D, Daniel MT, et al 1976 Proposals for the classification of the acute leukaemias (FAB cooperative group). British Journal of Haematology 33:451–458.

24. Bennett JM, Catovsky D, Daniel MT, et al 1985 Proposed revised criteria for the classification of acute myeloid leukemia. Annals of Internal Medicine 103:620–625.

25. Harris NL, Jaffe ES, Diebold J, et al 1999 World Health Organization classification of neoplastic diseases of the hematopoietic and lymphoid tissues: report of the Clinical Advisory Committee Meeting–Airlie House, Virginia, November 1997. Journal of Clinical Oncology 17:3835–3849.

26. Deal J, Hernandez AM, Pierre RV 1995 Ethylenediamine tetraacetic acid-associated leukoagglutination. American Journal of Clinical Pathology 103:338–340.

27. Howard MR, Smith RA 1999 Early diagnosis of septicaemia in preterm infants from examination of the peripheral blood films. Clinical and Laboratory Haematology 21:365–368.

28. Westerman DA, Evans D, Metz J 1999 Neutrophil hypersegmentation in iron deficiency anaemia: a case control study. British Journal of Haematology 107:512–515.

29. Gowland E, Kay HEM, Spillman JC, et al 1969 Agglutination of platelets by a serum factor in the presence of EDTA. Journal of Clinical Pathology 22:460–454.

30. Criswell KA, Breider MA, Bleavins MR 20901 EDTA-dependent platelet phagocytosis. A cytochemical, ultrastructural and functional characterization. American Journal of Clinical Pathology 115:376–384.

31. Stavem P, Berg K 1973 A macromolecular serum component acting on platelets in the presence of EDTA–"Platelet stain preventing factor." Scandinavian Journal of Haematology 10:202–208.

32. Crome PE, Barkhan P 1963 Platelet adherence to polymorphs. British Medical Journal ii:871.

33. Field EJ, Macleod I 1963 Platelet adherence to polymorphs. British Medical Journal ii:388.

34. Greipp PR, Gralnick HR 1976 Platelet to leucocyte adherence phenomena associated with thrombocytopenia. Blood 47:513–521.

35. Skinnider LF, Musclow CE, Kahn W 1978 Platelet satellitism: an ultrastructural study. American Journal of Hematology 4:179–185.

36. White LA Jr, Brubaker LH, Aster RH, et al 1978 Platelet satellitism and phagocytosis by neutrophils: association with antiplatelet antibodies and lymphoma. American Journal of Hematology 4:313–323.

37. Van Assendelft OW, McGrath C, Murphy RS, et al 1977 The differential distribution of leukocytes. In: Koepke JA (ed) CAP Aspen conference: differential leukocyte counting. College of American Pathologists, Northfield, IL.

6 Bone marrow biopsy

Imelda Bates

Biopsy of the bone marrow is an indispensable adjunct to the study of diseases of the blood and may be the only way in which a correct diagnosis can be made. Marrow can be obtained by needle aspiration, percutaneous trephine biopsy, or surgical biopsy. If performed correctly, bone marrow aspiration is simple and safe; it can be repeated many times and performed on outpatients. It seems to be safe in almost all circumstances, even when thrombocytopenic purpura is present. However, when there is a major disorder of coagulation, such as in haemophilia, it should never be attempted without appropriate cover and checking by coagulation factor assay prior to the procedure. Trephine biopsy is a little less simple, but it too can be performed on outpatients.

The disadvantage of bone marrow aspiration in comparison with trephine biopsy is that the arrangement of the cells in the marrow and the relationship between one cell and another is disrupted by the process of aspiration, and, in fibrotic marrows, blood rather than marrow may be aspirated. However, when marrow is aspirated, individual cells are well preserved. After staining, subtle differences between cells can be recognized to a far greater degree than is possible with sectioned material. The great value of trephine biopsy is that it can provide information about the structure of relatively large pieces of marrow. At the same time, morphological features of individual cells may be identified by making an imprint from the material obtained.

Studies on large numbers of cases have demonstrated that trephine biopsy specimens are superior to films of aspirated material in some circumstances (e.g., for diagnosing marrow involvement by lymphoma or nonhaematological neoplastic diseases). However, the simple procedure of marrow aspiration seldom fails to provide important information in patients who have a blood disease. The two techniques have important and complementary roles in clinical investigation.[1,2]

ASPIRATION OF THE BONE MARROW

Satisfactory samples of bone marrow can usually be aspirated from the sternum, iliac crest, or anterior or posterior iliac spines. In the majority of patients the procedure can be performed with local and oral analgesia without recourse to intravenous sedation.[3] The iliac spines have the advantage that if no material is aspirated, a trephine biopsy can be performed immediately. These sites, however, may be technically difficult in subjects who are obese or immobile, and puncture of the sternum occasionally may be necessary. The sternum should not be used in children. In adults, unless the needle is correctly inserted in the sternum, there is a danger of perforating the inner cortical layer and damaging the underlying large blood vessels and right atrium, with serious consequences.[4]

Performing a Bone Marrow Aspiration

Only needles designed for the purpose should be used for marrow aspiration (discussed later). The operator should always wear surgical gloves to obtain a biopsy of bone marrow and should take great care to avoid needlestick injuries. To perform a marrow aspiration, clean the skin in the area with 70% alcohol (e.g., ethanol) or 0.5% chlorhexidine (5% diluted 1 in 10 in ethanol). Infiltrate the skin, subcutaneous tissue, and periosteum overlying the selected site with a local anaesthetic such as 2–5 ml 2% lignocaine. Wait until anaesthesia has been achieved. With a boring movement, pass the needle perpendicularly into the cavity of the ilium at the centre of the oval posterior superior iliac spine or 2 cm posterior and 2 cm inferior to the anterior

superior iliac spine. When the bone has been penetrated, remove the stilette, attach a 1 or 2 ml syringe, and suck up marrow contents for making films. If a larger sample is needed, (e.g., for cytogenetic or immunophenotypic analysis), attach a second 5 or 10 ml syringe and aspirate a second sample. As a rule, material can be sucked into the syringe without difficulty; occasionally it may be necessary to reinsert the stilette, push the needle in a little further, and suck again. Failure to aspirate marrow—a "dry tap"—suggests bone marrow fibrosis or infiltration. Computed tomography–guided marrow sampling may be helpful in patients who are obese, in whom it is difficult to locate the iliac spine.[5]

Because bone marrow clots faster than peripheral blood, films should be made from the aspirated material without delay at the bedside. The remainder of the material may then be delivered into a bottle containing an appropriate amount of ethylenediaminetetra-acetic acid (EDTA) anticoagulant and used later to make more films. Preservative-free heparin should be used rather than EDTA if phenotyping or cytogenetic studies are needed. Some material can be preserved in fixative rather than anticoagulant for preparation of histological sections (p. 124). Fix some of the films in absolute methanol as soon as they are thoroughly dry for subsequent staining by a Romanowsky method or Perls' stain for iron. These films are also suitable for cytochemical staining (Chapter 13). If there has been a "dry tap," insert the stilette into the needle and push any material in the lumen of the needle onto a slide; in lymphomas and carcinomas, especially, sufficient material can be obtained to make a diagnosis.[6]

Puncture of the Ilium

The usual sites for puncture in adults are the posterior and, less commonly, the anterior iliac spine. If serial punctures are being performed, a different site should be selected for each to avoid aspirating marrow that has been diluted by haemorrhage resulting from previous punctures. The posterior iliac spine overlies a large marrow-containing area, and relatively large volumes of marrow can be aspirated from this site. Posterior iliac puncture can be carried out with the patient lying sideways, as for a lumbar puncture, or prone. The anterior superior iliac spine may be easier to locate in individuals who are very obese, and the bone overlying it is said to be thinner than that of the iliac crest.

Puncture of the Sternum

Puncture of the sternum must be performed with care to avoid pushing the aspiration needle through the bone. The usual site for puncture is the manubrium or the first or second parts of the body of the sternum. The manubrium is formed of rather denser bone than the body of the sternum, and, in elderly subjects at least, it tends to contain more fatty marrow than is found elsewhere in the sternum. The thickness of the cortex here varies from 0.2 mm to 5.0 mm, so it may be difficult to be certain that the needle point has reached the cavity of the bone.

The site for puncture of the manubrium should be about 1 cm above the sterno-manubrial angle and slightly to one side of the midline; if the body of the bone is to be punctured, this should be done opposite the second intercostal space slightly to one side of the midline. It is essential to use a needle with a guard that cannot slip, such as a Klima type. After piercing the skin and subcutaneous tissues, when the needle point reaches the periosteum, adjust the guard on the needle to allow it to penetrate about 5 mm further. If the guard cannot be advanced to this extent, it is not safe to proceed. Push the needle with a boring motion into the cavity of the bone. It is usually easy to appreciate when the cavity of the bone has been entered. Aspiration is then carried out as described earlier.

Puncture of Spinous Processes

Good samples of marrow may be obtained from adults by puncturing the spines of lumbar vertebrae. Puncture is not difficult because the bones lie superficially, but more pressure is required than for iliac or sternal puncture. Pass the needle into the spine of a lumbar vertebra slightly lateral to the midline in a direction at right angles to the skin surface, with the patient either sitting up or lying on his or her side as for a lumbar puncture.

Comparison of Different Sites for Marrow Puncture

There is considerable variation in the composition of cellular marrow withdrawn from adjacent or different sites. Aspiration from only one site may give misleading information; this is particularly true in aplastic anaemia because the marrow may be affected patchily.[7] In general, however, the overall cellularity, the haemopoietic maturation pathways, and the balance between erythropoiesis and leucopoiesis are similar at all sites. In practice, it is an advantage to have a choice of several sites for puncture, particularly when puncture at one site results in a "dry tap" or when only peripheral blood is withdrawn. Aspiration at a different site may yield cellular marrow or strengthen suspicion of a widespread change affecting the bone marrow, such as fibrosis or hypoplasia. In aplastic anaemia, several punctures may be necessary to arrive at the diagnosis.

ASPIRATION OF THE BONE MARROW IN CHILDREN

Iliac puncture, particularly in the region of the posterior spine, is usually the method of choice in children. Occasionally, in an older child who is obese, the posterior iliac spine cannot be felt. In this case, a satisfactory sample usually can be obtained from the anterior ilium. In small babies, marrow can be withdrawn from the medial aspect of the upper end of the tibia just below the level of the tibial tubercle. This site should be used with caution because it is vulnerable to fractures and laceration of the adjacent major blood vessels. In older children, the tibial cortical bone is usually too dense and the marrow within is normally less active. It must be remembered that sternal puncture in children should be avoided because the bone is thin and the marrow cavities are small.

MARROW PUNCTURE NEEDLES

Needles should be stout and made of hard stainless steel, about 7–8 cm in length, with a well-fitting stilette, and they must be provided with an adjustable guard. With reusable needles, the point of the needle and the edge of the bevel must be kept well sharpened. The most common reusable needles are the Salah and Klima needles (Fig. 6.1). A slightly larger needle with a T-bar handle at the proximal end was developed by Islam (Fig. 6.2); it provides a better grip, is more manoeuvrable, and is more successful for biopsies of excessively hard (e.g., osteosclerotic) or soft (e.g., profoundly osteoporotic) bone.[8] A modified version of the Islam needle has multiple holes in the distal portion of the shaft in addition to the opening at the tip to overcome sampling error when the marrow is not uniformly involved in a pathological lesion. Several types of disposable bone marrow aspiration and trephine biopsy needles are now available; their design is similar to the traditional reusable needles (Fig. 6.3).

PROCESSING OF ASPIRATED BONE MARROW

There is little advantage in aspirating more than 0.3 ml of marrow fluid from a single site for morphological examination because this increases peripheral blood dilution. If large amounts of marrow are needed for several tests, such as immunophenotyping, cytogenetics, and molecular studies, the syringe can be detached from the aspiration needle and the stilette can be replaced, leaving the aspiration needle in the bone. After the marrow smears have been prepared, the same or another syringe can be attached to the needle and another 5–10 ml of marrow can be aspirated.

It is good practice to obtain a sample of peripheral blood from the patient at the same time as the bone marrow so that both specimens can be

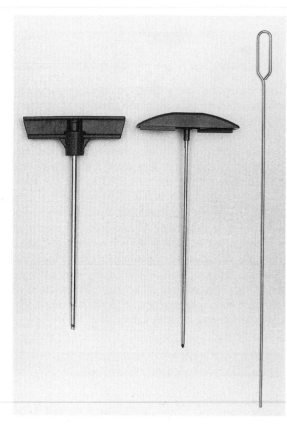

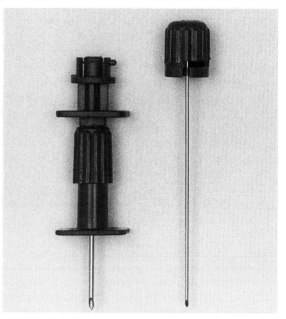

Fig 6.1 Disposable bone marrow needles. For aspiration (left) and trephine biopsy (right) (reduced ×0.75).

examined and stored together. This can be done simply by preparing some films from blood obtained from a finger prick after completing the bone marrow sampling or by venepuncture so that a full blood count can be obtained. The blood film should be permanently stored with the bone marrow films.

Preparing Films from Bone Marrow Aspirates

Make films, 3–5 cm in length, of the aspirated marrow using a smooth-edged glass spreader of not more than 2 cm in width (Fig. 6.4). The marrow fragments are dragged behind the spreader and leave a trail of cells behind them. Spreading should

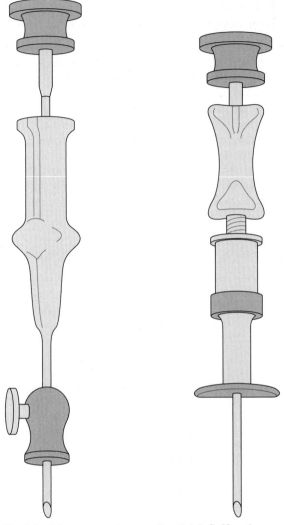

Fig 6.2   Marrow puncture needles. Salah (left) and Klima (right) (reduced ×0.75).

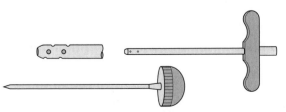

Fig 6.3   Islam's bone marrow aspiration needle. The dome-shaped handle and T-bar are intended to provide stability and control during operation.

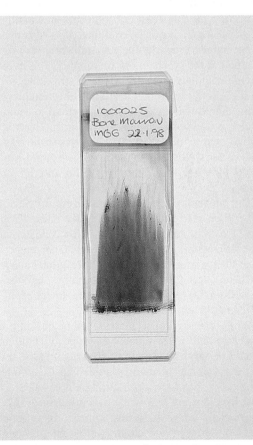

Fig 6.4   Film of aspirated bone marrow. The marrow particles are easily visible, mostly at the tail of the film (×1.5).

be towards the area to which the label is to be applied to avoid having particles dragged to the tip of the slide, where it is difficult to examine them. If there are insufficient fragments, they can be concentrated. This is not usually necessary for marrows that are very cellular such as in acute and chronic myeloid leukaemia and megaloblastic anaemia. Concentration of marrow can be achieved by delivering single drops of aspirate on to slides about 1 cm from one end. Most of the blood is quickly sucked off from the edge of the drop with the marrow syringe or a fine plastic pipette. The irregularly shaped marrow fragments tend to be left behind on the slide and can be lifted off with the spreader; smears can then be prepared as explained earlier.

After thorough drying, fix the films of bone marrow and stain them with Romanowsky dyes, as for peripheral blood films. However, a longer fixation time (at least 20 min in methanol) is essential for high-quality staining. If a film needs to be stained urgently, fix and stain one film only and permit the others to dry thoroughly. This avoids having all films showing artefacts resulting from fixation before thorough drying has been achieved. Films can also be stained by Perls' method to demonstrate the presence or absence of iron. Overnight drying may be necessary to achieve optimal results with a Perls' "dry tap" of sections; a normal range of 30–80% has been reported in the anterior iliac spine.

The preparation can be considered satisfactory only when marrow particles and free marrow cells can be seen in stained films. It is in the cellular trails that differential counts should be made, commencing from the marrow fragment and working back toward the head of the film; in this way, smaller numbers of cells from the peripheral blood are included in a differential count.

When the aspirated marrow is taken into an anticoagulant in a tube (e.g., dried EDTA) care should be taken that appropriate amounts are used for the volume of marrow to be anticoagulated. When films of marrow containing a gross excess of anticoagulant are spread (as when a few drops of marrow are added to a tube containing sufficient EDTA to prevent the clotting of 5 ml of blood), masses of pink-staining amorphous material may be seen and some of the erythroblasts and reticulocytes may clump together.

Concentration of bone marrow by centrifugation

Centrifugation can be used to concentrate the marrow cells and to assess the relative proportions of marrow cells, peripheral blood and fat in aspirated material. While concentration of poorly cellular samples is useful, especially when an abnormal cell is present in small numbers,[9] it is unnecessary when the aspirated material is of average or increased cellularity. Volumetric data, too, are of little value in individual patients because of the wide range of values encountered even in health. Methods for separation of marrow cells are described on page 69.

Preparation of films of post-mortem bone marrow

Films made of bone marrow obtained post-mortem are seldom satisfactory. If satisfactory results are to be achieved, the procedure must be carried out as soon after death as possible. When the marrow is spread in the ordinary way, the majority of the cells tend to break up and appear as smears. The rate and pattern of cellular autolysis during the first 15 hours after death has been studied, and the differences between the changes of post-mortem autolysis and those that occur in life as a result of blood diseases have been defined.[10] Blood cells are much better preserved if a small piece of marrow is suspended in 1–2 ml of 5% bovine albumin (1 volume 30% albumin, 5 volumes 9 g/l NaCl). The suspension is then centrifuged and the deposited marrow cells are resuspended in a volume of supernatant approximately equal to, or slightly less than, that of the deposit. Films are made of this suspension in the usual way.

EXAMINATION OF ASPIRATED BONE MARROW

Quantitative cell counts on aspirated bone marrow

A number of values for the cell content of aspirated normal bone marrow have been given in the literature.[11,12] The percentage of marrow in the sternum of healthy adults that is cellular rather than fatty is 48–79%. But quantitation of the cell content of aspirated marrow is not reliable in view of the tendency of the marrow to be aspirated in the form of particles of varying size as well as free cells, and the uncontrollable factor of dilution with peripheral blood, which according to some authors may amount to 40–100% in 0.25–0.5 ml bone marrow samples.

Quantitative cell counts on aspirated marrow are therefore difficult to interpret. For practical purposes, the degree of marrow cellularity can be assessed within broad limits as increased, normal, or reduced by inspection of a stained film containing marrow particles. As a rough guide, if less than 25% of the particle is occupied by haemopoietic cells, it is hypocellular, and if more than 75–80% is occupied, it is hypercellular. Less subjective quantitative measurement can be obtained by "point counting" of sections; a normal range of 30–80% has been reported in the anterior iliac spine.

Physiological variation in the cell content has to be taken into account. The cellularity of the marrow is affected by age. In adults, a smaller proportion of the marrow cavity is occupied by haemopoietic marrow than in children, and the proportion of fat cells to cellular marrow is increased. In one study, by means of point counting of sections from the iliac crest, the range of cellularity in children younger than 10 years was reported as 59–95% with a mean of 79%; at 30 years, the mean was 50%, and at 70 years, it was 30% with a range of 11–47%. The decrease in cellularity in elderly subjects is even more marked in the manubrium sterni. The marrow undergoes slight to moderate hyperplasia in pregnancy.

Differential Cell Counts on Aspirated Bone Marrow

For general purposes, it is not usually necessary to document the proportion of every stage of each cell type on the marrow slide. A 200–500-cell differential using the categories erythroid, myeloid, lymphoid, and plasma cells is generally adequate providing that a systematic scheme for examining the morphology of these, and all other, cells is also used. In some conditions, such as chronic myeloid leukaemia and myelodysplastic syndrome, detailed differential counts are important because the results may indicate prognosis and affect treatment.

Occasionally, it may be important to specifically count one cell type (e.g., blasts in acute leukaemia for assessing response to chemotherapy). Follow-up bone marrows should always be compared with previous bone marrow films to assess the course of a disease or the effect of treatment.

Sources of Error and Physiological Variations

Because of the naturally variegated pattern of the bone marrow, the irregular distribution of the marrow cells when spread in films, and the variable amount of dilution with blood, differential cell counts on marrow aspirated from normal subjects vary widely. Aspirating only a small volume and counting cells in the trails left behind marrow particles as they are spread on the slide minimizes the dilutional effect of blood. When there is an increase in associated reticulin, some cell types may resist aspiration or remain embedded in marrow fragments and will therefore be under-represented in the differential count. Megakaryocytes in particular are irregularly distributed and tend to be carried to the tail of the film. The chance aspiration of a lymphoid follicle would result in an abnormally high percentage of lymphocytes.[13]

Ideally, differential counts should be performed on sectioned material, but difficulties in identification make this impractical. Methacrylate embedding offers a better opportunity for correctly identifying cells. The incidence of the various cell types is usually expressed as percentages. The normal values for cell differentials in bone marrow (Table 6.1) can only be taken as an approximate guide.[11,12] The cellular composition of the bone marrow varies between normal infants, children, and young adults. Variation is marked in the first year, particularly so in the first month. The percentage of erythroblasts decreases from birth, and at 2–3 weeks they constitute only about 10% of the nucleated cells. Myeloid cells (granulocyte precursors) increase during the first 2 weeks of life, following which a sharp decrease occurs at about the 3rd week; however, by the end of the 1st month about 60% of the cells are myeloid. Lymphocytes constitute up to 40% of the nucleated cells in the marrow of small infants; the mean value at 2 years is approximately 20%, falling to about 15% during the rest of

Table 6.1 Normal ranges for differential counts on aspirated bone marrow

	95% Range	Mean[12]	Mean[11]
Myeloblasts	0–3	1.4	0.4
Promyelocytes	3–12	7.8	13.7*
Myelocytes (neutrophil)	2–13	7.6	–
Metamyelocytes	2–6	4.1	–
Neutrophils	22–46	32.1[M]; 37.4[W]	35.5
Myelocytes (eosinophil)	0–3	1.3	1.6
Eosinophils	0.3–4	2.2	1.7
Basophils	0–0.5	0.1	0.2
Lymphocytes	5–20	13.1	16.1
Monocytes	0–3	1.3	2.5
Plasma cells	0–3.5	0.6	1.9
Erythroblasts[†]	5–35	28.1[M]; 22.5[W]	23.5
Megakaryocytes	0–2	0.5	
Macrophages	0–2	0.4	2.0

*Includes all "immature neutrophils."
[†]Hammersmith Hospital data: Proerythroblasts, 0.5–5; early erythroblasts, 2–20; late erythroblasts, 2–10.
[M]Men
[W]Women.

childhood. The percentage of plasma cells is especially low from infancy up to the age of 5 years.

The hyperplasia that occurs in pregnancy affects both erythropoiesis and granulopoiesis, the latter proportionately less, although with some increase in the relative proportion of immature cells. The hyperplasia is maximal in the third trimester; a return to normal begins in the puerperium but is not completed until at least 6 weeks postpartum.

Cellular Ratios

Ratios based on a count of 200–500 cells can provide useful qualitative information. The myeloid:erythroid ratio has been widely used and is the ratio of neutrophil and neutrophil precursor cells to erythroid precursors. The inclusion of monocytes, eosinophils, and basophils is controversial but in practice makes little difference to the overall ratio, which varies from 2:1 to 4:1.[33] As an alternative, the leuco-erythrogenetic ratio can be calculated. For this, mature cells are excluded; the normal ratio has been reported as 0.56–2.67:1.[34] The myeloid:lymphoid ratio varies widely, 1–17:1, and the lymphoid:erythroid ratio has a similarly wide variation, 0.2–4.0:1.[35]

REPORTING BONE MARROW ASPIRATE FILMS

A systematic examination of the marrow aspirate, combined with knowledge of the clinical context, provides the best chance of arriving at a diagnosis. Choose several of the best spread stained films that contain easily visible marrow particles. Several particles should then be examined with a low-power (×10) objective to estimate whether the marrow is hypocellular, normocellular, or hypercellular (Fig. 6.5). Megakaryocytes and clumps of nonhaemopoietic cells (e.g., metastatic carcinoma cells) should be looked for at this stage of the examination; they are most often found toward the tail of the film.

Select for detailed examination—still using the ×10 objective—a highly cellular area of the film where the nucleated cells are well stained and well spread. Areas such as these can usually be found toward the tails of films behind marrow particles. The cells in these cellular areas should then be examined with a higher power (e.g., ×40) objective and subsequently, if necessary, with the ×100 oil-immersion objective. It is important always to examine marrows in a systematic fashion because it is easy to overlook subtle abnormalities. A suggested scheme for this is outlined below.

Systematic Scheme for Examining Bone Marrow Aspirate Films

Low Power (×10)
- **Determine cellularity** by examining several particles.
- **Identify megakaryocytes** and note morphology

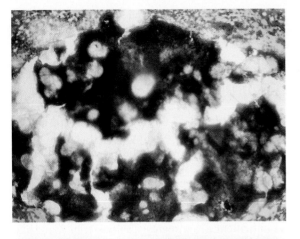

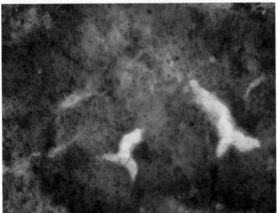

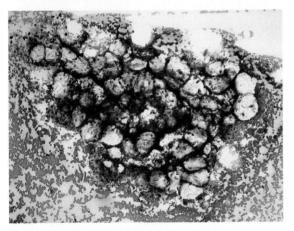

Figure 6.5   Film of aspirated bone marrow.
Photomicrographs of particles illustrating cellularity:
A: normal; B: hypercellular; and C: hypocellular.

and maturation sequence (higher power may be needed for smaller immature megakaryocytes and micromegakaryocytes).

- Look for clumps of **abnormal cells** that could indicate infiltration by metastatic tumour (higher power needed to examine content and morphology of clumps).

- Identify **macrophages** and examine at higher power for evidence of haemophagocytosis, malaria pigment, and bacterial or fungal infections that may be present in the cytoplasm. Higher power (×40, ×100 Oil Immersion)

- Identify all stages of **maturation of myeloid and erythroid cells.** This is usually easiest to achieve by starting with mature red cells and working backward to the most immature cells. Repeat the process for the myeloid series starting with mature neutrophils. Maturation abnormalities, such as giant pronormoblasts or evidence of dysfunctional maturation, including nuclear-cytoplasmic asynchrony, will suggest specific diagnoses such as parvovirus B19 infection, myelodysplastic syndrome, or megaloblastic anaemia, respectively. Changes in the proportion of primitive to mature myeloid cells may reflect response to treatment in leukaemia or recovery from agranulocytosis, and the actual percentage of blast cells may be of significance in the differentiation of refractory anaemias and in assessing leukaemia prognosis.

- Determine the **myeloid:erythroid** ratio. Whereas a lack of myeloid cells may be obvious without performing a formal differential count, it is easy to overlook an increase in erythroid cells, which might suggest blood loss or peripheral destruction.

- Perform a **differential count** (p. 121) using the categories erythroid, myeloid, lymphoid, plasma cell, and "others," simultaneously noting any morphological abnormalities. The normal lymphocyte percent in the marrow is 5–20%; moderate increases to 30–40%, which may indicate a significant disorder such as lymphoma, are not likely to be identified simply by rapidly surveying the slide. The proportion of lymphoid cells is an important indicator of prognosis in chronic lymphocytic leukaemia.[14] Plasma cells should be less than 2%; in plasma cell dyscrasias, they may be increased, occur in clumps, or have an abnormal morphological appearance.

- Look for areas of bone marrow **necrosis**.[15] In necrotic areas, the cells stain irregularly, with blurred outlines, cytoplasmic shrinkage, and nuclear pyknosis. Bone marrow necrosis may occur in sickle cell disease; it also occurs occasionally in lymphomas, acute lymphoblastic and chronic lymphocytic leukaemia, myeloproliferative diseases, and metastatic carcinoma, as well as in septicaemia, tuberculosis, and anorexia nervosa.[16] In patients with anorexia nervosa or cachexia, there may be gelatinous transformation of the ground substance of the marrow.[16]
- Assess the **iron content** of macrophages and look for iron granules in erythroid cells on a slide stained with a Perls' stain. At least seven particles should be examined to optimally assess a bone marrow aspirate for iron stores.[17] If fewer particles are available, a diagnosis of iron deficiency can only be tentative. In sideroblastic anaemia, the granules incompletely encircle the nucleus. Abnormal patterns of iron staining may also be seen in dyserythropoietic anaemias such as the thalassaemias.

Reporting Results

It is helpful to report bone marrow films on a printed form on which the report and conclusion can be set out in an ordered fashion (Fig. 6.6). Where a computerized reporting system is in use, it is useful to have a template with headings to ensure that the marrow reports are systematic and consistent. A list of the various descriptive comments that may be used should be provided in coded form to facilitate data entry. Report summaries should be intelligible to clinicians who are not haematology specialists.

PREPARATION OF SECTIONS OF ASPIRATED BONE MARROW FRAGMENTS

In situations where it is not possible to obtain a trephine biopsy (see below), the small fragments obtained by marrow aspiration can be fixed, stained, and examined. Such samples are useful for assessing cellularity and for detecting granulomas and tumour cells. If sections are required, it is convenient to let residual aspirated marrow clot within a plastic syringe and tease the sample out into the fixative once it has clotted.

PERCUTANEOUS TREPHINE BIOPSY OF THE BONE MARROW

Trephine biopsies of the bone marrow are invaluable in the diagnosis of conditions that yield a "dry tap" on bone marrow aspiration (e.g., myelofibrosis, infiltrations) or when disrupted architecture of the marrow is an important diagnostic feature (e.g., Hodgkin's disease, lymphoma). Like marrow aspirations, they can be carried out at the bedside or in outpatient departments. The posterior iliac spine is the usual site, although the anterior iliac spine can also be used. The posterior iliac spine is said to provide samples that are longer and larger, and the aspiration is less uncomfortable for the patient.[18]

The trephine specimen is obtained by inserting the biopsy needle into the bone and using a to-and-fro rotation to obtain a core of tissue. The main problems with this method are that the specimen may be crushed, thereby distorting the architecture, and it is difficult to detach the core of bone from inside the marrow space. Trephine biopsy needles, both reusable and disposable, have been specifically designed to overcome these problems. The Jamshidi needle has a tapering end to reduce crush artefact (Fig. 6.7), and the Islam trephine has a core-securing device (Fig. 6.8). If larger specimens are needed, trephine needles that have bores of 4–5 mm may be used. Other needles occasionally used for trephine biopsy specimens are a 2-mm bore "microtrephine" needle and a Vim–Silverman needle. However, compared with other needles, these yield smaller specimens of marrow that are prone to fracturing.

For the investigation of thrombocytopenia and neutropenia in small preterm neonates, sections of aspirated bone marrow can be obtained that allow assessment of marrow cellularity and architecture.[19] A 19G, half-inch Osgood needle* is introduced 2 cm below the tibial tuberosity. The trocar is removed and the hollow needle is advanced by twisting 2–3 mm into the marrow space. A syringe is used to

---

*Popper and Sons, New Hyde Park, New York.

Surname:_____ First Name: _____ Sex: _____ Date of birth: _____

Consultant:_____

Date taken: _____ Hospital No: _____ Lab No: _____

Clinical details:

WBC   Hb   MCV   Platelet count

Blood film:

Performed by: Aspiration Site: Ease of aspiration:

Particles:

Cellularity: M:E Ratio

Erythropoiesis:

Granulopoiesis:

Megakaryocytes:

Lymphocytes:

Plasma Cells:

Macrophages:

Other Cells:

Blast cells	Promyelocytes	Myelocytes and metamyelocytes	Neutrophils	Eosinophils
Basophils	Monocytes	Lymphocytes	Plasma cells	Erythroid

Storage iron: Siderotic granules:

Other tests to follow:

Conclusion:

Authorized by: Date:

Figure 6.6   Example of report form for bone marrow films.

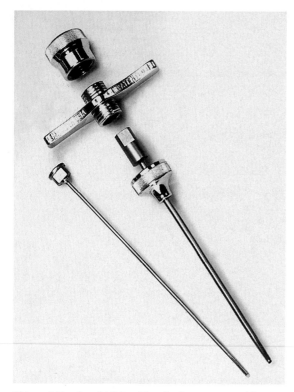

Figure 6.7   Jamshidi trephine for bone marrow biopsy.

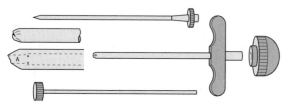

Figure 6.8   Islam trephine for bone marrow biopsy. The distal cutting edge is shaped to hold the core secure during extraction of the material.

apply suction to the needle until marrow appears; then the needle and syringe are withdrawn. The marrow clot is gently dislodged with the tip of a needle and placed into fixative. The specimen is processed as if it was an adult biopsy except that decalcification is not required.

Complications of Bone Marrow Biopsy

Bone marrow biopsy is generally a safe procedure, and serious adverse events occur in fewer than 0.05% of procedures.[20] The most common complication is bleeding, which can lead to significant morbidity, such as "gluteal compartment syndrome,"[21] and very rarely death. Bleeding is more often related to impairment of platelet function than to thrombocytopenia or a coagulation factor defect.[20]

Imprints from Bone Marrow Trephine Biopsy Specimens

Whenever a trephine biopsy is obtained, imprints can be taken before the specimen is transferred into fixative. This is particularly useful if the bone marrow aspirate is inadequate. The bony core is gently dabbed or rolled across the slide, which is then fixed and stained as for bone marrow smears (p. 63). This allows immediate examination of cells that fall out of the specimen onto the slide and may provide a diagnosis several days before the trephine biopsy specimen has been processed.

Processing of Bone Marrow Trephine Biopsy Specimens

The specimen should be fixed in 10% formal saline, buffered to pH 7.0, for 12–48 hours prior to decalcifying, dehydrating, and embedding in paraffin wax by the usual histological procedures. Cell shrinkage and distortion from the decalcification process may distort cellular detail. These disadvantages can be overcome by methyl methacrylate ("plastic") embedding. Details of the preparation of sections of bone marrow biopsies can be found in Bain et al.[22]

Staining of Sections of Bone Marrow Trephine Biopsy Specimens

Bone marrow sections should be routinely stained with haematoxylin and eosin (H&E) and a silver impregnation method for reticulin. Sections can also be stained with Romanowsky dyes such as May–Grünwald–Giemsa and for iron by Perls' re-

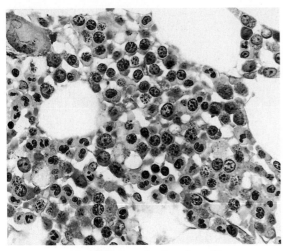

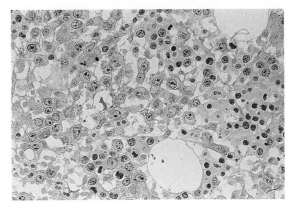

Figure 6.10   Photomicrograph of section of normal bone marrow. Iliac crest biopsy. Methacrylate embedding. Stained by May–Grünwald–Giemsa.

Figure 6.9   Photomicrograph of section of bone marrow. Iliac crest biopsy. Methacrylate embedding. Myeloblastic leukaemia. Stained by May–Grünwald–Giemsa.

action. H&E staining is excellent for demonstrating the cellularity and pattern of the marrow and for revealing pathological changes such as fibrosis or the presence of granulomata or carcinoma cells. Figure 6.9 shows the extent to which the cellularity of the marrow varies in health. Haemopoietic cells may be more easily identified in a Romanowsky-stained preparation (Figs. 6.10 and 6.11). Both paraffin- and plastic-embedded specimens are suitable for immunohistochemistry.

Silver impregnation stains the glycoprotein matrix, which is associated with connective tissue. The bone marrow always contains a small amount of this material, which is referred to as "reticulin" and is an early form of collagen. The reticulin content of iliac bone marrow is shown in Figure 6.12. An increase in marrow reticulin appears as an increase in the number and thickness of fibres. Increased reticulin deposition can occur in myeloproliferative disorders, particularly those associated with proliferation of megakaryocytes, and in lymphoproliferative disorders, secondary carcinoma with marrow infiltration, osseous disorders such as hyperparathyroidism and Paget's disease, and inflammatory reactions.[23] In myelofibrosis or myelosclerosis, a more "mature" form of collagen is present, which, unlike reticulin, is visible on H&E staining (Fig. 6.13).

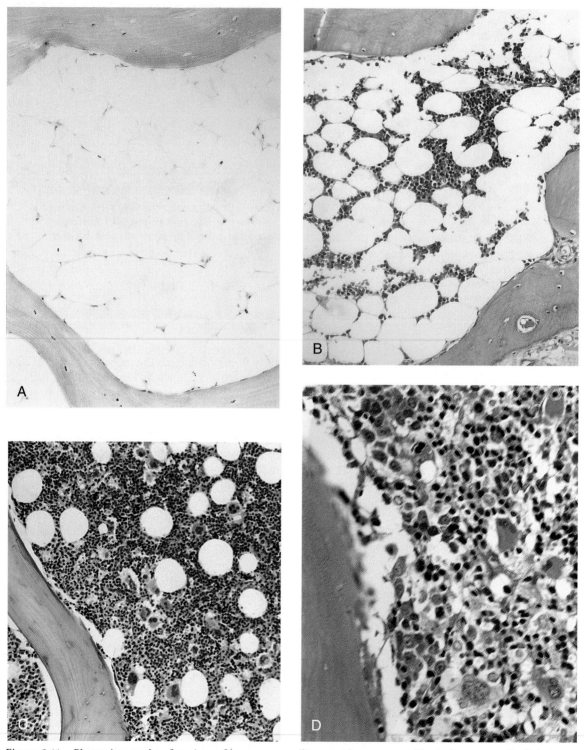

Figure 6.11   Photomicrographs of sections of bone marrow. Iliac crest bone marrow illustrating range of cellularity; A: hypocellular; B and C: normal cellularity; and D: hypercellular.

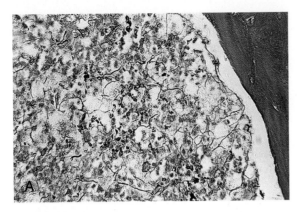

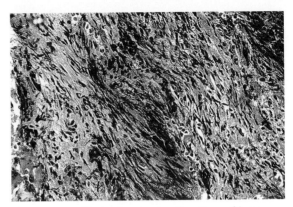

Figure 6.13   Photomicrographs of sections of bone marrow. Iliac crest biopsy; fibroblast proliferation, and collagen in myelofibrosis. Haematoxylin and eosin stain.

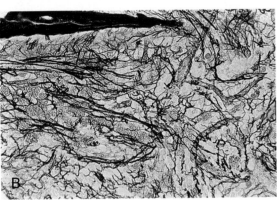

Figure 6.12   Photomicrographs of sections of bone marrow. Iliac crest biopsy. Stained for reticulin by silver impregnation method: A: normal; and B: chronic myelofibrosis.

REFERENCES

1. Bain BJ 2001 Bone marrow aspiration. Journal of Clinical Pathology 54:657–663.
2. Bain BJ 2001 Bone marrow trephine biopsy. Journal of Clinical Pathology 54:737–742.
3. Hall R. 2004 Results of bone marrow biopsy patient satisfaction survey at the Royal Bournemouth Hospital. British Journal of Haematology 125 (supp 1), Abstract 200, p. 62.
4. Marti J, Anton E, Valenti C 2004. Complications of bone marrow biopsy. British Journal of Haematology 124:555–563.
5. Devaliaf V, Tudor G. 2004 Bone marrow examination in obese patients. British Journal of Haematology 125:537–539.
6. Engeset A, Nesheim A, Sokolowski J 1979 Incidence of "dry tap" on bone marrow aspirations in lymphomas and carcinomas: diagnostic value of the small material in the needle. Scandinavian Journal of Haematology 22:417–422.
7. Ferrant A 1980 Selective hypoplasia of pelvic bone marrow. Scandinavian Journal of Haematology 25:12–18.
8. Jacobs P 1995 Choice of needle for bone marrow trephine biopsies. Hematology Reviews 9:163–168.
9. Fillola GM, Laharrague PF, Corberand JX 1992 Bone marrow enrichment technique for detection and characterization of scarce abnormal cells. Nouvelle Revue Française d'Hématologie 34:337–341.
10. Hoffman SB, Morrow GW Jr, Pease GL, et al 1964 Rate of cellular autolysis in postmortem bone marrow. American Journal of Clinical Pathology 41:281–286.
11. Den Ottolander GJ 1996 The bone marrow aspirate of healthy subjects. British Journal of Haematology 95:574–575.
12. Bain B 1996 The bone marrow aspirate of healthy subjects. British Journal of Haematology 94:206–209.
13. Maeda K, Hyun BH, Rebuck JW 1977 Lymphoid follicles in bone marrow aspirates. American Journal of Clinical Pathology 67:41–48.
14. Rozman C, Montserrat E, Rodriguez-Fernandez JM et al 1984 Bone marrow histologic pattern: the best single prognostic parameter in chronic lymphocytic leukemia—a multivariate survival analysis of 329 cases. Blood 64:642–648.
15. Kiraly JF, Wheby MS 1976 Bone marrow necrosis. American Journal of Medicine 60:361–368.
16. Smith RRL, Spivak JL 1985 Marrow cell necrosis in anorexia nervosa and involuntary starvation. British Journal of Haematology 60:525–530.

17. Hughes DA, Stuart-Smith SE, Bain BJ 2004. How should stainable iron in bone marrow films be assessed? Journal of Clinical Pathology 57:1038–1040.

18. Hernándes-Gaciá MT, Hernández-Nieto L, Pérez-González E et al 1993 Bone marrow trephine biopsy: anterior superior iliac spine versus posterior superior iliac spine. Clinical and Laboratory Haematology 15:15–19.

19. Sola M, Rimsza L, Christensen R 1999 A bone marrow biopsy technique suitable for use in neonates. British Journal of Haematology 107:458–460.

20. Bain B 2003 Bone marrow biopsy morbidity and mortality. British Journal of Haematology 121:949–951

21. Roth JS, Newman EC 2002. Gluteal compartment syndrome and sciatica after bone marrow biopsy: a case report and review of the literature. American Surgeon 68(9):791–794

22. Bain B, Clark DC, Lampert IO, Wilkins BS 2000 Bone marrow pathology, 3rd ed., Blackwell Science, Oxford.

23. McCarthy DM 1985 Fibrosis of the bone marrow: content and causes. British Journal of Haematology 59:1–7.

7 Iron deficiency anaemia and iron overload

Mark Worwood

IRON METABOLISM

The iron content of the body and its distribution among the various proteins is summarised in Table 7.1. Most of the iron is present in the oxygen-carrying protein of the red blood cell–haemoglobin. Iron turnover is also dominated by the synthesis and breakdown of haemoglobin. Haem is synthesised in nucleated red cells in the bone marrow by a pathway ending with the incorporation of iron into protoporphyrin IX by ferrochelatase. Haem breakdown takes place in phagocytic cells, largely those in the spleen, liver, and bone marrow. Iron is released from haem by haem oxygenase and is largely reused for haem synthesis. Every day about 30 mg of iron are used to make new haemoglobin, and most of this is obtained from the breakdown of old red cells.

Relatively little iron is lost from the body (about 1 mg/d in men), and these losses are not influenced by body iron content or the requirement of the body for iron. The body iron content is maintained by variation in the amount of iron absorbed. In women, menstruation and childbirth increase iron losses to about 2 mg/d. Iron absorption may not increase sufficiently to compensate for these iron losses, and this may eventually lead to the development of iron deficiency anaemia. In most men and postmenopausal women there is some "storage" iron. This is iron in ferritin, or its insoluble derivative haemosiderin, which is available for haem synthesis if necessary. Many young women and children have little or no storage iron.

The iron-binding protein, transferrin, is responsible for extracellular transport. Most cells obtain iron from transferrin, which binds to transferrin receptors on the cell surface. This is followed by internalisation into vesicles with release of iron into the cells and recycling of the apotransferrin (the protein without iron) into the plasma (Fig 7.1).

Dietary Iron Absorption

Iron absorption[1] depends on the amount of iron in the diet, its bioavailability, and the body's need for iron. A normal Western diet provides approximately 15 mg of iron daily. Of that iron, digestion within the gut lumen releases about half in a soluble form, from which only about 1 mg (5–10% of dietary iron) is transferred to the portal blood in a healthy adult male.

Table 7.1 Distribution of iron in the body (70-kg man)		
Protein	Location	Iron content (mg)
Haemoglobin	Red blood cells	3000
Myoglobin	Muscle	400
Cytochromes and iron sulphur proteins	All tissues	50
Transferrin	Plasma and extravascular fluid	5
Ferritin and haemosiderin	Liver, spleen, and bone marrow	100–1000

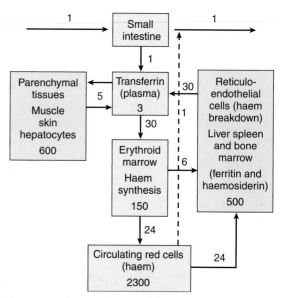

Figure 7.1 **Iron exchange within the body.** Numbers in boxes refer to amount of iron (mg) in the various compartments and the numbers alongside arrows indicate transfer in mg/d. The iron in parenchymal tissues is largely haem in muscle and ferritin/haemosiderin in hepatic parenchymal cells. The dotted line indicates the small loss of iron (9.5 mg) into the gut from red cells; the remaining iron loss is in exfoliated gut cells and bile.

Dietary and Luminal Factors

Much of the dietary iron is nonhaem iron derived from cereals (often fortified with additional iron), with a lesser, but well-absorbed, component of haem iron from meat and fish. With iron deficiency, the maximum iron absorption from a mixed Western diet is no more than 3–4 mg daily. This amount is much less in the predominantly vegetarian, cereal-based diets of most of the world's population.

Nonhaem iron is released from protein complexes by acid and proteolytic enzymes in the stomach and small intestine. It is maximally absorbed from the duodenum and less well from the jejunum, probably because the increasingly alkaline environment leads to the formation of insoluble ferric hydroxide complexes. Many luminal factors enhance (e.g., meat and vitamin C) or inhibit (e.g., phytates and tannins) nonhaem iron absorption. Therapeutic ferrous iron salts are well-absorbed (c 10–20%) on an empty stomach, but when taken with meals, absorption is reduced by the same dietary interactions that affect nonhaem food iron.

Iron Absorption at the Molecular Level

Several membrane transport proteins, regulatory proteins, and associated oxidoreductases involved in iron transport through the intestinal cell have been identified. Nonhaem iron is released from food as Fe^{3+} (ferric iron) and reduced to Fe^{2+} (ferrous iron) by a membrane-bound, ferrireductase, Dcytb. Iron is transported across the brush-border membrane by the metal transporter, DMT1. Some iron is incorporated into ferritin and lost when the cells are exfoliated. Iron destined for retention by the body is transported across the serosal membrane by ferroportin 1. Before uptake by transferrin, Fe^{2+} is oxidised to Fe^{3+} by hephaestin (a membrane protein homologous to the plasma copper-containing protein caeruloplasmin) or by plasma caeruloplasmin.

Haemoglobin and myoglobin are digested in the stomach and small intestine. Haem is initially bound by haem receptors at the brush border membrane and the iron is released intracellularly by haem oxygenase before entering the labile iron pool and following a common pathway with iron of nonhaem origin.

Regulation of Iron Absorption

Iron absorption may be regulated both at the stage of mucosal uptake and at the stage of transfer to the blood. As the epithelial cells develop in the crypts of Lieberkuhn, their iron status reflects that of the plasma (transferrin saturation) and this programmes the cells to absorb iron appropriately as they differentiate along the villus. Transfer to the plasma depends on the requirements of the erythron for iron and the level of iron stores.[2] This regulation is mediated directly by hepcidin, a peptide synthesized in the liver in response to iron and inflammation.[3]

Cellular Iron Uptake and Release[4]

Transferrin binds to the transferrin receptor (TfR) lining the cell. The two proteins bind strongly to form a high affinity complex, which initiates endocytosis of the local membrane. The resulting endosome contains the transferrin–transferrin receptor complex. The pH of the endosome is then reduced by a proton pump to induce a conformational change in holotransferrin, which releases its iron. Iron is transported into the cell via DMT1. This iron is then either stored as ferritin or used within the cell (e.g., for haemoglobin synthesis in erythroid precursors). The apotransferrin and the transferrin receptor return to the cell surface where they dissociate at neutral pH so that the cycle can start again.

The reticuloendothelial macrophages play a major role in recycling iron resulting from the degradation of haemoglobin from senescent erythrocytes. They engulf red blood cells and release the iron within using haem oxygenase. The iron is rapidly released to plasma transferrin or stored as ferritin. Little is known about the mechanism of release, but ferroportin 1 may be an essential component.

Iron Storage

All cells require iron for the synthesis of proteins but also have the ability to store excess iron.[5] There are two forms of storage iron: a soluble form, known as ferritin, and insoluble haemosiderin. Ferritin consists of a spherical protein (molecular mass 480,000) enclosing a core of ferric-hydroxy-phosphate, which may contain up to 4000 atoms of iron. Haemosiderin is a degraded form of ferritin in which the protein shells have partly degraded, allowing the iron cores to aggregate. Haemosiderin deposits are readily visualised with the aid of the light microscope as areas of Prussian-blue positivity after staining of tissue sections with potassium ferrocyanide in acid (p. 311). Ferritin is found in all cells and in the highest concentration in liver, spleen, and bone marrow.

Regulation of Iron Metabolism

The expression of a number of iron proteins involved in both transport and storage is largely controlled by posttranscriptional regulation by iron regulatory proteins (IRP1 and 2).[4] The conformation of these cytosolic, RNA-binding proteins is directly affected by the amount of iron within a cell, and they accordingly inhibit or enhance translation of several iron-containing proteins, thereby regulating their expression.

When the labile iron pool is deficient of iron, the IRP has an open binding site for iron responsive elements (IRE) present on the messenger RNA (mRNA) of some iron proteins. IREs consist of a base-paired stem interrupted by an unpaired cytosine, followed by an upper stem of five paired bases and a six-membered loop. When the labile iron pool is saturated with iron, the iron binds to the IRP 1 to produce a 4Fe-4S cluster, which blocks the IRE binding site and prevents the IRP binding to the IRE. In the presence of iron, IRP 2 (which is not an Fe-S protein) is degraded.

Different iron proteins are regulated by IRP in different ways, depending on where the IRE is located. If the IRE is at the 3′ UTR of the mRNA, IRP binding will stabilise translation by protecting the translation product from endonucleolytic cleavage (transferrin receptor and DMT1). If the IRE is at the 5′ UTR of the mRNA, IRP binding will inhibit the translation of mRNA. Both ferritin subunits have a 5′ UTR IRE. When iron is abundant, the IRP does not bind to the 5′ IRE so ferritin expression is not inhibited and excess iron can be stored adequately. When iron is scarce, the IRP binds to the IRE and inhibits ferritin synthesis.

Plasma Iron Transport

Almost all the iron in the plasma is tightly bound to transferrin. Delivery to cells requires specific binding to transferrin receptors. The plasma iron pool (transferrin-bound iron) is about 3 mg, although the daily turnover is more than 30 mg. In addition, smaller amounts of iron are carried in the plasma by other proteins.

Haptoglobin[6] is a serum glycoprotein that avidly binds haemoglobin released into the bloodstream by haemolysis. The haemoglobin–haptoglobin complex is rapidly removed from the plasma by a specific receptor, CD163, which is highly expressed on tissue macrophages.[7]

Hemopexin[8] is a plasma glycoprotein of molecular mass approximately 60 kDa that binds haem and transports the haem to cells by a process that involves receptor-mediated endocytosis of haemopexin with recycling of the intact protein.

In health, low concentrations of *ferritin* are found in the plasma and ferritin concentrations reflect the level of body iron stores. Much of this ferritin appears to be glycosylated and has a relatively low iron content.[9] Such ferritin has a relatively prolonged survival in the blood ($T_{1/2}$ of the order of 30 hours). Ferritin is also released into the circulation as a result of tissue damage (most strikingly after necrosis of the liver). Tissue ferritin is cleared rapidly from the circulation ($T_{1/2}$ in approximately 10 min) by the liver.

Nontransferrin iron describes a form of iron that is not bound to transferrin, is of low molecular mass, and can be bound by specific iron chelators.[10] Several assays have been described that have demonstrated such a fraction in plasma from patients with iron overload. The chemical form of this iron is unknown, but it is probably rapidly removed from the circulation by the liver.

IRON STATUS

Normal iron status implies a level of erythropoiesis that is not limited by the supply of iron and the presence of a small reserve of "storage iron" to cope with normal physiological needs.[11] The ability to survive the acute loss of blood (iron) that may result from injury is also an advantage. The limits of normality are difficult to define, and some argue that physiological normality is the presence of only a minimal amount of storage iron[12] but the extremes of iron deficiency anaemia and haemochromatosis are well understood.

Apart from too little or too much iron in the body, there is also the possibility of a maldistribution (Fig. 7.2). An example is anaemia associated with inflammation or infection where there is a partial failure of erythropoiesis and of iron release from the phagocytic cells in liver, spleen, and bone marrow, which results in accumulation of iron as ferritin and haemosiderin in these cells. Thus determination of iron status requires an estimate of the amount of haemoglobin iron (usually by measuring the haemoglobin concentration (Hb) in the blood; see Chapter 3) and the level of storage iron (measuring serum ferritin concentration). Iron deficiency should be suspected in hypochromic, microcytic anaemia, but in the early stages of iron deficiency red cells may be normocytic and normochromic. Another feature of iron deficiency is an increased concentration of protoporphyrin in the red cells; normally, there is a small amount, but defective haem synthesis caused by lack of iron results in an accumulation of a significant amount (mostly as zinc protoporphyrin) in the red cells.[13]

Additional assays are sometimes required. In genetic haemochromatosis, early iron accumulation is indicated by an increased transferrin saturation. The serum ferritin concentration increases only later as the level of stored iron increases. In the anaemia of chronic disease, patients often have normal serum ferritin concentrations even in the absence of storage iron in the bone marrow (p. 314). In this situation, the assay of serum transferrin receptor can detect tissue iron deficiency.

DISORDERS OF IRON METABOLISM

Clinical aspects of iron metabolism have been reviewed[14,15] and are summarised in Table 7.2. A guideline on genetic haemochromatosis is available.[16]

METHODS FOR ASSESSING IRON STATUS

The methods used to assess the level of iron status are summarised in Table 7.3. Some are not generally applicable but have value in the standardisation of indirect methods. The determinations of Hb and red cell indices are described in Chapter 3.

SERUM FERRITIN

With the recognition that the small quantity of ferritin in human serum (15–300 µg/l in healthy men) reflects body iron stores, measurement of serum ferritin has been widely adopted as a test for iron deficiency and iron overload. The first reliable method to be introduced was an immunoradiometric assay[17] in which excess radiolabelled antibody was reacted with ferritin, and antibody not

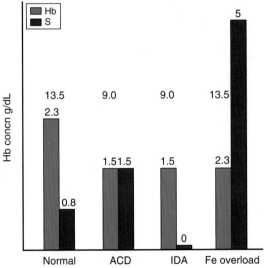

Figure 7.2 **Body iron distribution.** ACD: anaemia of chronic diseases; IDA: iron deficiency anaemia; Hb: haemoglobin iron; S: storage iron (ferritin and haemosiderin).

Table 7.2   Disorders of iron metabolism

Iron deficiency
Deficient intake
Diet of low bioavailability

Increased physiological requirements
Rapid growth in early childhood and in adolescence

Blood loss
Physiological (e.g., menstruation)
Pathological (e.g., gastrointestinal)

Malabsorption of iron
Reduced gastric acid secretion (e.g., after partial
gastrectomy)
Reduced duodenal absorptive area (e.g., in coeliac
disease)
Redistribution of iron

Macrophage iron accumulation
Inflammatory, infectious, or malignant diseases
("anaemia of chronic disease")
Iron overload

Increased iron absorption
Hereditary haemochromatosis—commonly homozygosity
for HFE C282Y but sometimes involving other genes
Massive ineffective erythropoiesis (e.g., severe
thalassaemia syndromes, sideroblastic anaemias)
Sub-Saharan iron overload ("Bantu siderosis")—only in
combination with increased dietary iron
Other rare inherited disorders (e.g., congenital
atransferrinaemia)
Inappropriate iron therapy (rare)

Multiple blood transfusions in refractory anaemias
Thalassaemia major
Aplastic anaemia
Myelodysplastic syndromes

bound to ferritin was removed with an immuno-adsorbent. This assay was supplanted by the two-site immunoradiometric assay,[18] which is sensitive and convenient. Since then the principle of this assay has been extended to nonradioactive labelling, including enzymes (enzyme-linked immunosorbent assay, or ELISA). Most current laboratory immunoassay systems for clinical laboratories include ferritin in the assay repertoire. Factors to be considered when selecting an immunoassay system

are discussed later. The method described in the next section is an ELISA. The most sophisticated equipment required is a microtitre plate reader.

IMMUNOASSAY FOR FERRITIN

Reagents and Materials

Ferritin

Ferritin may be prepared from iron-loaded human liver or spleen obtained at operation (spleen) or postmortem. The permission of the patient or the patient's relatives should be obtained for use in preparation of ferritin. Tissue should be obtained as soon as possible after death and may be stored at −20°C for 1 year. Remember the risk of infection when handling tissues and extracts. Ferritin is purified by methods that exploit its stability at 75°C. Further purification is obtained by precipitation from cadmium sulphate solution and gel-filtration chromatography.[19] Purity should be assessed by polyacrylamide gel electrophoresis,[20] and the protein content should be determined by the method of Lowry et al as described by Worwood.[20] Human ferritin may be stored at 4°C, at concentrations of 1–4 mg protein/ml, in the presence of sodium azide as a preservative, for up to 3 years. Such solutions should not be frozen. Ferritin, from human liver or spleen, may be obtained from several suppliers of laboratory reagents. This may be used as a standard after calibration against the international standard (see later).

Antibodies to Human Ferritin

High-affinity antibodies to human liver or spleen ferritin are suitable. Polyclonal antibodies may be raised in rabbits or sheep by conventional methods,[21] and the titre can be checked by precipitation with human ferritin.[20] An immunoglobulin G (IgG)-enriched fraction of antiserum is required for labelling with enzyme in the assay. The simplest method is to precipitate IgG with ammonium sulphate.[22] Monoclonal antibodies that are specific for "L" subunit–rich ferritin (liver or spleen ferritin) are also suitable. Suitable antibodies (including a preparation labelled with horseradish peroxidase) may be obtained from Dako Ltd., High Wycombe, Bucks, UK.

Table 7.3   Assessment of body iron status and confounding factors

Measurement	Reference range (adults)	Diagnostic use	Confounding factors
Haemoglobin concentration	M 13–17 g/dl F 12–15 g/dl	Defining anaemia and assessing its severity; response to a therapeutic trial of iron confirms iron deficiency anaemia.	Other causes of anaemia besides iron deficiency.

Red cell indices
    Mean cell volume
    Mean cell haemoglobin
	83–101 fl
	27–32 pg
		Low values indicate iron deficient erythropoiesis.	May be reduced in disorders of haemoglobin synthesis, other than iron deficiency (thalassaemia, sideroblastic anaemias, anaemia of chronic disease).

Tissue iron supply Serum iron[†]	10–30 μmol/l	Low values in iron deficiency, high values in iron overload.	Reduced in acute and chronic disease; labile, use of fasting morning sample reduces variability
Total iron binding capacity (TIBC)[†]	47–70 μmol/l	High values characteristic of tissue iron deficiency. Low values in iron overload. May also be calculated from transferrin concentration (Tf g/l $\times$ 25).	Rarely used on its own. Reliable reference ranges not available.
Transferrin saturation (TS) [iron/TIBC $\times$ 100]	16–50%	Low values in iron deficiency, high values in iron overload. Raised TS is an early indicator of iron accumulation in genetic haemochromatosis.	See serum iron (above).
Iron supply to the bone marrow Serum transferrin receptor (sTfR) Red cell zinc protoporphyrin (ZPP) Red cell ferritin ("L" type) % hypochromic red cells	2.8–8.5 mg/l* <80 μmol/mol Hb 3–40 ag/cell <6%	Reduced red cell ferritin, increased ZPP, sTfR, and % hypochromic red cells indicate impaired iron supply to the bone marrow. Useful for identifying early iron deficiency and, with a measure of iron stores, distinguishing this from anaemia of chronic disease (ACD). In ACD, sTfR only increases in the presence of tissue iron deficiency.	sTfR concentration related to extent of erythroid activity as well as iron supply to cells ZPP, red cell ferritin, and % hypochromic cells are stable measures determined at time of red cell formation. Values may not reflect current iron status. May be increased by other causes of impaired iron incorporation into haem (sideroblastic anaemias, lead poisoning, inflammation).

Table 7.3   Assessment of body iron status and confounding factors—cont'd

Measurement	Reference range (adults)	Diagnostic use	Confounding factors
Iron stores			
Serum ferritin	M 15–300 µg/l F 15–200 µg/l	Correlated with body iron stores from deficiency to overload.	Increased: as acute-phase protein and by release of tissue ferritin after organ damage (particularly liver disease). Decreased: vitamin C deficiency.
Tissue biopsy iron			
Liver (chemical assay)	3–33 µmol/g dry weight	Confirmation of iron overload.	Potential for sampling error on needle biopsy when <0.5 mg or liver is nodular.
Bone marrow (Perls' stain)	(Grade)	Graded as absent, present, or increased. Most commonly used to differentiate ACD from IDA.	Adequate sample required.
Quantitative phlebotomy	<2 g Fe	Treatment of genetic haemochromatosis.	
Urine chelatable Fe (after intramuscular injection of deferoxamine)	<2 mg/24h	Rarely used but may provide confirmation of iron overload.	
Imaging			
MRI (magnetic resonance imaging)		Becoming available both for hepatic and cardiac iron deposition.	Machines widely available but special analysis and software required.
SQID (superconducting quantum interface device)[111]		Quantitation of liver iron overload using magnetic properties of iron.	Not available in UK.

Modified from Pippard.[126]
*Units and reference ranges are specific to method.
†Slightly different values are given in Chapter 2, Table 2.2.

Conjugation of Antiferritin IgG Preparation to Horseradish Peroxidase[23]

1. Dissolve 4 mg of horseradish peroxidase (Sigma Type VI P-8375) in 1 ml of water and add 200 µl of freshly prepared 0.1 mol/l sodium periodate solution. The solution should turn greenish-brown. Mix gently by inverting and leave for 20 min at room temperature, mixing gently every 5 min. Dialyse overnight against 1 mmol/l sodium acetate buffer, pH 4.4.

2. Add 20 µl of 0.2 mol/l sodium carbonate buffer, pH 9.5, to a solution of antiferritin IgG fraction (8 mg in 1 ml). Add 20 µl of 0.2 mol/l sodium carbonate buffer, pH 9.5, to the horseradish peroxidase solution to increase the pH to 9.0–9.5 and immediately mix the 2 solutions. Leave at room temperature for 2 hours and mix by inversion every 30 min.

3. Add 100 µl of freshly prepared sodium borohydride solution (4 mg/ml in water) and let it stand at 4°C for 2 hours. Dialyse overnight against 0.1 mol/l borate buffer, pH 7.4.

4. Add an equal volume of 60% glycerol in borate buffer to the conjugate solution and store at 4°C.

Buffer A

Phosphate-buffered saline, pH 7.2, containing 0.05% Tween 20. Prepare a ×10 concentrated (1.5 mol/l) stock solution by dissolving sodium chloride, 80 g; potassium chloride, 2 g; anhydrous disodium phosphate, 11.5 g; and anhydrous potassium phosphate (KH2PO4), 2 g in 1 litre of water. Store at room temperature. Prepare Buffer A by diluting 100 ml of stock solution to 1 litre with water and adding 0.5 ml of Tween 20. Store at 4°C for up to 2 weeks.

Buffer B

Prepare by dissolving 5 g of bovine serum albumin (BSA; Sigma A-7030) in 1 litre of buffer A. Store at 4°C for up to 2 weeks.

Buffer C

Carbonate buffer, 0.05 mol/l, pH 9.6. Dissolve sodium carbonate, 1.59 g and sodium bicarbonate, 2.93 g in 1 litre of water and store at room temperature.

Buffer D

Citrate phosphate buffer, 0.15 mol/l, pH 5.0. Dissolve 21 g of citric acid monohydrate in 1 litre of water and store at 4°C. Dissolve 28.4 g of anhydrous disodium phosphate in 1 litre of water and store at room temperature. Prepare fresh buffer on the day of assay by mixing 49 ml of citric acid solution with 51 ml of phosphate solution.

Substrate Solution

Prepare immediately before use by adding 33 µl of hydrogen peroxide, 30%, to 100 ml of buffer D and mixing well. Add 1 tablet containing 30 mg of *o*-phenylenediamine dihydrochloride (Sigma P 8412) and mix.

Sulphuric Acid

Purchase as a 4M solution.

Preparation and Storage of a Standard Ferritin Solution

Dilute a solution of human ferritin to approximately 200 µg/ml in water. Measure the protein concentration by the method of Lowry after diluting further to 20–50 µg/ml. Then dilute the ferritin solution (approximately 200 µg/ml) to a concentration of 10 µg/ml in 0.05 mol/l sodium barbitone solution containing 0.1 mol/l NaCl, 0.02% NaN_3, and BSA (5 g/l) and adjusted to pH 8.0 with 5 mol/l HCl. Deliver 200 µl into 200 small plastic tubes, cap tightly, and store at 4°C for up to 1 year. For use, dilute in Buffer B to 1000 µg/l, then prepare a range of standard solutions between 0.2 and 25 µg/l. Calibrate this working standard against the World Health Organization (WHO) standard for the assay of serum ferritin 94/572, recombinant human L type ferritin. Information from www.nibsc.ac.uk.

Coating of Plates

Microtitre plates (96-well) for immunoassay are required. Do not use the outer wells until you have established the assay procedure and can check that all wells give consistent results. Coat the plates by adding to each well 200 µl of antiferritin IgG preparation diluted to 2 µg/ml in Buffer C. Cover the plate with a lid and leave overnight at 4°C. On the day of the assay, empty the wells by sharply inverting the plate and dry them by tapping briefly on paper towels. Block unreacted sites by adding 200 µl of 0.5% (w/v) BSA in Buffer C. After 30 min at room temperature, wash each plate three times by filling each well with Buffer A (using a syringe and needle) and emptying and draining as described earlier. Plates may be stored, dry, at 4°C for up to 1 week.

Preparation of Test Sera

Collect venous blood and separate the serum. Samples may be stored for 1 week at 4°C or for 2 years at –20°C. Plasma obtained from ethylene-diaminetetra-acetic acid (EDTA) or heparinized blood is also suitable. For assay, dilute 50 µl of serum to 1 ml with Buffer B. Further dilutions may be made in the same buffer if required.

Assay Procedure

The use of a multichannel pipette for rapid addition of solutions is recommended. Standards and sera, in duplicate, should be added to each plate within 20 min.

Add 200 µl of standard solution or diluted serum to each well. Cover the plate and leave at room temperature on a draught-free bench away from direct sunlight for 2 hours. Empty the wells by sharply inverting the plate and drain by standing them on paper towels with occasional tapping for 1 min. Wash three times by filling each well with Buffer A, leaving for 2 min at room temperature, and draining as described earlier. Dilute the conjugate in 1% BSA in Buffer A. The optimal dilution (of the order of 10^3–10^4 times) must be ascertained by experiment. Add 200 µl of diluted horseradish peroxidase conjugate to each well and leave the covered plate for a further 2 hours at room temperature. Wash three times with Buffer A. Add 200 µl of substrate solution to each well. Incubate the plate for 30 min in the dark. Stop the reaction by adding 50 µl of 4M sulphuric acid to each well. Read the absorbance at 492 nm within 30 min, using a microtitre plate reader. Alternatively, transfer 200 µl from each well to a tube containing 800 µl of water and read the absorbance in a spectrophotometer.

Calculation of Results

Calculate the mean absorbance for each point on the standard curve and plot against ferritin concentration using semilogarithmic paper. Read concentrations for the sera from this curve. If results are captured on a file and calculated with a computer program, the log-logit plot provides a linear dose response. For serum ferritin concentrations greater than 200 µg/l, reassay at a dilution of 100 times or greater. Control sera should be included in each assay.

Selecting an Assay Method

The following notes may be of use for those considering introducing a ferritin assay into a clinical laboratory using an immunoassay system.

1. *Limit of detection.* For some early radioimmunoassays, the limit of detection approached 10 µg/l, and this caused difficulties in using the assay for detection of iron deficiency. Most current assays have a lower limit of about 1 µg/l.
2. *The "high-dose hook."* This is a problem peculiar to labelled-antibody assays, particularly two-site immunoradiometric assays.[24] This causes sera with very high ferritin concentrations to give anomalous readings in the lower part of the

standard curve. Most current commercial assays are not affected. Because of the wide range of serum ferritin concentrations that may be encountered in hospital patients (0–40,000 µg/l), it is good practice to dilute and reassay any samples giving readings higher than the working range of the assay.

3. *Interference by non-ferritin proteins in serum.* This may occur with any method but particularly with labelled antibody assays. Serum proteins may inhibit the binding of ferritin to the solid phase when compared with the binding in buffer solution alone. Such an effect may be avoided by diluting the standards in a buffer containing a suitable serum or by diluting serum samples as much as possible. For example, in the assay described earlier, the sample is diluted 20 times with buffer. Another cause of error, which is difficult to detect, is interference by anti-Ig antibodies.[25] These antibodies bind to the animal immunoglobulins used to detect the antigen and form artefactual "sandwiches." Such antibodies are found in about 10% of patients and normal subjects. Interference may be reduced by adding the appropriate species of animal immunoglobulins to block the cross-reaction, but this is not always successful.[26] One solution is to use antibodies from different species as solid-phase and labelled antibodies. Thus one may use a polyclonal, rabbit antiferritin to coat plates in the ELISA with a polyclonal sheep antiferritin labelled with horseradish peroxidase as the second antibody. Rabbit serum (0.5%) replaces BSA in buffer B.
4. *Reproducibility.* Most assays are satisfactory. With microtitre plate assays there may be "edge" effects (differences between readings for inner and outer wells).
5. *Dilution of serum samples.* It should be established that both standard and serum samples dilute in parallel over a 100-fold range.
6. *Accuracy.* The use of the WHO standard ferritin preparation is recommended (see earlier discussion).

Evaluation reports are available from the U.K. Medicines and Healthcare products Regulatory Agency (MHRA; formerly the Medical Devices Agency) for the following systems: Abbott IMx, Abbott AxSYM, and Chiron ACS:180 (MDA/97/41);

Roche Elecsys 2010 (MDA/98/56) and Wallac Auto DELFIA (MDA/00/32) Beckman Coulter Access (MDA/00/18). All provided excellent assays for serum ferritin. The technology is developing rapidly, so reports are rarely available for newly introduced equipment.

Interpretation

The use of serum ferritin for the assessment of iron stores has become well-established.[27] In most normal adults, serum ferritin concentrations lie within the range of 15–300 µg/l. During the first months of life, mean serum ferritin concentrations change considerably, reflecting changes in storage iron concentration. Concentrations are lower in children (<15 years) than in adults and from puberty to middle life are higher in men than in women. In adults, concentrations of less than 15 µg/l indicate an absence of storage iron. Reference ranges quoted by kit manufacturers vary and this is partly a result of the selection of "normal" subjects. Sometimes subjects with iron deficiency are included, and sometimes they are excluded. The interpretation of serum concentration in many pathological conditions is less straightforward, but concentrations of less than 15 µg/l indicate depletion of storage iron. In children, mean levels of storage iron are lower and a threshold of 12 µg/l has been found to be appropriate for detecting iron deficiency.[28]

Iron overload causes high concentrations of serum ferritin, but these may also be found in patients with liver disease, infection, inflammation, or malignant disease. Careful consideration of the clinical evidence is required before concluding that a high serum ferritin concentration is primarily the result of iron overload and not a result of tissue damage or enhanced synthesis of ferritin. A normal ferritin concentration provides good evidence against iron overload but does not exclude genetic haemochromatosis. This is because haemochromatosis is a late-onset condition and iron stores may remain within the normal range for many years.

Serum ferritin concentrations are high in patients with advanced haemochromatosis, but the serum ferritin estimation should not be used alone to screen the relatives of patients or to assess reaccumulation of storage iron after phlebotomy. The early stages of iron accumulation are detectable by an increased serum iron concentration, a decreased unsaturated iron-binding capacity, and increased transferrin saturation; the serum ferritin concentration may be within the normal range. In this situation, the measurement of serum iron and total iron-binding capacity provides useful clinical information not given by the ferritin assay.

In patients with acute or chronic disease, interpretation of serum ferritin concentrations is less straightforward[29] and patients may have serum ferritin concentrations of up to 100 µg/l despite an absence of stainable iron in the bone marrow. Ferritin synthesis[30] is enhanced by interleukin-1— the primary mediator of the acute-phase response. In patients with chronic disease, the following approach should be adopted: low serum ferritin concentrations indicate absent iron stores, values within the normal range indicate either low or normal levels, and high values indicate either normal or high levels. In terms of adequacy of iron stores for replenishing haemoglobin in patients with anaemia, the degree of anaemia must also be considered. Thus a patient with an Hb of 100 g/l may benefit from iron therapy if the serum ferritin concentration is less than 100 µg/l because below this level there is unlikely to be sufficient iron available for full regeneration. Here measurement of serum transferrin receptor concentration may be of value (see p. 147).

Immunologically, plasma ferritin resembles the "L-rich" ferritins of liver and spleen and only low concentrations are detected with antibodies to heart or HeLa cell ferritin, ferritins rich in "H" subunits. The heterogeneity of serum ferritin on isoelectric focusing is largely the result of glycosylation and the presence of variable numbers of sialic acid residues and not variation in the ratio of H to L subunits.[31] Attempts to assay for "acidic" (or "H"-rich) isoferritins in serum as tumour markers have not been successful.[32,33] The iron content of serum ferritin is low,[31] and its measurement is not diagnostically useful.[34]

ESTIMATION OF SERUM IRON CONCENTRATION

Iron is carried in the plasma bound to the protein transferrin (molecular mass 78,000). This molecule binds two atoms of iron as Fe^{3+} and delivers iron to cells by interaction with the membrane transferrin receptor. The following method is a modification of that recommended by the International Council for Standardization in Haematology (ICSH) and is based on the development of a coloured complex when ferrous iron is treated with a chromogen solution.[35]

Reagents and Materials

All reagents must be of analytical grade with the lowest obtainable iron content.

Preparation of Glassware.

It is essential to avoid contamination by iron. If possible, use disposable plastic tubes and bottles. If glassware is to be used, wash in a detergent solution, soak in 2 mol/l HCl for 12 hours, and finally rinse in iron-free water.

Protein Precipitant

100 g/l trichloracetic acid (0.61 M) and 30 ml/l thioglycollic acid in 1 mol/l HCl. This solution may be stored in the dark for 2 months. Ascorbic acid is an alternative reducing agent, although there may be more interference from copper. However, any benefit from reduced copper interference is usually outweighed by the associated health and safety problems of working with thioglycollic acid. To 45 ml 1 mol/l HCl in a 50 ml screwcap tube add 5 ml 6.1 mol/l trichloracetic acid solution (Sigma 490–10). Add 200 mg ascorbic acid and mix. Make a fresh solution when required and discard after 4 hours.

Chromogen Solution

In 100 ml 1.5 mol/l sodium acetate dissolve 25 mg of ferrozine [monosodium 3-(2-pyridyl)-5, 6-bis(4-phenylsulphonic acid)-1, 2, 4-triazine]. Store in the dark for up to 4 weeks.

Iron Standard 80 *μ*mol/l

Add 22.1 ml of deionized water to a universal container (the easiest way is by weight). Add 200 μl of 2 mol/l HCl and mix. Add 100 μl of iron standard solution (1000 μg Fe/ml in 1% HCl, Aldrich No. 30, 595–2) and mix. Store for up to 2 months at room temperature.

Iron-Free Water

Use deionized water for the preparation of all solutions.

Method

Place 0.5 ml of serum (free of haemolysis), 0.5 ml of working iron standard, and 0.5 ml of iron-free water (as a blank), respectively, in each of three 1.5 ml plastic Eppendorf tubes with lids. Add 0.5 ml of protein precipitant to each and replace the lid. Mix the contents vigorously (e.g., with a vortex mixer), and allow to stand for 5 min. Centrifuge the tube containing the serum at 13,000 g for 4 min (in a microfuge) to obtain an optically clear supernatant. To 0.5 ml of this supernatant, and to 0.5 ml of each of the other mixtures, add 0.5 ml of the chromogen solution with thorough mixing. After standing for 10 min, measure the absorbance in a spectrophotometer against water at 562 nm. If a microcentrifuge is not available, use double the volume of serum and reagents in a 3 ml plastic tube with lid and centrifuge at 1500 g for 15 min in a bench centrifuge.

If EDTA-plasma is used, the colour develops more slowly and the preparation should be allowed to stand for at least 15 min before measuring the absorbance. The use of EDTA-plasma is not recommended. Iron chelators (e.g., deferoxamine) also delay colour development.[36]

Calculation

$$\text{Serum iron (μmol/l)} = \frac{(A_{562} \text{ test} - A_{562} \text{ blank})}{(A_{562}\text{standard} - A_{562}\text{blank})} \times 80$$

ALTERNATIVE PROCEDURE: SERUM IRON WITHOUT PROTEIN PRECIPITATION

This is a microtitre plate method developed from the assay of Persijn et al.[37]

Reagents and Materials

Iron Standard

80 μmol/l (see previous). Dilute with an equal volume of water to make the 40 μmol/l standard.

Phosphate–Ascorbate Buffer (Stock)

Add approximately 200 ml of deionized water to an acid-washed plastic beaker. Add 17.5 g sodium dihydrogen orthophosphate ($NaH_2PO_2 2H_2O$) to the water and dissolve fully by stirring (plastic stirrer). Adjust the pH to 4.9 using 2 M NaOH solution (2 g NaOH in 25 ml water). Make the volume up to 250 ml and add 25 ml of the buffer to 10 universal containers. Store for up to 1 month at room temperature. Prior to use, add 50 mg of ascorbic acid to each universal container required and shake to dissolve. Discard after 4 hours.

Chromogen Solution

Add 50 mg of ferrozine (see p. 142) to 25 ml deionized water, and shake to dissolve. Store for up to 1 month in the dark at room temperature.

Microtitre Trays

Microtitre trays should be optical grade, with flat-bottomed wells.

Control Serum

Suitable control sera are Lyphochek (Biorad).

Method

Add 80 μl of deionized water ("0") standard solution (40, 80 μmol/l), controls (C1, C2) and samples (S1, S2, etc.) to the microtitre plate (see plate map, Fig. 7.3).

Add 80 μl of phosphate-ascorbate buffer to each well, using a multichannel pipette. Tap the tray to mix. Leave for 20 min. During this time, take an initial absorbance reading of the tray at 560–570 nm on a microtitre plate reader. Add 40 μl of chromogen solution to each well, then tap the tray to mix. Cover with a film or lid. Incubate for 40 min at 37°C. Take a second absorbance reading. Calculate the net absorbance values.

Calculations

Calculate the difference in Absorbance (δA) between the final and initial readings for the water blank (δA_0), each standard (δA_{40}, δA_{80}) and serum sample (δA_{sample}).

The approximate values are 0.015–0.03 for the water blank (zero standard) and 0.25–0.28 for the 40 μmol Fe/l standard. Subtract the mean net value of the zero standard (δA_0) from each standard or sample (δA_{sample}). The net value of the 80 μmol/l standard should be 2× that of the 40 μmol/l standard.

Serum iron concentrations are:

$$\frac{\Delta A_{sample} - \Delta A_0 \times 40 \text{ μmol/l}}{\Delta A_{40} - \Delta A_0}$$

The data may be downloaded from the plate reader and imported into a suitable database or statistical program (e.g., Excel or Minitab) for these calculations.

Automated Methods

Procedures for measuring serum iron are available for most clinical chemistry analysers. A nonprecipitation method similar to that described earlier is

	1	2	3	4	5	6	7	8	9	10	11	12
A	0	80	C1	S1	S5	S9	S13	S17	S21	S25	S29	S33
B	0	80	C1	S1	S5	S9	S13	S17	S21	S25	S29	S33
C	0	80	C1	S2	S6	S10	S14	S18	S22	S26	S30	S34
D	0	80	C1	S2	S6	S10	S14	S18	S22	S26	S30	S34
E	40	0	C2	S3	S7	S11	S15	S19	S23	S27	S31	S35
F	40	0	C2	S3	S7	S11	S15	S19	S23	S27	S31	S35
G	40	0	C2	S4	S8	S12	S16	S20	S24	S28	S32	S36
H	40	0	C2	S4	S8	S12	S16	S20	S24	S28	S32	S36

Figure 7.3   Plate map for serum iron determination.

available from Randox Ltd (www.randox.com). The performance of several methods was reviewed by Tietz et al[38] who found differences between the various methods, particularly at low values of serum iron concentration. More recently Blanck et al[39] carried out an interlaboratory comparison and found no significant differences in results generated by methods currently in use. Variability across laboratories and across methods was low. Serum iron concentrations may be measured by atomic absorption spectroscopy, but this has the disadvantage of measuring any haem iron present as a result of haemolysis.

SERUM IRON CONCENTRATIONS IN HEALTH AND DISEASE[36]

Jacobs et al[40] measured serum iron concentrations in a random sample of 517 women and 499 men in the general population of Wales. Serum iron concentrations approximated to a normal distribution. The mean (± SD) of 16.1 ± 7.4 μmol/l in women was slightly lower than for men (18.0 ± 6.3 μmol/l). These figures do not refer to "iron replete" subjects because subjects with absent iron stores or with frank anaemia were included. Using the microtitre plate method described earlier, Jackson et al[41] determined serum iron concentrations in 10,500 blood donors from South Wales. For 1502 "first time" donors, mean age of 28 years, the mean (± SD) was 16.7 ± 6.0 μmol/l for men and 14.4 ± 6.7 μmol/l for women. Again subjects included potential donors who failed the screening test for anaemia and were not permitted to give blood on that occasion. In the first month of life mean concentration of serum iron is higher (22 μmol/l) than in adults, falls to about 12 μmol/l by the age of 1 year, and remains at that level throughout childhood.[42,43]

Measurement of the serum iron concentration alone provides little useful clinical information because, although methodological variation is low, there is considerable variation from hour to hour and day to day in normal individuals (see p. 151). Low concentrations are found in patients with iron deficiency anaemia; in chronic disease (including inflammation, infection, and cancer); and during the acute-phase response, including after surgery.

Therefore, low serum iron concentrations do not necessarily indicate an absence of storage iron. High concentrations are found in liver disease, hypoplastic anaemias, ineffective erythropoiesis, and iron overload.

IRON-BINDING CAPACITY, SERUM TRANSFERRIN, AND TRANSFERRIN SATURATION

Estimation of Total Iron-Binding Capacity

In the plasma, iron is bound to transferrin and the total iron-binding capacity (TIBC) is a measure of this protein. The additional iron-binding capacity of transferrin is known as the unsaturated iron-binding capacity (UIBC). The serum iron concentration plus the UIBC together give TIBC.

Iron-binding capacity is usually measured by adding an excess of iron and measuring the iron retained in solution after the addition of a suitable reagent such as light magnesium carbonate or an ion-exchange resin that removes excess iron. All methods are empiric, and none is completely satisfactory. The method described as follows was developed by the ICSH.[44]

Principle

Excess iron as ferric chloride is added to serum. Any iron that does not bind to transferrin is removed with excess magnesium carbonate. The iron concentration of the iron-saturated serum is then measured.

Reagents

Basic magnesium carbonate, $MgCO_3$, "light grade." *Saturating solution (100 μmol Fe/l).* Add 17.7 ml deionized water to a universal container (by weight is most convenient). Add 100 μl of 1 mol/l HCl. Add 100 μl of iron standard solution (see p. 142). Mix and store for up to 2 months at room temperature. The "saturating iron solution" contains 5.6 μg Fe/ml (100 μmol Fe/l).

Method

Place 0.5 ml of serum (EDTA-plasma should not be used) in a 1.5 ml Eppendorf tube and add 0.5 ml of saturating iron solution. Mix carefully by hand and leave at room temperature for 15 min. Use a plastic scoop or tube to add 100 mg (±15 mg) of light magnesium carbonate, and cap the tube. Shake vigorously and allow to stand for 30 min with occasional mixing. Centrifuge at 13,000 g for 4 min in a microcentrifuge. If the supernatant contains traces of magnesium carbonate, remove the supernatant and recentrifuge. Carefully remove 0.5 ml of the supernatant and treat as serum for the iron estimation described earlier. Multiply the final result by 2.

DETERMINATION OF UNSATURATED IRON-BINDING CAPACITY

The UIBC may be determined by methods that detect iron remaining, and able to bind to chromogen, after adding a standard and excess amount of iron to the serum.[37] The UIBC is the difference between the amount added and the amount binding to the chromogen.

Reagents and Materials

Saturating Solution 2000 μmol/l
Add 7.95 ml of deionized water to a universal container (by weight is most convenient). Add 1.0 ml of iron standard solution (see p. 142 HCl). Mix. Store for up to 2 months at room temperature.

Tris Buffer (Stock)
Add approximately 200 ml of deionized water to a weighed acid-washed plastic beaker. Add 6.8 g Tris to the water and fully dissolve by stirring with a plastic stirrer. Adjust the pH to 7.8 using 2 M HCl. Adjust the volume to 250 ml with water (by weight), mix, and add 24.5 ml (24.5 g) into universal containers. Store for up to 1 month at room temperature.

Tris–Ascorbate–Iron Buffer
Immediately prior to use, add 50 mg of ascorbic acid to each universal container of Tris buffer required and dissolve by mixing. Add 0.5 ml of the saturating solution (2000 μmol/l) and mix. Discard after 4 hours.

Chromogen Solution
See page 142.

Microtitre Trays
See page 143.

Control Serum
See page 143.

Method

Add 80 μl of deionized water ("0"), control (C1, C2), and sample (S1, S2, etc.) to the microtitre plate (see Fig. 7.4). Add 160 μl of Tris–ascorbate–iron buffer

	1	2	3	4	5	6	7	8	9	10	11	12
A	0	C1	S1	S5	S9	S13	S17	S21	S25	S29	S33	S37
B	0	C1	S1	S5	S9	S13	S17	S21	S25	S29	S33	S37
C	0	C1	S2	S6	S10	S14	S18	S22	S26	S30	S34	S38
D	0	C1	S2	S6	S10	S14	S18	S22	S26	S30	S34	S38
E	0	C2	S3	S7	S11	S15	S19	S23	S27	S31	S35	S39
F	0	C2	S3	S7	S11	S15	S19	S23	S27	S31	S35	S39
G	0	C2	S4	S8	S12	S16	S20	S24	S28	S32	S36	S40
H	0	C2	S4	S8	S12	S16	S20	S24	S28	S32	S36	S40

Figure 7.4   Plate map for UIBC determination.

to each well, using a multichannel pipette. Tap the tray to mix. Leave the tray for 20 min. During this time, take an initial reading ($A_{initial}$) of the $A_{560-570\ nm}$. Add 40 μl of chromogen solution to each sample and tap the tray to mix; cover with a film or lid. Incubate for 40 min at 37°C. Take a final absorbance reading (A_{final}).

Calculations

The saturating solution added to each well (160 μl) contains 6.4 nmol Fe. Calculate the absorbance reading corresponding to 6.4 nmol Fe from the mean value of the readings in column 1 as $A_{final} - A_{initial}$ (A_s). (Note: This absorbance reading should be within 5% of the 80 μmol/l value for the iron determination.)

Once A_s has been calculated, it is used in the following equation:

For controls 1 and 2 and samples:

$$UIBC = [1- (A_{final}- A_{initial})] / A_s \times 80\ \mu mol/l$$

Data may be imported into a database for calculation. As with the serum iron determination, protocols for clinical chemistry analysers sometimes include a method for UIBC.

Determination of total iron-binding capacity from UIBC:

$$TIBC = serum\ iron + UIBC\ (\mu mol/l)$$

Fully Automated Methods

A number of methods used to determine the TIBC using clinical chemistry analysers require a pre-treatment step. Direct (fully automated procedures) have been developed.[45] A nonprecipitation method (UIBC) similar to that described earlier is available from Randox Ltd. (www.randox.com).

SERUM TRANSFERRIN

An alternative approach is to measure transferrin directly by an immunological assay. This avoids some of the spuriously high values of TIBC found when the transferrin is saturated and nontransferrin iron is measured.[35] Rate immunonephelometric methods are rapid and precise.[46] There is generally a good correlation between the chemical and immunological TIBC,[47,48] although when TIBC was calculated as the sFe + UIBC, values were lower than the direct TIBC.[47,48] Transferrin concentrations (g/l) may be converted to TIBC (μmol/l) by multiplying by 25, and this factor appears to be appropriate in practice as well as theory.[49]

Normal Range of Transferrin and Total Iron-Binding Capacity

In health, the serum transferrin is c 2.0–3.0 g/l, and 1 mg of transferrin binds 1.4 μg of iron. The normal serum TIBC (mean ± SD) was 68.0 ± 12.6 μmol/l in a random sample of 517 women and 63.2 ± 9.1 μmol/l for 499 men.[40] For 890 first-time, female blood donors of mean age 27 years the mean TIBC (determined by the UIBC method described earlier) was 56.7 ± 12.1 μmol/l. In 612 first-time, male blood donors of mean age 28 years the mean was 54.2 ± 10 μmol/l (mean ± SD).[41] In both surveys the sample included some individuals with iron deficiency. Note the comment earlier about lower values given by the colorimetric UIBC method. The TIBC is increased in iron deficiency anaemia and in pregnancy; it is lower than normal in infections, malignant disease, and renal disease. In pathological iron overload, the TIBC of the serum is reduced.

Diagnostically, although a raised TIBC is characteristic of iron deficiency anaemia, the TIBC is usually used to calculate the transferrin saturation. The UIBC has attracted little diagnostic use, but is being evaluated as a screening test for iron overload in genetic haemochromatosis. In genetic haemochromatosis (subjects homozygous for *HFE* C282Y), a UIBC (determined as described earlier) of less than 20 μmol Fe/l was found in most men and in about 50% of women.[41] UIBC and transferrin saturation were equally sensitive and specific. For UIBC methods, optimum thresholds for detecting subjects with genetic haemochromatosis have varied. Murtagh et al[50] determined the optimum threshold to be 25.6 μmol/l (sensitivity 0.91 and specificity 0.95). In this case, fasting blood samples were taken. UIBC was as reliable as transferrin saturation in detecting HFE haemochromatosis in both reports.

TRANSFERRIN SATURATION

The transferrin saturation is the ratio of the serum iron concentration and the TIBC expressed as a percentage. If transferrin is measured immunologically, then the corresponding TIBC (µmol/l) may be calculated by multiplying the transferrin concentration (g/l) by 25. In a sample of the Welsh population,[40] the mean transferrin saturation in 499 men was 29.1 ± 11.0%; in 517 women it was 24.6 ± 11.8%. For first-time blood donors from South Wales the mean transferrin saturation was 31.1 ± 10.9% for 612 men and 25.5 ± 12.9% for 890 women. A transferrin saturation of less than 16% is usually considered to indicate an inadequate iron supply for erythropoiesis.[51] The most valuable use of calculating transferrin saturation is for the detection of genetic haemochromatosis. Even in the early stages of the development of iron overload,[41,52] an elevated transferrin saturation is indicative of the disorder (suggested thresholds vary but >55% for men and >50% for women are an appropriate compromise).[16]

Transferrin Index

Beilby et al[46] have recommended that the transferrin saturation is replaced by the "transferrin index." This is the serum iron concentration (µmol/l) divided by the transferrin concentration (determined immunologically and expressed as µmol/l). They claimed that the transferrin index had better precision than the transferrin saturation and showed greater specificity for detecting iron overload than the transferrin saturation. However, the transferrin index has attracted little use.

SERUM TRANSFERRIN RECEPTOR

Almost all cells in the body obtain iron from the plasma protein, transferrin, but transferrin has a very high affinity for iron at neutral pH and iron release takes place through a specific membrane receptor. The transferrin receptor consists of two identical, protein subunits of molecular mass 95 kDa. Transferrin binds to the receptor, the complex is internalized, and iron is released when the pH of the internal vesicles is reduced to about 5.5. After iron release, apotransferrin returns to the circulation and can undertake further cycles of iron uptake and delivery.[53] The cells that require the most iron are the nucleated red cells in the bone marrow, which synthesize haemoglobin, and these have the greatest number of transferrin receptors. Transferrin receptor synthesis is also controlled by iron supply. The mechanism involves IREs (see p. 134), iron regulatory elements at the 3' untranslated region of the receptor mRNA. In the absence of iron, an IRP binds to the RNA, thus stabilizing it and permitting synthesis of the peptide. In the presence of adequate iron concentrations, binding of iron by the IRP changes the conformation of the protein and prevents its binding to the mRNA. The mRNA is rapidly broken down, and synthesis of transferrin receptors is reduced. A second receptor, TFR2, also binds transferrin, but its synthesis is not regulated by IRPs.[54]

In 1986, Kohgo et al[55] reported that transferrin receptors were detectable in the plasma by immunoassay. Since then, there has been much investigation of the physiological and diagnostic significance of circulating transferrin receptors.[56] The protein is derived by proteolysis at the cell membrane and circulates bound to transferrin. Plasma concentrations reflect the number of cellular receptors and, in patients with adequate iron stores, the number of nucleated red cells in the bone marrow. Because the number of cellular transferrin receptors per cell increases in iron deficiency, concentrations also increase when erythropoiesis becomes iron limited. Table 7.4 summarises the conditions associated with reduced or elevated levels of circulating transferrin receptor.

Assays for the Serum Transferrin Receptor

There has been no agreement about the source of transferrin receptor as standard or as an antigen for the raising of antibodies. Transferrin receptors have been purified from placenta and from serum. The receptor may or may not be bound to transferrin as a standard or to raise antibodies. No "reference" method is therefore described here. Three enzyme immunoassay kits (Orion; Ramco; R&D) for the determination of serum transferrin receptor concentrations have been evaluated for the Medical

Table 7.4 Serum transferrin receptor (sTfR) concentrations in human disease

sTfR concentration	Condition
Increased	Increased erythroid proliferation:
	Autoimmune haemolytic anaemia
	Hereditary spherocytosis
	β Thalassaemia intermedia or major
	β Thalassaemia/HbE
	Haemoglobin H disease
	Sickle cell anaemia
	Polycythaemia vera
	Decreased tissue iron stores:
	Iron deficiency anaemia
Normal to increased	Idiopathic myelofibrosis
	Myelodysplastic syndrome
	Chronic lymphocytic leukaemia
Normal	Haemochromatosis (but see text)
	Acute and chronic myeloid leukaemia
	Most lymphoid malignancies
	Solid tumours
	Anaemia of chronic disease
Decreased	Chronic renal failure
	Aplastic anaemia
	Postbone marrow transplantation

Modified from Feelders et al.[53]

Devices Agency.[57] All have been approved for diagnostic purposes in the United States by the Food and Drug Administration. Assays for fully automated, diagnostic, immunoassay systems are now being introduced and offer improved sensitivity, reproducibility, and speed. One example is the Nichols Advantage system (www.nicholsdiag.com).

The different reference ranges in the available commercial assays reflect the differences in preparations of transferrin receptor used to raise antibodies and as a standard in the various assays. For the Orion, Ramco, and R&D kits Akesson et al[58] and Worwood et al[57] noted some assay drift but found acceptable intraassay coefficient of variance

(CV) values. The determined sensitivity was adequate for clinical purposes for the three assay systems. There are differences in units and absolute amounts for serum transferrin receptor concentrations. Four different units (nmol/l, g/ml, mg/l [ng/ml], and kU/l) and different normal ranges are in use.[59] At the present time serum transferrin receptor (sTfR) is not included in the national external quality control schemes for the UK (NEQAS) and the Welsh External Quality Assessment Scheme (WEQAS).

Reference Ranges

sTfR concentrations are high in neonates and decline until adult concentrations are reached at 17 years. Concentrations are similar in normal men and women, unlike serum concentrations, which are lower in premenopausal women than in men. During pregnancy sTfR levels increase, returning to nonpregnant values 12 weeks after delivery.[60] sTfR concentrations with different assay systems cannot be directly compared because reference ranges differ. At present it is necessary to either establish a reference range from a panel of healthy subjects or accept that recommended by the manufacturer.

Samples

The information provided by the manufacturers shows good recovery of standard and linearity but some problems with interference. Although serum is the preferred matrix, the R&D and Ramco assays give the same results with EDTA, heparin, and citrate plasma. Orion states that EDTA-plasma is not acceptable. It is recommended that sera are stored for no more than 2 days at room temperature, 7 days at 2–8°C, 6 months at –20°C, and 1 year at –70°C. Repeated freezing and thawing are not advisable. Moderate haemolysis is not a problem. There is no interference at serum bilirubin concentrations of less than 1700 μmol/l (R&D) or 280 μmol/l (Orion). However, Ramco noted that addition of bilirubin at a concentration of 17 μmol/l (10 μg/ml) caused a 16% increase in apparent serum transferrin receptor concentration. This represents a bilirubin concentration of only about twice the upper limit of normal.

Transferrin Receptor Concentrations in Diagnosis

Erythropoiesis

The function of the TfR in delivering iron to the immature red cell immediately suggested an application in the clinical laboratory for the assay of circulating TfR. The use of the assay to monitor changes in the rate of erythropoiesis has been explored by several authors.[61-63] When iron supply is not limiting, the assay can provide a replacement for ferrokinetic investigations that required the injection of radioactive iron.[64]

Iron Deficiency

The major application of the serum transferrin receptor assay has been to detect patients with an absence of stored iron (ferritin and haemosiderin in cells). When normal subjects are subjected to quantitative phlebotomy, serum ferritin concentrations decrease steadily as iron stores are depleted, but there is little change in sTfR concentration. As iron stores become exhausted (serum ferritin $<15\,\mu g/l$), sTfR levels increase and continue increasing as haemoglobin concentrations decrease.[65] In this study the increased rate of erythropoiesis during phlebotomy had little effect on sTfR levels as long as iron stores were adequate so that most of the increase in sTfR level must be the result of iron deficiency rather than increased erythropoiesis. However, the rate of phlebotomy was only 250 ml per week (about 500 ml per week is usually removed during treatment of haemochromatosis) and higher rates might cause an immediate increase in sTfR levels during phlebotomy. The Log[sTfR/serum ferritin] gives a linear relationship with storage iron that has considerable potential for assessing iron stores in epidemiological studies.[66] In infants (age 8–15 months) sTfR concentration increases as the severity of iron deficiency increases.[67]

Circulating transferrin receptor levels increased, not only in patients with simple iron deficiency, but also in patients with the anaemia of chronic disease who lack stainable iron in the bone marrow.[68] Detection of a lack of storage iron is difficult in patients with the anaemia of chronic disease because serum iron concentrations are low regardless of iron stores and serum ferritin concentrations, although reflecting the level of iron stores, are

higher than in patients not suffering from chronic disease (see page 141). However, in several studies the sTFR has not proved to be superior to serum ferritin for detecting iron deficiency.[119-125]

In both iron deficiency anaemia and the anaemia of chronic disease, sTfR levels are also influenced by changes in the rate of erythropoiesis. Ineffective erythropoiesis—an increase in the proportion of immature red cells destroyed within the bone marrow—increases in iron deficiency anaemia.[69] In the anaemia of chronic disease, erythropoiesis is normal or depressed[69]; nevertheless iron deficiency increases the number of receptors.[70]

Although it has been claimed that sTfR measurements provide a sensitive indicator of iron deficiency in pregnancy,[71] questions remain about the decreased erythropoiesis in early pregnancy because this may mask iron deficiency at this time[72] and increases in sTfR in later pregnancy appear to relate to increased erythropoiesis rather than iron depletion.[60] Measurement of sTfR did not enhance the sensitivity and specificity for the detection of iron deficiency anaemia in pregnant women from Malawi, where anaemia and chronic disease are very prevalent.[73]

Iron Overload

Normal concentrations of sTfR have been reported for patients with genetic haemochromatosis (although some had been venesected) and also for patients with African iron overload.[74] In contrast, lower mean values of sTfR were found in subjects with a raised transferrin saturation.[75,76] However, there is considerable overlap with the normal range of sTfR concentration, and measurement of sTfR in iron overload is unlikely to be of diagnostic value.

ERYTHROCYTE PROTOPORPHYRIN

Assay of erythrocyte protoporphyrin (EP)[13] has been performed for many years as a screening test for lead poisoning. More recently, there has been considerable interest in its use in evaluating the iron supply to the bone marrow. The "free" protoporphyrin concentration of red blood cells increases in iron deficiency. Usually, more than 95% is present as zinc protoporphyrin (ZPP). The original method required a chemical extraction and use of a fluorescence spectrometer. This has now been largely replaced, for detection of iron deficiency, by the direct measurement of the fluorescence of ZPP (μmol/mol haem) in an instrument called a haematofluorometer.

Analysers

Two dedicated analysers are available: the Proto Fluor Z from Helena Laboratories, Beaumont, Texas (www.helena.com) and a portable machine from Aviv Biomedical, Inc. (www.avivbiomedical.com). The machines should be operated exactly as described by the manufacturer. The small sample size (about 20 μl of venous or skin-puncture blood), simplicity, rapidity, and reproducibility within a laboratory are advantages. Furthermore, the test has an interesting retrospective application. Because it takes weeks for a significant proportion of the circulating red blood cells to be replaced with new cells, it is possible to make a diagnosis of iron deficiency anaemia some time after iron therapy has commenced. Chronic diseases that reduce serum iron concentration, but do not reduce iron stores, also increase protoporphyrin levels.[77]

Diagnostic Applications

The measurement of EP levels as an indicator of iron deficiency has particular advantages in paediatric haematology and in large-scale surveys in which the small sample size and simplicity of the test are important. The normal range in adults is less than 70 μmol/mol haem. Mean values in normal women are slightly higher than in men.[78] One potential confounder is the contribution of other fluorescent compounds (including drugs) in the plasma, and concentrations are lower if washed red cells are assayed.[79] Garrett and Worwood[80] found a mean (range) of 44 (30–68) μmol/mol haem in women and 41 (29–64) in men. However, washing is a tedious process and is rarely undertaken. Paediatric reference ranges have been determined in 6478 subjects (ages 0–17 years).[81] Mean ZPP values were higher in females than males and declined slightly with age. A diurnal variation was noted, with ZPP concentrations being higher between 18.00 and midnight. No explanation was offered.

The WHO[28] has recommended levels for the detection of iron deficiency. For children younger than age 5 years, levels should be greater than 61 μmol/mol haem; for all other subjects, levels should be greater than 70 μmol/mol haem. These are higher than the 97.5 percentile established from surveys of healthy children[81] and are based on the sensitivity and specificity for detecting the absence of storage iron.

Units

To convert between the various units used to express protoporphyrin levels, the following calculations apply:

$$\mu g \text{ EP/dl red cell} = \mu g \text{ EP/dl whole blood/haematocrit}$$

From μg EP/dl red cell to μg EP/g Hb
multiply by 0.037

From μg EP/dl red cell to μmol EP/mol haem
multiply by 0.87

These factors are based on an assumed normal mean cell haemoglobin concentration, although this may be measured in individual samples and an appropriate factor calculated.

Infection and inflammation, lead poisoning, and haemolytic anaemia all cause significant elevation of ZPP. Measurement of ZPP is most useful when iron deficiency is common and the other conditions are rare. In the general clinical laboratory, therefore, ZPP provides less information about iron storage levels in patients with anaemia than does the serum ferritin assay.[82]

Although blood samples may be taken at any time of day, fresh blood is required (samples must not be frozen) and the method has not been automated.

METHODOLOGICAL AND BIOLOGICAL VARIABILITY OF ASSAYS

The blood assays vary greatly in both methodological and biological stability. Haemoglobin concentrations are stable, and a simple and well-standardised method ensures relatively low day-to-day variation in individuals (Table 7.5). Automated cell counters

Table 7.5 Overall variability of assays for iron status (within subject, day–to-day coefficient of variance for healthy subjects)

Hb	Serum ferritin	Serum iron	TIBC	ZPP	STfR	Reference
	15 (M; F)					83
1.6 (F)	15 (M; F)					112
		29(F)				113
		27 (M)				114
3 (MF)						115
	15 (M; F)	29 (M; F)				116
	13 (M; F)*	33 (M; F)*	11 (M; F)*			117
4 (MF)	14 (M)	27 (M)				84
	26 (F)	28 (F)				
	27 (M; F)	29 (M; F)	7 (M; F)		14 (M; F)	94
	26 (F)V				14 (F)	86
	15 (M)V				12 (M)	
	28 (F)C				11(F)	
	12 (M)C				10 (M)	
				5 (M; F)		79
3 (F)†	11 (F)†	26 (F)†	4 (F)†		13 (F)†	118

F, female; M, male; STfR, serum transferrin receptor; TIBC, total iron-binding capacity; ZPP, zinc protoporphyrin.
*Patients with anaemia.
†70–79-year-old healthy women.
CCapillary blood
VVenous blood.

analyse at least 10,000 cells and thus increase precision. ZPP values also appear to be relatively stable. The more complicated procedures involved in immunoassays mean higher methodological variation for serum ferritin assays (CV of at least 5%) and this, coupled with some physiological variation, gives an overall CV for serum ferritin for an individual over a period of weeks of the order of 15%. There is, however, little evidence of any significant diurnal variation in serum ferritin concentration.[83] The serum iron determination is an example of extremes with reasonably low methodological variation coupled with extreme physiological variability, giving an overall "within subject" CV of approximately 30% when venous samples are taken at the same time of day. A diurnal rhythm has been reported with higher values in the morning than in late afternoon, when the concentration may fall to 50% of the morning value.[36] However, variations are not consistently diurnal.[83a] The circadian fluctuation is largely the result of variation in the release of iron from the reticuloendothelial system to the plasma. It should be noted that for the studies summarised in Table 7.5 the type of blood sample, length of study period, and statistical analysis vary. The somewhat higher variability for Hb and ferritin reported by Borel et al[84] may be a result of their use of capillary blood and plasma. Pootrakul et al[85] have demonstrated that mean plasma ferritin concentration is slightly higher in capillary specimens than venous specimens and that within and between sample variation was approximately 3-fold greater. Variability was less for capillary serum than plasma but still greater than for venous serum. However, the increased variability of capillary samples may be related to sampling technique because Cooper and Zlotkin[86] found little difference in variability between venous and capillary samples.

The effect of menstruation on iron-status indicators was examined in 1712 women aged 18–44 years from the Second National Health and Nutrition Examination Survey (NHANES II) after adjusting for potential confounders. Adjusted mean values of Hb, transferrin saturation, and serum ferritin were lowest for women whose blood was drawn during menses and highest for women examined in luteal or late luteal phase of the menstrual cycle (Hb, 130 vs. 133 g/l; transferrin saturation, 21.2% vs. 24.8%, $P < 0.01$ for both; serum ferritin, 17.2 vs. 24.0 µg/l, $P < 0.05$). The prevalence estimate of impaired iron status was significantly higher for women whose blood was drawn during the menstrual phase than for women whose blood was drawn during the luteal and late luteal phases. The authors concluded that cyclic variations in indicators of iron status are a potential source of error when iron status is assessed in large population surveys that include women of reproductive age.[87]

Starvation, or even fasting for a short period, can cause elevation of the serum ferritin concentration,[88] and vitamin C deficiency can reduce ferritin concentration.[89] Moderate exercise has little effect on serum ferritin concentration,[90] although exhausting exercise leads to increases in serum ferritin concentration as a result of muscle damage and inflammatory reactions.[91,92] Seasonal changes in red cell parameters have been reported[93] and Maes et al[94] found statistically significant seasonal patterns for serum iron, transferrin, serum ferritin, and sTfR. The peak–trough difference in the yearly variation, expressed as a percentage of the mean, was greatest for serum ferritin (39%) and least for sTfR and transferrin (12%).

These results have clear implications for the use of these assays in population studies.[95-97] For accurate diagnosis either a multiparameter analysis is required or several samples should be assayed. For haemoglobin, one sample is required for 95% confidence and 20% accuracy[98]; for sTfR, one sample was required,[86,99] but for ferritin one to three samples was required.[86,98] This is the number of days required to estimate the true average value of the indicator for a subject (i.e., within 20% of the true value 95% of the time).

PREDICTIVE VALUE OF INDICATORS OF IRON METABOLISM

The major diagnostic use of the various measures of iron status is in the differential diagnosis of hypochromic anaemia. The large amount of iron present as haemoglobin means that the degree of any anaemia must always be considered in assessing iron status. There is an overall reduction in body iron in iron deficiency anaemia. No single measurement of iron status is ideal for all clinical circumstances because all are affected by confounding factors (Table 7.3). The anaemia of chronic disorders is associated with normal or increased iron stores (normal or increased serum ferritin) accompanied by a reduced tissue iron supply (low serum iron and low to normal TIBC). Although the serum ferritin is an acute-phase reactant, values below 50 µg/l are usually associated with absent iron stores in rheumatoid arthritis, renal disease, and inflammatory bowel disease. Serum transferrin receptor levels may also provide valuable diagnostic information on iron deficiency in chronic disease.

Despite years of investigations, there is little reliable comparative information. The main reason for this is the difficulty of distinguishing between the presence and absence of storage iron. Most investigators have used the grade of storage iron in the bone marrow as a "gold standard." This is an invasive procedure and therefore limits drastically the number of patients investigated. It is often difficult to justify bone marrow aspiration to determine a patient's iron status and even more difficult in the case of normal volunteers. Furthermore, bone marrow aspiration followed by staining for iron is not a reproducible procedure. Observer error,[100] inadequate specimens, and lack of correlation with response to iron therapy[101] have been described. Demonstrating a response in Hb to oral iron therapy has been the method of choice in paediatric practice.

Iron Deficiency Anaemia in Adults

Almost all measures show a high sensitivity and specificity for distinguishing between subjects with iron deficiency and those with iron stores and normal haemoglobin levels in the absence of any other disease process. Guyatt et al[102] conducted a systematic review of the diagnostic value of the various laboratory tests for the diagnosis of iron deficiency. They concluded that serum ferritin was the most powerful test for simple iron deficiency and also for iron deficiency in hospital patients. However, this analysis did not include the transferrin receptor.

Detection of Iron Deficiency in Acute or Chronic Disease

Table 7.6 summarises a number of studies in which bone marrow iron was assessed and the sensitivity and specificity of various assays was compared. Despite very different results between studies, some general points may be made.

Conventional red cell parameters, mean cell volume (MCV), and mean cell haemoglobin do not distinguish between the presence or absence of bone marrow iron in patients with chronic disease. The serum iron concentration is almost invariably low in chronic disease and, although the TIBC (or transferrin concentration) is higher for patients with no storage iron, neither this measurement, nor the transferrin saturation derived from the serum iron and TIBC, provide useful discrimination.

In chronic disease serum ferritin concentration reflects storage iron levels but are higher than in normal subjects. It is necessary to set a threshold of 30–50 µg/l to distinguish between the presence and absence of storage iron. Even with this limit sensitivity is low.

Combinations of serum ferritin, erythrocyte sedimentation rate (ESR), or C-reactive protein (CRP) either in a discriminant analysis[99] or logistic regression[103] provide only marginal improvement in the ability to detect a lack of storage iron.

The serum transferrin receptor level discriminates between the presence and absence of storage iron, although there is disagreement as to whether the assay is superior to serum ferritin. Several studies

Table 7.6 Sensitivity/specificity of methods for diagnosis of iron deficiency in the presence of chronic disease

In adults, iron stores are determined by staining for iron in bone marrow. Optimum diagnostic thresholds selected vary.								
Test	1	2*	3*	4	5	6	7	8
References	119	120	68	121	123	124	125	
MCV	–	–	0.86	–	–	0.42/0.83	–	–
% Hypo	–	–	–	0.77/0.90	–	–	–	–
Serum iron	–	–	0.68	L	–	–	NS	–
TIBC	–	–	0.84[†]	L	–	–	–	–
% Saturation	–	–	0.79[†]	L	–	0.38–0.89	–	–
Serum ferritin	0.79/0.97	0.870	0.89	0.86/0.90	1.00/0.81	0.25/0.99	0.94/0.95	0.92/0.98
ZPP	0.74/0.94		–	L	–	–	–	–
STfR	0.63/0/81	0.704	0.98	L	1.00/0.84	0.71/0.74	0.61/0.68	0.92/0.84
sTfR/log ferritin	0.74/0.97	0.865	1.00	–	1.00/0.97	0.67/0.93	–	–

L, Lower sensitivity/specificity than serum ferritin, individually or in combination. The combination of ferritin and erythrocyte sedimentation rate or C-reactive protein did not improve efficiency. MCV, mean cell volume; TIBC, total iron-binding capacity; ZPP, zinc protoporphyrin; STfR, serum transferrin receptor.
References in Row 1: 1, 119; 2, 120; 3, 68; 4, 121; 5, 122; 6, 123; 7, 124; 8, 125.
*Area under receiver operating characteristics (ROC) curve.
[†]Transferrin concentration (equivalent to TIBC; see text).
[‡]Transferrin index (equivalent to % saturation; see text).

show that the sTfR/log$_{10}$ ferritin ratio provides superior discrimination to either test on its own. The use of Log ferritin decreases the influence of serum ferritin (and thus the acute-phase response) on the overall ratio. Although the Log[sTfR/ ferritin] is an excellent measure of iron stores in healthy subjects,[66] this transformation (i.e., after calculating the ratio of sTfR/ferritin) may not provide the best discrimination for clinical applications. When the assay of sTfR is readily available on high-throughput immunoanalysers the sTfR/log ferritin ratio may provide the best discriminator for identifying the coexistence of iron deficiency in chronic disease. However, this will also require standardisation of units and ranges for the various sTfR assays if the use of the ratio is to gain wide acceptance.

Functional Iron Deficiency

Functional iron deficiency is the situation in which iron stores are apparently adequate but iron supply for erythropoiesis remains inadequate. This often occurs during the treatment of patients with anaemia and renal failure with erythropoietin. The diagnostic question is to identify those patients with a functional iron deficiency who will require parenteral iron therapy to respond to erythropoietin with an acceptable increase in Hb. The percentage hypochromic erythrocytes is a good predictor of response.[104] Fishbane and colleagues[105] concluded that reticulocyte haemoglobin content (CHr) was a markedly more stable analyte than serum ferritin or transferrin saturation and it predicted functional iron deficiency more efficiently. They did not include percentage hypochromic cells in their analysis. Fernandez-Rodriguez and colleagues[106] assessed the sensitivity and specificity of ferritin, TIBC, transferrin saturation index, red blood cell ferritin, and sTfR in 63 patients with anaemia and chronic renal failure undergoing dialysis, who were not being treated with erythropoietin. Storage iron was assessed by bone marrow iron staining. For serum ferritin, a cut-off value of 121 g/l gave a sensitivity and specificity of 75%. Efficiency was lower for sTfR and RBC ferritin. MCV, transferrin saturation index, and TIBC showed the lowest values for sensitivity and specificity.

Iron Deficiency in Infancy and Childhood

In infants, thresholds for the diagnosis of iron deficiency and iron deficiency anaemia are not universally agreed. There are rapid changes in iron status in the first year of life as fetal haemoglobin is replaced by haemoglobin A. The serum ferritin concentration is a less useful guide to iron deficiency than in adults partly because of the rapid decline in concentration in the first 6 months and the low concentrations generally found in children older than 6 months of age. Domellof et al[107] have suggested revised cut-offs for iron deficiency, including serum ferritin and sTfR, for infants up to age 1 year.

In children the reason for detecting iron deficiency is to identify those who will respond to iron therapy. Margolis et al[108] found that the best predictor of response was the initial Hb, although sensitivity was only 66% and specificity was 60%. Serum ferritin, transferrin saturation, and erythrocyte protoporphyrin (EP) had even lower efficiencies, and combination of the various measures made little improvement. Hershko et al[109] studied children in villages from the Golan Heights (Israel) and concluded that EP was a more reliable index of iron deficiency than serum ferritin. They suggested that a significant incidence of chronic disease affected both ferritin and iron values. ZPP provides a useful indicator of iron-deficient erythropoiesis, although high values may indicate lead poisoning rather than iron deficiency. The small sample volume for ZPP determination is also an advantage in paediatric practice.

A report published in 2003 confirms the effect of low-level infection on measures of iron status. Abraham et al[110] studied 101 healthy, 11-month-old infants. On the morning of blood sampling, slight clinical signs of airway infection were observed for 42 infants. Extensive blood analyses were done, including high sensitivity C-reactive protein (CRP). CRP measured by the routine methods gave values of less than 6 mg/l for all infants, but with the high sensitivity assay values were higher for many infants with symptoms of airway infection. Serum iron concentration was depressed in these children and correlated significantly with CRP level. When a further blood sample was taken, serum ferritin concentration was higher for the children with the higher CRP level, serum iron was reduced, but sTfR and transferrin levels were unaffected.

Pregnancy

In early pregnancy serum ferritin concentrations usually provide a reliable indication of iron deficiency. Haemodilution in the second and third trimesters of pregnancy reduces the concentrations of all measures of iron status, and this means that the threshold values for iron deficiency established in nonpregnant women are not appropriate. In principle, determination of values as ratios (ZPP umol/mol haem, transferrin saturation, and sTfR/ferritin) should be more reliable. In healthy women who were not anaemic and who were supplemented with iron,[60] serum iron, TS, and sFn fell from the first to the third trimester and increased after delivery; TIBC increased during pregnancy and fell after delivery. sTfR concentrations showed a substantial increase (approximately twofold) during pregnancy, and this probably reflects increased erythropoiesis.[60] In contrast, Carriaga et al[71] reported that the mean sTfR concentration of pregnant women in the third trimester did not differ from that in nonpregnant women and that sTfR concentration was not influenced by pregnancy *per se*. Choi et al suggest that different assays and different ages in the control groups may explain this discrepancy.[60]

CONCLUSION

Body iron status usually may be assessed by considering the Hb, red cell indices, and serum ferritin concentration along with evidence of inflammation, infection, and liver disease. The sTfR may provide useful discrimination between the presence and absence of iron stores in the anaemia of chronic disease, but its use is hindered by the lack of agreement about units and reference ranges. Measurement of transferrin saturation is essential for evaluating iron accumulation in genetic haemochromatosis.

REFERENCES

1. Miret S, Simpson RJ, Mckie AT 2003 Physiology and molecular biology of dietary iron absorption. Annual Review of Nutrition 23:283–301.
2. Cavill I, Worwood M, Jacobs A. 1975 Internal regulation of iron absorption. Nature 256:328–329.
3. Ganz T, 2003 Hepcidin: a key regulator of iron metabolism and mediator of anemia of inflammation. Blood 102:783–788.
4. Hentze MW, Muckenthaler MU, Andrews NC 2004 Balancing acts: molecular control of mammalian iron metabolism. Cell 117:285–297.
5. Harrison PM, Arosio P 1996 Ferritins: Molecular properties, iron storage function and cellular regulation. Bba-Bioenergetics 1275:161–203.
6. Langlois MR, Delanghe JR 1996 Biological and clinical significance of haptoglobin polymorphism in humans. Clinical Chemistry 42:1589–600.
7. Kristiansen M, Graversen JH, Jacobsen C et al 2001 Identification of the haemoglobin scavenger receptor. Nature 409:198–201.
8. Tolosano E, Altruda F 2002 Hemopexin: structure, function, and regulation. DNA and Cell Biology 21:297–306.
9. Worwood M. 1990 Ferritin. Blood Reviews 4:259–269.
10. Hider RC 2002 Nature of nontransferrin-bound iron. European Journal of Clinical Investigation 32:50–54.
11. British Nutrition Foundation. Report of the Task Force 1995 Iron–Nutritional and Physiological Significance. Chapman and Hall, London.
12. Sullivan JL 1981 Iron and the sex difference in heart disease risk. Lancet 1:1293–1294.
13. Labbe RF, Vreman HJ, Stevenson DK 1999 Zinc protoporphyrin: a metabolite with a mission. Clinical Chemistry 45:2060–2072.
14. Hoffbrand AV, Worwood M 2005 Iron overload. In: Hoffband AV, Tuddenham E, Catovsky D (eds) Postgraduate Haematology. Blackwell Publishing, Oxford.
15. Worwood M, Hoffband AV 2005 Iron metabolism and iron deficiency. In: Hoffband AV, Tuddenham E, Catovsky D (eds) Postgraduate Haematology. Blackwell Publishing, Oxford.
16. Dooley J, Worwood, M. Guidelines on diagnosis and therapy: genetic haemochromatosis 2000

British Committee for Standards in Haematology. www.bcshguidelines.com.

17. Addison GM, Beamish MR, Hales CN et al 1972 An immunoradiometric assay for ferritin in the serum of normal subjects and patients with iron deficiency and iron overload. Journal of Clinical Pathology 25:326–329.

18. Miles LE, Lipschitz DA, Bieber CP, et al 1974 Measurement of serum ferritin by a 2-site immunoradiometric assay. Analytical Biochemistry 61:209–224.

19. ICSH (Expert Panel on Iron) 1985. Proposed international standard of human ferritin for the serum ferritin assay. British Journal of Haematology 61:61–63.

20. Worwood M 1980 Serum ferritin. In: Cook JD (ed) Iron, p. 59–89. Churchill Livingstone, New York.

21. Dresser DW. 1986 Immunization of experimental animals. In: Weir DM (ed) Handbook of Experimental Immunology, p. 8.1–8.21. Blackwell Science, Oxford.

22. Johnson GD, Holborow EJ 1986 Preparation and use of fluorochrome conjugates. In: Weir DM (ed) Handbook of Experimental Immunology, p. 28.1–28.21. Blackwell Science, Oxford.

23. Wilson MB, Nakane PK 1978 Recent developments in the periodate method of conjugating horseradish peroxidase (HRPO) to antibodies In: Knapp W, Houlbar K, Houlbar K (eds) Immunofluorescence and related staining techniques, p. 215–224. Elsevier/North-Holland, Amsterdam.

24. Perera P, Worwood M 1984 Antigen-binding in the 2-site immunoradiometric assay for serum ferritin—the nature of the hook effect. Annals of Clinical Biochemistry 21:393–397.

25. Boscato LM, Stuart MC 1988 Heterophilic antibodies: a problem for all immunoassays. Clinical Chemistry 34:27–33.

26. Zweig MH, Csako G, Benson CC et al 1987 Interference by anti-immunoglobulin-G antibodies in immunoradiometric assays of thyrotropin involving mouse monoclonal-antibodies. Clinical Chemistry 33:840–844.

27. Worwood M Ferritin in human tissues and serum [Review:167 refs] 1982 Clinics in Haematology 11:275–307.

28. World Health Organization 2001 Iron deficiency anemia. Assessment, prevention, and control. A guide for programme managers, www.who.int/nut/documents/ida_assessment_prevention_control.

29. Witte DL 1991 Can serum ferritin be effectively interpreted in the presence of the acute-phase response? Clinical Chemistry 37:484–485.

30. Rogers JT, Bridges KR, Durmowicz GP et al 1990 Translational control during the acute phase response. Ferritin synthesis in response to interleukin-1. Journal of Biological Chemistry 265:14572–14578.

31. Worwood M 1986 Serum ferritin. Clinical Science 70:215–220.

32. Cavanna F, Ruggeri G, Iacobello C et al 1983 Development of a monoclonal antibody against human heart ferritin and its application in an immunoradiometric assay. Clinica Chimica Acta 134:347–356.

33. Jones BM, Worwood M, Jacobs A 1980 Serum ferritin in patients with cancer: determination with antibodies to HeLa cell and spleen ferritin. Clinica Chimica Acta 106:203–214.

34. Nielsen P, Gunther U, Durken M et al 2000 Serum ferritin iron in iron overload and liver damage: correlation to body iron stores and diagnostic relevance. Journal of Laboratory and Clinical Medicine 135:413–418.

35. ICSH 1990 Revised recommendations for the measurement of serum iron in human blood. British Journal of Haematology 75:615–616.

36. Bothwell TH, Charlton RW, Cook JD, et al 1979 Iron metabolism in man. Blackwell Scientific Publications, Oxford.

37. Persijn J-P, van der Slik W, Riethorst A 1971 Determination of serum iron and latent iron-binding capacity (LIBC). Clinica Chimica Acta 35:91–98.

38. Tietz NW, Rinker AD, Morrison SR 1996 When is a serum iron really a serum iron? A follow-up study on the status of iron measurements in serum. Clinical Chemistry 42:109–111.

39. Blanck HM, Pfeiffer CM, Caudill SP et al 2003 Serum iron and iron-binding capacity: a round-robin interlaboratory comparison study. Clinical Chemistry 49:1672–1675.

40. Jacobs A, Waters WE, Campbell H et al 1969 A random sample from Wales III. Serum iron, iron binding capacity and transferrin saturation. British Journal of Haematology 17:581–587.

41. Jackson HA, Carter K, Darke C, et al 2001 HFE mutations, iron deficiency and overload in 10 500 blood donors. British Journal of Haematology 114:474–484.

42. Koerper MA, Dallman PR 1977 Serum iron concentration and transferrin saturation in the diagnosis of iron deficiency in children: normal developmental changes. Journal of Pediatrics 91:870–874.

43. Saarinen UM, Siimes MA 1977 Developmental changes in serum iron, total iron binding capacity

and transferrin saturation in infancy. Journal of Pediatrics 91:877.

44. International Committee for Standardization in Haematology 1978 The measurement of total and unsaturated iron binding capacity in serum. British Journal of Haematology 38:281–290.

45. Siek G, Lawlor J, Pelczar D et al 2002 Direct serum total iron-binding capacity assay suitable for automated analyzers. Clinical Chemistry 48:161–166.

46. Beilby J, Olynyk J, Ching S et al 1992 Transferrin index: an alternative method for calculating the iron saturation of transferrin. Clinical Chemistry 38:2078–2081.

47. Huebers HA, Eng MJ, Josephson BM et al 1987 Plasma iron and transferrin iron-binding-capacity evaluated by colorimetric and immunoprecipitation methods. Clinical Chemistry 33:273–277.

48. Yamanishi H, Iyama S, Yamaguchi Y et al 2003 Total iron-binding capacity calculated from serum transferrin concentration or serum iron concentration and unsaturated iron-binding capacity. Clinical Chemistry 49:175–178.

49. Gambino R, Desvarieux E, Orth M et al 1997 The relation between chemically measured total iron-binding capacity concentrations and immunologically measured transferrin concentrations in human serum. Clinical Chemistry 43:2408–2412.

50. Murtagh LJ, Whiley M, Wilson S et al 2002 Unsaturated iron binding capacity and transferrin saturation are equally reliable in detection of HFE hemochromatosis. American Journal of Gastroenterology 97:2093–2099.

51. Bainton DF, Finch CA 1964 The diagnosis of iron deficiency anemia. American Journal of Medicine 37:62–70.

52. Edwards CQ, Kushner JP 1993 Screening for hemochromatosis. New England Journal of Medicine 328:1616–1620.

53. Feelders RA, Kuiperkramer EPA, Vaneijk HG 1999 Structure, function and clinical significance of transferrin receptors. Clinical Chemistry and Laboratory Medicine 37:1–10.

54. Trinder D, Baker E 2003 Transferrin receptor 2: a new molecule in iron metabolism. International Journal of Biochemistry & Cell Biology 35:292–296.

55. Kohgo Y, Nishisato T, Kondo H et al 1986 Circulating transferrin receptor in human serum. British Journal of Haematology 64:277–281.

56. Cook JD 1999 The measurement of serum transferrin receptor. American Journal of the Medical Sciences 318:269–276.

57. Worwood M, Ellis RD, Bain BJ 2000 Three serum transferrin receptor ELISAs. MDA/2000/09. Her Majesty's Stationary Office, Norwich, UK.

58. Akesson A, Bjellerup P, Vahter M 1999 Evaluation of kits for measurement of the soluble transferrin receptor. Scandinavian Journal of Clinical & Laboratory Investigation 59:77–81.

59. Kuiperkramer EPA, Huisman CMS, Vanraan J et al 1996 Analytical and clinical implications of soluble transferrin receptors in serum. European Journal of Clinical Chemistry and Clinical Biochemistry 34:645–649.

60. Choi JW, Im MW, Pai SH 2000 Serum transferrin receptor concentrations during normal pregnancy. Clinical Chemistry 46:725–727.

61. Kohgo Y, Niitsu Y, Kondo H et al 1987. Serum transferrin receptor as a new index of erythropoiesis. Blood 70:1955–1958.

62. Huebers HA, Beguin Y, Pootrakul PN et al 1990 Intact transferrin receptors in human plasma and their relation to erythropoiesis. Blood 75:102–107.

63. Beguin Y, Clemons GK, Pootrakul P et al 1993 Quantitative assessment of erythropoiesis and functional classification of anemia based on measurements of serum transferrin receptor and erythropoietin. Blood 81:1067–1076.

64. Cavill I, Ricketts C 1980 Human iron kinetics. In: Jacobs A, Worwood M (eds) Iron in Biochemistry and Medicine II, p. 573, Academic Press, London.

65. Skikne B, Flowers CH, Cook JD 1990 Serum transferrin receptor: a quantitative measure of tissue iron deficiency. Blood 75:1870–1876.

66. Cook JD, Flowers CH, Skikne BS 2003 The quantitative assessment of body iron. Blood 101:3359–3364.

67. Olivares M, Walter T, Cook JD et al 2000 Usefulness of serum transferrin receptor and serum ferritin in diagnosis of iron deficiency in infancy. American Journal of Clinical Nutrition 72:1191–1195.

68. Punnonen K, Irjala K, Rajamaki A 1997 Serum transferrin receptor and its ratio to serum ferritin in the diagnosis of iron deficiency. Blood 89:1052–1057.

69. Kuiperkramer PA, Huisman CMS, Vandermolensinke J et al 1997 The expression of transferrin receptors on erythroblasts in anaemia of chronic disease, myelodysplastic syndromes and iron deficiency. Acta Haematologica 97:127–131.

70. Fitzsimons EJ, Houston T, Munro R et al 2002 Erythroblast iron metabolism and serum soluble transferrin receptor values in the anemia of rheumatoid arthritis. Arthritis & Rheumatism–Arthritis Care & Research 47:166–171.

71. Carriaga MT, Skikne BS, Finley B et al 1991 Serum transferrin receptor for the detection of iron deficiency in pregnancy. American Journal of Clinical Nutrition 54:1077–1081.

72. Akesson A, Bjellerup P, Berglund M et al 1998 Serum transferrin receptor: a specific marker of iron deficiency in pregnancy. American Journal of Clinical Nutrition 68:1241–1246.

73. Vandenbroek NR, Letsky EA, White SA et al 1998 Iron status in pregnant women: which measurements are valid? British Journal of Haematology 103:817–824.

74. Baynes RD, Cook JD, Bothwell TH et al 1994 Serum transferrin receptor in hereditary hemochromatosis and African siderosis. American Journal of Hematology 45:288–292.

75. Khumalo H, Gomo ZAR, Moyo VM et al 1998 Serum transferrin receptors are decreased in the presence of iron overload. Clinical Chemistry 44:40–44.

76. Looker AC, Loyevsky M, Gordeuk VR 1999 Increased serum transferrin saturation is associated with lower serum transferrin receptor concentration. Clinical Chemistry 45:2191–2199.

77. Hastka J, Lasserre JJ, Schwarzbeck A et al 1993 Zinc protoporphyrin in anemia of chronic disorders. Blood 81:1200–1204.

78. Yip R 1994 Changes in iron metabolism with age. In: Brock JH, Halliday JW, Pippard MJ et al (eds) Iron metabolism in health and disease, p. 427–448. WB Saunders, London.

79. Hastka J, Lasserre JJ, Schwarzbeck A et al 1992 Washing erythrocytes to remove interferents in measurements of zinc protoporphyrin by front-face hematofluorometry. Clinical Chemistry 38:2184–2189.

80. Garrett S, Worwood M 1994 Zinc protoporphyrin and iron deficient erythropoiesis. Acta Haematologica 191:21–25.

81. Soldin OP, Miller M, Soldin SJ 2003. Pediatric reference ranges for zinc protoporphyrin. Clinical Biochemistry 36:21–25.

82. Zanella A, Gridelli L, Berzuini A et al 1989 Sensitivity and predictive value of serum ferritin and free erythrocyte protoporphyrin for iron-deficiency. Journal of Laboratory and Clinical Medicine 113:73–78.

83. Dawkins S, Cavill I, Ricketts C et al 1979 Variability of serum ferritin concentration in normal subjects. Clinical & Laboratory Haematology 1:41–46.

83a. Dale JC, Burritt MF, Zinsmeister AR 2002 Diurnal variation of serum iron, iron-binding capacity, transferrin saturation and ferritin levels. American Journal of Clinical Pathology 117:802–808.

84. Borel MJ, Smith SM, Derr J et al 1991 Day-to-day variation in iron-status indices in healthy men and women. American Journal of Clinical Nutrition 54:729–735.

85. Pootrakul P, Skikne BS, Cook JD 1983 The use of capillary blood for measurements of circulating ferritin. American Journal of Clinical Nutrition 37:307–310.

86. Cooper MJ, Zlotkin SH 1996 Day-to-day variation of transferrin receptor and ferritin in healthy men and women. American Journal of Clinical Nutrition 64:738–742.

87. Kim I, Yetley EA, Calvo MS 1993 Variations in iron-status measures during the menstrual-cycle. American Journal of Clinical Nutrition 58:705–709.

88. Lundberg PA, Lindstedt G, Andersson T et al 1984 Increase in serum ferritin concentration induced by fasting. Clinical Chemistry 30:161–163.

89. Chapman RW, Gorman A, Laulicht M et al 1982 Binding of serum ferritin to concanavalin A in patients with iron overload and with chronic liver disease. Journal of Clinical Pathology 35:481–486.

90. Nikolaidis MG, Michailidis Y, Mougios V 2003 Variation of soluble transferrin receptor and ferritin concentrations in human serum during recovery from exercise. European Journal of Applied Physiology 89:500–502.

91. Fallon KE 2001 The acute phase response and exercise: the ultramarathon as prototype exercise. Clinical Journal of Sport Medicine 11:38–43.

92. Stupnicki R, Malczewska J, Milde K et al 2003 Day to day variability in the transferrin receptor/ferritin index in female athletes. British Journal of Sports Medicine 37:267–269.

93. Kristalboneh E, Froom P, Harari G et al 1993 Seasonal changes in red-blood-cell parameters. British Journal of Haematology 85:603–607.

94. Maes M, Bosmans E, Scharpe S et al 1997 Components of biological variation in serum soluble transferrin receptor: relationships to serum iron, transferrin and ferritin concentrations, and immune and haematological variables. Scandinavian Journal of Clinical Laboratory Investigation 57:31–41.

95. Dallman PR 1984 Diagnosis of anemia and iron-deficiency: analytic and biological variations of laboratory tests. American Journal of Clinical Nutrition 39:937–941.

96. Looker AC, Dallman PR, Carroll MD et al 1997 Prevalence of iron deficiency in the United States. Journal of the American Medical Association 277:973–976.

97. Wiggers P, Dalhoj J, Hyltoft Petersen P et al 1991 Screening for haemochromatosis: influence of analytical imprecision, diagnostic limit and prevalence on test validity. Scandinavian Journal of Clinical & Laboratory Investigation 51:143–148.

98. Lammikeefe CJ, Lickteig ES, Ahluwalia N et al 1996 Day-to-day variation in iron status indexes is similar for most measures in elderly women with and without rheumatoid arthritis. Journal of the American Dietetic Association 96:247–251.

99. Ahluwalia N, Lammikeefe CJ, Bendel RB et al 1995 Iron-deficiency and anemia of chronic disease in elderly women: a discriminant-analysis approach for differentiation. American Journal of Clinical Nutrition 61:590–596.

100. Bentley DP, Williams P 1974 Serum ferritin concentration as an index of storage iron in rheumatoid arthritis. Journal of Clinical Pathology 27:786–738.

101. Tessitore N, Solero GP, Lippi G et al 2001 The role of iron status markers in predicting response to intravenous iron in haemodialysis patients on maintenance erythropoietin. Nephrology Dialysis Transplantation 16:1416–1423.

102. Guyatt G, Oxman AD, Ali M et al 1992 Laboratory diagnosis of iron-deficiency anemia— an overview. Journal of General Internal Medicine 7:145–153.

103. Kotru M, Rusia U, Sikka M et al 2004 Evaluation of serum ferritin in screening for iron deficiency in tuberculosis. Annals of Hematology 83:95–100.

104. Macdougall IC, Cavill I, Hulme B et al 1992 Detection of functional iron-deficiency during erythropoietin treatment: a new approach. British Medical Journal 304:225–226.

105. Fishbane S, Shapiro W, Dutka P et al 2001 A randomized trial of iron deficiency testing strategies in hemodialysis patients. Kidney International 60:2406–2411.

106. Fernandez-Rodriguez AM, Guindeo-Casasus MC, Molero-Labarta T et al 1999 Diagnosis of iron deficiency in chronic renal failure. American Journal of Kidney Diseases 34:508–513.

107. Domellof M, Dewey KG, Lonnerdal B et al 2002 The diagnostic criteria for iron deficiency in infants should be reevaluated. Journal of Nutrition 132:3680–3686.

108. Margolis HS, Huntley HH, Bender TR et al 1981 Iron deficiency in children: the relationship between pretreatment laboratory tests and subsequent hemoglobin response to iron therapy. American Journal of Clinical Nutrition 34:2158–2168.

109. Hershko C, Baror D, Gaziel Y et al 1981 Diagnosis of iron-deficiency anemia in a rural-population of children: relative usefulness of serum ferritin, red-cell protoporphyrin, red-cell indexes, and transferrin saturation determinations. American Journal of Clinical Nutrition 34:1600–1610.

110. Abraham K, Muller C, Gruters A et al 2003 Minimal inflammation, acute phase response and avoidance of misclassification of vitamin A and iron status in infants: importance of a high-sensitivity C-reactive protein (CRP) assay. International Journal for Vitamin and Nutrition Research 73:423–430.

111. Brittenham GM 1988 Noninvasive methods for the early detection of hereditary hemochromatosis. [Review]. Annals of the New York Academy of Sciences 526:199–208.

112. Gallagher SK, Johnson LK, Milne DB 1989 Short-term and long-term variability of indexes related to nutritional-status. I. Ca, Cu, Fe, Mg, and Zn. Clinical Chemistry 35:369–373.

113. Statland BE, Winkel P 1977 Relationship of day-to-day variation of serum iron concentration to iron-binding capacity in healthy young women. American Journal of Clinical Pathology 67:84–90.

114. Statland BE, Winkel P, Bokieland H 1976 Variation of serum iron concentration in healthy young men: within day and day-to-day changes. Clinical Biochemistry 9:26–29.

115. Statland BE, Winn RK, Harris SC 1977 Evaluation of biologic sources of variation of leucocyte counts and other hematologic quantities using very precise automated analysers. American Journal of Clinical Pathology 69:48–54.

116. Pilon VA, Howantitz PJ, Howanitz JH et al 1981 Day-to-day variation in serum ferritin concentration in healthy subjects. Clinical Chemistry 27:78–82.

117. Romslo I, Talstad I 1988 Day-to-day variations in serum iron, serum iron binding capacity, serum ferritin and erythrocyte protoporphyrin concentrations in anaemic subjects. European Journal of Haematology 40:79–82.

118. Ahluwalia N 1998 Diagnostic utility of serum transferrin receptors measurement in assessing iron status. Nutrition Reviews 56:133–141.

119. van Tellingen A, Kuenen JC, de Kieviet W et al 2001 Iron deficiency anaemia in hospitalised patients: value of various laboratory parameters— differentiation between IDA and ACD. Netherlands Journal of Medicine 59:270–279.

120. Lee EJ, Oh EJ, Park YJ et al 2002 Soluble transferrin receptor (sTfR), ferritin, and sTfR/log ferritin index in anemic patients with nonhematologic malignancy and chronic inflammation. Clinical Chemistry 48:1118–1121.

121. Kurer SB, Seifert B, Michel B et al 1995 Prediction of iron deficiency in chronic inflammatory rheumatic disease anaemia. British Journal of Haematology 91:820–826.

122. Bultink IEM, Lems WF, de Stadt RJV et al 2001 Ferritin and serum transferrin receptor predict iron deficiency in anemic patients with rheumatoid arthritis. Arthritis and Rheumatism 44:979–981.

123. Means RT, Allen J, Sears DA et al 1999 Serum soluble transferrin receptor and the prediction of marrow iron results in a heterogeneous group of patients. Clinical & Laboratory Haematology 21:161–167.

124. Joosten E, Van Loon R, Billen J et al 2002 Serum transferrin receptor in the evaluation of the iron status in elderly hospitalized patients with anemia. American Journal of Hematology 69:1–6.

125. Mast AE, Blinder MA, Gronowski AM et al 1998 Clinical utility of the soluble transferrin receptor and comparison with serum ferritin in several populations. Clinical Chemistry 44:45–51.

126. Pippard MJ 2003 Iron-deficiency anemia, anemia of chronic disorders, and iron overload. In: Wickramasinghe SL, McCullough J (eds) Blood and bone marrow pathology, p. 203–228, Churchill Livingstone, London.

8 Investigation of megaloblastic anaemia— cobalamin, folate, and metabolite status

Malcolm Hamilton and Sheena Blackmore

Investigation of the vitamin B_{12} and folate status of individuals is not restricted to investigation of individuals with classical features of megaloblastic anaemia alone because neuropathy and neuro-psychiatric changes may occur in B_{12} deficiency in the absence of macrocytosis or anaemia.[1-4] The finding that folate supplementation reduced incidence of neural tube defects[5] highlighted the importance of defining optimum population folate levels. Increased plasma homocysteine and serum methylmalonic acid (MMA) levels have been advocated as sensitive indicators of folate and cobalamin deficiency[6] that may be subclinical, although widespread applicability of metabolite levels to routine laboratory practice was limited in the past as a result of technical difficulty in measurement. Elevated homocysteine level is an independent vascular disease risk factor[7] and is associated with risk of idiopathic venous thrombosis.[8] Implementing dietary supplementation with folate to reduce homocysteine levels, in an attempt to prevent myocardial infarction and stroke, is a factor in the development of homocysteine assays. Increased plasma homocysteine levels occur in both B_{12} and folate deficiency as a result of reduction in methionine synthesis and resultant homocysteine accumulation. Thus modern laboratory investigation of B_{12} and folate status now includes measurement of homocysteine. These investigations extend not only to individuals suspected of having specific clinical deficiencies or excess, but also to population studies for which the definition of analyte reference ranges is crucial.

The limitations of total serum B_{12} measurement have been highlighted by studies that showed poor specificity of only 50% (i.e., healthy persons with a low level or low cobalamin levels with no evidence of deficiency) and sensitivity of 95% (i.e., 5% clinically deficient with normal level).[9-11] Some authors have advocated measurement of metabolites such as methylmalonic acid (MMA) in serum or urine and plasma homocysteine to assist in the assessment of cobalamin status.[11] Although MMA measurement is still not widely available, requiring gas chromatography-mass spectrometry (GC-MS), plasma homocysteine measurement by high-performance liquid chromatography (HPLC) and commercial enzyme immunoassays are available. In addition, measurement of the physiologically active minor fraction of cobalamin—that is, holotranscobalamin[12,13] (B_{12} transcobalamin II complex)—is also commercially available* and, as a sensitive and early marker of cobalamin deficiency, may offer advantages over total serum B_{12} measurement, which predominantly comprises B_{12} transcobalamin I complex (haptocorrin). These additional diagnostic tools may facilitate more precise diagnosis in patients in whom prolonged therapy may have been initiated inappropriately and continued unnecessarily or, conversely, discontinued inappropriately because of lack of confidence in the original assessment.

HAEMATOLOGICAL FEATURES OF MEGALOBLASTIC ANAEMIA

Megaloblastic anaemia resulting from impaired DNA synthesis is characterised by the presence of megaloblastic red cell precursors in the bone marrow and occasionally also in the blood. Megaloblasts have a characteristic chromatin pattern (Fig. 8.1) and increased cytoplasm as a result of asynchrony of nuclear and cytoplasmic maturation with a relatively immature nucleus for the degree of cytoplasmic haemoglobinisation. The delay in nuclear maturation caused by delay in DNA synthesis resulting from lack of vitamin B_{12} or folate is also seen in all

lineages, particularly granulocytic marrow precursors with giant metamyelocytes (Fig. 8.2) and polylobed neutrophils with increased lobe size as well as number of nuclear segments (see Fig. 5.10, p. 83). In severe pernicious anaemia a progressive increase in mean red cell volume (MCV) up to 130 fl occurs, with oval macrocytes, poikilocytes, and hyper-

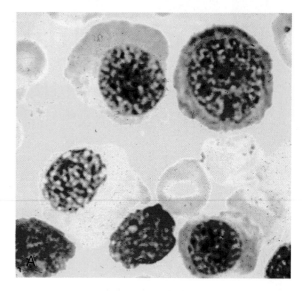

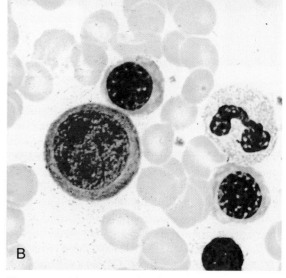

Figure 8.1 Photomicrographs of bone marrow films stained by May-Grünwald-Giemsa. A: Megaloblasts; B: Normoblasts for comparison.

---

*Axis Shield HoloTC RIA 50356/50349/50346. See product literature at www.axis-shield.com/product.

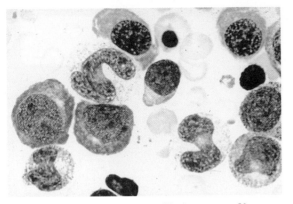

Figure 8.2   Photomicrograph of bone marrow film stained by May-Grünwald-Giemsa showing giant metamyelocytes.

segmentation of neutrophils (greater than 5% with more than 5 nuclear lobes).[14,15] The mean platelet volume is decreased, and there is increased platelet anisocytosis, as detected by the platelet distribution width (PDW). The MCV falls to 110–120 fl as megaloblastic change advances. Howell–Jolly bodies and basophilic stippling are seen in the red cells.

Differential Diagnosis of Macrocytic Anaemia

Macrocytic red cells are also seen in myelo-dysplasia, which can be suspected by the presence of hypogranular neutrophils or monocytosis. Excess alcohol consumption results in an increased MCV as a result of round macrocytes, although rarely does it go higher than 110 fl unless coexisting folate deficiency is present. Hypothyroidism, liver disease, aplastic anaemia, rare inherited orotic aciduria, or Lesch-Nyhan syndrome also have a high MCV. Automated reticulocyte counts facilitate detection of increased red cell turnover and high MCV as a result of haemolysis or bleeding. Coexisting iron deficiency or thalassaemia trait may mask macrocytic changes, although a high red cell distribution width indicates anisocytosis and the need for blood film review. Congenital dyserythropoietic anaemias type I and III and erythroleukaemia exhibit some features of megaloblastic erythropoiesis that are unrelated to B_{12} and folate. Drugs interfering with DNA synthesis (e.g., azathioprine, azidothymidine [AZT], or hydroxy-carbamide) result in macrocytosis and megaloblastic

erythropoiesis. Anticonvulsant therapy interferes with folate metabolism,[16] whereas the impact of oral contraceptives on folate absorption and metabolism is controversial.[17] Prolonged nitrous oxide anaes-thesia destroys methylcobalamin and causes acute megaloblastic change.[18]

INVESTIGATION FOR SUSPECTED COBALAMIN OR FOLATE DEFICIENCY

Microbiological cobalamin and folate assays and competitive radiodilution binding assays for measurement of cobalamin and folate, which were often performed together, have largely been replaced by separate analysis by automated binding assays. The application of a suitable testing strategy for patients suspected of having cobalamin or folate deficiency is shown in Tables 8.1–8.3.

Table 8.1 highlights the important clinical details that should be elicited by the clinician and submitted with the request to assist the laboratory in interpretation of the numeric results of cobalamin and folate assays. Ideally, test requests should not be accepted without this information, but this may not always be practical.

Table 8.2 lists the important laboratory investi-gations that should be performed—results must not be reported in isolation from other laboratory results and clinical details. If investigations are performed in different laboratories, authorization and release of results requires access to all laboratory data on the individual patient. Laboratory information systems should facilitate this cross-disciplinary access.

Table 8.3 provides a list of clinical and laboratory features for diagnosis of pernicious anaemia. These criteria avoid undue reliance on a single B_{12} assay, and should help clinicians to make a diagnosis even when critical tests are not available.

In view of the lack of specificity and sensitivity of serum cobalamin assays, and frequent lack of avail-ability of other diagnostic tests, basing the diagnosis of pernicious anaemia, which requires lifelong parenteral B_{12} therapy, solely on laboratory results, is not straightforward. A checklist of laboratory and clinical diagnostic criteria, as shown in Table 8.3, helps to achieve a greater degree of diagnostic certainty than any single diagnostic test and permits

Table 8.1   Significance of clinical details

Symptoms or signs	Possible significance
Tiredness, palpitations, pallor	Anaemia
Slight jaundice	Ineffective erythropoiesis
Neurological	
Cognitive impairment, optic atrophy, loss of vibration sense, joint position sense; plantar responses normal or abnormal; tendon reflexes depressed.	Cobalamin deficiency, subacute combined degeneration of the spinal cord, and sensor/motor peripheral neuropathies
Dietary and Gastrointestinal History	
Vegetarian or vegan; poor nutrition, (e.g., tea and toast diet in elderly or students); dietary fads	Low iron stores and iron deficiency Cobalamin deficiency in babies born to mothers who are vegans Folate deficiency (often with iron deficiency)
Weight loss, bloating, and steatorrhoea, particularly nocturnal bowel movements	Feature of folate deficiency and Crohn's disease
Mouth ulcers, abdominal pain, perianal ulcers, fistulae in Crohn's disease	Terminal ileal Crohn's—cobalamin deficiency
Glossitis, angular cheilosis and koilonychias, alcohol history	Cobalamin deficiency Coexisting iron deficiency Poor diet and interference with folate metabolism
History of Autoimmune Disease in Patient or Family	
Hypothyroidism, pernicious anaemia, or coeliac disease.	Increased likelihood of pernicious anaemia or coeliac disease
Surgery	
Gastrectomy/bowel resection	Cobalamin deficiency usually 2 years post gastrectomy Ileal disease resulting in cobalamin deficiency Blind loop syndromes
Physical Appearance	
Grey hair, blue eyes, vitiligo	Association with pernicious anaemia
Pregnancy	Increased iron and folate requirements. Cobalamin levels fall by 30% in 3rd trimester
Malabsorptive Syndrome	
Tropical sprue, bacterial overgrowth, fish tape worm in Scandinavian countries	Combined folate and iron deficiency Cobalamin deficiency
Drug History	See text
Other Haematological Disorders	
Myeloproliferative disorders, haemolytic anaemias, leukaemias	Increased folate utilisation may result in folate deficiency
Myeloma	Paraprotein interference with cobalamin assays resulting in falsely low cobalamin levels, which normalise on treatment of myeloma

Table 8.2   Laboratory tests in suspected cobalamin or folate deficiency

Diagnostic Tests	Diagnostic Features Suggestive of Cobalamin or Folate Abnormality	Will Help to Exclude	Pitfalls
Full blood count	Macrocytosis	–	Macrocytosis and anaemia may be absent despite neuropathy
Blood film	Oval macrocytes, hypersegmented neutrophils (>5% with >5 lobes) Howell–Jolly bodies suggests hyposplenism and therefore coeliac disease as a cause of the deficiency	Myelodysplastic syndrome (hypogranular or (hypolobulated neutrophils , dimorphic red cells) alcohol excess/liver disease (round macrocytes, target cells, stomatocytes), haemolytic anaemia (see Chapter 5)	Hypersegmented neutrophils are not invariably present; they may occur during cytotoxic therapy
Reticulocyte count	Absolute count low pretreatment	Reticulocyte response at day 6 post-therapy confirms response to B_{12} or folate therapy provided only low dose is given	Reticulocyte response may be blunted if inadequate iron stores
Bone marrow aspirate (including Perls' stain) before treatment or within 24 hours of cobalamin or folate therapy—indicated if severe, unexplained macrocytic anaemia	Megaloblastic erythropoiesis, giant metamyelocytes, hypersegmented neutrophils, sideroblasts infrequent	Myelodysplastic syndromes, aplastic anaemia	Megaloblastic change is not necessarily a result of deficiency; can be drug induced or as a feature of a myelodysplastic syndrome
Serum B_{12}	B_{12} <180 ng/l suggestive of cobalamin deficiency, may be a result of pernicious anaemia, veganism, or gastrectomy; in the absence of these causes, may result from malabsorption of protein-bound B_{12} (e.g., as a result of achlorhydria)	B_{12} <180 ng/l with no clinical signs or symptoms and normal MMA and homocysteine confirms falsely low B_{12}, which may be a result of folate deficiency; give folic acid and monitor B_{12} level unless neuropathy present	B_{12} >180 ng/l but presence of neuropathy or strong clinical suspicion of B_{12} deficiency requires a therapeutic trial or additional tests, such as MMA and homocysteine: if these are increased treat with B_{12} and monitor response by repeat metabolite levels at day 6; B_{12} deficiency is confirmed if levels fall on treatment
Serum folate	Low level, particularly if red cell folate also low		Subject to diurnal variation Low levels may result from recent deterioration in diet

Table 8.2   Laboratory tests in suspected cobalamin or folate deficiency—cont'd

Diagnostic Tests	Diagnostic Features Suggestive of Cobalamin or Folate Abnormality	Will Help to Exclude	Pitfalls
Red cell folate	Low level, particularly if B_{12} deficiency is excluded		Low red cell folate and high serum folate occur in cobalamin deficiency— treat with B_{12}
			Folate assays may exhibit different responses to folic acid, compared to MTHF Assays may not be optimised for haemolysate matrix. Definition of reference range requires reference method and population studies
Intrinsic factor antibody test (can be done as a reflex test when serum B_{12} is significantly reduced)	Positive in 50–60% of cases of pernicious anaemia and, when positive, obviates Schilling test		False positive (rare) Negative in 40–50% of cases of pernicious anaemia; if negative, proceed to Schilling test
Schilling test (Part I, basic test; Part II, with intrinsic factor; Part III, following course of antibiotics)	Part I <5% and part II normal or near normal confirms malabsorption as a result of lack of intrinsic factor (e.g., pernicious anaemia); Parts I and II abnormal, suggests malabsorption not resulting from intrinsic factor deficiency*		Invalid in renal failure; Part II may not correct in pernicious anaemia if intrinsic factor antibodies are present at high concentration in gastric juice
Upper gastrointestinal endoscopy and duodenal biopsy**	Villous atrophy in coeliac disease		
Serum gastrin or gastric juice pH	Raised serum gastrin or gastric juice pH of >6 confirms achlorhydria: if not present, diagnosis of pernicious anaemia is suspect		

Table 8.2 Laboratory tests in suspected cobalamin or folate deficiency—cont'd

Diagnostic Tests	Diagnostic Features Suggestive of Cobalamin or Folate Abnormality	Will Help to Exclude	Pitfalls
Serum MMA and/or plasma homocysteine, before treatment or before and 6 days after treatment[†]	Raised homocysteine in folate and B_{12} deficiency; raised MMA in B_{12} deficiency, which is helpful to confirm deficiency if B_{12} is low and IF antibodies are absent	Lack of significance of low B_{12} is indicated by normal MMA and homocysteine and no clinical signs	Both MMA and homocysteine are elevated in renal impairment

MMA, methylmalonic acid; MTHF, methyltetrahydrofolate.
*If Part II fails to correct, proceed to barium follow through or small bowel enema to diagnose ileal disease (e.g., Crohn's disease); Parts I and II abnormal, Part III normal indicates malabsorption resulting from bacterial overgrowth (e.g., blind loop syndrome).
**Upper gastrointestinal tract endoscopy also useful if dyspepsia develops in known pernicious anaemia so as to exclude gastric carcinoma.
[†]Plasma homocysteine assay is now widely available; in suspected B_{12} deficiency it provides a useful test of biochemical cobalamin deficiency. Correction of elevated levels after treatment provides confirmation of deficiency.

the diagnosis to be made even when a single diagnostic test is anomalous or unavailable. Clinical and other laboratory criteria thus provide additional supportive evidence of an autoimmune aetiology even if the more demanding diagnostic laboratory criteria are not met.

Clinical and Diagnostic Pitfalls in the Investigation of Cobalamin and Folate Deficiency

Serum folate is altered by acute dietary change and interruption of enterohepatic recycling; it can therefore be low without significant tissue deficiency.[19] This may be a particular problem in hospital inpatients. Red cell folate was originally advocated as correlating better with megaloblastic change[20] reflecting the folate status over the lifespan of the red cells (2–3 months), but a subsequent study suggested that little was to be gained by the addition of red cell folate analysis[21] because only 14% of patients with low serum folate also have low red cell folate levels.[19] Minor haemolysis *in vitro* may cause spurious elevation of serum folate levels. More than half of the patients with severe cobalamin deficiency have a low red cell folate resulting from the lack of cobalamin as a cofactor in the uptake of methyl

tetrahydrofolate (MTHF) monoglutamate by cells and in the synthesis of folate polyglutamates within cells,[22,23] with a corresponding normal or high serum folate. Treatment with cobalamin alone will correct the low red cell folate and high serum folate levels. Concern over the intermethod variability of red cell folate assays, and questions about the additional benefits[24] of measurement of both serum and red cell folate, have reduced the use of these assays. However, satisfactory results are possible if appropriate care is taken with preanalytical sample preparation and analysis. 5MTHF is a very labile substance, and the addition of ascorbate has reduced the coefficient of variation by half in serum folate assays in external quality assurance surveys.[76] The interplay between serum B_{12}, serum folate, and red cell folate and plasma homocysteine and MMA is shown in Table 8.4. In view of the limitations of both serum and red cell folate assays, it is prudent to measure both.

Investigation of Cobalamin Deficiency

The principle causes of cobalamin deficiency are shown in Table 8.5. If malabsorption is suspected, this requires further evaluation of intestinal absorption of B_{12} by the Schilling test (i.e., measurement of

Table 8.3 Combined clinical and laboratory checklist for diagnosis of pernicious anaemia

Diagnostic checklist to permit diagnosis of pernicious anaemia in patient with low B_{12} and not vegan or postgastrectomy	Laboratory criteria	Clinical criteria
Minor criteria	Macrocytosis Anaemia Raised plasma homocysteine Gastric pH above 6 Raised serum gastrin Positive gastric parietal cell antibody	Parasthesiae, numbness or ataxia Hypothyroidism Vitiligo Family history of pernicious anaemia or hypothyroidism
Major criteria	Low serum B_{12} (<180 ng/l) or raised serum methylmalonic acid in presence of normal renal function Megaloblastic anaemia not resulting from folate deficiency Positive intrinsic factor antibodies using high-specificity test.	
Reference standard criteria	Schilling test shows malabsorption of oral cyanacobalamin corrected by coadministration of intrinsic factor	

urinary excretion of radiolabelled oral B_{12} with and without administration of intrinsic factor [IF]). The Schilling test may be repeated after antibiotic therapy to demonstrate correction of malabsorption as a result of bacterial overgrowth in the blind loop syndrome.

Investigation of Folate Deficiency

Lack of a standardised method and an internationally recognised reference method makes it difficult to define folate deficiency with a clinical cutoff point above which no clinical or biochemical evidence of deficiency is present. Elevated levels of homocysteine have been found in elderly subjects,[25] indicating possible subclinical deficiency in the elderly at folate levels less than 4.8 nmol/l. The causes of clinical deficiency and supportive information or diagnostic tests are shown in Table 8.6.

Limitations of Cobalamin and Folate Assays for Diagnosis of Folate and Cobalamin Deficiencies

Because many patients with low serum B_{12} levels do not have demonstrable clinical or subclinical cobalamin deficiency, there appears to be a lack of specificity in cobalamin assays. The positive or negative predictive value of a low or normal result for serum folate or B_{12} may be improved by combination of the laboratory result with careful evaluation of other laboratory findings and clinical evaluation of the patient. An isolated abnormal result of serum folate, B_{12}, or whole blood folate should not be the sole criterion on which treatment decisions are based, and a repeat assay and other confirmatory and clinical evaluation are necessary prior to a diagnostic conclusion. Additional secondary testing with metabolite levels and monitoring of treatment response is recommended.

Table 8.4 Interaction between serum cobalamin, serum folate, red cell folate, plasma homocysteine, serum methylmalonic acid, urinary methylmalonic acid, and holotranscobalamin

Clinical status	Normal B_{12} and folate	B_{12} deficient	Folate deficient
Serum B_{12}*	Usually normal, but may be high in liver disease, myeloproliferative disorders, acute inflammation, recovery from autoimmune neutropenia Low in 25% of elderly subjects	Usually low, but up to 5% of patients with megaloblastic anaemia may have results within reference range	Usually normal, but low B_{12} may be seen in severe folate deficiency, which corrects when monotherapy with folic acid is given
Serum folate*	Usually normal	Usually normal; high serum folate may occur in B_{12} deficiency	Usually low, but normal levels are found with recent dietary improvement
Notes on red cell folate	Folate assays may exhibit different responses to folic acid[†] compared to MTHF.[‡] Assays may not be optimised for haemolysate matrix. Definition of reference range requires reference method and population studies.		
Red cell folate*	Usually normal	Low	Usually low, but normal in very acute deficiency state
Plasma homocysteine	Usually normal; but may be high in renal failure or in MTHFR C677T mutation. Levels may fall with folate supplements	High in B_{12} deficiency and in 50% of samples from patients with low B_{12} consistent with metabolic B_{12}-deficient state	High in folate deficiency—corrected with folic acid therapy
Serum methylmalonic acid	Usually normal; high in 10% normals or with high intake methionine or renal failure	High in B_{12} deficiency and in 50% of samples from patients with low B_{12} consistent with metabolic B_{12}-deficient state	Usually normal, but high in 5% of patients who are folate deficient
Urinary methylmalonic acid	Normal even in renal failure	High	Normal
Holotranscobalamin	Normal although lower levels in elderly	Low in B_{12} deficiency	Normal

*For normal reference values, see Chapter 2, p. 15.
[†]Pteroglutamic acid
[‡]Methyl tetrahydrofolate

Standards, Accuracy, and Precision of Folate and Cobalamin Assays

There are currently no internationally recognised reference methods for serum cobalamin measurement. Solid phase extraction and electrospray ionization tandem mass spectrometric measurement of the principle physiological form of folate (5-MTHF) has been proposed as a reference method for folate[26,27] against which serum or whole blood serum standards can be verified, and a whole blood folate standard has been developed in the United Kingdom (see p. 694).[28] Evaluation of commercial automated binding assays by recovery experiments has shown under-recovery of added 5MTHF and over-recovery of pteroylglutamic acid (PGA), whereas the proposed reference method shows close to 100% recovery and close agreement with the suitably calibrated microbiological assay.[77] Differential sensitivity of assays to pteroylglutamic acid and genetic variability in a

Table 8.5 Causes of cobalamin deficiency

Reduced intake	Supportive diagnostic information
Strict vegetarian/vegan Dietary fad that excludes dairy products and meat Breastfed babies of mothers who are vegetarian or cobalamin deficient Poor dietary intake in elderly	Dietary history Ethnic origin/culture
Malabsorption as a result of loss or inactivity of intrinsic factor	**Supportive information/diagnostic tests**
Addisonian pernicious anaemia	Diagnostic criteria for pernicious anaemia (see Table 8.3)
Gastrectomy (partial or total)	History of gastric surgery
Bacterial overgrowth or parasitic infestation of small bowel	Radiolabelled lactose breath tests for bacterial overgrowth Repeat Schilling test postantibiotic therapy
Pancreatic dysfunction failure of trypsin release of B_{12} from R binding proteins	Pancreatic function tests; exocrine pancreatic dysfunction results in false-positive Schilling part I test.
Malabsorption as a result of failure of B_{12}-intrinsic factor complex uptake in ileum Ileal resection	Radiological, enteroscopic, or capsule camera study of small bowel for Crohn's disease of terminal ileum, tuberculous ileitis
Congenital Imerslund-Gräsbeck syndrome	Subjects of Scandinavian origin
Tropical sprue	Small bowel biopsy
Zollinger-Ellison syndrome	Multiple gastric and duodenal ulcers Pancreatic adenoma on imaging
Food cobalamin malabsorption	**Supportive diagnostic information/tests**
Atrophic gastritis with achlorhydria Gastric surgery	Endoscopic and gastric biopsy findings
Abnormal transport proteins	**Supportive information /diagnostic tests**
Transcobalamin II deficiency	Megaloblastic anaemia in presence of normal cobalamin levels; transcobalamin II levels
Transcobalamin I deficiency results	No evidence of clinical deficiency but low serum cobalamin levels Possible fall in holotranscobalamin levels in elderly
Inborn errors of cobalamin metabolism	**Supportive information /diagnostic tests**
	Serum and urinary methylmalonic acid and metabolite measurement
Acquired drug effects	**Supportive information**
Nitrous oxide: chronic repeated exposure Colchicine: chronic usage impairs B_{12} uptake resulting from diarrhoea	Drug history

Table 8.6   Causes of folate deficiency—cont'd

Reduced intake	Supportive information/diagnostic tests
Poor diet particularly alcoholics (wine and spirits because beer contains folate) Elderly or students "tea and toast diet" Dietary fads Premature babies Unsupplemented parenteral nutrition	Dietary and alcohol history
Malabsorption	**Supportive information/diagnostic tests**
Coeliac disease (often with coexisting iron deficiency) Tropical sprue Small bowel resection, malabsorption syndromes	Antiendomyseal, antigliadin tests, antitissue transglutaminase. Small bowel biopsy
Drug effects	**Supportive information/diagnostic tests**
Sulphasalazine, methotrexate, trimethoprim-sulphamethoxazole, pyrimethamine, phenytoin, sodium valproate, oral contraceptives	Drug history Bone marrow aspiration
Hereditary hyperhomocysteinamia	
Homozygotes for C677T MTHFR have lower folate levels	
Increased folate turnover	
Pregnancy: progressive fall in 3rd trimester Increased requirements for breastfeeding Skin disease—severe psoriasis or exfoliation Haemodialysis Haemolysis: haemoglobinopathy, paroxysmal nocturnal haemoglobinuria, autoimmune haemolytic anaemia (see Chapters 11 and 12).	

proportion of *in vivo* formyl folates result in inter-method variability. The microbiological assay was the method used to assign a potency value to the British Standard for human serum B_{12}.[29] In practice, accuracy for serum and red cell folate and serum cobalamin is judged by comparative performance of specified methods in external quality assessment schemes. These have shown serum B_{12} intramethod and overall assay coefficients of variation (CV) of 4%–12% and up to 20% at clinically relevant levels; there is thus a substantial "grey" indeterminate range between normal and low values. Serum folate intramethod and intermethod CVs are between 8% and 20%, and higher CVs of up to 50% are seen for red cell folate assays. The causes of this variability include patient factors as well as preanalytical, analytical, and postanalytical factors, as discussed later.

Genetic Factors

A number of methylenetetrahydrofolate reductase polymorphisms have been described[30] that alter the proportion of formylfolate in serum, and this could be a potential source of differential response of a serum to different assays. Individuals homozygous for C677T genetic polymorphism have 25% higher plasma homocysteine levels than controls.[31] A genetic-nutrient interactive effect is noted in that the polymorphism confers a greater effect on homo-cysteine levels in those individuals with low folate levels. Cigarette smoking, age, renal disease, drugs including levodopa, and folate supplements all affect homocysteine levels.

Preanalytical Sample Preparation

Serum B_{12} is stable at room temperature and is not affected by sample handling, unless the sample is haemolysed. Folate is affected by recent dietary intake, and if possible fasting samples should be taken. However, this is difficult in practice and assumes that the reference range was also based on fasting samples. Marked loss of folate activity is observed as a result of light and temperature instability. Because red cells contain 30–50 times more folic acid than serum, even slight haemolysis will affect serum folate analysis. Thus, rapid transportation and separation prior to analysis, avoidance of storage at room temperature, and the storage of samples at 2–8°C for a maximum of 48 hours, or at –20°C for no longer than 28 days are all critical factors in the accuracy and precision of serum folate assays. Presence of lysis in a plasma or serum sample can be readily determined and may be quantified (p. 190).

The addition of either ascorbic acid or sodium ascorbate 5 mg/ml will stabilise folate in serum or haemolysates, extending sample storage times. Stabilisation of serum folate with sodium ascorbate added to the primary blood collection tube would improve the reproducibility of routine serum folate assays as shown in external quality control surveys,[76,77] but would necessitate introduction of separate B_{12} and folate sample tubes since ascorbate interferes with cobalamin analysis. EDTA plasma is unsuitable, and heparinized plasma may result in higher values. Samples must be fibrin free and free of bubbles.

Analytical Factors

Analytical sensitivity varies between methods: detection of serum B_{12} levels of 50 ng/l or less is preferable to lower limits for detection of 150 ng/l because this provides increased sensitivity at the clinically important lower end of the reference range. Analytical sensitivity in chemiluminescence assays is defined as the concentration of analyte that corresponds to the relative light units that are two standard deviations less than the mean relative light units of 20 replicates of the analyte zero standard. For many folate assays this is in the region of 0.3 ng/ml (0.68 nmol/l) or less.

Limitations and Interference

Ascorbic acid destroys vitamin B_{12}; therefore ascorbate-treated serum cannot be used for B_{12} assays. Methotrexate and folinic acid interfere with folate measurement because these drugs cross-react with folate-binding proteins. Minor degrees of haemolysis significantly increase serum folate values as a result of high red cell folate levels. Lipaemia with >2.25 mmol/l (2 g/l) of triglycerides and bilirubin >340 µmol/l (200 mg/l) may affect assays.

Postanalytical

The clinical interpretation of laboratory data should take account of the positive or negative predictive value of a result. The report should include a reference range, the derivation of which should be indicated. Food supplementation with folate or additional vitamin intake by populations has resulted in bimodal distributions of vitamin levels, further complicating definition of normality.

METHODS FOR COBALAMIN AND FOLATE ANALYSIS

Microbiological bioassays and radiodilution assays for serum B_{12} and folate[32] are still used, albeit by a decreasing minority of laboratories, although they are an important part of the evaluation of new automated methods and evaluation of new international standards. They are detailed in the 9th edition of this book.

Current methods are highly automated, heterogenous, solid-phase separation assays with chemiluminescence or fluorescence detection systems.

COMPETITIVE PROTEIN BINDING ASSAYS

General Principles

The majority of automated single-platform, multianalyte, random-access analysers allow assays for serum B_{12}, folate, and homocysteine by nonisotopic competitive protein binding or immunoassays. Second antibodies may be utilised as part of the separation procedures. These assays have been designed for serum assays, and the assay platforms may not be optimised for analysis of haemolysates.

SERUM B_{12} ASSAYS

Release from Endogenous Binders and Conversion of Analyte to Appropriate Form

Nearly 99% of serum B_{12} is bound to endogenous binding proteins (transcobalamins) and must be released from these before measurement. The release step utilises alkaline hydrolysis (NaOH at pH 12–13) in the presence of potassium cyanide (KCN) which converts cobalamin to the more stable cyancobalamin and dithiothreitol (DTT) to prevent rebinding of released B_{12}. Alkaline hydrolysis requires subsequent adjustment of pH to be optimal for the binding agent.

Binding of B_{12} to Kit Binder

The binding of B_{12} to kit binder is the competitive step of the assay in which serum-derived cyancobalamin competes with labelled cobalamin, which is usually complexed to a chemiluminescent or fluorescent substrate or an enzyme for limited binding sites on porcine intrinsic factor. Specificity for cobalamin is ensured by purification of the IF or by blocking contaminating corrinoid binders (R binders) by addition of excess blocking cobinamide. Specificity of pure and blocked IF can be demonstrated by the addition of cobinamide to sera. There should be no increase in assay value. Recombinant IF may offer enhanced specificity over chemically purified porcine IF. Other assays rely on an alkaline denaturation step to inactivate the endogenous binders. Assays must not be affected by the presence of high-titre antiintrinsic factor antibody in patient sera.

Separation of Bound and Unbound B_{12}

Following competitive binding, the separation of bound and unbound B_{12} is achieved by a number of electro- or physico-chemical and immunological methods. The *Roche Elecsys* utilises a electrochemiluminescence measuring cell in which the bound B_{12}–ruthenium IF, attached by biotin–streptavidin to paramagnetic microparticles, is temporarily immobilised on an electrode by a magnet. The *Abbott IMx* uses polymer microparticles (beads) coated with porcine IF to bind B_{12}, and the bound B_{12} is then immobilised by irreversible binding to a glass fibre matrix. These methods are designed to improve separation of bound and unbound B_{12}; they may utilise murine anti-intrinsic factor antibody-enzyme conjugates as part of the signal generation.

Signal Generation

The bound fraction is then detected by addition of chemiluminescent, fluorescent, or colorimetric enzyme substrates, which result in generation of fluorescence or light emission. There are two types of signal: flash, which is pH or electrically induced, and plateau, which is sustained. The initial rate of reaction or the area under the curve is used to calculate the result.

Electrochemiluminescence Immunoassay

In the *Roche Elecsys* and *E170* a voltage is applied to the electrode on which the bound B_{12}–ruthenium IF complexes have been immobilised by magnetic attraction and generate electrochemical luminescence, which is measured by the photomultiplier; the relative light units are inversely proportional to the sample B_{12} concentration. The signal that is produced is timed and integrated by the instrument's software.

Enzyme-Linked Fluorescence Generation

In the *Abbott Axsym* substrates such as 4-methylumbelliferyl phosphate are cleaved by an enzyme (i.e., alkaline phosphatase-ligand complex), and the resulting reaction generates fluorescence, the intensity of which is inversely proportional to the B_{12} concentration in the sample.

The *Bayer Centaur, ACS,* and the *Abbott Architect* use acridinium esters bound to B_{12}-IF complex coupled to paramagnetic particles; photons are emitted in response to pH change. The *Diagnostic Products Immulite 2000* uses adamantyl dioxatane phosphate as an alternative substrate, which is cleaved by alkaline phosphatase-labelled B_{12}-IF complex, resulting in generation of a plateau chemiluminescent signal. Although the *Bayer immuno 1* uses alkaline phosphatase–labelled complexes, the substrate is p-nitrophenyl phosphate and signal generation at 405 nm is strictly a colour formation reaction. The *Tosoh Eurogenetics* uses alkaline phosphatase/4 methylumbelliferyl phosphate, and *Beckman Coulter Access* uses alkaline phosphatase/dioxatane phosphate (Lumi-Phos) for signal generation.

Precise descriptions of the assay methods are given in the product literature.

SERUM FOLATE METHODS

The first methods used for measurement of serum folate were microbiological assays. Radioisotope dilution (RID) assays were subsequently developed and the newer commercial, automated, competitive-binding assays are based on similar principles. As with B_{12}, the use of the original microbiological and RID procedures for serum and red cell folate measurements has diminished. Definition of assay response to different forms of folate is crucial for interassay comparisons, particularly in view of the effect of dietary supplementation with folate.

Release from Endogenous Binders

Serum folate present as 5MTHF is released from endogenous binders ($^2/_3$ weakly bound to serum proteins and a minority to membrane-derived soluble folate receptors) by alkaline denaturation. DTT or monothioglycerol (MTG) is used in most folate assays to prevent reattachment of folate to the endogenous binders and to keep the folate in its reduced form.

Binding of Folate to Folate Binding Protein

β-Lactoglobulin, isolated from cow's milk, is commonly used as a binding agent in folate assays, i.e., folate binding protein (FBP). Unfortunately, these lactoglobulins are not specific for the attachment of 5MTHF, and will bind many forms of folate dependent on pH. These properties have been utilised for the standardisation of folate assay. The physiologically active form (5MTHF) is very unstable. Pteroylglutamic acid (PGA), present in vitamin supplements, is more stable, binds to FBP, and has been used as an alternative standard for the folate assays. Its use as a standard depends on the observation that the binding affinities for 5MTHF and PGA are equivalent at pH 9.3 ± 0.1. It is therefore essential that the pH must be strictly maintained at the binding stage of the procedure.[33] In most of these assays serum-derived folate competes with chemiluminescent or enzyme-labelled folate for limited sites on FBP. In the *Roche* methods the FBP is labelled with ruthenium and competition exists between endogenous and biotin-labelled folate.

Separation of Bound and Unbound Folate

Following competitive binding the separation of bound and unbound folate is achieved by a number of electro- or physico-chemical and immunological methods.

In the *Abbott Imx* ion capture assay, murine anti-FBP immunoglobulin G (IgG) results in negatively charged polyanion–folate complexes. These are captured electrostatically using a positively charged glass fibre matrix (charge imparted by high molecular-weight quarternary ammonium compound) that removes the bound fraction. The *Beckman Access* uses murine anti-FBP goat antimouse IgG coated on paramagnetic particles. *Diagnostic Products* uses murine anti-FBP coated on polystyrene beads with separation by centrifugation.

Signal Generation

Generation of electro-chemiluminescence, chemiluminescent, fluorescent, or light emission is similar to that for B_{12} methods. In assays where the bound B_{12} complex is labelled with chemiluminescent esters, signal is generated in response to pH change or electrically induced.

RED CELL FOLATE METHODS

Whereas *Lactobacillus casei* responds equally to both triglutamates and monoglutamates, the affinity of the FBP varies with the number of glutamate residues. Reproducible protein-binding assays for red cell folate can only be achieved by release and conversion of the protein-bound folate polyglutamates, mainly 5MTHF with four or five additional glutamate moieties, to a monoglutamate form. Adequate dilution of the red cells in hypotonic solution, a pH between 3.0–6.0 (ideally pH 4.5–5.2) for optimal conditions for plasma folate deconjugase (polyglutamate hydrolase), and ascorbic acid to stabilise the reduced forms are required.[34,35]

Haemolysate preparations for the newer assay platforms vary widely. The concentration of ascorbic acid varies from 0.09% to 1%, dilution factors from 1:5 to 1:31, and the duration of haemolysate preparation from 40 to 180 minutes. Some assays require the addition of protein and use bovine serum or human serum albumin, whereas others are aqueous only. The pH of lysing diluent varies from 3.0 to 4.0, and that of the deconjugase step from 4.0 to 6.8 (the final pH of the lysate after protein addition varies from 4.4 to 7.5). These various factors may help to explain the large intermethod differences detected in external quality assessment surveys. Inadequate lysis and deconjugation will give falsely low results.[36,37]

If a manufacturer's advice is not given, a suitable haemolysate method described below may be used. However, when the haemolysate is analysed using the serum folate methodology, this preparation method may not be suitable for all instruments.

Haemolysate Preparation

Red cell folate samples are usually collected in EDTA tubes and may be stored at 4°C for up to 48 hours prior to lysate preparation. The lysate is prepared by adding 0.1 ml of whole blood of known PCV to 1.9 ml. of 1 g/dl freshly prepared aqueous ascorbic acid, incubated at room temperature for 60 minutes, in the dark. The ascorbic acid stabilises the folate and the pH of 4.6 allows plasma folate deconjugase to deconjugate the polyglutamate forms to the monoglutamate form. Folate activity should be assayed straight away, or the lysate may be stored at 4°C for no more than 24 hours prior to analysis. Storage at –20°C for longer periods is permissible, but an approximately 10% decrease in activity is noted following a single freeze/thaw cycle. Whole blood in heparin, EDTA, or citrate–phosphate–dextrose (CPD) can be used in some, but not all, assays.

Calculation of Red Blood Cell Folate from Haemolysate Folate Result

1. Multiply the haemolysate folate value by the dilution factor (e.g., 21 if a 1:21 dilution) to obtain the folate concentration of whole blood in µg/l.
2. Divide the whole blood folate result in (1) by the PCV (l/l) and multiply by 100.
3. The result obtained in (2) should, if possible, be corrected for the serum folate value, which for patient populations taking supplemented dietary folate may now be quite significant, as is illustrated in the following worked example:

Corrected RBC folate (µg/l) =

$$\text{RBC folate µg/l} - \text{serum folate µg/l} \times \frac{(1-PCV)}{PCV}$$

e.g., when PCV is 0.45, RBC folate is 180 µg/l, and serum folate is 28 µg/l, then;
corrected RBC folate (µg/l) = 180 µg/l – 28 µg/l

$$\times \frac{(1 - 0.45)}{0.45} = 145.8 \text{ µg/l}$$

Many serum assays have an upper limit of 22–28 µg/l, and a sample must therefore also be diluted and retested to obtain accurate results. Serum folate is traditionally quoted as µg/l or ng/ml; to convert to SI units; µg/l × 2.265 = nmol/l and nmol/l × 0.44 = µg/l.

Serum B_{12} and Folate and Red Cell Folate Assay Calibration

For serum B_{12} methods, cobalamin is protein bound, and therefore standards either need to be lyophilised serum or an aqueous solution of cyancobalamin. Lyophilised standards are available from the National Institute for Biological Standards and Control (see p. 694). For serum folate analysis, 5MTHF is the physiologically active folate form and therefore should be used as the standard. However, 5MTHF is highly unstable, and historically PGA has been used as the primary calibrator either gravimetrically added to aqueous standards or used to assign values to secondary serum matrix standards. The principle underlying the use of PGA is dependent on the equimolar binding of 5MTHF or PGA at pH 9.3.[37] More recent work suggests the pH of equimolar binding may be nearer 8.9 than 9.3. Standards may be either aqueous or in a matrix of human protein.

Whole Blood Folate Standards

An international reference preparation for whole blood folates[28] is available from the National Institute for Biological Standards and Control (NIBSC) (see p. 694).

Primary Instrument Calibration

Currently, one manufacturer has chosen 5MTHF as their instrument calibrator, although this is referenced to aqueous gravimetric primary standards. Methods calibrated in this way should be optimised for the detection of 5MTHF and should not require the adjustment of the binding pH to 9.3. The majority of other manufacturers use gravimetric PGA calibrators or PGA values assigned to serum matrix calibrators referenced to older RID methods.

Internal Adjustment Calibration

Most automated assay systems use calibration curves that are stored on 2D barcode systems with each reagent lot. The barcode also contains the mathematic formulae for shifting or adjusting the observed responses to the master curve when the instrument requires routine calibration. The calibration interval within reagent lots usually varies from 7 to 28 days—stability varies up to 28 days. Most instruments require a 2-point calibration when changing lot numbers of primary reagent packs, when replacing system components, and when internal quality control results are out of range. Reagents should be discarded at the end of the stability intervals and should not be used beyond the expiry dates. Particular care should be taken to ensure calibrants are correctly mixed and homogenous. Aliquots of reagents may be stored at 2–8°C or at –20°C if permitted by the manufacturer.

Internal Quality Control

As a minimum requirement two levels of quality control material should be assayed daily when samples are being analysed. A choice of batch analysis, or true random access, may be preferred by the operator, although in view of folate in-

stability prolonged on-board times are to be avoided by consideration of the test repertoire for a given set of samples. Suitable controls are available commercially.*

METABOLITE TESTING OF THE COBALAMIN FOLATE METABOLIC PATHWAYS

Measurement of the metabolites that accumulate in the absence of cobalamin or folate has long been advocated as a more sensitive index of cobalamin or folate deficiency than total cobalamin or folate levels.[11] Deficiency of cobalamin leads to failure to convert methylmalonyl-coenzyme A (CoA) to succinyl-CoA by methylmalonyl-CoA mutase resulting in accumulation of methylmalonyl-CoA and its hydrolysis product MMA, which increases both in serum and urine. Cobalamin is also a co-factor in the action of methionine synthase, which converts homocysteine to methionine. 5MTHF is also involved in methionine synthesis by methylation of cobalamin. Low levels of cobalamin or folate thereby result in increased homocysteine and MMA in plasma and urine.

A study[38] of patient samples with serum B_{12} less than 170 ng/l showed raised MMA in 40% and raised homocysteine in 54%. This suggests that low B_{12} levels have only a 40%–54% specificity for a cobalamin deficiency state, although concurrent folate deficiency may have resulted in low cobalamin levels. If these patients have true B_{12} tissue deficiency, the elevated metabolite levels would be expected to fall to normal on treatment. This occurred in those patients with a raised MMA, suggesting that high MMA has a specificity for B_{12} deficiency in this preselected group of close to 100%. The homocysteine failed to correct in approximately half of those patients with raised levels, suggesting a lower specificity.

METHYLMALONIC ACID MEASUREMENT

Principle

Methylmalonic acid (MMA) is one of several dicarboxylic acids present in urine and plasma. Before

---

*Bio-Rad Laboratories.

separating MMA from other interfering substances it is necessary to obtain derivatives of these compounds. Urine concentration of MMA is higher than plasma concentration and needs to be normalised for urine creatinine concentration and corrected for the effects of renal impairment or dehydration.

Serum measurement offers added convenience, is unaffected by diet, and can use the same sample as that obtained for B_{12}.

Methods

Plasma or serum MMA is extracted, purified and, using *tert*-butyldimethylsilysl derivatives of MMA, measured by GC-MS. A deuterated stable isotope of MMA is used as an internal standard. The use of dycyclohexyl, another derivative of MMA, was described by Rasmussen.[39]

A method for screening for inborn errors of metabolism using 0-(2,3,4,5,6-pentafluorobenzyl) hydroxylamine HCl to derive oxoacids, followed by liquid partition chromatography, was described by Hoffman.[40] In more recent HPLC or capillary electrophoresis methods,[41,42] MMA can be derivatised using the fluorescent compound 1-pyrenyldiazomethane to yield a fluorescent monoester adduct. After separation by HPLC or capillary electrophoresis, short-chain dicarboxylic acids are quantified following laser-induced fluorescence activation.

Reference ranges for serum MMA measured by GC-MS and using mean ±3 SD of log transformed data are 53–376 nmol/l (Allen[43]) and 50–440 nmol/l (Rasmussen et al[44]).

HOMOCYSTEINE MEASUREMENT

Principle

Homocysteine is a disulphide amino acid present at low concentrations in cells (<1 µmol/l) and in plasma at 5–15 µmol/l.[45] Homocysteine has a reactive sulfhydryl group that forms disulphide bonds with homocysteine or cysteine or protein sulfhydryl groups to form the oxidized form of homocysteine: homocystine, homocysteine-cysteine mixed disulfide, or protein-bound homocysteine. The free homocysteine is <2% of plasma homocysteine, and 80% is as protein bound homocysteine; the remainder is homocystine or mixed disulfides. Reducing conditions convert all these species to homocysteine by reduction of disulfides; therefore total homocysteine is measured.

For quantitation, plasma homocysteine requires protein precipitation and reduction of disulphide bonds. The S-H group of homocysteine is derivatised using a thiol-specific reagent and the resulting adduct is detected. A variety of methods[46] have evolved from ion-exchange amino acid analyzers, radioenzymatic determination, capillary gas chromatography,[47] stable isotope dilution combined with capillary GC-MS,[48] liquid chromatography electrospray tandem mass spectrometry,[49] and HPLC methods using fluorochromophore detection. The increasing availability of benchtop GC-MS may permit wider application of stable-isotope dilution method.

HPLC kits using fluorochromophore detection systems are now available from *Drew Scientific* and *Bio-Rad*. After addition of internal standard the methods first reduce disulphide bonds followed by removal of protein and derivatising of the thiol groups. Separation requires reverse-phase HPLC using a C18-DB column and heptane sulphonic acid/methanol mobile phase at pH 1.9–2.0. Detection is by fluorescence of the fluorophore at λ_{ex} 385 nm and λ_{em} 515nm.

Development of enzyme immunoassays for homocysteine has dramatically changed the availability of its measurement in routine laboratories. These are discussed further in the following section.

Immunoassay for Homocysteine Measurement

Automated enzyme immunoassays[50] have now been developed by a number of manufacturers. Buffered DTT releases bound homocysteine and reduces homocystine and mixed disulphides to homocysteine. Enzymatic conversion of homocysteine to s-adenosyl homocysteine (sAH) is achieved by addition of adenosine and s-adenosyl hydrolase. In the *Axis-Shield, Bayer Centaur,* and *Diagnostic Products Immulite 2000* methods synthetically derived sAH is bound to the separator system (coated wells, paramagnetic particles, or polystyrene beads). Labelled murine anti-sAH is added, and in the presence of sample-derived sAH competes for binding to immobilised sAH. The concentration of labelled anti-sAH bound to the separation phase sAH is inversely proportional to the concentration of sAH derived from the original sample. An appropriate substrate and suitable conditions for colour, chemiluminescence, or fluorescence generation permit analyte quantitation. The enzyme immunoassay produces comparable results to GC-MS and some HPLC methods.[51-53]

HPLC Measurement of Homocysteine

The *Drew Scientific* HPLC reduces homocystine with 2-mercaptoethylamine, and uses a C18-DB reverse phase column, with heptane sulphonic acid/methanol for mobile phase, to produce ammonium fluoro-benzofurazan-4-sulphonate derivative, measured by fluorescence. Current precision in UKNEQAS surveys is 17% for HPLC and 5% for fluorescence polarisation immunoassay (unpublished information from UKNEQAS Coagulation, courtesy of E. Preston & T. Woods).

Preanalytical Variables in Homocysteine Testing

Plasma homocysteine is elevated in both B_{12} and folate deficiency and is elevated in individuals with a common genetic polymorphism of methylene-tetrahydrofolate reductase, C677T polymorphism, the homozygous form of which is present in 10% of Western populations and results in homocysteine levels 25% above the normal upper limit. Raised homocysteine level is an independent risk factor for vascular disease, including myocardial infarction and stroke.[7] Homocysteine levels are affected by age, renal disease, smoking, excessive coffee consumption, and drugs, including levodopa. Correction of elevated homocysteine levels in patients with cobalamin or folate deficiency by administration of one or both vitamins provides proof of a deficiency state, which may be subclinical.

Factors affecting albumin levels will alter homocysteine because it is protein bound, and venepuncture should not be performed after venous stasis or following the subject resting in supine position. Plasma is preferred because cells leak homocysteine, resulting in an increase of 10% during clot formation from uncoagulated samples. Even plasma will show an increase of 10% per hour at room temperature as a result of leakage from red cells.[54] Samples should be kept on ice and centrifuged as soon as possible, at least within 1 hour.

Dynamic Testing of Cobalamin Folate Metabolism

Measurement of metabolite response at 1 week following cobalamin or folate treatment provides the opportunity to perform an *in vivo* dynamic function test of the cobalamin–folate metabolic pathways and confirm a diagnosis of tissue deficiency of one vitamin or the other.

Another dynamic functional test of cobalamin–folate metabolism, utilised primarily in research laboratories, is the deoxyuridine suppression test,[55] in which failure of suppression by deoxyuridine of tritiated thymidine ^{3}H-TdR incorporation into DNA in cobalamin or folate deficient is corrected by treatment with the appropriate haematinic. The method was described in the 9th edition of this book.

Investigation of the Cause of Cobalamin Deficiency

Once cobalamin deficiency has been confirmed by the finding of an unequivocally low serum B_{12} result (with or without confirmatory raised metabolite levels and response to therapy), the aetiology of the low cobalamin should be elucidated as in Table 8.5. Gastric parietal cell antibodies are present in 90% of patients with pernicious anaemia, but this is of low specificity, being found in 15% of elderly subjects, and is therefore of little discriminatory use. Achlorhydria as a cause of cobalamin malabsorption may be suspected by the presence of raised gastrin levels.[56]

MEASUREMENT OF INTRINSIC FACTOR ANTIBODY

Principle

Two types of antibody to IF have been detected in the sera of patients with pernicious anaemia. Type I blocks the binding of B_{12} to IF, whereas type II prevents the attachment of IF or the IF-B_{12} complex to ileal receptors. Type II antibodies (precipitating antibodies) may be precipitated by IF-B_{12} complex and sodium sulphate at pH 8.3 in barbitone buffer. More than 60% of patients with pernicious anaemia are reported to have type I or type II antibodies.[57,58] Automated competitive binding assays are now available and have largely superceded radiodilution assays. A number of manufacturers are developing IF antibody assays for their multianalyte immunoassay platforms.

Assay methods have been reviewed,[57] and one method for detection of types I and II IF antibody based on radiodilution competitive binding was described in the 9th edition of this book.

Intrinsic Factor Antibody Kits

Radioisotopic competitive binding assay kits that detect blocking (type I) antibodies only are being superseded by automated competitive binding assays for inclusion in the test repertoire of these multianalyte platforms. An ELISA (enzyme-linked immunosorbent assay) kit that detects both type I and type II antibodies is available from a number of companies.

Principle of Binding Assay for Type I Intrinsic Factor Antibodies

Current methods for serum type I intrinsic factor antibodies (IFAb) are adaptations of the B_{12} competitive binding assays.

Patient serum is incubated with a binder, such as microcrystalline cellulose, that is coated with IF. IFAb type I, if present, will attach to the binder, reducing the number of available B_{12} binding sites. The labelled B_{12} occupies any free IF sites on the solid phase, which is then separated and counted. The solid phase is separated by centrifugation and decanting and is resuspended in the presence of ^{57}Co labelled B_{12}.

This method is potentially subject to interference from free B_{12} in the patient serum. Under normal circumstances 99% of B_{12} in serum is bound, but this type of method may be subject to interference if the patient has high levels of circulating free B_{12}, as might be the case following treatment with intramuscular B_{12}.

ELISA Methods for Type I and Type II Intrinsic Factor Antibodies

Serum is incubated in the presence of IF bound to a solid phase in such a way that both the type I and type II binding sites are available for binding IFAb.[58]

Excess unbound serum is removed and the solid phase is further incubated with conjugate-labelled (e.g., horseradish peroxidase) antihuman IgG. Unbound conjugate is removed and substrate is added to develop the signal, which is proportional to the amount of IFAb in the original serum. The specificity of the IF antibody assay will depend on the purity of the solid-phase IF. Purified porcine intrinsic factor or recombinant intrinsic factor are used in different ELISAs and the UKNEQAS Intrinsic factor antibody quality control surveys have shown variable positive rates for different types of ELISA, perhaps reflecting different sensitivities and specificity of patient sera.[78]

Interpretation

International reference and calibration material for IFAb is not available, and results of both types of methods are expressed in arbitrary units or as a ratio of a cutoff deemed as positive by each manufacturer. As a consequence of the use of arbitrary units and the requirement to detect both antibodies concurrently, independent quality control material is not available.

INVESTIGATION OF ABSORPTION OF B_{12}

In patients who are B_{12} deficient and who are IFAb negative, it is important to establish whether the capacity to absorb the vitamin is normal. Absorption tests should be reserved for those individuals in whom low B_{12} levels are a result of genuine tissue deficiency, confirmed by supportive laboratory or clinical findings (e.g., macrocytosis, hypersegmented neutrophils, megaloblastic anaemia, neuropathy, neuropsychiatric features, or elevation of cobalamin dependent metabolites) to avoid excessive investigation of "falsely low or indeterminate" serum B_{12} levels.

B_{12} absorption can simply be evaluated by therapeutic trial with an oral dose of 100 μg of cyanocobalamin and careful monitoring of haematological and clinical response. Tests based on measurement of urinary excretion are described in the following section.

URINARY EXCRETION (SCHILLING TEST)[59-61]

Principle

The capacity to absorb B_{12} normally is measured by administering a dose of B_{12} labelled by a radio-isotope of cobalt and measuring the percentage that is excreted in the urine. [58]Co (half-life 71 days) and [57]Co (half-life 270 days) are suitable isotopes.* [57]Co emits γ rays of several energies, the most important being of 122 keV, and no particulate energies are emitted. It can be used with larger tracer doses than [58]Co, and is the isotope of choice when a well-type scintillation counter is used. [58]Co can be used with all counting methods, but its counting efficiency is low, and relatively large amounts must be given to obtain adequate count rates. Cyanocobalamin is more stable than hydroxocobalamin and is the choice for labelling.

Method

Give an oral dose of 1.0 μg (37 kBq) of radioactive B_{12} (cyanocobalamin) in about 200 ml of water to a patient who has fasted overnight and, at the same time, give 1 mg of nonradioactive cyanocobalamin intramuscularly as a flushing dose. The patient should fast for a further 2 hours. Collect all the urine for 24 hours, and measure the radioactivity of this urine and of a standard that consists of an identical dose of radioactive B_{12} suitably diluted in water. Calculate the percentage dose excreted in the urine as follows:

$$\frac{\text{Total counts per min in 24 hr urine} \times 100}{\text{Counts per min in standard (=test dose)}}$$

It may be convenient to prepare 10 test doses at one time from the stock solution. Using sterile containers, do the following:

1. Dilute the contents to 100 ml in water.
2. Take 100 ml for the standard and dilute to 100 ml in water; this standard is a 1:10,000 dilution of the test dose.

3. Dispense the remainder in 10 ml volumes.
4. Store doses and standard at 4°C.
5. Mix the 24-hour urine collection well and estimate the radioactivity in equal volumes of urine and standard.
6. Calculate the percentage of the test dose excreted as follows:

$$\frac{\text{Urine counts per min} \times \text{urine volume (ml)} \times 100}{\text{Standard counts per min} \times \text{dilution of standard}}$$

Interpretation of Results

The normal urinary excretion is >10% of the test dose in the first 24 hours when cyanocobalamin is used as the flushing dose; in patients with pernicious anaemia or B_{12} deficiency associated with intestinal malabsorption the excretion is usually <5%, whereas in patients with inadequate dietary intake absorption will be normal. Results with hydroxocobalamin are generally higher than with cyanocobalamin.[61,62]

In pernicious anaemia, absorption can be increased by the addition of oral intrinsic factor, whereas in malabsorption resulting from an intestinal defect absorption there is failure of correction. The second test dose with IF* (part II Schilling test) may be given 48 hours after the first, provided a flushing intramuscular injection of B_{12} is given 24 hours after the first oral dose.

Potential Errors

Incomplete urine collection is a common cause of error. In renal disease where excretion may be delayed, urine should be collected for a further 24 hours. Deficiency of B_{12} or folate may cause temporary malabsorption of B_{12}.[63] Absorption tests should therefore be carried out when patients are B_{12} replete, or if results are discrepant the test should be repeated after 2 months. Achlorhydria as a result of atrophic gastritis or following partial gastrectomy has been shown to be associated with normal absorption of aqueous B_{12} but malab-

---

*Radioactive B_{12} is available from GE Healthcare/Amersham International: Vial CR3P consists of [58]Co-B_{12} (10 μg of B_{12} with activity of 0.37 MBq) and Vial CR51P is [57]Co-B_{12}.

*Human recombinant IF is available from Cobento Biotech A/S, DK8000, Aarhus C, Denmark. E-mail: info@cobento.dk; see Bor MV, Fedosov SN, Laursen NB, Nexø E 2003 Recombinant human IF expressed in plants is suitable for use in measurement of vitamin B_{12}. Clinical Chemistry 49:2081-2083.

sorption of protein bound B_{12}.[64] Addition of egg yolk or chicken serum has been used as a "food Schilling test."[65-67]

Whole Body Counting

Whole body counting requires specialised equipment, as described in Chapter 15. The principle is to count the absorption 14 days after administration of the dose and original counting. The percentage retained is usually >30% and often >50%, whereas in pernicious anaemia <20% is retained with a correction of 15% or greater after the addition of IF.

B_{12} BINDING CAPACITY OF SERUM OR PLASMA: TRANSCOBALAMIN MEASUREMENT

Principle

Transcobalamin I (TC I) binds 80% or more of the total serum B_{12}, and the B_{12}-TC I complex is known as holohaptocorrin. TC II is the minor but important transport protein that delivers B_{12} to the tissues. The B_{12}-TC II complex is known as holotranscobalamin (HoloTC) and 6–25% of total serum B_{12} is carried in this complex. HoloTC is believed to be the first B_{12} metabolite that decreases on inadequate B_{12} absorption. TC II and III are normally virtually unsaturated unless an individual is undergoing B_{12} treatment. TC II and III should therefore be measured prior to B_{12} treatment. TC I and III (R binders) are glycosylated proteins differing in their sugar moiety. Chronic myeloid leukaemia, myelofibrosis, and other myeloproliferative disorders are characterised by increased levels of TC I and therefore total serum B_{12}. Primary liver cancer (fibrolamellar hepatoma) is also associated with synthesis of large quantities of an abnormal form of TC I. It has been suggested that some low B_{12} levels without evidence of B_{12} deficiency may result from a decrease in R binder concentration.[68] Congenital absence of R binders TC I and III results in very low serum B_{12} but no evidence of B_{12} deficiency.[69] In congenital absence of TC II, which results in fulminating pancytopaenia and megaloblastosis within 2 months of birth, the serum B_{12} is normal, unsaturated B_{12} binding capacity is decreased as a result of absent TC II, and B_{12}

absorption is reduced; the deoxyuridine suppression test is abnormal and corrected by B_{12}.

UNSATURATED B_{12} BINDING CAPACITY AND TRANSCOBALAMIN IDENTIFICATION AND QUANTITATION

Measurement of unsaturated B_{12} binding capacity is rarely undertaken and is only available in reference laboratories. Details of the method were given in the 9th edition of this book. It is mainly of use for detection of transcobalamin I deficiency as a cause for very low serum B_{12} with no clinical features of cobalamin deficiency. It is also required for diagnosing the rare TC II deficiency. In addition, the assay has been used as a tumour marker for primary liver cancer.

Reference Ranges for Transcobalamins

The normal range for serum unsaturated B_{12} binding capacity is 670–1200 ng/l; for plasma collected into EDTA-sodium fluoride it is 505–1208 ng/l,[70] TC I 49–132 ng/l, TC II 402–930 ng/l, and TC III 80–280 ng/l.

HOLOTRANSCOBALAMIN ASSAYS

Principle

About 6–20% of B_{12} is bound to TC II forming the physiologically active complex HoloTC and in this form is taken up by cells. Levels of Holotranscobalamin (HoloTC) B_{12} are 30–160 pmol/l. The remainder of the serum B_{12} is bound to haptocorrin, or TC I. Haptocorrin is involved in the transport of B_{12} to the liver and enterohepatic circulation thereof. Haptocorrin also binds B_{12} in the gastric contents, and B_{12} is released from haptocorrin by pancreatic proteases prior to capture by IF. HoloTC is thought to be the first metabolite to decrease following reduced intake or absorption of B_{12}.[12,13,71] A commercial assay is available from Axis-Shield (see footnote on p. 162). The clinical utility of this approach has yet to be fully defined, and the merits of HoloTC compared to metabolite measurement remain to be clarified. It may be a sensitive marker of cobalamin malabsorption.[72] Quantitation of transcobalamin saturation may enhance its utility.

HoloTC Radioimmunoassay

The HoloTC radioimmunoassay[73] uses magnetic microspheres coated with monoclonal antibody to human transcobalamin to capture transcobalamin, and achieves separation from haptocorrin by magnetic separator. A ^{57}Co B_{12} tracer together with a reducing and a denaturing agent are then added to destroy the HoloTc linkage. When the B_{12} binder containing IF is added the free B_{12} and tracer compete for binding. The unbound tracer is removed by centrifugation, and the bound fraction is measured using a gamma counter. The measured radioactivity reflects the competition between tracer and vitamin B_{12} bound to transcobalamin (i.e., HoloTC). The concentration of vitamin B_{12} in the sample is calculated from a calibration curve using recombinant human HoloTC. An 0.4 ml sample is required, the coefficient of variation is less than 10%, assay limit of detection is 10 pmol, and assay time is 4 hours.

Quantitation of Transcobalamin Saturation

Nexo and colleagues[74,75] described a method permitting measurement of total TC and HoloTC. The method uses B_{12} modified by acid treatment and bound to magnetic beads, which can then be used to remove unsaturated TC or apoTC from serum. The remaining HoloTC is then measured by ELISA. Thus the total and HoloTC can be measured and the TC saturation (HoloTC/Total TC) can be quantitated.

In a study of 137 healthy blood donors the reference range for HoloTC was 40–150 pmol/l. 10% of circulating TC is saturated with a reference range of 5–20%. 15–50% of B_{12} is bound to TC. In subjects who are B_{12} deficient, HoloTC was 2–34 pmol/l and the TC saturation was 0.4–3%, well below the reference interval, providing a clear cutoff from normal sera. Nexo's method combines a sensitive ELISA[74] for TC with a simple procedure for removal of the unsaturated TC or apoTC.

ACKNOWLEDGMENTS

Helpful discussion and advice was provided by Ian McDowell, Andrew Gorringe, Rachel Still, Stuart Moat, Richard Ellis, Professor Mark Worwood, and the Cardiff Health Hospital B_{12} Group. Thanks also to Mrs. Shirley Hamilton for encouragement in completing the chapter.

REFERENCES

1. Waters AH Mollin DL 1963 Observations on the metabolism of folic acid in pernicious anaemia. British Journal of Haematology 9:319–327.
2. Jewsbury ECO 1954 Subacute combined degeneration of the cord and achlorhydric peripheral neuropathies without anaemia. Lancet 3:307–312.
3. Healton EH, Savage DG, Brust JCM, et al 1991 Neurologic aspects of cobalamin deficiency. Medicine 70:229–245.
4. Lindenbaum J, Healton EB, Savage DG, et al 1988 Neuropsychiatric disorders caused by cobalamin deficiency in the absence of anaemia or macrocytosis. New England Journal of Medicine 318:1720–1728.
5. Rush D 1992 Folate supplements prevent recurrence of neural tube defects. FDA Dietary supplement Task Force. Nutrition Reviews 50:22–28.
6. Savage DG, Lindenbaum J, Stabler SP, et al 1994 Sensitivity of serum methylmalonic acid and total homocysteine for diagnosing cobalamin and folate deficiencies. American Journal of Medicine 96:239–246.
7. Nygard O, Vollset, SE Refsum H, et al 1999 Total homocysteine and cardiovascular disease. Journal of Internal Medicine 246:425–454.
8. Ridker PM, Hennekens CH, Selhub J, et al 1997 Interrelation of hyperhomocystinaemia, factor V Leiden, and risk of future venous thromboembolism. Circulation 95:1777–1782.
9. Stabler SP, Allen RH, Savage DG, et al 1990 Clinical spectrum and diagnosis of cobalamin deficiency. Blood 76:871–881.
10. Moelby L, Rasmussen K, Jensen MK, et al 1990 The relationship between clinically confirmed cobalamin deficiency and serum methylmalonic acid. Journal of Internal Medicine 228:373–378.
11. Green R 1995 Metabolite assays in cobalamin and folate deficiency. Balliere's Clinical Haematology 8:533–566.
12. Herzlich B, Herbert V 1988 Depletion of serum holotranscobalamin. II. An early sign of negative vitamin B_{12} balance. Laboratory Investigations 58:332–337.
13. Ulleland M, Eilertsen I, Quadros EV, et al 2002 Direct assay for cobalamin bound to

Transcobalamin (holotranscobalamin) in serum. Clinical Chemistry 48:526–532.

14. Chanarin I 1969 The Megaloblastic Anaemias p. 348, Blackwell Scientific, Oxford.

15. Lindenbaum J, Nath BJ 1980 Megaloblastic anaemia and neutrophil hypersegmentation. British Journal of Haematology 44:511–513.

16. Rose M, Johnson I 1978 Reinterpretation of the haematological effects of anti-convulsant treatment Lancet 1:1349–1350.

17. Shojania AM, Hornady GJ 1982 Oral contraceptives: effect of folate and B_{12} metabolism. Canadian Medical Association Journal 126:244–247.

18. Lassen HCA, Henriksen A, Neukirch F, et al 1956 Treatment of tetanus: severe bone marrow depression after prolonged nitrous oxide anaesthesia. Lancet 270:527–530.

19. Chanarin I 1979 The megaloblastic anaemias, 2nd ed., p.193, Blackwell, Oxford.

20. Hoffbrand AV Newcombe BFA, Mollin DL 1966 Method of assay of red cell folate activity and the value of the assay as a test for folate deficiency. Journal of Clinical Pathology 19:17–28.

21. Phekoo K, Williams Y, Schey SA, et al 1994 Folate assays serum or red cell? Journal of the Royal College of Physicians of London 31:291–295.

22. Lavoie A, Tripp E, Hoffbrand AV 1974 The effect of vitamin B_{12} deficiency on methylfolate metabolism and pteroylpolyglutamate synthesis in human cells. Clinical Science and Molecular Medicine 47:617–630.

23. Perry J, Lumb M, Laundy M, et al 1976 Role of vitamin B_{12} in folate coenzyme synthesis. British Journal of Haematology 32:243–248.

24. Jaffe JP, Schilling RE 1991 Erythrocyte folate levels: a clinical study. American Journal of Hematology 36:116–121.

25. Selhub J, Jacques PF, Wilson PWF, et al 1993 Vitamin status and input as primary determinants of homocystinaemia in an elderly population. Journal of the American Medical Association 270:2693–2698.

26. Nelson B, Pfeiffer CM, Margolis S, et al 2004 Solid-phase extraction-electrospray ionization mass spectrometry for the quantification of folate in human plasma or serum. Analytical Biochemistry 325:41–51.

27. Pfeiffer CM, Fazili Z, McCoy L, et al W Gunter 2004 Determination of folate vitamers in human serum by stable isotope dilution tandem mass spectrophotometry and comparison with radioassay and microbiologic assay. Clinical Chemistry 50:423–432.

28. Thorpe S, Sands D, Heath AB, et al 2004 An international standard for whole blood folate: evaluation of a lyophilised haemolysate in an international collaborative study. Clinical Chemistry and Laboratory Medicine 42:533–539.

29. Curtis AD, Mussett MV, Kennedy DA 1986 British Standard for human serum vitamin B_{12}. Clinical and Laboratory Haematology 8:135–147.

30. Bagley PJ, Selhub J 1998 A common mutation in the methylenetetrahydrofolate reductase gene is associated with an accumulation of formylated tetrahydrofolates in red blood cells. Proceedings of the National Academy of Science 95:13217–13220.

31. Jacques PF, Bostom AG, Williams RR, et al 1996 Relation between folate status, a common mutation in methylenetetrahydrofolate reductase and plasma homocysteine concentrations. Circulation 93:7–9.

32. O'Broin SD, Kelleher BP 1992 Microbiological assay on microtitre plates of folate in serum and red cells. Journal of Clinical Pathology 45 344–347.

33. Givas J, Gutcho S 1975 pH dependence of the binding of folate to milk binder in radioassay of folates. Clinical Chemistry 21:427–428.

34. Bain BJ, Wickramasinghe SN, Broom GW, et al 1984 Assessment of the value of a competitive protein binding radioassay of folic acid in the detection of folic acid deficiency. Journal of Clinical Pathology 37:888–894.

35. Omer A 1969 Factors influencing the release of assayable folate from erythrocytes. Journal of Clinical Pathology 22:217–221.

36. Netteland B, Bakke OM 1977 Inadequate sample preparation as a source of error in determination of erythrocyte folate by competitive binding radioassay. Clinical Chemistry 23:1505–1506.

37. Shane B, Tamura T, Stokstad ELR 1980 Folate assay: a comparison of radioassay and microbiological methods. Clinica Chimica Acta 100:13–19.

38. Gorringe AP, Ellis R, McDowell IFW, et al 2004 Role of serum methylmalonic acid, homocysteine and transcobalamin II in the diagnosis of vitamin B_{12} deficiency [Abstract 77]. British Journal Haematology 125 (Suppl 1):12.

39. Rasmussen K 1989 Solid phase sample extraction for rapid determination of methylmalonic acid in serum and urine by a stable isotope dilution method. Clinical Chemistry 35:260–264.

40. Hoffman G, Aramaki S, Blum-Hoffman E, et al 1989 Quantitative analysis for organic acids in biological sample: batch isolation followed by gas chromatographic-mass spectrometric analysis. Clinical Chemistry 35:587–595.

41. Schneede J, Ulleland PM 1993 An automated assay for methylmalonic acid in serum and urine based

on derivatization with 1-pyrenyldiazomethane, liquid chromatography and fluorescence detection. Clinical Chemistry 39:392–393.

42. Schneede J, Ulleland PM 1995 Application of capillary electrophoresis with laser-induced fluorescence detection for routine determination of methylmalonic acid in human serum. Analytical Chemistry 67:812–819.

43. Allen RH, Stabler SP, Savage DG, et al 1990 Diagnosis of cobalamin deficiency. I. Usefulness of serum methylmalonic acid and total homocysteine concentrations. American Journal of Hematology 34:90–98.

44. Rasmussen K, Moller J, Ostergaard K, et al 1990 Methylmalonic acid concentrations in serum of normal subjects: biological variability and effect of oral l-isoleucine loads before and after intramuscular administration of cobalamin. Clinical Chemistry 36:1295–1299.

45. Ulleland PM, Refsum H, Stabler SP, et al 1993 Total homocysteine in plasma or serum: methods and clinical applications. Clinical Chemistry 39:1764–1779

46. Rasmussen K Moller J 2001 Methodologies of testing. In: Carmel R Jacobsen DW (eds) Homocysteine in health and disease, p. 9–20, Cambridge University Press, Cambridge.

47. Kataoka H, Takagi K, Makita M 1995 Determination of total plasma homocysteine and related aminothiols by gas chromatography with flame photometric detection. Journal of Chromatography B: Biomedical Applications 664:421–425.

48. Stabler SP, Marcell PD, Podell ER, et al 1987 Quantitation of total homocysteine, total cysteine, and methionine in normal serum and urine using capillary gas chromatography-mass spectrometry. Analytical Biochemistry 162:185–196.

49. Magera MJ, Lacey JM, Casetta B, et al 1999 Method for the determination of total homocysteine in plasma and urine by stable isotope dilution and electrospray tandem mass spectrometry. Clinical Chemistry 45:1517–1522.

50. Shipchandler MT, Moore EG 1995 Rapid fully automated measurement of plasma homocysteine with the Abbott Imx analyzer. Clinical Chemistry 41:991–994.

51. Pfeiffer CM, Twite D, Shih J, et al 1999 Method comparison for total plasma homocysteine between the Abbott Imx analyzer and an HPLC assay with internal standardization. Clinical Chemistry 45:152–153.

52. Pfeiffer CM, Huff DL, Smith SJ, et al Comparison of plasma total homocysteine measurements in 14 laboratories: an international study. Clinical Chemistry 45:1261–1288.

53. Nexo E, Engbaek F, Ueland PM, et al 2000 Evaluation of novel assays in clinical chemistry: quantification of plasma total homocysteine. Clinical Chemistry 46:1150–1156.

54. Andersson A, Isaksson A, Hultberg B 1992 Homocysteine export from erythrocytes and its implications for plasma sampling. Clinical Chemistry 38:1311–1315.

55. Wickramasinghe SN, Matthews JH 1988 Deoxyuridine suppression: biochemical basis and diagnostic applications. Blood Reviews 2:168–177.

56. Slingerland DW, Cararelli JA, Burrows BA, et al 1984 The utility of serum gastrin levels in assessing the significance of low serum B_{12} levels. Archives of Internal Medicine 144:1167–1168.

57. Shackleton PJ, Fish DI, Dawson DW 1989 Intrinsic factor antibody tests. Journal of Clinical Pathology 42:210–212.

58. Waters HM, Smith C, Howarth JE, et al 1989. A new enzyme immunoassay for the detection of total type I and type II intrinsic factor antibody. Journal of Clinical Pathology 42:307–312.

59. Schilling RF 1953 Intrinsic factor studies. II. The effect of gastric juice on the urinary excretion of radioactivity after the oral administration of radioactive vitamin B_{12}. Journal of Laboratory and Clinical Medicine 42:860–866.

60. International Committee for Standardization in Haematology 1981 Recommended method for the measurement of vitamin B_{12} absorption. Journal of Nuclear Medicine 22:1091–1093.

61. Wallis J, Clark DM, Bain BJ 1986 The use of hydroxocobalamin in the Schilling test. Scandinavian Journal of Haematology 37:337–340.

62. England JM, Snashall EA, De Silva PM 1981 Comparison of the DICOPAC with the conventional Schilling test. Journal of Clinical Pathology 34:1191–1192.

63. Herbert V 1969 Transient (reversible) malabsorption of vitamin B_{12}. British Journal of Haematology 17:213–219.

64. Gozzard DI, Dawson DW, Lewis MJ 1987 Experiences with dual protein bound aqueous vitamin B_{12} absorption test in subjects with low serum B_{12} concentrations. Journal of Clinical Pathology 40:633–637.

65. Doscherholmen A, McMahon J, Ripley D 1978 Inhibitory effect of eggs in vitamin B_{12} absorption: description of a simple ovalbumin [57]Co-vitamin B_{12}

absorption test. British Journal of Haematology 33:261–272.

66. Doscherholmen A, Slivis S, McMahon J 1983 Dual Schilling test for measuring absorption of food bound and free vitamin B_{12} simultaneously. American Journal of Clinical Pathology 80:490–495.

67. Dawson DW, Sawers AH, Sharma RK 1984 Malabsorption of protein bound vitamin B_{12} British Medical Journal 288:675–678.

68. Carmel R 1988 R-binder deficiency: a clinically benign cause of cobalamin deficiency. Journal of the American Medical Association 250:1886–1890.

69. Jacob E, Herbert V 1975 Measurement of unsaturated "granulocyte-related" (TCI and TCIII) and "liver-related" (TCII) binders by instant batch separation using a microfine precipitate of silica (QUSO G32). Journal of Laboratory and Clinical Medicine 88:505–512.

70. Scott JM, Bloomfield FJ, Stebbins R, et al 1974 Studies on derivation of transcobalamin III from granulocytes: enhancement by lithium and elimination by fluoride of in vitro increments in vitamin B_{12}-binding capacity. Journal of Clinical Investigation 53:228–239.

71. Nexo E, Christensen A, Hvas Ab, et al 2002 Quantification of holotranscobalamin, a marker of vitamin B_{12} deficiency. Clinical Chemistry 48 561–562.

72. Lindgren A, Kilander A, Bagge E, et al 1999 Holotranscobalamin: a sensitive marker of cobalamin malabsorption. European Journal of Clinical Investigation 29:321–329.

73. Ulleland M, Eilertsen I, Quadros EV, et al 2002 Direct assay for cobalamin bound to transcobalamin (holotranscobalamin) in serum. Clinical Chemistry 48:526–532.

74. Nexo E, Christensen A, Petersen TE, et al 2000 Measurement of transcobalamin by ELISA. Clinical Chemistry 46:1643–1649.

75. Nexo E, Christensen A, Hvas A, et al 2002 Quantification of holotranscobalamin, a marker of vitamin B_{12} deficiency. Clinical Chemistry 48:561–562.

76. Blackmore S, Lee A, Hamilton MS 2005 The impact of sample stabilisation with sodium ascorbate on the analysis of serum folate in the UKNEQAS Haematinics surveys. Clinica Chimica Acta 355 UKNP 1.3 S459.

77. Blackmore S, Pfeiffer C, Hamilton MS, et al 2005 Recoveries of folate species from serum pools sent to participants of the UKNEQAS Haematinics scheme in February and March 2004. Clinica Chimica Acta 355 UKNP 1.2 S459.

78. Lee A, Blackmore S, Hamilton MS 2005 A new external quality assessment (EQA) Scheme for Intrinsic factor antibody (IFAb) assays: a key diagnostic criterion for pernicious anaemia. Clinica Chimica Acta 355 UKTP 4.42 S297.

9 Laboratory methods used in the investigation of the haemolytic anaemias

S. Mitchell Lewis and David Roper

Normally, red cells undergo lysis at the end of their lifespan of about 120 days. In haemolytic anaemia, the red cell lifespan is shortened. The causes can be divided into three groups:

1. Defects within red cells from dysfunction of enzyme-controlled metabolism, abnormal haemoglobins, and thalassaemias
2. Loss of structural integrity of red cell membrane and cytoskeleton in hereditary spherocytosis, elliptocytosis, paroxysmal nocturnal haemo-globinuria (PNH), and immune and drug-associated antibody damage
3. Damage by outside factors such as mechanical trauma, microangiopathic conditions, thrombotic thrombocytopenic purpura, and chemical toxins

At the end of a normal lifespan, red cells are destroyed within the reticulo-endothelial system in the spleen, liver, and bone marrow. In some haemolytic anaemias, the haemolysis may occur predominantly in the reticulo-endothelial system (extravascular) and the plasma haemoglobin (Hb) concentration is barely increased. In other disorders, a major degree of haemolysis takes place within the bloodstream (intravascular haemolysis): the plasma Hb increases substantially, and in some cases the amount of Hb so liberated may be sufficient to lead to Hb being excreted in the urine (haemoglobinuria). However, there is often a combination of both mechanisms. The two pathways by which Hb derived from effete red cells is metabolized are illustrated in Figure 9.1.

INVESTIGATION OF HAEMOLYTIC ANAEMIA

The clinical and laboratory phenomena of increased haemolysis reflect the nature of the haemolytic mechanism, where the haemolysis is taking place and the response of the bone marrow to the anaemia resulting from the haemolysis, namely, erythroid hyperplasia and reticulocytosis.

The investigation of patients suspected of suffering from a haemolytic anaemia comprises several distinct stages: recognizing the existence of increased haemolysis; determining the type of haemolytic mechanism; and making the precise diagnosis. In practice, the procedures are often telescoped because the diagnosis in some instances may be obvious to the experienced observer from a glance down the microscope at the patient's blood film.

The following practical scheme of investigation is recommended. In each group, tests are listed in order of importance and practicability.

Is there evidence of increased haemolysis?

1. Hb estimation; reticulocyte count; inspection of a stained blood film for the presence of spherocytes, elliptocytes, irregularly contracted cells, schistocytes, or auto-agglutination (see Chapter 5)
2. Test for increased unconjugated serum bilirubin and urinary urobilinogen excretion; measurement of haptoglobin or haemopexin
3. Detection of urinary Hb or haemosiderin

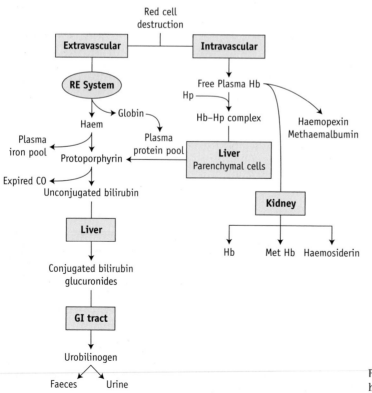

Figure 9.1 Catabolic pathway of haemoglobin.

What is the type of haemolytic mechanism?

1. Direct antiglobulin test (DAT) with broad-spectrum serum
2. Osmotic fragility and glycerol lysis test
3. Measurement of Hb in urine; plasma Hb; Schumm's test

What is the precise diagnosis?

1. If a hereditary haemolytic anaemia is suspected:

a. Osmotic-fragility determination after 24 hours of incubation at 37°C; red cell instability at 45°C; screening test for red cell glucose-6-phosphate dehydrogenase (G6PD) deficiency; red cell pyruvate kinase assay; assay of other red cell enzymes involved in glycolysis; estimation of red cell glutathione (see Chapter 10).
b. Estimation of % Hb A2 and % Hb F; electrophoresis for abnormal Hb; tests for sickling; tests for unstable Hb; blood count parameters, especially mean cell volume (MCV) and mean cell Hb (MCH); gene analysis (see Chapter 12).
c. Demonstration of the proteins of the red cell membrane and cytoskeleton (spectrin, etc.) by gel electrophoresis and by specific radioimmunoassay.

2. If an autoimmune acquired haemolytic anaemia is suspected:

a. Direct antiglobulin test using anti-immunoglobulin and anticomplement sera; tests for autoantibodies in the patient's serum; titration of cold agglutinins; Donath–Landsteiner test; electrophoresis of serum proteins; demonstration of thermal range of autoantibodies; tests for agglutination and/or lysis of enzyme-treated cells by autoantibodies; tests for lysis of normal cells by autoantibodies (see Chapter 11).

3. If the haemolytic anaemia is suspected of being drug induced:

a. Screening test for red cell G6PD; glutathione stability test; staining for Heinz bodies; identification of methaemoglobin (Hi) and sulphaemoglobin (SHb); tests for drug-dependent antibodies.

4. If mechanical stress is suspected:

a. Red cell morphology; platelet count; renal function tests; coagulation screen; fibrinogen assay; test for fibrinogen/fibrin degradation products (see Chapter 16).

5. In obscure cases:

a. Investigations for PNH (e.g., acidified serum test [Ham's test], sucrose lysis test) (see Chapter 11).
b. Measurement of lifespan of patient's red cells (see Chapter 15).
c. If splenectomy is contemplated, determination of sites of haemolysis by radionuclide imaging (see Chapter 15).

PLASMA HAEMOGLOBIN

Methods for estimation of plasma Hb are based on (a) peroxidase reaction and (b) direct measurement of Hb by spectrometry. In the peroxidase method, the catalytic action of haem-containing proteins brings about the oxidation of tetramethylbenzidine* by hydrogen peroxide to give a green colour, which changes to blue and finally to reddish violet. The intensity of reaction may be compared in a spectrometer with that produced by solutions of known Hb. Hi and Hb are measured together.

A pink tinge to the plasma is detectable by eye when the Hb is higher than 200 mg/l. When the plasma Hb is >50 mg/l, it can be measured as haemiglobincyanide (HiCN) or oxyhaemoglobin by a spectrometer at 540 nm[1] (see p. 26). Lower concentrations can also be measured reliably provided that the spectrometer plots of concentration/absorbance give a linear slope passing through the origin. This facility is provided by the Low Hb HemoCue, which can reliably measure plasma Hb at or higher than 100 mg/l.[2]

Sample Collection

Every effort must be made to prevent haemolysis during the collection and manipulation of the blood. For this, it is possibly preferable to use a syringe rather than an evacuated tube system. A clean

---

*This is an analogue of benzidene that can be used with the standard safety precautions for handling any toxic chemicals; benzidene itself is a carcinogenic substance, the use of which is prohibited in many countries.

venipuncture is essential; a plastic syringe and relatively wide-bore needle should be used. When the required amount of blood has been withdrawn, the needle should be detached with care and 9 volumes of blood should be added to 1 volume of 32 g/l sodium citrate. Haemolysis may be reduced to a minimum if the blood is collected through a wide-bore needle direct into a siliconized centrifuge tube containing heparin and the plasma is separated without delay.

Peroxidase Method[3]

Reagents
Benzidine Compound
Dissolve 1 g of 3,3′,5,5′-tetramethylbenzidine in 90 ml of glacial acetic acid and make up to 100 ml with water. The solution will keep for several weeks in a dark bottle at 4°C.

Hydrogen Peroxide
Dilute 1 volume of 3% ("10 vols") H_2O_2 with 2 volumes of water before use.

Acetic Acid
Use 100 g/l glacial acetic acid.

Standard
A blood sample of known Hb content is diluted with water to a final concentration of 200 mg/l. It is convenient to use an HiCN standard solution as the source of Hb.

Method

Add 20 µl of plasma to 1 ml of the benzidine reagent in a large glass tube. At the same time, set up a control tube, in which 20 µl of water are substituted for the plasma, and a standard tube, containing 20 µl of the Hb standard. Add 1 ml of the H_2O_2 solution to each tube, and mix the contents well.

Allow the mixture to stand at about 20°C for 20 min, and then add 10 ml of the acetic acid solution to each tube; after mixing, allow the tubes to stand for a further 10 min. Compare the coloured solutions at 600 nm, using the colour developed by the control tube as a blank. If the Hb of the plasma to be tested is abnormally high, it can be measured by the method used with whole blood (described later).

Spectrophotometric Method

From a normal blood sample, prepare an 80 g/l haemolysate (see p. 28).

Dilute 1:100 with phosphate buffer, pH 8, to obtain a Hb concentration of 800 mg/l. By 6 consecutive double dilutions with phosphate buffer, make a set of 7 lysate standards with values from 800 to 12.5 mg/l.

Read the absorbance of each solution at 540 nm, with water as a blank. Prepare a calibration graph by plotting the readings of absorbance (on y axis) against Hb concentration (on x axis) on arithmetic graph paper, and draw the slope. Check that the slope is linear.

Read the absorbance of the plasma directly at 540 nm with a water blank, and read the Hb concentration from the calibration graph. If absorbance is greater than the maximum value plotted on the graph, repeat the reading with a sample diluted with buffer.

When this modification of the HemoCue haemoglobinometer is available (see p. 189), fill the special cuvette with plasma and carry out the test in accordance with the instructions that are provided.

Normal Range

The normal range is 10–40 mg/l; lower levels may be obtained when blood is collected into a siliconized centrifuge tube with heparin (as previously discussed).

Significance of Increased Plasma Haemoglobin
Hb liberated from the intravascular or extravascular breakdown of red cells interacts with the plasma haptoglobins to form a Hb–haptoglobin complex,[4] which, because of its size, does not undergo glomerular filtration, but it is removed from the circulation by, and degraded in, reticulo-endothelial cells. Hb in excess of the capacity of the haptoglobins to bind it passes into the glomerular filtrate; it is then partly excreted in the urine in an uncomplexed form, resulting in haemoglobinuria, and partly reabsorbed by the proximal glomerular tubules where it is broken down into haem, iron, and globin. The iron is retained in the cells and eventually excreted in the urine (haemosiderin). The haem and globin are reabsorbed into the plasma.

The haem complexes with albumin forming methaemalbumin and with haemopexin (see p. 194); the globin competes with Hb to form a complex with haptoglobin. In effect, the plasma Hb level is significantly increased in haemolytic anaemias when haemolysis is sufficiently severe for the available haptoglobin to be fully bound. The highest levels are found when haemolysis takes place predominantly in the bloodstream (intravascular haemolysis). Thus, marked haemoglobinaemia, with or without haemoglobinuria, may be found in PNH, paroxysmal cold haemoglobinuria, the cold-haemagglutinin syndrome, blackwater fever, march haemoglobinuria, other mechanical haemolytic anaemias (e.g., that after cardiac surgery). In warm-type autoimmune haemolytic anaemias, sickle cell anaemia, and severe β thalassaemia, the plasma Hb level may be slightly or moderately increased, but in hereditary spherocytosis, in which haemolysis occurs predominantly in the spleen, the levels are normal or only very slightly increased.

Haem within the proximal tubular epithelium undergoes further degradation to bilirubin with liberation of iron, some of which is retained intracellularly bound to proteins as ferritin and haemosiderin. When haemolysis is severe, the excess of Hb that occurs in the glomerular filtrate will lead to an accumulation of intracellular haemosiderin in the glomerular tubular cells; when these cells slough, haemosiderin will appear in the urine (see p. 195).

The presence of excess Hb in the plasma is a reliable sign of intravascular haemolysis only if the observer can be sure that the lysis has not been caused during or after the withdrawal of the blood. It is also necessary to exclude colouring of the plasma from certain foods and food additives.

Increased levels may occur as a result of violent exercise, as well as in runners and joggers from mechanical trauma caused by continuous impact of the soles of the feet with hard ground.[4]

SERUM HAPTOGLOBIN

Haptoglobin is a glycoprotein that is synthesized in the liver. It consists of two pairs of α chains and two pairs of β chains. With haemolysis, free Hb readily dissociates into dimers of α and β chains; the α chains bind avidly with the β chains of haptoglobin

in plasma or serum to form a complex that can be differentiated from free Hb by column chromatographic separation or by its altered rate of migration in the α_2 position on electrophoresis.

Direct measurement of haptoglobin is also possible by turbidimetry or nephelometry and by radial immunodiffusion.[5] The methods described below are cellulose acetate electrophoresis and radial immunodiffusion.

Electrophoresis Method[6,7]

Principle
Known amounts of Hb are added to serum. The Hb–haptoglobin complex is separated by electrophoresis on cellulose acetate; the presence of bound and free Hb is identified in each sample, and the amount of haptoglobin is estimated by noting where free Hb appears.

Reagents
Buffer (pH 7.0, ionic strength 0.05)
$Na_2HPO_4.H_2O$ 7.1g/l, 2 volumes; $NaH_2PO_4.H_2O$ 6.9g/l, 1 volume. Store at 4°C.

Haemolysates
Prepare as described on page 283. Adjust the Hb to 30 g/l with water, and dilute this preparation further with water to obtain a batch of solutions with Hb concentrations of 2.5, 5, 10, 20, and 30 g/l. These solutions are stable at 4°C for several weeks.

Stain
Dissolve 0.5 g of *o*-dianisidine (3,3′-dimethoxybenzidine) in 70 ml of 95% ethanol; prior to use, add together 10 ml of acetate buffer, pH 4.7 (sodium acetate 2.92 g, glacial acetic acid 1 ml, water to 1 litre), 2.5 ml of 3% (10 volumes) H_2O_2 and water to 100 ml.

Clearing Solution
Glacial acetic acid 25 ml, 95% ethanol 75 ml.

Acetic Acid Rinse
Glacial acetic acid, 50 ml/l.

Method
Serum is obtained from blood allowed to clot undisturbed at 37°C. As soon as the clot starts to

retract, remove the serum by pipette and centrifuge it to rid it of suspended red cells. The serum may be stored at −20°C until used.

Mix well 1 volume of each of the diluted haemolysates with 9 volumes of serum. Allow to stand for 10 min at room temperature.

Impregnate cellulose acetate membrane filter strips (12 × 2.5 cm) in buffer solution, and blot to remove all obvious surface fluid. Apply 0.75 ml samples of the serum-haemolysate mixtures across the strips as thin transverse lines. As controls, include strips with serum alone and Hb lysate alone. Electrophorese at 0.5 mA/cm width. Good separation patterns about 5–7 cm in length should be obtained in 30 min (Fig. 9.2).

After electrophoresis is completed, immerse the membranes in freshly prepared o-dianisidine stain for 10 min. Then rinse with water and immerse in 50 ml/l acetic acid for 5 min. Remove the membranes and place in 95% ethanol for exactly 1 min. Transfer the membranes to a tray containing freshly prepared clearing solution and immerse for exactly

30 sec. While they are still in the solution, position the membranes over a glass plate placed in the tray. Remove the glass plate with the membranes on it, drain the excess solution from the membranes, transfer the glass plate to a ventilated oven preheated to 100°C, and allow the membranes to dry for 10 min.

Interpretation

The patterns of free Hb and Hb–haptoglobin complex migration are shown in Figure 9.2. Hb–haptoglobin complex appears in the α_2 globulin position. When there is more Hb than can be bound to the haptoglobin, the free Hb migrates in the β globulin position. The amount of haptoglobin present in the serum is determined semi-quantitatively as between the lowest concentration of Hb, which shows only a free Hb band, and the adjacent strip, which shows a band of Hb–haptoglobin complex. In the total absence of haptoglobin, an Hb band alone will be seen even at 2.5 g/l. In severe intravascular haemolysis with depleted haptoglobin, some of the haem may bind in the β globulin position to haemopexin (see below) and some to serum albumin to form methaemalbumin.

The concentration of haptoglobin can be determined quantitatively with a densitometer. The test is carried out as described earlier, but only one haemolysate is required with an Hb of 30–40 g/l. After the plate has cooled, the membranes are scanned by a densitometer at 450 nm with a 0.3-mm slit width. The density of the haptoglobin band is calculated as a fraction of the total Hb in the electrophoretic strip:

$$\text{Haptoglobin (g/l)} = \text{Haptoglobin fraction} \times \text{Hb (g/l)}$$

Radial Immunodiffusion (RID) Method

Principle

The test serum samples and reference samples of known haptoglobin concentration are dispensed into wells in a plate of agarose gel containing a monospecific antiserum to human haptoglobin. Precipitation rings form by the reaction of haptoglobin with the antibody; the diameter of each ring is proportional to the concentration of haptoglobin in the sample.

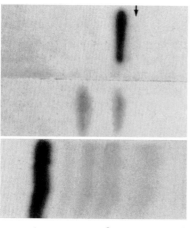

A α_1 α_2 β

Figure 9.2   Demonstration of serum haptoglobin. A: Serum from case of haemolytic anaemia with no haptoglobin: the added haemoglobin is demonstrated as a band in the β-globulin position. B: Normal serum with added haemoglobin: there are bands in the β-globulin (Hb) and α_2-globulin (Hb–haptoglobin complex) positions, respectively. The line of origin is indicated by the arrow. The pattern of serum electrophoresis is shown below (A, albumin; α_1, α_2, and β, components of globulin).

Reagents

Single Diffusion Plates*

Dissolve agarose (20 g/l) in boiling phosphate buffered water, pH 7.4 (p. 691). Allow to cool to 50°C. Add 5% sheep or goat antihuman haptoglobin antiserum diluted in buffered water, pH 7.4. Mix well but without creating bubbles. Pour the gel onto thin plastic trays (plates) to a thickness of less than 1 mm. After the gel has set, cut out a series of wells about 2 mm in diameter, about 2 cm apart. Extract the core by a pipette tip with a negative pressure pump. Cover the plates with fitted lids, and store in sealed packets at 4°C until used.

Reference Sera

Preparations of human serum with stated haptoglobin concentration are available commercially. They should be stored at 4°C.

Test Serum

Test serum can be kept at 4°C for 2–3 days, but if it is not used within this time, store at –20°C. Thaw completely, and mix well immediately before use.

Method

Allow the plate (in its sealed packet) and the sera to equilibrate at room temperature for 15 min. Remove the lid from the plate. Check for moisture; if present, allow to evaporate. Add 5 ml of each serum into one of the wells in the plate. Stand for about 10 min to ensure that the serum is completely absorbed into the gel. Then cover the plate, return it to its container, and reseal the packet. Leave on a level surface at room temperature for 18 hours. From measurements of the reference sera, construct a reference curve on log-linear graph paper by plotting haptoglobin concentration on the vertical axis (logarithmic scale) and the diameter of the rings on the horizontal scale (linear scale). Measure the diameter of the precipitation ring formed by the test serum and express concentration in g/l (Fig. 9.3).

Normal Ranges[5]

By direct measurement, results are expressed as haptoglobin concentration; slightly different normal

*Gel plates containing the antiserum are available commercially.

reference values have been reported for the different methods:

RID: 0.8–2.7 g/l
Nephelometry: 0.3–2.2 g/l
Turbidimetry: 0.5–1.6 g/l

When measured as Hb-binding capacity, in normal sera haptoglobins will bind 0.3–2.0 g/l of Hb. With this wide range of values there are no obvious sex differences, but in both men and women levels increase after the age of 70 years.

Significance

Haptoglobins begin to be depleted when the daily Hb turnover exceeds about twice the normal rate.[8] This occurs irrespective of whether the haemolysis is predominantly extravascular or intravascular; but rapid depletion, often with the formation of

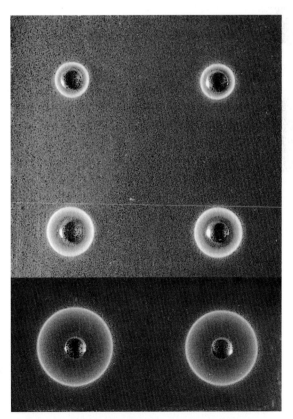

Figure 9.3 Demonstration of serum haptoglobin. Radial immunodiffusion: A: low; B: normal; and C: increased concentrations.

methaemalbumin, occurs as a result of small degrees of intravascular haemolysis, even when the daily total Hb turnover is not increased appreciably above normal. Low concentrations of haptoglobins, in the absence of increased haemolysis, may be found in hepatocellular disease and are characteristic of congenital ahaptoglobinaemia, which occurs in about 2% of Whites and a larger number of Blacks.[9] Low concentrations may also be found in megaloblastic anaemias, probably because of increased haemolysis, and following haemorrhage into tissues.

The haptoglobin–Hb complex is cleared by the reticulo-endothelial system, mainly in the liver. The rate of removal is influenced by the concentration of free Hb in the plasma: at levels below 10 g/l, the clearance $T_{1/2}$ is 20 min; at higher concentrations, clearance is considerably slower.

Increased haptoglobin concentrations may be found in pregnancy, chronic infections, malignancy, tissue damage, Hodgkin's disease, rheumatoid arthritis, systemic lupus erythematosus, and biliary obstruction and as a consequence of steroid therapy or the use of oral contraceptives. Under these circumstances, a normal haptoglobin concentration does not exclude haemolysis.

SERUM HAEMOPEXIN

Haemopexin is a β_1 glycoprotein of molecular weight 70,000, synthesized in the liver. It has a transport function. Haem derived from Hb, which fails to bind to haptoglobin, complexes with either haemopexin or albumin. The former has a much higher affinity, and only when all the haemopexin has been used up will the haem combine with albumin to form methaemalbumin. The haem–haemopexin complex is eliminated from the circulation (e.g., by the liver Kupffer cells).

Haem binds in a 1:1 molar ratio to haemopexin; 6 μg/ml of free haem is required to deplete the normal binding levels of haemopexin. In normal adults of both sexes, its concentration is 0.5–1.15 g/l (by nephelometry) or 0.5–1.5 g/l (by electrophoresis)[5]; there is less in newborn infants, about 0.3 g/l, but adult levels are reached by the end of the first year of life. In severe intravascular haemolysis, when haptoglobin is depleted, haemopexin is low or absent and plasma methaemalbumin is elevated. With less severe haemolysis, although haptoglobin is likely to be reduced or absent, haemopexin may be normal or only slightly lowered. Haemopexin seems to be disproportionately low in thalassaemia major, and low levels may be found in certain pathological conditions other than haemolytic disease, namely, renal and liver diseases. The concentration is increased in diabetes mellitus, infections, and carcinoma.[8]

Haemopexin can be measured by the same methods as for haptoglobin with radial immunodiffusion[8] or electrophoresis.[10]

EXAMINATION OF PLASMA (OR SERUM) FOR METHAEMALBUMIN

A simple but not very sensitive method is to examine the plasma using a hand spectroscope.

Free the plasma from suspended cells and platelets by centrifuging at 1200–1500 g for 15–30 min. Then view it in bright daylight with a hand spectroscope using the greatest possible depth of plasma consistent with visibility. Methaemalbumin gives a rather weak band in the red (at 624 nm) (Fig. 9.4). Because HbO$_2$ is usually present as well, its characteristic bands in the yellow–green may also be visible. The position of the methaemalbumin absorption band in the red can be readily differentiated from that of Hi by means of a reversion spectroscope.

Presumptive evidence of the presence of small quantities of methaemalbumin, giving an absorption band too weak to recognize, can be obtained

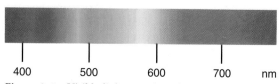

Figure 9.4   Visible light spectrum showing wavelengths of the colours of the spectrum. This ranges from 380 to 780 nm. Fraunhofer lines should be seen at approximately 431 nm, 486nm, 518 nm, 527 nm, 589 nm, 656 nm, and 687 nm.

by extracting the pigment by ether and then converting it to an ammonium haemochromogen, which gives a more intense band in the green (Schumm's test).

Schumm's Test

Method
Cover the plasma (or serum) with a layer of ether. Add a one-tenth volume of saturated yellow ammonium sulphide and mix it with the plasma. Then view it with a hand spectroscope. If methaemalbumin is present, a relatively intense narrow absorption band at 558 nm will be seen in the green.

Significance of Methaemalbuminaemia
Methaemalbumin is found in the plasma when haptoglobins are absent in haemolytic anaemias in which lysis is predominantly intravascular. It is a haem–albumin compound formed subsequent to the degradation of Hb liberated into plasma. It remains in circulation until the haem is transferred from albumin to the more highly avid haemopexin.

Quantitative Estimation by Spectrometry

To 2 ml of plasma (or serum) add 1 ml of iso-osmotic phosphate buffer, pH 7.4. Centrifuge the mixture for 30 min at 1200–1500 g, and measure its absorbance in a spectrophotometer at 569 nm. Add about 5 mg of solid sodium dithionite to the supernatant diluted plasma. Shake the tube gently to dissolve the dithionite and leave for 5 min to allow complete reduction of the methaemalbumin. Remeasure the absorbance. The difference between the two readings represents the absorbance due to methaemalbumin; its concentration can be read from a calibration graph.

Calibration Graph
Prepare solutions containing 10–100 mg/l methaem-albumin by dissolving appropriate amounts of haemin (bovine or equine) in a minimum volume of 40 g/l human serum albumin. Measure the absorbance of each solution in a spectrophotometer at 569 nm, and draw a graph from the figures obtained.

DEMONSTRATION OF HAEMOSIDERIN IN URINE

Method
Centrifuge 10 ml of urine at 1200 g for 10–15 min. Transfer the deposit to a slide, spread out to occupy an area of 1–2 cm, and allow to dry in the air. Fix by placing the slide in methanol for 10–20 min and then stain by the method used to stain blood films for siderocytes (p. 312). Haemosiderin, if present, appears in the form of isolated or grouped blue-staining granules, usually from 1–3 μm in size (Fig. 9.5); they may be both intracellular and extra-cellular. If haemosiderin is present in small amounts, and especially if distributed irregularly on the slide, or if the findings are difficult to interpret, the test should be repeated on a fresh sample of urine collected into an iron-free container and centrifuged in an iron-free tube. (For the preparation of iron-free glassware, see p. 695.)

Significance of Haemosiderinuria
Haemosiderinuria is a sequel to the presence of Hb in the glomerular filtrate. It is a valuable sign of intravascular haemolysis because the urine will be found to contain iron-containing granules even if there is no haemoglobinuria at the time. However, haemosiderinuria is not found in the urine at the onset of a haemolytic attack even if this is accom-

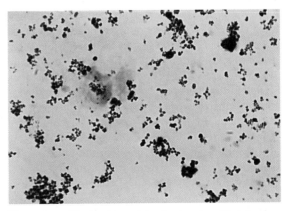

Figure 9.5 Photomicrograph of urine deposit stained by Perls' reaction.

panied by haemoglobinaemia and haemoglobinuria because the Hb has first to be absorbed by the cells of the renal tubules. The intracellular breakdown of Hb liberates iron, which is then re-excreted. Haemosiderinuria may persist for several weeks after a haemolytic episode.

CHEMICAL TESTS OF HAEMOGLOBIN CATABOLISM

Measurement of serum or plasma bilirubin, urinary urobilin, and faecal urobilinogen can provide important information in the investigation of haemolytic anaemias. In this section, their interpretation and significance in haemolytic anaemias will be described, but because currently the tests are seldom performed in a haematology laboratory, for details of the techniques readers are referred to textbooks of clinical chemistry.[5]

Serum Bilirubin

Bilirubin is present in serum in two forms: as unconjugated prehepatic bilirubin and bilirubin conjugated to glucuronic acid. Normally, the serum bilirubin concentration is <17 μmol/l (10 mg/l) and mostly unconjugated. As illustrated in Figure 9.1, when there is increased red cell destruction, the protoporphyrin gives rise to an increased amount of unconjugated bilirubin and carbon monoxide. The bilirubin is then conjugated in the liver, and this bilirubin glucuronide is excreted into the intestinal tract. Bacterial action converts bilirubin glucuronide to urobilin and urobilinogen. In haemolytic anaemias, the serum bilirubin usually lies between 17 and 50 μmol/l (10–30 mg/l) and most is unconjugated. Sometimes the level may be normal, despite a considerable increase in haemolysis. Levels >85 μmol/l (50 μg/l) and/or a large proportion of conjugated bilirubin suggest liver disease. In haemolytic disease of the newborn (HDN), the bilirubin level is an important factor in determining whether an exchange transfusion should be carried out because high values of unconjugated bilirubin are toxic to the brain and can lead to kernicterus. In normal newborn infants, the level often reaches 85 μmol/l, whereas in infants with HDN levels of 350 μmol/l are not uncommon and need to be urgently reduced by exchange transfusion. Moderately raised serum bilirubin levels are frequently found in dyshaemopoietic anaemias (e.g., pernicious anaemia), where there is ineffective erythropoiesis. Although part of the bilirubin comes from red cells that have circulated, a major proportion is derived from red cell precursors in the bone marrow that have failed to complete maturation.

Total bilirubin can be measured by direct reading spectrophotometry at 454 (or 461) and 540 nm; the former are the selected wavelengths for bilirubin, whereas the latter automatically corrects for any interference by free Hb. The instrument can be standardised with bilirubin solutions of known concentration or with a coloured glass standard. Another direct reading method is by reflectance photometry on a drop of serum that is added to a reagent film.

An alternative "wet chemistry" method is by the reaction with aqueous diazotized sulphanilic acid. A red colour is produced, which is compared in a photoelectric colorimeter with that of a freshly prepared standard or read in a spectrophotometer at 600 nm. Only conjugated bilirubin reacts directly with this aqueous reagent; unconjugated bilirubin, which is bound to albumin, requires either the addition of ethanol to free it from albumin or an accelerator such as methanol or caffeine to enable it to react. A positive urine spot test indicates a condition in which there is an elevated serum conjugated bilirubin. There is also a simple optical method, the Lovibond Comparator (Tintometer Ltd), in which the colour produced by reaction with sulphanilic acid is matched against the colours of a set of glass standards in a disk.

Bilirubin is destroyed by exposure to direct sunlight or any other source of ultraviolet (UV) light, including fluorescent lighting. Solutions are stable for 1–2 days if kept at 4°C in the dark.

Urobilin and Urobilinogen

Urobilin and its reduced form urobilinogen are formed by bacterial action on bile pigments in the intestine. The excretion of faecal urobilinogen in health is 50–500 μmol (30–300 mg) per day. It is increased in patients with a haemolytic anaemia. Quantitative measurement of faecal urobilinogen should, in theory, provide an estimate of the total rate of bilirubin production. This is, however, a crude method of assessing rates of haemolysis, and minor degrees are more reliably demonstrated by red cell lifespan studies. Urobilinogen excretion is also increased in dyshaemopoietic anaemias such as pernicious anaemia because of ineffective erythropoiesis.

The amount of urobilinogen in the urine in health is up to 6.7 μmol (4 mg) per day. However, these measurements are method dependent, and laboratories should establish their own normal reference values. This is not a reliable index of haemolysis, as excessive urobilinuria can be a consequence of liver dysfunction as well as of increased red cell destruction.

For estimation in the faeces, the bile-derived pigments (stercobilin) are reduced to urobilinogen, which is extracted with water. The solution is then treated with Ehrlich's dimethylaminobenzaldehyde reagent to produce a pink colour, which can be compared with either a natural or an artificial standard in a quantitative assay.

Qualitative Test for Urobilinogen and Urobilin in Urine

Schlesinger's Zinc Test

To 5 ml of urine, add 2 drops of 0.5 mol/l iodine to convert urobilinogen to urobilin. After mixing the sample and then leaving it standing on the bench for 1–2 min, add 5 ml of a 100 g/l suspension of zinc acetate in ethanol and centrifuge the mixture. A green fluorescence becomes apparent in the clear supernatant if urobilin or urobilinogen is present. If a spectroscope is available, the fluid may be examined for the broad absorption band (caused by urobilin) at the green–blue junction (see Fig. 9.4). Urobilinogen can also be detected in freshly voided urine by commercially available reagent strip methods.

PORPHYRINS

Haem synthesis is initiated by succinyl coenzyme A and glycine, activated by the rate-limiting enzyme ALA-synthase. This produces δ-aminolaevulinic acid (ALA), which is the precursor of the porphyrins (Fig. 9.6). The three porphyrins of clinical importance in humans are as follows: protoporphyrin,

uroporphyrin, and coproporphyrin together with their precursor ALA. Protoporphyrin is widely distributed in the body, and, in addition to its main role as a precursor of haem in Hb and myoglobin, it is a precursor of cytochromes and catalase. Uroporphyrin and coproporphyrin, which are precursors of protoporphyrin, are normally excreted in small amounts in urine and faeces. Red cells normally contain a small amount of coproporphyrin (5–35 nmol/l) and protoporphyrin (0.2–0.9 μmol/l). Deranged haem synthesis (e.g., in sideroblastic anaemias or lead toxicity) and iron deficiency anaemia result in an increased concentration of protoporphyrin in the red cells

Appropriate tests are usually performed in clinical chemistry laboratories, including sophisticated methods for measuring red cell porphyrins, as

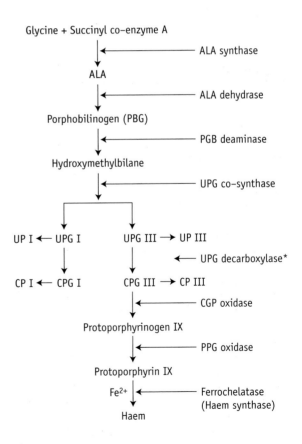

*acts on both isomer I and isomer III

Figure 9.6   Biosynthesis of porphyrin. See Table 9.1 for explanation of abbreviations.

described in an Association of Clinical Pathology Best Practice document.[11] Simple qualitative screening tests for urinary porphobilinogen and urinary porphyrin are described later. Urinary porphobilinogen will help to diagnose the acute forms of porphyria, particularly when the patient is symptomatic, and this test can lead to a definite diagnosis in a critical clinical situation.

Demonstration of Porphobilinogen in Urine

Principle
Ehrlich's dimethylaminobenzaldehyde reagent reacts with porphobilinogen to produce a pink aldehyde compound, which can be differentiated from that produced by urobilinogen by the fact that the porphobilinogen compound is insoluble in chloroform.

Ehrlich's Reagent
Dissolve 0.7 g of *p*-dimethylaminobenzaldehyde in a mixture of 150 ml of 10 mol/l HCl and 100 ml of water.

Method
Specimens must be protected from light, and the test is best carried out on freshly passed urine. Mix a few ml of urine and an equal volume of Ehrlich's reagent in a large test tube. Add 2 volumes of a saturated solution of sodium acetate. The urine should then have a pH of about 5.0, giving a red reaction with Congo red indicator paper.

If a pink colour develops in the solution, add a few ml of chloroform and shake the mixture thoroughly to extract the pigment. The colour due to urobilinogen or indole will be extracted by the chloroform, whereas that owing to porphobilinogen will not and remains in the supernatant aqueous fraction. A kit is available for a semiquantitative test using ion-exchange resin (Trace Laboratories; in the United Kingdom from Alpha Laboratories). When present, the concentration of porphobilinogen in the urine may be estimated quantitatively by a test kit method (Biorad) or by spectrophotometry at 555 nm.

Aminolaevulinic Acid

When ALA is present in the urine, it can be concentrated with acetyl acetone. It then reacts with Ehrlich's

reagent in the same way as porphobilinogen to give a red solution with an absorbance maximum at 553 nm. It can be separated from porphobilinogen by ion-exchange resins and estimated quantitatively by a spectrometric method.

Demonstration of Porphyrins in Urine

Principle
Porphyrins exhibit pink–red fluorescence when viewed by UV light (at 405 nm). Uroporphyrin can be distinguished from coproporphyrin by the different solubilities of the two substances in acid solution.

Method
Mix 25 ml of urine with 10 ml of glacial acetic acid in a separating funnel, and extract twice with 50 ml volumes of ether. Set the aqueous fraction (Fraction 1) aside. Wash the ether extracts in a separating funnel with 10 ml of 1.6 mol/l HCl and collect the HCl fraction (Fraction 2). View both fractions in UV light (at 405 nm) for pink–red fluorescence. Its presence in Fraction 1 indicates uroporphyrin; its presence in Fraction 2 indicates coproporphyrin. The presence of the porphyrins should be confirmed spectroscopically (described later).

If uroporphyrin has been demonstrated, the reaction can be intensified by the following procedure. Adjust the pH of Fraction 1 to 3.0–3.2 with 0.1 mol/l HCl and extract the fraction twice with 50 ml volumes of ethyl acetate. Combine the extracts and extract 3 times with 2 ml volumes of 3 mol/l HCl. View the acid extracts for pink–red fluorescence in UV light and spectroscopically for acid porphyrin bands.

Spectroscopic Examination of Urine for Porphyrins

Spectroscopic examination of urine for porphyrins is carried out on extracts, made as described earlier, or on urine that is acidified with a few drops of 10 mol/l HCl. If porphyrins are present, a narrow band will appear in the orange at 596 nm and a broader band will appear in the green at 552 nm (see Fig. 9.4). Qualitative tests are adequate for screening purposes. Accurate determinations require spectrophotometry or chromatography. Porphyrins are stable in ethylenediaminetetra-acetic acid (EDTA) blood for up to 8 days at room temperature if protected from light. Urine should be collected in a brown bottle, or if in a clear container, kept in a light-proof bag. If the urine is rendered alkaline to pH 7–7.5 with sodium bicarbonate, porphyrins will not be lost for several days at room temperature.

Significance of Porphyrins in Blood and Urine

Normal red cells contain <650 nmol/l of protoporphyrin and <64 nmol/l of coproporphyrin.[11] Increased amounts are present during the first few months of life. At all ages, there is an increase in red cell protoporphyrin in iron deficiency anaemia or latent iron deficiency, lead poisoning, thalassaemia, some cases of sideroblastic anaemia, and the anaemia of chronic disease. Zinc protoporphyrin is also elevated in these conditions (see p. 149).

Normally, a small amount of coproporphyrin is excreted in the urine (<430 nmol/ day). This is demonstrable by the qualitative test described earlier, the intensity of pink–red fluorescence being proportional to the concentration of coproporphyrin. The excretion of coproporphyrin is increased when erythropoiesis is hyperactive (e.g., in haemolytic anaemias and polycythaemia), in pernicious anaemia, and in sideroblastic anaemias. It is high in liver disease; renal impairment results in diminished excretion. In lead poisoning, there is an increase in red cell protoporphyrin and coproporphyrin, with excretion of exceptionally high levels of urinary ALA, coproporphyrin III, and uroporphyrin I.

Normally, porphobilinogen cannot be demonstrated in urine, and only traces of uroporphyrin (<50 nmol/day), not detectable by the qualitative test described earlier, are present.[11] ALA excretion is normally <40 mmol/day; it is increased in lead poisoning.

The increase in urinary coproporphyrin excretion occurring in the previously mentioned conditions is known as *porphyrinuria*. There is no increase in uroporphyrin excretion. The porphyrias, however, are a group of disorders associated with abnormal porphyrin metabolism.

There are several forms of porphyria, caused by specific enzyme defects, each with a different clinical effect and pattern of excretion of porphyrin and precursors[12] (Table 9.1). The most common type is acute intermittent porphyria, in which the defect in the enzyme porphobilinogen deaminase presents in one of three ways:

Type 1: Decreased enzyme activity together with reduced amount of the enzyme in the red cells
Type 2: Decreased enzyme activity in lymphocytes and liver cells but normal red cell activity
Type 3: Reduced red cell enzyme activity but normal amount of enzyme in the red cells

The different mutations of the porphobilinogen deaminase in the three types can be identified by DNA hybridization using specific oligonucleotides.[13] Other acute forms are variegate and coproporphyria.

The most common hepatic type is *porphyria cutanea tarda;* which results in photosensitivity, dermatitis, and often hepatic siderosis; it is the result of a defect in uroporphyrinogen decarboxylase. In this and other porphyrias associated with photosensitive dermatitis (see Table 9.1) plasma porphyrins are elevated. There are two erythropoietic types: *congenital erythropoietic porphyria,* caused by defective uroporphyrinogen cosynthase, and *erythropoietic protoporphyria,* caused by defective ferrochelatase. In the former, uroporphyrin and coproporphyrin are present in red cells and urine in increased amounts; in the latter, increased protoporphyrin is found in the red cells, but the urine is normal. In erythropoietic porphyria, haemolytic anaemia may occur.

ABNORMAL HAEMOGLOBIN PIGMENTS

Methaemoglobin (Hi; also called MetHb), sulphaemoglobin (SHb), and carboxyhaemoglobin (HbCO) are of clinical importance, and each has a characteristic absorption spectrum demonstrable by simple spectroscopy or, more definitely, by spectrometry. If the absorbance of a dilute solution of blood (e.g., 1 in 200) is measured at wavelengths between 400 and 700 nm, characteristic absorption spectra are obtained[14–16] (Fig. 9.7 and Table 9.2). In practice, the abnormal substance represents usually only a fraction of the total Hb (except in carbon monoxide poisoning), and its identification and accurate measurement may be difficult. Hi can be measured more accurately than SHb.

Absorption spectroscopy is a method by which a substance can be characterized by the wavelengths

Table 9.1 Distribution of porphyrins in red cells, urine and faeces in different forms of porphyria

Disease	Clinical effect	Enzyme defect*	Red cells	Urine	Faeces
ALA dehydratase deficiency porphyria	(a)	ALA dehydratase (porpobilinogen synthase)	ZnP ALA	CPIII	–
Acute intermittent porphyria	(a)	PBG deaminase	–	PBG ALA	–
Congenital erythropoietic porphyria	(b)	UPG III cosynthase	UP I C PI ZnP	UP I CP I	UP I CP I
Acquired cutaneous hepatic porphyria (symptomatic)	(b)	UPG decarboxylase	–	UP I CP III	–
Hereditary coproporphyria	(a), (b)	CPG oxidase	–	CP III	CP III
Variegate porphyria (South African genetic)	(a), (b)	PPG oxidase	–	PBG[†] ALA[†]	CP III PP
Erythropoietic protoporphyria	(b)	Ferrochelatase	PP	–	PP

*See Figure 9.6.
[†]Mainly during acute attacks.
(a) Gastrointestinal and/or nervous system disorders.
(b) Photosensitive dermatitis.
ALA, α-aminolaevulinic acid; PBG, porphobilinogen; UP, uroporphyrin; CP, coproporphyrin; PP, protoporphyrin; UPG, uroporphyrinogen; CPG, coproporphyrinogen; PPG, protoporphyrinogen; ZnP, Zinc protoporphyrin.

at which the colour spectrum is absorbed when light is passed through a solution of the substance. The specific absorption bands are identifiable by their positions (Fig 9.4).

Spectroscopic Examination of Blood for Methaemoglobin and Sulphaemoglobin

Method

Dilute blood 1 in 5 or 1 in 10 with water and then centrifuge. Examine the clear solution, if possible in daylight, using a hand spectroscope. It is important that the greatest possible depth or concentration of solution consistent with visibility should be examined and that a careful search should be made (with varying depths or concentrations of solution) for absorption bands in the red part of the spectrum at 620–630 nm. If bands are seen in the red, add a drop of yellow ammonium sulphide to the solution. A band caused by Hi, but not that caused by SHb, will disappear. For comparison, lysed blood may be treated with a few drops of potassium ferricyanide (50 g/l) solution, which will cause the formation of Hi; SHb may be prepared by adding to 10 ml of a 1 in 100 dilution of blood 0.1 ml of a 1g/l solution of phenylhydrazine hydrochloride and a drop of water that has been previously saturated with hydrogen sulphide. The spectra of the unknown and the known pigments may then be compared in a reversion spectroscope. The absorption band in the red caused by Hi is at 630 nm (compare with methaemalbumin at 624 nm) (see Fig. 9.4).

Hi and SHb are formed intracellularly; they are not found in plasma except under very exceptional circumstances (e.g., when their formation is associated with intravascular haemolysis).

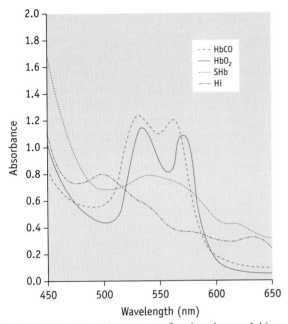

Figure 9.7   Absorption spectra of various haemoglobin pigments. HbCO, carboxyhaemoglobin; HbO$_2$, oxyhaemoglobin; SHb, sulphaemoglobin; Hi, methaemoglobin.

Table 9.2 Positions in spectrum for optimal absorbance of haemoglobin derivatives in absorption spectrometry (in nm)*	
Oxyhaemoglobin	542, 577
Deoxygenated haemoglobin:	431, 556
Carboxyhaemoglobin:	538, 568
Methaemoglobin:	500, 630
Sulphaemoglobin:	620
Methaemalbumin	624
Haemochromogen	
(Schumm's test)	558

* Some approximations where slightly different figures have been reported in different studies.

Measurement of Methaemoglobin[14,15]

Principle

Hi has a maximum absorption at 630 nm. When cyanide is added, this absorption band disappears and the resulting change in absorbance is directly proportional to the concentration of Hi. Total Hb in the sample is then measured after complete conversion to HiCN by the addition of ferricyanide-cyanide reagent. The conversion will measure oxyhaemoglobin and Hi but not SHb. Thus, the presence of a large amount of SHb will result in an erroneously low measurement of total Hb. Turbidity of the haemolysate can be overcome by the addition of a nonionic detergent.

Reagents

Phosphate buffer: 0.1 mol/l, pH 6.8
Potassium cyanide: 50 g/l
Potassium ferricyanide: 50 g/l
Nonionic detergent: 10 ml/l [Triton X-100* or Nonidet P40†]

Method

Lyse 0.2 ml of blood in a solution containing 4 ml of buffer and 6 ml of detergent solution. Divide the lysate into two equal volumes (A and B). Measure the absorbance of A in a spectrophotometer at 630 nm (D_1). Add 1 drop of potassium cyanide solution and measure the absorbance again, after mixing (D_2). Add 1 drop of potassium ferricyanide solution to B, and after 5 min, measure the absorbance at the same wavelength (D_3). Then add 1 drop of potassium cyanide solution to B and after mixing make a final reading (D_4). All the measurements are made against a blank containing buffer and detergent in the same proportion as present in the sample.

Calculation

$$\text{Hi (\%)} = \frac{D_1 - D_2}{D_3 - D_4} \times 100$$

The test should be carried out within 1 hour of collecting the blood. After dilution, the buffered lysate can be stored for up to 24 hours at 2–4°C without significant autooxidation of Hb to Hi.

*Aldrich
†For example, VWR International, Merck, BDH, Eurolab

Screening Method for Sulphaemoglobin

Principle

An absorbance reading at 620 nm measures the sum of the absorbance of oxyhaemoglobin and SHb in any blood sample. In contrast to oxyhaemoglobin, the absorption band caused by SHb is unchanged by the addition of cyanide. The residual absorbance, as read at 620 nm, is therefore proportional to the concentration of SHb. The absorbance of the oxyhaemoglobin alone at 620 nm can only be inferred from a reading at 578 nm, and a conversion factor, A^{578}/A^{620}, has to be determined experimentally for each instrument on a series of normal blood samples.[16,17] The absorbance of SHb is obtained by subtracting the absorbance of the oxyhaemoglobin from that of the total Hb. This provides an approximation only, but it may be regarded as adequate for clinical purposes in the absence of a more reliable method.

Method

Mix 0.1 ml of blood with 10 ml of a 20 ml/l solution of a nonionic detergent (Triton X-100 or Nonidet P40; see footnote p. 201). Record the absorbance (A) at 620 nm (total Hb). Add 1 drop of 50 g/l potassium cyanide, and after letting it stand for 5 min, record A at 620 nm and at 578 nm.

Calculation

$$SHb\ (\%) = \frac{2 \times A^{620}\ SHb}{A^{620}\ HbO_2}$$

$$\text{where } A^{620}\ HbO_2 = \frac{\text{Absorbance read at 578 nm}}{\text{Conversion factor,}}$$

$$\text{and } A^{620}\ SHb = A^{620}\ \text{total Hb} - A^{620}\ HbO_2$$

Significance of Methaemoglobin and Sulphaemoglobin in Blood

Hi is present in small amounts in normal blood and constitutes 1–2% of the total Hb. Its concentration is very slightly higher in infants, especially in premature infants, than in older children and adults. An excessive amount of Hi occurs as the result of oxidation of Hb by drugs and chemicals such as phenacetin, sulphonamides, aniline dyes, nitrates, and nitrites.

The Hi produced by drugs is chemically normal, and the pigment can be reconverted to oxyhaemoglobin by reducing agents such as methylene blue.

Other (rare) types of methaemoglobinaemia are caused by inherited deficiency of the enzyme NADH-Hi reductase and by inherited Hb abnormalities (types of Hb M). The absorption spectra of the Hb Ms differ from that of normal Hi, and they react slowly and incompletely with cyanide; their concentration cannot be estimated by the method of Evelyn and Malloy.[14] Methaemoglobinaemia leads to cyanosis which becomes obvious with as little as 15g/l of Hi, that is, about 10%.

SHb is usually formed at the same time as methemoglobin; it represents a further and irreversible stage in Hb degradation. It is present as a rule at a much lower concentration than is Hi.

Demonstration of Carboxyhaemoglobin

Principle

Oxyhaemoglobin, but not HbCO, is reduced by sodium dithionite, and the percentage of HbCO in a mixture can be determined by reference to a calibration graph.

Calibration graph

Dilute 0.1 ml of normal blood in 20 ml of 0.4 ml/l ammonia and divide into two parts. To each add 20 mg of sodium dithionite. Then bubble pure carbon monoxide into one for 2 min, so as to provide a 100% solution of HbCO.

Add various volumes of the HbCO solution to the reduced Hb solution to provide a range of concentrations of HbCO. Within 10 min of adding the dithionite, measure the absorbance of each solution at 538 nm and 578 nm. Plot the quotient A^{538}/A^{578} on arithmetic graph paper against the % HbCO in each solution.

Method[16,17]

Dilute 0.1 ml of blood in 20 ml of 0.4 ml/l ammonia and add 20 mg of sodium dithionite. Measure the absorbance in a spectrophotometer at 538 nm and 578 nm within 10 min. Calculate the quotient A^{538}/A^{578} and read the % HbCO in the blood from the calibration curve[16] or calculate it from the equation.[16]

$$\% \ HbCO = \frac{\{2.44 \times A^{538}\}}{A^{578}} - 2.68$$

Significance of Carboxyhaemoglobin in Circulating Blood

Carbon monoxide has an affinity for Hb *c* 200 times that of oxygen. This means that even low concentrations of carbon monoxide rapidly lead to the formation of HbCO. Less than 1% of HbCO is present in normal blood and up to 10% in smokers.[17,18] There is also an increased production, and excretion in the lungs, in haemolytic anaemias. A high concentration in blood from inhalation of the gas causes tissue anoxia and may lead to death. However, recovery can take place because HbCO dissociates in time in the presence of high concentrations of oxygen.

Identification of Myoglobin in Urine

Myoglobin is the principal protein in muscle, and it may be released into the circulation when there is cardiac or skeletal muscle damage. Some may be excreted in the urine where its concentration can be measured by a specific and relatively sensitive radioimmunoassay.[19] Because the absorption spectra of myoglobin and Hb are similar, although not identical, it is not possible to distinguish them readily by spectroscopy or spectrometry, but they can be separated by column chromatography.[20] Normally, men have less than 80 μg/l and women have less than 60 μg/l, increasing slightly in old age, whereas children have very low values.[5]

REFERENCES

1. Moore GL, Ledford ME, Merydith A 1981 A micromodification of the Drabkin hemoglobin assay for measuring plasma hemoglobin in the range of 5 to 2000mg/dl. Biochemical Medicine 26:167–173.
2. Morris LD, Pont A, Lewis SM 2001 Use of a new HemoCue system for measuring haemoglobin at low concentrations. Clinical and Laboratory Haematology 23:91–96.
3. Standefer JC, Vanderjogt D 1977 Use of tetramethyl benzidine in plasma hemoglobin assay. Clinical Chemistry 23:749–751.
4. Davidson RJL 1969 March or exertional haemoglobinuria. Seminars in Hematology 6:150–161.
5. Burtis CA, Ashwood ER 2000 NW Tietz's Fundamentals of Clinical Chemistry. 5th Edition. Saunders, Philadelphia.
6. Brus I, Lewis SM 1959 The haptoglobin content of serum in haemolytic anaemia. British Journal of Haematology 5:348–355.
7. Valeri CR, Bond JC, Flower K, et al. 1965 Quantitation of serum hemoglobin-binding capacity using cellulose acetate membrane electrophoresis. Clinical Chemistry 11:581–588.
8. Nagel RL, Gibson QH 1971 The binding of hemoglobin to haptoglobin and its relation to subunit dissociation of hemoglobin. Journal of Biological Chemistry 246:69–73.
9. Hanstein A, Muller-Eberhard U 1968 Concentration of serum hemopexin in healthy children and adults and in those with a variety of hematological disorders. Journal of Laboratory and Clinical Medicine 71:232–239.
10. Heide K, Haupt H, Störiko K, et al. 1964 On the heme-binding capacity of hemopexin. Clinica Chimica Acta 10:460–469.
11. Deacon AC, Elder GH 2001 Frontline tests for the investigation of suspected porphyria: ACP Best Practice No. 165. Journal of Clinical Pathology 54:500–507.
12. Bottomley SS, Muller-Eberhard U 1988 Pathophysiology of heme synthesis. Seminars in Haematology 25:282–302.
13. Sassa S 1996 Diagnosis and therapy of acute intermittent porphyria. Blood Reviews 10:53–55.
14. Van Kampen EJ, Zijlstra WG 1965 Determination of hemoglobin and its derivates. Advances in Clinical Chemistry 8:141–187.
15. Zijlstra WG, Buursma A, van Assendelft OW 2003 Visible and near infrared absorption spectra of human and animal haemoglobin: determination and applications. VSP Publishers, Zeist, Netherlands.
16. Zwart A, van Kampen EJ, Zijlstra WG 1986 Results of routine determination of clinically significant hemoglobin derivatives by multicomponent analysis. Clinical Chemistry 32:972–978.
17. Shields CE 1971 Elevated carbon monoxide level from smoking in blood donors. Transfusion (Philadelphia) 11:89–93.
18. Russell MAH, Wilson C, Cole PV, et al. 1973 Comparison of increases in carboxyhaemoglobin after smoking "extra mild" and "non mild" cigarettes. Lancet ii:687–690.
19. Stone MJ, Willerson JT, Waterman MR 1982 Radioimmunoassay of myoglobin. Methods in Enzymology 84:172–177.
20. Cameron BF, Azzam SA, Kotite L, et al. 1965 Determination of myoglobin and hemoglobin. Journal of Laboratory and Clinical Medicine 65:883–890.

10 Investigation of the hereditary haemolytic anaemias: membrane and enzyme abnormalities

David Roper and Mark Layton

The various initial steps to be taken in the investigation of a patient suspected of having a haemolytic anaemia are outlined in Chapter 9, and the changes in red cell morphology that may be found in haemolytic anaemias are illustrated in Chapter 5. This chapter describes procedures useful in investigating haemolytic anaemias suspected of resulting from defects within the red cell membrane or deficiency of enzymes important in red cell metabolism.

The precise identification of an enzyme defect is beyond the scope of most haematology laboratories; it may require the isolation and purification of the enzyme and the determination and delineation of its kinetic and structural properties. In a service laboratory, it is sufficient to identify the general nature of the defect, whether it be in the membrane or the metabolic pathways of the red cell. In the case of putative metabolic defects, an attempt should be made, where possible, to pinpoint the enzyme involved. The first part of this chapter describes screening tests for spherocytosis, including hereditary spherocytosis (HS), and for glucose-6-phosphate dehydrogenase (G6PD) deficiency. The later sections of the chapter describe specific enzyme assays and the measurement of 2,3-diphospho-glycerate (2,3-DPG) and reduced glutathione (GSH).

Most of the enzyme assays have been standardized by the International Council for Standardization in Haematology (ICSH). Commercial kits are also available for some quantitative assays and screening tests. These are noted in the relevant sections.

INVESTIGATION OF MEMBRANE DEFECTS

The osmotic fragility test gives an indication of the surface area/volume ratio of erythrocytes. Its greatest usefulness is in the diagnosis of hereditary spherocytosis. The test may also be used in screening for thalassaemia. Red cells that are spherocytic, for whatever cause, take up less water in a hypotonic solution before rupturing than do normal red cells.

Other tests that demonstrate red cell membrane defects include glycerol lysis time; cryohaemolysis; autohaemolysis; and, more specifically, membrane protein analysis.

OSMOTIC FRAGILITY, AS MEASURED BY LYSIS IN HYPOTONIC SALINE

Principle

The method to be described is based on that of Parpart et al.[1]

Small volumes of blood are mixed with a large excess of buffered saline solutions of varying concentration. The fraction of red cells lysed at each saline concentration is determined colorimetrically. The test is normally carried out at room temperature (15–25°C).

Reagents

Prepare a stock solution of buffered sodium chloride, osmotically equivalent to 100 g/l (1.71 mol/l) NaCl, as follows: Dissolve NaCl, 90 g; Na_2HPO_4, 13.65 g (or $Na_2HPO_42H_2O$, 17.115 g); and $NaH_2PO_4.2H_2O$, 2.34 g in water. Adjust the final volume to 1 litre. This solution will keep for months at 4°C in a well-stoppered bottle. Salt crystals may form on storage and must be thoroughly redissolved before use.

In preparing hypotonic solutions for use, it is convenient to make first a 10 g/l solution from the 100 g/l NaCl stock solution by dilution with water. Dilutions equivalent to 9.0, 7.5, 6.5, 6.0, 5.5, 5.0, 4.0, 3.5, 3.0, 2.0, and 1.0 g/l are convenient concentrations. Intermediate concentrations such as 4.75 and 5.25 g/l are useful in critical work, and an additional 12.0 g/l dilution should be used for incubated samples.

It is convenient to make up 50 ml of each dilution. The solutions keep well at 4°C if sterile, but should be inspected for moulds before use and discarded if moulds develop.

Method

Heparinized venous blood or defibrinated blood may be used; oxalated or citrated blood is not suitable because of the additional salts added to it. The test should be carried out within 2 hours of collection with blood stored at room temperature or within 6 hours if the blood has been kept at 4°C.

1. Deliver 5.0 ml of each of the 11 saline solutions into 12 × 75 mm test tubes. Add 5.0 ml of water to the 12th tube.
2. Add to each tube 50 μl of well-mixed blood, and mix immediately by inverting the tubes several times, avoiding foam.
3. Leave the suspensions for 30 min at room temperature. Mix again, and then centrifuge for 5 min at 1200 g.
4. Remove the supernatants and estimate the amount of lysis in each using a spectrometer at a wavelength setting of 540 nm or a photoelectric colorimeter provided with a yellow–green (e.g., Ilford 625) filter. Use as a blank the supernatant from tube 1 (osmotically equivalent to 9 g/l NaCl).

5. Assign a value of 100% lysis to the reading with the supernatant of tube 12 (water), and express the readings from the other tubes as a percentage of the value of tube 12. Plot the results against the NaCl concentration (Fig. 10.1).

Notes

1. The measurement of osmotic fragility is a simple procedure that requires a minimum of equipment. It will yield gratifying results if carried out carefully.
2. The blood must be delivered into the 12 tubes with great care. The critical point is not that the amount be exactly 50 µl, but rather that the amount added to each tube must be the same. Two methods are recommended:
   a. Using an automatic pipette, after aspirating the blood gently, wipe the outside with tissue paper, taking care not to suck out any blood from the inside of the tip by capillary action. The blood is then delivered into the saline solution and the pipette is rinsed in and out several times until no blood is visible inside its tip.

      The tip has to be changed before moving on to the next tube. This procedure takes time and may result in an increased exposure for the first few tubes. It is therefore advisable to start the timing only after the addition of the sample to the first tube.

   b. Using a Pasteur pipette with a perfectly flat end, 1 mm in diameter, suck up about 1 ml of blood, avoiding any bubbles, and wipe the outside of the pipette. With the pipette held vertically above tube 1, deliver a single drop (about 50 µl) without the blood touching the wall of the tube. Then deliver single drops into the remaining 11 tubes.

      Method b appears to be primitive, but with practice it is perfectly satisfactory; it is also more economical and much faster than method a. With either method, the best way to test its accuracy is to do a preliminary test by delivering the blood into several tubes all containing the same saline solution (e.g., either 3.0 or 1.0 g/l). The readings with the supernatants should be all within 5% of each other.

3. If the amount of blood available is limited (e.g., from babies), and the spectrometer takes 1 ml cuvettes, the volumes can be scaled down to 1 ml of saline solution and 10 µl of blood. However, to deliver 10 µl of blood reproducibly is not easy. With method b, a Pasteur pipette or capillary pipette with a much smaller diameter, calibrated to give 10 µl drops of blood, would have to be used. It is then more difficult to maintain accuracy. Method a may be preferable in this case.
4. With the method using 50 µl of blood and with non-anaemic blood, the reading for 100% lysis will

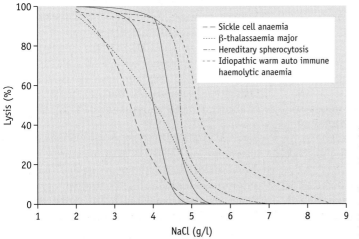

Figure 10.1   Osmotic fragility curves. Osmotic fragility curves of patients suffering from the following: sickle cell anaemia, β-thalassaemia major, hereditary spherocytosis, and "idiopathic" warm autoimmune haemolytic anaemia. The normal range is indicated by the unbroken lines

be about 0.7. With a modern spectrometer, any figure between 0.5 and 1.5 is acceptable. If the value is less than 0.5, the test should be repeated using more blood or less saline (the reverse if the reading is higher than 1.5). With photoelectric colorimeters, values higher than 0.5 are often not very accurate.

5. When transferring the supernatant from a tube to the spectrometer cuvette, care has to be taken not to disturb the pellet. If it is well packed, the supernatant can simply be poured from the tube into the cuvette; with a spectrometer provided with an automatic suction device, this is usually satisfactory. Alternatively, a plastic Pasteur pipette should be used.

6. Even when a normal range has been established, it is essential always to run a normal control sample along with that of the patients to be tested to check, for example, the saline solutions.

The sigmoid shape of the normal osmotic fragility curve indicates that normal red cells vary in their resistance to hypotonic solutions. Indeed, this resistance varies gradually (osmotically) as a function of red cell age, with the youngest cells being the most resistant and the oldest cells being the most fragile. The reason for this is that old cells have a higher sodium content and a decreased capacity to pump out sodium.

Osmotic Fragility after Incubating the Blood at 37°C for 24 Hours

Method
Defibrinated blood should be used, care being taken to ensure that sterility is maintained.

Incubate 1 ml or 2 ml volumes of blood in sterile 5-ml bottles. It is advisable to set up the samples in duplicate in case one has become infected, as indicated by gross lysis and change in colour.

After 24 hours, if no infection is evident, pool the contents of the duplicate bottles after thoroughly mixing the sedimented red cells in the overlying serum and estimate the fragility as previously described.

Because the fragility may be markedly increased (Fig. 10.2), set up additional hypotonic solutions containing 7.0 g/l and 8.0 g/l NaCl. In addition, use

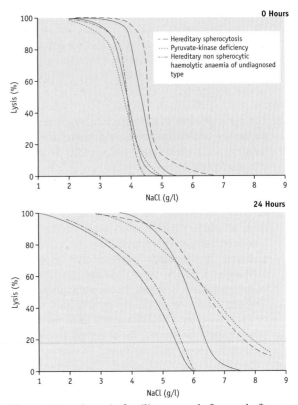

Figure 10.2 Osmotic fragility curves before and after incubating blood at 37°C for 24 hours. From patients suffering from the following: hereditary spherocytosis, pyruvate-kinase deficiency, and hereditary non-spherocytic haemolytic anaemia of undiagnosed type. The normal range is indicated by the unbroken lines.

a solution equivalent to 12.0 g/l NaCl because sometimes, as in HS, lysis may take place in 9.0 g/l NaCl. In this case, use the supernatant of the tube containing 12.0 g/l NaCl as the blank in the colorimetric estimation.

The incubation fragility test is conveniently combined with the estimation of the amount of spontaneous autohaemolysis (see p. 213).

Factors Affecting Osmotic Fragility Tests

In carrying out osmotic fragility tests by any method, three variables capable of markedly affecting the results must be controlled, quite apart from the accuracy with which the saline solutions have been made up. These are as follows:

1. The relative volumes of blood and saline
2. The final pH of the blood in saline suspension
3. The temperature at which the tests are carried out

A proportion of 1 volume of blood to 100 volumes of saline is chosen because the concentration of blood is so small that the effect of the plasma on the final tonicity of the suspension is negligible. When weak suspensions of blood in saline are used, it is necessary to control the pH of the hypotonic solutions, and it is for this reason that phosphate buffer is added to the saline. Even so, small differences will be found between the fragility of venous blood and maximally aerated (i.e., oxygenated) blood. For the most accurate results, it is recommended that the blood should be mixed until bright red. Finally, it is ideal for tests to be carried out always at the same temperature, although for most purposes room temperature is sufficiently constant.

The extent of the effect of pH and temperature on osmotic fragility was well illustrated in the paper of Parpart et al.[1] The effect of pH is more important: a shift of 0.1 of a pH unit is equivalent to altering the saline concentration by 0.1 g/l, the fragility of the red cells being increased by a decrease in pH. An increase in temperature decreases the fragility, an increase of 5°C being equivalent to an increase in saline concentration of about 0.1 g/l.

Lysis is virtually complete at the end of 30 min at 20°C, and the hypotonic solutions may be centrifuged at the end of this time.

Further details of the factors that affect and control haemolysis of red cells in hypotonic solutions were given by Murphy.[2]

Recording the Results of Osmotic Fragility Tests

In the past, osmotic fragility most often has been expressed in terms of the highest concentration of saline at which lysis is just detectable (initial lysis or minimum resistance) and the highest concentration of saline in which lysis appears to be complete (complete lysis or maximum resistance). It is, however, useful also to record the concentration of saline causing 50% lysis (i.e., the median corpuscular fragility [MCF]) and to inspect the entire fragility curve (Fig. 10.1). The findings in health are summarized in Table 10.1.

Table 10.1   Osmotic fragility in health (at 20°C and pH 7.4)

	Fresh blood (g/l NaCl)	Blood incubated 24 hours, 37°C (g/l NaCl)
Initial lysis	5.0	7.0
Complete lysis	3.0	2.0
MCF (50% lysis)	4.0–4.45	4.65–5.9

MCF, median corpuscular fragility.

Alternative Methods of Recording Osmotic Fragility
Two simple alternative methods of recording the results quantitatively are available: The data may be plotted on probability paper or increment-haemolysis curves can be drawn. Both methods emphasize heterogeneity of the cell population with respect to osmotic fragility. If the observed amounts of lysis of normal blood are plotted on the probability scale against concentrations of saline, an almost straight line can be drawn through the points; the line is only skewed where lysis is almost complete. This method enables the MCF to be read off with ease.

In disease, tailed curves also skew the line to varying degrees at the other end of the probability plot. To obtain increment-haemolysis curves, the differences in lysis between adjacent tubes are plotted against the corresponding saline concentrations. Definitely bimodal curves may be obtained during recovery from a haemolytic episode.[3]

Interpretation of Results

The osmotic fragility of freshly taken red cells reflects their ability to take up a certain amount of water before lysing. This is determined by their volume-to-surface area ratio. The ability of the normal red cell to withstand hypotonicity results from its biconcave shape, which allows the cell to increase its volume by about 70% before the surface membrane is stretched; once this limit is reached lysis occurs.[4] Spherocytes have an increased volume-to-surface area ratio; their ability to take in water before stretching the surface membrane is thus more limited than normal and they are therefore particularly susceptible to osmotic lysis.

The increase in osmotic fragility is a property of the spheroidal shape of the cell and is independent of the cause of the spherocytosis. Characteristically, osmotic fragility curves from patients with HS who have not been splenectomized show a "tail" of very fragile cells (Fig. 10.3). When plotted on probability paper, the graph indicates two populations of cells: the very fragile and the normal or slightly fragile. After splenectomy the red cells are more homogeneous, the osmotic fragility curve indicating a more continuous spectrum of cells, from fragile to normal.

Decreased osmotic fragility indicates the presence of unusually flattened red cells (leptocytes) in which the volume-to-surface area ratio is decreased. Such a change occurs in iron deficiency anaemia and thalassaemia in which the red cells with a low mean cell haemoglobin (MCH) and mean cell volume (MCV) are unusually resistant to osmotic lysis (see Fig. 10.1). A simple one-tube osmotic fragility is a useful screening test for β thalassaemia and some haemoglobinopathies in countries with a high incidence of these abnormalities (see p. 683). Reticulocytes and red cells from patients who have been splenectomized also tend to have a greater amount of membrane compared with normal cells and are osmotically resistant. In liver disease, target cells may be produced by passive accumulation of lipid, and these cells, too, are resistant to osmotic lysis.[5]

The osmotic fragility of red cells after incubation for 24 hours at 37°C is also a reflection of their volume-to-surface area ratio, but the factors that alter this ratio are more complicated than in fresh red cells. The increased osmotic fragility of normal red cells, which occurs after incubation (see Fig. 10.2), is mainly caused by swelling of the cells associated with an accumulation of sodium that exceeds loss of potassium. Such cation exchange is determined by the membrane properties of the red cell, which control the passive flux of ions, and the metabolic competence of the cell, which determines the active pumping of cations against concentration gradients. During incubation for 24 hours, the metabolism of the red cell becomes stressed and the pumping mechanisms tend to fail, one factor being a relative lack of glucose in the medium.

The osmotic fragility of red cells that have an abnormal membrane, such as those of HS and hereditary elliptocytosis (HE), increases abnormally after incubation (Fig. 10.2). Similar results occur in hereditary stomatocytosis.[6a] The results with red cells with a glycolytic deficiency, such as those of pyruvate kinase (PK) deficiency, are variable. In severe deficiencies, osmotic fragility may increase substantially (see Fig. 10.2), but, in other cases, the fragility may decrease owing to a greater loss of potassium than gain of sodium. In thalassaemia major and minor, osmotic fragility is frequently markedly reduced after incubation, again owing to a marked loss of potassium.[7] A similar, although usually less marked, change is seen in iron deficiency anaemia.

To summarise, measurement of red cell osmotic fragility provides a useful indication as to whether a patient's red cells are normal because an abnormal result invariably indicates abnormality. The reverse is, however, not true (i.e., a result that is within the normal range does not mean that the red cells are normal). The findings in some important haemolytic anaemias are summarised in Table 10.2.

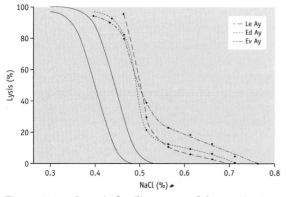

Figure 10.3   Osmotic fragility curves of three patients suffering from hereditary spherocytosis belonging to the same family (brother, sister and uncle [Le Ay]). The area between the unbroken lines represents the normal range.

FLOW CYTOMETRIC (DYE BINDING) TEST

Principle

The osmotic fragility test lacks specificity and sensitivity and fails to detect atypical or mild HS. Moreover, it can be affected by factors unrelated to

Table 10.2 Osmotic fragility in haemolytic anaemias: a summary

Condition	Notes
A. Associated with increased osmotic fragility (OF)	
Hereditary spherocytosis (HS)	Entire curve may be "shifted to the right," or most of it may be within the normal range but with a "tail" of fragile cells. Curve within normal range in 10–20% of cases. After incubation for 24 hours, abnormalities usually more marked, but still some false-negative results. Splenectomy does not affect MCF but reduces the tail of fragile cells
Hereditary elliptocytosis (HE)	As in HS, but in general changes less marked. Abnormal OF usually correlates with severity of haemolysis (i.e., OF is normal in nonhaemolytic HE)
Hereditary stomatocytosis	As in HS with large osmotically fragile cells with low MCHC
Other inherited membrane abnormalities	Results variable; with milder disorders curve more likely to be abnormal after incubation for 24 hours
Autoimmune haemolytic anaemia	Tail of fragile cells roughly proportional to number of spherocytes; rest of curve normal (or even left-shifted on account of high reticulocytosis)
B. Associated with decreased OF	
Thalassaemia	MCF decreased in all forms of thalassaemia, except in some α-thalassaemia heterozygotes; usually the entire curve is left-shifted
Enzyme abnormalities	OF usually normal (anaemia originally referred to as hereditary nonspherocytic), but tail of highly resistant cells may be seen on account of high reticulocyte court. After incubation for 24 hours, there may be a tail of fragile cells
Hereditary xerocytosis	Increased resistance to osmotic lysis and increased MCHC
Iron deficiency	Curve shifted to left, wholly or partly, depending on proportion of hypochromic red cells

OF, osmotic fragility; HE, hereditary elliptocytosis; HS, hereditary spherocytosis; MCF, median corpuscular fragility; MCHC, mean cell haemoglobin concentration.

red cell cytoskeletal defects; for example, positive results may be obtained for red cells from patients who are pregnant or who have immune or other haemolytic anaemias or renal failure. The flow cytometric (dye binding) test of King and colleagues[8] measures the fluorescent intensity of intact red cells labelled with eosin-5-maleimide (EMA), which reacts covalently with Lys-430 on the first extracellular loop of Band 3 protein. The N-terminal cytoplasmic domain of Band 3 interacts with ankyrin and protein 4.2, which in turn cross-link with the spectrin-based cytoskeleton and stabilises the membrane lipid bilayer.[9] Deficiency or abnormality of Band 3 may result in decreased fluorescence. This is seen in HS red cells but has also been observed in cases of Southeast Asian ovalocytosis, congenital dyserythropoietic anaemia Type II, and the stomatocytic variant cryohydrocytosis. Blood samples in ethylenediaminetetraacetic acid (EDTA) may be analysed for up to 48 hours after collection provided they have been stored in the refrigerator.

Reagents

EMA.

EMA is light sensitive and must be kept in the dark, preferably wrapped in aluminium foil and stored at 4°C. Prepare a stock solution by dissolving 1 mg in 1 ml of phosphate buffered saline (PBS). Mix well and store in 200 µl aliquots at –20°C.

Bovine serum albumin (30%) solution (BSA).
Available commercially. Dilute to 0.5% with PBS.

PBS.
See p. 691.

Method

Thaw a tube of stock EMA solution in the dark at room temperature and dilute with an equal volume of PBS to obtain a working solution of 0.5 mg/ml. Mix 5 μl of washed packed red cells with 25 μl of EMA working solution in a plastic microfuge tube. Set up control tubes from blood of normal individuals and perform all tests in duplicate. Leave a rack with the tubes in a cupboard in the dark at room temperature for 30 min. Mix and return to the cupboard for a further 30 min.

Then, spin the tubes in a bench-top microfuge for 5–10 sec and remove the supernatant dye carefully with a fine-tip pipette.

Wash the labelled red cells three times with 500 μl PBS containing 0.5% BSA. The third wash should be colourless. If it is still pink, suggesting that traces of dye particle remain in the tube, discard the sample and repeat the cell labelling procedure.

Resuspend the packed red cells in 500 μl of the PBS–BSA wash solution. Transfer 100 μl of the cell suspension into a plastic flow cytometer tube and add 1.4 ml of wash solution. Keep the cell suspensions in the dark by wrapping in aluminium foil until use. Count each sample for 15,000 events in the gated red cell area.

Interpretation of Results

Results should be expressed as a ratio of mean value of the test to control sample. Each laboratory should set the reference range and cut-off values for its own instrument. In our laboratory a ratio of 0.8 or more is regarded as normal.

GLYCEROL LYSIS-TIME TESTS

The osmotic fragility test is somewhat cumbersome and requires 2 ml or more of whole blood. It is thus not suitable for use in newborn babies or as a population screening test. In 1974 Gottfried and Robertson[10] introduced a glycerol lysis-time (GLT) test, a one-tube test, to measure the time taken for 50% haemolysis of a blood sample in a buffered hypotonic saline–glycerol mixture. The original method had greater sensitivity in the osmotic-resistant range, but it also could identify most patients with HS by a shorter GLT_{50}. Better identification of HS blood from normal was obtained by 24-hour incubation of samples and by modifying the glycerol reagent.[11] Zanella et al modified the original test further by decreasing the pH.[12] There is some loss of specificity for HS with the acidified glycerol lysis-time test (AGLT) compared with the original method, but in practice this loss is unimportant.

Acidified Glycerol Lysis-Time Test[12]

Principle

Glycerol present in a hypotonic buffered saline solution slows the rate of entry of water molecules into the red cells so that the time taken for lysis may be more conveniently measured. Like the osmotic fragility test, differentiation can be made between spherocytes and normal red cells.

Reagents

Phosphate buffered saline.
Add 9 volumes of 9.0 g/l (154 mmol/l) NaCl to 1 volume of 100 mmol/l phosphate buffer (2 volumes of 14.9 g/l Na_2HPO_4 added to 1 volume of 13.61 g/l KH_2PO_4). Adjust the pH to 6.85 ± 0.05 at room temperature (15–25°C). This adjustment must be accurate.

Glycerol reagent (300 mmol/l).
Add 23 ml of glycerol (27.65 g AR grade) to 300 ml of PBS and bring the final volume to 1 litre with water.

Method

Add 20 μl of whole blood, anticoagulated with EDTA, to 5.0 ml of PBS, pH 6.85. Mix the suspension carefully.

Transfer 1.0 ml to a standard 4 ml cuvette of a spectrometer equipped with a linear-logarithmic recorder. Fix the wavelength at 625 nm and start the recorder. Add 2.0 ml of the glycerol reagent rapidly to the cuvette with a 2 ml syringe or automatic pipette and mix well.

The rate of haemolysis is measured by the rate of fall of turbidity of the reaction mixture. The results are expressed as the time required for the optical density to fall to half the initial value ($AGLT_{50}$). The test can also be carried out using a colorimeter and stopwatch.

Results

Normal blood takes more than 30 min (1800 sec) to reach the $AGLT_{50}$. The time taken is similar for blood from normal adults, newborn infants, and cord samples. In patients with HS, the range of the $AGLT_{50}$ is 25–150 sec. A short $AGLT_{50}$ may also be found in chronic renal failure, chronic leukaemias, and autoimmune haemolytic anaemia; it also may be found in some pregnant women.[12]

Significance of the AGLT

The same principles apply as with the osmotic fragility test. Cells with a high volume-to-surface area ratio resist swelling for a shorter time than normal cells. This applies to all spherocytes, whether the spherocytosis is caused by HS or other mechanisms. The test is particularly useful in screening family members of patients with HS where morphological changes are too small to indicate clearly whether the disorder is present.

CRYOHAEMOLYSIS

Principle

Whereas osmotic fragility is abnormal in any condition where spherocytes occur, it has been suggested that cryohaemolysis is specific for HS.[13] This appears to result from the fact that the latter is dependent on factors that are related to molecular defects of the red cell membrane rather than to changes in the surface area-to-volume ratio. The test can be carried out on EDTA blood up to 1 day old.

Reagent

Buffered 0.7 mol/l sucrose.
23.96 g sucrose in 100 ml of 50 mmol/l phosphate buffer, pH 7.4. This can be stored frozen in 2 ml aliquots in tubes ready for use.

Method[13]

1. Centrifuge the blood and wash the red cells three times with cold (4°C) 9 g/l NaCl. Make a suspension of 50–70% cells in the saline and keep on ice until tested.
2. Prepare 2 ml volumes of reagent, thawing if frozen, and stand for 10 min in a 37°C waterbath to equilibrate.
3. Pipette 50 µl of the cell suspension into each of 2 tubes of the warmed reagent, vortex immediately for a few seconds, and then incubate for exactly 10 min at 37°C.
4. Without delay, transfer the tubes to an icebath for another 10 min, vortex for a few seconds, and then centrifuge to sediment the remaining cells. Transfer some of the supernatant to a clean tube.
5. Prepare a 100% haemolysate solution by pipetting 50 µl of the original sample into 2 ml of water. Centrifuge and dilute 200 µl of the supernatant in 4 ml of water.
6. Read absorbance at 540 nm of the test and the 100% lysis samples.

Calculation

$$\% \text{ cryohaemolysis} = \left[\frac{A^{540} \text{ test}}{A^{540} \text{ haemolysate}} \right] \times 21$$

Interpretation

Streichman et al[13] report the range of cryohaemolysis in normal subjects to be 3–15%, whereas in hereditary spherocytosis there is >20% lysis. However, it is recommended that individual laboratories establish their own reference values for the method. Increased lysis is not exclusive to hereditary spherocytosis and may be observed in hereditary stomatocytosis.

AUTOHAEMOLYSIS: SPONTANEOUS HAEMOLYSIS DEVELOPING IN BLOOD INCUBATED AT 37°C FOR 48 HOURS

The autohaemolysis test is useful as an initial screen in suspected cases of haemolytic anaemia. It provides information about the metabolic competence of the red cells and helps to distinguish membrane and enzyme defects if the results of the tests are taken together with other observations such as morphology, inheritance, and the presence or absence of associated clinical disorders.[14]

Principle

Aliquots of blood are incubated both with and without sterile glucose solution at 37°C for 48 hours. After this period, the amount of spontaneous haemolysis is measured colorimetrically.

Method

It is essential to use aseptic techniques in setting up the autohaemolysis test to maintain sterility throughout the incubation period.

Use sterile defibrinated blood and deliver four 1-ml or 2-ml samples into sterile 5 ml capped bottles. Retain a portion of the original sample; separate and store this as the preincubation serum.

Add to 2 of the bottles 50 or 100 µl of sterile 100 g/l glucose solution so as to provide a concentration of glucose in the blood of at least 30 mmol/l. Make sure that the caps of the bottles are tightly closed, and place the series of bottles in the incubator at 37°C. A sample from a known normal individual should be run in parallel as a control.

After 24 hours, thoroughly mix the content by gentle swirling. After incubating for 48 hours, inspect the samples for signs of infection, thoroughly mix again, then from each bottle remove a sample for the estimation of the packed cell volume (PCV) and haemoglobin (Hb) concentration and centrifuge the remainder to obtain the supernatant serum.

Estimate the spontaneous lysis by means of a colorimeter or a spectrometer at 540 nm.

As a rule, it is convenient to make a 1 in 10 dilution of the incubated serum in cyanide-ferricyanide (Drabkin's) solution (see p. 27), unless there is marked haemolysis, when a 1 in 25 or 1 in 50 dilution is more suitable. A corresponding dilution of the preincubation serum is used as a blank, and a 1 in 100 or 1 in 200 dilution of the whole blood in Drabkin's solution indicates the total amount of Hb present and serves as a standard.

Calculate the percentage lysis, allowing for the change in PCV resulting from the incubation as follows:

$$\text{Lysis (\%)} = \frac{R_t - B}{R_0} \times \frac{D_o}{D_t} \times (1 - PCV_t) \times 100$$

where R_o = reading of diluted whole blood; R_t = reading of diluted serum at 48 hours; B = reading of blank; PCV_t = packed cell volume at time T; D_o = dilution of whole blood (e.g., 1 in 200 = 0.005); and D_t = dilution of serum (e.g., 1 in 10 = 0.1).

The reading at time t is multiplied by $(1 - PCV_t)$ so as to give the concentration that would be found if the liberated Hb was dissolved in whole blood (i.e., in both plasma and red cell compartments), not in the plasma compartment alone.

Normal Range of Autohaemolysis

Lysis at 48 hours: without added glucose, 0.2–2.0%; with added glucose, 0–0.9%.

The results obtained are sensitive to slight differences in technique, and each laboratory should use a carefully standardized procedure and establish its own normal range. If the amount of liberated Hb is small, it is more accurate (although more time consuming) to measure lysis by a chemical method rather than by a direct spectrometric method (see p. 189). It can also be measured directly by a simple and rapid procedure with a *HemoCue Plasma/Low Hb system.*[15]

Significance of Increased Autohaemolysis

Little or no lysis takes place when normal blood is incubated for 24 hours under sterile conditions, and the amount present after 48 hours is small.[14] If glucose is added so that it is present throughout the incubation, the development of lysis is markedly slowed. The amount of autohaemolysis that occurs after 48 hours with and without glucose is determined by the properties of the membrane and the metabolic competence of the red cell. In membrane disorders such as HS, the rate of glucose consumption is increased to compensate for an increased cation leak through the membrane.[6b] During the 48-hour incubation, glucose is therefore used up relatively rapidly so that energy production fails more quickly than normal unless glucose is added. This is one factor that contributes to the increased rate of autohaemolysis in HS. Usually, but not always, the addition of glucose to the blood decreases the rate of autohaemolysis in HS. This was referred to as Type-1 autohaemolysis.[14] When the utilisation of glucose via the glycolytic pathway is impaired, as in PK deficiency, the rate of autohaemolysis at 48 hours is usually increased and glucose fails to correct or may even aggravate lysis (Type-2 autohaemolysis).[6c] Although a similar result may be seen in severe HS (Type B), in the absence of spherocytosis failure of glucose to diminish autohaemolysis is a strong indication of a glycolytic block. Blood from patients with G6PD deficiency or other disorders of the pentose phosphate pathway may undergo a slight increase in autohaemolysis (without additional glucose), which is corrected by the addition of glucose. Commonly, the result is normal, but examination of the incubated blood may show an increase in methaemoglobin (Hi) (discussed later). Not all glycolytic enzyme deficiencies give a Type-2 reaction so that a Type-1 result does not exclude the possibility of such a defect.

In the acquired haemolytic anaemias, the results of the autohaemolysis test are variable and generally not very helpful in diagnosis. In the autoimmune haemolytic anaemias, lysis may be increased in the absence of additional glucose but the effect of added glucose is unpredictable. In paroxysmal nocturnal haemoglobinuria (PNH), the autohaemolysis of aerated defibrinated blood is usually normal.

Autohaemolysis may be increased in haemolytic anaemias caused by oxidant drugs or when there are defects in the reducing power of the red cell. Heinz bodies, Hi, or both will be detectable at the end of incubation. Normally, red cells produce less than 4% Hi after 48 hours incubation and Heinz bodies are not seen. Red cells containing an unstable Hb also contain Heinz bodies at the end of the incubation period and increased amounts of Hi.

The nucleosides adenosine, guanosine, and inosine, like glucose, diminish the rate of auto-haemolysis when added to blood. Remarkably, adenosine triphosphate (ATP) strikingly retards haemolysis in PK deficiency, although glucose itself is ineffective.[16] ATP does not pass the red cell membrane.

The autohaemolysis test lacks specificity. This has drawn much criticism on the test, including the suggestion that it has no place in the screening of blood for inherited defects.[17] The best way to detect metabolic defects in red cells is undoubtedly to measure glucose consumption, lactate production, and the contribution to metabolism of the pentose phosphate pathway. These measurements are, unfortunately, difficult and are likely to be undertaken only by specialized laboratories. The autohaemolysis test does provide some information about the metabolic competence of the red cells and helps to distinguish membrane defects from enzyme defects.

In summary, we feel that the autohaemolysis test is still useful in the investigation of patients who have or who may have chronic haemolytic anaemia for the following reasons:

1. If the result is entirely normal, an intrinsic red cell abnormality is unlikely.
2. If abnormal haemolysis is fully corrected by glucose, a metabolic abnormality is unlikely and a membrane abnormality is likely.
3. If abnormal haemolysis shows little or no correction by glucose, a metabolic abnormality is likely, provided that obvious features of sphero-cytosis are not present on the blood film.

Thus, in our experience a combination of red cell morphology with the results of the autohaemolysis tests makes it possible to differentiate membrane abnormalities from enzyme deficiencies in the vast majority of cases.

MEMBRANE PROTEIN ANALYSIS

Defects of red cell membrane proteins that constitute the cytoskeleton are associated with congenital haemolytic anaemias accompanied by characteristic morphological features. Their analysis is generally only possible in the setting of a reference laboratory. Sodium dodecyl sulfate (SDS) - polyacrylamide gel electrophoresis of the membranes will identify qualitative and quantitative alterations in the specific proteins. Densitometry of protein bands on the gel gives an overall profile, showing spectrin, ankyrin, Band 3 (the anion transport protein), and protein 4.2. Spectrin variants may be detected after limited trypsin digestion of spectrin extracted from the red cell membranes; an increase in spectrin dimer is indicative of an unstable tetramer, leading to susceptibility to red cell fragmentation in hereditary elliptocytosis and hereditary pyropoikilocytosis.[18]

Membrane protein defects implicated in hereditary haemolytic anaemias are listed in Table 10.3.

Table 10.3 Haemolytic anaemias associated with defects of red cell membrane proteins[18]

Band	Protein	Haemolytic anaemia
1	α Spectrin	HE, HS, HPP
2	β Spectrin	HE, HS
2.1	Ankyrin	HS
3	Anion exchanger	HS, SAO, CDAII
4.1	Protein 4.1	HE
4.2	Pallidin	HS
7	Stomatin	HSt
PAS-1	Glycophorin A	CDAII
PAS-2	Glycophorin C	HE

CDAII, congenital dyserythropoietic anaemia Type II; HE, hereditary elliptocytosis; HPP, hereditary pyropoikilocytosis; HS, hereditary spherocytosis; HSt, hereditary stomatocytosis; SAO, southeast Asia ovalocytosis.

DETECTION OF ENZYME DEFICIENCIES IN HEREDITARY HAEMOLYTIC ANAEMIAS

It is feasible for most haematology laboratories to identify the enzyme deficiencies of G6PD and PK and to indicate where the probable defect lies in less common disorders. Detailed investigation of the aberrant enzymes and of the metabolism of the abnormal cells is probably best undertaken by specialised laboratories. Comprehensive accounts of methods available for studying red cell metabolism are to be found in Beutler's *Red Cell Metabolism, a Manual of Biochemical Methods*[19] and in the ICSH recommendations.[20]

There are two stages in the diagnosis of red cell enzyme defects: first, screening procedures and second, specific enzyme assays. The simple nonspecific screening procedures such as the osmotic fragility and autohaemolysis tests, which have already been described, may indicate the presence of a metabolic disorder, and simple biochemical tests are available to show whether the disorder is in the pentose phosphate or the Embden–Meyerhof pathways; these intermediate stages of glycolysis are illustrated in Figure 10.4.

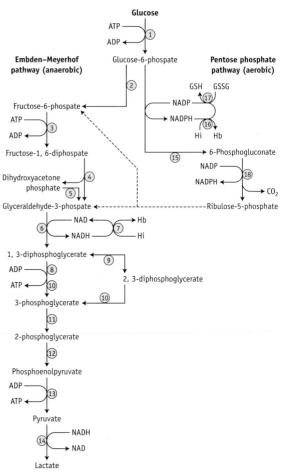

Figure 10.4 Schematic representation of red cell glycolytic pathways. The enzymes are indicated as follows: 1: hexokinase; 2: glucosephosphate isomerase; 3: phosphofructokinase; 4: aldolase; 5: triose phosphate isomerase; 6: glyceraldehyde-3-phosphate dehydrogenase; 7: NADH-methaemoglobin reductase; 8: phosphoglycerate kinase; 9: diphosphoglyceromutase; 10: diphosphoglycerate phosphatase; 11: phosphoglyceromutase; 12: enolase; 13: pyruvate kinase; 14: lactate dehydrogenase; 15: glucose-6-phosphate dehydrogenase; 16: NADPH-methaemoglobin reductase; 17: glutathione reductase; 18: 6-phosphogluconate dehydrogenase. NADH, reduced form of nicotine adenine dinucleotide; NADPH, reduced form of nicotine adenine dinucleotide phosphate.

These investigations may be augmented by quantitation of the major red cell metabolites 2,3-DPG, ATP, and GSH, which are present at millimolar concentrations and which can be assayed conveniently by spectrometric techniques. Metabolic block in the Embden–Meyerhof pathway is most accurately pinpointed by measurement of the concentration of glycolytic intermediates with demonstration of accumulation of metabolites proximal and depletion of metabolites distal to the defective step (Fig. 10.4). These assays, which are generally confined to specialized laboratories, must be performed on deproteinised red cell extracts immediately after preparation.

Screening Tests for G6PD Deficiency and other Defects of the Pentose Phosphate Pathway

Many variants of the red cell enzyme, G6PD, have been detected, and the methods used to identify variants have been standardised.[21] Inheritance is sex-linked because the enzyme is controlled by one gene locus in the X chromosome. Variants that have deficient activity produce one of several types of clinical disorders. The two most common variants are the Mediterranean type, which has very low activity and which may lead to favism (i.e., acute intravascular haemolysis following the ingestion of broad beans), and the A- type found in Black populations in West Africa and the United States, which leads to primaquine sensitivity. Both groups are susceptible to haemolysis produced by oxidant drugs and infections.

Much less frequently, a chronic non-spherocytic haemolytic anaemia is produced by rare variants of the enzyme. Severe neonatal jaundice with anaemia occurs in about 5% of patients who have major deficiencies of enzyme activity.

G6PD deficiency in hemizygous (male) or homozygous (female) individuals may be readily detected by screening tests, but it is more difficult to detect heterozygous (female) carriers. Other defects of the pentose phosphate pathway (see p. 216) also lead to deficiency in the reducing power of the red cell. The clinical syndromes associated with these defects include intravascular haemolysis, with or without methaemoglobinaemia, in response to oxidative drugs.

G6PD catalyses the oxidation of glucose-6-phosphate (G6P) to 6-phosphogluconate (6PG) with the simultaneous reduction of nicotine adenine dinucleotide phosphate (NADP) to reduced NADP (NADPH):

$$\text{G6P} + \text{NADP} \xrightarrow{\text{G6PD}} \text{6PG} + \text{NADPH}$$

In a second, consecutive, oxidative reaction 6PG is converted to 6-phosphogluconolactone, with reduction of a further molecule of NADP to NADPH. The lactone then undergoes decarboxylation to ribulose 5-phosphate through a reaction catalysed by a specific lactonase, but that can also take place spontaneously. Thus the overall reaction catalysed by 6PG dehydrogenase (6PGD) can be written as follows:

$$\text{6PG} + \text{NADP} \xrightarrow{\text{6PGD}} \text{6PGD Ru5P} + \text{CO}_2 + \text{NADPH}$$

The release of CO_2 drives the reaction to the right so that in practice the pathway is not reversible.

NADPH is an important reducing compound for the conversion of oxidised glutathione (GSSG) to GSH (see Fig. 10.4) and, under conditions of stress, the reconversion of Hi to Hb. Screening tests for G6PD deficiency depend on the inability of cells from deficient subjects to convert an oxidised substrate to a reduced state. The substrates used may be the natural one of the enzyme, NADP, or other naturally occurring substrates linked by secondary reactions to the enzyme—for example, GSSG or Hi or artificial dyes such as methylene blue. The reaction is demonstrated by fluorescence,[22] colour change when a dye is used,[23] or deposit of a dye (e.g., a blue ring of formazan from diphenyltetrazolium bromide in the presence of phenazine methosulphate).[24]

Which screening test is used in any particular laboratory will depend on a number of factors such as cost, time required, temperature and humidity, and availability of reagents. Two tests that are commonly used and that are generally reliable are described here.

Fluorescent Screening Test for G6PD Deficiency

The method of fluorescent screening test for G6PD deficiency is that of Beutler and Mitchell[22] modified as recommended by ICSH.[20]

Principle

NADPH, generated by G6PD present in a lysate of blood cells, fluoresces under long-wave ultraviolet (UV) light. In G6PD deficiency, there is an inability to produce sufficient NADPH; this results in a lack of fluorescence.

Reagents

D-Glucose-6-phosphate.
10 mmol/l. Dissolve 305 mg of the disodium salt, or an equivalent amount of the potassium salt, in 100 ml of water.

NADP⁺.
7.5 mmol/l. Dissolve 60 mg of $NADP^+$, disodium salt, in 10 ml of water.

Saponin.
750 mmol/l (10 g/l).

Tris-HCl buffer.
pH 7.8. See page 692.

Oxidized glutathione (GSSG) 8 mmol/l
Dissolve 49 mg of GSSG in 10 ml of water.

Mix the reagents in the following proportion: 2 volumes of G6P, 1 volume of $NADP^+$, 2 volumes of saponin, 3 volumes of buffer, 1 volume of GSSG, and 1 volume of water.

The combined reagent is stable at –20°C for 2 or more years and for at least 2 months if kept at 4°C. Azide may be added to prevent growth of contaminants without loss of activity. Dispense 100 μl volumes into appropriate small tubes and keep at –20°C ready for use.

Method

Thaw out sufficient tubes to set up test and controls. Allow reagent to reach room temperature before use.

Add 10 μl of whole blood, either anticoagulated (EDTA, heparin, ACD [acid–citrate–dextrose], or CPD [citrate–phosphate–dextrose]) or added before clotting, to 100 μl volumes of the reagent mixture and keep at room temperature (15–25°C).

Apply 10 μl of the reaction mixture on to a Whatman No. 1 filter paper at the beginning of the reaction and again after 5–10 min. A shorter interval may be appropriate at a high ambient temperature (c 25–30°C). Allow to air dry

thoroughly before examining the spots under UV light. Record whether fluoresence is present (+) or absent (–). Always set up samples of normal blood and known G6PD-deficiency blood in parallel.

If the samples are to be collected away from the laboratory, place about 10 μl of blood on Whatman No. 1 filter paper and allow it to dry. Cut out the disc of dried blood in the laboratory and add it to the reaction mixture. A sample of normal blood should always be tested as a positive fluorescence (i.e., normal) control.

The test can be carried out on blood stored in ACD (provided it is sterile) for up to 21 days at 4°C and for about 5 days at room temperature.

Interpretation

Fluorescence is produced by NADPH formed from $NADP^+$ in the presence of G6PD. Some of the NADPH produced is oxidised by GSSG, but this reaction, catalyzed by glutathione reductase, is normally slower than the rate of NADPH production. Red cells with less than 20% of normal G6PD activity do not cause fluorescence.

Like all screening tests, this method is useful when large numbers of samples are to be tested, but the result must be interpreted with caution in an individual patient. The main causes of erroneous interpretations are as follows:

1. *False-normal.* If there is reticulocytosis, a vivid fluorescence may be seen with a genetically G6PD-deficient blood sample because young red cells have more G6PD activity. If the test is carried out during an acute haemolytic episode, the patient's blood should be retested when the reticulocyte count has returned to normal.
2. *False-deficient.* If the patient is anaemic, very little fluorescence may be seen despite the G6PD being genetically normal, simply because there are relatively few red cells in the 10 μl of blood used.

Although it is possible to correct for either or both of these contingencies, if in doubt, it is best to proceed directly to a quantitative enzyme assay (discussed later).

The test is meant to give only a + or – (normal or deficient) result by comparison with the controls, and it does not make sense to grade by eye the intensity of fluorescence. If a control G6PD-deficient sample is not available, the appearance of the "zero time" spot can be used for reference. The threshold for a "deficient" result can be worked out by making dilutions of a normal blood sample in saline and is best set by regarding as deficient the fluorescence obtained when G6PD activity is 20% of normal or less (corresponding to a 1 in 5 dilution of normal blood). This means that very mildly deficient variants, and a substantial proportion of heterozygotes (see p. 220), will be missed. However, clinically important haemolysis is unlikely to occur in subjects who have more than 20% G6PD activity, and therefore this seems an appropriate (although arbitrary) threshold for a diagnostic laboratory. Because the test depends on visual inspection, it is best to select the time of incubation in relation to ambient temperature in preliminary trials. NADPH production is a cumulative process. Therefore, given enough time, a G6PD-deficient sample will fluoresce. The time allowed for the reaction should be one at which the contrast in fluorescence between a G6PD-normal and a G6PD-deficient sample is maximal.

METHAEMOGLOBIN REDUCTION TEST[23]

Principle

Sodium nitrite converts Hb to Hi. When no methylene blue is added, methaemoglobin persists, but incubation of the samples with methylene blue allows stimulation of the pentose phosphate pathway in subjects with normal G6PD levels. The Hi is reduced during the incubation period. In G6PD-deficient subjects, the block in the pentose phosphate pathway prevents this reduction.

Reagents

Sodium nitrite.
180 mmol/l.

Dextrose.
280 mmol/l. Dissolve 5 g of AR dextrose and 1.25 g of $NaNO_2$ in 100 ml of water.

Methylene blue.
0.4 mmol/l. Dissolve 150 mg of methylthionine chloride (methylene blue chloride, Sigma) in 1 litre of water.

Nile blue sulphate.
22 mg in 100 ml of water. This may be used as an alternative to methylene blue.

The reagents may be used in a variety of ways to suit the convenience of the laboratory. A batch of tubes may be prepared in advance of use by mixing equal volumes of the reagents (sodium nitrite with methylene blue or Nile blue sulphate) and pipetting 0.2 ml of the combined reagent into individual glass tubes. Glass tubes must be used because plastic may adsorb some reagents. The contents of the tubes are allowed to evaporate to dryness at room temperature (15–25°C) or in an oven at a temperature not exceeding 37°C. The tubes must then be tightly stoppered. The reagent will keep for 6 months at room temperature. The reagents may, however, be used fresh, without drying.

Method

Use anticoagulated blood (EDTA or ACD) and test the samples preferably within 1 hour of collection if left on the bench or within 6 hours if kept at 4°C. Blood in ACD, however, can be stored for up to 1 week but will be unsatisfactory if there is any haemolysis. With blood from patients who are severely anaemic, adjust the PCV to 0.40 ± 0.05.

Add 2 ml of blood to the tube containing 0.2 ml of the combined reagent either freshly prepared or dried. Close the tube with a stopper and gently mix the contents by inverting it 15 times.

Prepare control tubes by adding 2 ml of blood to a similar tube without reagents (normal reference tube) and to a tube containing 0.1 ml of sodium nitrite–dextrose mixture without methylene blue ("deficient" reference tube).

Incubate the samples at 37°C for 90 min. If the blood has been heparinized, incubation should be continued for 3 hours.

After the incubation, pipette 0.1 ml volumes from the test sample, the normal reference tube, and the deficient reference tube into 10 ml of water in separate, clear glass test tubes of identical diameter. Mix the contents gently. Compare the colours in the different tubes (see next section).

Interpretation

Normal blood yields a colour similar to that in the normal reference tube (i.e., a clear red). Blood from deficient subjects gives a brown colour similar to that in the deficient reference tube. Heterozygotes give intermediate reactions.

Although this method takes longer than the fluorescent test, its advantages include the fact that it is extremely inexpensive and that the only equipment required is a waterbath. In addition, the test can be complemented by cytochemical analysis that lends itself to detecting G6PD deficiency in patients with reticulocytosis and in heterozygotes.

Detection of Heterozygotes for G6PD Deficiency

Females heterozygous for G6PD deficiency have two populations of cells, one with normal G6PD activity and the other with deficient G6PD activity. This is the result of inactivation of one of the two X chromosomes in individual cells early in the development of the embryo. All progeny cells (i.e., somatic cells) in females will have the characteristics of only the active X chromosome.[25] The total G6PD activity of blood in the female will depend on the proportion of normal to deficient cells. In most cases, the activity will be between 20% and 80% of normal. However, a few heterozygotes (about 1%) may have almost only normal or almost only G6PD-deficient cells.

Screening tests for G6PD deficiency fail to demonstrate most heterozygotes. The deficient red cells may, however, be identified in blood films by a cytochemical elution procedure (see next section).

Test Kits

Several commercial kits are available for detection of G6PD deficiency. A fluorescent spot test (previously Sigma 103) and a test based on reduction of the dye dichloroindophenol to a colourless state in the presence of phenazine methosulphate (previously Sigma 400) are available commercially.*

The Quantase kit[†] is a photometric method for use on whole blood or dried blood spots; NADPH produced by oxidation of G6P to 6PG is measured by an increase in absorption at 340 nm.

---

*Trinity Biotech, Oxford X14 4TF; see their Web site for product list.
[†]Quantase Ltd., Cumbernauld, Scotland.

Each test or batch of tests should include a normal and a G6PD-deficient sample. Sheep blood is a useful source of naturally deficient blood. Where possible, participation in an external quality assessment (or proficiency testing) scheme is also recommended (see p. 667).

CYTOCHEMICAL TESTS FOR DEMONSTRATING DEFECTS OF RED CELL METABOLISM

Cytochemical methods have been developed by means of which some of these defects are demonstrable in individual cells. Thus tests have been described for demonstrating red cells deficient in G6PD.[26-28] The principle on which the methods are based is that red cells are treated with sodium nitrite to convert their oxyhaemoglobin (HbO_2) to methaemoglobin (Hi). In the presence of G6PD, Hi reconverts to HbO_2, but in G6PD deficiency, Hi persists. The blood is then incubated with a soluble tetrazolium compound (MTT), which will be reduced by HbO_2 (but not by Hi) to an insoluble formazan form.

Attempts have been made to improve the reliability of the test for detecting heterozygotes (e.g., by controlled slight fixation of the red cells and accelerating the reaction with an exogenous electron carrier [1-methoxyphenazine metho-sulphate]).[29] These cytochemical procedures are not more sensitive in the demonstration of G6PD deficiency than are the simple screening tests described above. They may, however, be useful in genetic studies and when assessing G6PD activity in women[30]; they may be the only way to detect deficiency in the heterozygous state.

Demonstration of G6PD-Deficient Cells

Reagents
Sodium nitrite.
0.18 mol/l (12.5 g/l). The solution must be stored in a dark bottle and made up monthly.

Incubation medium.
9 g/l NaCl, 4 ml; 50 g/l glucose, 1.0 ml; 0.3 mol/l phosphate buffer pH 7.0, 2.0 ml; 0.11 g/l Nile blue sulphate, 1.0 ml; water, 2.0 ml.

MTT tetrazolium.
5g/l of 3-(4,5-dimethyl-thiazolyl-1-2)-2,5 diphenyl-tetrazolium bromide in 9 g/l NaCl.

Hypotonic saline.
6 g/l NaCl.

Method[26]

Venous blood collected into ACD should be used. The test should be carried out within 8 hours of collection, and the blood should be kept at 4°C until it is tested. Centrifuge the blood at 4°C for 20 min at 1200–1500 g.

Discard the supernatant and add 0.5 ml of the packed red cells to 9 ml of 9 g/l NaCl and 0.5 ml of sodium nitrite solution contained in a 15 ml glass centrifuge tube. Incubate at 37°C for 20 min. Centrifuge at 4°C for 15 min at appoximately 500 g, then discard the supernatant fluid without disturbing the buffy coat and uppermost layer of red cells. Wash the cells three times in cold saline. After the last washing, remove the buffy coat, mix the packed cells well, and transfer 50 ml to a glass tube containing 1 ml of the incubation medium. Incubate the suspension undisturbed at 37°C for 30 min. Then add 0.2 ml of MTT solution, shake gently, and incubate at 37°C for 1 hour. Resuspend the cells thoroughly. Place one drop adjacent to one drop of hypotonic saline on a glass slide, mix the drops thoroughly, and cover with a coverglass.

Examine the red cells with an oil-immersion objective, noting the presence of formazan granules (Fig. 10.5).

Interpretation

When G6PD activity is normal, all the red cells are stained. In G6PD hemizygotes, the majority of the red cells are unstained. In heterozygotes, mosaicism is usually seen; usually 40–60% of the cells are unstained, so the proportion may be much less, and in extreme cases only as few as 2–3% may be unstained.

PYRIMIDINE-5′-NUCLEOTIDASE SCREENING TEST

Pyrimidine-5′-nucleotidase (P5N) was first described by Valentine et al[31] as a cytosolic enzyme in human

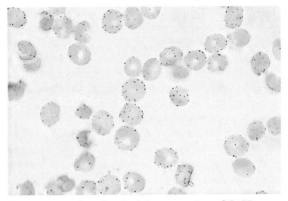

Figure 10.5   Cytochemical demonstration of G6PD (glucose-6-phosphate dehydrogenase). Normal blood; positive reaction with formazan granules in the red cells.

red cells. Deficiency of P5N-1 (uridine monophosphate hydrolase-1), which shows autosomal recessive inheritance, is associated with congenital haemolytic anaemia. Heterozygotes are clinically and haematologically normal and typically have about half the normal red cell P5N activity. Homozygous P5N deficiency, in which enzyme activity is generally 5–15% of normal, results in a chronic nonspherocytic haemolytic anaemia. This is characterized by mild to moderate haemolysis, pronounced basophilic stippling visible in up to 5% of red cells, and marked increase in both red cell glutathione and pyrimidine nucleotides. Osmotic fragility is normal. The rate of autohaemolysis is increased with little or no reduction in lysis by added glucose.[6]

P5N deficiency appears to be a comparatively rare cause of hereditary nonspherocytic haemolytic anaemia. Because lead is an inhibitor of P5N, an acquired deficiency occurs in lead toxicity, and this may be important in the pathogenesis of the associated anaemia. The ultimate diagnostic test is a quantitative assay of P5N activity; but the finding of supranormal levels of red cell nucleotides (mostly pyrimidines) is strongly suggestive and can be used for screening.

Activity of P5N may be measured by a colorimetric method[31] or by a radiometric method.[32] For the screening of P5N deficiency, the method recommended by ICSH is the determination of the UV spectra of a blood extract.[33]

Principle

The nucleotide pool of normal red cells consists largely (>96%) of purine (adenine and small amounts of guanine) derivatives. The levels of cytidine and uridine are normally extremely low. However, in P5N-deficient cells, more than 50% of this pool consists of pyrimidine nucleotides.

In acidic solutions, cytidine nucleotides have an absorbance maximum at approximately 280 nm, whereas adenine, guanine, and uridine nucleotides absorb maximally at 260 nm. The ratio of absorbance at 260 nm to absorbance at 280 nm reflects the relative abundance of cytidine nucleotides; the absorbance ratio is lower when pyrimidine derivatives are higher.

Reagents

Sodium chloride solution
NaCl, 9 g/l.

Perchloric acid
4%. 28.6 ml of a 70% perchloric acid solution are diluted to a final volume of 500 ml with water.

Glycine buffer
1 mol/1 pH 3.0. 7.51 g of glycine are dissolved in about 80 ml of water, the pH is adjusted to 3.0 with concentrated hydrochloric acid (HCl) and the solution is made up to a final volume of 100 ml with water.

Method[33]

For a sample preparation centrifuge blood freshly collected in EDTA at 1200 g for 5 min, remove the plasma, and wash the cells three times with ice-cold 9 g/l NaCl solution. Add 1 ml of a 50% suspension of the washed red cells to 4 ml of ice-cold 4% perchloric acid (PCA) solution, and then shake vigorously for 30 sec. Transfer the clear supernatant obtained after centrifugation at 1200 g for 15 min to a small test tube. Prepare a sham extract by adding 1 ml of 9 g/l NaCl to 4 ml of 4% PCA solution.

Add 500 µl of water and 300 µl of 1 mol/l glycine buffer to each of two cuvettes. To correct for optical differences between the cuvettes, read the sample cuvette against the blank at 260 and at 280 nm, giving readings B^{260} and B^{280}. Add 200 µl of the red cell extract to the sample cuvette and 200 µl of the sham extract to the blank cuvette. With the spectrometer zeroed at 260 nm on the blank cuvette, read the sample cuvette to obtain the value S^{260}. Repeat the process at 280 nm to obtain the reading S^{280}.

The A^{260}/A^{280} absorbance ratio (R) is calculated by subtracting the cuvette blank readings (positive or negative) at 260 and 280 nm from the readings obtained on the red cell extract when blanked against the sham extract:

$$R = \frac{S^{260} - B^{260}}{S^{280} - B^{280}}$$

Interpretation

The A^{260}/A^{280} absorbance ratio of freshly collected washed red cells has been reported to be 3.11 ± 0.41 (mean ± SD). Absorbance ratios of less than 2.29 imply that the concentration of cytidine nucleotide is increased and suggest a reduced level of P5N. Selective accumulation of pyrimidines owing to putative defect in CDP choline phosphotransferase has been reported in rare patients with a disorder that resembles P5N deficiency characterized by haemolytic anaemia and basophilic stippling.

Samples showing a significantly reduced absorbance ratio should have a specific assay for P5N carried out.[34] This is likely to require referral to a reference laboratory where a nucleotide profile may also be undertaken. Nucleotide extraction followed by radiolabelling and separation by high-performance liquid chromatography can be performed. The nucleotides have characteristic UV absorption spectra and retention times, which permit subsequent radiodetection and quantification.

RED CELL ENZYME ASSAYS

As is illustrated in Figure 10.4, a large number of enzymes play a part in the metabolism of glucose in the red cell, and genetically determined variants of almost all the enzymes are known to occur. This means that in investigating a patient suspected of suffering from a hereditary enzyme-deficiency haemolytic anaemia, multiple enzyme assays may be needed to identify the defect. In practice, however, G6PD deficiency and PK deficiency should be excluded first because of the relative frequency (common in the case of G6PD, not rare in the case of PK) with which variants of these enzymes are associated with deficiency and increased haemolysis.

Many methods are available for assaying each enzyme, and for this reason the ICSH has produced simplified methods suitable for diagnostic purposes.[35] These methods are not necessarily the most appropriate for detailed study of the kinetic properties of the variant enzymes, but they are relatively simple to set up and allow comparison of results between different laboratories.

General Points of Technique

Collection of Blood Samples

Blood samples may be anticoagulated with heparin (10 iu/ml blood), EDTA (1.5 mg/ml blood), or ACD (for formulae and volumes see pp. 689–690). In any of these anticoagulants, all normal enzymes are stable for 6 days (and most for 20 days) at 4°C and for 24 hours at 25°C. However, enzyme variants in samples from patients may be less stable. Therefore, we recommend that ACD is used as anticoagulant and that the samples are tested promptly. Ideally, samples of blood should be transferred to central laboratories in tubes surrounded by wet ice at 4°C. Frozen samples are unsuitable because the cells are lysed by freezing. Further details of enzyme stability were given by Beutler.[19] Approximately 1 ml of blood is required for each enzyme assay.

Separation of Red Cells from Blood Samples

Leucocytes and platelets generally have higher enzyme activities than red cells. Moreover, with many enzyme deficiency, notably PK deficiency, the decrease in enzyme activity may be much less pronounced in leucocytes and platelets than in red cells, or it even may be absent. It is, therefore, necessary to prepare red cells as free from contamination as possible. Various methods are suitable (see ICSH[35]); two are described in the following.

Washing the Red Cells

Centrifuge the anticoagulated blood at 1200–1500 g for 5 min and remove the plasma together with the buffy coat layer.

Resuspend the cells in 9 g/l NaCl (saline) and repeat the procedure three times. This will remove about 80–90% of the leucocytes.

This simple method is adequate in most instances when more complicated manoeuvres are impractical, but it has the disadvantage that some of the reticulocytes and young red cells are lost together with the buffy coat. In addition, the remaining leucocytes may still be sufficient to cause misleading results—for instance, in PK deficiency. Therefore, ideally the following method should be adopted.

Filtration through Microcrystalline Cellulose Mixtures

Pure red cell suspensions can be made from whole blood by filtering the blood through a mixed bed of microcrystalline cellulose (mean size 50 μm) and α-cellulose. Mix approximately 0.5 g of each type of cellulose with 20 ml of ice-cold saline; this gives sufficient slurry for 3–5 columns. The barrel of a 5 ml syringe is used as a column. The outlet of the syringe is blocked with absorbent cotton wool, equal in volume to the 1 ml mark on the barrel. Pour the well-shaken slurry into the column to give a bed volume of 1–2 ml after the saline has run through. Wash the bed with 5 ml of saline to remove any "fines." When the saline has run through, pipette 1–2 ml of whole blood onto the column, taking care not to disturb the bed. Collect the filtrate, and once the blood has completely run into the bed, wash the column through with 5–7 ml of saline. The column should be made freshly for each batch of enzyme assays and used promptly.

By this method, about 99% of the leucocytes and about 90% of the platelets are removed. About 97% of the red cells are recovered, and reticulocytes are not removed selectively. The procedure should not alter the age or size of distribution of the recovered red cells compared to native blood. This should be checked with each new batch of cellulose by counting reticulocytes.

Wash the cells collected from the column twice in 10 volumes of ice-cold saline and finally resuspend them in the saline to give a 50% suspension.

Determine the Hb and/or red cell count in a sample of the suspension.

Preparation of Haemolysate

Mix 1 volume of the washed or filtered suspension with 9 volumes of lysing solution consisting of 2.7 mmol/l EDTA, pH 7.0, and 0.7 mmol/l 2-mercaptoethanol (100 mg of EDTA disodium salt and 5 µl of 2-mercaptoethanol in 100 ml of water); adjust the pH to 7.0 with HCl or NaOH.

Ensure complete lysis by freeze-thawing. Rapid freezing is achieved using a dry-ice acetone bath or methanol that has been cooled to –20°C. Thawing is achieved in a waterbath at 25°C or simply in water at room temperature. Usually the haemolysate is ready for use without further centrifugation, but a 1-min spin in a microfuge is recommended to remove any turbidity (this may be unsuitable for some red cell enzymes that are stroma-bound). Dilutions, when necessary, are carried out in the lysing solution. The haemolysate should be prepared freshly for each batch of enzyme assays. Most enzymes in haemolysates are stable for 8 hours at 0°C, but it is best to carry out assays immediately. G6PD is one of the least stable enzymes in this haemolysate, and its assay should be conducted within 1 or 2 hours of the lysate being prepared. The storing of frozen cells or haemolysates is not recommended; it is preferable to store whole blood in ACD.

Control Samples

Control samples should always be assayed at the same time as the test samples even when a normal range for the various enzymes has been established.

Take the control samples of blood at the same time as the test samples and treat them in the same way. When receiving samples from outside sources, always ask for a normal "shipment control" to be included.

Reaction Buffer

The ICSH recommendation is for a Tris-HCl/EDTA buffer that is appropriate for all the common enzyme assays. The buffer consists of 1 mol/l Tris-HCl and 5 mmol/l Na$_2$EDTA, the pH being adjusted to 8.0 with HCl.

Dissolve 12.11 g of Tris (hydroxymethyl) methylamine and 168 mg of Na$_2$ EDTA in water; adjust the pH to 8.0 with 1 mol/l HCl, and bring the volume to 100 ml at 25°C.

Only two assays will be described in detail—those for G6PD and PK. However, the principles of these assays apply to all other enzyme assays. The assays are carried out in a spectrometer at a wavelength of 340 nm unless otherwise indicated. A final reaction

mixture of 1.0 ml (or 3.0 ml) is suitable, the quantities given in the text being for 1.0 ml reaction mixtures unless otherwise stated. All dilutions of auxiliary enzymes are made in the lysing solution, and all working materials should be kept in an icebath until ready for use. The assays are carried out at a controlled temperature, 30°C being the most appropriate. Cuvettes loaded with the assay reagents should be preincubated at this temperature for 10 min before starting the reaction. In most cases, the reaction is started by the addition of substrate. Many spectrometers have a built-in or attached recorder, by which the absorbance changes can be conveniently measured. If no recorder is available, visual readings should be made every 60 sec. In any case, the reaction should be followed for 5–10 min, and it is essential to ensure that during this time the change in absorbance is linear with time.

G6PD Assay

The reactions involving G6PD have already been described (p. 216). The activity of the enzyme is assayed by following the rate of production of NADPH, which, unlike NADP, has a peak of UV light absorption at 340 nm.

Method

The assays are carried out at 30°C, the cuvettes containing the first four reagents and water being incubated for 10 min before starting the reaction by adding the substrate, as shown in Table 10.4. Commercial kits are also available.*

The change in absorbance following the addition of the substrate is measured over the first 5 min of the reaction. The value of the blank is subtracted from the test reaction, either automatically or by calculation.

Calculation of Enzyme Activity

The activities of the enzymes in the haemolysate are calculated from the initial rate of change of NADPH accumulation:

G6PD activity in the lysate (in mol/ml)

$$= \Delta A/min \times \frac{10^3}{6.22}$$

*Trinity Biotech, OX14 4TF.

Table 10.4   Glucose-6-phosphate dehydrogenase assay

Reagents	Assay (μl)	Blank (μl)
Tris-HCl EDTA buffer, pH 8.0	100	100
MgCl₂, 100 mmol/l	100	100
NADP, 2 mmol/l	100	100
1:20 Haemolysate	20	20
Water	580	680
Start reaction by adding: G6P, 6 mmol/l	100	–

EDTA, ethylenediaminetetra-acetic acid; NADP, G6P, glucose-6-phosphate.

where 6.22 is the mmol extinction coefficient of NADPH at 340 nm and 10^3 is the factor appropriate for the dilutions in the reaction mixture. Results are expressed per 10^{10} red cells, per ml red cells, or per g Hb by reference to the respective values obtained with the washed red cell suspension. However, the ICSH recommendation is to express values per g Hb, and it is ideal to determine the Hb concentration of the haemolysate directly. When doing this, use a haemolysate to Drabkin's solution ratio of 1:25.

G6PD is very stable, and, with most variants, venous blood may be stored in ACD for up to 3 weeks at 4°C without loss of activity.

Some enzyme-deficient variants lose activity more rapidly, and this will cause deficiency to appear more severe than it is. Therefore, for diagnostic purposes, a delay in assaying well-conserved samples should not be a deterrent.

Normal Values

The normal range for G6PD activity should be determined in each laboratory. If the ICSH method is used, values should not differ widely from the given values. Results are expressed in enzyme units (eu)*, which are the μmoles of substrate converted per min.

For adults, these values are 8.83 ± 1.59 eu/g Hb at 30°C. However, newborns and infants may have enzyme activity that deviates appreciably from the adult value.[35,36] In one study, the newborn mean activity was about 150% of the adult mean.[37]

Interpretation of Results

In assessing the clinical relevance of a G6PD assay, three important facts must be kept in mind:

1. The gene for G6PD is on the X-chromosome, and therefore males, having only one G6PD gene, can be only either normal or deficient hemizygotes. By contrast, females, who have two allelic genes, can be either normal homozygotes or heterozygotes with "intermediate" enzyme activity or deficient homozygotes.
2. Red cells are likely to haemolyse on account of G6PD deficiency only if they have less than about 20% of the normal enzyme activity.
3. G6PD activity falls off markedly as red cells age. Therefore, whenever a blood sample has a young red cell population, G6PD activity will be higher than normal, sometimes to the extent that a genetically deficient sample may yield a value within the normal range. This usually, but not always, will be associated with a high reticulocytosis.

In practice, the following notes may be useful:

1. In males, diagnosis does not present difficulties in most cases because the demarcation between normal and deficient subjects is sharp. There are very few acquired situations in which G6PD activity is decreased (one is pure red cell aplasia where there is reticulocytopenia), whereas an increased G6PD activity is found in all acute and chronic haemolytic states with reticulocytosis. Therefore a G6PD value below a well-established normal range always indicates G6PD deficiency. A value in the low-normal range in the face of reticulocytosis should also raise the suspicion of G6PD deficiency because with reticulocytosis G6PD activity should be *higher* than normal. In such suspicious cases, G6PD deficiency can be confirmed by repeating the assay when the reticulocytosis has subsided, or by assaying older red cells after density fractionation, or by conducting family studies.
2. In females, all the same criteria apply, with the added consideration that heterozygosity can

*Enzyme units

never be rigorously ruled out by a G6PD assay; for this purpose, the cytochemical test described on page 220 is more useful than a spectrometric assay, and a counsel of perfection is to use the two in conjunction with each other and with family studies. However, in most cases, a normal value in a female means that she is a normal homozygote, and a value of less than 10% of normal means that she is a deficient homozygote (Table 10.5); but a few heterozygotes may fall in either of these ranges because of the "extreme phenotypes" that can be associated with an unbalanced ratio of the mosaicism consequent on X-chromosome inactivation. Any value between 10% and 90% of normal usually means a heterozygote, except for the complicating effect of reticulocytosis. As far as the clinical significance of heterozygosity for G6PD deficiency is concerned, it is important to remember that, because of mosaicism, a fraction of red cells in heterozygotes (on the average, 50%) is as enzyme-deficient as in a hemizygous male and therefore susceptible to haemolysis. The severity of potential clinical complications is roughly proportional to the fraction of deficient red cells. Therefore, within the heterozygote range, the actual value of the assay (or the proportion of deficient red cells estimated by the cytochemical test) correlates with the risk of haemolysis. During an acute episode, heterozygotes may be missed if their deficient red cells have undergone haemolysis, thus leaving only the normal population in circulation. This can occur before a reticulocyte response becomes apparent and may result in G6PD activity within the normal range.

Identification of G6PD Variants

There are many variants of G6PD in different populations with enzyme activities ranging from nearly 0 to 500% of normal activity (see full details in reference 38). Classification and provisional identification of variants are based on their physicochemical and enzymic characteristics.[39] Criteria were laid down by a World Health Organization scientific group[21] for the minimum requirements for identification of such variants, and these recommendations have now been revised.[40] The tests are carried out on male hemizygotes and are as follows:

- Red cell G6PD activity
- Electrophoretic migration
- Michaelis constant (K_m) for G6PD
- Relative rate of utilization of 2-deoxyG6P (2dG6P)
- Thermal stability

The full amino-acid sequence of G6PD has been established, and definitive identification can be made by sequence analysis at the DNA level.[41,42] Diagnosis of G6PD deficiency by molecular analysis may be clinically useful when a patient has received a large volume of transfused blood or when a reticulocytosis results in a normal enzyme assay level; also, females who are heterozygous deficient can readily be identified (see Chapter 21).

Table 10.5 Glucose-6-phosphate dehydrogenase in various clinical situations (activity in enzyme units [eu] per g haemoglobin)			
Male genotypes	Gd+	Gd-	
Female genotypes	Gd+/Gd+	Gd-/Gd-	Gd+/Gd-
In health	7–10	<2	2–7
In increased haemolysis unrelated to G6PD deficiency	15	4	4–9
During recovery from G6PD-related anaemia	–	6.5	6–10

G6PD, glucose-6-phosphate dehydrogenase.
The values quoted are examples.
Gd+ designates an allele encoding normal G6PD; *Gd-* designates an allele encoding a variant associated with G6PD deficiency.

PYRUVATE KINASE ASSAY

Many variants of PK have deficient enzyme activity *in vivo*.[43,44] In most cases, deficient activity can be identified by simple enzyme assay. However, PK activity in red cells is subject to regulation by a number of effector molecules. With some PK variants, the maximum velocity (V_{max}) of the enzyme is normal or nearly so, but at the low-substrate concentrations found *in vivo* PK activity may be sufficiently low to cause haemolysis, either because affinity for the substrates, phospho-enolpyruvate (PEP) and ADP, is low or because binding of the important allosteric ligand, fructose-1,6-diphosphate, is altered. Some of these unusual variants can be identified by carrying out the enzyme assay not only under standard conditions but also at low substrate concentrations. Functional PK deficiency can also be identified by finding high concentrations of the substrates immediately above the block in the glycolytic pathway, particularly 2,3-DPG.[45] (For measurement of 2,3-DPG, see p. 230.)

PK deficiency is inherited as an autosomal recessive condition.

Method

The preparation of haemolysate, buffer, and lysing solution is exactly the same as for the G6PD assay. In the PK assay, it is particularly important to remove as many contaminating leucocytes and platelets as possible because these cells may be unaffected by a deficiency affecting the red cells and may contain high activities of PK. The principle of the assay is as follows:

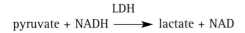

The pyruvate so formed is reduced to lactate in a reaction catalysed by lactate dehydrogenase (LDH) with the conversion of NADH (reduced form of nicotine adenine dinucleotide) to NAD:

$$\text{pyruvate} + \text{NADH} \xrightarrow{\text{LDH}} \text{lactate} + \text{NAD}$$

To ensure that this secondary reaction is not rate limiting, LDH is added in excess to the reaction mixture and the PK activity is measured by the rate of fall of absorbance at 340 nm.

The reaction conditions are established in a 1 ml cuvette at 30°C by adding all the reagents shown in Table 10.6 except the substrate PEP to the cuvette

Table 10.6 Reagents for pyruvate kinase assay

Reagents	Assay (μl)	Blank (μl)	Low-S (μl)
Tris-HCl EDTA buffer, pH 8.0	100	100	100
KCl 1 mol/l	100	100	100
MgCl₂ 100 mmol/l	100	100	100
NADH 2 mmol/l	100	100	100
ADP, neutralized 30 mmol/l	50	–	20
LDH 60 u/ml	100	100	100
1:20 haemolysate	20	20	20
Water	330	380	455
PEP 50 mmol/l	100	100	5

Low-S, low-substrate conditions; EDTA, ethylenediaminetetra-acetic acid; NADH, reduced form of nicotine adenine dinucleotide; ADP, adenine diphosphate; LDH, lactate dehydrogenase; PEP, phosphoenolpyruvate:

and incubating them at 30°C for 10 min before starting the reaction by the addition of the PEP.

The amounts to be added for low-substrate conditions are also shown in Table 10.6.

The change in absorbance (A) is measured over the first 5 min and the activity of the enzyme in micromoles of NADH reduced/min/ml haemolysate is calculated as follows:

$$\frac{\Delta A/\text{min}}{6.22} \times 10$$

where 6.22 is the millimolar extinction coefficient of NADH at 340 nm.

Express results as for G6PD.

A blank assay should be carried out to be certain that the LDH is free of PK activity. Use the 2-mercapto-ethanol-EDTA stabilizing solution (p. 223) in place of haemolysate for both the blank and system mixtures. If no change in absorbance is observed, indicating that the LDH is free of contaminating PK, it is unnecessary to recheck on subsequent assays. Otherwise, the blank rate must be subtracted in computing the true enzyme activity each time.

Normal Values

As with all enzyme assays, a normal range should be determined for each laboratory. Values should, however, not be widely different between laboratories if the ICSH methods are used. The normal range of PK activity at 30°C is 10.3 ± 2 eu/g Hb. At a low-substrate concentration, the normal activity is 15 ± 3% of that at the high-substrate concentration. Mean neonatal value is about 140% that of adults.[37]

Interpretation of Results

PK, like G6PD, is an age-dependent red cell enzyme. But unlike G6PD deficiency, PK deficiency is usually associated with chronic haemolysis. Therefore, patients in whom PK deficiency is suspected almost invariably have a reticulocytosis, and if their PK level is below the normal range, they can be considered to be PK deficient. Thus, once the technique and normal values are well established in a laboratory, and provided shipment controls are always included, the main problem is of underdiagnosis rather than of overdiagnosis of PK deficiency. One way to pick up abnormal variants has been included in the method recommended (i.e., the use of low-substrate concentrations). Even so, PK deficiency may be missed because marked reticulocytosis may increase PK activity markedly. This means that a PK activity in the normal range in the presence of a marked reticulocytosis is highly suspicious of inherited PK deficiency (because with reticulocytosis the activity ought to be *higher* than normal). In such cases, the importance of family studies cannot be overemphasized. Heterozygotes have about 50% of the normal PK activity, sometimes less, but they do not suffer from haemolysis. Therefore, the heterozygous parents of a patient may have a red cell PK activity lower than that of their homozygous PK-deficient offspring; this finding may clinch the diagnosis. In this context, assay of an alternative red cell age-dependent enzyme (e.g., G6PD or hexokinase) may be a useful aid to interpretation.

ESTIMATION OF REDUCED GLUTATHIONE[46]

The red cell has a high concentration of the sulphydryl containing tripeptide, GSH. An important function of GSH in the red cell is the detoxification of low levels of hydrogen peroxide, which may form spontaneously or as a result of drug administration. GSH may also function in maintaining the integrity of the red cell by reducing sulphydryl groups of Hb, membrane proteins, and enzymes that may have become oxidised. Maintenance of normal levels of GSH is a major function of the hexose mono-phosphate shunt. Reduction of GSSG (oxidized glutathione) back to the functional GSH is linked to the rate of reduction of $NADP^+$ in the initial step of the shunt.

Principle

The method described is based on the development of a yellow colour when 5,5′-dithiobis (2-nitrobenzoic acid) (Ellman's reagent, DTNB) is added to sulphydryl compounds. The colour that develops is fairly stable for about 10 min, and the reaction is little affected by variation in temperature.

The reaction is read at 412 nm. GSH in red cells is relatively stable, and venous blood samples anti-coagulated with ACD maintain GSH levels for up to 3 weeks at 4°C. GSH is slowly oxidized in solution, so only fresh lysates should be used for the assay.

Reagents

Lysing solution.
Disodium EDTA, 1 g/l.

Precipitating reagent.
Metaphosphoric acid (sticks), 1.67 g; disodium EDTA, 0.2 g; NaCl, 30 g; water to 100 ml.

Solution is more rapid if the reagents are added to boiling water and the volume is made up after cooling. This solution is stable for at least 3 weeks at 4°C. If any EDTA remains undissolved, the clear supernatant should be used.

Disodium hydrogen phosphate.
300 mmol/l. $Na_2HPO_4.12H_2O$, 107.4 g/l, or $Na_2 HPO_4.2H_2O$, 53.4 g/l or anhydrous Na_2HPO_4, 4.6 g/l.

DTNB reagent.
Dissolve 20 mg of DTNB in 100 ml of buffer, pH 8.0. Trisodium citrate, 34 mmol/l (10 g/l) or Tris/HCl (p. 692), are suitable buffers.

The solution is stable for up to 3 months at 4°C.

Glutathione standards.

When standard curves are constructed, suitable dilutions are made from a 1.62 mmol/l (50 mg/dl) stock solution of GSH.

The stock solution should be made freshly with degassed (boiled) water or saline for each run as GSH oxidizes slowly in solution.

Method

Add 0.2 ml of well-mixed, anticoagulated blood of which the PCV, red cell count, and Hb have been determined, to 1.8 ml of lysing solution and allow to stand at room temperature for no more than 5 min for lysis to be completed.

Add 3 ml of precipitating solution, mix the solution well, and allow to stand for a further 5 min.

After remixing, filter through a single-thickness Whatman No. 42 filter paper.

Add 1 ml of clear filtrate to 4 ml of freshly made Na_2HPO_4 solution. Record the absorbance at 412 nm (A_1). Then add 0.5 ml of the DTNB reagent, and mix well by inversion.

The colour develops rapidly and remains stable for about 10 min. Read its development at 412 nm in a spectrometer (A_2).

A reagent blank is made using saline or plasma instead of whole blood.

If assays are carried out frequently, it is not necessary to construct standard curves for each batch. They are, however, essential initially to calibrate the apparatus used and should be done regularly to check the suitability of the reagents. Suitable dilutions of GSH are achieved by substituting 5, 10, 20, and 40 µl of the 1.62 mmol/l stock solution (make up to 0.2 ml with lysing solution) for the blood in the reaction.

Calculation

Determination of Extinction Coefficient (ε)

The molar extinction coefficient of the chromophore at 412 nm is 13600. This only applies when a narrow band wavelength is available. When a broader waveband is used, the extinction coefficient is lower.

The system may be calibrated by comparing the extinction absorbance in the test system (D_2) with that obtained in a spectrometer with a narrow band at 412 nm (D_1). The derived correction factor, E_1, is given by D_1/D_2 and is constant for the test system.

Calculation of GSH Concentration

The amount of GSH in the cuvette sample (GSH_c) is given by the following:

$$\Delta A^{412} \times \frac{E_1}{\varepsilon} \times 5.5 \ \mu mol$$

The concentration of GSH in the whole blood sample is as follows:

$$\frac{GSH_c \times 5}{0.2} \ \mu mol/ml$$

The unit is often expressed in terms of mg/dl of red cells. The molecular weight of GSH is 307. Thus, GSH in mg/dl packed red cells is given by the following:

$$\frac{GSH_c \times 5}{0.2} \times \frac{1}{PCV} \times 307 \times 100$$

Normal Range

The normal range may be expressed in a number of ways (e.g., 6.57 ± 1.04 µmol/g Hb or 223 ± 35 µmol (or 69 ± 11 mg)/dl packed red cells). Neonatal mean value is about 150% that of adults.[37]

Significance

Glutathione replenishment in mature red cells is accomplished through the consecutive action of two enzymes: γ-glutamylcysteine synthetase and glutathione synthetase. Although very rare, hereditary deficiency of either enzyme virtually abolishes the synthesis of GSH. The deficient cells are very prone to oxidative destruction and are short lived, resulting in a nonspherocytic haemolytic anaemia.

Increases in GSH have been described in various conditions such as dyserythropoiesis, myelofibrosis, P5N deficiency, and other rare congenital haemolytic anaemias of unknown aetiology.

Glutathione Stability Test

Principle

In normal subjects, incubation of red cells with the oxidising drug acetylphenylhydrazine has little effect on the GSH content because its oxidation is reversed by glutathione reductase, which in turn relies on G6PD for a supply to NADPH. Therefore, in subjects who are G6PD deficient, the stability of GSH is significantly reduced.

Reagents

Acetylphenylhydrazine.
670 mmol/l. Dissolve 100 mg in 1 ml of acetone.

Transfer 0.05 ml volumes (containing 5 mg of acetylphenylhydrazine) by pipette to the bottom of 12×75 mm glass tubes. Dry the contents of the tubes in an incubator at 37°C, stopper, and store in the dark until used.

Method

Venous blood, anticoagulated with EDTA, heparin, or ACD, may be used; it may be freshly collected or previously stored at 4°C for up to 1 week.

Add 1 ml to a tube containing acetylphenyl-hydrazine and place another 1 ml in a similar tube not containing the chemical. Invert the tubes several times, and then incubate them at 37°C.

After 1 hour, mix the contents of the tubes once more and incubate the tubes for a further 1 hour. At the end of this time, determine and compare the GSH concentration in the test sample and in the control sample.

Interpretation

In normal adult subjects, red cell GSH is lowered by not more than 20% by incubation with acetylphenylhydrazine. In subjects who are G6PD deficient, it is lowered by more than this: in heterozygotes (females), the fall may amount to about 50%, whereas in hemizygotes (males) the fall is often much greater and almost all may be lost.

The test is not specific for G6PD deficiency, and other rare defects of the pentose phosphate pathway may give abnormal results.

Glutathione and Glutathione Stability in Infants

During the first few days after birth, the red cells have a normal or high content of GSH. On the addition of acetylphenylhydrazine, the GSH is unstable in both normal infants and infants who are G6PD deficient. In normal infants, however, the instability can be corrected by the addition of glucose and, by the time the normal infant is 3–4 days old, the cells behave like adult cells.[47,48]

2,3-DIPHOSPHOGLYCERATE

The importance of the high concentration of 2,3-DPG in the red cells of man was recognized at about the same time by Chanutin and Curnish[49] and Benesch and Benesch.[50] 2,3-DPG binds to a specific site in the β chain of Hb, and it decreases its oxygen affinity by shifting the balance of the so-called T and R conformations of the molecule. The higher the concentration of 2,3-DPG, the greater the partial pressure of oxygen (pO_2) needed to produce the same oxygen saturation of Hb. This is reflected in a 2,3-DPG-dependent shift in the oxygen dissociation curve.

Measurement of the concentration of 2,3-DPG in red cells may also be useful in identifying the probable site of an enzyme deficiency in the metabolic pathway. In general, enzyme defects cause an increase in the concentration of metabolic intermediates above the level of the block and a decrease in concentration below the block. Thus 2,3-DPG is increased in PK deficiency and decreased in hexokinase deficiency. In most other disorders of the glycolytic pathway, however, the 2,3-DPG concentration is normal because increased activity through the pentose phosphate pathway allows a normal flux of metabolites through the triose part of the glycolytic pathway.

Measurement of Red Cell 2,3-Diphosphoglycerate

Various methods have been used to assay 2,3-DPG. Krimsky[51] used the catalytic properties of 2,3-DPG in the conversion of 3-phosphoglycerate (3PG) to 2-phosphoglycerate (2PG) by phosphoglycerate mutase (PGM). At very low concentrations of 2,3-DPG, the rate of conversion is proportional to the concentration of 2,3-DPG. This method is elegant and extremely sensitive but too cumbersome for routine use. A fluorimetric method was described by Lowry et al,[52] and this has been modified for spectrometry. Rose and Liebowitz[53] found that glycolate-2-phosphate increased the 2,3-DPG phosphatase activity of PGM, and a quantitative assay of the substrate, 2,3-DPG, was evolved on this basis.

Principle

2,3-DPG is hydrolysed to 3PG by the phosphatase activity of PGM stimulated by glycolate-2-phosphate. This reaction is linked to the conversion of NADH to NAD by glyceral-dehyde-3-phosphate dehydrogenase (Ga3PD) and phosphoglycerate kinase (PGK):

$$2,3\text{-DPG} \xrightarrow[\text{(glycolate-2-phosphate)}]{\text{2,3-DPG phosphatase}} 3\text{PG} + \text{Pi}$$

$$3\text{PG} + \text{ATP} \xrightarrow{\text{PGK}} 1,3\text{-DPG} + \text{ADP}$$

$$1,3\text{-DPG} + \text{NADH} \xrightarrow{\text{Ga3PD}} \text{Ga3P} + \text{Pi} + \text{NAD+}$$

The fall in absorbance at 340 nm, as NADH is oxidized, is measured.

Reagents

Triethanolamine buffer.
0.2 mol/l, pH 8.0.
   Dissolve 9.3 g of triethanolamine hydrochloride in *c* 200 ml of water; then add 0.5 g of disodium EDTA and 0.25 g of $MgSO_4.7H_2O$. Adjust the pH to 8.0 with 2 mol/l KOH (approximately 15 ml) and make up the volume to 250 ml with water.

ATP, sodium salt.
20 mg/ml. Dissolved in buffer, this is stable for several months when frozen.

NADH, sodium salt.
10 mg/ml. When dissolved in buffer, this is relatively unstable and should be made freshly each day.

Glyceraldehyde-3-phosphate dehydrogenase/ Phosphoglycerate kinase.
   Mixed crystalline suspension in ammonium sulphate.

Phosphoglycerate mutase.
   Crystalline suspension from rabbit muscle in ammonium sulphate (c 2500 u/ml).

Glycolate-2-phosphate.
   2-Phosphoglycolic acid, 10 mg/ml. After dissolving in water, this is stable for several months if kept frozen.

Method

Freshly drawn blood in EDTA or heparin may be used. If there is an unavoidable delay in starting the assay, blood (4 volumes) should be added to CPD anticoagulant (1 volume) and stored at 4°C. A control blood sample should be taken at the same time.
   2,3-DPG levels are stable for 48 hours if the blood is stored in this way. The Hb, red cell count, and PCV should be measured on part of the sample. It is not necessary to remove leucocytes or platelets.

Deproteinization.
Add 1 ml of blood to 3 ml of ice-cold 80 g/l trichloracetic acid (TCA) in a 10 ml conical centrifuge tube.
   Shake the tube vigorously, preferably on an automatic rotor mixer, and then allow to stand for 5–10 min for complete deproteinization. The shaking is important; otherwise some of the precipitated protein will remain on the surface of the mixture.
   Centrifuge at about 1200 g for 5–10 min at 4°C to obtain a clear supernatant. The 2,3-DPG in the supernatant is stable for 2–3 weeks when stored at 4°C; it is stable indefinitely if frozen.

Table 10.7		
	Test	Blank
Triethanolamine buffer	2.50 ml	2.50 ml
ATP	100 µl	100 µl
NADH	100 µl	100 µl
Deproteinized extract	250 µl	–
Ga-3-PD/PGK mixture	20 µl	20 µl
PGM	20 µl	20 µl
Water	–	250 µl
	3.00 ml	3.00 ml

Reaction

Deliver the reagents into a silica or high-quality glass cuvette, with a 1 cm light path. The quantities in Table 10.7 are for a 4 ml cuvette:

Warm the mixtures at 30°C for 10 min and record the absorbance of both test and blank mixtures at 340 nm. Then start the reaction by the addition of 100 μl of glycolate-2-phosphate.

Remeasure the absorbance (at 35 min) of the test and blank mixtures on completion of the reaction.

Make further measurements after a further 5 min to make sure the reaction is complete.

Only one blank is required for each batch of test samples.

Calculation

2,3-DPG (μmol/ml blood)

$$= (\Delta A \text{ test} - \Delta A \text{ blank}) \times \frac{3.10}{6.22} \times 16$$

$$= (\Delta A \text{ test} - \Delta A \text{ blank}) \times 8 = D$$

where 3.10 = the volume of reaction mixture, 6.22 = mmolar extinction coefficient of NADH at 340 nm, and 16 = dilution of original blood sample (1 ml in 3.0 ml of TCA, 0.25 ml added to cuvette).

The results of 2,3-DPG assays are best expressed in terms of Hb content or red cell volume. Thus, if the result of the previous calculation is represented by D, then:

$$\frac{D \times 1000}{(Hb)} = 2,3\text{-DPG in μmol/g Hb}$$

or

$$\frac{D \times 1000}{(Hb)} \times \frac{64}{1000} = 2,3\text{-DPG in μmol/μmol Hb}$$

and

$$D \times \frac{1}{PCV} = 2,3\text{-DPG in μmol/ml (packed) red cells,}$$

where Hb = Hb in g/l of whole blood and 64 is the molecular weight of Hb $\times 10^{-3}$.

The molar ratio of 2,3-DPG to Hb in normal blood is about 0.75:1.

Normal Range

The normal range is 4.5–5.1 μmol/ml packed red cells or 10.5–16.2 μmol/g Hb. Neonatal values are about 20% lower than adult.[37]

Each laboratory should determine its own normal range.

Significance of 2,3-DPG Concentration

An increase in 2,3-DPG concentration is found in most conditions in which the arterial blood is undersaturated with oxygen, as in congenital heart and chronic lung diseases, in most acquired anaemias, at high altitudes, in alkalosis, and in hyperphosphataemia. Decreased 2,3-DPG levels occur in hypophosphataemic states and in acidosis.

Acidosis, which shifts the oxygen dissociation curve to the right, causes a fall in 2,3-DPG, so that the oxygen dissociation curve of whole blood from patients with chronic acidosis (such as patients in diabetic coma or precoma) may have nearly normal dissociation curves. A rapid correction of the acidosis will lead to a major shift of the curve to the left (i.e., to a marked increase in the affinity of Hb for oxygen, which may lead to tissue hypoxia). Caution should therefore be exercised in correcting acidosis. Measurement of oxygen dissociation is described below.

From the diagnostic point of view, the main importance of 2,3-DPG determination is (a) in haemolytic anaemias and (b) in the interpretation of changes in the oxygen affinity of blood.

1. As already mentioned, increased or decreased 2,3-DPG may be associated with glycolytic enzyme defects, and increased 2,3-DPG (up to 2 to 3 times normal) is particularly characteristic of most patients with PK deficiency. Although this finding certainly cannot be regarded as diagnostic, a normal or low 2,3-DPG makes PK deficiency most unlikely.
2. Whenever a shift in the oxygen dissociation curve is observed and an abnormal Hb with altered oxygen affinity is suspected, determination of 2,3-DPG is essential. Indeed, there is a simple correlation between 2,3-DPG level and p_{50}, from which it is possible to work out whether any change in p_{50} is explained by an altered level of 2,3-DPG.[54]

2,3-DPG levels are generally slightly lower than normal in HS, and this probably accounts for the slight erythrocytosis that is sometimes seen after splenectomy. Extremely low red cell 2,3-DPG concentration associated with erythrocytosis has been reported in a kindred with complete 2,3-diphosphoglycerate mutase deficiency.[55]

OXYGEN DISSOCIATION CURVE

The oxygen dissociation curve is the expression of the relationship between the partial pressure of oxygen and oxygen saturation of Hb. Details of this relationship and the physiological importance of changes in this relationship were worked out in detail at the beginning of this century by the great physiologists Hüfner, Bohr, Barcroft, Henderson, and many others. Their work was summarised by Peters and Van Slyke in *Quantitative Clinical Chemistry, Volume 1.*[56] The relevant chapters of this book have been reprinted, and it would be difficult to improve their description of the importance of the oxygen dissociation curve.

> The physiological value of Hb as an oxygen carrier lies in the fact that its affinity for oxygen is so nicely balanced that in the lungs Hb becomes 95%–96% oxygenated, whereas in the tissues and capillaries it can give up as much of the gas as is demanded. If the affinity were much less, complete oxygenation in the lungs could not be approached; if it were greater, the tissues would have difficulty in removing from the blood the oxygen they need. Because the affinity is adjusted as it is, both oxyhaemoglobin and reduced Hb exist in all parts of the circulation but in greatly varied proportions.

Measuring the Oxygen Dissociation Curve

Determination of the oxygen dissociation curve depends on two measurements: pO_2 with which the blood is equilibrated and the proportion of Hb that is saturated with oxygen. Methods for determining the dissociation curve fall into three main groups:

1. The pO_2 is set by the experimental conditions and the percentage saturation of Hb is measured.
2. The percentage saturation is predetermined by mixing known proportions of oxygenated and deoxygenated blood and the pO_2 is measured.
3. The change in oxygen content of the blood is plotted continuously against pO_2 during oxy-

genation or deoxygenation and the percentage saturation is calculated.

The multiplicity of methods available for measuring the oxygen dissociation curve suggests that no method is ideal. The advantages and disadvantages of the various techniques have been reviewed.[57,58] The standard method with which new methods are compared is the gasometric method of Van Slyke and Neill.[59] This method is slow, demands considerable expertise, and is not suitable for most haematology laboratories. Commercial instruments are now available for performing the test and drawing the complete oxygen dissociation curve.* Such analysers are extremely quick and accurate and are therefore ideal for laboratories performing multiple determinations. Approximate measurement of oxygen saturation of Hb can also be obtained at the bedside by noninvasive pulse oximetry.

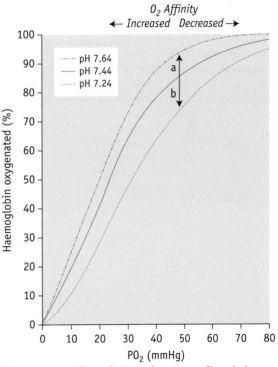

Figure 10.6   Effect of pH on the oxygen dissociation curve.

---

*For example, Hemox-Analyzer, TCS Scientific Corporation.

Interpretation

Figure 10.6 shows the sigmoid nature of the oxygen dissociation curve of Hb A and the effect of hydrogen ions on the position of the curve. A shift of the curve to the right indicates decreased affinity of the Hb for oxygen and hence an increased tendency to give up oxygen to the tissues; a shift to the left indicates increased affinity and so an increased tendency for Hb to take up and retain oxygen. Hydrogen ions, 2,3-DPG, and some other organic phosphates such as ATP shift the curve to the right. The amount by which the curve is shifted may be expressed by the $p_{50}O_2$ (i.e., the partial pressure of oxygen at which the Hb is 50% saturated).

The oxygen affinity, as represented by the $p_{50}O_2$, is related to compensation in haemolytic anaemias[60]; 1 g of Hb can carry about 1.34 ml of O_2. Figure 10.7 shows the O_2 dissociation curves of Hb A and Hb S plotted according to the volume of oxygen contained in 1 litre of blood when the Hb concentrations is 146 g/l and 80 g/l, respectively. The $p_{50}O_2$ of Hb A is given as 26.5 mm Hg (3.5 kPa) and Hb S as 36.5 mm Hg (4.8 kPa). It will be seen that in the change from arterial to venous saturation, the same volume of oxygen is given up despite the difference in Hb concentration. Patients with a high $p_{50}O_2$ achieve a stable Hb at a lower level than normal, and this should be taken into account when planning transfusion for these patients.

Bohr Effect

An increase in CO_2 concentration produces a shift to the right (i.e., a decrease in oxygen affinity). This effect, originally described by C. Bohr,[61] is mainly a result of changes in pH, although CO_2 itself has some direct effect. The Bohr effect is given a numeric value, $\Delta \log p_{50}O_2 / \Delta$ pH, where $\Delta \log p_{50}O_2$ is the change in $p_{50}O_2$ produced by a change in pH (Δ pH). The normal value of the Bohr effect at physiological pH and temperature is about 0.45.

Hill's Constant ("n")

Hill's constant ("n") represents the number of molecules of oxygen that combine with one molecule of Hb.[62] Experiments showed that the value was 2.6 rather than the expected 4. The explanation for this lies in the effect of binding 1 molecule of oxygen by Hb on the affinity for binding further oxygen molecules by Hb, the so-called allosteric effect of haem–haem interaction: "n" is a measure of this effect and the calculation of the "n" value helps in identifying abnormal Hbs, the molecular abnormality of which leads to abnormal haem–haem interaction.[63]

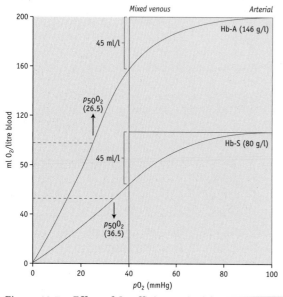

Figure 10.7   Effect of O_2 affinity on O_2 delivery to tissues.

REFERENCES

1. Parpart AK, Lorenz PB, Parpart ER, et al 1947 The osmotic resistance (fragility) of human red cells. Journal of Clinical Investigation 26:636–640.
2. Murphy JR 1967 The influence of pH and temperature on some physical properties of normal erythrocytes and erythrocytes from patients with hereditary spherocytosis. Journal of Laboratory and Clinical Medicine 69:758–775.
3. Suess J, Limentani D, Dameshek W, et al 1948 A quantitative method for the determination and charting of the erythrocyte hypotonic fragility. Blood 3:1290–1303.
4. Jacob HS, Jandl JH 1964 Increased cell membrane permeability in the pathogenesis of hereditary spherocytosis. Journal of Clinical Investigation 43:1704–1720.

5. Cooper RA 1970 Lipids of human red cell membrane normal composition and variability in disease. Seminars in Hematology 7:296–322.

6. Dacie Sir John 1985 The haemolytic anaemias, Vol. 1. The hereditary haemolytic anaemias, part 1. Churchill Livingstone, Edinburgh. (a) p 292, (b) p 146, (c) p 352.

7. Gunn RB, Silvers DN, Rosse WF 1972 Potassium permeability in β-thalassaemia minor red blood cells. Journal of Clinical Investigation 51:1043–1050.

8. King M-J, Behrens J, Rogers C et al 2000 Rapid flow cytometric test for the diagnosis of membrane cytoskeleton-associated haemolytic anaemia. British Journal of Haematology 111:924–933.

9. Golan DE, Corbett JD, Korsgren C et al 1996 Control of band 3 lateral and rotational mobility by band 4.2 in intact erythrocytes: release of band 3 oligomers from low affinity binding sites. Biophysical Journal 70:1534–1542.

10. Gottfried EL, Robertson NA 1974 Glycerol lysis time as a screening test for erythrocyte disorders. Journal of Laboratory and Clinical Medicine 83:323–333.

11. Gottfried EL, Robertson NA 1974 Glycerol lysis time of incubated erythrocytes in the diagnosis of hereditary spherocytosis. Journal of Laboratory and Clinical Medicine 84:746–751.

12. Zanella A, Izzo C, Rebulla P, et al 1980 Acidified glycerol lysis test: a screening test for spherocytosis. British Journal of Haematology 45:481–486.

13. Streichman S, Gescheidt Y 1998 Cryohemolysis for the detection of hereditary spherocytosis: correlation studies with osmotic fragility and autohemolysis. American Journal of Hematology 58:206–210.

14. Selwyn JG, Dacie JV 1954 Autohemolysis and other changes resulting from the incubation in vitro of red cells from patients with congenital hemolytic anemia. Blood 9:414–438.

15. Morris LD, Pont A, Lewis SM 2001 Use of the HemoCue for measuring haemoglobin at low concentrations. Clinical and Laboratory Haematology 23:91–96.

16. de Gruchy GC, Santamaria JN, Parsons IC, et al 1960 Nonspherocytic congenital hemolytic anemia. Blood 16:1371–1397.

17. Beutler E 1978 Why has the autohemolysis test not gone the way of the cephalin floculation test? Blood 51:109–110.

18. Palek J, Jarolim P 1993 Clinical expression and laboratory detection of red blood cell membrane protein mutations. Seminars in Hematology 30:249–283.

19. Beutler E 1984 Red cell metabolism. A manual of biochemical methods, 2nd ed., Grune & Stratton, Orlando.

20. Beutler E, Blume KG, Kaplan JC, et al 1979 International Committee for Standardization in Haematology. Recommended screening test for glucose-6-phosphate dehydrogenase (G-6-PD) deficiency. British Journal of Haematology 43:465–477.

21. World Health Organization Scientific Group 1967 Standardization of procedures for the study of glucose-6-phosphate dehydrogenase. Technical Report Series, No. 366. WHO, Geneva.

22. Beutler E, Mitchell M 1968 Special modification of the fluorescent screening method for glucose-6-phosphate dehydrogenase deficiency. Blood 32:816–818.

23. Brewer GJ, Tarlov AR, Alving AS 1962 The methemoglobin reduction test for primaquine-type sensitivity of erythrocytes. A simplified procedure for detecting a specific hypersusceptibility to drug hemolysis. Journal of the American Medical Association 180:386–388.

24. Fujii H, Takahashi K, Miwa S 1984 A new simple screening method for glucose-6-phosphate dehydrogenase deficiency. Acta Haematologica Japonica 47:185–188.

25. Lyon MF 1961 Gene action in the X-chromosomes of the mouse (*Mus musculus* L.). Nature (London) 190:372–373.

26. Fairbanks VF, Lampe LT 1968 A tetrazolium-linked cytochemical method for estimation of glucose-6-phosphate dehydrogenase activity in individual erythrocytes: applications in the study of heterozygotes for glucose-6-phoshate dehydrogenase deficiency. Blood 31:589–603.

27. Gall JC, Brewer GJ, Dern RJ 1965 Studies of glucose-6-phosphate dehydrogenase activity of individual erythrocytes: the methemoglobin-elution test for identification of females heterozygous for G6PD deficiency. American Journal of Human Genetics 17:350–363.

28. Tönz O, Rossi E 1964 Morphological demonstration of two red cell populations in human females heterozygous for glucose-6-phosphate dehydrogenase deficiency. Nature (London) 202:606–607

29. Kleihauer E, Betke K 1963 Elution procedure for the demonstration of methaemoglobin in red cells of human blood smears. Nature (London) 199:1196–1197

30. Vogels IMC, Van Noorden CJF, Wolf BHM et al 1986 Cytochemical determination of heterozygous glucose-6-phosphate dehydrogenase deficiency in

erythrocytes. British Journal of Haematology 63:402–405

31. Valentine WN, Fink K, Paglia DE, et al 1974 Hereditary haemolytic anaemia with human erythrocyte pyrimidine 5′-nucleotidase deficiency. Journal of Clinical Investigation 54:866–879.

32. Torrance J, West C, Beutler E 1977 A simple radiometric assay for pyrimidine 5′-nucleotidase. Journal of Laboratory and Clinical Medicine 90:563–568.

33. International Committee for Standardization in Haematology 1989 Recommended screening test for pyrimidine 5′-nucleotidase deficiency. Clinical and Laboratory Haematology 11:55–56.

34. Fairbanks LD, Jacomelli G, Micheli V et al 2002 Severe pyridine nucleotide depletion in fibroblasts from Lesch-Nyhan patients. Biochemical Journal 366:265–272.

35. International Committee for Standardization in Haematology 1977 Recommended methods for red-cell enzyme analysis. British Journal of Haematology 35:331–340.

36. Konrad PN, Valentine WN, Paglia DE 1972 Enzymatic activities and glutathione content of erythrocytes in the newborn. Comparison with red cells of older normal subjects and those with comparable reticulocytosis. Acta Haematologica 48:193–201.

37. Oski FA 1969 Red cell metabolism in the newborn infant: V. Glycolytic intermediates and glycolytic enzymes. Pediatrics 44:84–91.

38. Luzzatto L, Mehta A 1989 Glucose-6-phosphate dehydrogenase deficiency. In: Scriver CR, Beaudet A, Sly WS, Valle D (eds) The metabolic basis of inherited disease, pp. 2237–2265. McGraw-Hill, New York.

39. Yoshida A, Beutler E, Motulsky AG 1971 Human glucose-6-phosphate dehydrogenase variants. Bulletin of the World Health Organization 45:243–253.

40. World Health Organization Scientific Group on Glucose-6-Phosphate Dehydrogenase 1990 Bulletin of the World Health Organization, 67:601.

41. Vulliamy TJ, D'urso M, Battistuzzi G et al 1988 Diverse point mutations in the human glucose-6-phosphate dehydrogenase gene cause enzyme deficiency and mild or severe hemolytic anemia. Proceedings of the National Academy of Sciences of the USA 85:5171–5175.

42. Beutler E 1989 Glucose-6-phosphate dehydrogenase: new perspectives. Blood 73:1397–1401.

43. Miwa S, Fujii H, Takegawa S, et al 1980 Seven pyruvate kinase variants characterised by the ICSH recommended methods. British Journal of Haematology 45:575–583.

44. Miwa S, Nakashima K, Ariyoshi K et al 1975 Four new pyruvate kinase (PK) variants and a classical PK deficiency. British Journal of Haematology 29:157–169.

45. International Committee for Standardization in Haematology 1979 Recommended methods for the characterisation of red cell pyruvate kinase variants. British Journal of Haematology 43:275–286.

46. Beutler E, Duron O, Kelly B 1963 Improved method for the determination of blood glutathione. Journal of Laboratory and Clinical Medicine 61:882–888.

47. Lubin BH, Oski FA 1967 An evaluation of screening procedures for red cell glucose-6-phosphate dehydrogenase deficiency in the newborn infant. Journal of Pediatrics 70:488–492.

48. Zinkham WH 1959 An in-vitro abnormality of glutathione metabolism in erythrocytes from normal newborns: mechanism and clinical significance. Pediatrics 23:18–32.

49. Chanutin A, Curnish RR 1967 Effect of organic and inorganic phosphates on the oxygen equilibrium of human erythrocytes. Archives of Biochemistry and Biophysics 121:96–102.

50. Benesch R, Benesch RE 1967 The effect of organic phosphates from the human erythrocyte on the allosteric properties of haemoglobin. Biochemical and Biophysical Research Communications 26:162–167.

51. Krimsky I 1965 D-2,3-diphosphoglycerate. In: Bergmeyer HU (ed) Methods of enzymatic analysis. Academic Press, New York.

52. Lowry OH, Passonneau JV, Hasselberger FX, et al 1964 Effect of ischemia on known substrates and cofactors of the glycolytic pathway in brain, p 238. Journal of Biological Chemistry 239:18–30.

53. Rose ZB, Liebowitz J 1970 Direct determination of 2,3-diphosphoglycerate. Annals of Biochemistry and Experimental Medicine 35:177–180.

54. Duhm J 1971 Effects of 2,3-diphosphoglycerate and other organic phosphate compounds on oxygen affinity and intracellular pH of human erythrocytes. Pflügers Archiv für die gesampte Physiologie des Menschen und der Tiere 326:341–356.

55. Rosa R, Prehu MO, Beuzard Y, et al 1978 The first case of a complete deficiency of diphosphoglycerate mutase in human erythrocytes. Journal of Clinical Investigation 62:907–915.

56. Peters JP, Van Slyke DD 1931 Hemoglobin and oxygen. In: Quantitative clinical chemistry, vol. 1. Interpretations, p 525. Williams & Wilkins, Baltimore.

57. Bellingham AJ, Lenfant C 1971 Hb affinity for O_2 determined by O_2-Hb dissociation analyser and mixing technique. Journal of Applied Physiology 30:903–904.
58. Torrance JD, Lenfant C 1969 Methods for determination of O_2 dissociation curves, including Bohr effect. Respiration Physiology 8:127–136.
59. Van Slyke DD, Neill JM 1924 The determination of gases in blood and other solutions by vacuum extraction and manometric measurement. Journal of Biological Chemistry 61:523–573.
60. Bellingham AJ, Huehns ER 1968 Compensation in haemolytic anaemias caused by abnormal haemoglobins. Nature (London) 218:924–926.
61. Bohr C, Hasselbach K, Krogh A 1904 Ueber einen in biologischer Beziehung wichtigen Einfluss, den die Kohlensäurespannung des Blutes auf dessen Sauerstoffbindungübt. Skandinavisches Archiv für Physiologie 16:402.
62. Hill AV 1910 The possible effect of the aggregation of the molecules of haemoglobin on its dissociation curves. Journal of Physiology 40:4.
63. Bellingham AJ 1972 The physiological significance of the Hill parameter 'n'. Scandinavian Journal of Haematology 9:552–556.

11 Acquired haemolytic anaemias

Barbara J. Bain and Nay Win

ASSESSING THE LIKELIHOOD OF ACQUIRED HAEMOLYTIC ANAEMIA

Haemolytic anaemia may be suspected from either clinical or laboratory abnormalities. Suggestive clinical features include anaemia, jaundice, and splenomegaly. Other relevant clinical features that should be sought are a history of autoimmune disease, recent blood transfusion, recent infection, exposure to drugs or toxins, the presence of a cardiac prosthesis, and risk of malaria.

The basic laboratory investigations when a haemolytic anaemia is suspected are listed in Chapter 9. In this chapter tests are described that are more specific for the diagnosis of acquired haemolytic anaemia.

ASSESSMENT OF THE BLOOD FILM AND COUNT IN SUSPECTED ACQUIRED HAEMOLYTIC ANAEMIA

If haemolytic anaemia is suspected, a full blood count, reticulocyte count, and blood film should always be performed. The blood count shows a reduced haemoglobin concentration (Hb) and, usually, an increased mean cell volume (MCV). The increased MCV is attributable to the fact that reticulocytes, which may constitute a significant proportion of total red cells, are larger than mature red cells. The abnormalities that may be detected in the blood film and their possible significance in acquired haemolytic anaemia are shown in Table 11.1. Abnormalities detected in the blood film will

Table 11.1 Abnormalities that may be detected on blood film examination and their possible significance

Morphological abnormality observed on blood film examination	Type of acquired haemolytic anaemia suggested
Schistocytes	Fragmentation syndromes including microangiopathic haemolytic anaemia and mechanical haemolytic anaemia
Spherocytes	Autoimmune, alloimmune, or drug-induced immune haemolytic anaemia, burns, paroxysmal cold haemoglobinuria, *Clostridium welchii* sepsis
Microspherocytes	Burns, fragmentation syndromes
Irregularly contracted cells	Oxidant damage, Zieve's syndrome
Marked red cell agglutination	Cold-antibody–induced haemolytic anaemia
Minor red cell agglutination	Warm autoimmune haemolytic anaemia, paroxysmal cold haemoglobinuria
Hypochromia, microcytosis, and basophilic stippling	Lead poisoning
Erythrophagocytosis	Paroxysmal cold haemoglobinuria
Atypical lymphocytes	Cold-antibody–induced haemolytic anaemia associated with infectious mononucleosis or, less often, other infections
Lymphocytosis with mature small lymphocytes and smear cells	Autoimmune haemolytic anaemia associated with chronic lymphocytic leukaemia
Thrombocytopenia	Autoimmune haemolytic anaemia, thrombotic thrombocytopenic purpura, microangiopathic haemolytic anaemia associated with disseminated intravascular coagulation, paroxysmal nocturnal haemoglobinuria
Neutropenia	Paroxysmal nocturnal haemoglobinuria
No specific red cell features	Paroxysmal nocturnal haemoglobinuria

direct further investigations. For example, a Heinz body preparation would be relevant if irregularly contracted cells were present. Similarly, a direct antiglobulin test (DAT) would be indicated if the blood film showed spherocytes. Various inherited forms of haemolytic anaemia enter into the differential diagnosis of suspected acquired haemolytic anaemia. Thus spherocytes could be attributable to hereditary spherocytosis as well as to autoimmune or alloimmune haemolytic anaemia. Haemolysis with irregularly contracted cells could be attributable not only to oxidant exposure but also to an unstable haemoglobin, homozygosity for haemoglobin C, or glucose–6-phosphate dehydrogenase deficiency.

IMMUNE HAEMOLYTIC ANAEMIAS

Acquired immune-mediated haemolytic anaemias are the result of autoantibodies to a patient's own red cell antigens or alloantibodies in a patient's circulation, either present in the plasma or completely bound to red cells (e.g., transfused or neonatal red cells). Alloantibodies may be present in a patient's plasma and react with antigens on transfused donor red cells to cause haemolysis. Alloantibodies may also occur in maternal plasma and cause haemolytic disease of the newborn. Autoimmune haemolytic anaemia (AIHA) may be "idiopathic" or secondary, associated mainly with lymphoproliferative disorders and autoimmune diseases, particularly systemic lupus erythematosus. AIHA may also follow atypical (*Mycoplasma pneumoniae)* pneumonia or infectious mononucleosis and other viral infections. Paroxysmal cold haemoglobinuria (PCH) also belongs to this group of disorders. Occasionally, drugs may give rise to a haemolytic anaemia of immunological origin that closely mimics idiopathic AIHA both clinically and serologically. This was a relatively common occurrence with α-methyldopa, a drug that is now used very infrequently, but it also occurs occasionally with other drugs. A larger range of drugs give rise to an antibody that is directed primarily against the drug and only secondarily involves the red cells. This is an uncommon occurrence. Such drugs include penicillin, phenacetin, quinidine, quinine, the sodium salt of *p*-aminosalicylic acid, salicylazosulphapyridine, and cephalosporins.[1]

Types of Autoantibody

The diagnosis of an AIHA requires evidence of anaemia and haemolysis and demonstration of autoantibodies attached to the patient's red cells (i.e., a positive DAT [see p. 247]. A positive DAT may also be caused by the presence of *allo*antibodies (e.g., owing to a delayed haemolytic transfusion reaction), so details of any transfusion in the past months must be sought.

Autoantibodies can often be demonstrated free in the serum of a patient suffering from an AIHA. The ease with which the antibodies can be detected depends on how much antibody is being produced, its affinity for the corresponding antigen on the red cell surface, and the effect that temperature has on the adsorption of the antibody, as well as on the technique used to detect it. The autoantibodies associated with AIHA can be separated into two broad categories depending on how their interaction with antigen is affected by temperature: warm antibodies, which are able to combine with their corresponding red cell antigen readily at 37°C, and cold antibodies, which cannot combine with antigen at 37°C but form an increasingly stable combination with antigen as the temperature falls from 30–32°C to 2–4°C.

Cases of AIHA can similarly be separated into two broad categories according to the temperature characteristics of the associated autoantibodies: warm-type AIHA and the less frequent cold-type AIHA. The relative frequency of the two categories is illustrated in Table 11.2.[2]

Warm Autoantibodies

The most common type of warm autoantibody is an immunoglobulin G (IgG), which behaves *in vitro* very similarly to an Rh alloantibody; indeed many IgG autoantibodies have Rh specificity. IgA and IgM warm autoantibodies are much less common, and when present they are usually formed in addition to an IgG autoantibody (Table 11.3).[3]

Frequently, patients with warm-type AIHA have complement adsorbed onto their red cells, and the red cells are therefore agglutinated by antisera specific for complement or a complement component such as C3d (see Table 11.3). In these cases, the complement is probably not being bound by an IgG antibody but is on the cell surface as the result of the action of small and otherwise undetected amounts of IgM autoantibody.

Sometimes, patients with warm-type AIHA appear to have complement only on the red cell surface. This is more difficult to interpret because weak reactions of this type are not uncommon in patients with a variety of disorders in whom there is little evidence of increased red cell destruction. In some patients, this may be the result of the binding to the red cells of circulating immune complexes.

Warm autoantibodies free in the patient's serum are best detected by means of the indirect antiglobulin test (IAT) or by the use of enzyme-treated (e.g., trypsinized or papainized) red cells. (Antibodies that agglutinate unmodified cells directly *in vitro* are seldom present.) Not infrequently, antibodies that agglutinate enzyme-treated cells, sometimes at high titres, are present in the sera of patients in whom the IAT using unmodified cells is negative (Table 11.4). Occasionally, too, they are present in the sera of patients in whom the DAT is negative.

Antibodies in serum that can be shown to lyse (rather than simply agglutinate) unmodified red cells at 37°C in the presence of complement (warm haemolysins) are rarely demonstrable.[4a] If they are present, the patient is likely to suffer from extremely severe haemolysis. Antibodies in serum that lyse as well as agglutinate enzyme-treated cells but do not affect unmodified cells are, however, quite common. Their specificity is uncertain—they

Table 11.2   Relative incidence of different types of autoimmune haemolytic anaemia[2]

	Males	Females	Total
Warm antibodies			
"Idiopathic"	46	65	111
Associated with drugs (mostly α-methyldopa)	1	10	11*
Secondary			
Associated with:			
Lymphomas	14	23	37
Systemic lupus erythematosus	1	15	16
Other possible or probable autoimmune disorders	8	13	21
Infections and miscellaneous	9	4	13
Ovarian teratoma	0	1	1
Totals	79	131	210
Cold antibodies			
"Idiopathic" (CHAD)[†]	16	22	38
Secondary			
Associated with:			
Atypical or *Mycoplasma pneumonia* infection	5	18	23
Infectious mononucleosis	1	1	2
Lymphoma	3	4	7
Paroxysmal cold haemoglobinuria			
"Idiopathic"	7	1	8
Other secondary	4	3	7
Totals	36	49	85

*It should be noted that since this study was done the use of α-methyldopa has declined and this is now a rare cause of haemolytic anaemia.
†CHAD, chronic cold haemagglutinin disease. Although is often regarded as "idiopathic," it is actually consequent on an occult lymphoproliferative disorder, which leads to production of a cold agglutinin by a clone of neoplastic cells.

are not anti-Rh—and their presence is not necessarily associated with increased haemolysis.

Cold Autoantibodies

Cold autoantibodies are nearly always IgM in type. *In vivo* the majority do not cause haemolysis, although a minority can cause chronic intravascular haemolysis, the intensity of which is characteristically influenced by the ambient temperature. The resultant clinical picture is generally referred to as the cold haemagglutinin syndrome or disease (CHAD). Haemolysis results from destruction of the red cells by complement that is bound to the red cell surface by the antigen–antibody reaction, which takes place in the blood vessels of the exposed skin where the temperature is 28–32°C or less. The cold autoantibody in CHAD is monoclonal because this

syndrome is the result of a low-grade lymphoproliferative disorder.

The red cells of patients suffering from CHAD characteristically give positive antiglobulin reactions only with anticomplement (anti-C′) sera. (The C′ notation is used to distinguish anticomplement antibodies from anti-C antibodies of the Rh system.) This is because of red cells that have irreversibly adsorbed sublytic amounts of complement; it is a sign, therefore, of an antigen–antibody reaction that has taken place at a temperature below 37°C. The complement component responsible for the reaction with anti-C′ sera is the C3dg derivative of C3 (see p. 492).

In vitro, a cold-type autoantibody will often lyse normal red cells at 20–30°C in the presence of fresh human complement, especially if the cell–serum

Table 11.3 Direct antiglobulin test in warm–antibody autoimmune haemolytic anaemia: incidence of different reactions to specific antiglobulin sera[3]

Anti-IgG	Anti-IgA	Anti-IgM	Anti-C′	No. of patients	(%)
+	–	–	–	43	36
–	+	–	–	3	2
+	+	–	–	4	3
+	–	–	+	52	43
+	–	+	+	6	5
–	–	–	+	13	11
				121	100

Ig, immunoglobulin.

mixture is acidified to pH 6.5–7.0; it will usually lyse enzyme-treated red cells readily in unacidified serum, and agglutination and lysis of these cells may still occur at 37°C. Most of these cold-type autoantibodies have anti-I specificity (i.e., they react strongly with the vast majority of adult red cells and only weakly with cord-blood red cells). A minority are anti-i and react strongly with cord-blood cells and weakly with adult red cells. Rarely, the antibodies have anti-Pr or anti-M specificity and react with antigens on the red cell surface that are destroyed by enzyme treatment.

Another quite distinct, but rarely met with, type of cold antibody is the Donath–Landsteiner (D–L) antibody. This is an IgG and has anti-P specificity. The clinical syndrome the antibody produces is referred to as PCH.

PCH is caused by a biphasic IgG autoantibody, usually with anti-P specificity, and is commonly seen as acute condition in children. This antibody

Table 11.4 Results of testing for free autoantibodies in the sera of 210 patients with warm-antibody autoimmune haemolytic anaemia[2]

Indirect antiglobulin test (IAT)	Agglutination of enzyme-treated red cells at 37°C	Lysis of enzyme-treated red cells at 37°C	Agglutination of normal red cells at 20°C	No. and percentage of patients in group	
+	+	+	+	4	
+	+	+	–	16	
+	+	–	–	64	41%
+	–	–	–	2	
+	–	–	+	1	
–	+	+	+	16	
–	+	+	–	31	40%
–	+	–	–	29	
–	+	–	+	7	
–	–	–	–	39	19%

Notes
1. In 41% of the patients, the IAT was positive, and in 80% of the patients, the tests with enzyme-treated cells were positive (in half of these patients, the IAT was negative).
2. In 19% of the patients, all tests were negative.
3. In 13% of the patients, normal red cells were agglutinated at 20°C, probably by cold agglutinins.

binds to the red cells in the cold but activates complement and causes haemolysis on rewarming to 37°C. Cases may be idiopathic or can be secondary to acute viral infection in children.

The DAT is positive for complement only. Negative antibody screen by the standard IAT at 37°C is a common finding in a suspected case of PCH because of the low thermal amplitude nature of the autoantibody. If the antibody investigation is carried out at a lower temperature in PCH cases, pan-reactive cold antibodies may be detected because the majority of autoantibodies show anti-P specificity with thermal amplitude range up to 15–24°C. Usually the antibody titre is low (less than 64), even when investigated at 4°C.

Some of the characteristics of IgG, IgM, and IgA antibodies are listed in Table 11.5.

The clinical, haematological, and serological aspects of the AIHAs have been summarized by Dacie[4] and others.[5-9]

Table 11.5 Main characteristics of IgG, IgM, and IgA autoantibodies			
	IgG	IgM	IgA
Molecular weight (daltons)	146,000	970,000	160,000
Sedimentation constant (s)	7	19	7
Number of heavy-chain subclasses	4	1	2
Cross placenta	Yes	No	No
Cause activation of complement	Yes	Yes	No
Cause monocyte/ macrophage attachment	Yes	No	No
Number of antigen-binding sites	2	5 or 10	2
Types of AIHA produced	Warm; PCH	Usually cold	Warm

Ig, immunoglobulin; AIHA, autoimmune haemolytic anaemia; PCH, paroxysmal cold haemoglobinuria.

Methods of Investigation

Many of the methods used in the investigation of a patient suspected of suffering from AIHA are described in Chapter 19. Detailed description is given here of precautions to be taken when collecting blood samples from patients and of methods of particular value in the investigations.

Collection of Samples of Blood and Serum

To determine the true thermal amplitude or titre of cold agglutinins requires that the blood sample is collected and maintained strictly at 37°C until serum and cells are separated. This can be achieved by collecting venous (clotted and EDTA sample) blood and keeping it warmed at 37°C—ideally in an insulated thermos, but usually, in practice, by placing the sample tube in a beaker containing water at 37°C.

The red cells are available for antibody elution, and the serum can be examined for free antibody or other abnormalities. The clotted sample should then be centrifuged to separate the serum at 37°C (e.g., in an ordinary centrifuge into the buckets of which has been placed water warmed to 37–40°C). The EDTA sample is used for the DAT and other tests involving the patient's red cells. If the autoantibody in a par-ticular case is known to be warm in type, the blood may be separated at room temperature; otherwise, as already indicated, this should be carried out at 37°C. When samples are sent by post, it is best to send separately: (a) serum (separated at 37°C) and (b) whole blood added to ACD or CPD solution. Sterility must be maintained.

Storage of Samples

Samples of patient's blood, while keeping quite well in ACD or CPD at 4°C, are more difficult to preserve than normal red cells. In particular, if marked spherocytosis is present, considerable lysis develops on storage. However, satisfactory eluates can be made from washed red cells that are frozen at –20°C for weeks or months.

The patient's serum should be stored at –20°C or below in small (1–2 ml) volumes. If complement is to be titrated and the titration is not performed immediately, the serum should be frozen as soon as practicable at –70°C or below.

Scheme for Serological Investigation of Haemolytic Anaemia Suspected to be of Immunological Origin

It is important to consider which are the most useful tests to carry out and the order in which they should be done. A suggested scheme has been set out in the form of answers to questions.[10] Whereas some information may be helpful in classifying the type of AIHA, the single most important practical consideration is to determine whether, in addition to an autoantibody, there is any underlying alloantibody present. This should be identified before transfusion is undertaken to avoid a delayed haemolytic transfusion reaction that would compound existing haemolysis.

1. **Are the patient's red cells "coated" by immunoglobulins or complement (indicating an antigen-antibody reaction)?**

   Perform a DAT using a polyspecific "broad-spectrum" reagent, which contains both anti-IgG and anti-C'. (If the DAT is negative, it is unlikely, although not impossible, that the diagnosis is AIHA. See DAT-negative AIHA, p. 248.)

2. **If the DAT is positive, are immunoglobulins or complement adsorbed to the red cells?**

   Repeat the DAT using monospecific sera (p. 501) (i.e., anti-IgG and anti-C3d).

3. **If immunoglobulins are present on the red cells, is there antibody specificity?**

   Prepare eluates from the patient's red cells. Test these later (see number 6).

4. **What is the patient's blood group?**

   Determine the patient's ABO and Rh D and Kell type. The Rh phenotype is particularly important in warm-type AIHA; other antigens must be determined if alloantibodies are to be differentiated from autoantibodies (see p. 491).

5. **Is there free antibody in the serum? How does it react, and at what temperatures and by what methods can it be demonstrated? Is there any underlying alloantibody present?**

   Screen the serum with two or three red cell suspensions suitable for routine pretransfusion antibody screening (see p. 532) looking for agglutination and lysis at 37°C by the IAT (p. 502). If positive, identify the antibody using an antibody identification panel.

   a. If an alloantibody is identified, blood lacking the corresponding antigen must be selected for transfusion.

   b. If no alloantibody is identified in the serum or plasma, it is safe to assume there is no alloantibody present, unless the patient has been transfused in the last month; in the latter case, a red cell eluate is required because an alloantibody may be bound to the recently transfused cells and there may not be free antibody detectable in the serum/plasma.

   c. If the autoantibody is pan-reacting (i.e., is reacting against all panel cells), antibody adsorption tests are needed to remove the autoantibody so as to identify any underlying alloantibody. If the patient has not had a transfusion within the last 3 months, a ZZAP autoadsorption test is appropriate (see p. 251). If the patient has had a transfusion within the last 3 months, differential alloadsorption tests are needed. However, if the patient has had a transfusion within the last month, an eluate is required, irrespective of results of adsorption tests.

6. **If there is a warm autoantibody, what is the specificity of the autoantibody?**

   Test the serum also at 20°C against antibody-screening cells to show whether cold or warm antibodies, or a mixture of the two, are present in the serum.

   Test the eluate against the antibody identification panel of red cells by IAT and by using enzyme-treated red cells (p. 498). Titration of autoantibody may be useful in the presence of a strong alloantibody.

   Titrate the serum/plasma by the methods that have given positive results in the screening test using the same panel of red cells (see number 5a).

7. **If there is a cold antibody:**

   a. **Has the antibody any specificity? Is it an autoantibody or an alloantibody? What is its titre?**

   b. **What is the thermal range of the antibody?**

   Test the serum/plasma against a panel of O cells at 20°C, including A_1, A_2, B, cord cells, and patient's own cells. If an autoantibody is found, titrate at 4°C with ABO compatible adult

(I) cells, cord-blood (i) cells, the patient's cells, and adult (i) cells (if possible):

a. Determine the highest temperature at which autoagglutination of the patient's whole blood takes place (p. 255).

b. Titrate the patient's serum/plasma at 20°C, 30°C, and 37°C with pooled O adult cells, O cord cells, patient's own cells, and the panel of cells described earlier. If there was any agglutination or lysis at 37°C in the screening test (5(a)), titrate with the appropriate cells at this temperature.

c. If PCH is suspected, carry out the direct and two-stage indirect Donath–Landsteiner tests (p. 255).

8. **Is a drug suspected as the cause of the haemolytic anaemia?**

a. If a penicillin-induced haemolytic anaemia is suspected, test for antibodies using cells pre-incubated with the appropriate drug (p. 258).

b. If haemolysis induced by other drugs is suspected, add the drug in solution to a mixture of the patient's serum, normal cells, and fresh normal serum (p. 259). Look for agglutination of normal and enzyme-treated cells, and use the IAT.

9. **Are there any other serological abnormalities?**

Consider carrying out the following tests: serum protein electrophoresis and quantitative estimation of immunoglobulins, estimation of complement, tests for antinuclear factor, a screening test for heterophile antibodies (infectious mononucleosis screening test), and a test for mycoplasma antibodies.

The suggested scheme summarises what may be done by way of serological investigation of a patient suspected of having AIHA. Close collaboration between clinician and laboratory helps in deciding what tests should be done in any particular case.

Detection of Incomplete Antibodies by Means of the Direct Antiglobulin (Coombs) Test

Principle

As already described, the DAT involves testing the patient's cells without prior exposure to antibody *in vitro*. For the investigation of cases of AIHA, antiglobulin reagents specific for IgG, IgM, IgA,C3c, and C3d can be used.

Precautions

A blood sample in EDTA is preferred. (If a clotted sample is used, complement could be bound by normal incomplete cold antibody and give a false-positive result with anti-C3d.) Certain precautions are necessary when investigating a patient with possible AIHA. If a cold-reacting autoantibody is present, the patient's red cells should be washed four times in a large volume of saline* warmed to 37°C to wash off cold antibodies and obtain a smooth suspension of cells; there is no risk of washing off adsorbed complement components. However, the washing process should be accomplished as quickly as possible and the test should be set up immediately afterward because bound warm antibody occasionally elutes off the cells when they are washed, and false-negative results may be obtained. If for any reason the washing process has to be interrupted once it has begun, the cell suspension should be placed at 4°C to slow down the dissociation of the antibody.

Method

A spin tube technique, as described on page 502, is recommended.

Make a 2–5% suspension of red cells that have been washed four times in saline. Add 1 volume (drop) of the cell suspension to 2 volumes (drops) of antiglobulin reagent. Centrifuge for 10–60 sec. Refer to reagent manufacturer's instructions for specific details.

Examine for agglutination after gently resuspending the button of cells. A concave mirror and good light help in macroscopic readings. If the result appears to be negative, confirm this microscopically.

Each DAT or batch of tests should be carefully controlled as previously described.

Check negative results with the polyspecific antihuman globulin (AHG) or anti-IgG reagents by the addition of IgG-sensitized cells and anti-C' by the addition of complement-coated cells.

DAT Using Column Agglutination Technology

A card of several microtubes enables multiple sample testing. The microtubes contain a solid-phase matrix and the antiglobulin reagent to which patient's red cells are added. During centrifugation,

---

*Throughout this chapter, "saline" refers to 9 g/l NaCl buffered to pH 7.0.

unagglutinated cells pass to the tip of the tube, but agglutinates fail to pass through the gel, which acts as a sieve. As the antiglobulin reagent is already present in the microtubes, no washing or addition of IgG-coated cells to negative tests is required. Refer to individual manufacturer's instructions for details of methods for performing the tests.

Significance of Positive Direct Antiglobulin Test

A positive DAT anaemia does not necessarily mean that the patient has autoimmune haemolytic anaemia.[2,3,11] The causes of a positive test include the following:

1. An autoantibody on the red cell surface with or without haemolytic anaemia
2. An alloantibody on the red cell surface, as for example in haemolytic disease of the newborn or after an incompatible transfusion
3. Antibodies provoked by drugs adsorbed to the red cell (p. 257)
4. Normal globulins adsorbed to the red cell surface as the result of damage by drugs (e.g., some cephalosporins)
5. Complement components alone
   a. About 10–11% of patients with warm AIHA have red cells with positive DAT as a result of C3 coating alone[12] (Table 11.3).
   b. Cold haemagglutinin disease/paroxysmal cold haemoglobinuria
   c. Drug-dependent immune haemolytic anemia (complement-induced lysis)
   d. Adsorption of immune complexes to the red cell surface. This may be the mechanism of the (usually weak) reactions that are found in approximately 8% of hospital patients suffering from a wide variety of disorders (see below)
6. Passive infusion of alloantibodies in donor plasma/derivatives that react with recipient's red cells
   a. Transfusion of group O platelets with high titre anti-A,B to group A or B recipient.
   b. Intravenous immunoglobulin may contain ABO or anti-D antibodies.[13]
      In one study of patients treated with intravenous immunoglobulin after bone marrow transplantation, 49% of recipients developed a positive DAT and 25% had a positive antibody screen (passively transfused anti-A, -B, -D, or –K) of short duration (2–5 days).
7. Antibodies produced by passenger lymphocytes in solid organ transplant and bone marrow transplantation.[14,15]
   Passenger lymphocytes of donor origin produce antibodies directed against ABO or other antigens on the recipient's cells, causing a positive DAT.
8. Nonspecific binding of immunoglobulins (nonantibody) to red cells in patients with hypergammaglobulinemia or multiple myeloma and in recipients of antilymphocyte globulin and antithymocyte globulin[16]
   Szymanski et al[17] used an AutoAnalyser and used Ficoll and PVP to enhance agglutination by an anti-IgG serum highly diluted (usually to 1 in 5000) in 0.5% bovine serum albumin. In this sensitive system, the strength of agglutination was positively correlated with the serum γ-globulin concentration, being subnormal in hypogammaglobulinaemia and supranormal in hypergammaglobulinaemia.
   Similar findings were observed in patients with multiple myeloma. Nonspecific binding of IgG to red cells was related to the level of monoclonal protein in the patient's serum.[18]
   Usually, in patients with hypergammaglobulinaemia in whom the DAT is positive, attempts to demonstrate antibodies in eluates fail (i.e., eluates are nonreactive).[19,20]
9. Cross-reacting antiphospholipid antibodies adsorbing nonspecifically on to red cell membrane and binding to phospholipid epitopes. Positive DAT as a result of antiphospholipid antibodies has been documented in patients with primary antiphospholipid syndrome and antiphospholipid syndrome with systemic lupus erythematosus.[21] It has also been described in healthy blood donors.[22]
10. Incidental findings of positive DAT with no clear correlation between DAT and anaemia. A positive DAT is a common finding in patients with sickle cell disease because of abnormal amounts of IgG coated on red cells. There was no correlation between the amount of IgG on the patient's red cells and the severity of anaemia.[23]

There was an association between an elevated blood urea nitrogen and a positive DAT. Urea may alter the red cell membrane and enhance nonspecific IgG adsorption.[24]

11. Sensitization *in vitro* if a sample other than EDTA is used. If, for instance, clotted or defibrinated normal blood is allowed to stand in a refrigerator at 4°C, or even at room temperature, and the antiglobulin test is subsequently carried out, the reaction may be positive because of the adsorption of incomplete cold antibodies and complement from normal sera.[4b] Samples of blood taken into EDTA or ACD and subsequently chilled do not give this type of false-positive result because the anticoagulant inhibits the complement reaction.

12. False-positive agglutination may occur with a silica gel derived from glass.[25] Also, albeit rarely, the DAT has been positive with the blood of apparently perfectly healthy individuals (e.g., blood donors). Such occurrences have not been satisfactorily explained (see below).

Positive DATs in Normal Subjects

The occurrence of a clearly positive DAT in an apparently healthy subject is a rare but well-known phenomenon. Worlledge[11] reported a prevalence in blood donors of approximately 1 in 9000. In a later report, Gorst et al[26] estimated that the prevalence was approximately 1 in 14,000 with an increasing likelihood of a positive test with increasing age. Their report, and subsequent reports,[17,27] suggest that the finding of a positive DAT, using an anti-IgG serum, in an apparently healthy person is usually of little clinical significance and that, although overt AIHA may subsequently develop, this is infrequent. In some such individuals the DAT eventually becomes negative.

Positive DATs in Hospital Patients

In contrast to the rarity of positive DATs in healthy people, positive tests are much more frequent in hospital patients. Worlledge[11] reported that the red cells of 40 out of 489 blood samples (8.9%) submitted for routine tests were agglutinated by anti-C′ sera. Only one sample was agglutinated by an anti-IgG serum, and this had been obtained from a patient being treated with α-methyldopa. Freedman[28] reported a similar incidence—7.8% positive tests with

anti-C′ sera. Lau et al[29] used anti-IgG sera only. The tests were seldom positive (0.9% positive out of 4664 tests). The probable explanation for the relatively high incidence of positive tests with anti-C′ sera is that the reaction is between anti-C′ antibodies and immune complexes adsorbed to the red cells.

False-Negative Antiglobulin Test Results

There are several causes of false-negative test results:

1. Failure to wash the red cells properly—the antisera may then be neutralized by immunoglobulins or complement in the surrounding serum or plasma (p. 503).
2. Excessive agitation at the reading stage—this may break up agglutinates, leading to a false-negative result.
3. The use of impotent antisera so that weakly sensitized cells are not detected.
4. The use of antisera lacking the antibody corresponding to the subclass of immunoglobulin responsible for the red cell sensitization.
5. The presence of an antibody that is readily dissociable and is eluted in the washing process.

These phenomena are largely negated by the use of column agglutination technology.

DAT-Negative Autoimmune Haemolytic Anaemia

Most hospital blood banks use polyspecific "broad-spectrum" AHG reagent for screening for diagnosis of AIHA. These reagents contain antibody to human IgG and the C3d component of human complement and have little activity against IgA and IgM proteins. The incidence of IgA-only warm AIHA has been reported as 0.2% to 2.7%,[30] and the diagnosis may be missed if such polyspecific AHG is used for the DAT screen. In approximately 2–6% of patients who present with the clinical and haematological features of AIHA, the DAT is negative on repeated testing.[11,31,32]

Low-affinity IgG autoantibodies dissociate from the red cells during the washing phase if a tube technique is used, resulting in a negative DAT. Alternatively, there may be few IgG molecules coating the red cells, and this number may fall below the threshold of detection, which is 300–4000 molecules per red blood cell if a tube technique is used. In such cases, a positive DAT may be demonstrated by a more sensitive technique, such as a column agglutination method, an enzyme-linked immunoabsorbant assay or flow cytometry.[33-35]

If polyspecific AHG is used and the DAT remains negative with clinical evidence of haemolysis, a more sensitive technique should be used for further investigation.

The DiaMed DAT gel card, which contains a set of monospecific AHG reagents (i.e., anti-IgG, -IgA, -IgM, -C3c, -C3d, and an inert control) can be used. Because there is no washing phase, this permits the detection of low-affinity IgG, IgA, and IgM antibodies. A gel card can also pick up the rare IgA-only autoimmune haemolytic anaemia.

Preparing and Testing a Concentrated Eluate

The eluate technique concentrates low levels of immunoglobulin present on the red cell surface so that antibody may then be detected by screening the eluate with group O red cells by the IAT. Elution techniques reverse or neutralize the binding forces that exist between the red cell antigens and the antibody coating the cells. This may be achieved by several techniques (e.g., heat, alterations to the pH).

Manual Direct Polybrene Test

The following method[36] is modified from that of Lalezari and Jiang.[37] Polybrene is a polyvalent cationic molecule, hexadimethrine bromide, that can overcome the electrostatic repulsive forces between adjacent red cells, bringing the cells closer together. When low levels of IgG are present on the red cell surface, antibody linkage of adjacent red cells is enhanced. The Polybrene is then neutralized using a negatively charged molecule such as trisodium citrate. Sensitized red cells remain agglutinated after neutralization of the Polybrene. Unsensitized red cells will disaggregate after neutralization.

Reagents

Polybrene stock. 10% Polybrene in 9 g/l NaCl, pH 6.9 (saline).
Working Polybrene solution. Dilute the stock Polybrene solution 1 in 250 in saline.
Resuspending solution. 60 ml of 0.2 mol/l trisodium citrate added to 40 ml of 50 g/l dextrose.

Washing solution. 50 ml of 0.2 mol/l trisodium citrate in 950 ml of saline.
Low-ionic medium. 50 g/l dextrose containing 2 g/l disodium ethylenediamine tetraacetate. Adjust the pH of half the batch to 6.4. Store the remainder at the original pH (approx. 4.9); use this to repeat tests that are negative using low-ionic medium at pH 6.4.

Method

Ensure that all reagents are at room temperature.

Positive Control
Dilute an IgG anti-D in normal group AB serum. Find a dilution that gives a positive result with papainized cells but is negative by the IAT on standard testing with group O, D positive red cells (a dilution of 1 in 10,000 is often suitable).

Negative Control
Normal group AB serum that fails to agglutinate papainized group O, Rh D positive red cells.

1. Wash the cells four times in saline and make 3–5% suspensions of test and normal group O RhD red cells in saline.
2. Set up three 75 × 10 mm tubes as shown in Table 11.6. Leave at room temperature for 1 min.
3. Add 1 drop of working Polybrene solution to each tube and mix gently. Leave for 15 sec at room temperature.
4. Centrifuge for 10 sec at 1000 g. Decant, taking care to remove all the supernatant.
5. Leave for 3–5 min at room temperature before adding 2 drops of resuspending solution and mixing gently. Within 10 sec aggregates will dissociate leaving true agglutination in the positive tubes.
6. Read macroscopically after 10–60 sec. Check all negative results microscopically and compare with the negative control.
7. Repeat negative tests using low-ionic medium at the lower pH (about 4.9).

If the direct Polybrene test is negative, a supplementary antiglobulin test may be performed by washing the cells twice in the washing solution and testing with an anti-IgG antiglobulin reagent.

Table 11.6   Setting up a direct manual polybrene test

	Test	Positive control	Negative control
AB serum*	2	0	2
Dilute anti-D in AB serum*	0	2	0
3–5% test cells*	1	0	0
3–5% normal 0 Rh (D) cells*	0	1	1
Low ionic medium	0.6 ml	0.6 ml	0.6 ml

*Drops.

Determination of the Blood Group of a Patient with AIHA

ABO Grouping

No difficulty should be encountered in ABO grouping patients with warm-type AIHA using monoclonal reagents, but the presence of cold agglutinins may cause difficulties. The cells should in all cases be washed in warm (37°C) saline. They should then be groupable without any problem; the reactions must, however, be controlled with normal AB serum. Reverse grouping should be performed strictly at 37°C. Warm the known A_1, B, and 0 cells to 37°C before adding them to the patient's serum at 37°C. Read the results macroscopically.

Rh D Grouping

When the DAT is positive, monoclonal anti-D reagents should be used; if cold agglutinins are present, perform the test at 37°C. Appropriate controls should be included (see p. 527).

Demonstration of Free Antibodes in Serum

The sera of patients suffering from AIHA often contain free autoantibodies. However, free autoantibody is also often found with no haemolysis. As a result of improved reagent sensitivity, any clinically significant IgG complement-binding antibodies will be detected by current antibody screening methods.

Identification by Adsorption Techniques of Coexisting Alloantibodies in the Presence of Warm Autoantibodies

Adsorption techniques for the detection of alloantibodies present in the sera or eluates of patients with suspected or proved AIHA can be helpful in the following situations:

1. In screening for coexisting alloantibodies in patients with AIHA who have been pregnant or previously transfused and are found to have a pan-reactive antibody in their serum
2. In differentiating between autoantibodies and alloantibodies in the eluate of recently transfused patients with AIHA
3. In investigating haemolytic transfusion reactions owing to red cell alloantibodies in patients with AIHA

In some cases of AIHA, an underlying alloantibody may be detected by titrating the patient's serum and eluate against a panel of phenotyped reagent red cells. However, a high-titre autoantibody may mask the alloantibody; hence the need for adsorption techniques, especially in the situations outlined earlier.

Use of ZZAP Reagent in Autoadsorption Techniques

"ZZAP" reagent is a mixture of dithiothreitol and papain.[38] It dissociates an autoantibody already coating the patient's red cells and enzyme treats them, thus increasing the amount of autoantibody that can subsequently be adsorbed onto the patient's cells *in vitro*.

Reagents

Dithiothreitol (DTT), 0.2 mol/l.
Papain, 1%.
Phosphate-buffered saline (PBS), pH 6.8–7.2.

Prepare a suitable volume of ZZAP by making up the reagents in the following ratio: 0.2 mol/l DTT 5 volumes; and 1% papain 1 volume.
Check the pH and adjust to pH 6.0–6.5 using one drop at a time of 0.2 mol/l HCl or 0.2 mol/l NaOH.

Method

1. Add 2 volumes of ZZAP to 1 volume of packed red cells that have been washed four times. Incubate at 37°C for 30 min, mixing occasionally.
2. After incubation, wash the cells four times in saline, packing hard after the last wash.
3. Divide the cells into two equal volumes. To one volume, add an equal volume of the serum to be adsorbed. Incubate at 37°C for 1 hour.
4. Centrifuge at 1000 g. Remove the serum and add to the remaining volume of cells.
5. Repeat the adsorption procedure.
6. Remove the adsorbed serum and store at –20°C or below for alloantibody screening or cross-matching, which may be performed by standard techniques.

Notes

The autoadsorption techniques should only be used in the following circumstances:

1. When the patient has not had a transfusion in the previous 3 months because the presence of transfused red cells may allow the adsorption of alloantibody as well as autoantibody
2. When at least 2–3 ml of packed red cells are available from the patient
3. When the autoantibodies present react well with enzyme-treated red cells. If they do not, heat elution should be substituted for ZZAP treatment. Heat elution may be performed by shaking the washed cells for 5 min in a 56°C waterbath and then washing the cells.

Alloadsorption Using Papainized R_1R_1, R_2R_2, and rr Cells

The method of alloadsorption using papainized R_1R_1, R_2R_2, and rr cells may be used when autoadsorption is not appropriate—for instance, when the patient has had a transfusion in the previous 3 months or when less than 2–3 ml of the patient's red cells are available.

1. Select three group O antibody screening cells, which individually lack some of the blood-group antigens that commonly stimulate the production of clinically significant antibodies (e.g., c, e, C, E, K, Fy^a, Fy^b, Jk^a, Jk^b, S, s) (Table 11.7).

2. Papainize 2 ml of packed cells from each sample after washing the cells in saline four times.
3. Add to 1 ml of each sample of washed, packed, papainized cells, 1 ml of the patient's serum. Incubate for 20 min at 37°C.
4. Centrifuge to pack the cells. Remove the supernatant serum and add it to the second 1 ml volume of papainized cells. Incubate for 1 hour at 37°C.
5. Centrifuge again to pack the cells. Remove the supernatant and store at –20°C or below for further testing (e.g., alloantibody screening and cross-matching).

Method for Testing Alloadsorbed Sera

For alloantibody screening each adsorbed serum is tested against a panel of phenotyped red cells by the IAT. For cross-matching each adsorbed serum must be tested separately against the donor red cells by the IAT, using undiluted serum.

Example of Alloantibody Detection Using the Alloadsorption Technique in a Recently Transfused Patient with AIHA

The patient's serum when first tested against a panel of group O phenotyped red cells revealed only pan-reactive antibodies. In contrast, three absorbed sera, A, B, and C, obtained by adsorbing the patient's serum with three selected phenotyped samples of group O cells, were shown to contain anti-E and anti-Jk^a when tested against a panel of phenotyped group O cells using the IAT. The results of testing the adsorbed sera, A, B, and C, are shown in Table 11.7. The patient's red cell phenotype was R_1r Jk (a–b–).

Explanation of the Results of Testing Alloadsorbed Sera, A, B, and C

1. Because the R_1R_1-adsorbing cells were negative for the E and Jk^a antigens, adsorbed serum A could contain anti-E and anti-Jk^a. Testing the adsorbed serum A against the panel of cells suggested that this was the case.
2. Because the R_2R_2-adsorbing cells were positive for the E antigen but negative for the Jk^a antigen, adsorbed serum B could contain anti-Jk^a but not anti-E. Testing adsorbed serum B against the panel of cells confirmed the presence of anti-Jk^a.
3. Because the rr-adsorbing cells were negative for the E antigen but positive for the Jk^a antigen,

Table 11.7   Testing an alloabsorbed serum against a phenotyped panel of red cells

No.	Rh	M	N	S	s	P_1	Lu_a	Le_a	Le_b	K	Kp_a	Fy_a	Fy_b	Jk_a	Jk_b	Serum A	Serum B	Serum C
	Red cell phenotypes															Results of IAT		
1.	R_1R_1	+	+	+	+	+	−	−	−	+	−	+	+	+	+	1+	1+	−
2.	R_1R_1	+	−	−	+	−	+	−	+	−	−	+	+	+	+	1+	3+	−
3.	R_2R_2	+	+	+	+	+	+	+	−	−	−	−	+	−	+	1+	−	3+
4.	R_1R_2	+	+	+	−	+	−	−	+	−	−	−	+	+	−	1+	4+	1+
5.	r′r	+	−	+	+	+	−	−	+	−	−	+	+	−	+	−	−	−
6.	r″r	+	+	+	−	+	−	−	+	−	−	+	−	+	+	2+	2+	2+
7.	rr	+	+	−	+	+	−	−	−	+	−	+	+	+	−	2+	2+	−
8.	rr	+	−	+	+	+	−	+	−	−	−	+	−	+	−	1+	2+	(+)
9.	rr	−	+	−	+	+	−	+	−	−	+	+	+	+	+	2+	2+	−
10.	R_1R_2	−	+	+	+	−	−	−	+	+	−	−	+	+	−	1+	3+	2+

Phenotype of cells selected for absorption of serum

				Absorbed serum
1. R_1R_1,	C^w +, K −,	Fy(a + b −),	Jk(a − b +), M +, N −,s −	Serum A
2. R_2R_2,	C^w −, K−,	Fy (a − b +),	Jk(a − b +), M +, N +, s +	Serum B
3. rr,	C^w K+,	Fy(a + b −),	Jk(a + b −), M +, N −, s−	Serum C

IAT, indirect antiglobulin test.

adsorbed serum C could contain anti-E but not anti-Jk[a]. Testing adsorbed serum C against the panel of cells confirmed the presence of anti-E.

4. Because the phenotype of the patient's own red cells was R_1r, Jk (a– b–), the anti-E and anti-Jk[a] detected in the alloadsorbed sera must be alloantibodies. Blood for transfusion should be E-negative, Jk[a]-negative.

Additional Notes on Adsorption Techniques

1. If the patient has had a transfusion in the past month, an eluate must also be tested because alloantibody may be present on red cells but not in serum/plasma.
2. If the patient's serum contains a haemolytic antibody, EDTA should be added to prevent the uptake of complement and subsequent lysis of the cells used for adsorption. Add 1 volume of neutral EDTA (potassium salt) (see p. 690) to 9 volumes of serum. More commonly, a plasma sample is used.
3. It is often useful to alloadsorb both serum and eluate to differentiate between autoantibodies and allo-antibodies, particularly if the autoantibody is the mimicking type described by Issitt.[9]
4. If the autoantibody does not react with papainized cells, do *not* papainize the cells for adsorption.

Elution of Antibodies from Red Cells

The selection of any elution technique is often based on personal choice and the availability of the necessary reagents and equipment. However, heat elution techniques are best used for the elution of primary cold reactive (IgM) antibodies such as anti-A, anti-N, anti-M, anti-I, and IgG anti-A and anti-B antibodies associated with ABO hemolytic disease of the newborn (HDN). The Lui freeze and thaw technique (see below) may also be used for investigation of ABO HDN. Commercially prepared kits that alter the pH of the red blood cells are equally effective and circumvent the hazards of using organic solvents. Refer to the manufacturer's instructions for details. Methods for heat elution and Lui's elution techniques are given below. Commercial kits are now widely available.

Notes

1. A large volume of red blood cells is required to obtain enough eluate for testing.

2. The red blood cells must be washed at least 6X, and the last wash must be kept for testing to ensure removal of all free antibody.
3. Depending on the elution technique used, the prepared eluate may be frozen if testing is not possible immediately after preparation.

Heat Elution[39]

Mix equal volumes of washed packed cells and saline or 6% bovine serum albumin (BSA). Incubate at 56°C for 5 min. Agitate periodically. Centrifuge to pack the red cells. Remove the supernatant (the eluate), which may be haemoglobin stained. Test the eluate by appropriate techniques in parallel with the last wash from the red cells.

Freeze and Thaw Elution (Lui)[40]

Mix 0.5 ml of washed packed red cells with 3 drops of PBS or AB serum. Stopper the tube and rotate to coat the glass surface with red cells. Place at –20°C for 10 min. Thaw the red cells rapidly in a 37°C waterbath. Remove the stopper and centrifuge to sediment red cell stroma. Remove the supernatant and test in parallel with the last wash from the red cells by appropriate techniques.

Screening Eluates

The eluate and the saline of the last wash (control) are first screened against two or three samples of washed normal group O cells to see if they contain any antibodies using the IAT. If anti-A or anti-B is suspected, include A_1 and B cells. To 4–6 drops of eluate and control, add 2 drops of a 2% suspension by *normal ionic strength saline* (NISS).

Incubate for $1–1^1/_2$ hours at 37°C. Wash four times and, using optimal dilutions of anti-IgG, carry out the IAT by the tube method.

If the control preparation (the supernatant saline from the last washing) gives positive reactions, the possibility that an eluate contains serum antibody has to be considered.

Determination of the Specificity of Warm Autoantibodies in Eluates and Sera

When tested against a phenotyped panel, about two-thirds of autoantibodies appear to have Rh specificity, and in about half of these cases specificity against a particular antigen can be demonstrated.[2,6,9] Within the Rh system, anti–e-like is the most common specificity. D - - and Rh_{null} cells are an advantage.

The other one-third of autoantibodies may show specificity against other very high incidence antigens (e.g., Wr^b and En^a), and rarely other blood-group specificities are involved. It is essential to differentiate between autoantibodies and alloan-tibodies, especially if transfusion is being considered. The presence of alloantibodies in addition to auto-antibodies is suggested by any discrepancy between the serum and eluate results.

As already mentioned, the presence of alloan-tibodies in a serum complicates the determination of the specificity of an autoantibody, and it can be argued that it would be better to test only the eluted autoantibody and to leave the serum strictly alone. However, only a small volume of an eluate may be available, especially in patients who are anaemic, and it is generally wise to test both serum and eluate. The procedure is the same for both.

Titration of Warm Antibodies in Eluates or Sera

The methods used are those described in Chapter 19. The exact technique chosen, and the red cells used, should be those that have given the clearest results in the screening tests. Titration of the eluate can be useful in the presence of a pan-reacting autoantibody to exclude an underlying alloantibody.

In investigating cold autoantibodies, the following tests may sometimes provide clinically useful information:

Determination of the Specificity of Cold Autoantibodies

High-titre cold autoantibodies have a well-defined blood-group specificity, which is very often within the I/i system.[9,41,42] Because the I antigen is poorly developed in cord-blood red cells, whereas the i antigen is well developed, group O cord-blood red cells should be included in the panel used to test for I/i specificity. Adult cells almost always have the I antigen well expressed, but the strength of the antigen varies, and it is of considerable advantage to have available adult cells known to possess strong I antigen. (The rare adult i cells, if available, may also be used.)

Titration of Cold Antibodies

If the screening test is positive for cold auto-agglutinins, titrate as follows.

Prepare doubling dilutions of the serum in saline ranging from 1 in 1 to 1 in 512, and add 1 drop of each serum dilution into three series of (12 × 75 mm) tubes so that three replicate titrations can be made. Add 1 drop of a 2% suspension of pooled saline-washed adult group O (I) cells to the first row, 1 drop of cord-blood group O (i) cells to the second row, and 1 drop of the patient's own cells to the third row. Mix and leave for several hours at 4°C. Before reading, place pipettes and a tray of slides at 4°C. Read macroscopically at room temperature using chilled slides.

Normal Range

Using sera from normal White adults and normal adult I red cells, the cold-agglutinin titre at 4°C is 1 to 32; and with cord-blood (i) cells the titre is 0 to 8. In chronic CHAD, the end-point may not have been reached at a dilution of 1 in 512; if that is the case, further dilutions should be prepared and tested.

If a cold agglutinin is present at a raised titre, the presence of a cold alloantibody has to be excluded. In this case, the patient's own red cells will be found to react *much* less strongly than do normal adult I red cells. It should be noted that in CHAD the patient's cells commonly react less strongly than do normal adult I cells (Table 11.8).

Cold Agglutinin Titration Patterns

The presence of high-titre cold agglutinins in a patient's serum will be indicated by the screening procedure described earlier. To demonstrate that the agglutinins are autoantibodies, it is necessary to show that the patient's own cells are also agglutinated. The titre using the patient's cells is usually less (one-half or one-fourth) than that of control normal adult red cells (Table 11.8).

In CHAD, whether "idiopathic" or secondary to mycoplasma pneumonia or lymphoma, the auto-antibodies usually have anti-I specificity (Patient A.G. in Table 11.8).

In rare cases of haemolytic anaemia associated with infectious mononucleosis, an autoantibody of anti-i specificity has been demonstrated (Patient F.B. in Table 11.8), and this specificity, too, has been

Thermal Range of Donath–Landsteiner Antibody

The highest temperature at which D–L antibodies are usually adsorbed onto red cells is about 18°C. Hence little or no lysis can be expected unless the cell–serum suspension is cooled below this temperature. Chilling in crushed ice results in maximum adsorption of the antibody and leads to the binding of complement, which brings about lysis when the cell suspension is subsequently warmed at 37°C. Hence the "cold-warm" biphasic procedure necessary for lysis to be demonstrated with a typical D–L antibody.

Specificity of the Donath–Landsteiner Antibody

The D–L antibody appears to have a well-defined specificity within the GLOB blood-group system, namely, anti-P. However, in practice, almost all samples of red cells are acted upon because the cells that will not react (P^k and pp) are extremely rare.[45] Cord-blood cells are lysed to about the same extent as are adult P_1 and P_2 cells.

Treatment of Serum with 2-Mercaptoethanol or Dithiothreitol

Weak solutions of 2-mercaptoethanol (2-ME) or dithiothreitol (DTT) destroy the inter-chain sulphydryl bonds of gamma-globulins. IgM antibodies treated in this way lose their ability to agglutinate red cells while IgG antibodies do not.[9] IgA antibodies may or may not be inhibited depending upon whether or not they are made up of polymers of IgA. Since almost all autoantibodies are either IgM or IgG, treatment of serum or an eluate with 2-ME or DTT gives a reliable indication of the Ig class of autoantibody under investigation.[9,46]

Method

2-Mercaptoethanol

To 1 volume of undiluted serum add 1 volume of 0.1 mol/l 2-ME in phosphate buffer, pH 7.2 (see p. 691).

As a control, add a volume of the serum to the phosphate buffer alone. Incubate both at 37°C for 2 hours. Then titrate the treated serum and its control with the appropriate red cells.

If IgG antibody is present, the antibody titration in the control serum will be the same as that of the treated serum. However, if the antibody is IgM, the treated serum will fail to agglutinate the test cells or will agglutinate them to a much lower titre compared with the control untreated serum.

The control must remain active to show that the absence of agglutination is the result of reduction of IgM antibody and not dilution.

Dithiothreitol

0.01 mol/l DTT can be used in place of 0.1 mol/l 2-ME in the previous method.

Drug-Induced Haemolytic Anaemias of Immunological Origin

As already mentioned, acquired haemolytic anaemias may develop as the result of immunological reactions consequent on the administration of certain drugs.[6,47–49] Clinically, they often closely mimic AIHA of "idiopathic" origin, and for this reason a careful enquiry into the taking of drugs is a necessary part of the interrogation of any patient suspected of having an acquired haemolytic anaemia.

Two immunological mechanisms leading to a drug-induced haemolytic anaemia are recognized. These mechanisms can be referred to as "drug-dependent immune" and "drug-induced autoimmune." Both types of antibody may be present in some patients.[50,51] In a unifying concept, the target orientation of these antibodies covers a spectrum in which the primary immune response is initiated by an interaction between the drug or its metabolites and a component of the blood cell membrane to create a neoantigen.[52] Drug-dependent antibodies bind to both the drug and the cell membrane but not to either separately. If the drug is withdrawn, the immune reaction subsides. It has been postulated that in the case of the autoantibodies, the greater part of the neoantigen is sufficiently similar to the normal cell membrane to allow binding without the drug being present. Similar mechanisms have been described for drug-induced immune thrombocytopenia and neutropenia of immunological origin (p. 509).

In drug-dependent immune haemolytic anaemia, the drug is required in the *in vitro* system for the antibodies to be detected. The red cells become damaged by one of two mechanisms:

1. *Complement lysis.* A typical history is for haemolysis, which may be severe and intra-

vascular, to follow the readministration of a drug with which the patient has previously been treated and for the haemolysis to subside when the offending drug is withdrawn. The DAT is likely to become strongly positive during the haemolytic phase, the patient's red cells being agglutinated by anti-C′ and sometimes by anti-IgG.

Drugs that have been shown to cause haemolysis by the previously explained mechanism include quinine, quinidine and rifampicin, chlorpropamide, hydrochlorothiazide, nomifensine, phenacetin, salicylazosulphapyridine, the sodium salt of *p*-aminosalicylic acid, and stibophen. Petz and Branch listed 25 drugs reported to have brought about haemolysis by this mechanism.[48]

2. *Extravascular haemolysis.* This is brought about by IgG antibodies that usually do not activate complement, or if they do, not beyond C3. The DAT will be positive with anti-IgG and sometimes also with anti-C′.

The haemolytic anaemia associated with prolonged high-dose penicillin therapy is caused by the previously mentioned mechanism, and other penicillin derivatives, as well as cephalosporins and tetracycline, may cause haemolysis in a similar fashion. Haemolysis ceases when the offending drug has been identified and withdrawn.

Cephalosporins, in addition to causing the formation of specific antibodies, may alter the red cell surface so as to cause nonspecific adherence of complement and immunoglobulins. This may lead to a positive DAT but is seldom associated with increased haemolysis, although where it occurs it can be very severe.

Drug-Induced Autoimmune Haemolytic Anaemias

In the case of drug-induced autoimmune haemolytic anaemias, the antibody reacts with the red cell in the absence of the drug (these are sometimes referred to as "drug-independent antibodies"). The anti–red cell autoantibodies seem to be serologically identical to those of "idiopathic" warm-type AIHA. When the drug was widely used, the great majority of cases followed the use of the antihypertension drug α-methyldopa. The red cells are coated with IgG, and the serum contains autoantibodies that characteristically have Rh specificity.

Other drugs that have been reported to act in a similar fashion to α-methyldopa include L-dopa, chlordiazepoxide, mefenamic acid, flufenamic acid, and indomethicin.[2]

Typical serological features of the different types of drug-induced haemolytic anaemia of immunological origin are summarized in Table 11.9.

Detection of Antipenicillin Antibodies

The characteristic features of penicillin-induced haemolytic anaemia are as follows:

1. Haemolysis occurs only in patients receiving large doses of a penicillin for long periods (e.g., weeks).
2. The DAT is strongly positive with anti-IgG reagents.
3. The patient's serum and antibody eluted from the patient's red cells react *only* with penicillin-treated red cells—they do not react with normal untreated red cells.

Reagents

Barbitone buffer. 0.14 mol/l, pH 9.5 (see p. 690).
Penicillin solution. 0.4 g of penicillin G dissolved in 6 ml of barbitone buffer.

Penicillin-Coated Normal Red Cells

Wash group O reagent red cells three times in saline and make approximately 15% suspension in saline to which a one-tenth volume of barbitone buffer has been added. Add 2 ml of the red cell suspension to 6 ml of penicillin solution and incubate at 37°C for 1 hour. Then wash four times in saline and make 2% red cell suspensions in saline (for tube tests).

Control Normal Red Cells

Control normal red cells should be treated in exactly the same way as the penicillin-coated red cells except that the 6 ml of penicillin solution is replaced by 6 ml of barbitone buffer.

Method

Antipenicillin antibodies can be detected by the IAT in the usual way using the penicillin-coated red cells in place of normal unmodified cells. However, three extra controls are necessary.

Table 11.9 Serological features of the different types of drug-induced haemolytic anaemia of immunological origin

Mechanism	Prototype drug	DAT	IAT		
			No drug	Serum + drug	Eluate + drug
Drug Dependent Antibody:					
(a) C' activation	Quin(id)ine	C'*	Neg	C'*	Neg
(b) No C' activation	Penicillin	IgG	Neg	IgG	IgG
Autoantibody	α-Methyldopa	IgG	IgG		

*Occasionally also IgG.

1. Red cells that have not been exposed to penicillin should be added to the patient's serum.
2. Penicillin-treated red cells should be added to two normal sera known not to contain anti-penicillin antibodies (*negative controls).*
3. Penicillin-treated red cells should be added to a serum (if one is available) known to contain antipenicillin antibodies (*positive control).*

Cephalosporin can be used in a similar way to sensitize red cells. Control (2) is particularly important when drugs such as cephalosporins are used because overexposure *in vitro* to these drugs can lead to positive results with normal sera.

Note
Some drugs do not dissolve easily; incubation at 37°C, crushing tablets with a pestle and mortar, and vigorous shaking of the solution may help.

High-titre IgG antipenicillin antibodies often cause direct agglutination of penicillin-treated red cells in low dilutions of serum. The antibodies can be differentiated from IgM agglutinating antibodies by treatment with 2-ME or DTT (p. 257).

Detection of Antibodies Against Drugs Other Than Penicillin

In a patient with an immune haemolytic anaemia whose serum and red cell eluate does *not* react with normal red cells and who is receiving a drug or drugs other than penicillin or a penicillin derivative, antibodies that react with red cells only in the presence of the suspect drugs or drugs should be looked for in the following way.

The patient's serum and red cell eluates should be tested with normal and enzyme-treated group O red cells, carrying out the tests with and without the drug that the patient is receiving. The approach is essentially empirical. A saturated solution of the drug or its metabolite should be prepared in saline, and the pH should be adjusted to 6.5–7.0.

Set up 6 tubes containing the patient's serum and the drug solution in the proportions shown in Table 11.10, and add 1 drop of a 50% saline suspension of group O cells to each tube. Incubate at 37°C for 1 hour, and examine for agglutination and lysis. Wash the red cells four times in saline, and carry out an IAT using anti-IgG and anti-C' separately.

Interpretation

Tubes 1 and 2 test the patient's serum (? drug-dependent antibody) and normal red cells in the presence of the drug (Tube 1) and without the drug (Tube 2). Tubes 3 and 4 test the effect of added complement on the previous reactions. Tubes 5 and 6 without the patient's serum act as controls for tubes 3 and 4.

OXIDANT-INDUCED HAEMOLYTIC ANAEMIA

Oxidant-induced haemolytic anaemia should be suspected when the blood film of a patient exposed to an oxidant drug or chemical shows irregularly contracted cells. A Heinz-body test (see p. 315) is confirmatory. The oxidant may also cause methaemoglobinaemia or sulphaemoglobinaemia,

Table 11.10 Investigation of a suspected drug-induced immune haemolytic anaemia

	Tube no.					
	1	2	3	4	5	6
Patient's serum (drops)	10	10	5	5	0	0
Fresh normal serum (drops)	0	0	5	5	10	10
Drug solution volumes (drops)	2	0	2	0	2	0
Saline volumes (drops)	0	2	0	2	0	2
50% normal group O cells volumes (drops)	1	1	1	1	1	1

both of which can be confirmed by spectroscopy (see p. 198) or co-oximetry. The differential diagnosis of haemolysis induced by an exogenous oxidant includes other causes of haemolysis with irregularly contracted cells (e.g., Zieve's syndrome), glucose–6-phosphate dehydrogenase (G6PD) deficiency, and the presence of an unstable haemoglobin. In Zieve's syndrome (haemolysis associated with alcohol excess, fatty liver, and hyperlipidaemia), the plasma may be visibly lipaemic; if this syndrome is suspected, further investigations should include liver function test and serum lipid measurements.

MICROANGIOPATHIC AND MECHANICAL HAEMOLYTIC ANAEMIAS

Microangiopathic or mechanical haemolytic anaemia should be suspected when a blood film shows red cell fragments. Examination of the blood film is, in fact, the most important laboratory procedure in making this diagnosis. Because haemolysis is intravascular, useful confirmatory tests include serum haptoglobin estimation (see p. 191) and, when the condition is chronic, a Perls' stain of urinary sediment to detect the presence of haemosiderin (p. 195). Because a microangiopathic haemolytic anaemia is often part of a more generalized syndrome consequent on microvascular damage, other tests are also indicated in unexplained cases. They include tests of renal function, a platelet

count, and a coagulation screen including tests for D-dimer or fibrin degradation products (p. 434). Tests for verotoxin-secreting *E. coli* are indicated in cases of microangiopathic haemolytic anaemia with renal failure. If available, quantification of von Willebrand's factor-cleaving protease (ADAMTS13) is indicated in suspected thrombotic thrombocytopenic purpura.

PAROXYSMAL NOCTURNAL HAEMOGLOBINURIA

Paroxysmal nocturnal haemoglobinuria (PNH) is an acquired clonal disorder of haemopoiesis in which the patient's red cells are abnormally sensitive to lysis by normal constituents of plasma. In its classical form, it is characterized by haemoglobinuria during sleep (nocturnal haemoglobinuria), jaundice, and haemosiderinuria. Not uncommonly, however, PNH presents as an obscure anaemia without obvious evidence of intravascular haemolysis, or it develops in a patient suffering from aplastic anaemia or more rarely from myelofibrosis or chronic myeloid leukaemia.[53,54]

PNH red cells are unusually susceptible to lysis by complement.[55,56] This can be demonstrated *in vitro* by a variety of tests (e.g., the acidified-serum [Ham],[57] sucrose,[58] thrombin,[59] cold-antibody lysis,[60] inulin,[61] and cobra-venom[62] tests). In the acidified-serum, inulin, and cobra-venom tests, complement is activated via the alternative pathway, whereas in the cold-antibody test, and probably in the thrombin test, complement is activated by the classical sequence initiated through antigen–antibody interaction. In the sucrose lysis test, a low ionic strength is thought to lead to the binding of IgG molecules non-specifically to the cell membrane and to the subsequent activation of complement via the classical sequence. In addition, the alternative pathway appears to be activated.[63] In each test, PNH cells undergo lysis because of their greatly increased sensitivity to lysis by complement.

Minor degrees of lysis may be observed in the cold-antibody lysis and sucrose tests with the red cells from a variety of dyserythropoietic anaemias (e.g., aplastic anaemia, megaloblastic anaemia, and myelofibrosis).[64,65] Weak positive results in these tests thus have to be interpreted with care. PNH red cells, however, almost always undergo considerable lysis in these tests.

A characteristic feature of a positive test for PNH is that not all the patient's cells undergo lysis, even if the conditions of the test are made optimal for lysis (Fig. 11.1). This is because only a proportion of any patient's PNH red cell population is hypersensitive to lysis by complement. This population varies from patient to patient, and there is a direct relationship between the proportion of red cells that can be lysed (in any of the diagnostic tests) and the severity of *in vivo* haemolysis.

The phenomenon of some red cells being sensitive to complement lysis and some being insensitive was studied quantitatively by Rosse and Dacie, who obtained two-component complement sensitivity curves in a series of patients with PNH.[56] Later, Rosse reported that in some cases three populations of red cells could be demonstrated.[66,67]

1. Very sensitive (type III) cells, 10–15 times more sensitive than normal cells
2. Cells of medium sensitivity (type II), 3–5 times more sensitive than normal cells
3. Cells of normal sensitivity (type I)

In vivo the proportion of type III cells parallels the severity of the patient's haemolysis.

PNH is an acquired clonal disorder[68] resulting from a somatic mutation occurring in a haemopoietic stem cell. It has been demonstrated that a proportion of granulocytes, platelets, and lymphocytes are also part of the PNH clone.[69,70] The characteristic feature of cells belonging to the PNH clone is that they are deficient in several cell-membrane–bound proteins including red cell acetylcholineesterase,[71–73] neutrophil alkaline phosphatase,[74–76] CD55 (decay accelerating factor or DAF),[77–78] homologous restriction factor (HRF),[55,79] and CD59 (membrane inhibitor of reactive lysis or MIRL),[80–82] among others. CD55, CD59, and HRF all have roles in the protection of the cell against complement-mediated attack. CD59 inhibits the formation of the terminal complex of complement, and it has been established that the deficiency of CD59 is largely responsible for the complement sensitivity of PNH red cells. PNH type III red cells have a complete deficiency of CD59, whereas PNH type II red cells have only a partial deficiency, and it is this difference that accounts for

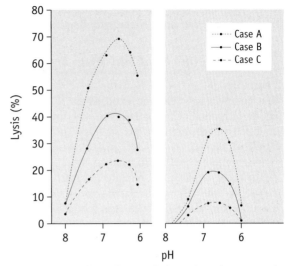

Figure 11.1   Effect of pH on lysis in vitro of paroxysmal nocturnal haemoglobinuria (PNH) red cells by human sera. The red cells of three patients of different sensitivity and two fresh normal sera, one serum being more potent than the other, were used.

their variable sensitivities to complement.[83,84] The analysis of these deficient proteins on PNH cells by flow cytometry, particularly of the red cells and neutrophils, has become a useful research and diagnostic tool but is only applicable in centres with a significant number of patients requiring investigation for PNH. By comparing the proportion of cells with deficient CD59 to the percentage lysis in the Ham test, it has been possible to assess the sensitivity of the Ham test. The standard Ham test is reasonably good at estimating the proportion of PNH red cells as long as they are PNH type III cells and comprise less than 20% of the total. In cases in which the PNH cells are type II and more than 20% are present, the standard Ham test significantly underestimates the proportion of PNH red cells. The standard Ham test can be negative when there are less than 5% PNH type III cells or less than 20% PNH type II cells. When the Ham test is supplemented with magnesium, to optimize the activation of complement, the percentage lysis gives a more accurate estimation of the proportion of PNH cells (Fig. 11.2).[85]

Certain chemicals, in particular sulphydryl compounds, can act on normal red cells *in vitro* so as to increase their complement sensitivity. In this way, PNH-like red cells can be created in the laboratory and can be used as useful reagents.

Acidified-Serum Lysis Test (Ham Test)

Principle

The patient's red cells are exposed at 37°C to the action of normal or the patient's own serum suitably acidified to the optimum pH for lysis (pH 6.5–7.0) (Table 11.11).

The patient's red cells can be obtained from defibrinated, heparinized, oxalated, citrated, or EDTA blood, and the test can be satisfactorily carried out even on cells that have been stored at 4°C for up to 2–3 weeks in ACD or Alsever's solution, if kept sterile. The patient's serum is best obtained by defibrination because in PNH if it is obtained from

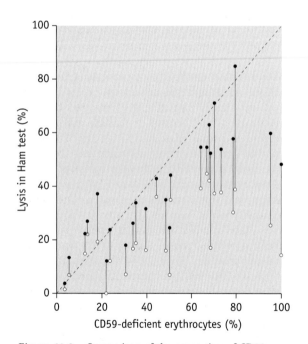

Figure 11.2 Comparison of the proportion of CD59-deficient red cells with the lysis in the Ham test. The percentage lysis in the Ham test with added magnesium (●) and without added magnesium (○) is plotted against the proportion of CD59-deficient red cells in the same samples from 25 patients with paroxysmal nocturnal haemoglobinuria (PNH). (With thanks to P. Hillmen, M. Bessler, D. Roper, and L. Luzzatto, unpublished observation.)

blood allowed to clot in the ordinary way at 37°C or at room temperature, it will almost certainly be markedly lysed. Normal serum should similarly be obtained by defibrination, although serum derived from blood allowed to clot spontaneously at room temperature or at 37°C can be used. Normal serum known to be strongly lytic to PNH red cells is to be preferred to patient's serum, the lytic potentiality of which is unknown. However, if the test is positive using normal serum, it is important, particularly if the patient appears not to be suffering from overt intravascular haemolysis, to obtain a positive result using the patient's serum to exclude hereditary erythroid multinuclearity associated with a positive acidified-serum test (HEMPAS) (see p. 264). The variability between the sera of individuals in their capacity to lyse PNH red cells is shown in Figure 11.1. The activity of a single individual's serum also varies from time to time,[86] and it is always important to include in any test, as a positive control, a sample of known PNH cells or artificially created "PNH-like" cells (see p. 266).

The sera should be used within a few hours of collection. Their lytic potency is retained for several months at −70°C, but at 4°C, and even at −20°C, this deteriorates within a few days.

Method

Deliver 0.5 ml samples of fresh normal serum, group AB or ABO compatible with the patient's blood, into 6 (3 pairs) of 75 × 12 mm tubes. Place two tubes at 56°C for 10–30 min to inactivate complement. Keep the other 2 pairs of tubes at room temperature and add to the serum in 2 of the tubes one-tenth volumes (0.05 ml) of 0.2 mol/l HCl. Add similar volumes of acid to the inactivated serum samples. Then place all the tubes in a 37°C waterbath.

While the serum samples are being dealt with, wash samples of the patient's red cells and of control normal red cells (compatible with the normal serum) twice in saline and prepare 50% suspensions in the saline. Then add one-tenth volumes of each of these cell suspensions (0.05 ml) to one of the tubes containing unacidified fresh serum, acidified fresh serum, and acidified inactivated serum, respectively. Mix the contents carefully and leave the tubes at 37°C. Centrifuge them after about 1 hour.

Add 0.05 ml of each cell suspension to 0.55 ml of water so as to prepare a standard for subsequent

Table 11.11   The acidified–serum lysis test with added magnesium

	Test (ml)		Controls (ml)			
Reagent	1	2	3	4	5	6
Fresh normal serum	0.5	0.5	0	0.5	0.5	0
Heat-inactivated normal serum	0	0	0.5	0	0	0.5
0.2 mol/l HCl	0	0.05	0.05	0	0.05	0.05
50% patient's red cells	0.05	0.05	0.05	0	0	0
50% normal red cells	0	0	0	0.05	0.05	0.05
*Magnesium chloride (250 mmol/l; 23.7 g/l)	0.01	0.01	0.01	0.01	0.01	0.01
Lysis (in a positive modified test)	Trace (2%)	+++ (30%)	–	–	–	–

*Only for modified test.

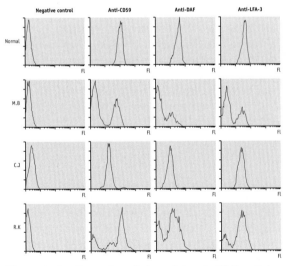

Figure 11.3   Expression of glycosylphosphatidylinositol (GPI)-linked proteins on the red cells in paroxysmal nocturnal haemoglobinuria (PNH). Flow cytometry of the erythrocytes from a normal control and three patients with PNH stained with a negative control antibody and antibodies to several GPI-linked proteins. M.B: two populations; normal and absent GPI-linked proteins. C.J: mainly reduced GPI-linked proteins, but there is also a very small normal component present. R.K: three populations; normal, reduced, and absent GPI-linked proteins. Fl: fluorescence intensity.

quantitative measurement of lysis and retain 0.5 ml of serum for use as a blank. For the measurement of lysis, deliver 0.3 ml volumes of the supernatants of the test and control series of cell–serum suspensions and of the blank serum and of the lysed cell suspension equivalent to 0% and 100% lysis, respectively, into 5 ml of 0.4 ml/l ammonia or Drabkin's reagent. Measure the lysis in a photoelectric colorimeter using a yellow–green (e.g., Ilford 625) filter or in a spectrometer at a wavelength of 540 nm.

If the test cells are from a patient with PNH, they will undergo definite, although incomplete, lysis in the acidified serum. Much less lysis, or even no lysis at all, will be visible in the unacidified serum. No lysis will be brought about by the acidified inactivated serum. The normal control sample of cells should not undergo lysis in any of the three tubes.

In PNH, 10–50% lysis is usually obtained when lysis is measured as liberated haemoglobin. Exceptionally, there may be as much as 80% lysis or as little as 5%.

The red cells of a patient who has had a transfusion will undergo less lysis than they would have before the transfusion because the normal transfused cells do not have increased sensitivity to lysis. In PNH, it is characteristic that a young cell (reticulocyte-rich) population, such as the upper red cell layer obtained by centrifugation, undergoes more lysis than the red cells derived from mixed whole blood.

Acidified-Serum Test Lysis with Additional Magnesium (Modified Ham Test)

Principle

The sensitivity of the Ham test can be improved by the addition of magnesium to the test to enhance the activation of complement.

Method

The method is identical to that for the standard Ham test (see above) with the addition of 10 μl of 250 mmol magnesium chloride (final concentration = 4 mmol) to each tube prior to the incubation (Table 11.11).

Significance of the Acidified-Serum Lysis Test

A positive acidified-serum test, carried out with proper controls, denotes the PNH abnormality, and PNH cannot be diagnosed unless the acidified-serum test is positive. The addition of magnesium chloride increases the sensitivity of the acidified-serum test.

When the acidified-serum test is positive, a direct antiglobulin test (p. 501) should also be carried out. If this is positive, it could be the result of a lytic antibody that has given a false-positive acidified-serum test. This can be confirmed by appropriate serological studies. In such complex cases flow cytometry after reaction of the red cells with anti-CD59 is recommended because it is a more definitive test for PNH (see below).

The only disorder other than PNH that may appear to give a clearcut positive test result is a rare congenital dyserythropoietic anaemia, congenital dyserythopoietic anaemia type II or HEMPAS.[87,88] In contrast to PNH, however, HEMPAS red cells undergo lysis in only a proportion (about 30%) of normal sera; moreover, they do not undergo lysis in the patient's own acidified serum and the sucrose lysis test is negative. In HEMPAS, the expression of glycosylphosphatidylinositol (GPI)-linked proteins, such as CD55 and CD59, is normal. Lysis in HEMPAS appears to be a result of the presence on the red cells of an unusual antigen, which reacts with a complement-fixing IgM antibody ("anti-HEMPAS") present in many, but not in all, normal sera.[88]

Heating at 56°C inactivates the lytic system and, if there is lysis in inactivated serum, the test cannot be considered positive. Markedly spherocytic red cells or effete normal red cells may lyse in acidified serum, probably owing to the lowered pH, and such cells may also lyse in acidified inactivated serum.

PNH red cells are not unduly sensitive to lysis by a lowered pH *per se*. The addition of the acid adjusts the pH of the serum-cell mixture to the optimum for the activity of the lytic system. As is shown in Figure 11.1, it is possible to construct pH-lysis curves, if different concentrations of acid are used. The optimum pH for lysis is between pH 6.5 and 7.0 (measurements made after the addition of the red cells to the serum).

Sucrose Lysis Test

An iso-osmotic solution of sucrose (92.4 g/l) is required.[89] This can be stored at 4°C for up to 3 weeks.

For the test, set up two tubes, one containing 0.05 ml of fresh normal group AB or ABO-compatible serum diluted in 0.85 ml of sucrose solution and the other containing 0.05 ml of serum diluted in 0.85 ml of saline. Add to each tube 0.1 ml of a 50% suspension of washed red cells. After incubation at 37°C for 30 min, centrifuge the tubes and examine for lysis. If lysis is visible in the sucrose-containing tube, measure this in a photo-electric colorimeter or a spectrometer as described earlier, using the tube containing serum diluted in saline as a blank and a tube containing 0.1 ml of the red cells suspension in 0.9 ml of 0.4 ml/l ammonia in place of the sucrose–serum mixture as a standard for 100% lysis.

Interpretation

The sucrose lysis test is based on the fact that red cells absorb complement components from serum at low ionic concentrations.[86,90] PNH cells, because of their great sensitivity, undergo lysis but normal red cells do not. The red cells from some patients with leukaemia[64] or myelofibrosis may undergo a small amount of lysis, almost always <10%; in such cases, the acidified-serum test is usually negative and PNH should not be diagnosed. In PNH, lysis usually varies from 10% to 80%, but exceptionally may be as little as 5%. Sucrose lysis and acidified-serum lysis of PNH red cells are fairly closely correlated. The sucrose lysis test is usually negative in HEMPAS.

Flow Cytometry Analysis of the GPI-Linked Proteins on Red Cells

Principle

The patient's red cells are stained with a fluorescein-labelled antibody that is specific for one of several GPI-linked proteins—for example, CD55 (decay accelerating factor), CD58 (leucocyte function antigen-3), or CD59 ("protectin")—which are deficient in PNH red cells. The stained cells are then analysed with a flow cytometer. In some laboratories where facilities are available, flow cytometry has replaced the Ham test as the primary method for the diagnosis of PNH.

The patient's red cells can be obtained in any of the anticoagulants described for the Ham test. The cells, if taken into ACD, can be stored for 2–3 weeks prior to analysis. Fluorescein-conjugated anti-CD59* gives excellent results when used for red cell analysis. It is important to use the conjugated antibody because staining with unconjugated anti-CD59 followed by a fluorescein-conjugated second layer antibody may result in artefact, probably owing to red cell agglutination. There is no suitable anti-CD55 antibody commercially available at present. Anti-CD58* gives reproducible results for red cell analysis, but the level of CD58 expression on PNH type-II cells is higher than that of many other GPI-linked proteins, and thus studying CD58 expression is useful but not ideal.[91]

Method

Chill 1×10^6 cells in 50 μl of PBS on ice with 50 μl of monoclonal antibody for 30 min. Wash twice in PBS + azide (200 mg/l), and then chill with fluorescein-labelled goat antimouse antibody on ice in the dark for 30 min. Wash twice in PBS+azide, and then fix with approximately 0.5 ml of 1% formaldehyde in Isoton II (Beckman–Coulter). Analysis is performed using a flow cytometer. A negative control antibody should always be used to assess the fluorescence of cells lacking the antigen. The cells from a normal subject should be stained as an additional control to verify that negative cells in the test sample are true PNH cells and not artefactual.

Other Immunological Techniques

The GPI-linked proteins such as CD59 can also be studied by a modification of the gel technology used for blood grouping.

Flow Cytometry Analysis of the GPI-Linked Proteins on Neutrophils

Principle

A proportion of the patient's neutrophils have been demonstrated to be part of the PNH clone in all patients with PNH. GPI-linked proteins that are suitable for analysis include CD16, CD24, CD55, CD59, and CD67.[92,93] There are available numerous fluorescein-conjugated antibodies to CD16 that are suitable for use in this analysis—for example, fluorescein-conjugated anti-Leu-11a (Beckman–Coulter) or fluorescein-conjugated anti-CD59 (Cymbus Biosciences).

Method

The patient's neutrophils are obtained by collecting blood, anticoagulating with preservative-free heparin (10 iu/ml), and obtaining a buffy coat. The formation of a buffy coat can be accelerated by adding 1 ml of 6% hetastarch in 0.9% sodium chloride (Hespan, DuPont) to 10 ml of blood. Then $1–2 \times 10^6$ cells are analysed. It is important that all the subsequent staining and washing are performed at 4°C to minimize nonspecific staining. Chill the cells in 50 μl of PBS on ice with 50 μl of monoclonal antibody (MoAb) for 30 min. Wash twice in PBS + 0.1% BSA (PBS + BSA), and then chill with fluorescein-labelled goat antimouse antibody on ice in the dark for 30 min. Wash twice in PBS + BSA, and then fix with approximately 0.5 ml of 1% formaldehyde in Isoton II (Beckman–Coulter). For conjugated antibodies, a single incubation step only is required followed by a wash and then fixing prior to analysis. Analysis is performed using a flow cytometer. Appropriate normal controls and negative controls should always be tested in parallel to the patient's samples.

A negative control antibody should always be used to assess the fluorescence of cells lacking the antigen. The cells from a normal subject should be

---

*MEM 43, Cymbus Bioscience Ltd, Southampton, UK.

*BRIC5, Bioproducts Laboratories, UK, used at 20 μg/ml.

stained as an additional control to verify that negative cells in the test sample are true PNH cells and not an artefact.

Significance of Flow Cytometric Analysis

The presence of a population of cells with a deficiency of more than one GPI-linked protein is diagnostic of PNH (Fig. 11.3). It is important to analyse more than one protein because there are extremely rare cases in which an inherited deficiency of one protein has been described (i.e., the Inab phenotype,[94-96] a deficiency of CD55 owing to a defect of the structural gene encoding this protein, and inherited deficiency of CD59[97] due to a defect in the gene encoding CD59). Analysis of the expression of CD59 on erythrocytes allows the identification of PNH type II as well as PNH type III red cells. This is important because, although patients with only PNH type II red cells do not usually suffer from significant haemolysis, they may suffer some of the complications of PNH, such as thrombosis. The analysis of neutrophils for GPI-linked proteins is more difficult than red cell analysis. It is, however, probably more sensitive because the proportion of abnormal neutrophils is usually higher than the proportion of PNH red cells because of the reduced survival of PNH red cells compared to normal cells and because of the effect of transfusions. Thus flow cytometry applied to neutrophils is a more sensitive method for the diagnosis of PNH than methods relying on the complement sensitivity of PNH red cells.

PNH-Like Red Cells

By treating normal red cells with certain chemicals, it is possible to increase their complement sensitivity so that they take on many of the characteristics of PNH cells.[98] The chemicals include sulphydryl compounds such as L-cysteine, reduced glutathione, 2-aminoethyl-*iso*-thiouronium bromide (AET), and 2-mercaptobenzoic acid.[99] AET- and 2-mercaptobenzoic acid-treated cells can be used conveniently as a positive control for *in vitro* lysis tests for PNH.[100]

Preparation of AET Cells

Prepare an 8 g/l solution of AET and adjust its pH to 8.0 with 5 mol/l NaOH. Collect normal blood into ACD and wash it ×2 in 9 g/l NaCl. Add 1 volume of the packed cells to 4 volumes of the AET solution in a 75 × 12 mm tube, which is then stoppered. Mix the contents gently and place the tube at 37°C for 10–20 min; the optimal time of incubation varies between red cell samples. Then wash the cells repeatedly with large volumes of saline until the supernatant is colourless. The red cells are now ready to use.[101]

Summary of Testing for PNH

The Ham test remains the main diagnostic test for PNH. If carried out with additional magnesium chloride and performed with the necessary controls, it is more sensitive than the unmodified test and remains specific for the diagnosis of PNH. The inclusion of a further test, such as the sucrose lysis test, is optional. The use of flow cytometry gives a better estimate of the size of the PNH clone and identifies the type of red cell abnormality. However, more experience and expensive equipment are required to perform flow cytometry reliably than is necessary to perform a Ham test. Flow cytometry is a useful diagnostic test in certain circumstances, especially when the patient is heavily transfused, and it becomes necessary to analyze neutrophils and when following a patient after bone marrow transplantation. Flow cytometry may also be useful in the follow-up of groups of patients with aplastic anaemia because clonal evolution into PNH may be detected at an earlier stage. For laboratories already using gel technology for blood grouping and antibody screening, this technique provides a simple method for screening red cells for deficiency of GPI-linked protein.

REFERENCES

1. Arndt PA, Leger RM, Garratty G 1999 Serology of antibodies to second and third generation cephalosporins associated with immune hemolytic anaemia and/or positive direct antiglobulin tests. Transfusion 39:1239–1246.
2. Dacie JV, Worlledge SM 1969 Auto-immune hemolytic anaemias. Progress in Hematology 6:82–120.
3. Dacie JV 1975 Auto-immune hemolytic anemias. Archives of Internal Medicine 135:1293–1300.

4. Dacie J 1992 The haemolytic anaemias vol 3. The auto-immune haemolytic anaemias, 3rd ed. (a) p 136, (b) p 276. Churchill Livingstone, Edinburgh.

5. Pirofsky B 1969 Autoimmunization and the autoimmune hemolytic anemias. Williams & Wilkins, Baltimore.

6. Petz LD, Garratty G 1980 Acquired immune hemolytic anemias. Churchill Livingstone, New York.

7. Sokol RJ, Hewitt S 1985 Autoimmune hemolysis: a critical review. CRC Critical Reviews in Oncology/Hematology 4:125–154.

8. Sokol RJ, Hewitt S, Booker DJ, et al 1985 Enzyme linked direct antiglobulin tests in patients with autoimmune haemolysis. Journal of Clinical Pathology 38:912–914.

9. Issitt PD 1985 Serological diagnosis and characterization of the causative autoantibodies. Methods in Hematology 12:1–45.

10. Engelfriet CP, von dem Borne AEG, Beckers D, et al 1974 Auto-immune haemolytic anaemia: serological and immunochemical characteristics of the auto-antibodies: mechanisms of cell destruction. Series Haematologica VII:328–347.

11. Worlledge SM 1978 The interpretation of a positive direct antiglobulin test (Review). British Journal of Haematology 39:157–162.

12. Sokol RJ, Hewitt S, Stamps BK 1981 Autoimmune haemolysis: An 18-year study of 865 cases referred to a regional transfusion centre. British Medical Journal 282:2023–2027.

13. Robertson VM, Dickson LG, Romond EH, et al 1987 Positive antiglobulin tests due to intravenous immunoglobulin in patients who received bone marrow transplant. Transfusion 27:28–31.

14. Ramsey G 1991 Red cell antibodies arising from solid organ transplants. Transfusion;31:76–86.

15. Petz LD 1987 Immunohematologic problems associated with bone marrow transplantation. Transfusion Medicine Reviews 1:85–100.

16. Shulman JA, Petz LD 1996 Red cell compatibility testing: clinical significance and laboratory methods. In: Petz LD, Swisher SN, Kleinman S, et al eds. Clinical practice of transfusion medicine, 3rd ed. p.199–244. New York: Churchill Livingstone.

17. Szymanski IO, Odgren PR, Fortier NL, et al 1980 Red blood cell associated IgG in normal and pathologic states. Blood 55:48–54.

18. Clark JA, Tranley PC, Wallas CH 1992 Evaluation of patients with positive direct antiglobulin tests and non-reactive eluates discovered during pretransfusion testing. Immunohaematology 8:9–12.

19. Heddle NM, Kelton JG, Turchyn KL, et al 1988 Hypergammaglobulinemia can be associated with a positive direct antiglobulin test, a nonreactive eluate, and no evidence of hemolysis. Transfusion 28:29–33.

20. Huh YO, Liu FJ, Rogge K, et al 1988 Positive direct antiglobulin test and high serum immunoglobulin G levels. American Journal of Clinical Pathology 90:197–200.

21. Vianna JL, Ordi-Ros J, Lopez-Soto A, et al 1994 Comparison of the primary and secondary antiphospholipid syndrome: A European Multicenter Study of 114 patients. American Journal of Medicine 96:1–9.

22. Win N, Islam SIAM, Peterkin MA, et al 1997 Positive direct antiglobulin test due to antiphospholipid antibodies in normal healthy blood donors. Vox Sanguinis 72:182–184.

23. Petz LD, Yam P, Wilkinson L, et al 1984 Increased IgG molecules bound to the surface of red blood cells of patients with sickle cell anemia. Blood 64:301–4.

24. Toy PT, Chin CA, Reid ME, et al 1985 Factors associated with positive direct antiglobulin tests in pretransfusion patients: a case control study. Vox Sanguinis 49:215–220.

25. Stratton F, Renton PH 1955 Effect of crystalloid solutions prepared in glass bottles on human red cells. Nature (London) 175:727.

26. Gorst DW, Rawlinson VI, Merry AH, et al 1980 Positive direct antiglobulin test in normal individuals. Vox Sanguinis 38:99–105.

27. Bareford D, Longster G, Gilks L, et al 1985 Follow-up of normal individuals with a positive antiglobulin test. Scandinavian Journal of Haematology 35:348–353.

28. Freedman J 1979 False-positive antiglobulin tests in healthy subjects. Journal of Clinical Pathology 32:1014–1018.

29. Lau P, Haesler WE, Wurzel HA 1976 Positive direct antiglobulin reaction in a patient population. American Journal of Clinical Pathology 65:368–375.

30. Sokol RJ, Booker DJ, Stamps R, et al 1997 IgA red cell autoantibodies and auto-immune hemolysis. Transfusion 37:175–181.

31. Chaplin H Jr 1973 Clinical usefulness of specific antiglobulin reagents in autoimmune hemolytic anemia. Progress in Hematology 8:25–49.

32. Worlledge SM, Blajchman MA 1972 The autoimmune haemolytic anaemias. British Journal of Haematology 23 (Suppl): 61–69.

33. Lai M, Rumi C, D'onofrio G, et al 2002 Clinically significant auto-immune hemolytic anemia with a

negative direct antiglobulin test by routine tube test and positive by column agglutination method. Immunohematology 18:112–116.

34. Sokol RJ, Hewitt S, Booker DJ, et al 1987 Small quantities of erythrocyte bound immunoglobulins and auto-immune haemolysis. Journal of Clinical Pathology 40:254–257.

35. Garratty G, Arndt PA 1999 Application of flow cytofluorometry to red blood cell immunology. Cytometry 38:259–267.

36. Owen I, Hows J 1990 Evaluation of the manual Polybrene technique in the investigation of autoimmune hemolytic anemia. Transfusion 30:814–818.

37. Lalezari P, Jiang AC 1980 The manual Polybrene test: a simple and rapid procedure for detection of red cell antibodies. Transfusion 20:206–211.

38. Branch DR, Petz LD 1999 Detecting alloantibodies in patients with autoantibodies. Transfusion 39:6–10.

39. Landsteiner K, Miller CP Jr 1925 Serological studies on the blood of primates. II. The blood groups in anthropoid apes. Journal of Experimental Medicine 42:853–862.

40. Eicher CA, Wallace ME, Frank S, et al 1978. The Lui elution: a simple method of antibody elution. Transfusion 18: 647–652.

41. Roelcke D 1989 Cold agglutination. Transfusion Medicine Review 3:140–166.

42. Wiener AS, Unger LJ, Cohen L, et al 1956 Type-specific cold auto-antibodies as a cause of acquired hemolytic anemia and hemolytic transfusion reactions: biologic test with bovine red cells. Annals of Internal Medicine 44:221–240.

43. Wolach B, Heddle N, Barr RD, et al 1981 Transient Donath-Landsteiner haemolytic anaemia. British Journal of Haematology 48:425–434.

44. Petz LD, Garratty G 2004 Acquired Immune Haemolytic Anaemias, 2nd ed. p. 224, Churchill Livingstone, New York.

45. Worlledge SM, Rousso C 1965 Studies on the serology of paroxysmal cold hemoglobinuria (PCH) with special reference to a relationship with the P blood group system. Vox Sanguinis 10:293–298.

46. Freedman J, Masters CA, Newlands M, et al 1976. Optimal conditions for the use of suphydryl compounds in dissociating red cell antibodies. Vox Sanguinis 30, 231–239.

47. Habibi B 1987 Drug-induced immune haemolytic anaemias. Baillières Clinical Immunology and Allergy 1:343–356.

48. Petz LD, Branch DR 1985 Drug-induced immune haemolytic anemias. Methods in Haematology 12:47–94.

49. Habibi B 1985 Drug induced red blood cell autoantibodies co-developed with drug specific antibodies causing haemolytic anaemias. British Journal of Haematology 61:139–143.

50. Salama A, Gottsche B, Mueller-Eckhardt C 1991 Autoantibodies and drug- or metabolite-dependent antibodies in patients with diclofenac-induced immune haemolysis. British Journal of Haematology 77:546–549.

51. Salama C, Mueller-Eckhardt C 1987 Cianidanol and its metabolites bind tightly to red cells and are responsible for the production of auto- and/or drug-dependent antibodies against these cells. British Journal of Haematology 66:263266.

52. Salama A, Mueller-Eckhardt C 1992 Immune-mediated blood dyscrasias related to drugs. Seminars in Hematology 29:54–63.

53. Dacie JV, Lewis SM 1972 Paroxysmal nocturnal haemoglobinuria: clinical manifestations, haematology and nature of the disease. Series Haematologica 5:3–23

54. Sirchia G, Lewis SM 1975 Paroxysmal nocturnal haemoglobinuria. Clinics in Haematology 4:199–229.

55. Hansch GM, Schonermark S, Roeicke D 1987 Paroxysmal nocturnal hemoglobinuria type III: lack of an erythrocyte membrane protein restricting the lysis by C5b–9. Journal of Clinical Investigation 80:7–12.

56. Rosse WF, Dacie JV 1966 Immune lysis of normal human and paroxysmal nocturnal hemoglobinuria (PNH) red blood cells. 1. The sensitivity of PNH red cells to lysis by complement and specific antibody. Journal of Clinical Investigation 45:736–748.

57. Ham TH, Dingle JH 1939 Studies on destruction of red blood cells. II. Chronic hemolytic anemia with paroxysmal nocturnal hemoglobinuria: certain immunological aspects of the hemolytic mechanism with special reference to serum complement. Journal of Clinical Investigation 18:657–672

58. Hartmann RC, Jenkins DE Jr, Arnold AB 1970 Diagnostic specificity of sucrose hemolysis test for paroxysmal nocturnal hemoglobinuria. Blood 35:462–475.

59. Crosby WH 1950 Paroxysmal nocturnal hemoglobinuria. A specific test for the disease based on the ability of thrombin to activate the hemolytic factor. Blood 5:843–846.

60. Dacie JV, Lewis SM, Tills D 1960 Comparative sensitivity of the erythrocytes in paroxysmal nocturnal haemoglobinuria to haemolysis by

acidified normal serum and by a high-titre cold antibody. British Journal of Haematology 6:362–371.

61. Brubaker LH, Schaberg DR, Jefferson DH, et al 1973 A potential rapid screening test for paroxysmal nocturnal hemoglobinuria. New England Journal of Medicine 288:1059–1060.

62. Kabakci T, Rosse WF, Logue GL 1972 The lysis of paroxysmal nocturnal haemoglobinuria red cells by serum and cobra factor. British Journal of Haematology 23:693–705.

63. Logue GL, Rossi WF, Adams JP 1973 Mechanisms of immune lysis of red blood cells in vitro. I. Paroxysmal nocturnal hemoglobinuria cells. Journal of Clinical Investigation 52:1129–1137.

64. Catovsky D, Lewis SM, Sherman D 1971 Erythrocyte sensitivity to in-vitro lysis in leukaemia. British Journal of Haematology 21:541–550.

65. Lewis SM, Dacie JV, Tills D 1961 Comparison of the sensitivity to agglutination and haemolysis by a high-titre cold antibody of the erythrocytes of normal subjects and of patients with a variety of blood diseases including paroxysmal nocturnal haemoglobinuria. British Journal of Haematology 7:64–72.

66. Rosse WF 1973 Variations in the red cells in paroxysmal nocturnal haemoglobinuria. British Journal of Haematology 24:327–342.

67. Rosse WF, Adams JP, Thorpe AM 1974 The population of cells in paroxysmal nocturnal haemoglobinuria of intermediate sensitivity to complement lysis: significance and mechanism of increased immune lysis. British Journal of Haematology 28:281–290.

68. Oni SB, Osunkoya BO, Luzzatto L 1970 Paroxysmal nocturnal hemoglobinuria: evidence for monoclonal origin of abnormal red cells. Blood 36:145–152.

69. Kinoshita T, Medof ME, Silber R, et al 1985 Distribution of decay-accelerating factor in the peripheral blood of normal individuals and patients with paroxysmal nocturnal hemoglobinuria. Journal of Experimental Medicine 162:75–92.

70. Nicholson-Weller A, Spicier DB, Austen KF 1985 Deficiency of the complement regulating protein "decay accelerating factor" on membranes of granulocytes, monocytes, and platelets in paroxysmal nocturnal hemoglobinuria. New England Journal of Medicine 312:1091–1097.

71. Auditore JV, Hartmann RC 1959 Paroxysmal nocturnal hemoglobinuria: II. Erythrocyte acetylcholinesterase defect. American Journal of Medicine 27:401–410.

72. Chow F-L, Telen MJ, Rosse WF 1985 The acetylcholinesterase defect in paroxysmal nocturnal hemoglobinuria: evidence that the enzyme is absent from the cell membrane. Blood 66:940–945.

73. De Sandre G, Ghiotto G 1960 An enzymic disorder in the erythrocytes of paroxysmal nocturnal haemoglobinuria: a deficiency in acetylcholinesterase activity. British Journal of Haematology 6:39–42.

74. Beck WS, Valentine WN 1965 Biochemical studies on leucocytes. II. Phosphatase activity in chronic lymphatic leucemia, acute leucemia and miscellaneous hematologic conditions. Journal of Laboratory and Clinical Medicine 38:245–253.

75. Hartmann RC, Auditore JV 1959 Paroxysmal nocturnal hemoglobinuria I. Clinical studies. American Journal of Medicine 27:389–400.

76. Lewis SM, Dacie JV 1965 Neutrophil (leucocyte) alkaline phosphatase in paroxysmal nocturnal haemoglobinuria. British Journal of Haematology 11:549–556.

77. Nicholson-Weller A, March JP, Rosenfield SI, et al 1983 Affected erythrocytes of patients with paroxysmal nocturnal hemoglobinuria are deficient in the complement regulatory protein, decay accelerating factor. Proceedings of the National Academy of Sciences of the U.S.A. 80:5066–5070.

78. Pangburn MK, Schreiber RD, Müller-Eberhard HF 1983 Deficiency of an erythrocyte membrane protein with complement regulatory activity in paroxysmal nocturnal hemoglobinuria. Proceedings of the National Academy of Sciences U.S.A. 80:5430–5434.

79. Zalman LS, Wood LM, Frank MM, et al 1987 Deficiency of the homologous restriction factor in paroxysmal nocturnal hemoglobinuria. Journal of Experimental Medicine 165:572–577.

80. Davies A, Simmons DL, Hale G, et al 1989 CD59 and LY-6-like protein expressed in human lymphoid cells, regulates the action of the complement membrane attack complex on homologous cells. Journal of Experimental Medicine 170:637–654.

81. Holguin MH, Wilcox LA, Bernshaw NJ, et al 1989 Relationship between the membrane inhibitor of reactive lysis and the erythrocyte phenotypes of paroxysmal nocturnal hemoglobinuria. Journal of Clinical Investigation 84:1387–1394.

82. Holguin MH, Fredrick NJ, Bernshaw LA, et al 1989 Isolation and characterization of a

membrane protein from normal human erythrocytes that inhibits reactive lysis of the erythrocytes of paroxysmal nocturnal hemoglobinuria. Journal of Clinical Investigation 84:7–17.

83. Rosse WF, Hoffman S, Campbell M, et al 1991 The erythrocytes in paroxysmal nocturnal haemoglobinuria of intermediate sensitivity to complement lysis. British Journal of Haematology 79:99–107.

84. Shichishima T, Terasawa T, Hashimoto C, et al. 1991 Heterogenous expression of decay accelerating factor and CD59/membrane attack complex inhibition factor on paroxysmal nocturnal haemoglobinuria (PNH) erythrocytes. British Journal of Haematology 78:545–550.

85. May JE, Rosse WF, Frank MM 1973 Paroxysmal nocturnal hemoglobinuria: alternative-complement-pathway-mediated lysis induced by magnesium. New England Journal of Medicine 289:705–709.

86. Packman CH, Rosenfeld SI, Jenkins DE Jr, et al 1979 Complement lysis of human erythrocytes. Differing susceptibility of two types of paroxysmal nocturnal hemoglobinuria cells to C5b-9. Journal of Clinical Investigation 64:428–433.

87. Crookston JH, Crookston MC, Burnie KL, et al 1969 Hereditary erythroblastic multinuclearity associated with a positive acidified-serum test: a type of congenital dyserythropoietic anaemia. British Journal of Haematology 17:11–26.

88. Verwilghen RL, Lewis SM, Dacie JV 1973 HEMPAS: congenital dyserythropoietic anaemia (type II). Quarterly Journal of Medicine 42:257–278.

89. Hartmann RC, Jenkins DE Jr 1966 The "sugar water" test for paroxysmal nocturnal hemoglobinuria. New England Journal of Medicine 275:155–157.

90. Mollison PL, Polley MJ 1964 Uptake of γ-globulin and complement by red cells exposed to serum at low ionic strength. Nature (London) 203:535.

91. Hillmen P, Hows JM, Luzzatto L 1992 Two distinct patterns of glycosylphosphatidylinositol (GPI) linked protein deficiency in the red cells of patients with paroxysmal nocturnal haemoglobinuria. British Journal of Haematology 80:399–405.

92. Plesner T, Hansen NE, Carlsen K 1990 Estimation of PI-bound proteins on blood cells from PNH patients by quantitative flow cytometry. British Journal of Haematology 75:585–590.

93. van der Schoot CE, Huizinga TWJ, van't Veer-Korthof ET, et al 1990 Deficiency of glycosyl-phosphatidylinositol-linked membrane glycoproteins of leukocytes in paroxysmal nocturnal hemoglobinuria, description of a new diagnostic cytofluorometric assay. Blood 76:1853–1859.

94. Merry AH, Rawlinson VI, Uchikawa M, et al 1989 Studies on the sensitivity to complement-mediated lysis of erythrocytes (Inab phenotype) with a deficiency of DAF (decay accelerating factor). British Journal of Haematology 73:248–253.

95. Merry AH, Rawlinson VI, Uchikawa M, et al 1989 Lack of abnormal sensitivity to complement-mediated lysis in erythrocytes deficient only in decay accelerating factor. Biochemical Society Transactions 17:514.

96. Telen MJ, Green AM 1989 The Inab phenotype: characterization of the membrane protein and complement regulatory defect. Blood 74:437–441.

97. Yamashina M, Ueda E, Kinoshita T, et al 1990 Inherited complete deficiency of 20-kilodalton homologous restriction factor (CD59) as a cause of paroxysmal nocturnal hemoglobinuria. New England Journal of Medicine 323:1184–1189.

98. Sirchia G, Ferrone S 1972 The laboratory substitutes of the red cell of paroxysmal nocturnal haemoglobinuria (PNH): PNH-like red cells. Series Haematologica 5:137–175.

99. Francis DA 1983 Production of PNH-like red cells using 2-mercaptobenzoic acid. Medical Laboratory Sciences 40:33–38.

100. Sirchia G, Marubini E, Mercuriali F, et al 1973 Study of two in vitro diagnostic tests for paroxysmal nocturnal haemoglobinuria. British Journal of Haematology 24:751–759.

101. Sirchia G, Ferrone S, Mercuriali F 1965 The action of two sulfhydryl compounds on normal human red cells. Relationship to red cells of paroxysmal nocturnal hemoglobinuria. Blood 25:502–510.

12 Investigation of abnormal haemoglobins and thalassaemia

Barbara Wild and Barbara J. Bain

THE HAEMOGLOBIN MOLECULE

Human haemoglobin is formed from two pairs of globin chains each with a haem group attached. Seven different globin chains are synthesized in normal subjects; four are transient embryonic haemoglobins referred to as Hb Gower 1, Hb Gower 2, Hb Portland 1, and Hb Portland 2. Hb F is the predominant haemoglobin of fetal life and comprises the major proportion of haemoglobin found at birth. Hb A is the major haemoglobin found in adults and children. Hb A_2 and Hb F are found in small quantities in adult life (approximately 2–3.3% and 0.2–1.0%, respectively). The adult proportions of Hbs A, A_2, and F are usually attained by 6–12 months of age.

The individual chains synthesised in postnatal life are designated α, β, γ, and δ. Hb A has two α chains and two β chains ($α_2 β_2$); Hb F has two α chains and two γ chains ($α_2 γ_2$), and Hb A_2 has two α chains and two δ chains ($α_2 δ_2$). The α chain is thus common to all three types of haemoglobin molecules.

α Chain synthesis is directed by two α genes, α 1 and α 2, on chromosome 16, and β and δ chain synthesis by single β and δ genes on chromosome 11. γ Chain synthesis is directed by two genes, $^Gγ$ and $^Aγ$, also on chromosome 11. The globin genes are shown diagrammatically in Figure 12.1.

The four chains are associated in the form of a tetramer: the $α_1 β_1$ (and equivalent $α_2 β_2$) contact is the strongest and involves many amino acids with many interlocking side chains; the $α_1 β_2$ (and equivalent $α_2 β_1$) contact is less extensive, and the contacts between similar chains are relatively weak. The binding of a haem group into the haem pocket in each chain is vital for the oxygen-carrying capacity of the molecule and stabilises the whole molecule. If the haem attachment is weakened, the globin chains dissociate into dimers and monomers.

There are many naturally occurring, genetically determined variants of human haemoglobin (more than 750)[1] and although many are harmless, some have serious clinical effects. Collectively, the clinical syndromes resulting from disorders of haemoglobin synthesis are referred to as "haemoglobinopathies." They can be grouped into three main categories:

1. Those owing to structural variants of haemoglobin, such as Hb S.
2. Those owing to failure to synthesise one or more of the globin chains of haemoglobin at a normal rate, as in the thalassaemias.
3. Those owing to failure to complete the normal neonatal switch from fetal haemoglobin (Hb F) to adult haemoglobin (Hb A). These comprise a group of disorders referred to as hereditary persistence of fetal haemoglobin (HPFH).

An individual can also have a combination of more than one of these abnormalities.

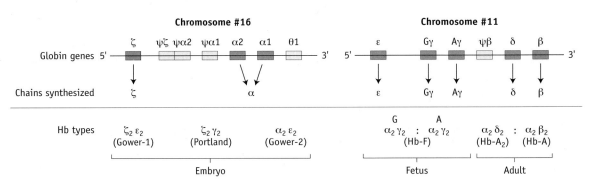

Figure 12.1 Location of the α-globin gene cluster on chromosome 16 and that of the β-globin gene cluster on chromosome 11. The black boxes represent functional genes. The α and γ globin genes are duplicated; the two α globin genes have the same product, whereas the products of the two g globin genes are slightly different ($^G γ = γ$ 136Gly; $^A γ = γ$ 136Ala).

STRUCTURAL VARIANTS OF HAEMOGLOBIN

Alterations in the structure of haemoglobin are usually brought about by point mutations affecting one or, in some cases, two or more bases, coding for amino acids of the globin chains. An example of such a point mutation is Hb S caused by the substitution of valine for glutamic acid in position 6 of the β-globin chain ($\beta6^{Glu \rightarrow Val}$). Less commonly, structural change is caused by shortening or lengthening of the globin chain. For example, five amino acids are deleted in the β chain of Hb Gun Hill, whereas in Hb Constant Spring 31 amino acids are added to the α chain. Mutations associated with a frame shift can also lead to synthesis of a structurally abnormal haemoglobin, which may be either shorter or longer than normal. There may also be combinations of segments of β and γ or δ chains resulting in hybrid haemoglobins; the β and δ combinations are known as the Lepore and anti-Lepore haemoglobins, respectively.

Many variant haemoglobins are haematologically and clinically silent because the underlying mutation causes no alteration in the function, solubility, or stability of the haemoglobin molecule. Many of these variants are separated using electrophoresis or chromatography, but some are not and remain undetected. Some structural variants are associated with severe clinical phenotypes in the homozygous or even heterozygous state; these mutations affect the physical or chemical properties of the haemoglobin molecule, resulting in changes in haemoglobin solubility, stability, or oxygen-binding properties. Some of these variants separate on electrophoresis or chromatography, whereas others do not. It is fortunate that the common haemoglobin variants that have clinical or genetic significance (e.g., Hbs S, C, D^{Punjab}, E, and O^{Arab}) are readily detectable by electrophoretic and chromatographic techniques.

Haemoglobins with Reduced Solubility

Hb S

By far the most common haemoglobin variant in this group is sickle haemoglobin or Hb S. As a result of the replacement of glutamic acid by valine in position 6 of the β chain, Hb S has poor solubility in the deoxygenated state and can polymerize with-in the red cells. The red cell shows a characteristic shape change because of polymer formation and becomes distorted and rigid, the so-called sickle cell (p. 102, Fig. 5.72). In addition, intracellular polymers lead to red cell membrane changes, generation of oxidant substances, and abnormal adherence of red cells to vascular endothelium.

Clinical syndromes associated with common structural variants and those owing to their interaction with β thalassaemia are shown in Table 12.1.

Sickle Cell Disease

Sickle cell disease[2] (also called disorder) is a collective name for a group of conditions causing clinical symptoms that are characterized by the formation of sickle red cells. It is common in people originating from Africa, but it is also found in considerable numbers of people of Indian, Arabic, and Greek descent.

The homozygous state or sickle cell anaemia (β genotype SS) causes moderate to severe haemolytic anaemia. The main clinical disability arises from repeated episodes of vascular occlusion by sickled red cells resulting in acute crises and eventually in end-organ damage. The clinical severity of sickle cell anaemia is extremely variable. This is partly due to the effects of inherited modifying factors, such as interaction with β thalassaemia or increased synthesis of Hb F, and partly to socioeconomic conditions and other factors that influence general health.[2]

Sickle cell trait (β genotype AS), the heterozygous state, is very common, affecting millions of people worldwide. There are no associated haematological abnormalities. *In vivo* sickling occurs only at very high altitudes and at low oxygen pressures. Spontaneous haematuria, owing to sickling in the renal papillae, is found in about 1% of people with sickle cell trait.

Other Forms of Sickle Cell Disease

Sickle cell/Hb C disease is a compound heterozygous state for Hbs S and C. The abbreviation "SC disease" is ambiguous and should be avoided; however, the term Hb SC disease is acceptable. This compound heterozygous state usually results in a milder form of sickle cell disease.

Table 12.1 Clinical Syndromes Encountered with β^S and β^C Variants

Hb	Genotype	Name	Clinical Problems
S	β^A/β^S	Sickle cell trait	None
	β^S/β^S	Sickle cell anaemia	Severe haemolytic anaemia, vaso-occlusive episodes
C	β^A/β^C	C trait	None
	β^C/β^C	C disease	Occasional mild anaemia, increased incidence of gallstones
D^{Punjab}	β^A/β^D	D trait	None
	β^D/β^D	D disease	Occasional mild anaemia
O^{Arab}	$\beta^A/\beta^{O\ Arab}$	O trait	None
	$\beta^{O\ Arab}/\beta^{O\ Arab}$	O disease	Haemolytic anaemia
Interactions	β^S/β^C	SC disease	Mild anaemia, vaso-occlusive problems
	$\beta^S/\beta^{D\ Punjab}$	SD disease	As for sickle cell anaemia
	$\beta^S/\beta^{O\ Arab}$	SO disease	As for sickle cell anaemia
	β^{Othal}/β^S	Sickle-β^0 thal	As for sickle cell anaemia
	β^{+thal}/β^S	Sickle-β^+ thal	Mild sickle cell disease
	β^{thal}/β^C	C/β thal	Mild haemolytic anaemia
	β^{thal}/β^D	D/β thal	Mild haemolytic anaemia
	$\beta^{thal}/\beta^{O\ Arab}$	O/β thal	Thalassaemia intermedia

Sickle β/thalassaemia arises as a result of inheritance of one Hb S and one β thalassaemia gene. Africans and Afro-Caribbeans with this condition are often heterozygous for a mild β^+ thalassaemia allele resulting in the production of about 20% of Hb A. This gives rise to a mild sickling disorder. Inheritance of Hb S and β^0 thalassaemia trait is associated with severe sickle cell disease. Interaction of Hb S with haemoglobin D^{Punjab} (Hb $D^{Los\ Angeles}$) or with Hb O^{Arab} gives rise to severe sickle cell disease.[2]

Hb C

Hb C is the second most common structural haemoglobin variant in people of African descent. The substitution of glutamic acid in position 6 of the β chain by lysine results in a haemoglobin molecule with a highly positive charge, decreased solubility, and tendency to crystallise. However, Hb C does not give a positive sickle solubility test. Heterozygotes are asymptomatic, but target cells and irregularly contracted cells may be present in blood films. Homozygotes may have mild anaemia with numerous target cells and irregularly contracted cells (p. 90 Fig. 5.32). Interaction with β^0 and β^+ thalassaemia trait results in mild or moderate haemolytic anaemia.

Other Sickling Haemoglobins

In addition to Hb S, there are nine haemoglobins (Hb $S^{Antilles}$, Hb $C^{Ziquinchor}$, Hb C^{Harlem}, Hb $S^{Providence}$, Hb S^{Oman}, Hb S^{Travis}, Hb $S^{South\ End}$, Hb $S^{Jamaica\ Plain}$, Hb $S^{Cameroon}$) that have both the β6 glutamic acid to valine mutation and an additional single point mutation in the β globin chain. These haemoglobins also have a positive solubility test because they have a reduced solubility but generally exhibit different electrophoretic and chromatographic properties from Hb S. They have clinical significance similar, but not necessarily identical, to Hb S: for example, Hb $S^{Antilles}$ is associated with an even greater propensity to sickling than Hb S.

Unstable Haemoglobins

Amino-acid substitutions close to the haem group, or at the points of contact between globin chains, can affect protein stability and result in intracellular precipitation of globin chains. The precipitated globin chains attach to the red cell membrane giving rise to Heinz bodies, and the associated clinical syndromes were originally called the *congenital Heinz body haemolytic anaemias*. Changes in membrane properties may lead to haemolysis, often aggravated by oxidant drugs. There is considerable heterogeneity in the haematological and clinical effects of unstable haemoglobins. Many are almost silent and are detected only by specific tests, whereas others are severe, causing haemolytic anaemia in the heterozygous state. Hb Köln is the most common variant in this rare group of disorders.[3,4]

Haemoglobins with Altered Oxygen Affinity

Haemoglobin variants with altered oxygen affinity are a rare group of variants that result in increased or reduced oxygen affinity.[5] Mutations that *increase* oxygen affinity are generally associated with benign lifelong erythrocytosis. This may be confused with polycythaemia vera and may be inappropriately treated with cytotoxic drugs or P^{32}.

Haemoglobin variants with *decreased* oxygen affinity are, with the exception of Hb S, even less common and are usually associated with mild anaemia and cyanosis. However, owing to the reduced oxygen affinity, these patients are not functionally anaemic despite the reduced Hb. The low steady-state haemoglobin concentration in Hb S homozygotes is, at least in part, a result of its reduced affinity.

Measurement of oxygen dissociation is described on page 233.

Hb M

The Hb M group is another rare group of variants.[6] Such haemoglobins have a propensity to form methaemoglobin, generated by the oxidation of ferrous iron in haem to ferric iron, which is incapable of binding oxygen. Despite marked cyanosis, there are few clinical problems. Most are associated with substitutions that disrupt the normal six-ligand state of haem iron.

Methaemoglobinaemia is also found in congenital NADH methaemoglobin reductase deficiency, as well as after exposure to oxidant drugs and chemicals (nitrates, nitrites, quinones, chlorates, phenacetin, dapsone, and many others).

THALASSAEMIA SYNDROMES

The thalassaemia syndromes[7] are a heterogeneous group of inherited conditions characterised by defects in the synthesis of one or more of the globin chains that form the haemoglobin tetramer. The clinical syndromes associated with thalassaemia arise from the combined consequences of inadequate haemoglobin production and of unbalanced accumulation of one type of globin chain. The former causes anaemia with hypochromia and microcytosis; the latter leads to ineffective erythropoiesis and haemolysis. Clinical manifestations range from completely asymptomatic microcytosis to profound anaemia that is incompatible with life and can cause death in *utero* (Table 12.2). This clinical heterogeneity arises as a result of the variable severity of the primary genetic defect in haemoglobin synthesis and the coinheritance of modulating factors, such as the capacity to synthesize increased amounts of Hb F.

Thalassaemias are generally inherited as alleles of one or more of the globin genes located on either chromosome 11 (for β, γ, and δ chains) or on chromosome 16 (for α chains). They are encountered in every population in the world but are most common in the Mediterranean littoral and near equatorial regions of Africa and Asia. Gene frequencies for the α and β thalassaemias on a global basis range from 1% to more than 80% in areas where malaria is endemic.[8]

β Thalassaemia Syndromes

Many different mutations cause β thalassaemia and related disorders.[9] These mutations can affect every step in the pathway of globin gene expression: transcription, processing of the messenger ribonucleic acid (mRNA) precursor, translation of mature mRNA, and preservation of post-translational integrity of the β chain. More than 200 mutations have been described.[10] Most types of β thalassaemia are the result of point mutations affecting the globin gene, but some large deletions are also known. Certain mutations are particularly common in some communities. This helps to simplify prenatal diagnosis, which is carried out by detection or exclusion of a particular mutation in fetal DNA.

The effect of different mutations varies greatly. At one end of the spectrum are a group of rare mutations, mainly involving exon 3 of the β globin gene, which are so severe that they can produce the clinical syndrome of thalassaemia intermedia in the

Table 12.2   Clinical syndromes of thalassaemia

Clinically asymptomatic

Silent carriers

α thalassaemia trait (some cases)

Rare forms of β thalassaemia trait

Thalassaemia Minor (low MCH and MCV, with or without mild anaemia)

α^+ thalassaemia trait (some cases)

α^0 thalassaemia trait

α^+/α^+ homozygotes

β^0 thalassaemia trait

β^+ thalassaemia trait

β thalassaemia trait

Some cases of Hb E/β thalassaemia

Thalassaemia intermedia (transfusion independent)

Some β^+/β^+ thalassaemia homozygotes

Interaction of β^0/β^0, β^0/β^+ or β^+/β^+ with α thalassaemia

Interaction of β^0/β or β^+/β with triple α

Hb H disease

α^0/Hb Constant Spring thalassaemia

$\beta^0/\delta\beta$ or $\beta^+/\delta\beta$ thalassaemia compound heterozygotes

δβ/δβ thalassaemia

Some cases of Hb E/β thalassaemia and Hb Lepore/β thalassaemia

Rare cases of heterozygotes for β thalassaemia mutation, particularly involving exon 3 ("dominant β thalassaemia")

Thalassaemia major (transfusion dependent)

β^0/β^0 thalassaemia

β^+/β^+ thalassaemia

β^0/β^+ thalassaemia

Some cases of β^0/Hb Lepore and β^+/Hb Lepore thalassaemia

Some cases of β^0/Hb E and β^+/Hb E thalassaemia

MCH, mean cell haemoglobin; MCV, mean cell volume.

heterozygous state. At the other end are mild alleles that produce thalassaemia intermedia in the homozygous or compound heterozygous state, and some that are so mild that they are completely haematologically silent, with normal mean cell volume (MCV) and Hb A_2 in the heterozygous state. In between are the great majority of β^+ and β^0 alleles, which cause β thalassaemia major in the homozygous or compound heterozygous state and in the heterozygous state give rise to a mild anaemia

(or Hb at the low end of the normal range), with microcytic, hypochromic indices and raised Hb A_2.[11]

β Thalassaemia major is a severe, transfusion-dependent, inherited anaemia. There is a profound defect of β chain production. Excess α chains accumulate and precipitate in the red cell precursors in the bone marrow resulting in ineffective erythropoiesis. The few cells that leave the marrow are laden with precipitated α chains and are rapidly removed by the reticuloendothelial system. The constant erythropoietic drive causes massive expansion of bone marrow and extramedullary erythropoiesis. If untreated, 80% of children with β thalassaemia die within the first 5 years.

Heterozygotes for β thalassaemia alleles usually have either a normal haemoglobin with microcytosis or a mild microcytic hypochromic anaemia; Hb A_2 is elevated and Hb F is sometimes also elevated. Laboratory features of various β thalassaemia syndromes are shown in Table 12.3.

α Thalassaemia Syndromes[12]

There are four syndromes of α thalassaemia: α^+ thalassaemia trait, where one of the two globin genes on a single chromosome fails to function; α^0 thalassaemia trait, where two genes on a single chromosome fail to function; Hb H disease, with three genes affected; and Hb Bart's hydrops fetalis, where all four are defective. These syndromes are usually a result of deletions of one or more genes, although approximately 20% of the mutations described are nondeletional. α^+Thalassaemia is particularly common in Africa, and α^0 thalassaemia is common in Southeast Asia. The laboratory features are shown in Table 12.3.

Hb Bart's hydrops fetalis occurs mainly in people from Southeast Asia but is also occasionally observed in people from Greece, Turkey, and Cyprus. An affected fetus will be stillborn or will die shortly after birth. Severe anaemia and oedema are the hallmarks of this condition. Women carrying a hydropic fetus have a high incidence of complications of pregnancy. Prenatal diagnosis should be offered for women at risk of having a fetus with Hb Bart's hydrops fetalis.

Hb H disease gives rise to haemolytic anaemia; patients rarely require transfusion or splenectomy.

α^0 *Thalassaemia trait* is characterized by micro-

Table 12.3   Laboratory findings in thalassaemia

Phenotype	Genotype	Usual MCV	Usual MCH	Hb A_2	Hb H inclusions
α Thalassaemia					
α thalassaemia trait	-α/αα (α$^+$/α)	N	N	N or ↓	-
α thalassaemia trait	-α/-α or −−/αα	N or↓	N or↓	N or ↓	+
Hb H Disease					
Mild	−−/-α (α^0/α+)	↓	↓	N or ↓	+++
Severe	−−/α^{T}α (α^0/α^T)	↓	↓	N or ↓	+++
Hb Bart's hydrops fetalis	−−/−− (α^0/α^0)	↓	↓	-	-
(α Thalassaemia major)					
β Thalassaemia					
β thalassaemia trait	β^0/β or β$^+$/β	↓	↓	↑	-
δβ thalassaemia trait	δβ^0/β	↓	↓	N or ↓	-
β thalassaemia trait with normal Hb A_2	β$^+$/β	↓	↓	N	-
Hb Lepore trait	Hb Lepore/β	↓	↓	N or ↓	-
β thalassaemia intermedia	Heterogeneous	↓	↓	↑, N or ↓	-
β thalassaemia major	β^0/β^0, β^0/β$^+$, β$^+$/β$^+$	↓	↓	↑, N or ↓	

MCV, mean cell volume; MCH, mean cell haemoglobin; N, normal.

cytic, hypochromic indices. The haemoglobin level may be normal or slightly reduced. α$^+$ Thalassaemia trait can be completely silent, or there may be borderline microcytosis with a slightly reduced or normal mean cell haemoglobin concentration (MCHC). Haematologically, homozygosity for α$^+$ thalassaemia trait resembles heterozygosity for α^0 thalassaemia trait, but the genetic implications are very different. Both α$^+$ thalassaemia trait and α^0 thalassaemia trait are more difficult to diagnose than β thalassaemia trait because there is no characteristic elevation in Hb A_2, and Hb H bodies are frequently not demonstrated. Definitive diagnosis of the α thalassaemia trait is more reliably made with the use of DNA techniques or globin chain biosynthesis studies.

Thalassaemic Structural Variants

These are abnormal haemoglobins characterized by both a biosynthetic defect and an abnormal structure, such as the Lepore haemoglobins (Table 12.4).

Increased Hb F in Adult Life

Haemoglobin production in man is characterized by two major switches in the haemoglobin composition of the red cells. During the first 3 months of gesta-tion, human red cells contain embryonic haemo-globins (see p. 273), whereas during the last 6 months of gestation, red cells contain predominantly fetal haemoglobin. The major transition from fetal to adult haemoglobin synthesis occurs in the perinatal period, and by the end of the first year of life red cells have a haemoglobin composition that usually remains constant throughout adult life. The major haemoglobin is then Hb A, but there are small amounts of Hb A_2 and Hb F. Only 0.2–1.0% of total haemoglobin in human red cells is Hb F, and it is restricted to a few cells called "F" cells. Both the number of F cells and the amount of Hb F per cell can be increased in various conditions, particularly if there is rapid bone marrow regeneration.[13]

The general organization of human globin gene clusters is shown in Figure 12.1. The products of two γ genes differ in only one amino acid: ^{G}γ has glycine in position 136, whereas ^{A}γ has alanine. In fetal red cells, the ratio of ^{G}γ to ^{A}γ is approximately 3:1; in adult red cells, it is approximately 2:3.

In recent years there has been much interest in the attempts to manipulate the fetal switch pharma-cologically. If it were possible to reactivate Hb F synthesis reliably beyond the perinatal period, both β thalassaemia major and sickle cell disease would be ameliorated.

Table 12.4 Thalassaemic structural variants*

Haemoglobin	Structure	When heterozygous	When homozygous	In combination with other haemoglobinopathies[17,18]
Lepore	Combination of δ and β chains owing to unequal crossover	Microcytosis, mild anaemia	Thalassaemia major or intermedia	With β thalassaemia gives thalassaemia major or intermedia
E[†]	$\beta^{26Glu \rightarrow Lys}$ resulting in abnormal messenger RNA	Microcytosis, mild anaemia	Microcytosis, mild anaemia	With β thalassaemia gives thalassaemia major or intermedia
Constant Spring	Elongated α chain owing to incorporation of 31 extra amino acids	Microcytosis, mild anaemia	Microcytosis, mild anaemia	With α^0 gives Hb H disease

*Many other thalassaemic structural variants have been described but are much rarer than the three shown in this table.
[†]13–30% frequency in Cambodia, Thailand, Vietnam, and some parts of China.

Inherited Abnormalities That Increase Hb F Concentration

More than 50 mutations that increase Hb F synthesis have been described.[13,14] They result in one of two phenotypes, HPFH or δβ thalassaemia; differentiation between these two types is not always simple but has clinical relevance. In general, HPFH has a higher percentage of Hb F and much more balanced chain synthesis. The most common, the African type of HPFH, is associated with a high concentration of Hb F (15–45%), pancellular distribution of Hb F on Kleihauer staining, and normal red cell indices. Mutations causing increased synthesis of Hb F are mostly deletions, but some nondeletion mutations have also been described. In contrast, subjects with δβ thalassaemia have lower levels of Hb F accompanied by microcytic, hypochromic indices. The major clinical significance of these abnormalities is their interaction with β thalassaemia and Hb S. Compound heterozygotes for either of these conditions and HPFH have much milder clinical syndromes than the homozygotes for haemoglobin S or β thalassaemia. Compound heterozygotes for either of these conditions and δβ thalassaemia have a condition much closer in severity to the homozygous states.

Increased Hb F is also found in many other haematological conditions, including congenital red cell aplasia and congenital aplastic anaemia (Blackfan-Diamond and Fanconi's anaemia, respectively), in juvenile chronic myelomonocytic leukaemia (previously designated juvenile chronic myeloid leukaemia), and in some myelodysplastic syndromes. A small but significant increase in Hb F may occur in the presence of erythropoietic stress (haemolysis, bleeding, recovery from acute bone marrow failure) and in pregnancy.

INVESTIGATION OF PATIENTS WITH A SUSPECTED HAEMOGLOBINOPATHY

Investigation of a person at risk of a haemoglobinopathy encompasses the confirmation or exclusion of the presence of a structural variant, thalassaemia trait, or both. If a structural haemoglobin variant is present, it is necessary to ascertain the clinical significance of the particular variant so that the patient is appropriately managed. If it is confirmed that thalassaemia trait is present, it is not usually necessary to determine the precise mutation present because the clinical significance is usually negligible. The exception to this is an antenatal patient whose partner has also been found to have thalassaemia trait. If prenatal diagnosis is being considered, it may be necessary to undertake mutation analysis to predict fetal risk accurately and to facilitate prenatal diagnosis (see p. 317).

Because the inheritance of a haemoglobinopathy *per se* has genetic implications, it is important that genetic counselling is available for these patients.

In the majority of patients, the presence of a haemoglobinopathy can be diagnosed with sufficient accuracy for clinical purposes from knowledge of the patient's ethnic origin and clinical history (including family history) and the results of physical examination combined with relatively simple haematological tests. Initial investigations should include determination of haemoglobin concentration and red cell indices. A detailed examination of a well-stained blood film should be carried out. In some instances, a reticulocyte count and a search for red cell inclusions give valuable information. Assessment of iron status by estimation of serum iron and total iron-binding capacity and/or serum ferritin is sometimes necessary to exclude iron deficiency. Other important basic tests are haemoglobin electrophoresis or chromatography, a sickle solubility test, and measurement of Hb A_2 and Hb F percentage. In cases of common haemoglobin variants and classical β thalassaemia trait, accurate data from these tests will facilitate a reliable diagnosis without the need for more sophisticated investigations. However, definitive diagnosis of some thalassaemia syndromes can only be obtained using DNA technology (see p. 309 and p. 557). Similarly, in particular situations, haemoglobin variants will require unequivocal identification by the use of DNA technology or protein analysis by mass spectrometry.[15] Individuals or families who require such investigation must be carefully selected on the basis of family history and on the results of the basic investigations described later in this chapter. Large-scale screening programmes are increasingly being undertaken in some countries where individual case histories and the results of other laboratory tests are not usually available. The problems of such programmes are discussed on page 296.

The majority of errors occurring in the detection and identification of a haemoglobinopathy are the result of either failure to obtain correct laboratory data or failure to interpret data correctly. In this chapter, a sequence of investigations is proposed based on procedures that should be available in the laboratory of any major hospital. Automated high-performance liquid chromatography (HPLC) is increasingly replacing haemoglobin electrophoresis as the initial investigative procedure in laboratories analysing large numbers of samples. Isoelectric focusing (IEF) is, in general, used only to a limited extent, mainly for neonatal screening or in specialist laboratories, and it is only briefly described here.

Laboratory investigation of a suspected haemoglobinopathy should follow a defined protocol, which should be devised to suit individual local requirements. The data obtained from the clinical findings, blood picture, and electrophoresis or HPLC will usually indicate in which direction to proceed. The investigation for a structural variant is described in the first section, and that for a suspected thalassaemia syndrome is described in the second section of this chapter. Screening tests for thalassaemia trait and haemoglobin E trait that may be especially applicable in under-resourced areas are described in Chapter 27.

LABORATORY DETECTION OF HAEMOGLOBIN VARIANTS

A proposed scheme of investigation is shown in Figure 12.2, and a list of procedures follows:[15,16]

1. Blood count and film examination (p. 280)
2. Collection of blood and preparation of haemolysates (p. 281)
3. Cellulose acetate electrophoresis, Tris buffer, pH 8.5 (p. 282)
4. Citrate agar or acid agarose gel electrophoresis, pH 6.0 (p. 284)
5. Automated HPLC (pp. 284–285)
6. IEF (p. 285)
7. Globin chain electrophoresis, pH 8.0 and 6.3 (pp. 288–290)
8. Tests for Hb S (p. 292)
9. Detection of unstable haemoglobins (p. 294)
10. Detection of Hb Ms (p. 295)
11. Detection of altered affinity haemoglobins (p. 295)
12. Differentiation of common structural variants (p. 296)

13. Neonatal screening (p. 293)
14. Tests, such as zinc protoporphyrin estimation, to exclude iron deficiency as a cause of microcytosis (see Chapter 7)
15. Molecular techniques (see Chapter 21)
16. Procedures for use in under-resourced laboratories (see Chapter 27)

Blood Count and Film

The blood count, including Hb and red cell indices, provides valuable information useful in the diagnosis of both α and β thalassaemia interactions with structural variants (see Chapter 3). A film examination may reveal characteristic red cell changes such as target cells in Hb C trait, sickle cells in sickle cell disease, and irregularly contracted cells in the presence of an unstable haemoglobin (see Chapter 5).

Discriminant functions using various formulae have been proposed as a basis for further testing for thalassaemia,[17,18] but we do not advise their use. Although such functions and formulae do indicate whether thalassaemia or iron deficiency is more likely, they may lead to individuals who have both iron deficiency *and* thalassaemia trait not being tested promptly. Generally this is not a problem, and indeed it may be preferable to keep the patient under observation until iron deficiency has been treated and then to reassess the likelihood of thalassaemia trait. However, many of the patients who require testing for thalassaemia are women who are already pregnant. In such patients the likely delay in testing is unacceptable. Moreover, these formulae do not appear to have been validated for use during pregnancy. For these reasons, we advise that whenever genetic counselling might be required,

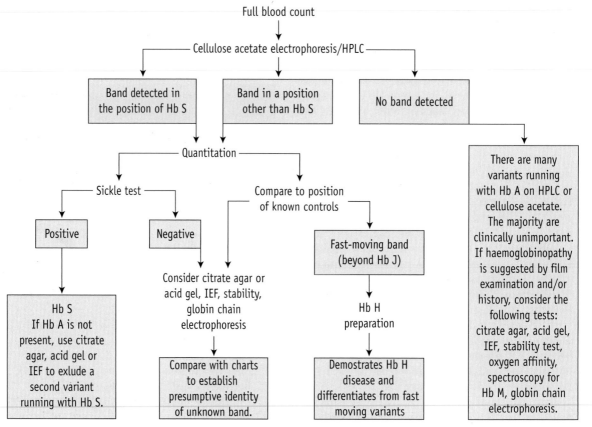

Figure 12.2   Suggested scheme of investigation for structural variants.

testing for β thalassaemia trait should be carried out in all individuals with an MCH of less than 27 pg, and screening for α thalassaemia trait should be carried out in those individuals with an MCH of less than 25 pg who belong to an ethnic group in which α^0 thalassaemia is prevalent.[11]

Collection of Blood and Preparation of Haemolysates

EDTA is the most convenient anticoagulant because it is used for the initial full blood count and film (see Chapter 1), although samples taken into any anticoagulant are satisfactory. Cells freed from clotted blood can also be used.

Preparation of Haemolysate for Qualitative Haemoglobin Electrophoresis

See individual methods.

Preparation of Haemolysate for the Quantification of Haemoglobins and Stability Tests

Preparation of haemolysate for the quantification of haemoglobins and stability tests can be used for qualitative electrophoresis and is necessary for quantitation of Hb A_2 and F or variant haemoglobins by elution. It is also essential for reliable stability tests and globin electrophoresis.

Lyse 2 volumes of washed packed cells in 1 volume of distilled water, and then add 1 volume of carbon tetrachloride (CCl_4). Alternatively, lyse by freezing and thawing, then add 2 volumes of CCl_4. Shake the tubes vigorously for approximately 1 min, then centrifuge at 1200 g (3000 rev/min) for 30 min at 4°C. Transfer the supernatant to a clean sample container and adjust the Hb to 100 ± 10 g/l with water. If an unstable Hb is suspected, organic solvents should be avoided.

Note: Whole blood samples are best stored as washed, packed cells frozen as droplets in liquid nitrogen and subsequently stored at –20°C, –70°C, or over liquid nitrogen. Alternatively, haemolysates may also be frozen at –20°C, –70°C, or over liquid nitrogen.

Control Samples

Interpretation of migration patterns of test samples is undertaken by comparison to migration and sepa-
ration of known abnormal haemoglobins used as control materials. Ideally, a mixture of Hbs A, F, S, and C should be included on each electrophoretic separation. This material can be prepared as follows:

1. The control can be made from either the combination of a sickle cell trait sample (Hb A + Hb S) combined with a Hb C trait sample (Hb A + Hb C) and normal cord blood (Hb F + Hb A) or the combination of normal cord blood with a sample from a person with Hb SC disease (Hb S + Hb C).
2. Prepare lysates by the method given for a purified haemolysate.
3. Mix equal volumes of the lysates together, and add a few drops of 0.3 mol/l KCN (20 g/l).
4. Analyze samples by electrophoresis to assess quality.
5. Aliquot and store frozen.

Note: Repeated freezing and thawing should be avoided.

Lyophilised controls are stable for considerably longer than liquid and can be purchased from commercial sources.

Quality Assurance

Because the haemoglobinopathies are inherited conditions, some of which carry considerable clinical and genetic implications, precise documentation and record keeping are of paramount importance.[19] The use of cumulative records when reviewing a patient's data is very useful because it of itself constitutes an aspect of quality assurance. In some situations, repeat sampling, family studies, or both may be required to elucidate the nature of the abnormality in an individual.

In-house standard operating procedures should be followed carefully, particularly in this field of haematology, where a small difference in technique can make a significant difference in the results obtained and can lead to misdiagnosis. Many of the techniques described have attention drawn to specific technical details that are important for ensuring valid results.[23]

It is necessary to use reference standards and control materials in each of the analyses undertaken and in some cases to use duplicate analysis to demonstrate precision. There are international standards for HbF and HbA$_2$ (see p. 694), whereas in some countries national reference preparations are also available from national standards institutions. These are extremely valuable because the target values have been established by collaborative studies. Control materials can be prepared in-house or obtained commercially. Samples stored as whole blood at 4°C can be used reliably for several weeks. All laboratories should confirm the normal range for their particular methods, and the normal range obtained should not differ significantly from published data.

All laboratories undertaking haemoglobin analysis should participate in an appropriate proficiency testing programme (p. 663). In the United Kingdom, the National External Quality Assessment Scheme (NEQAS) provides samples for sickle solubility tests; for detection and quantitation of variant haemoglobins; and for quantitation of Hbs A$_2$, F, and S.

National and international guidelines have been published for all aspects of the investigations given here.[11,20-25]

Cellulose Acetate Electrophoresis at Alkaline pH

Haemoglobin electrophoresis at pH 8.4–8.6 using cellulose acetate membrane is simple, reliable, and rapid. It is satisfactory for the detection of most common clinically important haemoglobin variants.[22,24,25]

Principle

At alkaline pH, haemoglobin is a negatively charged protein and when subjected to electrophoresis will migrate toward the anode (+). Structural variants that have a change in the charge on the surface of the molecule at alkaline pH will separate from Hb A. Haemoglobin variants that have an amino acid substitution that is internally sited may not separate, and those that have an amino acid substitution that has no effect on overall charge will not separate by electrophoresis.

Equipment

Electrophoresis tank and power pack. Any horizontal electrophoresis tank that will allow a bridge gap of 7 cm. A direct current power supply capable of delivering 350 V at 50 mA is suitable for both cellulose acetate and citrate agar electrophoresis.

Wicks of filter or chromatography paper.
Blotting paper.
Applicators. These are available from most manufacturers of electrophoresis equipment, but fine microcapillaries are also satisfactory.
Cellulose acetate membranes. Plastic-backed membranes (7.6 × 6.0 cm) are recommended for ease of use and storage.
Staining equipment.

Reagents

Electrophoresis buffer. Tris/EDTA/borate (TEB) pH 8.5. Tris-(hydroxymethyl)aminomethane (Tris), 10.2 g, EDTA (disodium salt), 0.6 g, boric acid, 3.2 g, water to 1 litre. The buffer should be stored at 4°C and can be used up to 10 times without deterioration.
Wetting agent. For example, Zip-prep solution (Helena Laboratories): 1 drop of Zip-prep in 100 ml water.
Fixative/stain solution. Ponceau S, 5 g, trichloroacetic acid, 7.5 g, water to 1 litre.
Destaining solution. 3% (v/v) acetic acid, 30 ml, water to 1 litre.
Haemolyzing reagent. 0.5% (v/v) Triton X-100 in 100 mg/l potassium cyanide.

Method

1. Centrifuge samples at 1200 g for 5 min. Dilute 20 μl of the packed red cells with 150 μl of the haemolyzing reagent. Mix gently and leave for at least 5 min. If purified haemolysates are used, dilute 40 μl of 10 g/dl haemolysate with 150 μl of lysing reagent.

2. *With the power supply disconnected,* prepare the electrophoresis tank by placing equal amounts of TEB buffer in each of the outer buffer compartments. Wet two chamber wicks in the buffer, and place one along each divider/bridge support ensuring that they make good contact with the buffer.

3. Soak the cellulose acetate by lowering it slowly into a reservoir of buffer. Leave the cellulose acetate to soak for at least 5 min before use.

4. Fill the sample well plate with 5 μl of each diluted sample or control and cover with a 50-mm coverslip or a "short" glass slide to prevent evaporation. Load a second sample well plate with Zip-prep solution.

5. Clean the applicator tips immediately prior to

use by loading with Zip-prep solution and then applying them to a blotter.

6. Remove the cellulose acetate strip from the buffer and blot twice between two layers of clean blotting paper. Do not allow the cellulose acetate to dry.

7. Load the applicator by depressing the tips into the sample wells twice, and apply this first loading onto some clean blotting paper. Reload the applicator and apply the samples to the cellulose acetate.

8. Place the cellulose acetate plates across the bridges, with the plastic side uppermost. Place two glass slides across the strip to maintain good contact. Electrophorese at 350 V for 25 min.

9. After 25 min electrophoresis, immediately transfer the cellulose acetate to Ponceau S and fix and stain for 5 min.

10. Remove excess stain by washing for 5 min in the first acetic acid reservoir and for 10 min in each of the remaining two. Blot once, using clean blotting paper, and leave to dry.

11. Label the membranes and store in a protective plastic envelope.

Interpretation and Comments

Figure 12.3 shows the relative electrophoretic mobilities of some common haemoglobin variants at pH 8.5 on cellulose acetate. Satisfactory separation of Hbs C, S, F, A, and J is obtained (Fig. 12.4). In general Hbs S, D, and G migrate closely together as do Hbs C, E, and O^{Arab}. Differentiation between these haemoglobins can be obtained by using acid agarose gels, citrate agar electrophoresis, HPLC, or IEF. However, there are slight differences in mobility between Hbs S, Lepore, and D^{Punjab} and also between Hbs C and E; optimization of the technique will facilitate detection of the difference. Generally, the Lepore Hbs and Hb D^{Punjab} migrate slightly anodal to Hb S (i.e., they are slightly faster than S); Hb C migrates slightly cathodal to Hb E (i.e., it is slightly slower than E).

All samples showing a single band in either the S or C position should be analysed further using acid agarose or citrate agar gel electrophoresis, HPLC, or IEF to exclude the possibility of a compound heterozygote such as SD, SG, CE, or CO)^{Arab}.

The quality of separation resulting from this procedure is affected primarily by both the amount of haemoglobin applied and the positioning of the origin. Also, delays between application of the sample and commencement of the electrophoresis, delay in staining after electrophoresis, or inadequate blotting of the acetate prior to application will cause poor results. This technique is sensitive enough to separate Hb F from Hb A and to detect Hb A$_2$ variants.

If an abnormal haemoglobin is present, the detection of a Hb A$_2$ variant band in conjunction with the abnormal fraction is evidence that the variant is an α chain variant. Globin electrophoresis at both acid and alkaline pH is also useful in elucidating which globin chain is affected. However, with the more ready availability of HPLC, it is less often needed.

When an abnormal haemoglobin is found, it may be of diagnostic importance to measure the percentage of the variant; this can be done by the electrophoresis with elution procedure for Hb A$_2$ estimation given on page 300. Quantitation of Hb S is often clinically useful, both in patients with sickle

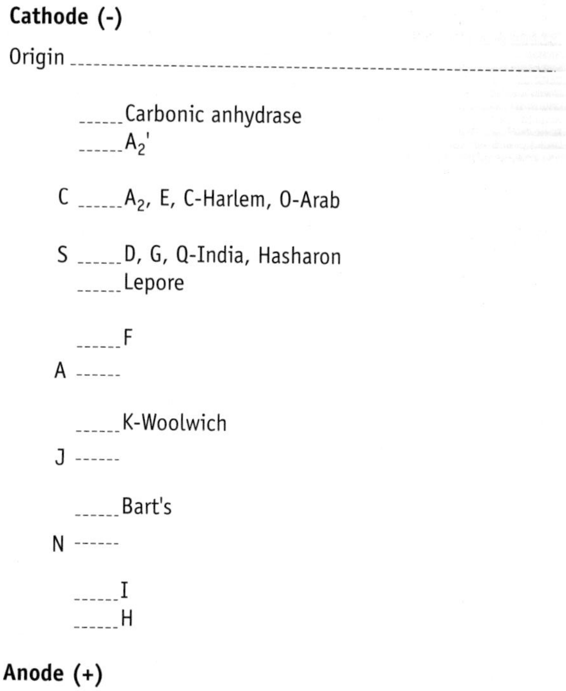

Cathode (-)

Origin --

      ------Carbonic anhydrase
      ------A$_2$'

C ------A$_2$, E, C-Harlem, O-Arab

S ------D, G, Q-India, Hasharon
      ------Lepore

      ------F

A ------

      ------K-Woolwich

J ------

      ------Bart's

N ------

      ------I
      ------H

Anode (+)

Figure 12.3   Schematic representation of relative mobilities of some abnormal haemoglobins. Cellulose acetate pH 8.5.

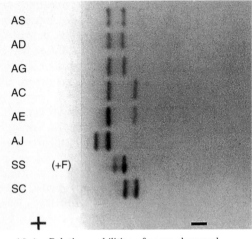

AS

AD

AG

AC

AE

AJ

SS   (+F)

SC

+   **−**

Figure 12.4   Relative mobilities of some abnormal haemoglobins. Cellulose acetate pH 8.5.

cell disease who are being treated by transfusion and for the diagnosis of conditions in which Hb S is coinherited with α and β thalassaemia, as outlined in Table 12.5. Quantitation of Hb S can be done with HPLC, electrophoresis with elution or by microcolumn chromatography.

Citrate Agar Electrophoresis at pH 6.0

Equipment[26,27]

Electrophoresis tank and power pack. Any horizontal electrophoresis tank that will allow a bridge gap of 7 cm. A direct current power supply capable of delivering 350 V at 50 mA is suitable for both cellulose acetate and citrate agar electrophoresis.

Cooling bars (Helena Laboratories).

Perspex trays, 80 × 100 × 2 mm.

Wicks of sponge, filter paper, or chromatography paper.

Applicators. These are available from most manufacturers of electrophoresis equipment, but fine microcapillaries are also satisfactory.

Reagents

Difco Bacto-agar.

Lysing reagent. 0.5% (v/v) Triton X-100 in 100 mg/l potassium cyanide.

Buffer

Stock buffer. Trisodium citrate dihydrate, 73.5 g; 0.5 mol/l citric acid, 34.0 ml; water to 1 litre.

Working buffer. Dilute stock buffer 1 in 5 with water. Prepare on day of use.

5 g/dl potassium cyanide. Potassium cyanide, 0.5 g, distilled water to 100 ml.

Dianisidine stain. 3% Hydrogen peroxide (10 vol), 1.0 ml; 1% sodium nitroprusside (nitroferricyanide), 1.0 ml; 3% acetic acid, 10.0 ml; 0.2% o-dianisidine in methanol, 5.0 ml. Prepare mixture just before use.

Wetting agent. For example, Zip-prep solution (Helena Laboratories); 1 drop in 100 ml water.

3% Acetic acid. 120 ml glacial acetic acid made up to 4 litres with water.

Gel-Bond or similar support.

Method

1. Centrifuge sample (1200 g for 5 min). Dilute 20 μl of packed red cells with 300 μl of haemolysing reagent. Mix gently and leave for at least 5 min. For cord-blood samples, dilute 20 μl of packed red cells with 150 μl of the lysing reagent. For purified haemolysates, dilute 20 μl of 10 g/dl haemolysate with 150 μl of lysing reagent.

2. *With the power supply disconnected,* place equal volumes working buffer in each of the outer buffer compartments. Wet two sponge wicks in the buffer and place one in each compartment against the divider. Place two frozen cooling sticks in each central chamber. If cooling bars or ice packs are not available, run the electrophoresis at 4°C.

3. Add 0.5 g agar to 50 ml working buffer. Heat to approximately 95°C, stirring gently until the agar has dissolved. Allow to cool to 60°C; add 0.5 ml of 5 g/dl potassium cyanide. Pipette approximately 10 ml into each of 4 Perspex trays (80 × 100 × 2 mm) and allow to stand for about 15 min at room temperature until set. These gels may be kept for 1 week at 4°C in a sealed plastic bag. Allow gels to come to room temperature before use.

4. Fill the sample well plate with 5 μl of each sample and cover with a 6 cm coverslip or glass slide. Load a second sample well plate with Zip-prep solution. Clean the applicator tips by loading with Zip-prep solution and then applying them

Table 12.5   Results of laboratory investigations in interactions of Hb S and α or β thalassaemia in adults

	MCV	% S	% A	% A$_2$	% F
AS	N	35–38	62–65	<3.5	<1
SS	N	88–93	0	<3.5	5–10
S/β^0 thalassaemia	L	88–93	0	>3.5	5–10
S/β$^+$ thalassaemia	L	50–93	3–30	>3.5	1–10
S/HPFH	N	65–80	0	<3.5	20–35
AS/α$^+$ thalassaemia	N/L	28–35	62–70	<3.5	<1
AS/α^0 thalassaemia	L	20–30	68–78	<3.5	<1
SS/α thalassaemia	N/L	88–93	0	<3.5	1–10

MCV, mean cell volume; N, normal; L, low; HPFH, hereditary persistence of fetal haemoglobin.

to blotting paper. Load the applicator, and apply this first loading onto some clean blotting paper. Reload the applicator and apply the samples to the agar gel.

5. Place gel plate in an inverted position in the electrophoresis tank so that the gel is in contact with sponge wicks, and run at a constant voltage of 50 V for 60 min.

6. After 60 min, disconnect from power supply, remove gel, and apply the stain solution by layering onto the agar using a Pasteur pipette. Allow to stain for 10 min at room temperature.

7. Wash in three changes of 3% acetic acid, float gels onto the hydrophilic side of a piece of Gel Bond, and leave to dry. These mounted gels may then be kept indefinitely.

Interpretation and Comments

Figure 12.5 shows the relative electrophoretic mobilities of some common haemoglobin variants at pH 6.0 on citrate agar.

Agarose Gel Electrophoresis

Agarose gels are commercially available as substitutes for both alkaline and acid separation systems. They are simple to use and particularly useful in laboratories that process small numbers of samples.

Reagents and Method

The manufacturer's method should be followed.

Interpretation

With acid agarose systems, the principle of the test is the same as that of citrate agar electrophoresis at the same pH, but it should be noted that there are significant differences in mobility of some variant haemoglobins. With alkaline systems, in general the same separation patterns are obtained, but where individual application notes are available these should be used for reference. Because not all kits provide these, laboratories may need to build up their own data on known variants.

Automated High-Performance Liquid Chromatography

Automated cation-exchange HPLC[28] is being used increasingly as the initial diagnostic method in haemoglobinopathy laboratories with a high workload.[29] Both capital and consumable costs are higher than with haemoglobin electrophoresis, but labour costs are less; overall costs may be similar.[30] In comparison with haemoglobin electrophoresis, HPLC has four advantages:

1. The analysers are automated and thus utilise less staff time and permit processing of large batches.

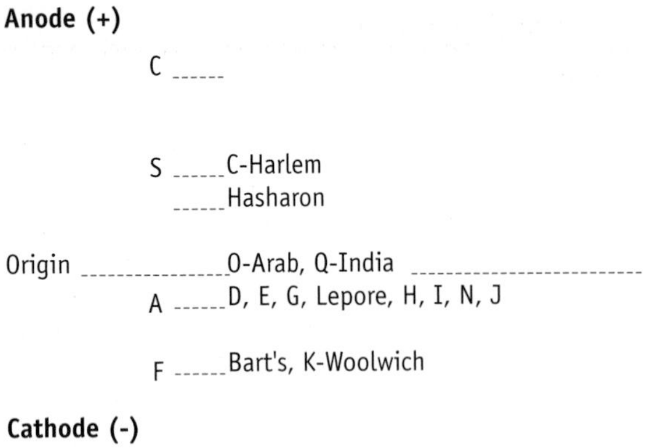

Anode (+)

C ------

S ------C-Harlem
------Hasharon

Origin --------------O-Arab, Q-India --------------------------
A ------D, E, G, Lepore, H, I, N, J

F ------Bart's, K-Woolwich

Cathode (-)

Figure 12.5   Schematic representation of relative mobilities of some abnormal haemoglobins. Citrate agar pH 6.0.

2. Very small samples (5 μl) are sufficient for analysis; this is especially useful in paediatric work.
3. Quantification of normal and variant haemoglobins is available on every sample.
4. A provisional identification of a larger proportion of variant haemoglobins can be made.

Principle

HPLC depends on the interchange of charged groups on the ion exchange material with charged groups on the haemoglobin molecule. A typical column packing is 5 μm spherical silica gel. The surface of the support is modified by carboxyl groups to have a weakly cationic charge, which allows the separation of haemoglobin molecules with different charges by ion exchange. When a haemolysate containing a mixture of haemoglobins is adsorbed onto the resin, the rate of elution of different haemoglobins is determined by the pH and ionic strength of any buffer applied to the column. With automated systems now in use, elution of the charged molecules is achieved by a continually changing salt gradient; fractions are detected as they pass through an ultraviolet/visible light detector and are recorded on an integrating computer system. Analysis of the area under these absorption peaks gives the percentage of the fraction detected. The time of elution (retention time) of any normal or variant haemoglobin present is compared with that of known haemoglobins, providing quantification of both normal haemoglobins (A, F, and A_2) and many variants.

Figure 12.6 shows a schematic representation of an HPLC system, and Figure 12.7 shows a chromatogram of a mixture of different haemoglobins. Systems are available from various manufacturers.

Method

The manufacturer's procedure should be followed. To prolong the life of the column it is important to follow the manufacturer's instructions with regard to the concentration of haemoglobin in the sample to be injected.

Interpretation and Comments

Results are accurate and reproducible, but as with every method of haemoglobin analysis, controls should be run with every batch. If the system is being used for the detection of haemoglobin variants, elution times can be compared with those of known controls; actual times, however, are affected by the batch of buffer and column, the age of the column, and the laboratory temperature. A better comparison can be obtained using the relative elution time, which is calculated by dividing the elution time of the variant with that of the main Hb A fraction. It should be noted that Hb A is separated into its component fractions of A_0 and A_1, and the A_1 fraction frequently subdivides into several peaks. Skill is required in interpretation of the results because various normal and abnormal haemoglobins may have the same retention time and a glycosylated variant haemoglobin will have a different retention time from the nonglycosylated form. HPLC usually separates Hbs A, A_2, F, S, C, D^{Punjab}, and $G^{Philadelphia}$ from each other.[29,31] However, both Hb E and Hb Lepore co-elute with haemoglobin A_2 (as other haemoglobins co-elute with A, S, and F). The retention time of glycosylated and other derivatives of Hb S can be the same as those of Hb A_0 and A_2. For example, derivatives of haemoglobin S co-elute with haemoglobin A_2, so that percentages of A_2 by this method are inaccurate and therefore do not have the same significance as percentage of haemoglobin A_2 measured by alternative methods.[32] For these reasons, and because there are more than 750 variants identified, HPLC can never definitively identify any haemoglobin. It is important to analyse variants found using second-line techniques, such as a sickle solubility test, alkaline and acid electrophoresis, or iso-electric focusing.

HPLC is also applicable for the quantification of Hb A_{1c} for the monitoring of diabetes mellitus; to make optimal use of staff and equipment, this procedure is sometimes carried out in haematology laboratories. In fact, an increased glycosylated fraction is not infrequently noted when HPLC is performed for investigation of a suspected haemoglobinopathy.[33] Unless the patient is already known to suffer from diabetes mellitus, this abnormality should be drawn to the attention of clinical staff.

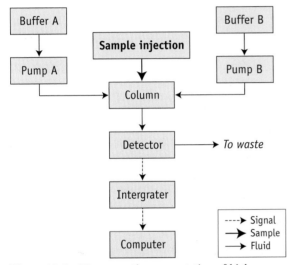

Figure 12.6 Diagrammatic representation of high-performance liquid chromatography (HPLC) showing the flow of sample and buffers.

Isoelectric Focusing

Principle
IEF utilizes a matrix containing carrier ampholytes of low molecular weight and varying isoelectric points (pI). These molecules migrate to their respective pIs when a current is applied, resulting in a pH gradient being formed; for haemoglobin analysis, a pH gradient of 6–8 is usually used. Haemoglobin molecules migrate through the gel until they reach the point at which their individual pIs equal the corresponding pH on the gel. At this point, the charge on the haemoglobin is neutral, and migration ceases. The pH gradient counteracts diffusion, and the haemoglobin variant forms a discrete narrow band.[34,35]

Method
Pre-prepared plates of either polyacrylamide or agarose gel can be obtained from various manufacturers. For the exact method, the manufacturer's instructions should be followed.

Interpretation and Comments
IEF is satisfactory for analysis of haemolysates, whole blood samples, or dried blood spots. The use of dried blood spots is suitable for samples that have to be transported long distances and where only a few drops of blood can be obtained. Whereas IEF has the advantage that it separates more variants than cellulose acetate, it also has the disadvantage that it separates haemoglobin into its post-translational derivatives. For instance, Hb F separates into F_1 (acetylated F) and F_{II}; Hb A can produce five

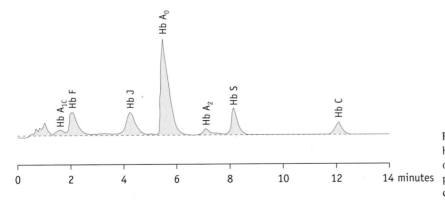

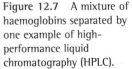

Figure 12.7 A mixture of haemoglobins separated by one example of high-performance liquid chromatography (HPLC).

bands—A_0, A_1, A(αmet), A(βmet), and A($\alpha\beta$met)— and similarly for other haemoglobins. This makes interpretation more difficult. Identification of variants is still only provisional using IEF, and second-line methods should be used for further analysis.

Figure 12.8 shows the relative isoelectric points of some common haemoglobin variants, and Figure 12.9 shows the separation obtained.

Globin Chain Electrophoresis

Principle

Electrophoresis of globin chains[36,37] is used to establish which chain is affected (i.e., α or β or γ). This information is useful in further predicting the nature of the variant and possible interactions.

Alkaline Globin Chain Electrophoresis, pH 8.0

Reagents

Add 2 ml concentrated hydrochloric acid to 98 ml of acid acetone that has been cooled to –20°C. The reagent should be prepared just before use.

Buffer

Stock buffer. Diethyl barbituric acid, 36.8 g, 1 mol/l sodium hydroxide solution, 120 ml. Dissolve the diethyl barbituric acid in 1500 ml of boiling distilled water. Allow to cool to room temperature and adjust pH to 8.0 with 1 mol/l NaOH. Make up to a final volume of 2 litres. Store at room temperature.

Working buffer. Stock buffer, 600 ml, urea, 360 g, DL-dithiothreitol (DTT), 60 mg. Prepare on day of use.

Stain solvent. Glacial acetic acid, 400 ml, methanol, 1800 ml, distilled water, 1800 ml.

Amido black stain. Stain solvent, 1 litre, amido black (Naphthol black), 0.4 g.

Diethyl ether.

Equipment

Electrophoresis tank and power pack. Any horizontal electrophoresis tank that will allow a bridge gap of 7 cm. A direct current power supply capable of delivering 350 V at 50 mA is suitable for both cellulose acetate and citrate agar electrophoresis.

Wicks of filter or chromatography paper.

Blotting paper.

Applicators. These are available from most manufacturers of electrophoresis equipment, but fine microcapillaries are also satisfactory.

Cellulose acetate membranes. Plastic backed membranes (7.6 × 6.0 cm) are recommended for ease of use and storage.

Staining equipment.

Glass centrifuge tubes.

Method

1. With a whole blood sample, wash the cells twice in 9 g/l NaCl and lyse by adding an equal volume of water to the washed, packed cells. Purified haemolysates are also suitable.
2. Add 20 ml of the haemolysate to 10 ml of cold acid acetone in a glass centrifuge tube, dispersing the haemoglobin rapidly by flushing with the pipette.
3. Centrifuge at 700 g for 10 min in a refrigerated centrifuge.
4. With a Venturi pump, remove all but a small amount of the supernatant acid acetone. Avoid contamination of the pipette by the globin pellet. Resuspend the globin pellet by means of a vortex mixer.
5. Add 10 ml of cold acetone forcefully to thoroughly disperse the globin.
6. Centrifuge at 700 g for 5 min in a refrigerated centrifuge.
7. Repeat steps 4 to 6.
8. Remove the acetone and resuspend the globin. Add 10 ml of diethyl ether and agitate forcefully to disperse the globin.
9. Centrifuge at 700 g for 5 min in a refrigerated centrifuge.
10. Dry the globin to a cream-coloured pellet by sucking air over the globin with a Pasteur pipette attached to a Venturi pump. The globin can be stored at –20°C until tested. Dissolve each of the globin pellets in 200 ml of working buffer before use.
11. *With the power supply disconnected,* prepare the electrophoresis tank by placing 100 ml of working buffer in each of the outer buffer compartments. Soak two paper wicks and place one along each of the dividers.
12. Carefully lower cellulose acetate plate(s) into a reservoir of working buffer. Allow to soak for at least 1 hour before use.

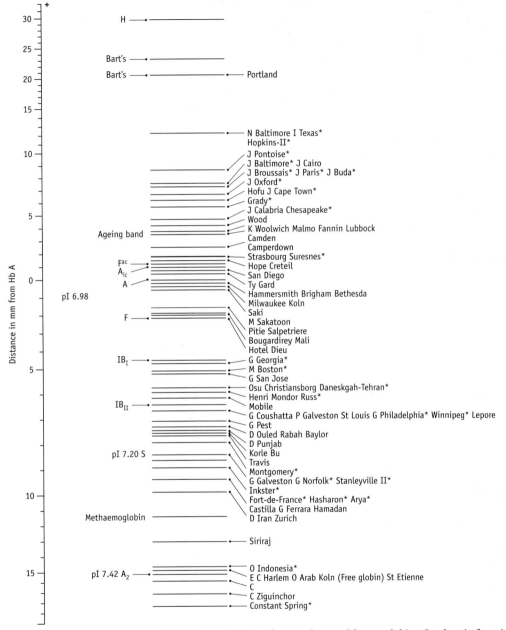

Figure 12.8   Schematic representation of relative mobilities of some abnormal haemoglobins. Isoelectric focusing. Note the presence of two bands for haemoglobin Bart's. The scale in mm is not linear. *Indicates α chain mutations. (Reproduced with permission from Basset et al.[33])

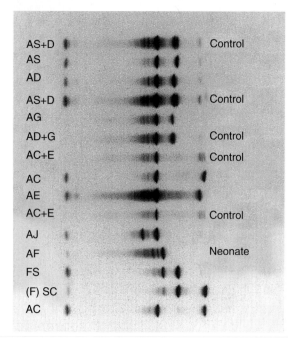

AS+D — Control
AS
AD
AS+D — Control
AG
AD+G — Control
AC+E — Control
AC
AE
AC+E — Control
AJ
AF — Neonate
FS
(F) SC
AC

Figure 12.9 Relative mobilities of some abnormal haemoglobins. Isoelectric focusing. The controls are mixtures of various haemoglobins.

13. Place 5 μl of the patient and control globin samples in a sample well plate.
14. Remove the cellulose acetate from the working buffer and blot between two layers of clean blotting paper until nearly dry.
15. Load the sample applicator and apply onto clean blotting paper; reload and apply onto the cellulose acetate in the central position.
16. Place the cellulose acetate plate in the electrophoresis tank with two microscope slides across each plate to maintain contact with the wicks.
17. Electrophorese at 200 V for 1 hour.
18. On completion of the electrophoresis, place the plate into the amido black stain solution and leave to fix and stain for 10 min.
19. Destain the plates in stain solvent, leaving for 5–10 min in each reservoir until the background is clear.
20. Remove the plates from the solvent and allow to dry between two clean sheets of blotting paper.

Interpretation and Comments

Normal α chains migrate toward the cathode, and normal β chains migrate toward the anode. The relative migration of globins from the test samples are compared to both the known controls and the mobilities of the test samples on cellulose acetate electrophoresis. The relative mobilities of some abnormal α and β chains are shown in Figure 12.10.

Acid Globin Chain Electrophoresis, pH 6.3

Reagents

Lysing solution. 40% w/v tetrasodium EDTA stock, 0.25 ml, 10 g/dl potassium cyanide (KCN) stock, 1.0 ml, water to 100 ml.

30% citric acid. Citric acid, 30 g, make up to 100 ml with water.

Buffers

Stock TEB buffer, pH 8.5. Tris, 10.2 g, EDTA, 0.6 g, boric acid, 3.2 g.

TEB-urea soaking buffer, pH 6.3. Stock TEB buffer, 138 ml, distilled water, 282 ml, urea, 216 g. Dissolve the urea in the diluted TEB buffer, then adjust the pH to 6.3 with 30% citric acid. Prepare on day of use.

TEB-urea-merceptoethanol working buffer, pH 6.3. Stock TEB buffer, 490 ml, urea, 250 g. Dissolve the urea in the TEB buffer, then adjust the pH to 6.3 with 30% citric acid. *It is essential that TRIS-sensitive electrodes are used in the pH adjustment.* Save 2 ml of this buffer to use later as sample diluent, then add 5.6 ml of 2-mercaptoethanol to the remainder of the buffer, while stirring. Prepare on day of use.

Ponceau S (0.5% in 7.5% trichloroacetic acid). Ponceau S, 20 g, trichloroacetic acid, 300 ml, water to 4 litres. Store at room temperature.

3% acetic acid. Glacial acetic acid, 120 ml, water to 4 litres. Store at room temperature.

9 g/l NaCl.

Equipment

Electrophoresis tank and power pack. Any horizontal electrophoresis tank that will allow a bridge gap of 7 cm. A direct current power

Cathode (−)

TEB-Urea-Citrate pH 6.3   TEB-Urea pH 8.0

$\qquad$ α G-Philadelphia
$\qquad$ α A
                                      $\qquad$ α G-Philadelphia
                                      $\qquad$ α A
                                      $\qquad$ β C
$\qquad$ α I
$\qquad$ β E
$\qquad$ β C $\qquad$ β E, δ A$_2$
                                      $\qquad$ β O-Arab
$\qquad$ δ A$_2$
                                      $\qquad$ α I

$\qquad$ β S, O-Arab $\qquad$ β S
$\qquad$ β D-Punjab, G-Coushatta $\qquad$ β D-Punjab, G-Coushatta
$\qquad$ β A

                                      $\qquad$ β A, γ F
$\qquad$ γ F $\qquad$ β K-Woolwich
$\qquad$ β K-Woolwich, J-Baltimore $\qquad$ β J-Baltimore
                                      $\qquad$ β N-Seattle

$\qquad$ β N-Seattle

Origin $\qquad\qquad\qquad\qquad\qquad\qquad$ Origin

Anode (+)

Figure 12.10   Schematic representation of relative mobilities of some globin chains.

supply capable of delivering 350 V at 50 mA is suitable for both cellulose acetate and citrate agar electrophoresis.

Wicks of filter paper or chromatography paper.

Blotting paper.

Applicators. These are available from most manufacturers of electrophoresis equipment, but fine microcapillaries are also satisfactory.

Cellulose acetate membranes. Plastic-backed membranes (7.6 × 6.0 cm) are recommended for ease of use and storage.

Staining equipment.

Method

1. Wash at least 40 μl of packed red cells twice in 9 g/l NaCl. Add 20 μl of washed, packed cells to 60 μl of lysing solution, mix gently, and leave for 5 min. Transfer 20 μl of this lysate to a tube containing 20 μl of fresh TEB-urea working buffer, then add 4 ml 2-mercaptoethanol immediately before use. Purified haemolysates may also be used.

2. *With the power supply disconnected,* prepare the electrophoresis tank by placing 50 ml of TEB-urea-mercaptoethanol working buffer in each of the outer buffer compartments. Soak and position a paper wick along each divider.

3. Soak the cellulose acetate membrane plate(s) overnight in TEB-urea soaking buffer.

4. Blot the plate(s) and transfer to 600 ml of TEB-urea-mercaptoethanol working buffer. Leave to soak for between 30 min and 1 hour.

5. Place 5 μl of the patient and control samples in a sample well plate.

6. Remove the cellulose acetate from the working buffer and blot between two sheets of clean blotting paper until nearly dry.

7. Load the sample applicator and apply onto clean blotting paper; reload and apply the samples onto the cellulose acetate in the central position.

8. Place the cellulose acetate plate in the electrophoresis tank with the cellulose acetate in contact with the anode and cathode wicks. Place two microscope slides onto the back of the plate to maintain contact with the wicks.

9. Electrophorese at 150 V for 2 hours.

10. Prepare the staining equipment by filling the first reservoir with Ponceau S solution and three more reservoirs with 3% acetic acid.

11. On completion of the electrophoresis, place the plate into the Ponceau S stain solution and leave to fix and stain for 5 min.
12. Remove excess stain by immersing the plates into 3% acetic acid, leaving for 5–10 min in each reservoir until the background is clear. Do not agitate the plate in the acetic acid because the cellulose acetate becomes very fragile and easily peels off the backing plastic.
13. Remove the plates from the acetic acid and allow to dry between two clean sheets of blotting paper.

Results

Normal α chains migrate toward the cathode, and normal β chains migrate toward the anode. The relative migration of globins from the test samples are compared to both the known controls and the mobilities of the test samples on cellulose acetate electrophoresis. The relative mobilities of some abnormal α and β chains are shown in Figure 12.10.

TESTS FOR Hb S

Tests to detect the presence of Hb S depend on the decreased solubility of this haemoglobin at low oxygen tensions.

Sickling in Whole Blood

The sickling phenomenon may be demonstrated in a thin wet film of blood (sealed with a petroleum jelly/paraffin wax mixture or with nail varnish). If Hb S is present, the red cells lose their smooth, round shape and become sickled. This process may take up to 12 hours in Hb S trait, whereas changes are apparent in homozygotes and compound heterozygotes after 1 hour at 37°C. These changes can be hastened by the addition of a reducing agent such as sodium dithionite as follows:

Reagents

Disodium hydrogen phosphate (Na₂HPO₄). 0.114 mol/l (16.2 g/l).
Sodium dithionite (Na₂S₂O₄). 0.114 mol/l (19.85 g/l). Prepare freshly just before use.
Working solution. Mix 3 vol of Na_2HPO_4 with 2 vol of $Na_2S_2O_4$ to obtain a pH of 6.8 in the resultant solution. Use immediately.

Method

Add 5 drops of the freshly prepared reagent to 1 drop of anticoagulated blood on a slide. Seal between slide and coverglass with a petroleum jelly/ paraffin wax mixture or with nail varnish. Sickling takes place almost immediately in sickle cell anaemia and should be obvious in sickle cell trait within 1 hour (Fig. 12.11). A test on a positive control of Hb A plus Hb S must be performed at the same time.

Hb S Solubility Test

Principle

Sickle cell haemoglobin is insoluble in the deoxygenated state in a high molarity phosphate buffer. The crystals that form refract light and cause the solution to be turbid.[38]

Reagents

Phosphate buffer. Anhydrous dipotassium hydrogen phosphate, 215 g, anhydrous potassium dihydrogen phosphate, 169 g, sodium dithionite, 5 g, saponin, 1 g, water to 1 litre.

Note: Dissolve the K_2HPO_4 in water before adding the KH_2PO_4, then add the dithionite and finally the saponin. This solution is stable for 7 days. Store refrigerated.

Method

1. Pipette 2 ml of reagent into three 12×75 mm test tubes.
2. Allow the reagent to warm to room temperature.
3. Add 10 μl of packed cells (from EDTA-anti-coagulated blood) to one tube, 10 μl of packed cells from a known sickle cell trait subject as a positive control to the second tube, and 10 μl packed cells from a normal subject as a negative control to the final tube.
4. Mix well and leave to stand for 5 min.

Note: The blood reagent mixture should be light pink or red. A light orange colour indicates that the reagent has deteriorated.

5. Hold tube 2.5 cm in front of a white card with narrow black lines and read for turbidity, in comparison with the positive and negative control samples.

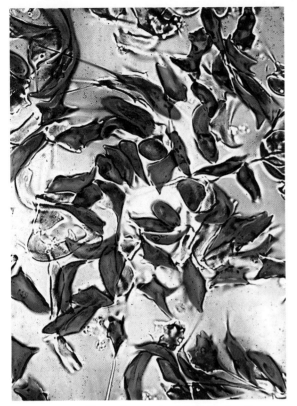

Figure 12.11   Photomicrograph of sickled red cells.
Sickle cell anaemia. Sealed preparation of blood. Fully
sickled filamentous forms predominate.

6. If the test appears to be positive, centrifuge at
1200 g for 5 min. A positive test will show a dark
red band at the top, whereas the solution below
will be pink or colourless.

Interpretation and Comments

A positive solubility or sickling test indicates the
presence of Hb S and as such is useful in the differential diagnosis of Hbs D and G, which migrate with
Hb S on cellulose acetate electrophoresis at alkaline
pH. Positive results are also obtained on samples
containing the rare haemoglobins that have both
the Hb S mutation and an additional mutation in
the β chain. A positive solubility test merely indicates
the presence of a sickling haemoglobin and does not
differentiate between homozygotes, compound
heterozygotes, and heterozygotes. In an emergency,
it may be necessary to decide if an individual suffers

from sickle cell disease before the haemoglobin
electrophoresis results are available. In these circumstances, if the solubility test is positive, a provisional diagnosis of sickle cell trait can be made if
the red cell morphology is normal on the blood film.
If the blood film shows any sickle or target cells,
irrespective of the Hb, a provisional diagnosis of
sickle cell disease should be made; many patients
with sickle cell/Hb C compound heterozygosity will
have a normal Hb. Remember that the sickle test is
likely to be negative in infants with sickle cell disease.

False-positive results have been reported in severe
leucocytosis; in hyperproteinaemia (such as multiple
myeloma); and in the presence of an unstable
haemoglobin, especially after splenectomy. The use
of packed cells, as described in this method, minimizes
the problem of false-positive results caused by
hyperproteinaemia and hyperlipidaemia.

False-negative results can occur in patients with
a low Hb, and the use of packed cells will overcome
this problem. False-negative results may also occur
if old or outdated reagents are used and if the
dithionite/buffer mixture is not freshly made. False-
negative results are likely to be found in infants
younger than age 6 months and in other situations
(e.g., posttransfusion) in which the Hb S level is less
than 20%.

All sickle tests, whether positive or negative, must
be confirmed by electrophoresis or HPLC at the
earliest opportunity.

NEONATAL SCREENING

Cord-blood or a heel-prick sample should be tested
from all babies at risk of sickle cell disease or
β thalassaemia major (i.e., where the mother has a
gene for Hb S, C, D^{Punjab}, E, O^{Arab}, Lepore, or β or δβ
thalassaemia trait). If a cord-blood specimen is used,
it is important that the sample is collected by
venipuncture of the cleaned umbilical vein to avoid
contamination with maternal blood because even
small quantities of maternal blood can cause a case
of sickle cell disease to be misdiagnosed as sickle
cell trait.

In areas where the frequency of haemoglobinopathies is high, universal neonatal screening
should be undertaken where possible. In England,
universal screening is currently being set up to

cover the whole of the country.[39] The screening programme is linked to the existing dried blood spot screening programme in place for phenylketonuria and congenital hypothyroidism. The same dried blood spot sample is tested for sickle cell disease and thalassaemia major.

Dried blood spot samples are tested using HPLC and IEF—HPLC is typically the first-line test, and abnormalities are confirmed by IEF. Haemoglobin electrophoresis is not recommended for the analysis of dried blood spots. Analysis of cord-blood samples is undertaken as a clinician-led request rather than for general screening. If umbilical cord-blood samples are used, they can be examined using haemoglobin electrophoresis using cellulose acetate at alkaline pH, citrate agar at acid pH,[22] or HPLC or IEF. If any abnormality is detected, a confirmatory technique should also be undertaken.

Babies provisionally diagnosed as having Hbs SS, SC, SD[Punjab], SO[Arab], or Sβ thalassaemia should be retested within 6–8 weeks of birth. After confirmation of the diagnosis, they should be followed in a paediatric clinic, immediately started on prophylactic penicillin to prevent pneumococcal infections, and appropriately managed in the long term.[3] Babies with β thalassaemia major will also be detected by the routine screening protocol; Hb A is either absent or greatly reduced at birth and when the babies are retested. The diagnosis of β thalassaemia trait cannot be reliably made until 12 months of age unless DNA techniques are used (see p. 561).

DETECTION OF AN UNSTABLE HAEMOGLOBIN

Haemoglobin variants exhibit a wide variety of instability but the clinically unstable haemoglobins can be detected by both the heat stability test and the isopropanol test.[40] However, minor degrees of instability that have little or no clinical significance may need other techniques. The unstable haemoglobins are frequently silent using electrophoretic or chromatographic techniques, and tests for haemoglobin instability are essential in the detection or exclusion of an unstable haemoglobin.

Several methods are available for the demonstration of haemoglobin instability. Samples analyzed should be as fresh as possible and certainly less than 1 week old. Controls should be of the same age as the test sample; a normal cord-blood sample can be used as a positive control. The isopropanol test uses chemically prepared controls.

Heat Stability Test

Principle

When haemoglobin in solution is heated, the hydrophobic van der Waals bonds are weakened and the stability of the molecule is decreased.[41,42] Under controlled conditions, unstable haemoglobins precipitate, whereas stable haemoglobins remain in solution.

Reagent

Tris-HCl buffer, pH 7.4, 0.05M. Tris, 6.05 g, water to 1 litre. Adjust the pH to 7.4 with concentrated HCl. See note on page 290 concerning Tris-sensitive electrodes.

Method

1. Add 0.2 ml of lysate, freshly prepared by the purified haemolysate method given on page 281, to a tube containing 1.8 ml of buffer. The negative control is obtained from a fresh normal sample.
2. Place the tubes in a waterbath at 50°C. Examine the tubes at 60, 90, and 120 min for precipitation.

Interpretation and Comments

A major unstable haemoglobin will have undergone marked precipitation at 60 min and profuse flocculation at 120 min. The normal control may show some (fine) precipitation at 60 min, but this should be minimal.

Isopropanol Stability Test

Principle

When haemoglobin is dissolved in a solvent such as isopropanol, which is more nonpolar than water, the hydrophobic van der Waals bonds are weakened and the stability of the molecule is decreased. Under controlled conditions, unstable haemoglobins precipitate, whereas stable haemoglobins remain in solution. This method has the advantage that it does not require a 37°C waterbath, and positive controls can be made by modification of the reagent buffer.[43]

Reagents

Tris-HCl buffer, pH 7.4, 0.1 mol/l. Tris, 12.11 g, water to 1 litre. Adjust the pH to 7.4 with concentrated HCl. See note on page 293 concerning Tris-sensitive electrodes.

Isopropanol buffer, 17%. Make 17 volumes of isopropanol up to 100 volumes with tris-HCl buffer. The 17% isopropanol buffer solution may be stored in a tightly stoppered glass bottle for 3 months at 4°C.

Positive controls. These are buffers produced by adding small amounts of zinc to the standard 17% isopropanol buffer. For the strongest positive control (5+), add 0.6 mmol/l zinc acetate, and for the weaker positive control (1+), add 0.1 mmol/l zinc acetate to the buffer. Samples containing haemoglobin E or haemoglobin F can also be used as weak positive controls.

Method

1. Prepare oxyhaemoglobin haemolysates from test and normal control samples as given on page 283.
2. Pipette 2.0 ml of the standard isopropanol buffer into two tubes, followed by 2.0 ml of the 1+ and 5+ control solutions, respectively, into two further tubes.
3. Add 0.2 ml of test sample to the first tube. Add 0.2 ml normal control sample into the three remaining tubes.
4. Place the tubes in a waterbath at 37°C for 30 min. Examine the tubes at 5, 20, and 30 min for turbidity and fine flocculation.

Interpretation and Comments

A normal sample will remain clear until 30 min, when a slight cloudiness may appear. Some unstable haemoglobins will show clearly observable precipitation even after 5 min incubation, whereas milder variants will not show precipitation until 20 min.

Positive results may be given by samples containing as little as 10% Hb F or by samples containing increased methaemoglobin as a result of prolonged storage. If the normal sample undergoes premature precipitation, check the temperature of the waterbath because it is likely to be higher than 37°C.

False-negative results should be avoided by continuing the incubation until the normal control undergoes precipitation.

DETECTION OF HB MS

Methaemoglobin (Hi) has iron present in the ferric form. Inherited variants of haemoglobin that undergo oxidation to methaemoglobin more readily than Hb A are referred to as Hb Ms. This is one of the causes of a very rare condition, congenital methaemoglobinaemia. The other cause of inherited methaemoglobinaemia is methaemoglobin reductase deficiency (see p. 202). Methaemoglobin levels vary but may be as high as 40% of the total haemoglobin. Methaemoglobinaemia *per se* may also be caused by oxidant chemicals.

Methaemoglobin variants may be detected by haemoglobin electrophoresis at pH 7, but almost all can be distinguished from methaemoglobin A (Hi A) by their absorption spectra. Each methaemoglobin has its own distinct absorption spectrum. Hi A has two absorption peaks at 502 nm and 632 nm, whereas the peak absorbances for the variant Hb Ms are at different wavelengths (Fig. 12.12).

Reagent

Potassium ferricyanide. 0.1mol/l.

Method

1. Lyse washed red cells from a blood sample of known Hb A and of the test sample with water to give haemoglobin concentration of about 1 g/l.
2. Convert the haemoglobin to Hi by the addition of 5 μl of potassium ferricyanide solution to each ml of haemolysate.
3. Leave for 10 min at room temperature.
4. Record the spectrum of Hi A using an automatic scanning spectrometer.
5. Compare to the spectrum of Hi in the test sample.

DETECTION OF ALTERED AFFINITY HAEMOGLOBINS

Electrophoretic and chromatographic techniques are frequently unsuccessful in separating these abnormal haemoglobins and cannot be relied on for detection because the amino acid substitution often does not involve a change in charge.

The most informative investigation is the measurement of the oxygen dissociation curve (p. 232). The most significant finding is a decreased

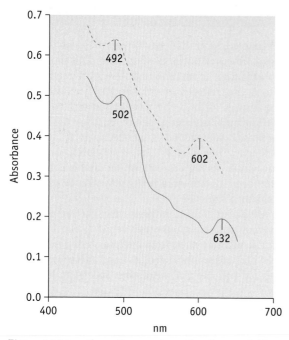

Figure 12.12   Absorption maxima of methaemoglobins in the range of 450–650 nm. Normal methaemoglobin is shown by a solid line; Hb M Saskatoon is shown by a dotted line. (Reproduced with permission from Lehmann H, Huntsman KG 1974 Man's haemoglobins, 2nd ed. p. 214. North-Holland, Amsterdam.

Hill's constant ("n" value) because this can only come about by a change in the structure of the haemoglobin. The p_{50} may be either increased (low-affinity haemoglobin) or decreased (high-affinity haemoglobin). High-affinity haemoglobins result in an increase in Hb level, whereas low-affinity haemoglobins result in a decrease in Hb level. The p_{50} alone may be affected by other factors such as the high concentration of 2,3-DPG in pyruvate kinase deficiency. Aspects of this are discussed in Chapter 10.

DIFFERENTIAL DIAGNOSIS OF COMMON HAEMOGLOBIN VARIANTS

Suggested methods for differential diagnosis are given in Table 12.6, and Figure 12.13 gives a comparison of some common variants using different techniques.

INVESTIGATION OF SUSPECTED THALASSAEMIA

A suggested scheme of investigations is shown in Figure 12.14; the methods used are listed in the following.

1. Estimates of Hb A_2 between 3.3% and 3.8% need careful assessment and should be repeated using a second method.
2. Hb A_2 values in α thalassaemia trait are usually below 25%. Some types of β thalassaemia trait have normal Hb A_2 values.

Methods for Investigation of Thalassaemia

1. Full blood count with red cell indices and blood film and, in selected cases, reticulocyte count.
2. Hb A_2 measurement by cellulose acetate electrophoresis with elution (p. 298).
3. Hb A_2 measurement of microcolumn chromatography (p. 299).
4. Automated HPLC (p. 301).
5. Quantitation of Hb F (p. 302 or HPLC).
6. Assessment of the distribution of Hb F (p. 305).
7. Assessment of iron status (p. 306).
8. Demonstration of red cell inclusion bodies (p. 307).
9. DNA analysis (p. 308).

Blood Count and Film

The blood count, including haemoglobin and red cell indices, provides valuable information useful in the diagnosis of both α and β thalassaemia. In classical cases, there will be an elevation in the red cell count, accompanied by a decrease in MCV and MCH. The MCHC and red cell distribution width (RDW) are often normal in thalassaemia trait, whereas in iron-deficiency anaemia they are more likely to be increased. The blood film may show features such as target cells, basophilic stippling, and microcytosis in the absence of hypochromia, which point to a diagnosis of thalassaemia trait. Anisochromasia, which is a feature of iron deficiency, is not usual in α and β thalassaemia trait, although it may be seen in haemoglobin H disease. Haemoglobin H disease is also characterized by marked poikilocytosis. The reticulocyte count is increased in haemoglobin H disease.

Table 12.6 Methods helpful in the differential diagnosis of common structural variants

Initial Finding on cellulose acetate electrophoresis	Most likely variant	Differentiation
Band in position of Hb S	Hb S, D, G-Philadelphia, Lepore	Blood count, quantitation, solubility test, citrate agar/acid gel electrophoresis, IEF, HPLC
Band in position of Hb C	Hb C, E, O-Arab	Quantitation, citrate agar/acid gel electrophoresis, IEF, HPLC
Very fast band	Hb I, H	H bodies

IEF, isoelectric focusing; HPLC, high-performance liquid chromatography.

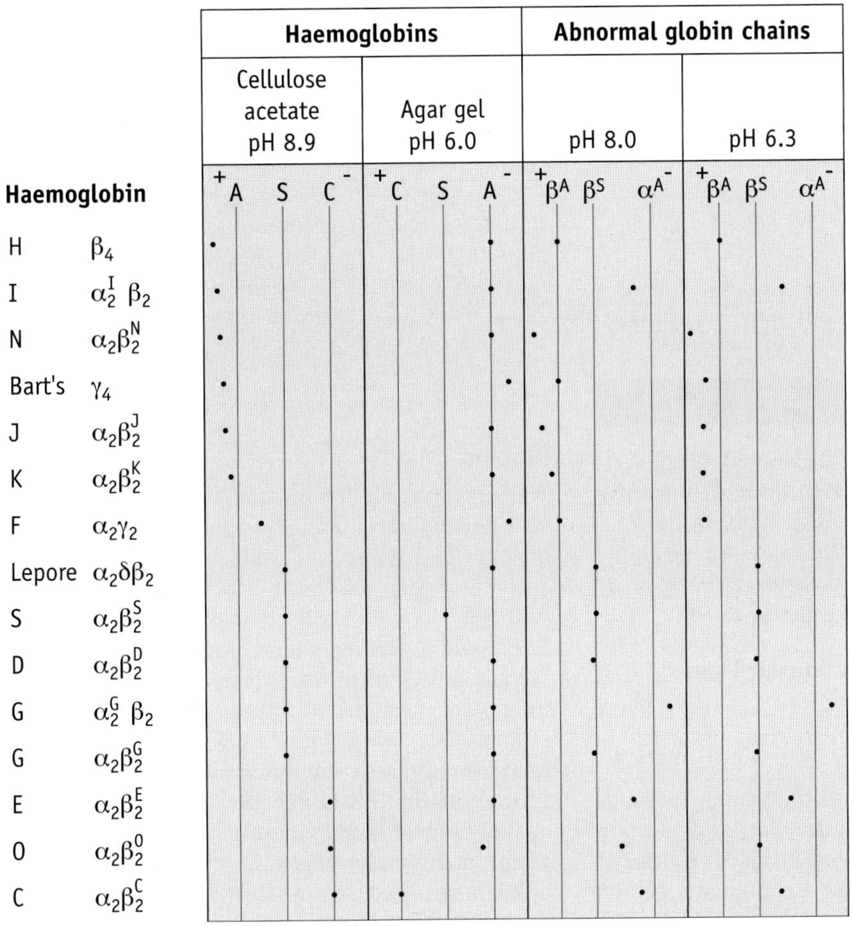

Figure 12.13 Comparison of the relative mobilities of some abnormal haemoglobins by different methods. The position of Hbs A, S, and C and their corresponding chains are indicated by the vertical lines. (Adapted from ICSH.[22])

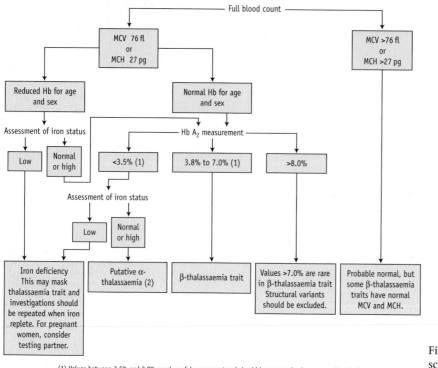

Figure 12.14   Suggested scheme of investigation for thalassaemia.

(1) Values between 3.5% and 3.8% need careful assessment and should be repeated using a second method.
(2) A₂ values in α-thalassaemia are usually below 2.5%. some types of β-thalaessamia trait have normal Hb A₂ values

QUANTITATION OF Hb A₂

An increased HbA_2 level is characteristic of heterozygous β thalassaemia, and its accurate measurement is required for the diagnosis or exclusion of β thalassaemia trait. Estimations may be made by elution after cellulose acetate electrophoresis or by chromatography, either microcolumn or HPLC.

Measurement of Hb A₂ by Elution from Cellulose Acetate

Principle

Haemolysate is separated into its component fractions by alkaline electrophoresis on cellulose acetate membrane. The relative proportions of the separated fractions are quantitated by spectrometry of the eluates of the separated fractions.[44,45]

Equipment

Electrophoresis tank and power pack. See page 284.
Wicks of double filter paper or chromatography paper.
Cellulose acetate membranes (78 × 150 mm).

Reagent

TEB buffer, pH 8.5. Tris(hydroxymethyl) methylamine, 40.8 g; disodium EDTA, 2.4 g; orthoboric acid, 12.8 g; water to 4 litres.

Method

1. Prepare a purified haemolysate from washed red cells as described on page 283. The haemolysate may be kept at 4°C for up to 1 week before analysis.
2. *With the power supply disconnected,* pour equal amounts of TEB buffer into both the anode and the cathode chambers. Cut lengths of filter or chromatography paper, soak them in the buffer chamber, and place them along the bridge supports as wicks. Set the bridge gap to 7 cm.
3. Soak the cellulose acetate by carefully floating the cellulose acetate sheet onto the surface of the buffer, making sure that no air bubbles are trapped underneath it. When the sheet has absorbed the

buffer, submerge the sheet. Leave for at least 5 min, remove, and blot carefully between two sheets of blotting paper.

4. Position the cellulose acetate across the bridge supports so that the long end of the sheet is on the anodal side. Using a ruler as a guideline, apply 30 μl of lysate to each sheet 1 cm from the cathode in a single line. Leave 1 cm margin at each end of the application line.

5. Run at a constant voltage of 250 V until separation is complete. This will take approximately 60 min, and there should be at least a 1 cm gap between the A and A₂ bands at the end of the run. Check the separation at 40 min, ensuring that the Hb A (or variant such as Hb H, Hb J, or Hb N) does not travel onto the wicks. Check again at 5–10 min thereafter. Samples with a variant band between the A and A₂ bands will take up to 30 min longer to obtain satisfactory separation.

6. Remove the sheet, holding it carefully at the anodal wick contact; do not place on a work surface. Cut off and discard the cellulose acetate that has been in contact with the cathodal wick. Cut a "blank" strip of approximately 2 cm wide from the cathodal end of one sheet (do not use cellulose acetate that includes the application line). Cut out the Hb A₂ section, cutting the band into pieces approximately 1 cm square directly into a clean universal container. Cut out any variant band in the same way and finally cut out the Hb A band.

7. Add 4 ml of distilled water to both the blank and Hb A₂ containers, and add 16 ml water to the Hb A container. Variant bands are usually eluted in 8 ml of water, although this may vary.

8. Mix the eluates for 20 min, and mix again by inversion just before measuring the absorbance.

9. Read the absorbance of the blank against water at 415 nm. This reading should be less than 0.005. Read the absorbances of the haemoglobin solutions at 415 nm against the cellulose acetate blank.

Calculation

$$\% \text{ Hb A}_2 = \frac{\text{Absorbance of Hb A}_2 \times 100}{\text{Absorbance of Hb A}_2 + (\text{Absorbance of Hb A} \times 4)}$$

Interpretation and Comments

For interpretation of results and normal ranges, see page 302. Duplicate values obtained should be within 0.2%. This method is inaccurate in the presence of Hb C, Hb E, and Hb O^{Arab} because they do not separate from Hb A₂.

The procedure is useful for the measurement of haemoglobin variants: in these cases, the volume of water used for elution should be adjusted to the apparent quantity of the variant as judged on electrophoresis. Particular care must be taken when cutting strips on which a variant of haemoglobin (e.g., Hb S) is present because the separation between Hb S and Hb A₂ is less certain.

To obtain accurate and precise results, use the same cuvette when reading the blank, Hb A₂, and Hb A absorbance of each sample. Read the blank, Hb A₂, and Hb A in that order to minimize the effects of carryover. Some types of cellulose acetate are unsuitable for elution; this can be detected by a very high blank reading. The haemoglobin concentration of the haemolysate is important: the absorbance reading of the haemoglobin A₂ must be at least 0.1 absorbance unit because low values will give inaccurately low Hb A₂ results.

Measurement of Hb A₂ by Microcolumn Chromatography

Principle

Microcolumn chromatography depends on the interchange of charged groups on the ion exchange cellulose with charged groups on the haemoglobin molecule. When a mixture of haemoglobins is adsorbed onto the cellulose, a particular haemoglobin component may be eluted from the column using a buffer (developer) with a specific pH and/or ionic strength, whereas other components (either a single haemoglobin or a mixture of haemoglobins) may be eluted by changing the pH or ionic strength of the developer. The separation of haemoglobin components depends on the pH and/or ionic strength of the developers used for the equilibration of the column and for the elution, the type of cellulose, the volume of the sample added, the size of the column, the gradient, flow rates, and temperature. The following methods use the anion exchanger diethylaminoethyl (DEAE) cellulose (Whatman DE-

52 microgranular pre-swollen), with Tris-HCl developers[46] or glycine-KCN developers.[47]

Measurement of Hb A_2 by Microcolumn Chromatography with Tris-HCL Buffers[46]

Reagents

DE-52 ion exchange cellulose (Whatman).
Stock buffer 1.0 mol/l Tris. Tris, 121.1 g; water to 1 litre. See note on page 293 concerning tris-sensitive electrodes.
Working buffer 1. KCN, 200 mg; stock buffer, 100 ml; water to 2 litres; adjust to pH 8.5 with concentrated HCl.
Working buffer 2. KCN, 200 mg; stock buffer, 100 ml; water to 2 litres; adjust to pH 8.3 with concentrated HCl.
Working buffer 3. KCN, 200 mg; stock buffer, 100 ml; water to 2 litres; adjust to pH 7.0 with concentrated HCl.

Important: If the buffers are stored at 4°C, they must be allowed to come to room temperature before use.

Method

1. Prepare the slurry by adding 10 g of DE-52 to 200 ml of buffer 1. Mix gently, and allow the cellulose to settle. Decant the supernatant and add a further 200 ml of buffer 1, mix gently for 10 min, then adjust the pH of the thoroughly suspended cellulose to 8.5 with concentrated HCl. Allow the cellulose to settle, remove the supernatant, and resuspend in a further 200 ml of buffer 1. Mix gently for 10 min and ensure the pH is 8.5. Allow to settle and remove enough buffer so that the settled cellulose constitutes about half the total volume.
2. Secure short-form pipettes vertically in a support rack. Place either a 3 mm glass bead or a small piece of cotton wool in the tapered part of the pipette to act as a support for the slurry.
3. Fill the pipettes with thoroughly suspended cellulose slurry and allow the column to pack to a height of 5–6 cm.
4. Dilute 1 drop of haemolysate (100 g/l) with 5 drops of buffer 1.
5. When the excess buffer has drained from the column, gently apply the diluted lysate to the top

of the column and allow it to be adsorbed onto the resin. Do not allow the surface of the column to dry out.

6. Apply 8 ml buffer 2 gently to the column with a 10–15 cm length of polythene tubing attached to the top of the pipette acting as a reservoir. Collect the eluate in a 10 ml flask and make the volume up to 10 ml with buffer 2.
7. Elute the remaining Hb A, using 10 ml of buffer 3; collect the eluate and make the volume up to 25 ml with the remaining buffer 3.
8. Read the absorbance of the eluted haemoglobins at 415 nm in a spectrometer, using water as a blank.

Calculate the Hb A_2 as follows:

$$\% \text{ Hb } A_2 = \frac{A^{415} \text{ Hb } A_2 \times 100}{A^{415} \text{ Hb } A_2 + (2.5 \times A^{415} \text{ Hb } A)}$$

Interpretation and Comments

For interpretation and normal ranges, see page 302. The technique is inappropriate in the presence of haemoglobin variants (see below). Factors affecting quality assurance include the concentration of haemoglobin applied to the column—excess haemoglobin will cause contamination of the Hb A_2 fraction with Hb A. An inadequate amount of haemoglobin will result in an eluate with an absorbance too low for accurate measurement.

The flow rate of the column may be adjusted by altering the height of the reservoir above the column. A flow rate of 10–20 ml/hour is satisfactory. Raising the reservoir increases the flow rate but broadens the Hb A_2 band on the column, which will not affect quantitation providing there is adequate separation. To elute the Hb A_2 band, 8 ml of buffer 2 should be used; the greater part of that should elute between 4 and 6 ml.

Measurement of Hb A_2 by +Microcolumn Chromatography with Glycine-Potassium Cyanide Developers

The method described as follows is suitable for samples containing variants such as Hb S. The elution of Hb A_2 is dependent on the pH of the ion exchanger and on the molarity of the developer.[47]

Reagents

Developer A. Glycine, 15.0 g, KCN, 0.1 g, water to 1 litre.
Developer B. NaCl, 9.0 g, water to 1 litre.
DE-52 ion exchange cellulose (Whatman).

Method

1. Prepare the slurry by adding 50 g of DE-52 to 250 ml of developer. Mix gently, then allow to settle and remove the supernatant. Repeat this process at least twice, then adjust the pH of the thoroughly suspended cellulose to 7.6 with 0.1 mol/l HCl.

If the slurry is made too acidic, it should be discarded because any attempt to readjust it would increase the total ionic concentration and therefore alter the elution pattern. The slurry may be stored for up to 4 weeks, but the pH should be checked and, if necessary, readjusted before use.

2. Secure short-form pipettes vertically in a support rack. Place either a 3 mm glass bead or a small piece of cotton wool in the tapered part of the pipette to act as a support for the slurry.
3. Fill the pipette with thoroughly suspended DE-52 slurry, and allow the column to pack under gravity to a height of about 6 cm.
4. Check each batch of columns with a Hb AS haemolysate. The Hb A_2 should elute in the first 3–4 ml, and the Hb S should elute in the next 15–20 ml of the developer.
5. Dilute 1 drop of lysate (100 g/l) with 6 drops of water.
6. When all the excess buffer has drained from the column, gently apply the diluted lysate to the top of the column, and allow it to be adsorbed onto the resin. Do not allow the surface of the column to dry out.
7. Apply developer A gently to the column with a piece of polythene tubing attached to the top of the pipette acting as a reservoir. About 3–4 ml of developer should be used to elute the Hb A_2 band. Collect the eluate in a 5 ml flask, and make the volume up to 5 ml with developer A.
8. Elute the remaining Hb A, or Hb S + Hb A, using 15–20 ml of developer B; collect the eluate and make the volume up to 25 ml with developer B. If, at any stage, the flow through the column stops, it should be discarded.

9. Read the absorbance of the eluted haemoglobins at 415 nm in a spectrometer, using water as a blank.

Calculate the Hb A_2 as follows:

$$\% \ Hb \ A_2 = \frac{A^{415} \ Hb \ A_2 \times 100}{A^{415} \ Hb \ A_2 + (5 \times A^{415} \ Hb \ A)}$$

Modification for the Measurement of Hb S

To estimate the percentage of Hb S and the remaining haemoglobin as well as that of Hb A_2, Hb A_2 is eluted in the first 3–4 ml with developer A, Hb S is eluted in the next 15–20 ml of the same developer A, and the remaining haemoglobin is eluted with developer B. The eluate containing Hb A_2 is diluted to 5 ml, and the eluates containing Hb S and the remaining haemoglobin are diluted to 25 ml. To ensure elution of all the Hb A_2 in the first 3–4 ml, and all the Hb S in the next 15–20 ml, the pH of the ion exchanger may need adjustment following a test chromatogram.[47]

Interpretation and Comments

Hb A_2 percentages tend to be very slightly lower using the Tris buffer system, but with either procedure there should be a distinction between normal and classical β thalassaemia trait subjects.[46] An advantage of the glycine-KCN method is less sensitivity to minor changes in the pH of the developer; also it may be used for samples containing Hb S.

It should be noted that measurement of Hb A_2 in the presence of Hb S is not usually a very useful test. It is not necessary in order to distinguish sickle cell trait from sickle cell/β⁺ thalassaemia and is not always reliable in distinguishing sickle cell anaemia from sickle cell/β⁰ thalassaemia because there is often interaction with α thalassaemia trait. In these circumstances, family studies can be extremely helpful.

Measurement of Hb A_2 by High-Performance Liquid Chromatography

The principle of HPLC has been explained on page 285. When this technology is used as the primary method for detecting variant haemoglobins, simultaneous quantitation of Hb A_2 and Hb F means that it can replace three separate traditional methods:

haemoglobin electrophoresis, quantitation of Hb A_2, and quantification of Hb F. Each laboratory should establish its own reference range for the quantitation of Hb A_2 by this method, which should be similar to published ranges. Because the quantitation of Hb A_2 may be inaccurate in the presence of certain variant haemoglobins, such as Hb E, Hb Lepore, and Hb S^{32}, each chromatogram should always be inspected. Inspection will also permit identification of specimens with a split A_2 band as the result of heterozygosity for a δ chain variant. If the quantity of a haemoglobin with the retention time of Hb A_2 is higher than expected, an alternative technique should be applied to confirm its identity because a peak labelled as Hb A_2 can be Hb E or another haemoglobin that elutes with Hb A_2.

INTERPRETATION OF Hb A_2 VALUES

Hb A_2 values should be interpreted in relation to a reference range established in each individual laboratory using blood samples from the local population with a normal Hb and red cell indices.[11,48-51] The standard operating procedure for the relevant method should be strictly followed and 95% reference ranges should be determined. Ranges may differ slightly between methods and between laboratories. For example, in one of our laboratories the range determined for microcolumn chromatography was 2.2–3.3%, whereas in the other it was 2.3–3.5%. Technical variables affecting the range may include the use of packed cells rather than whole blood. Results obtained by HPLC analysis may be 0.1–0.2% higher than the results obtained by electrophoresis with elution. Once a reference range is determined, there is still a practical problem with borderline results, given that repeat estimates may vary by 0.1–0.2%. We recommend that Hb A_2 levels of 3.4–3.7% be regarded as borderline and that the assay should be repeated both on the same sample and on a fresh sample. There is also evidence that Hb A_2 is elevated in patients with HIV.[52,53]

When assays are being performed for genetic counselling, it can be useful to investigate the partner whenever borderline results are obtained.

The Hb A_2 percentage should be interpreted with knowledge of the Hb and red cell indices (Table 12.7).

QUANTITATION OF Hb F

Hb F may be estimated by several methods based on its resistance to denaturation at alkaline pH, by HPLC, or by an immunological method.[54] Of the alkaline denaturation methods, that of Betke et al[55] is reliable for small amounts (<10–15%) of Hb F, whereas for levels of more than 50%, and in cord blood, the method of Jonxis and Visser[56] is preferable; however, this method is not reliable at levels of less than 10%.

Immunological methods have been devised to measure Hb F by immunodiffusion,[57] for which commercial kits are available,* and by enzyme-linked immunoassay (ELISA).[58]

Modified Betke Method for the Estimation of Hb F

Principle
To measure the percentage of Hb F in a mixture of haemoglobins,[55] sodium hydroxide is added to a lysate and, after a set time, denaturation is stopped by adding saturated ammonium sulphate. The ammonium sulphate lowers the pH and precipitates the denatured haemoglobin. After filtration, the quantity of undenatured (unprecipitated) haemoglobin is measured. The proportion of alkali-resistant (fetal) haemoglobin is then calculated as a percentage of the total amount of haemoglobin present.

Equipment
Filter paper. Whatman No. 42.
Vortex mixer.
Glass tubes.

Reagents
Cyanide solution. Potassium cyanide, 25 mg; potassium ferricyanide, 100 mg. Dissolve in 500 ml distilled water. Store in a dark bottle.
Saturated ammonium sulphate solution. Bring 1 litre of water to the boil and add ammonium sulphate until the solution is saturated. Cool and equilibrate at 20°C before use.
1.2 mol/l Sodium hydroxide. Sodium hydroxide 4.8 g; distilled water to 100 ml. Prepare monthly. Equilibrate at 20°C before use.

*Helena Laboratories, Beaumont, Texas, USA.

Table 12.7   Interpretation of Hb A$_2$ values

Hb A2 Range (%)	Interpretation
>7.0	Hb A$_2$ values of >7.0% are extremely rare Exclude a structural variant Repeat Hb A$_2$ estimation Rare β thalassaemia mutations
3.8–7.0	β thalassaemia trait, unstable haemoglobin
3.4–3.7	Severe iron deficiency in β thalassaemia trait Additional δ chain variant with β thalassaemia trait (Total A$_2$ must be measured) Interaction of α and β thalassaemia Rare β thalassaemia mutations Presence of Hb S, making accurate measurement difficult Interaction of α thalassaemia and Hb S Analytical error; repeat analysis

2.0–3.3	Normal
	δ β thalassaemia (if Hb F elevated)
	Rare cases of
	    β thalassaemia trait, including coexisting
	    β and δ thalassaemia and coexisting
	    β and α thalassaemia
	α thalassaemia trait

<2.0	δ β thalassaemia (if Hb F elevated) α thalassaemia trait Hb H disease Additional δ chain variant present (total Hb A$_2$ must be measured) δ thalassaemia Iron deficiency

Method

1. Prepare a lysate as described on page 281. The lysate may be stored at 4°C for up to 1 week before use.
2. Add 0.25 ml lysate to 4.75 ml cyanide solution to make a solution of haemiglobincyanide (HiCN).
3. Transfer 2.8 ml of the haemiglobincyanide solution to a glass test tube and allow to equilibrate at 20°C.
4. Blow in 0.2 ml of 1.2 mol/l of NaOH and mix on a vortex mixer for 2–3 sec.
5. After exactly 2 min, blow in 2 ml saturated ammonium sulphate solution and mix on a vortex mixer. Leave tubes to stand for 5–10 min at 20°C.
6. Filter twice through the same Whatman No. 42 filter paper, using a clean test tube to collect the filtrate each time. If the filtrate is not completely clear, filter again through the same paper. This filtrate contains the alkali-resistant haemoglobin.
7. To measure the total haemoglobin, transfer 0.4 ml of the haemiglobincyanide solution from step 2 into another tube and add 13.9 ml of water.
8. Read the absorbance of the alkali-resistant and total haemoglobin at 420 nm against a water blank.
9. Calculate the percentage alkali-resistant haemoglobin as follows:

$$\% \text{ Alkali-resistant haemoglobin} = \frac{A^{420} \text{ alkali-resistant Hb}}{A^{420} \text{ total Hb} \times 20} \times 100$$

Interpretation and Comments

Elevation of Hb F has a variety of causes (see page 306). In very exceptional situations, other abnormal haemoglobins will also exhibit resistance to alkali, giving high results. It is imperative that haemoglobin electrophoresis or HPLC is done on these samples tested for Hb F to exclude the possibility of an unusual variant being present.

A normal and a raised Hb F control should be tested with every batch of samples. The raised Hb F control should ideally contain between 5 and 15% Hb F, and this can be prepared from a mixture of cord and adult blood. Each laboratory must verify its own normal range, which should not differ significantly from published values; for adults the range is 0.2–1.0%.

Zago et al[59] reported variability in the capacity of different batches of filter paper to absorb haemoglobin from the filtrate, which caused low results. It is necessary to equilibrate the temperature of the reagents to 20°C and to control the reaction temperature to 20°C to obtain accurate and reproducible results.

Method of Jonxis and Visser

Principle

The increased resistance of Hb F to denaturation by alkali is detected by recording the change in absorption at 576 nm in each min, caused by the addition of ammonium hydroxide.[56] At this wavelength, the absorption of oxyhaemoglobin differs from that of the alkali haemochromogen that is formed on denaturation.

When the logarithm of the percentage of haemoglobin remaining undenatured is plotted against time, a straight line is obtained. By extrapolation to time zero, the percentage of Hb F in the original sample can be calculated.

Reagents

Ammonium hydroxide solution. NH$_4$OH, 100 g, water to 1 litre.

Sodium hydroxide solution 0.06 mol/l. Sodium hydroxide, 2.4 g, water to 1 litre.

Method

1. All reagents should be allowed to reach room temperature before use. Add 0.1 ml of blood or lysate (100 g/l) to 10 ml of water and mix.
2. Add 2 drops of ammonium hydroxide solution and mix.
3. Measure the absorbance in a spectrophotometer at 576 nm (A$_B$).
4. Add 0.1 ml of the same blood or lysate to 10 ml of sodium hydroxide solution; then add 2 drops of ammonium hydroxide solution and mix thoroughly.
5. Measure the absorbance in a spectrometer at 576 nm at every min for 15 min (A$_T$); then incubate the solution at 37°C for 15 min, cool to room temperature, and measure the absorbance (A$_E$). The ratio A$_B$:A$_E$ should be constant.
6. Calculate the percentage of undenatured haemoglobin at each min as follows:

$$\frac{A_T^{576} - A_E^{576}}{A_B^{576} - A_E^{576}} \; (\times \, 100)$$

Plot the percentage on the logarithmic scale of semilogarithmic paper against time. This should produce a straight line from which the original amount of Hb F at time zero can be found by extrapolation.

Interpretation and Comments

Comments regarding controls and normal ranges given for the Betke method are also applicable to this method. In addition, the Jonxis and Visser method requires an accurate spectrometer because the maximum absorption peak at 576 nm is very narrow and the difference in extinction between oxyhaemoglobin and alkali haemochromogen is relatively small.

For interpretation of results, see page 306.

Radial Immunodiffusion

The radial immunodiffusion procedure[57] can be used for the quantitation of Hb F. The principle is based on an antibody–antigen reaction; the anti-Hb F is incorporated into the gel support medium resulting in the formation of a visible opaque precipitin ring.

The square of the diameter of this ring is directly proportional to the concentration of Hb F. A standard curve must be prepared from samples containing known levels of Hb F plotted against their haemoglobin concentrations. Helena Laboratories market a kit containing prepared plates, a microdispenser, and a measuring device.

The method is simple, but the formation of the precipitin rings requires at least 18 hours of incubation at room temperature. For this reason, rapid diagnostic work is not possible. Care must be taken with sample application because damage to the plate wells results in asymmetric precipitin rings and erroneous measurements.

ASSESSMENT OF THE INTRACELLULAR DISTRIBUTION OF Hb F

Differences in the intracellular distribution of Hb F are used to differentiate between heterozygotes for $\delta\beta$ thalassaemia and the classical African type of HPFH. In the former, it can be shown that not all red cells contain Hb F (heterocellular distribution), whereas in the latter every cell contains Hb F (pancellular distribution), although there is some variability in content from cell to cell. It has been suggested that a heterocellular distribution may be more apparent than real and merely reflects that high levels of Hb F tend to give a more pancellular distribution than lower levels. For this reason, results should be treated with caution and not used to make a diagnosis in isolation.

Two techniques have been widely used for demonstrating intracellular Hb F distribution. The most frequently used is the acid elution test of Kleihauer[60] that was originally developed for the detection of fetal red cells in the maternal circulation following transplacental haemorrhage. This method is described on page 317. Less frequently used is the more sensitive immunofluorescent technique described in the following.

Immunofluorescent Method

Principle
Anti-Hb F antibody binds specifically and quantitatively to Hb F in fixed red cells. These cells can be identified after treatment with a second fluorescent-labelled antibody directed against the anti-Hb F.[14]

Equipment
Glass slides.
Coplin jars.

Microscope. Equipped with accessories for ultraviolet (UV) fluorescence.
Moist chamber. Made from a Petri dish with moistened filter paper in the bottom.

Reagents
Phosphate buffered saline (PBS), pH 7.1. See page 691.
Rabbit antihuman Hb F serum. Dilute the antiserum 1 in 64 in PBS; store in small aliquots at –20°C. Stable for several months.
Sheep (or goat) antirabbit immunoglobulin labelled with fluorescein isothiocyanate. Dilute 1 in 32 in PBS; store in small aliquots at –20°C. Stable for several months.
Fixative. Acetone, 90 ml, methanol, 10 ml.

Method
1. Prepare thin blood films and allow to dry overnight.
2. Fix for 5 min at room temperature, shake off excess fixative, and rinse immediately in PBS. If the films are too thick, they will peel off at this stage.
3. Rinse the slides in water and allow to dry.
4. Layer 5 µl of the anti-Hb F antisera onto the slide.
5. Incubate in the moist chamber at 37°C for 30 min or at room temperature for 60 min.
6. Rinse the slides thoroughly in PBS to remove any unbound antiserum.
7. Rinse the slides in water and allow to dry.
8. Layer 5 µl of the antirabbit antisera onto the slide.
9. Incubate in the moist chamber at 37°C for 30 min or at room temperature for 60 min.
10. Rinse the slides thoroughly in PBS to remove any unbound antiserum.
11. Rinse the slides in water and allow to dry.
12. Examine microscopically using a ×40 objective and filters suitable for use with fluorescein isothiocyanate. To quantitate the number of Hb F-containing cells, count the total number of cells in a field under white light using an eyepiece grid, then the number of stained cells under the UV light. If the level of Hb F is less than 10%, at least 2000 cells should be counted.

Comments

In normal adults, from 0.1 to 7.0% of cells show detectable fluorescence. The proportion of positive cells correlates well with the percentage of Hb F as measured by alkali denaturation at levels between 0.5% and 5.0%. As little as 1 pg of Hb F per cell can be detected, giving much greater sensitivity than the acid elution method. This increased sensitivity, however, may make a heterocellular distribution appear pancellular if the proportion of Hb F if greater than 10%.[54]

Interpretation of Hb F values[11,14]

Hb F Range (%)	Interpretation
0.2–1.0	Normal results
1.0–5.0	In approximately 30% of β thalassaemia traits
	Some heterozygotes for a variant haemoglobin
	Some homozygotes for a variant haemoglobin
	Some compound heterozygotes for a variant haemoglobin and β thalassaemia
	Some individuals with haematological disorders (aplastic anaemia, myelodysplastic syndromes, juvenile myelomonocytic leukaemia)
	Some pregnant women (second trimester)
	Sporadically in the general population, particularly in Afro-Caribbeans (representing heterozygosity for nondeletional HPFH)
5.0–20.0	Occasional cases of β thalassaemia trait
	Some homozygotes for a variant haemoglobin
	Some compound heterozygotes for a variant haemoglobin and β thalassaemia
	Some types of heterozygous HPFH δβ thalassaemia
15.0–45.0	Heterozygous HPFH African type (usually more than 20%)
	Some cases of β thalassaemia intermedia
>45.0	β thalassaemia major
	Some cases of β thalassaemia intermedia
	Neonates
>95.0	Homozygous African-type (deletional) HPFH
	Some neonates (particularly if premature)

ASSESSMENT OF IRON STATUS IN THALASSAEMIA

Concurrent iron deficiency makes the diagnosis of thalassaemia trait more difficult because it masks the typical blood picture and can reduce Hb A_2 synthesis.[48,49,51] In β thalassaemia trait, dependent on the severity of the anaemia, the Hb A_2 value may be reduced to borderline or even to normal levels (3.0–3.5%). However, in many patients with β thalassaemia trait and iron deficiency, the Hb A_2 will still be raised.

Whenever possible, individuals should not be investigated for the presence of thalassaemia trait if they are iron deficient. Iron stores are usually replete after 3–4 months of treatment with iron. However, if a pregnant woman is suspected of having a thalassaemia trait, it is not possible to wait for the correction of iron deficiency to establish the diagnosis. The woman and her partner should be tested without delay with DNA analysis of globin genes being carried out if both are suspected of having thalassaemia trait (see Chapter 21. p. 562).

In addition to traditional methods for iron assessment, such as measurement of serum ferritin or serum iron plus total iron-binding capacity, estimation of zinc protoporphyrin (see pp. 149 and 199) is of potential value. This test can be carried out on an EDTA sample within a haematology laboratory and is a measure of iron incorporation at the cellular level.

RED CELL INCLUSIONS

The most important red cell inclusions found in the haemoglobinopathies are Hb H inclusion bodies (precipitated β chain tetramers) found in α thalassaemia,[61] α chain inclusions found in β thalassaemia major,[7,62] and Heinz bodies found in unstable haemoglobin diseases.[42,63]

Precipitated α chains are found in the cytoplasm of nucleated red cell precursors of patients with β thalassaemia major; they can be demonstrated by supravital staining of the bone marrow with methyl violet (as can Heinz bodies) and appear as irregularly shaped bodies close to the nucleus of normoblasts. After splenectomy they may also be found in the peripheral blood normoblasts and reticulocytes. Heinz bodies (insoluble denatured globin chains) form as a result of exposure to oxidant drugs or chemicals and develop spontaneously in glucose-6-phosphate dehydrogenase (G6PD) deficiency and in the unstable haemoglobin diseases. They are usually only seen in the peripheral blood after splenectomy. When caused by the presence of an unstable haemoglobin, they may be demonstrated in the peripheral blood of patients with an intact spleen if their blood is kept at 37°C for 24–48 hours. The use of methyl violet and of brilliant cresyl blue in the demonstration of precipitated α chain and Heinz bodies is described on p. 315.

Demonstration of Hb H Inclusion Bodies

Reagent
Staining solution. 1.0% brilliant cresyl blue or New methylene blue. New batches of stain must be tested with a known positive control because the redox action of the dyes may vary from batch to batch.

Method
1. Mix 2 vol of fresh blood (within 24 hours of collection) with 1 vol of staining solution.
2. Incubate at 37°C for 2 hours or at room temperature for 4 hours.
3. Resuspend the cells and spread a thin blood film.
4. Examine the film as for a reticulocyte count. The inclusion bodies appear as multiple greenish-blue dots, like the pitted pattern on a golf ball (p. 316). They can be readily distinguished from reticulocytes, which exhibit uneven reticular material or infrequent fine dots.

Interpretation and Comments
In α⁺ thalassaemia trait, only a very occasional H body (1:1000 to 1:10,000) is usually seen; they are more numerous in α⁰ thalassaemia, but the number of cells developing inclusions is not reliable in differentiating the various gene deletion patterns seen in α thalassaemia, and the absence of demonstrable inclusions does not preclude a diagnosis of α thalassaemia trait. This test is most useful in Hb H disease, where inclusions are usually found in more than 30% of red cells.

FETAL DIAGNOSIS OF GLOBIN GENE DISORDERS

Prenatal diagnosis of globin gene disorders[20] is carried out if the fetus is at risk of thalassaemia major or a severe form of sickle cell disease such as sickle cell anaemia. Two approaches to fetal diagnosis are available: globin chain synthesis (used if the putative father is not available) and DNA analysis. DNA can be obtained from a chorionic villus sample or from amniotic fluid. Methods used for DNA analysis are described in Chapter 21.

When a potentially at-risk couple is detected, they will require counselling, and if a fetal diagnosis is requested, it is necessary to confirm the parental haemoglobin phenotype. The family or parental blood samples are sent to the diagnostic centre, and the timing of fetal sampling is arranged.

Sample Requirements

Blood samples for globin chain synthesis have to be fresh (received within a few hours of collection) and transported at 4°C. Blood samples for DNA analysis can be sent by overnight delivery without refrigeration but must be processed, at the latest, within 3 days of collection. Ten ml of blood in EDTA or heparin are required from each parent. If restriction fragment length polymorphism (RFLP) linkage analysis is required, the following additional samples are needed: blood from either a homozygous normal or affected child, or from a heterozygous child and one set of grandparents, or if no child is available, blood from both sets of grandparents. The samples must be carefully and clearly labelled, and the family tree must be drawn. Particulars of all haematological tests must be given.

Chorionic villus samples must be dissected free of any maternal tissue and sent by urgent overnight delivery in tissue culture medium or, preferably, in a special buffer obtainable from the DNA diagnostic laboratory. Amniotic fluid samples (15–20 ml are needed) must be received within 24 hours of collection. If a longer transit time is unavoidable, the amniocytes should be resuspended in tissue culture medium.

The laboratory performing DNA analysis for disorders of globin chain synthesis must be given accurate information on the precise ethnic origin of family members so that optimal use is made of the DNA available for diagnosis.

It is essential that follow-up data are obtained on all cases that have undergone fetal diagnosis. This should include tests on cord blood or heel prick sample at birth and a test at 6 months to confirm the carrier state. Whenever possible, DNA analysis of the child's globin genes should be carried out.

REFERENCES

1. Hardison R, Miller W (Updated) Globin gene server. www.globin.cse.psu.edu.
2. Serjeant GR, Sergeant BE 2001 Sickle cell disease, 3rd ed. Oxford University Press, Oxford.
3. Dacie JV 1988 The haemolytic anaemias, vol 2: The hereditary haemolytic anaemias, 3rd ed. p 322. Churchill Livingstone, Edinburgh.
4. White JM 1974 The unstable haemoglobin disorders. Clinics in Haematology 3:333–356.
5. Stephens AD 1977 Annotation: Polycythaemia and high affinity haemoglobins British Journal of Haematology 36:153–159.
6. Kiese M 1974 Methemoglobinemia: A complete treatise. CRC Press, Cleveland, OH.
7. Weatherall DJ, Clegg JB 2001 The thalassaemia syndromes, 4th ed. Blackwell Science, Oxford.
8. Flint J, Harding RM, Boyce AJ, Clegg JB 1998. The population genetics of haemoglobinopathies. Baillière's Clinical Haematology, 11:1–51.
9. Thein SL 1998 β-thalassaemia. Baillière's Clinical Haematology, 11:91–126
10. Thein SL 2000 β thalassaemia. Fifth Congress of the European Haematology Association. In: Green AR (ed), Educational Book, Birmingham, p. 132–137
11. British Committee for Standards in Haematology 1994 Guidelines for the investigation of the α and β thalassaemia traits. Journal of Clinical Pathology 47:289–295.
12. Higgs DR 1993 β-Thalassaemia. Baillière's Clinical Haematology, 6:117–150.
13. Wood WG 1993 Increased Hb F in adult life. Baillière's Clinical Haematology, 6:177–213.
14. Wood WG, Stamatoyannopoulos G, Lim G, et al 1975 F cells in the adult: normal values and levels in individuals with hereditary and acquired elevations of Hb F. Blood 46:671–682.
15. Wild BJ, Green BN, Cooper EK et al 2001 Rapid identification of hemoglobin variants by electrospray ionization mass spectrometry. Blood Cells, Molecules and Diseases 27:691–704.
16. Wild BJ, Bain BJ 2004 Detection and quantitation of normal haemoglobins: an analytical review. Annals of Clinical Biochemistry 41:1–15.
17. Lafferty JD, Crowther MA, Ali MA, et al 1996 The evaluation of various mathematical RBC indices and their efficacy in discriminating between thalassemic and non-thalassemic microcytosis. American Journal of Clinical Pathology 106:201–205.
18. Eldibany MM, Totonchi KF, Joseph NJ, et al 1999 Usefulness of certain red blood cell indices in diagnosing and differentiating thalassemia trait from iron deficiency anemia. American Journal of Clinical Pathology 111:676–682.
19. Stephens AD, Wild BJ 1990 Quality control in haemoglobinopathy investigations. Methods in Hematology 22:72–85.

20. British Committee for Standards in Haematology 1988 Guidelines for haemoglobinopathy screening. Clinical and Laboratory Haematology 10:87–94.
21. British Committee for Standards in Haematology 1994 Guidelines for fetal diagnosis of globin gene disorders. Journal of Clinical Pathology 47:199–204.
22. International Committee for Standardization in Haematology 1988 Recommendations for neonatal screening for haemoglobinopathies. Clinical and Laboratory Haematology 10:335–345.
23. British Committee for Standards in Haematology Working Party of the General Haematology Task Force 1998 The laboratory diagnosis of haemoglobinopathies. British Journal of Haematology 101:783–792.
24. International Committee for Standardization in Haematology 1978 Simple electrophoretic system for presumptive identification of abnormal hemoglobins. Blood 52:1058–1064.
25. International Committee for Standardization in Haematology 1978 Recommendations for a system for identifying abnormal hemoglobins. Blood 52:1065–1067.
26. Schneider RG 1974 Identification of hemoglobin by electrophoresis. In: Schmidt RM, Huisman THJ, Lehmann H (eds) The detection of hemoglobinopathies, p.11. CRC Press, Cleveland, OH.
27. Marder VJ, Conley CL 1959 Electrophoresis of hemoglobin on agar gel. Frequency of hemoglobin D in a Negro population. Bulletin of the Johns Hopkins Hospital 105:77–88.
28. Schroeder WA, Shelton JB, Shelton JR 1980 Separation of hemoglobin peptides by high performance liquid chromatography HPLC. Hemoglobin 4:551–559.
29. Wild BJ, Stephens AD 1997 The use of automated HPLC to detect and quantitate haemoglobins. Clinical and Laboratory Haematology 19:171–176.
30. Phelan L, Bain BJ, Roper D, et al 1999 An analysis of relative costs and potential benefits of different policies for antenatal screening for β thalassaemia trait and variant haemoglobins. Journal of Clinical Pathology 52:697–700.
31. Riou J, Godart CM, Hurtrel D, et al 1997 Cation-exchange HPLC evaluated for presumptive identification of hemoglobin variants. Clinical Chemistry 43:34–39.
32. Head CE, Conroy M, Jarvis M et al 2004 Some observations on the measurement of haemoglobin A_2 and S percentages by high performance liquid chromatography in the presence and absence of thalassaemia. Journal of Clinical Pathology 57:276–280.
33. Millar CM, Phelan L, Bain BJ 2002 Diabetes mellitus diagnosed following request for haemoglobin electrophoresis. Lancet 117:778.
34. Righetti PG, Gianazza E, Bianchi-Bosisio A, et al 1986 The hemoglobinopathies: conventional isoelectric focusing and immobilized pH gradients for hemoglobin separation and identification. Methods in Hematology 15:47–71.
35. Basset P, Beuzard Y, Garel MC, et al 1978 Isoelectric focusing of human hemoglobins: its application to screening to characterization of 70 variants and to study of modified fractions of normal hemoglobins. Blood 51:971–982.
36. Ueda S, Schneider RG 1969. Rapid identification of polypeptide chains of hemoglobin by cellulose acetate electrophoresis of hemolysates. Blood 34:230–235.
37. Schneider RG 1974 Differentiation of electrophoretically similar hemoglobins ì such as S, D, G and P or A_2, C, E and O by electrophoresis of the globin chains. Clinical Chemistry 20:1111–1115.
38. Evatt BL, Gibbs WN, Lewis SM, et al 1992 Fundamental diagnostic hematology: Anemia, 2nd ed. U.S. Department of Health and Human Services, Atlanta and World Health Organization, Geneva.
39. NHS Sickle cell and thalassemia screening programme. www.kcl-phs.org.uk/haemscreening.
40. Carrell RW 1986 The hemoglobinopathies: methods of determining hemoglobin instability (unstable hemoglobins). Methods in Haematology 15:109–124.
41. Grimes AJ, Meisler A 1962 Possible cause of Heinz bodies in congenital Heinz body anaemia. Nature 194:190–191.
42. Grimes AJ, Meisler A, Dacie JV 1964 Congenital Heinz-body anaemia: further evidence on the cause of Heinz-body production in red cells. British Journal of Haematology 10:281–290.
43. Carrell RW, Kay R 1972 A simple method for the detection of unstable haemoglobins. British Journal of Haematology 23:615–619.
44. Marengo-Rowe AJ 1965 Rapid electrophoresis and quantitation of hemoglobins on cellulose acetate. Journal of Clinical Pathology 18:790–792.
45. International Committee for Standardization in Haematology 1978 Recommendations for selected methods for quantitative estimation of Hb A2 and for Hb A2 reference preparation. British Journal of Haematology 38:573–578.
46. Efremov GD, Huisman THJ, Bowman K, et al 1974 Microchromatography of hemoglobins: II A rapid

method for the determination of Hb A2. Journal of Laboratory and Clinical Medicine 83:657–664.

47. Huisman THJ, Schroeder WA, Brodie AR, et al 1975 Microchromatography of hemoglobins III. A simplified procedure for the determination of hemoglobin A2. Journal of Laboratory and Clinical Medicine 86:700–702.

48. Kattamis C, Panayotis L, Metaxotou-Mavromati A, et al 1972 Serum iron and unsaturated iron binding capacity in β thalassaemia trait: their relation to the levels of Hb A, A2 and F. Journal of Medical Genetics 9:154–159.

49. Alperin JB, Dow PA, Peteway MB 1977 Hemoglobin A2 levels in health and various hematological disorders. American Journal of Clinical Pathology 67:219–226.

50. Efremov GD 1986 The hemoglobinopathies: quantitation of hemoglobins by microchromatography. Methods in Hematology 15:72–90.

51. Wasi P, Na-Nakorn S, Pootrakul S, et al 1969 Alpha- and beta-thalassemia in Thailand. Annals of New York Academy of Sciences 165:60–82.

52. Routy J, Monte M, Beaulieu R, et al 1993 Increase of haemoglobin A2 in human immuno-deficiency virus-1-infected patients treated with zidovudine. American Journal of Hematology 43:86–90.

53. Howard J, Henthorn JS, Murphy S, et al 2005 Implications of increased haemoglobin A2 values in HIV positive women in the antenatal clinic, Journal of Clinical Pathology 58:556–558.

54. Felice AE 1986. The hemoglobinopathies: quantitation of fetal hemoglobin. Methods in Hematology 15:91–108.

55. Betke K, Marti HR, Schlicht L 1959 Estimation of small percentage of foetal haemoglobin. Nature 184:1877–1878.

56. Jonxis JHP, Visser HKA 1956 Determination of low percentages of fetal hemoglobin in blood of normal children. American Journal of Diseases of Children 92:588–591.

57. Chudwin DS, Rucknagel DL 1974 Immunological quantification of hemoglobins F and A2. Clinica Chimica Acta 50:413–418.

58. Makler MT, Pesce AJ 1980 ELISA assay for measurement of hemoglobin A and hemoglobin F. American Journal of Clinical Pathology 74:673–676.

59. Zago MA, Wood WG, Clegg JB, et al 1979. Genetic control of F-cells in human adults. Blood 53:977–986.

60. Kleihauer E 1974 Determination of fetal hemoglobin: elution technique. In: Schmidt RM, Huisman THJ, Lehmann H (eds) The detection of hemoglobinopathies, p.20, CRC Press, Cleveland, OH.

61. Weatherall DJ 1983 The thalassemias: haematologic methods. Methods in Haematology 6:27–30.

62. Fessas P 1963 Inclusions of hemoglobin in erythroblasts and erythrocytes of thalassemia. Blood 21:21–32.

63. White JM, Dacie JV 1971 The unstable hemoglobins ì molecular and clinical features. Progress in Hematology 7:69–102.

13 Erythrocyte and leucocyte cytochemistry

David Swirsky and Barbara J. Bain

ERYTHROCYTE CYTOCHEMISTRY

Siderocytes and Sideroblasts

Siderocytes are red cells containing granules of nonhaem iron; they were originally described by Grüneberg[1] in small numbers in the blood of normal rat, mouse, and human embryos and in large numbers in mice with a congenital anaemia. The granules are formed of a water-insoluble complex of ferric iron, lipid, protein, and carbohydrate. This siderotic material (or haemosiderin) reacts with potassium ferrocyanide to form a blue compound, ferriferrocyanide; this reaction is the basis of a positive Prussian blue (Perls') reaction. The material also stains by Romanowsky dyes and then appears as basophilic granules, which have been referred to as "Pappenheimer bodies" (Fig. 13.1).[2] By contrast, ferritin, which is a water-soluble nonhaem compound of iron with the protein apoferritin, is not detectable by Perls' reaction. Ferritin is normally present in all cells in the body, whereas, in health, haemosiderin is mainly found in macrophages in the bone marrow, liver (Kupffer cells), and spleen; when the body is overloaded with iron, as in haemochromatosis or transfusional haemosiderosis, excess iron is also found in other tissues.

Iron is transported in plasma attached to a β globulin, transferrin, and passes selectively to the bone marrow, where the iron-transferrin complex binds to transferrin receptors on the surface of the erythroblast; the iron is released from transferrin and enters the cell. Most of the iron is rapidly converted to haem partly in the cytosol and partly in the mitochondria. The nonhaem residue is in the form of ferritin. Degradation of the ferritin turns some of it into haemosiderin, which can be visualized under the light microscope as golden-yellow refractile particles in phagocytic cells; when stained by Perls' reaction, haemosiderin is blue.

In health, siderotic granules can normally be seen, in preparations stained by Perls' reaction, in the cytoplasm of many of the erythroblasts of human bone marrow and in marrow reticulocytes.[3] However, they are not normally seen in human peripheral blood red cells. After splenectomy, siderocytes can always be found in the peripheral blood, often in large numbers. The reason for this is probably because reticulocytes, after delivery from the marrow, are normally sequestered for a time in the spleen, and there they complete haem synthesis, utilizing, for this purpose, the iron stored in their cytoplasm within the siderotic granules. After splenectomy, this stage of reticulocyte maturation

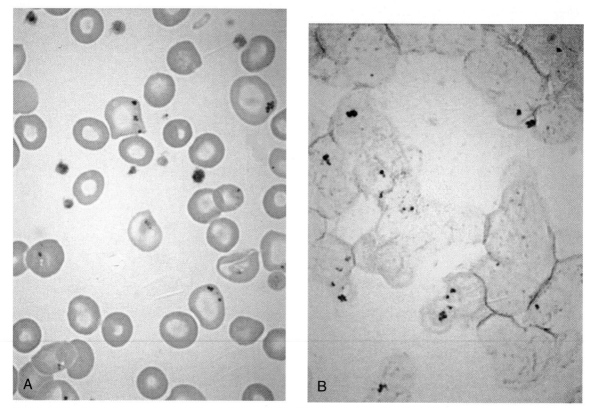

Figure 13.1 Siderotic granules and "Pappenheimer bodies." Photomicrographs of erythrocytes in a peripheral blood film from a patient with a myelodysplastic syndrome (refractory anaemia with ring sideroblasts) who had had a splenectomy showing Pappenheimer bodies: May-Grünwald–Giemsa *(A)*; and siderotic granules: Perls' reaction *(B)*.

has to take place in the bloodstream, with the result that, even in an otherwise healthy person, a small percentage of siderocytes can then be found in the peripheral blood. The spleen is also probably able to remove large siderotic granules—as may be found in disease—from red cells by a process of pitting,[4] and in its absence such granules persist in the red cells throughout their lifespan.

Method of Staining Siderotic Granules

Air dry films of peripheral blood or bone marrow and fix with methanol for 10–20 min. When they are dry, place the slides in a solution of 10 g/l potassium ferrocyanide in 0.1 mol/l HCl made by mixing equal volumes of 47 mmol/l (20 g/l) potassium ferrocyanide and 0.2 mol/l HCl immediately before use.

Leave the slides in the solution for about 10 min at about 20°C. Wash well in running tap water for 20 min, rinse thoroughly in distilled water, and then counterstain with 1 g/l aqueous neutral red or eosin for 10–15 sec. Care must be taken to avoid contamination by iron that may have been present on the slides or in staining dishes. Prepare the glassware by soaking in 3 mol/l HCl before washing (see p. 695). For quality control, a positive bone marrow film should always be stained together with the test films.

Prussian-blue staining can be applied to films that have previously been stained by Romanowsky dyes, even after years of storage. It is advisable to let the films stand in methanol overnight to remove most of the Romanowsky stain. The film should be checked before carrying out Perls' reaction to ensure that there is no residual blue staining that could obscure Prussian-blue staining. Sundberg and Bromann described a technique whereby films were stained first by a Romanowsky dye (Wright's stain) and then overstained by the acid–ferrocyanide method.[5] This can give beautiful pictures, but the small blue-stained iron-containing granules tend to be masked in young erythroblasts by the general basophilia of the cell cytoplasm. Hayhoe and Quaglino described a method for combined periodic acid–Schiff (PAS) and iron staining.[6] This may be helpful in the investigation of abnormal erythropoiesis in which the erythroblasts give a positive PAS reaction (see p. 323). A rapid method has been described for demonstrating siderotic granules by staining with 1% bromochlorphenol blue for 1 min.[7] Iron-containing granules stain dark purple.

Significance of Siderocytes

Siderocytes contain one or two (rarely many) small, unevenly distributed iron-containing granules that stain a Prussian-blue colour. There are normally a few very small scattered siderotic granules in about 40% of late erythroblasts.[3] They stain faintly and may be difficult to see by light microscopy. The percentage of erythroblasts recognizable as sideroblasts is increased in haemolytic anaemias and megaloblastic anaemias and in haemochromatosis and haemosiderosis, in proportion to the degree of saturation of transferrin (i.e., to the amount of iron available). A disproportionate increase in the percentage of erythroblasts that are sideroblasts occurs when the synthesis of haemoglobin is impaired, in which case the siderotic granules are both more numerous and larger than normal (Fig. 13.2). When there is a defect in haem synthesis, the granules are deposited in mitochondria and frequently appear to be arranged in a collar around the nucleus (Fig. 13.3) giving the "ring sideroblasts" characteristic of sideroblastic anaemias. In contrast, the distribution of the granules within the cell tends to be mainly normal in conditions in which globin synthesis alone is affected (e.g., in thalassaemia) or when there is iron overload.

There are several types of sideroblastic anaemia. These include the congenital (hereditary) type, pyridoxine (vitamin B$_6$) deficiency (rarely), sideroblastic anaemia caused by B$_6$ antagonists (e.g., drugs used in antituberculosis therapy), and secondary sideroblastic anaemia in alcoholism and lead poisoning. The presence of ring sideroblasts is a defining feature of refractory anaemia with ring

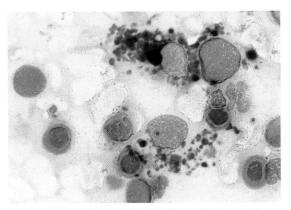

Figure 13.2   Pathological sideroblasts. Thalassaemia. There is massive accumulation of iron-containing granules in normoblasts and phagocytic cells. Perls' reaction.

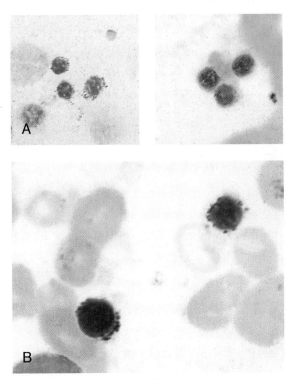

Figure 13.3   Pathological sideroblasts. Sideroblastic anaemias. Accumulation of iron-containing granules in normoblasts, arranged characteristically around the nucleus. A: Hereditary type; B: myelodysplastic syndrome. Perls' reaction.

sideroblasts[8] and refractory cytopenia with multi-lineage dysplasia and ring sideroblasts, two of the World Health Organization (WHO) categories of myelodysplastic syndrome (MDS). They may also occur in other categories of MDS. Ring sideroblasts are not uncommon in other haematological neoplasms, including idiopathic myelofibrosis and acute myeloid leukaemia (AML), particularly erythroleukaemia and the WHO categories of therapy-related AML and AML with multilineage myelodysplasia.

In sideroblastic anaemia as a feature of a haematological neoplasm, erythroblasts at all stages of maturity may be loaded with siderotic granules, whereas in the secondary sideroblastic anaemias and in the hereditary types, the more mature cells seem most affected.

In addition to the siderotic granules within erythroblasts, haemosiderin can normally be seen in marrow films as accumulations of small granules, lying free or in macrophages in marrow fragments.[9] The amount of haemosiderin will be markedly increased in patients with increased iron stores, whereas haemosiderin is absent in iron deficiency anaemia (Fig. 13.4). In practice, staining to demonstrate iron stores in marrow fragments and siderotic granules in erythroblasts is a simple and valuable diagnostic procedure and should be applied to marrow films as a routine.

In chronic infections, and in other examples of "anaemia of chronic disease," the iron stores may be increased, with much siderotic material in macrophages but little or none visible in erythroblasts. Markedly excessive iron in macrophages is also a feature of thalassaemia intermedia and major and some dyserythropoietic anaemias. Conversely, absence of iron is diagnostic of iron deficiency or iron depletion (the latter term indicating the state in

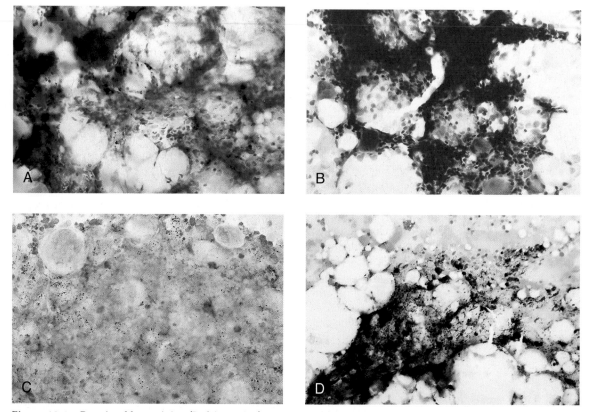

Figure 13.4 Prussian-blue staining (Perls' reaction) on aspirated bone marrow particles to demonstrate iron stores. A: normal, B: absent, C: increased, and D: grossly increased.

which storage iron is absent but anaemia is not yet evident). One study has shown that to establish the absence of stainable iron, at least seven particles must be examined, if necessary using more than one slide for this purpose.[10] There is no cytochemical method of demonstrating ferritin; methods of assay are described in Chapter 7.

Haemoglobin Derivatives

Heinz Bodies in Red Cells

Heinz, in 1890, was the first to describe in detail inclusions in red cells developing as the result of the action of acetylphenylhydrazine on the blood.[11] It is now known that Heinz bodies can be produced by the action on red cells of a wide range of aromatic nitro- and amino-compounds, as well as by inorganic oxidizing agents such as potassium chlorate. They also occur when one or other of the globin chains of haemoglobin is unstable. In man, the finding of Heinz bodies is a sign of either chemical poisoning, drug intoxication, glucose-6-phosphate dehydrogenase (G6PD) deficiency, or the presence of an unstable haemoglobin (e.g., Hb Köln). When of chemical or drug origin, Heinz bodies are likely to be visible in red cells only if the patient has been splenectomized previously or when massive doses of the chemical or drug have been taken. When owing to an unstable haemoglobin, they are rarely visible in freshly withdrawn red cells except after splenectomy. They may nevertheless develop *in vitro* in presplenectomy blood if it is incubated for 24–48 hours.[12] Heinz bodies are a late sign of oxidative damage and represent an end-product of the degradation of haemoglobin. Reviews dealing with Heinz bodies include those by Jacob[13] and by White.[14]

Demonstration of Heinz Bodies

Unstained Preparations

Heinz bodies may be seen as refractile objects in dry, unstained films, if the illumination is cut down by lowering the microscope condenser; they also can be seen by dark-ground illumination or phase-contrast microscopy. However, it is preferable to look for them in stained preparations (see below). In size they vary from 1 to 3 μm. One or more may be present in a single cell. They are usually close

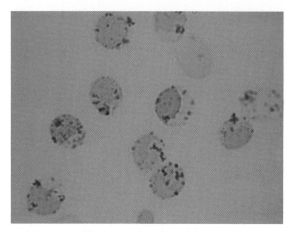

Figure 13.5 Glucose-6-phosphate dehydrogenase deficiency. Many of the cells contain large Heinz bodies. Stained supravitally by methyl violet. (Courtesy of Mr. David Roper.)

to the cell membrane and may cause a protrusion of the membrane; in wet preparations, they may move around within the cells in a slow Brownian movement.

The degradation product of an unstable haemoglobin (e.g., Hb Köln) exhibits green fluorescence when excited by blue light at 370 nm in a fluorescence microscope.[15]

Stained Preparations

Dissolve approximately 0.5 g of methyl violet in 100 ml of 9 g/l NaCl and filter. Add 1 volume of blood (in any anticoagulant) to 4 volumes of the methyl violet solution and allow the suspension to stand for about 10 min at room temperature. Then prepare films and allow them to dry or view the suspension of cells between slide and coverglass. The Heinz bodies stain an intense purple (Fig 13.5).

Heinz bodies also stain with other basic dyes. Brilliant green stains them well, and none of the stain is taken up by the remainder of the red cell.[16] Rhodanile blue (5 g/l solution in 10 g/l NaCl) stains them rapidly[17] (i.e., within 2 min), at which time reticulocytes are only weakly stained. Compared with methyl violet, Heinz bodies stain less intensely with brilliant cresyl blue or New methylene blue. Nevertheless, they may be readily seen as pale blue bodies in a well-stained reticulocyte preparation, if the preparation is not counterstained.

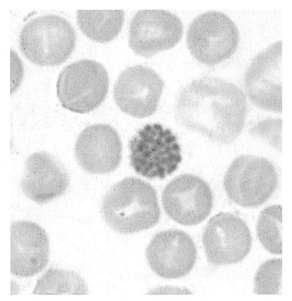

Figure 13.6   Denaturation of Hb H by brilliant cresyl blue. The round bodies consist of precipitated Hb H.

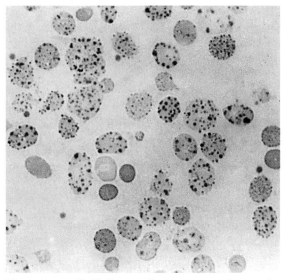

Figure 13.7   Hb H disease. Almost every erythrocyte is affected.

If permanent preparations are required, fix the vitally stained films by exposure to formalin vapour for 5–10 min. Then counterstain the fixed films with 1 g/l eosin or neutral red, after thoroughly washing in water. If films are fixed in methanol, Heinz bodies are decolourized.

In β thalassaemia major, methyl violet staining of the bone marrow will demonstrate precipitated α chains. These appear as large irregular inclusions in late normoblasts, usually single and closely adhering to the nucleus. If such patients are splenectomized, inclusions are also found in reticulocytes and mature red blood cells.

Demonstration of Haemoglobin H Inclusions

Patients with α thalassaemia, who form haemoglobin H (β_4), have red cells in which multiple blue–green spherical inclusions develop on exposure to brilliant cresyl blue or New methylene blue as in reticulocyte preparations[18] (Fig. 13.6). This is mainly a feature of haemoglobin H disease, but small numbers of similar cells may be seen in α thalassaemia trait, particularly, but not only, in α^0 thalassaemia trait.

Method

Mix together in a small tube as for staining reticulocytes (p. 36) equal volumes of fresh blood or blood

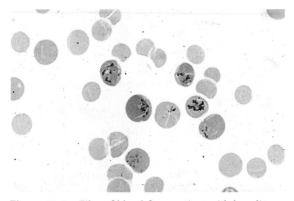

Figure 13.8   Film of blood from patient with hereditary spherocytosis. There is an increased number of reticulocytes. Stained supravitally by brilliant cresyl blue.

collected into ethylenediaminetetra-acetic acid (EDTA) and 10 g/l brilliant cresyl blue or 20 g/l New methylene blue in iso-osmotic phosphate buffer pH 7.4. Leave the preparation at 37°C for 1–3 hours, and make films at intervals during this time. Allow the films to dry, and examine them without counterstaining. Haemoglobin H precipitates as multiple pale-staining greenish-blue, almost spherical, bodies of varying size (Fig. 13.7), which can be clearly differentiated from the darker-staining reticulofilamentous material of reticulocytes (Fig. 13.8).

The number of cells containing inclusions varies according to the type of α thalassaemia. In α^0 thalassaemia trait, only 0.01–1.0% of the red cells contain inclusions, but this finding provides a significant clue to diagnosis. In haemoglobin H disease (e.g., resulting from α^0 thalassaemia/α^+ thalassaemia compound heterozygosity, $--/-\alpha\alpha$), as a rule at least 10% of the cells develop inclusions and, in some cases, the percentage is considerably greater.

When few cells are affected, they will be easier to detect in an enriched preparation.[19] Fill 2–3 capillary tubes with the blood and centrifuge for 5 min in a microhaematocrit centrifuge. Then score the tubes just below the buffy coat layer and also about 1 cm further down; break them at the score marks and carefully transfer the broken-off segments into a small tube. Add 1 drop of stain and incubate at 37°C for 3 hours before making a film.

It should be noted that a haemoglobin H preparation is not recommended when precise diagnosis of the type of α thalassaemia trait is required (e.g., in antenatal diagnosis). DNA analysis is then indicated (see p. 560).

Carboxyhaemoglobin and Methaemoglobin

Carboxyhaemoglobin- and methaemoglobin-containing cells can be demonstrated cytochemically. These methods are described by Kleihauer.[20] They have little practical value in modern practice.

Fetal Haemoglobin

An acid-elution cytochemical method that was introduced by Kleihauer et al[21] is a sensitive procedure to identify individual cells containing haemoglobin F even when few are present. Their detection in the maternal circulation has provided valuable information on the pathogenesis of haemolytic disease of the newborn.

The identification of cells containing haemoglobin F depends on the fact that they resist acid elution to a greater extent than do normal cells; thus, in the technique described in the following, they appear as isolated, darkly stained cells among a background of palely staining ghost cells. The occasional cells that stain to an intermediate degree are less easy to evaluate; some may be reticulocytes because these also resist acid elution to some extent. The following method, in which elution is carried out at pH 1.5, is recommended.[22]

Reagents

Fixative. 80% ethanol.

Elution solution. Solution A: 7.5 g/l haematoxylin in 90% ethanol. Solution B: FeCl$_3$, 24 g; 2.5 mol/l HCl, 20 ml; doubly distilled water to 1 litre.
For use, mix well 5 vols of A and 1 vol of B. The pH is approximately 1.5. The solution can be used for about 4 weeks; if a precipitate forms, the solution should be filtered.

Counterstain. 1 g/l aqueous erythrosin or 2.5 g/l aqueous eosin.

Method

Prepare fresh air-dried films. Immediately after drying, fix the films for 5 min in 80% ethanol in a Coplin jar. Then rinse the slides rapidly in water and stand them vertically on blotting paper for about 10 min to dry. Next, place the slides for 20 sec in a Coplin jar containing the elution solution. Then wash the slides thoroughly in water, and finally place them in the counterstain for 2 min. Rinse in tap water and allow them to dry in the air. Fetal cells stain red and adult ghost cells stain pale pink (Fig. 13.9). Films prepared (a) from a mixture of cord blood and adult blood and (b) from normal adult blood should be stained alongside the test films as positive and negative controls, respectively.

A number of modifications of the Kleihauer method have been proposed. In one, New methylene blue is incorporated in the buffer solution, the

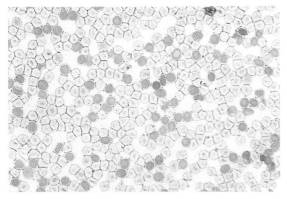

Figure 13.9   Cytochemical demonstration of fetal haemoglobin. Acid elution method. The preparation consists of a mixture of cord and normal adult blood. The darkly staining cells are fetal cells.

reaction time is prolonged, and buffer is used for washing the films.[23] The advantage of this technique is that reticulocytes stain blue, whereas cells containing haemoglobin F stain pink.

An immunofluorescent staining method has been developed based on the use of a specific antibody against haemoglobin F, which does not react with haemoglobin A.[24] By using a double-labelling procedure with rhodamine-labelled antibody against γ globin and a fluorescein-labelled antibody against β globin, it is possible to detect the presence of haemoglobin F and haemoglobin A in the same cell.[25]

Haemoglobin S and Other Haemoglobin Variants

Immunodiffusion with specific antibodies has been used for the identification of haemoglobin S, haemoglobin A_2, and haemoglobin F in red cells.[26,27] An alternative method is by detection of cells after labelling the cells with fluorescein isothiocyanate (FITC).[26] By a double-labelling method similar to that described earlier, it is possible to identify haemoglobin S as well as another haemoglobin in individual cells.

LEUCOCYTE CYTOCHEMISTRY

Leucocyte cytochemistry encompasses the techniques used to identify diagnostically useful enzymes or other substances in the cytoplasm of haemopoietic cells. These techniques are particularly useful for the characterization of immature cells in the AMLs and the identification of maturation abnormalities in the myelodysplastic syndromes and myeloproliferative disorders. There are many variations in the staining techniques, as discussed in the recommendations of an Expert Panel of the International Committee (now Council) for Standardization in Haematology.[28,29] Detailed reference works discussing the theoretical and practical aspects of cytochemistry are available.[30] The use of cytochemistry to characterise lymphoproliferative disorders has been largely superseded by immunological techniques (see Chapter 14). The results of cytochemical tests should always be interpreted in relation to Romanowsky stains and immunological techniques. Control blood or marrow slides should always be stained in parallel to ensure the quality of the staining. The principal uses of cytochemistry are as follows:

1. To characterize the blast cells in acute leukaemias as myeloid
2. To identify granulocytic and monocytic components of acute myeloid leukaemia (AML)
3. To identify unusual lineages occasionally involved in clonal myeloid disorders (e.g., basophils and mast cells)
4. To detect cytoplasmic abnormalities and enzyme deficiencies in myeloid disorders (e.g., myeloperoxidase-deficient neutrophils in myelodysplasia or acute leukaemia, neutrophil alkaline phosphatase-deficient neutrophils in chronic myeloid leukaemia [CML]).

Myeloperoxidase

Myeloperoxidase (MPO) is located in the primary and secondary granules of neutrophils and their precursors, in eosinophil granules, and in the azurophilic granules of monocytes. The MPO in eosinophil granules is cyanide resistant, whereas that in neutrophils and monocytes is cyanide sensitive. MPO splits H_2O_2, and in the presence of a chromogenic electron donor forms an insoluble reaction product. Various benzidine substitutes have been used, of which 3,3′-diaminobenzidine (DAB) is the preferred chromogen.[31,32] The reaction product is stable, insoluble, and nondiffusible. Staining can be enhanced by immersing the slides in copper sulphate or nitrate, but this is generally not required in normal diagnostic practice. Alternative nonbenzidine–based techniques use 4-chloro-1-naphthol (4CN)[33] or 3-amino-9-ethylcarbazole.[34] The former gives very crisp staining but is soluble in some mounting media and immersion oil; the latter shows some diffusibility and does not stain as strongly as DAB.

Method with 3,3′-Diaminobenzidine

Reagents

Fixative. Buffered formal acetone (BFA) (p. 692).

Substrate. 3,3′-DAB (Sigma D-8001).*

Buffer. Sorensen's phosphate buffer pH 7.3 (p. 692).

Hydrogen peroxide (H_2O_2, 30% w/v.).

Counterstain. Aqueous haematoxylin.

---

*This and all other Sigma products from Sigma-Aldrich.

Method

1. Fix air-dried smears for 30 sec in cold BFA.
2. Rinse thoroughly in gently running tap water and air dry.
3. Incubate for 10 min in working substrate solution. Thoroughly mix 30 mg DAB in 60 ml buffer, add 120 μl H_2O_2, and mix well.
4. Counterstain with haematoxylin for 1–5 min, rinse in running tap water, and air dry.

Technical Considerations

MPO is not inhibited by heparin, oxalate, or EDTA anticoagulants. Films should be made within 12 hours of blood collection. Staining is satisfactory on slides kept at room temperature for at least a week. The DAB should be stored frozen at −20°C in 1 ml aliquots of 30 mg in 1 ml of buffer. For optimum results, it is essential to dissolve the DAB thoroughly in the buffer and to ensure the reagents in the incubation mixture are well mixed. The stain is robust and not strictly pH dependent, with identical results being obtained when using buffers ranging in pH from 7.0 to 9.0. The counterstaining time should be adjusted to the minimum time to give clear nuclear detail. Methyl green is an alternative counterstain, giving excellent contrast with the DAB reaction product, but nuclear detail is more difficult to discern.

Results and Interpretation

The reaction product is brown and granular (Fig. 13.10A). Red cells and erythroid precursors show diffuse brown cytoplasmic staining. The most primitive myeloblasts are negative, with granular positivity appearing progressively as they mature toward the promyelocyte stage. The positivity may be localized to the Golgi region. Promyelocytes and myelocytes are the most strongly staining cells in the granulocyte series, with positive (primary) granules packing the cytoplasm. Metamyelocytes and neutrophils have progressively fewer positive (secondary) granules. Eosinophil granules stain strongly, and the large specific eosinophil granules are easily distinguished from neutrophil granules. Eosinophil granule peroxidase is distinct biochemically and immunologically from neutrophil peroxidase. Monoblasts and monocytes may be negative or positive. When positive, the granules are smaller than in neutrophils and diffusely scattered

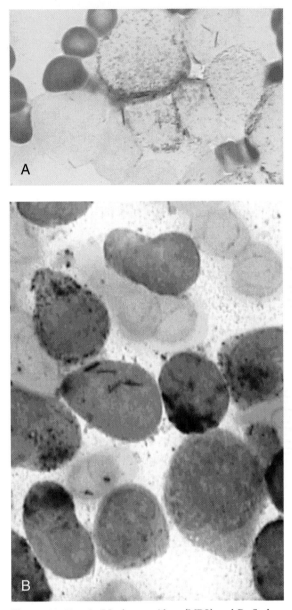

Figure 13.10   A: Myeloperoxidase (MPO) and B: Sudan black B (SBB). Bone marrow in acute myeloid leukaemia (FAB M1). Myeloperoxidase staining shows Auer rods and cytoplasmic granular staining, whereas with SBB localised positive reaction in the blast cells is more definite and Auer rods are prominent.

throughout the cytoplasm. MPO activity is present in basophil granules but is not demonstrable in mature basophils by the DAB reaction described earlier.

Pathological Variations

Rare individuals have congenital deficiency of neutrophil MPO. All stages of the neutrophil lineage, from the myeloblast onward, are negative. In these individuals, the eosinophils stain normally. Other individuals have an MPO deficiency confined to eosinophils or monocytes. Dysplastic neutrophils may be MPO negative. Auer rods stain well with DAB and are seen more frequently on MPO staining than on Romanowsky-stained films.

Sudan Black B

Sudan black B (SBB) is a lipophilic dye that binds irreversibly to an undefined granule component in granulocytes, eosinophils, and some monocytes. It cannot be extracted from the stained granules by organic dye solvents and gives comparable information to that of MPO staining.[35] The currently used staining solution is essentially that described by Sheehan and Storey.[36]

Reagents

Fixative. 40% formaldehyde solution.

Stain. SBB (Sigma No. S 2380) 0.3 g in 100 ml absolute ethanol.

Phenol buffer. Dissolve 16 g crystalline phenol in 30 ml absolute ethanol. Add to 100 ml distilled water in which 0.3 g $Na_2HPO_4.12H_2O_2$ has been dissolved.

Working stain solution. Add 40 ml buffer to 60 ml SBB solution.

Counterstain. May–Grünwald–Giesma or Leishman stain (see p. 63).

Method

1. Fix air-dried smears in formalin vapour as follows. Place a small square of filter paper in the bottom of a Coplin jar. Add 2 drops of 40% formalin, put on the lid, and leave for 15 min to allow vaporization. Place the slides in the Coplin jar and replace the lid. After 5–10 min, remove the slides and stand on end for 15 min to "air wash."
2. Immerse the slides in the working stain solution for 1 hour in a Coplin jar with a lid on.
3. Transfer slides to a staining rack and immediately flood with 70% alcohol. After 30 sec, tip the 70% alcohol off and flood again for 30 sec. Repeat three times in total.
4. Rinse in gently running tap water and air dry.
5. Counterstain without further fixation with Leishman stain or May–Grünwald–Giemsa.

Technical Considerations

Buffered formol acetone fixation for 30 sec is a satisfactory alternative to formalin vapour. The working stain solution should be replaced after 4 weeks. Bone marrow smears with fatty spicules containing lipid-soluble SBB benefit from a 5-sec swirl in xylene followed by rinsing in running tap water and air drying prior to counterstaining. The Romanowsky counterstain gives excellent cytological detail of all cells present.

Results and Interpretation

The reaction product is black and granular. The results are essentially similar to those seen with MPO staining, both in normal and leukaemic cells (Fig. 13.10B and 13.15B). MPO-negative neutrophils are also SBB negative. The only notable difference is in eosinophil granules, which have a clear core when stained with SBB. Rare cases (1–2%) of acute lymphoblastic leukaemia (ALL) show nongranular smudgy positivity not seen with MPO staining.[37] Basophils are generally not positive but may show bright red/purple metachromatic staining of the granules.

Neutrophil Alkaline Phosphatase

Alkaline phosphatase activity is found predominantly in mature neutrophils, with some activity in metamyelocytes. Although demonstrated as a granular reaction product in the cytoplasm, enzyme activity is associated with a poorly characterized intracytoplasmic membranous component distinct from primary or secondary granules.[38] Other leucocytes are generally negative, but rare cases of lymphoid malignancies show cytochemically demonstrable activity.[39] Bone marrow macrophages are positive. Early methods of demonstrating alkaline phosphatase relied on the use of glycerophosphate or other phosphomonoesters as the substrate at alkaline pH, with a final black reaction product of lead sulphide.[40] Azo-dye techniques are simpler, giving equally good results. These methods use substituted naphthols as the substrate, and it is the liberated naphthol rather than phosphate that is used to combine with the azo-dye to give the final reaction product.[41-43]

Reagents

Fixative. 4% formalin methanol. Add 10 ml 40% formalin to 90 ml methanol. Keep at −20°C or in the freezer compartment of a refrigerator. Discard after 2 weeks.

Substrate. Naphthol AS phosphate (Sigma N-5625). Store in freezer.

Buffer. 0.2 mol/l Tris buffer pH 9.0 (see p. 692).

Stock substrate solution. Dissolve 30 mg naphthol AS phosphate in 0.5 ml N,N-dimethylformamide (Sigma D-4551). Add 100 ml 0.2 mol/l Tris buffer, pH 9.1. Store in a refrigerator at 2–4°C. The solution is stable for several months.

Coupling azo-dye. Fast Blue BB salt (Sigma F-0250). Store in freezer.

Counterstain. Neutral red, 0.02% aqueous solution.

Method

1. Fix freshly made air-dried blood films for 30 sec in cold 4% formalin methanol.
2. Rinse with tap water and air dry.
3. Prepare working substrate solution by allowing 40 ml of stock substrate solution to warm to room temperature. Add 24 mg of Fast Blue BB and mix thoroughly until dissolved. Incubate slides for 15 min.
4. Wash in tap water and air dry.
5. Counterstain for 3 min in 0.02% aqueous neutral red, rinse briefly, and air dry.

Technical Considerations

N,N-dimethylformamide may dissolve some types of plastic; therefore a glass tube should be used to dissolve the substrate. Blood films should be made soon after blood collection, preferably within 30 min because neutrophil alkaline phosphatase (NAP) activity decreases rapidly in EDTA-anticoagulated blood. Once spread, the blood film should be stained within 6 hours. Control films with a predictably high score (see later)—for example, from a patient with reactive neutrophilia or a pregnant woman—should be made, if possible, from fresh blood samples also. The technical aspects of blood film preparation and the effects of fixation on NAP activity are discussed by Kaplow.[44] The normal range for healthy adults should be established in individual laboratories using a standard staining technique and consistent scoring criteria (see later).

Results and Interpretation

The reaction product is blue and granular. The intensity of reaction product in neutrophils varies from negative to strongly positive, with coarse granules filling the cytoplasm and overlying the nucleus (Fig. 13.11). An overall score is obtained by assessing the stain intensity in 100 consecutive neutrophils, with each neutrophil scored on a scale of 1–4 as follows:

0 Negative, no granules
1 Occasional granules scattered in the cytoplasm
2 Moderate numbers of granules
3 Numerous granules
4 Heavy positivity with numerous coarse granules crowding the cytoplasm, frequently overlying the nucleus

The overall possible score will range between 0 and 400 per 100 cells. Reported normal ranges show

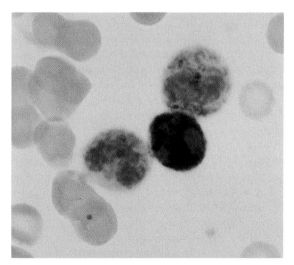

Figure 13.11   Neutrophil alkaline phosphatase. A strongly positive (4+) and moderately positive (3+ and 2+) intensity of reaction are shown.

some variations, owing possibly in part to variations in scoring criteria and methodology: 13–160 (mean 61)[44]; 14–100 (mean 46)[45]; 37–98 (mean 68)[46]; 11–134 (mean 48).[47] A normal range should therefore be established in each laboratory.

In normal individuals, it is rare to find any neutrophils with a score of 3, and a score of 4 should not be present. There is some physiological variation in NAP scores. Newborn babies, children, and pregnant women have high scores, and premenopausal women have, on average, scores one-third higher than those of men.[38] In pathological states, the most significant diagnostic use of the NAP score is in CML. In the chronic phase of the disease, the score is almost invariably low, usually zero. Transient increases may occur with intercurrent infection. In myeloid blast transformation or accelerated phase, the score rises. Low scores are also commonly found in paroxysmal nocturnal haemoglobinuria (PNH) and the very rare condition of hereditary hypophosphatasia. There are many causes of a raised NAP score, notably in the neutrophilia of infection, polycythaemia vera, leukaemoid reactions, and Hodgkin's disease. In aplastic anaemia, the NAP score is high, but it falls if PNH supervenes. With the greater use of cytogenetic and molecular genetic techniques to confirm the diagnosis of CML, the NAP score is needed much less often.

Acid Phosphatase Reaction

Cytochemically demonstrable acid phosphatase is ubiquitous in haemopoietic cells. The staining intensity of different cell types is somewhat variable according to the method used. Its main diagnostic use is in the diagnosis of T-cell ALL and hairy cell leukaemia.[48,49] These diseases are more reliably diagnosed and characterised by immunophenotyping when this is available (see Chapter 14). The unmodified acid phosphatase stain is now largely redundant but the tartrate-resistant acid phosphatase stain is still useful for confirmation of the diagnosis of hairy cell leukaemia when immunophenotyping is not available. The pararosaniline method given in the following section, modified from Goldberg and Barka,[50] is recommended for demonstrating positivity in T lymphoid cells. Use of Fast Garnet GBC as coupler may be preferred for the demonstration of tartrate-resistant acid phosphatase activity.[28,49]

Reagents

Fixative. Methanol, 10 ml; acetone, 60 ml; water, 30 ml; and citric acid, 0.63 g. Adjust to pH 5.4 with 1 mol/l NaOH before use.

Buffer pH 5.0. Sodium acetate trihydrate, 19.5 g, sodium barbiturate, 29.5 g, water to 1 litre (Michaeli's veronal acetate buffer).

Substrate solution. 25 mg naphthol AS-BI phosphate (Sigma N 2125) dissolved in 2.5 ml N,N-dimethylformamide.

Sodium nitrite. 4% $NaNO_2$ aqueous solution.

Coupling reagent.

1. Stock pararosaniline. Dissolve 1 g pararosaniline (Sigma No. P-7632) in 25 ml warm 2 mol/l HCl. Filter when cool. Store at room temperature in the dark. Stable for 2 months.
2. 4% sodium nitrite solution. Dissolve 200 mg sodium nitrite in 5 ml distilled water. Stable for 1 week at 4–10°C.
3. Hexazotised pararosaniline. Mix equal volumes of pararosaniline and 4% sodium nitrite together 2 min before use.

Counterstain. 1% Aqueous methyl green or aqueous haematoxylin.

Tartaric acid L(+) (Sigma T1807).

Working solution A. Mix 92.5 ml of buffer with 2.5 ml of substrate solution. Add 32.5 ml of distilled water and then add 4 ml of hexazotised pararosaniline. Mix well, and adjust pH to 5.0 using 1 mol/l NaOH.

Working solution B. Add 375 mg of crystallin L(+)-tartaric acid to 50 ml of working solution A; the final concentration is then 50 mmol/l.

Method

1. Air dry films for several hours (24 hours if possible).
2. Fix for 10 min in methanol/acetone/citric acid, rinse in tap water, and air dry.
3. Incubate for 1 hour at 37°C in working solutions A (acid phosphatase reaction) or incubate 2 films in working solutions A and B, respectively (tartrate-resistant acid phosphatase reaction).
4. Rinse in tap water and air dry.

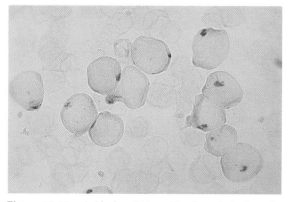

Figure 13.12   Acid phosphatase. T-cell acute leukaemia with intense localised staining.

5. Counterstain in 1% aqueous methyl green or aqueous haematoxylin for 5 min.
6. Rinse in tap water and mount wet in warmed glycerin jelly.

Results and Interpretation

The reaction product is red with a mixture of granular and diffuse positivity (Fig. 13.12). In T cells, acid phosphatase is an early differentiation feature. Almost all acute and chronic T-lineage leukaemias show strong activity. In T-lineage ALL, the activity is usually highly localized (polar). Granulocytes are strongly positive. Monocytes, eosinophils, and platelets show variable positivity. In the bone marrow, macrophages, plasma cells, and megakaryocytes are strongly positive.

In hairy cell leukaemia the majority of leukaemic cells react equally positively in the presence and absence of tartaric acid (Fig. 13.13).

When immunophenotyping is available, the unmodified acid phosphatase reaction is redundant. If a full range of appropriate monoclonal antibodies is available, the acid phosphatase reaction is also redundant.

Periodic Acid-Schiff Reaction

Periodic acid specifically oxidizes 1–2 glycol groups to produce stable dialdehydes. These dialdehydes give a red reaction product when exposed to Schiff's reagent (leucobasic fuchsin). Positive reactions occur with carbohydrates, principally glycogen, but also monosaccharides, polysaccharides, glyco-

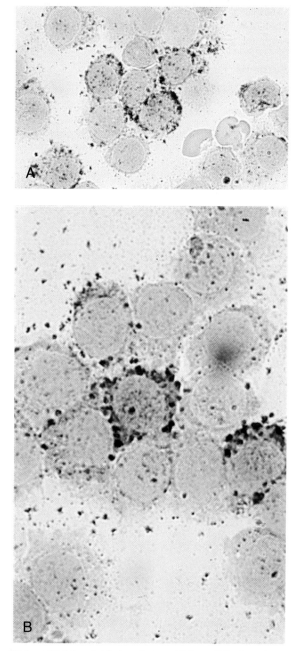

Figure 13.13   Acid phosphatase. Hairy cell leukaemia acid phosphatase *(A)* and tartrate-resistant acid phosphatase *(B)*.

proteins, mucoproteins, phosphorylated sugars, inositol derivatives, and cerebrosides.[51] Glycogen can be distinguished from other positively reacting substances by its sensitivity to diastase digestion. In haemopoietic cells, the main source of positive reactions is glycogen.

Reagents

Fixative. Methanol.

1% periodic acid. $HIO_4.2H2O$, 10 g/l in distilled water.

Schiff's reagent. Dissolve 5 g basic fuchsin in 500 ml of hot distilled water. Filter when cool. Saturate with SO_2 gas by bubbling for 1–12 hours in a fume cupboard. Shake vigorously with 2 g activated charcoal for 1 min in a conical flask in a fume cupboard and filter immediately through a large Whatman No. 1 filter into a dark bottle. The reagent is stable for 6 months at room temperature, stored in the dark.

Counterstain. Aqueous haematoxylin.

Method

1. Fix films for 15 min in methanol.
2. Rinse in gently running tap water and air dry.
3. If required, expose fixed control films to digestion in diastase (100 mg in 100 ml of 0.9 g/l NaCl) for 20–60 min at room temperature.
4. Flood slides with 1% periodic acid for 10 min.
5. Rinse in running tap water for 10 min and air dry.
6. Immerse in Schiff's reagent for 30 min in a Coplin jar with a lid (the Schiff's reagent can be returned to the stock bottle).
7. Rinse in running tap water for 10 min and air dry.
8. Counterstain in aqueous haematoxylin for 5–10 min.

Technical Considerations

Formalin vapour (5 min), formalin/ethanol (10 ml 40% formalin/90 ml ethanol) (10 min), or buffered formalin acetone (45 s) are satisfactory alternative fixatives. Previously fixed, iron-stained, or Romanowsky-stained smears can be overstained with the PAS reaction satisfactorily. Romanowsky-stained smears can be partly decolourized by soaking in methanol for 1 hour prior to step 4. The intensity of the reaction product depends on the quality of the Schiff's reagent. Normal neutrophils should always stain intensely red, and deterioration

of the Schiff's reagent can be detected by examination of control normal films. Some methods recommend rinsing in a dilute sodium metabisulphite HCl solution ("SO_2 water") after step 6, but this is not necessary with good-quality Schiff's reagent.

Results and Interpretation

The reaction product is red, with intensity ranging from pink to bright red (Figs. 13.14 and 13.15C). Cytoplasmic positivity may be diffuse or granular. Granulocyte precursors show diffuse weak positivity, with neutrophils showing intense confluent granular positivity. Eosinophil granules are negative, with diffuse cytoplasmic positivity. Basophils may be negative but often show large irregular blocks of positive material not related to the granules. Monocytes and their precursors show variable diffuse positivity with superimposed fine granules, often at the periphery of the cytoplasm. Normal erythroid precursors and red cells are negative. Megakaryocytes and platelets show variable, usually intense, diffuse positivity with superimposed fine granules, coarse granules, and large blocks. Of peripheral lymphocytes, 10–40% show granular positivity with negative background cytoplasm, with no detectable differences between T and B cells.[52,53] When immunophenotyping is available, the PAS reaction is redundant for the diagnosis of ALL. It can still be useful in AML and MDS to identify abnormal erythroblasts and dysplastic megakaryocytes and to demonstrate the cytoplasmic blush that helps to confirm a diagnosis of acute promyelocytic leukaemia.

Esterases

Leucocyte esterases are a group of enzymes that hydrolyse acyl or chloroacyl esters of α-naphthol or naphthol AS. Li et al[54] identified nine esterase isoenzymes using polyacrylamide gel electrophoresis of leucocyte extracts from normal and pathological cells. The gels were stained in parallel with cell smears. The isoenzymes fell into two groups: bands 1, 2, 7, 8, and 9 corresponded to the "specific" esterase of neutrophils, staining specifically with naphthol AS-D chloroacetate esterase (chloroacetate esterase, CAE), whereas bands 3, 4, 5, and 6 corresponded to "nonspecific" esterase (NSE), staining with α-naphthyl acetate esterase (ANAE) and α-

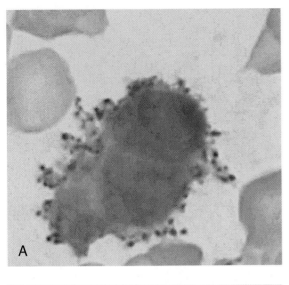

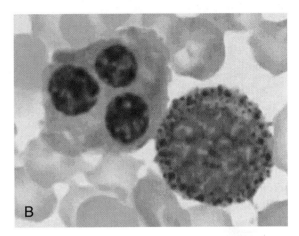

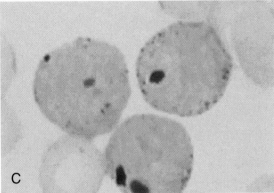

Figure 13.14   Periodic acid–Schiff stain. A: Dysplastic micromegakaryocytes with diffuse cytoplasmic staining and some coarse granules; B: dyserythropoiesis with diffuse staining in a trinucleate normoblast and coarse granular and diffuse staining in a proerythroblast; and C: acute lymphoblastic leukaemia with blasts showing block positivity.

naphthyl butyrate esterase (butyrate esterase, ANBE). Band 4 was best demonstrated by ANBE and band 5 by ANAE. The NSEs are inhibited by sodium fluoride (NaF). Naphthol AS acetate and naphthol AS-D acetate react with both specific and nonspecific esterases, but only the reaction with the NSEs is inhibited by NaF. The methods using parallel slides with and without NaF are not generally used anymore because it is usually more informative to perform a combination of chloroacetate esterase and one of the "nonspecific" esterase stains on a single slide. The combined methods have the advantage of demonstrating pathological double staining of individual cells. All the esterase stains can be performed using a variety of coupling reagents, each of which gives a different coloured reaction product. The methods outlined as follows have been chosen for their simplicity and reliability.

Naphthol AS-D Chloroacetate Esterase[28]

Reagents

Fixative. Buffered formal acetone (p. 692).

Buffer. 66 mmol/l phosphate buffer pH 7.4 see p. 691.

Naphthol AS-D chloroacetate substrate solution. Dissolve 0.1 g of naphthol AS-D chloracetate (Sigma N-0758) in 40 ml N,N-dimethyl-formamide (Sigma D-4254). Keep refrigerated.

Working substrate solution. Add 2 ml of naphthol AS-D chloroacetate stock solution to 38 ml of

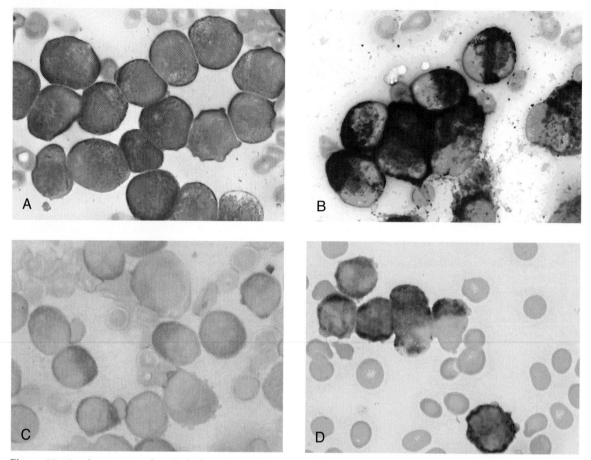

Figure 13.15   Acute promyelocytic leukaemia. A: May–Grünwald–Giemsa stain shows hypergranular promyelocytes with scattered Auer rods; B: Sudan black B with strongly stained cytoplasm; C: Periodic acid–Schiff staining shows diffuse cytoplasmic blush; and D: Chloroacetate esterase gives strong cytoplasmic staining.

66 mmol/l phosphate buffer pH 7.4. Mix well. Add 0.4 ml of freshly prepared hexazotised New fuchsin. Mix well.

Coupling reagent.

1. Hexazotised New fuchsin. Dissolve 4 g of New fuchsin in 100 ml of 2N HCl.
2. Sodium nitrite solution 0.3 mol/l. Dissolve 2.1 g of sodium nitrite ($NaNO_2$) in 100 ml of water.
3. Immediately prior to using, add 0.2 ml of the hexazotised New fuchsin to 0.4 ml sodium nitrite, mix well, and leave for 1 min before adding to substrate solution.

Counterstain. Aqueous haematoxylin

Method

1. Fix air-dried smears in cold buffered formalin acetone for 30 sec.
2. Rinse in gently running tap water and air dry.
3. Immerse the slides in the working substrate solution in a Coplin jar for 5–10 min.
4. Rinse in running tap water and air dry.
5. Counterstain in aqueous haematoxylin for 1 min.
6. "Blue" in running tap water for 1 min and air dry.

Technical Considerations

The CAE stain is robust and reliable. A satisfactory alternative to New fuchsin is 40 mg of Fast blue BB, but it requires thorough vigorous mixing with the substrate solution. The incubation time is important because most haemopoietic cells show some scattered granular staining if the incubation is prolonged. Hydrolysis of the substrate is rapid, with staining virtually complete within 3–5 min.

Results and Interpretation

The reaction product is bright red (Fig. 13.15D). It is confined to cells of the neutrophil series and mast cells. Cytoplasmic CAE activity appears as myeloblasts mature to promyelocytes. Positivity in myeloblasts is rare, but promyelocytes and myelocytes stain strongly, with reaction product filling the cytoplasm. Later cells stain strongly but less intensely. It is therefore useful as a marker of cytoplasmic maturation in myeloid leukaemias. In acute promyelocytic leukaemia, the cells show heavy cytoplasmic staining. The characteristic multiple Auer rods stain positively, often with a hollow core. It is rare to see CAE-positive Auer rods in other forms of AML except in cases with the t(8;21) translocation.[55]

α-Naphtyl Butyrate Esterase

Reagents

Fixative. Buffered formalin acetone.

Buffer. 100 mmol/l Phosphate buffer (Sorensen's) pH 8.0.

Substrate stock solution. α-Naphthyl butyrate (Sigma N-8125) 100 µl in 5 ml acetone. The solution should be stored at –20°C and is stable for at least 2 months.

Coupling reagent. Fast Garnet GBC (Sigma F 8761) 15 mg.

Counterstain. Aqueous haematoxylin.

Method

1. Fix air-dried smears in buffered formalin acetone for 30 sec. Rinse in gently running tap water and air dry.
2. Add the Fast Garnet GBC to 50 ml buffer and mix well.
3. Add 0.5 ml of the α-naphthyl butyrate/acetone solution and mix well.
4. Pour the incubation medium into a Coplin jar containing the fixed slides and incubate for 20–40 min.
5. Rinse thoroughly by running tap water into the Coplin jar until clear.
6. Air dry and counterstain in aqueous haematoxylin for 1–5 min.

Technical Considerations

The reaction product is soluble in immersion oil and synthetic mounting media. If slides are to be looked at repeatedly, they should be mounted in an aqueous mounting medium (e.g., Apathy's gum-arabic mountant or glycerin/gelatin). There may be batch-to-batch variation of the Fast Garnet GBC. Staining can be controlled by removing the control slide from the incubation medium after 20 min and examining it wet under a low-power (e.g., ×20) objective, returning it to the incubation medium while still wet. When the monocytes show as dark brown, staining is complete. Hexazotised pararosaniline is an alternative coupling reagent, which gives an insoluble brown reaction product and is suitable for mounting in synthetic mounting media.[54]

Results and Interpretation

The reaction product is brown and granular (Fig. 13.16). The majority of monocytes (>80%) stain strongly, the remainder showing some weak staining. Negative monocytes are rare. Neutrophils, eosinophils, basophils, and platelets are negative. B lymphocytes are negative and T lymphocytes are unreliably stained. In the bone marrow, monocytes, monocyte precursors, and macrophages stain

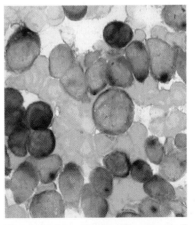

Figure 13.16 Nonspecific esterase. Positive *(brown)* reaction in acute monocytic leukaemia (FAB M5).

strongly. α-Naphthyl butyrate is more specific for identifying a monocytic component in AML than α-naphthyl acetate (see later).

α-Naphthyl Acetate Esterase

Reagents

Fixative. Buffered formalin acetone.

Buffer. 66 mmol/l phosphate buffer pH 6.3.

Substrate solution. Dissolve 100 mg α-naphthyl acetate (Sigma N-8505) in 5 ml ethylene monomethyl ether. Store at 4–10°C.

Coupling reagent.

1. Stock pararosaniline. Dissolve 1 g pararosaniline (Sigma No. P-7632) in 25 ml warm 2 mol/l HCl. Filter when cool. Store at room temperature in the dark. Stable for 2 months.
2. 4% sodium nitrite solution. Dissolve 200 mg sodium nitrite in 5 ml distilled water. Keep stable for 1 week at 4–10°C.
3. Hexazotised pararosaniline. Mix equal volumes of pararosaniline and 4% sodium nitrite together 1 min before use.

Incubation medium. Add 2 ml of the α-naphthyl acetate solution to 38 ml of the 66 mmol/l phosphate buffer pH 6.3 and mix well. Add 0.4 ml of freshly prepared hexazotised pararosaniline and mix well.

Counterstain. Aqueous haematoxylin.

Method

1. Fix air-dried smears in cold buffered formalin acetone for 30 sec.
2. Rinse in running tap water and air dry.
3. Immerse the slides for 30–60 min in the incubation medium in a Coplin jar.
4. Rinse in gently running tap water in the Coplin jar until clear and air dry.
5. Counterstain in aqueous haematoxylin for 2–5 min.

Technical Considerations

Fast Blue BB 80 mg can be substituted as a coupling reagent. This gives a dark green/brown granular reaction product, which is soluble in mounting media and immersion oil. The haematoxylin staining time should be adjusted to give clear nuclear detail without overstaining to obscure nucleoli and chromatin texture.

Results and Interpretation

The reaction product is diffuse red/brown in colour. Normal and leukaemic monocytes stain strongly. Normal granulocytes are negative, but in myelodysplasia or AML may give positive reactions of varying intensity. Megakaryocytes stain strongly, and leukaemic megakaryoblasts may show focal or diffuse positivity. Most T lymphocytes and some T lymphoblasts show focal "dotlike" positivity, but immunophenotyping has superseded cytochemistry for identifying and subcategorising T cells. Leukaemic erythroblasts may show focal or diffuse positivity.

Sequential Combined Esterase Stain Using ANAE and CAE

Reagents

As earlier.

Method

1. Follow the method and steps 1–4 listed earlier for α-naphthyl acetate stain, rinse in tap water, and air dry.
2. Without further fixation, prepare the naphthol AS-D chloroacetate incubation medium as explained previously, substituting 10 mg Fast Blue BB (Sigma No. F 0250) for hexazotised New fuchsin, and incubate for 10 min.
3. Rinse in tap water and counterstain with aqueous haematoxylin for 1–3 min.

Technical Considerations

Fast Blue BB is relatively insoluble, and the chloroacetate incubation medium should be mixed vigorously before use.

Results and Interpretation

The ANAE gives a brown reaction product, and the CAE gives a granular bright blue product (Fig. 13.17). Staining patterns are identical to those seen with the two stains used separately. The double-staining technique avoids the need to compare results from separate slides and reveals aberrant staining patterns. In myelomonocytic leukaemias, cells staining with both esterases may be present. In myelodysplasia and AML with dysplastic granulo-

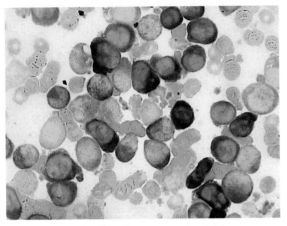

Figure 13.17   Combined esterase stain. Acute myelomonocytic leukaemia with almost equal numbers of chloroacetate esterase *(blue)* and nonspecific esterase *(brown)* positive cells.

cytes, double staining of individual cells may be present. This may be helpful when the diagnosis MDS is not otherwise certain, but the same abnormal pattern may be seen in nonclonal dysplastic states such as megaloblastic anaemia.

Single Incubation Double Esterase (Naphthol AS-D Choloroacetate and α-Naphthyl Butyrate)[56]

Reagents

Fixative. Buffered formalin acetone.

Buffer. 100 mmol/l phosphate buffer pH 8.0 (Sorensen's).

Substrates.

1. 2.5 mg naphthol AS-D chloroacetate (Sigma N-0758) in 1 ml acetone.
2. 4 mg α-naphthyl butyrate (Sigma N-8000) in 1 ml acetone.

Coupling reagent. Fast Blue BB salt (Sigma No. F-0250).

Counterstain. Aqueous haematoxylin.

Method

1. Fix air-dried smears in buffered formalin acetone for 30 sec.
2. Rinse in tap water and air dry.

3. Dissolve 80 mg Fast Blue BB in 50 ml phosphate buffer by vigorous mixing.
4. Add naphthol AS-D chloroacetate and mix well.
5. Add α-naphthyl butyrate and mix well.
6. Incubate slides for 10–15 min in a Coplin jar in the dark.
7. Flush the Coplin jar with running tap water until clear.
8. Air dry the slides.
9. Counterstain in aqueous haematoxylin for 1 min, rinse, and air dry.

Technical Considerations

Steps 4 and 5 should be carried out rapidly. Staining can be extended to 30 min if necessary to ensure maximal ANBE staining, but at longer incubation times some nonspecific granular CAE staining may occur.

Results and Interpretation

The CAE reaction product is bright blue (granulocytes); the ANBE product is dark green/brown (monocytes). ANBE does not stain megakaryocytes or T cells as strongly as α-naphthyl acetate. Lam et al suggest the use of hexazotised pararosaniline as coupling reagent in a single incubation combined esterase, which gives contrasting bright red and brown reaction products.[57]

In AML, the stain is useful for identifying monocytic and granulocytic components.

Toluidine Blue Stain

Toluidine blue staining is useful for the enumeration of basophils and mast cells. It binds strongly to the granules in these cells and is particularly useful in pathological states in which the cells may not be easily identifiable on Romanowsky stains. In AML, CML, and other myeloproliferative disorders, basophils may be dysplastic and poorly granular, as may the mast cells in some forms of acquired mastocytosis.

Reagents

Toluidine blue 1% w/v in methanol. Add 1 g of toluidine blue (BDH 34077) to 100 ml methanol and mix for 24 hours on a roller or with a magnetic flea. The stain is stable indefinitely at room temperature. Keep tightly stoppered.

Method

1. Place air-dried smears on a staining rack and flood with the toluidine blue solution.
2. Incubate for 5–10 min.
3. Rinse briefly in gently running tap water until clear, and air dry.

Results and Interpretation

The granules of basophils and mast cells stain a bright red/purple and are discrete and distinct (Fig. 13.18). Nuclei stain blue and cells with abundant RNA may show a blue tint to the cytoplasm. Although toluidine blue is said to be specific for these granules, with >10 min incubation, the primary granules of promyelocytes are stained red/purple. However these are smaller and finer than the mast cell or basophil granules and easily distinguished.

Cytochemical Reactions and Leukaemia Classification

Myelodysplastic Syndromes and Acute Myeloid Leukaemia

MDS is an acquired clonal preleukaemic bone marrow disorder characterized largely by a cellular or hypercellular marrow, peripheral cytopenias, and variable morphological abnormalities of the haemo-poietic cells. The classification system proposed by the French–American–British (FAB) cooperative group

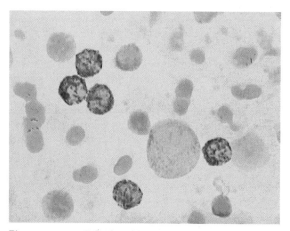

Figure 13.18   Toluidine blue. Chronic myeloid leukaemia in accelerated phase. There are five strongly positive basophils.

in 1982[58] was widely used for many years but is now being superseded by the WHO classification (see Chapter 23). A Perls' reaction for haemosiderin is essential for the demonstration of ring sideroblasts. Other cytochemical evidence of dysplasia includes double staining of cells with chloroacetate and ANAE, the presence of SBB- or MPO-negative neutrophils, and the presence of Auer rods (SBB and MPO).

In AML, cytochemistry is helpful in defining monocytic cells (ANAE and ANBE), identifying Auer rods, and demonstrating dysplasia (as mentioned earlier).

Acute Lymphoblastic Leukaemia

The modern diagnosis and classification of ALL is by cytology, followed by immunophenotyping (see Chapter 14). If immunophenotyping is not available, cytochemistry remains important. It should be noted that, on Romanowsky staining, lymphoblasts may rarely contain fine azurophil granules. However, Auer rods are never seen and MPO and CAE are negative, whether or not fine granules are present. Occasionally granules give a weak reaction with SBB. Although not lineage specific, the pattern of any PAS positivity may be helpful.[30] In ALL, 95% of cases of show positive blocks or granules of bright red PAS-positive material. This may be present in very few blasts (<1%) or the majority. The critical difference from granular or block positivity in other leukaemic cells is the glass-clear background cytoplasm in lymphoblasts. Myeloblasts, monoblasts, leukaemic erythroblasts, and megakaryoblasts all show some degree of diffuse cytoplasmic positivity, and occasionally block positivity is seen. Acid phosphatase staining is more likely to give focal positivity in T-cell than B-cell acute leukaemias, but the difference is not clear enough to be of diagnostic certainty and focal positivity is sometimes also seen in the erythroblasts of erythroleukaemia. Esterase staining is generally unhelpful; some T-cell cases show focal positivity with ANAE, but this is not specific.

Chronic Myeloproliferative Disorders

Although low NAP scores are typical in chronic phase CML and high scores are usually found in other myeloproliferative disorders, the finding of a high NAP score is too nonspecific to be of diagnostic help.

Chronic Lymphoproliferative Disorders

Chronic lymphoproliferative disorders are now characterised by immunophenotyping. The reactions for acid hydrolases (acid phosphatase, ANAE, β-glucuronidase, and β-glucosaminidase) show focal positivity in most T-cell disorders but are negative in B-cell disorders. The tartrate-resistant acid phosphatase reaction for hairy cell leukaemia is the only cytochemical stain that is sufficiently specific to still be regarded as diagnostically useful (in the absence of immunophenotyping).

REFERENCES

1. Grüneberg H 1941 Siderocytes: a new kind of erythrocyte. Nature (London) 148:114–115.
2. Pappenheimer AM, Thompson KP, Parker DD, et al 1945 Anaemia associated with unidentified erythrocytic inclusions after splenectomy. Quarterly Journal of Medicine 14:75–100.
3. Kaplan E, Zuelzer WW, Mouriquand C 1954 Sideroblasts: a study of stainable nonhemoglobin iron in marrow normoblasts. Blood 9:203–213.
4. Crosby WH 1957 Siderocytes and the spleen. Blood 12:165–170.
5. Sundberg RD, Bromann H 1955 The application of the Prussian blue stain to previously stained films of blood and bone marrow. Blood 10:160–166.
6. Hayhoe FGJ, Quaglino D 1960 Refractory sideroblastic anaemia and erythraemic myelosis: possible relationship and cytochemical observations. British Journal of Haematology 6:381–387.
7. Kass L, Eickholt MM 1978 Rapid detection of ringed sideroblasts with bromchlorphenol blue. American Journal of Clinical Pathology 70:738–740.
8. Bennett JM 1986 Classification of the myelodysplastic syndromes. Clinics in Haematology 15:909–923.
9. Rath CE, Finch CA 1948 Sternal marrow hemosiderin: a method for the determination of available iron stores in man. Journal of Laboratory and Clinical Medicine 33:81–86.
10. Hughes DA, Stuart-Smith SE, Bain BJ 2004 How should stainable iron in bone marrow films be assessed? Journal of Clinical Pathology 57:1038–1040.
11. Heinz R 1890 Morphologische Veränderungen der rother Blutkörperchen durche Gifte. Virchows Archiv 122:112.
12. Dacie JV, Grimes AJ, Meisler A, et al 1964 Hereditary Heinz-body anaemia: a report of studies on five patients with mild anaemia. British Journal of Haematology 10:388–402.
13. Jacob HS 1970 Mechanisms of Heinz body formation and attachment to red cell membrane. Seminars in Hematology 7:341–354.
14. White JM 1976 The unstable haemoglobins. British Medical Bulletin 32:219–222.
15. Eisinger J, Flores J, Tyson JA, et al 1985 Fluorescent cytoplasm and Heinz bodies of hemoglobin Köln erythrocytes: evidence for intracellular heme catabolism. Blood 65:886–893.
16. Schwab MLL, Lewis AE 1969 An improved stain for Heinz bodies. American Journal of Clinical Pathology 51:673.
17. Simpson CF, Carlisle JW, Mallard L 1970 Rhodanile blue: a rapid and selective stain for Heinz bodies. Stain Technology 45:221–223.
18. Gouttas A, Fessas Ph, Tsevrenis H, et al 1955 Description d'une nouvelle variété d'anémie hémolytique congénitale. Sang 26:911–919.
19. Lin CK, Gau JP, Hsu HC, et al 1990 Efficacy of a modified technique for detecting red cell haemoglobin H inclusions. Clinical and Laboratory Haematology 12:409–415.
20. Kleihauer E, Betke K 1963 Elution procedure for the demonstration of methaemoglobin in red cells of human blood smears. Nature (London) 199:1196–1197.
21. Kleihauer E, Braun H, Betke K 1957 Demonstration von fetalem Hämoglobin in den Erythrocyten eines Blutausstrichs. Klinische Wochenschrift 35:637–638.
22. Nierhaus K, Betke K 1968 Eine vereinfachte Modifikation der säuren Elution für die cytologische Darstellung von fetalem Hämoglobin. Klinische Wochenschrift 46:47.
23. Clayton EM, Felhaus WD, Phythyon JM 1963 The demonstration of fetal erythrocytes in the presence of adult red blood cells. American Journal of Clinical Pathology 40:487–490.
24. Tomoda Y 1964 Demonstration of foetal erythrocytes by immunofluorescent staining. Nature (London) 202:910–911.
25. Thorpe SJ, Huehns EG 1983 A new approach for the antenatal diagnosis of β-thalassaemia: a double labelling immunofluorescence microscopy technique. British Journal of Haematology 53:103–112.
26. Headings V, Bhattacharya S, Shukla S, et al 1975 Identification of specific hemoglobins within individual erythrocytes. Blood 45:263–271.

27. Papayannopoulou Th, McGuire TC, Lim G, et al 1976 Identification of haemoglobin S in red cells and normoblasts using fluorescent anti-Hb antibodies. British Journal of Haematology 34:25–31.

28. Shibata A, Bennett JM, Castoldi GL, et al 1985 Recommended methods for cytological procedures in haematology. Clinical and Laboratory Haematology 7:55–74.

29. International Council for Standardization in Haematology 1993 Procedures for the classification of acute leukaemias. Leukemia and Lymphoma 11:37–48.

30. Hayhoe FGJ, Quaglino D 1988 Haematological cytochemistry, 2nd ed. Churchill Livingstone, Edinburgh.

31. Graham RC, Karnovsky MJ 1966 The early stages of absorption of injected horseradish peroxidase in the proximal tubules of mouse kidney: ultrastructural cytochemistry by a new technique. Journal of Histochemistry and Cytochemistry 14:291–302.

32. Novikoff AB, Goldfischer S 1969 Visualization of peroxisomes (microbodies and mitochondria with diaminobenzidine). Journal of Histochemistry and Cytochemistry 17:675–680.

33. Elias JM 1980 A rapid sensitive myeloperoxidase stain using 4-chloro-1-naphthol. American Journal of Clinical Pathology 73:797–799.

34. Graham RC, Lundholm U, Karnovsky MJ 1965 Cytochemical demonstration of peroxidase activity with 3-amino-9-ethylcarbazole. Journal of Histochemistry and Cytochemistry 13:150–152.

35. Lillie RD, Burtner HJ 1953 Stable sudanophilia of human neutrophil leucocytes in relation to peroxidase and oxidase. Journal of Histochemistry and Cytochemistry 1:8–26.

36. Sheehan HL, Storey GW 1974 An improved method of staining leucocyte granules with Sudan Black B. Journal of Pathology and Bacteriology 49:580.

37. Stass SA, Pui C-H, Mel Vin S, et al 1984 Sudan black B positive acute lymphoblastic leukaemia. British Journal of Haematology 57:413–421.

38. Rosner F, Lee SL 1965 Endocrine relationships of leukocyte alkaline phosphatase. Blood 5:356–369.

39. Poppema S, Elema JD, Halie MR 1981 Alkaline phosphatase positive lymphomas: a morphologic, immunologic and enzyme histochemical study. Cancer 47:1303–1312.

40. Gomori G 1952 Microscopic histochemistry: principles and practice. University of Chicago Press, Chicago.

41. Kaplow LS 1955 A histochemical procedure for localizing and evaluating leucocyte alkaline phosphatase activity in smears of blood and marrow. Blood 10:1023–1029.

42. Kaplow LS 1963 Cytochemistry of leukocyte alkaline phosphatase: use of complex naphthol AS phosphates in azo-dye coupling technics. American Journal of Clinical Pathology 39:439–449.

43. Rustin GJS, Wilson PD, Peters TJ 1979 Studies on the subcellular localisation of human neutrophil alkaline phosphatase. Journal of Cell Science 36:401–412.

44. Kaplow LS 1968 Leukocyte alkaline phosphatase cytochemistry: applications and methods. Annals of the New York Academy of Sciences 155:911.

45. Hayhoe FGJ, Quaglino D 1958 Cytochemical demonstration and measurement of leucocyte alkaline phosphatase in normal and pathological states by modified azo-dye coupling technique. British Journal of Haematology 4:375–389.

46. Rutenberg AB, Rosales CL, Bennett JM 1965 An important histochemical method for the demonstration of leukocyte alkaline phosphatase activity: clinical applications. Journal of Laboratory and Clinical Medicine 65:698–705.

47. Bendix-Hansen K, Helleberg-Rasmussen I 1985 I. Evaluation of neutrophil alkaline phosphatase: untreated myeloid leukaemia, lymphoid leukaemia and normal humans. Scandinavian Journal of Haematology 34:264–269.

48. Yam LT, Li CY, Lam KW 1971 Tartrate-resistant acid phosphatase isoenzyme in the reticulum cells of leukemic reticuloendotheliosis. New England Journal of Medicine 284:357.

49. Li CY, Yam LT, Lam KW 1970 Acid phosphatase isoenzyme in human leucocytes in normal and pathologic conditions. Journal of Histochemistry and Cytochemistry 18:473–481.

50. Goldberg AF, Barka T 1962 Acid phosphatase activity in human blood cells. Nature 195:297.

51. Hotchkiss RD 1948 A microchemical reaction resulting in the staining of polysaccharide structures in fixed tissue preparations. Archives of Biochemistry 16:131–141.

52. Higgy KE, Burns GF, Hayhoe FGJ 1977 Discrimination of B, T and null lymphocytes by esterase cytochemistry. Scandinavian Journal of Haematology 18:437–438.

53. Quaglino D, Hayhoe FGJ 1959 Observations on the periodic acid-Schiff reaction in lymphoproliferative diseases. Journal of Pathology and Bacteriology 78:521–532.

54. Li CY, Yam LT, Lam KW 1973 Esterases in human leucocytes. Journal of Histochemistry and Cytochemistry 21:1.

55. Swirsky DM, Li YS, Matthews JG, et al 1983 Translocation in acute granulocytic leukaemia: cytological, cytochemical and clinical features. British Journal of Haematology 56:199–213.

56. Swirsky DM 1984 Single incubation double esterase cytochemical reaction using a single coupling reagent. Journal of Clinical Pathology 37:1187–1190.

57. Lam KW, Li CY, Yam LT 1985 Simultaneous demonstration of non-specific esterase and chloro-acetate esterase in human blood cells. Stain Technology 60:169–172.

58. Bennett JM, Catovsky D, Daniel M-T, et al 1982 Proposals for the classification of the myelodysplastic syndromes. British Journal of Haematology 51:189–199.

14 Immunophenotyping

Estella Matutes, Ricardo Morilla, and Daniel Catovsky

INTRODUCTION

Since the development of the hybridoma technology in the 1970s, there have been major advances in the immunophenotypic characterization of haemopoietic malignancies, and this, in turn, has resulted in a better understanding of normal haemopoietic differentiation. Prior to the availability of monoclonal antibodies (McAbs), it was possible to distinguish B from T lymphocytes and from early lymphoid precursor cells by the expression of surface or cytoplasmic immunoglobulins in B lymphocytes; the ability to form rosettes with sheep erythrocytes (E-rosettes) in T lymphocytes; and the expression of the nuclear enzyme, terminal deoxynucleotidyl transferase (TdT), in lymphoid precursors. Over the last two decades, the application of new technology has had a major impact on the diagnosis of acute and chronic leukaemias, has provided clues to the pathogenesis of these disorders, and has made possible monitoring small numbers of residual leukaemic cells. Beyond its diagnostic value, some chimeric McAbs, such as those recognising the CD20, CD52, and CD33 antigens, are used *in vivo* as therapeutic tools; therefore, their estimation in the leukaemic cells has become an important clinical issue.

In addition to the availability of a large number of McAbs that identify antigens in haemopoietic cells that are lineage-specific or are restricted to particular levels of differentiation, a number of immunological techniques have been developed that permit the following:

1. Detection of both membrane and cytoplasmic or nuclear antigens by flow cytometry in previously fixed and stabilized cells
2. Simultaneous double, triple, and quadruple immunostaining with directly labelled McAb with different fluorochromes
3. Analysis of whole blood or bone marrow specimens without requiring the separation of mononuclear cells
4. Quantification of the number of molecules of an antigen at a single-cell level
5. Analysis or quantification of selected cell populations, such as the estimation of CD34 stem cells by applying gating strategies using CD45-labelled cells

Although the important diagnostic role of immunophenotyping is well-recognised, results should always be interpreted in the light of morphology and other relevant clinical and laboratory data.

This chapter includes descriptions of the following:

1. Techniques currently used for immunophenotyping
2. Panels of markers useful for the diagnosis of acute leukaemia and chronic lymphoproliferative disorders and the rationale for their selection
3. Immunophenotypic profiles that characterize the different types of acute leukaemias and chronic lymphoproliferative disorders
4. New McAbs (e.g., against the tumour-suppressor gene product p53, CD38, ZAP-70, and cyclin D1), which are relevant for prognosis and differential diagnosis between lymphoid disorders
5. Strategies to detect minimal residual disease (MRD) by immunophenotyping

METHODS FOR THE STUDY OF IMMUNOLOGICAL MARKERS

There are several ways of testing cell markers:

1. Flow cytometry to test suspensions of viable cells or fixed cells
2. Immunocytochemistry to examine cells on cytospin-made slides or directly on blood or bone marrow films
3. Immunohistochemistry to study cells in frozen or paraffin-embedded sections from bone marrow biopsy specimens or other haemopoietic tissues

The first two methods are used in haematology laboratories dealing with analysis of leukaemic samples, and the last is used, as a rule, in histopathology laboratories.

Preparation of the Specimens and Cell Separation

Immunophenotyping can be performed on isolated mononuclear cells as described later in the chapter or on whole blood specimens using lysing solutions.

The mononuclear cell fraction contains lymphocytes, monocytes, blasts, and other mononuclear cells (according to the sample). Methods for separating mononuclear cells include density gradient centrifugation with Ficoll-Triosil, Hypaque, or Lymphoprep. When necessary, platelets can also be excluded by defibrinating the blood before separation.

Lymphoprep Method of Separation (Nycomed)

Dilute 10 ml of anticoagulated (e.g., heparinised or ethylenediaminetetra-acetic acid [EDTA]-anticoagulated) blood with an equal volume of phosphate buffered saline (PBS), pH 7.3 (p. 691) or Hanks' solution. Add 10 ml of the diluted blood, drop by drop, to 7.5 ml of Lymphoprep and then centrifuge for 30 min at 2000 rpm (approximately 500 g; see p. 695). There are three layers visible: a layer of mononuclear cells in the middle and red cells and neutrophils at the bottom. After removing the plasma, pipette the mononuclear cell layer into another tube and wash three times with Hanks' solution or tissue culture medium.

Lysing Method

Blood and bone marrow samples are treated with a hypotonic erythrocyte lysing solution of commercial NH_4Cl^- bases containing reagents. These are often supplied by the manufacturers of McAb (e.g., FACS lysing solution, BD Biosciences). The samples are treated at the time of incubation with the McAb (see below) without loss of fractions of mononuclear cells. The time of incubation with the lysing reagent is important because prolonged exposure may alter the forward and side light scatter (FSC/SSC) patterns, whereas exposure that is too brief leaves red cells intact, resulting in excess debris and inaccurate results.

Prior to incubation with the lysing solution, the white cell count of the blood or bone marrow specimen should be estimated and, if necessary, the sample should be diluted to a maximum white cell concentration of $25–30 \times 10^6$ cells/ml.

Flow Cytometry Methods

Immunophenotyping on cell suspensions is the method for detecting membrane antigens in viable cells and cytoplasmic and nuclear antigens in previously fixed and stabilized cells. If a flow cytometer is not available, reading can also be performed by fluorescence microscopy. Both flow cytometry and fluorescence microscopy permit simultaneous detection of membrane and nuclear or cytoplasmic antigens by means of double or triple immunostaining.

Detection of Membrane Antigens

Direct Immunofluorescence

For direct immunofluorescence (double staining) (Fig. 14.1) label tubes with the name of the patient,

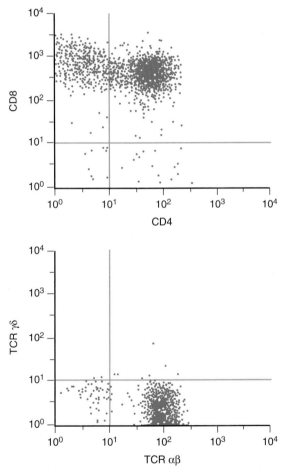

Figure 14.1   Double direct immunofluorescence staining. **Upper:** Dot plot showing the coexpression of CD4 and CD8 in cells from a case of T-cell prolymphocytic leukaemia. **Lower:** Dot plot showing that the majority of lymphocytes express in the membrane the T-cell receptor (TCR) αβ complex and are negative with McAb against the TCR γδ complex.

type of specimen, laboratory number, and the combination of fluorochrome-conjugated McAb including isotopic controls. The latter are mouse immunoglobulin (Ig) of the same isotope as the McAb but with no antigen specificity.

Pipette 100 μl of the specimen (whole peripheral blood or bone marrow) into a tube.

Add the appropriate McAb combination labelled with fluorescein (FITC), phycoerythrin (PE), or a third colour tamden dye (Cy5.PE) for instruments with one laser with excitation at 488 nm. There are more than a dozen fluorochromes that can be used for immunophenotyping, and indeed, some analyses use 11 colours. The limitations on which fluorochromes can be used will depend on the number of lasers available and detectors in the instrument. The volume of the McAb ranges from 5 to 20 μl, according to the manufacturer's instructions.

Incubate at room temperature for 15 min.

Add 1 ml of lysing solution (commercially available from the manufacturer) and leave for 10 min at room temperature. Centrifuge for 5 min at 2000 rpm and discard the supernatant.

Add 2 ml of PBS (pH 7.3) containing 0.02% sodium azide, 0.02% bovine serum albumin (BSA), and 0.01% EDTA (PBS-azide-BSA). Centrifuge for 5 min at 2000 rpm and discard supernatant.

Add 2 ml of PBS-azide-BSA or Hanks' solution, centrifuge for 5 min at 2000 rpm, and discard the supernatant.

Resuspend the cells in 0.2–0.5 ml of sheath fluid solution (e.g., Isoton, Beckman Coulter).

Read on a flow cytometer or by fluorescence microscopy after mounting the cells on a slide.

Indirect Immunofluorescence (Single Staining)

Label tubes with the name of the patient, type of specimen, laboratory number, and the McAb.

Add 100 μl of the specimen (whole blood or bone marrow).

Add the appropriate McAb (first layer nonlabelled antibody). The volume ranges from 5 to 20 μl, according to the manufacturer's instructions. Incubate at room temperature for 15 min.

Add 2 ml of PBS-azide-BSA or Hanks' solution and centrifuge for 5 min at 2000 rpm.

Discard supernatant and repeat this step once more.

Following the manufacturer's instructions, add the appropriate volume and concentration of the second layer, which is usually a goat or a rabbit antimouse Ig F(ab)2 fragment.

Incubate for 15 min at room temperature.

Add 1 ml of lysing solution (commercially available from the McAb manufacturer) for 10 min at room temperature. Centrifuge for 5 min at 2000 rpm and discard the supernatant.

Add 2 ml of PBS-azide-BSA, centrifuge for 5 min at 2000 rpm, and discard the supernatant after centrifugation.

Resuspend the cells in 0.25–0.5 ml of sheath fluid solution (e.g., Isoton) provided by the manufacturer.

Read on a flow cytometer or by fluorescence microscopy.

Detection of Surface Immunoglobulin

Surface Ig heavy and light chains can be detected by means of double or triple immunostaining. The object is to demonstrate clonality of a B-cell population. Double staining uses double colour conjugated polyclonal anti-kappa and anti-lambda labelled with different fluorochromes in a single tube (Fig. 14.2) or combines a FITC-labelled B-cell marker (e.g., CD19) and a PE-labelled anti-light chain, either anti-kappa or anti-lambda. The triple colour immunostaining combines a FITC-conjugated anti-kappa, PE-conjugated anti-lambda, and a B-cell marker (e.g., CD19) labelled with a third colour in a single tube.

The immunostaining of surface Ig differs from the method used to detect other surface antigens by McAb. The reason is that soluble serum Ig coats the surface of cells, mainly monocytes but also lymphocytes, and interferes with the detection of Ig, giving rise to misleading results, either false positive or false negative. To overcome this problem, cells have to be washed with Hanks' solution or PBS prior to incubating with the anti-kappa and anti-lambda reagents.

There are two methods suitable for detecting surface Ig in blood and bone marrow cells, according to whether a PBS wash or a lysing procedure is used as the first step.

Method 1 (PBS Wash as First Step, No Lysing)

Label tubes with the name of the patient, type of specimen, laboratory number, and the McAb.

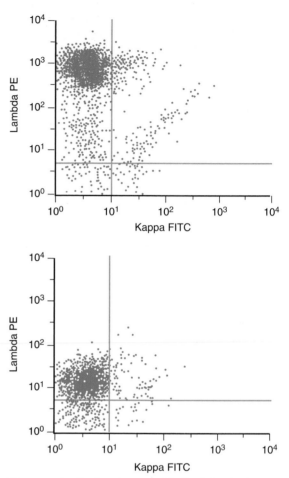

Figure 14.2 Surface immunoglobulin light chain staining. **Upper:** Dot plot showing strong expression of lambda light chain in a case of follicular lymphoma. **Lower:** By contrast to the upper case, weak/dim expression of lambda light chain in a case of chronic lymphocytic leukaemia. Cells are negative with anti-kappa in both cases.

Pipette 100 μl of the specimen (blood or bone marrow) into a tube.

Add 2 ml of PBS-azide-BSA kept at 37°C and centrifuge for 5 min at 2000 rpm. Using a pipette, carefully discard the supernatant. Repeat the procedure and resuspend the specimen in 50 μl of PBS-azide-BSA.

Add the appropriate McAb combination, e.g., anti-kappa and anti-lambda or CD19 and anti-kappa. The volume of the McAb is usually between 5 and 20 μl, according to the manufacturer's instructions.

Incubate at room temperature for 15 min.

Add 1 ml of lysing solution (commercially available from most McAb manufacturers) and incubate for 10 min at room temperature.

Add 1 ml of PBS-azide-BSA or Hanks' solution, centrifuge for 5 min at 2000 rpm, and discard the supernatant. Repeat this step.

Resuspend cells in 0.2–0.5 ml of sheath fluid solution (e.g., Isoton).

Read on a flow cytometer or by fluorescence microscopy.

Method 2 (Lysing as First Step)

Label tubes with the name of the patient, type of specimen, laboratory number, and the McAb.

Pipette 100 µl of the specimen (whole blood or bone marrow).

Add 2 ml of lysing solution, incubate for 10 min at room temperature, and wash twice in PBS-azide-BSA.

Add the appropriate volume of McAb combination, according to the manufacturer's recommendations.

Incubate for 15 min at 4°C. Add 2 ml of PBS-azide-BSA or Hanks' solution, centrifuge for 5 min at 2000 rpm, and discard the supernatant. Repeat this step.

Resuspend cells in 0.2–0.5 ml of sheath fluid (e.g., Isoton) and read on a flow cytometer.

Detection of Intracellular Antigens

There are several commercially available kits containing solutions to fix and stabilize cells to detect cytoplasmic or nuclear antigens. Overall, these reagents have little or no effect on the light scatter pattern, although their reliability and consistency for detecting particular nuclear and cytoplasmic antigens may vary.[1,2]

The kits contain two solutions: solution A is the fixing agent based on a paraformaldehyde solution and solution B is a stabilising agent based on a combination of a lysing solution and a detergent.

The methods follow the manufacturer's kit instructions. Details that follow are for the method using Fix and Perm (Caltag, Burlingame, CA, USA).

Method

Label tubes with the name of the patient, type of specimen, laboratory number, and the McAb.

Pipette 100 µl of the specimen (whole blood or bone marrow) into a tube.

Add 100 µl of solution A (fixative) and incubate at room temperature for 15 min.

Wash twice in PBS-azide-BSA by centrifuging for 5 min at 2000 rpm.

Add 100 µl of solution B (stabilising agent) and the appropriate amount of fluorochrome-conjugated McAb.

Incubate at room temperature for 15 min.

Wash twice in PBS-azide-BSA, centrifuging for 5 min at 2000 rpm.

Resuspend in 0.2–0.5 ml of sheath fluid solution (e.g., Isoton).

Read on a flow cytometer.

Simultaneous Detection of Cytoplasmic/Nuclear and Membrane Antigens

Method

The first step in simultaneous detection of cytoplasmic/nuclear and membrane antigens (Fig. 14.3) involves immunostaining for detecting the membrane antigen, followed by cytoplasmic or nuclear antigen detection.

Label tubes with the name of the patient, type of specimen, laboratory number, and the McAb.

Pipette 100 µl of specimen (whole blood or bone marrow) into a tube.

Add the appropriate fluorochrome-conjugated McAb, usually PE, to detect the membrane antigen.

Incubate at room temperature for 15 min.

Add 15 µl of solution A (fixative) and incubate at room temperature for 15 min. Continue with the steps described earlier.

Add 1 ml of PBS-azide-BSA or Hanks' solution, centrifuge for 5 min at 2000 rpm, and discard the supernatant.

Multicolour Flow Cytometry

Advances in flow cytometry hardware and software and the development of new dyes have resulted in the routine use of multicolour and multiparametric flow cytometry. This approach has advantages over double and triple colour measurements in the detection of minimal residual disease in acute myeloid leukaemia (AML) and in acute lymphoblastic

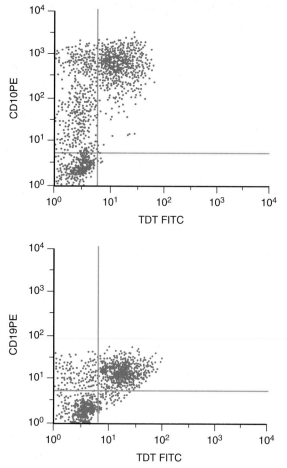

Figure 14.3   Simultaneous detection of membrane and nuclear antigens. **Upper:** Dot plot illustrating the coexpression of CD10 in the cell membrane and nuclear terminal deoxynucleotidyl transferase (TdT) in chronic lymphocytic leukaemia (CLL). **Lower:** Coexpression of membrane CD19 and nuclear TdT in the same case.

leukaemia (ALL) (e.g., using CD45/CD19/CD10 and TdT), the enumeration of the proportion of clonal plasma cells in multiple myeloma, and the detection in the leukaemic cells of certain molecules that are widely expressed in normal blood cells (e.g., ZAP-70 in chronic lymphocytic leukaemia).

Quantification of Antigens

Quantification is defined as the measurement of the intensity of staining of cells by flow cytometry to provide an absolute value for the light intensity it measures.[3,4]

Quantification of fluorescence is performed by comparing cell fluorescence with an external standard. By using different commercially available beads, it is now possible to measure the quantity of fluorescence relative to the peak channel obtained by flow cytometry using a standard curve for its calculation. Fluorescence quantification can be expressed in terms of antibody binding capacity (ABC) or molecules equivalent soluble fluorochrome (MESF).

The method involves either indirect immunofluorescence or direct immunofluorescence. Because the latter is simpler, it is the method generally used in routine practice. It comprises four separate steps:

1. Choice of quantification kit
2. Staining of cells and beads
3. Acquisition of data
4. Quantification—calculation of the ABC or MESF values

There are three essential requirements for successful quantification, namely (a) the McAb has to be applied at saturating amounts both for the beads and the cells in the specimen; (b) the same reagent from a specified company and at the same dilution should be used for the test and for any subsequent tests; and (c) the instrument fluorescence setting should be maintained unchanged once the beads have been run, and analysis of the unknown sample should be carried out at the same settings.

The type of bead depends on the procedure used for the sample preparation. The beads are commercially available in kits, which usually comprise two tubes. One tube contains four types of beads with four different levels of fluorescence uptake: one very dim, one very bright, and two intermediate; the other tube contains a blank (e.g., nonfluorescent beads) (Fig. 14.4).

1. Choice of Quantification Kit

Direct Immunofluorescence
QSC (Quantum Simply Cellular, Sigma-Aldrich) are beads coated with goat antimouse Ig that are used to quantify direct immunofluorescence and to measure the ABC when saturated with the same fluorochrome-conjugated McAb as used in the cell

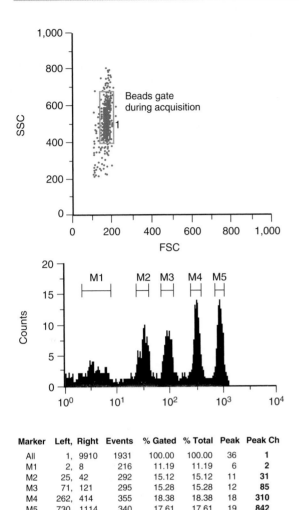

Marker	Left, Right	Events	% Gated	% Total	Peak	Peak Ch
All	1, 9910	1931	100.00	100.00	36	1
M1	2, 8	216	11.19	11.19	6	2
M2	25, 42	292	15.12	15.12	11	31
M3	71, 121	295	15.28	15.28	12	85
M4	262, 414	355	18.38	18.38	18	310
M5	730, 1114	340	17.61	17.61	19	842

Figure 14.4 Beads for antigen quantification. **Upper:** Gate used for the acquisition of the beads to eliminate doublets. **Lower:** Beads fluorescence intensity showing five peaks: blank (M1); dim (M2); bright (M5); and intermediate (M3 and M4).

sample. Each level of the standard can bind to a certain amount of mouse Ig. The beads require separate calibration for each McAb.

Indirect Immunofluorescence

QIFIKIT (Dako Cytomation) are beads coated with McAb that mimic McAb-bearing cells. Because these receptors bind to the secondary antibody used to stain both the cells and the beads they require only one calibration per experiment.[4]

Direct and Indirect Immunofluorescence

FCSC (Quantum beads) (Bangs Laboratories, Indiana, USA) are coated with known molecules of fluorochrome and are available conjugated to FITC or PE to measure the MESF. The fluorescence of the cells is compared to that of standard molecules of fluorochrome.

2. Staining of Cells and Beads

After the quantification beads have been set up, begin the staining of cells by one of the methods described in the following section, depending on the antigen to be quantified. This could be a membrane, nuclear or cytoplasmic antigen, or combinations of two of them.

Direct Immunofluorescence

Label a 5 ml round-bottom tube as the McAb to be quantified with beads.

Add 50 μl of QSC beads and 10 μl of the McAb to the appropriate tubes and incubate for 1 hour at 4°C.

Add 2 ml of PBS-azide-BSA to each tube and centrifuge for 5 min at 2000 rpm. Discard the supernatant and resuspend in 250 μl of sheath fluid (e.g., Isoton).

Indirect Immunofluorescence

Label a 5 ml round-bottom tube as beads.

Add 100 μl of beads and the secondary antibody (antimouse Ig) to the tube with the beads and stain for 1 hour at 4°C.

Add 2 ml of PBS-azide-BSA to each tube and centrifuge for 5 min at 2000 rpm. Discard the supernatant and resuspend in 250 μl of Isoton.

Direct and Indirect Immunofluorescence

Label a 5 ml round-bottom tube as Quantum beads.

Add 100 μl of beads and stain for 1 hour at 4°C.

Then add 2 ml of PBS-azide-BSA to each tube and centrifuge for 5 min at 2000 rpm.

Discard the supernatant and resuspend in 250 μl of sheath fluid (e.g., Isoton).

3. Acquisition of Data

The first step involves acquisition of data relating to the beads on a flow cytometer. The data from a single tube with beads are sufficient for quantification with FCSC Quantum beads and QIFIKIT beads. With QSC, where a tube is run for each McAb, the tube with the beads for that particular McAb should be run first followed by all the relevant tubes with beads for each of the different McAbs.

To bring the beads into the FSC/SSC dot plot, the SSC voltage must be decreased more than for cells. There may be some doublets if the tube is not shaken vigorously, and these are excluded by placing a tight gate around the beads and acquiring the data only for these gated beads. The instrument should be set up so that the fluorescence signal of the tube with the blank (unlabelled) beads is located in the region between 0 and 10^1 and four other peaks of fluorescence are seen along the axis of the relevant fluorochrome. When the fluorescence voltage is established, these settings should be maintained throughout the rest of the analysis of the unknown samples. With QSC, the appropriate settings for each individual McAb must be used.

The data for the samples are then obtained. With the FCSC Quantum Cellular and QIFIKIT, only one set of beads is required because the same fluorescence standard curve can be used for the different McAbs to be quantified (e.g., CD5, CD19, CD4, CD8). With QSC, one set of fluorescence beads is stained for each McAb. The samples for a particular McAb should be run with the fluorescence settings obtained from beads stained with the corresponding McAb, so that one fluorescence standard curve should be obtained for each McAb. Thus, one curve is required with CD5-stained beads for all CD5-stained samples; one curve is required with CD19-stained beads for CD19-stained samples, and so on.

4. Quantification: Calculation of ABC or MESF Values

Relevant software is provided with the quantification kits. These programs are user friendly and take into account the make of the instrument, the voltage used for the sample, the fluorochrome used, and the source of the McAb. When the data obtained from the flow cytometer are entered, a standard curve is automatically produced. The standard calibration curve is produced when the values of the peak channels of the blank and the other four peaks obtained from the flow cytometer are entered into the program. The known number of molecules of fluorochrome obtained from the supplier of the beads is also entered into the program. The peak values for the unknown sample and one of the negative control samples are obtained by running them at the same fluorescence setting as the beads. When the peak value obtained with the sample is entered into the program, the ABC/MESF value of the unknown sample is calculated and the data are saved. For the final estimation of the ABC or MESF, the ABC or MESF value of the control tube is subtracted from the ABC or MESF value of the marker.

Immunocytochemistry

The most common immunocytochemical techniques are the immunoperoxidase (IP) and the alkaline phosphatase antialkaline phosphatase (APAAP) methods.[5,6] These detect both membrane and intracellular antigens prior to fixation of the preparation. The APAAP method is suitable for use on blood and bone marrow films and permits good preservation of cell morphology. IP is simpler than APAAP and is useful for the study of mature and immature lymphoid cells, but bone marrow samples containing myeloid cells with endogenous peroxidase may give a false-positive reaction unless steps are taken to inhibit the endogenous peroxidase activity. Unfortunately, these procedures may affect cell morphology and thus defeat one of the purposes of the test.

Immunoperoxidase

The IP method can be carried out with directly labelled antibodies (e.g., antihuman Ig conjugated with peroxidase) or by indirect methods using two or three layers. The first layer is a McAb (mouse Ig); the second layer is an antimouse Ig antibody conjugated with horseradish peroxidase; a third layer is a complex of peroxidase and antiperoxidase, which binds to the second layer and is used to reinforce the reaction. The reaction is completed by testing for peroxidase, using diaminobenzidine (DAB).

Method

Prepare cytocentrifuge slides and allow them to dry for at least 6–8 hours at room temperature. If not used immediately, they should be wrapped in aluminium foil and stored at −20°C. Before testing, frozen material must be thawed at room temperature for 30 min. Make a ring around the chosen area using a diamond pencil.

Fix the slides in pure acetone for 10 min. If they have been kept at room temperature for more than 3 days, fix them for only 5 min.

Dry in air and then surround the marked area with a silicone ring (Dako pen* or Sigmacote**).

Incubate for 30 min in a moist chamber with 30 μl of McAb diluted in PBS. The dilution of the McAb should be titrated in the individual laboratory for each batch of reagent, using known positive and negative controls.

Wash (flush) carefully with PBS (pH 7.3). Without allowing the slides to dry, add the second layer antibody immediately after the second wash.

Incubate for 30 min with 30 μl of peroxidase-conjugated rabbit antimouse Ig antibody (Dako) diluted 1:20 in PBS (pH 7.3) containing 2% human AB serum.

Wash (flush) carefully with PBS (pH 7.3) twice as indicated earlier.

Incubate for 30 min in a moist chamber with 30 μl of peroxidase-labelled swine antirabbit antibody (Dako) diluted 1:20 in PBS (pH 7.3) containing 2% human AB serum.

Wash (flush) carefully with PBS (pH 7.3) twice as explained earlier.

Prepare an IP solution of 30 mg of DAB with 30% hydrogen peroxide in 50 ml of PBS; filter and pour into a coupling jar. Immerse the slides in this solution and incubate for 10 min at room temperature in the dark.

Note that the peroxidase substrate (DAB) is carcinogenic and must be handled with safety precautions, using a fume cupboard and gloves. As an alternative safer procedure, tablets of DAB, which are available commercially (Dako), can be diluted in PBS as explained earlier.

Rinse in distilled water.
Counterstain with Harris haematoxylin for 10–20 sec.
Wash in tap water for 2 min.
Wipe off excess water, let the slides dry in the air, and mount with DPX (disterene resine dibutylphthalate in xylene).

---

*Dako Cytomation.
**Sigma-Aldrich.

For assessment of the reactivity with anti-TdT or other rabbit polyclonal antibody, carry out an additional incubation for 30 min with a mouse anti-rabbit Ig antibody diluted 1:20 in PBS (pH 7.3) with 2% human AB serum prior to the incubation with the second layer of peroxidase-conjugated rabbit antimouse Ig antibody.

Interpretation

A positive reaction is identified by light microscopy as a dark brown deposit.

Immunoalkaline Phosphatase Antialkaline Phosphatase

The APAAP method involves several steps that can be applied to peripheral blood and bone marrow films. The stages include incubation with the McAb, incubation with a rabbit antimouse Ig antibody, and incubation with immune complexes of APAAP. The second and third steps can be repeated to reinforce the reaction.

Method

Make films or cytocentrifuge slides and let them dry for at least 6–8 hours. If not used immediately, wrap the slides in aluminium foil and store at –20°C. If frozen, thaw at room temperature for 30 min before carrying out the test.

Make a ring around the chosen area using a diamond pencil. To test more than one McAb in the same slide, several rings can be marked.

Fix in pure cold acetone for 10 min. If the slides have been kept at room temperature for more than 72 hours, fix them for only 5 min.

Allow to dry in the air.

When using peripheral blood or bone marrow films, wash around the encircled areas with a cotton stick wet with PBS to remove the adjacent red blood cells.

Surround the marked areas with a silicone ring (Dako pen or Sigmacote).

Incubate for 30 min with 30 μl of McAb diluted in Tris buffered saline (TBS) 0.05 mol/l, pH 7.6. The appropriate dilution of the McAb must be determined by titrating each batch of reagent, using known positive and negative controls.

For all subsequent procedures, the slides must not be allowed to dry and incubation must be carried out in a moist chamber.

Wash (flush) carefully with TBS 0.05 mol/l and, immediately after the wash, add 20 µl of the second layer consisting of a rabbit antimouse Ig (Dako) diluted in TBS 0.05 mol/l with 2% human AB serum.

Incubate for 30 min at room temperature in a moist chamber.

Wash (flush) again with TBS.

Incubate for 45 min with 100 µl of mouse APAAP complexes (Dako) diluted 1:60 in TBS 0.05 mol/l.

Wash (flush) again with TBS.

Cover the circles with the filtered APAAP developing solution for 15–20 min.

Rinse in distilled water.

Counterstain with Harris haematoxylin for 10–20 sec.

Wash in tap water for 2 min.

Wipe off excess water and mount with Glycergel (Dako) or another water-soluble mounting medium.

Do not use DPX to cover preparations because the reaction will be faint or will become negative.

For estimation of the reactivity with anti-TdT or other polyclonal rabbit antibody, carry out a further incubation step with a mouse antirabbit Ig antibody diluted 1:20 in TBS prior to the incubation with the second layer.

Buffers

TBS 0.05 M, pH 7.6 (to wash and dilute McAb). Make a stock solution with 60.57 g of tris-hydroxymethyl-methylamine in 500 ml of distilled water. Adjust pH to 7.6 with 385 ml of 1 N HCl. Add distilled water to 1 litre and store at 4°C.

To prepare the working solution, dilute the stock solution 1:10 in 9 g/l NaCl.

TBS 0.1 M, pH 8.2 (to dilute the substrate). Make a stock solution with 1.21 g of Tris and 80 ml of water. Adjust pH to 8.2 with 4.8 ml of 1 N HCl. Add water to 100 ml (this solution can be stored for 1 month at 4°C).

Developing solution (substrate). Mix, in the following order, 20 mg of naphthol AS-MX phosphate (Sigma-Aldrich), 2 ml of N,N-dimethylformamide (Merck), 98 ml of Tris buffer 0.1 mol/l, and 24 mg of levamisole (Sigma-Aldrich).

Store in glass flasks at −20°C in 5 ml aliquots.

Thaw immediately before use; add 5 mg of fast red TR salt (Sigma-Aldrich) per vial and filter.

The developing solution is also available commercially as a kit.

Immunological Markers in Acute Leukaemia

Panel of McAb Useful for Diagnosis and Classification

Although there are a large number of McAb-recognizing antigens of haemopoietic cells, for practical reasons a well-defined set of reagents needs to be selected for the study of cases of acute leukaemia. The set of markers described here have been largely selected in accordance with the recommendations of the European Group for the Immunological Classification of Leukaemias (EGIL) and the British Committee for Standards in Haematology.[7,8]

An initial McAb panel should help to distinguish AML from ALL and further classify ALL into B- or T-cell lineage (Table 14.1). This panel is constituted as follows:

1. B-lymphoid markers: CD19, CD10, and cytoplasmic CD22 and CD79a
2. T-lymphoid markers: CD2, CD7, and cytoplasmic CD3
3. Myeloid markers: CD13, CD33, CD117, and cytoplasmic myeloperoxidase (anti-MPO)
4. Nonlineage specific markers, which are expressed in haemopoietic progenitor cells: CD34, HLA-Dr, and TdT

Two aspects that need to be considered are the degree of lineage specificity of the antigen and whether it is expressed in the membrane or the cytoplasm. Some markers are highly specific and sensitive for a particular lineage (e.g., CD3 for T cells, CD79a for B cells, and anti-MPO for myeloid cells), whereas others (e.g., CD10, CD13, or CD7) are less lineage specific. Nevertheless, the latter may support the lymphoid or myeloid commitment in cases that are negative with the most specific markers or when results are equivocal. The second aspect to take into account when performing immunophenotyping is that the most specific markers are either expressed earlier in the cytoplasm than in the membrane during cell differentiation (e.g., CD3), or they are only detectable in the cyto-

Table 14.1   Panel of monoclonal antibodies for the diagnosis of acute leukaemias

	ALL		AML
	B-lineage	**T-lineage**	
First-line	CD19, CD22, CD79a, CD10*	CD7, CD2, cyCD3	CD13, CD33, CD117, anti-MPO
		TdT, HLA-Dr, CD34	
Second-line	cymu,* SmIg	CD1a, CD5, CD4, CD8, anti-TCR	CD41, CD42, CD61, anti-glycophorin A

*CD10 and cymu are not essential for a diagnosis of B-lineage ALL, but they are important in paediatric cases to identify common-ALL, pro-B-ALL, and pre-B-ALL.
Optional markers: CD14, antilysozyme, CD36.
ALL, acute lymphoblastic leukaemia; AML, acute myeloid leukaemia; CD, cluster of differentiation; cy, cytoplasmic; MPO, myeloperoxidase; TdT, terminal deoxynucleotidyl transferase; SmIg, surface immunoglobulin; TCR, T-cell receptor.

plasm (e.g., anti-MPO, CD79a), or both.[9–11] Markers against haemopoietic precursors such as TdT or CD34, although not essential in routine practice, are helpful when problems of differential diagnosis arise between acute leukaemias and large cell lymphomas in leukaemic phase.

A second set of McAb is necessary to classify ALL further into the various subtypes and to identify rare cases of AML derived from cells committed to the megakaryocytic and erythroid lineages. This set comprises cytoplasmic and membrane Ig staining in B-lineage ALL; CD1a, CD4, CD5, CD8, and anti-TCR in T-lineage ALL; and, in AML, antibodies that detect membrane glycoproteins present in platelets and megakaryocytes or glycophorin A expressed by erythroid precursors.[7,12]

Identification of cell reactivity with other McAb may include CD14, antilysozyme, and CD36. Although CD14 and antilysozyme are not specific for acute monoblastic leukaemias, both are more frequently expressed during monocytic differentiation. CD36 is often expressed in poorly differentiated erythroid leukaemias. Although this marker is not specific for erythroid precursors, being expressed also in monoblasts and megakaryocytic cells, when considered together with reactivity with other McAb (e.g., negative for HLA-Dr, antiplatelet McAb, and CD13/CD33), it is highly indicative of erythroid acute leukaemia.

McAbs against nonhaemopoietic cells rarely need to be investigated when performing immunophenotyping for the diagnosis of acute leukaemias. However, rare cases of neuroblastoma or oat cell carcinoma can mimic acute leukaemia in the bone marrow, and in such cases antineuroblastoma McAb and the pan-leucocyte marker CD45 may help in establishing the correct diagnosis.

Other markers that are useful for the characterisation of acute leukaemias, although not routinely used, are the following:

1. A McAb that recognizes the altered distribution of promyelocytic protein (PML) in cases of AML-M3 with t(15;17). Although PML is expressed in normal myeloid cells and in blasts from AML other than M3, the pattern of expression—for example, multiparticulate or cytoplasmic in the cases with t(15;17)—is different from that of normal myeloid cells or myeloblasts of other types of AML. The latter are either negative with anti-PML or have the protein expressed in larger nuclear bodies. The reactivity with anti-PML needs to be assessed under fluorescence microscopy or light microscopy with an immunocytochemical technique.[13,14]

2. The McAbs 7.1/NG2 and NG1 that are preferentially expressed in a subset of pro-B or early B-cell ALL with 11q23 rearrangement[15] and in a proportion of AML with features of monocytic differentiation (irrespective of the presence of 11q23 rearrangement).[16–18]

3. The McAb CD56 to identify rare cases of blastic/aggressive natural killer (NK) cell leukaemia in cases without evidence of myeloid and lymphoid commitment with specific cell markers.

Immunological classification of acute leukaemias

There are two major differentiation lineages in the lymphoid system, B and T, and lymphoblastic leukaemias arise from B- or T-precursor cells. Table 14.2 illustrates that only a few McAbs react positively with the most immature lymphoblasts; with maturation, however, more McAbs become reactive. Thus, to demonstrate all cases of leukaemia of a particular lineage, it is important always to include in the battery of McAbs those that will detect the most immature cells. B-lineage ALL is defined by the expression of at least two B-cell antigens, CD79a, CD19, and/or CD22; T-lineage ALL is defined by the expression of nuclear TdT and CD3. CD7 is also consistently positive in T-ALL. However, the expression of CD7 does not by itself define T-ALL because this McAb is positive in about 20% of cases of AML.

B- and T-lineage ALL can be further subclassified on the basis of cell differentiation or maturation (Table 14.2). Although this subclassification is not essential for diagnosis, it is important because of the correlation between certain B-lineage subtypes and molecular cytogenetic and clinical features.

B-lineage ALL can be classified into four subtypes: pro-B-ALL (previously designated null-ALL), common-ALL (see Fig. 14.3), pre-B-ALL, and mature B-ALL (Table 14.2). There is some correlation between these immunological subtypes and molecular genetics and prognosis. The majority of infant ALL with t(4;11)(q21;q23) and/or rearrangement of the MLL gene at 11q23 are pro-B-ALL and often express CD15, whereas the common-ALL phenotype is associated with hyperdiploidy or t(12;21) involving the TEL gene, both associated with a good prognosis. The t(1;19)(q23;p13) is more common in the subset of pre-B-ALL. "Mature B-ALL" (L3 ALL) is not classified as ALL in the World Health Organization (WHO) classification but is included in the group of high-grade, non-Hodgkin's lymphomas because it corresponds to the leukaemic manifestation of Burkitt's lymphoma.[19]

T-lineage ALL can also be subdivided into several subgroups according to the stage of differentiation of the lymphoblasts. In the most immature form or pro-T-ALL, blasts only express CD7 and cytoplasmic CD3; in pre-T-ALL, there is also expression of CD2 or CD5; cortical T-ALL is defined by the expression of CD1a; and in the rare mature T-ALL, blasts express membrane as well as cytoplasmic CD3 (Table 14.2). T-cell-associated antigens such as CD2, CD5, CD4, CD8, and TCR are expressed with variable frequency in the cortical and mature T-ALL; for instance, coexpression of CD4 and CD8, a phenotype characteristic of normal cortical thymocytes, is frequent in cortical T-ALL. In addition, mature T-ALL can be subclassified in two subgroups on the basis of the membrane expression of the T-cell receptor (TCR) complex molecules, $\alpha\beta$ or $\gamma\delta$.

Table 14.2   Immunological classification of acute leukaemias

Acute lymphoblastic leukaemias (ALL) (TdT+)

B-cell precursor (CD19+ and/or CD79a+ and/or CD22+)
    pro-B-ALL (no expression of other B-cell markers)
    common-ALL (CD10+, cytoplasmic IgM–)
    pre-B-ALL (cytoplasmic IgM+)
    mature B-ALL* (surface Ig+)
T-cell precursor (cytoplasmic CD3+, CD7+)†
    pro-T-ALL (no expression of other T-cell markers)
    pre-T-ALL (CD2+ and/or CD5+)
    cortical T-ALL (CD1a+)
    mature T-ALL (membrane CD3+)

Acute myeloid leukaemias (AML)

AML (M0–M5) (anti-MPO+ and/or CD13+, and/or CD33+ and/or CD117+)
Pure erythroid leukaemia (antiglycophorin A+, antiblood group antigen+, CD36+)
Megakaryoblastic leukaemias (CD41+, CD42+, CD61+).

Miscellaneous

Biphenotypic acute leukaemias (coexpression of myeloid and lymphoid markers)†
Myeloid antigen positive ALL
Lymphoid antigen positive AML
Dendritic cell leukaemias
Blastic natural killer cell leukaemias

*Mature B-ALL of the French–American–British classification is typically TdT negative.
†CD4 and CD8 are variably expressed.
‡Scores for biphenotypic acute leukaemia are described in Table 14.3.
TdT, terminal deoxynucleotidyl transferase; Ig, immunoglobulin; MPO, myeloperoxidase.

AML can be defined immunologically by the expression of two or more myeloid markers: CD13, CD33, CD117, and anti-MPO in the absence of lymphoid markers.[7] The most specific marker for the myeloid lineage is anti-MPO followed by CD117; as a rule, both are negative in ALL.[20] There is no marker that allows the distinction between the various French–American–British (FAB) subtypes of AML.[21] However, some McAb may be preferentially positive in certain AML subtypes such as CD14 and antilysozyme in cases with monocytic differentiation, absence of HLA-Dr expression in M3 AML, or expression of CD19 in M2 AML. Furthermore, immunological markers are essential for the diagnosis of poorly differentiated myeloid leukaemias or M0 AML in which blasts do not show myeloid features by morphology or cytochemistry.[22,23]

In poorly differentiated leukaemias in which the first panel of lymphoid and myeloid markers does not show positive results, McAb against platelet glycoproteins Ib, the complex IIb/IIIa and IIIa (e.g., CD41, CD42, and CD61), should be tested to confirm or exclude the diagnosis of acute megakaryoblastic leukaemia,[7,12] and McAb to glycophorin A or to the red blood cell groups such as Gerbich should be used to confirm or exclude erythroid leukaemias.

Immunophenotyping enables recognition of an unusual form of acute leukaemia designated acute biphenotypic or acute mixed lineage leukaemia. This leukaemia accounts for 5% of cases and is characterised by the coexpression of a constellation of myeloid and lymphoid antigens in the blast cells (Table 14.3). The lack of agreement among various workers on the definition of biphenotypic leukaemia has made it difficult to establish whether this constitutes a distinct clinicopathological entity. We have described a scoring system[24,25] that has been adopted by the EGIL group with some modifications,[7] which aims to distinguish biphenotypic acute leukaemias from cases of ALL or AML with aberrant expression of a marker from another lineage. This scoring is based on the number and lineage specificity of the lymphoid and myeloid markers expressed by the blast cells and has been modified and adopted by WHO.[26] The most specific markers score 2, e.g., CD3 for the T-lymphoid lineage, CD79a, Ig and CD22 for the B-lymphoid lineage, and MPO for the myeloid lineage.[7,24,25,26]

Table 14.3 Scoring system for the diagnosis of biphenotypic acute leukaemias*

Score	B-lymphoid	T-lymphoid	Myeloid
2	CD79a cyCD22 cyIgM	CD3 anti-TCR αβ anti-TCR γδ	anti-MPO
1	CD19 CD20 CD10	CD2 CD5 CD8 CD10	CD117 CD13 CD33 CD65
0.5	TdT CD24	TdT CD7	CD14 CD15

*Biphenotypic acute leukaemia is defined when scores for the myeloid and one of the lymphoid lineages are >2 points. Each marker scores the corresponding point. Cases of ALL or AML with expression of myeloid or lymphoid markers, respectively, but with scores less than 2.5 have been described as myeloid antigen+ ALL and lymphoid antigen+ AML. In contrast to biphenotypic acute leukaemias, they do not seem to be cytogenetically or prognostically different from ALL or AML with no aberrant antigen expression.
MPO, myeloperoxidase; TCR, T-cell receptor; TdT, terminal deoxynucleotidyl transferase.

The origin of the leukaemic cells in the biphenotypic acute leukaemias is unknown. Indeed, WHO considers these leukaemias together with acute undifferentiated leukaemias under the umbrella of acute leukaemias of ambiguous lineage.[26]

In addition to ALL and AML there are exceedingly rare types of acute leukaemia that nevertheless are increasingly recognised. These comprise leukaemias derived from dendritic cells in which cells express CD56, CD4, CD123, HLA-Dr, and CD68[27] and aggressive NK cell leukaemias.[28]

Immunological Markers in Chronic Lymphoproliferative Disorders

Immunophenotyping is essential for the diagnosis and characterisation of the lymphoproliferative disorders. Immunological markers enable one to distinguish lymphoblastic leukaemias and lymphoblastic lymphomas, which are TdT-positive, from mature or chronic lymphoid diseases, which are consistently TdT-negative. Immunophenotyping also demonstrates whether the malignant cells are of B- or T-lymphoid nature and demonstrates clonality in the

B-cell cases. Markers may also be useful to confirm or establish the diagnosis of certain entities that show distinct immunological profiles and others, may provide prognostic information.

Panel of McAb for Diagnosis and Classification

The diagnosis of a B- or T-cell disorder requires a small battery of McAb. It is convenient to use a two-step procedure with an initial panel applicable to all cases and a second panel based on the results with the first panel and the tentative diagnosis by clinical features and/or cell morphology (Table 14.4).[8,29]

The first panel of markers is intended to distinguish B-cell from T-cell disorders, to demonstrate B-cell clonality, to confirm the diagnosis of CLL, and to confirm or exclude a non-CLL B-cell neoplasm. It comprises immunostaining with anti-kappa and anti-lambda, CD2 (T-cell marker), CD5 (a marker of T-cells and a subset of B-cells), and four McAbs that detect antigens in subsets of B-cells: CD23, FMC7, CD79b against the β chain of the B-cell receptor and membrane CD22. With the two latter reagents, as well as surface Ig, assessment of the fluorescence intensity is important to distinguish between CLL and other B-cell disorders (Fig. 14.5). The results obtained with this set of McAbs can be combined into a scoring system (Table 14.5) to establish the diagnosis of CLL and to distinguish CLL cases with atypical morphology and CLL with increased numbers of prolymphocytes (CLL/PL) from other B-cell diseases such as B-cell prolymphocytic leukaemia (B-PLL) and B-cell lymphomas in leukaemic phase.[29] The characteristic profile of CLL is weak surface immunoglobulin (SmIg), CD5+, CD23+, FMC7−, and weak or negative CD79b and CD22.[29-32] FMC7 has been shown to recognise an epitope of CD20, and it has been suggested that this marker could be replaced by CD20 in the diagnostic scoring system for CLL. However, data show that replacement of FMC7 by CD20 results in a decrease in sensitivity of the scoring because most cases of CLL express CD20 weakly.[33] Nevertheless, although CD20 is not particularly useful for diagnosis, it should be incorporated into the panel of markers for chronic lymphoid disorders because it is used increasingly as a therapeutic tool in these conditions.

When the marker profile using the first-line panel of McAb yields a B-cell phenotype not typical of CLL, a second panel of McAb can be used. This is selected in light of the review of the cell morphology, clinical information, or other laboratory features. For example, estimation of the cell reactivity with four McAbs (CD11c, CD25, CD103, and HC2) is useful to distinguish hairy cell leukaemia (HCL) from other disorders with circulating villous cells that may be confused with HCL, such as SLVL, also known as splenic marginal zone lymphoma, or marginal zone lymphoma and the HCL variant. Cells from the majority of HCL cases coexpress the three or four of the markers mentioned earlier, whereas SLVL and cells from HCL variant are positive with one or at most two of these markers.[34] More recently, another McAb, CD123, that recognises the β chain of the interleukin 3 receptor has been shown to be useful in distinguishing HCL from SLVL and the variant form of HCL. CD123 is consistently expressed in HCL cells, whereas it is negative in the other two conditions.[35] Therefore CD123 could replace HC2 in a routine setting because the latter McAb is not commercially available.

When the first-line panel of markers suggests a T-cell phenotype (CD2+, CD5+/−), expression of other T-cell markers such as CD3, CD7, CD4, and CD8 may need to be investigated. CD25 may be used in cases of suspected adult T-cell leukaemia lymphoma. When markers do not indicate either B lineage or T lineage, testing for NK cell markers should be considered.

Unusual situations may occur in the case of plasma cell leukaemia, in which the cells are

---

Table 14.4 Panel of monoclonal antibodies for the diagnosis of lymphoid disorders

	B cell	T cell
First-line	SmIg (kappa/lambda), CD19, CD23, FMC7, mCD79b, mCD22, CD5*	CD2, CD5*
Second-line	CD11c, CD25, CD103, CD123, CD38, CD138, CyIg	CD3, CD4, CD7, CD8

*B-cell subset and T-cell marker.
Optional markers: CD25, CD79a, and natural killer associated (e.g., CD16, CD56, CD57, and CD11b).
CyIg, cytoplasmic immunoglobulin; SmIg, surface immunoglobulin.

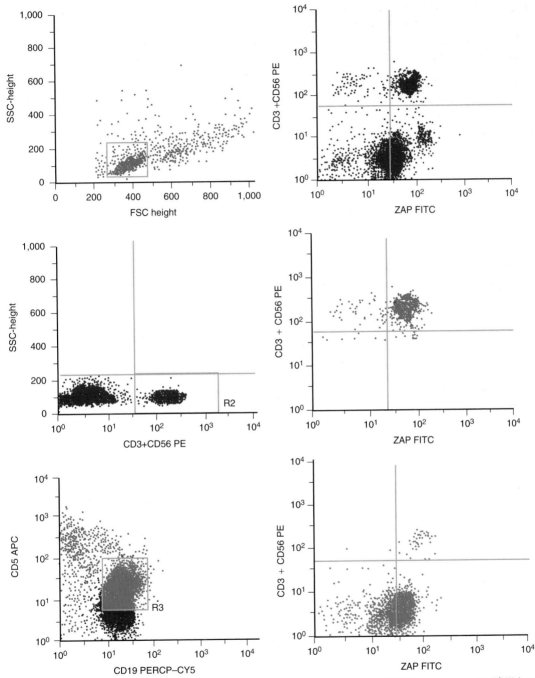

Figure 14.5   Flow cytometry dot plots using a four-colour method to detect ZAP-70 expression in T/NK lymphocytes and chronic lymphocytic leukaemia (CLL) lymphocytes. **Upper plots:** Gate on the whole lymphocyte population (*left*) and the expression of ZAP-70 (*right*). **Middle plots:** Gate on CD3/CD56-positive cells, which represent T and natural killer cells (*left*) and the expression of ZAP-70 in this population (*right*). **Lower plots:** Gate on CD5/CD19 positive cells (CLL cells) (left) and the expression of ZAP-70 in this subset (*right*).

Table 14.5 Scoring system for the diagnosis of chronic lymphocytic leukaemia (CLL)*

Marker	Points	
	1	0
CD5	Positive	Negative
CD23	Positive	Negative
FMC7	Negative	Positive
SmIg[†]	Weak	Moderate/strong
CD22/CD79b[†]	Weak/negative	Moderate/strong

*Scores for CLL range from 3 to 5, whereas in the other B-cell disorders they range from 0 to 2.
[†]Membrane expression.

negative with all T-cell and the majority of B-cell markers including surface Ig expression; cells express Ig only in the cytoplasm (with light chain restriction) and are positive with CD38 and CD138 and negative for CD45. In this situation a triple flow cytometry stain using CD45, CD38, and cytoplasmic Ig light chains is useful. Normal and malignant plasma cells may also express CD79a, a cytoplasmic epitope of the α chain of the B-cell receptor.

Other markers that have diagnostic and prognostic value in chronic lymphoid disorders are described below.

Anti-cyclin D1

McAbs that detect cyclin D1 are preferentially expressed in cells from mantle cell lymphoma (MCL) cases and in other cases of lymphoma in which cells carry the t(11;14)(q13;q32).[36,37] These antibodies are mainly used on tissue sections by immunohisto-chemistry or on cytospin preparations with immuno-cytochemistry, but it is also possible to estimate the expression of cyclin D1 by flow cytometry with the McAb 5D4 after stabilization and fixation of the cells. The sensitivity and specificity of cyclin D1 staining by flow cytometry is around 80%, and therefore the flow cytometry staining for this cyclin needs to be considered in a diagnostic setting when mantle cell lymphoma needs to be ruled out.[38]

p53 Protein

The p53 protein marker can be detected in cells by immunocytochemistry and flow cytometry with specific antibodies. There is a good correlation between p53 expression and deletions or point mutations of the *TP53* gene. It therefore appears that there is no need for gene sequencing to be done on a routine basis because flow cytometry, fluorescence *in situ* hybridization (FISH), or both provide accurate information of the p53 status.[39] Although not essential for diagnosis, this test may be useful as a prognostic indicator because of its correlation with resistance to therapy and disease progression in patients with CLL, B-PLL, and other B-cell disorders.[40,41]

CD38 and ZAP-70 Expression

CD38 and ZAP-70 are two markers shown to have a major prognostic impact in CLL. The expression of CD38 has emerged as a prognostic factor indepen-dent of the immunoglobulin heavy chain (IgVH) mutational status.[42] CD38 should be assessed by a triple colour flow cytometry method to ensure that the expression is evaluated in the leukaemic cells. Although the first reports used thresholds of 20–30% CD38+ cells to consider this marker as positive, it has become apparent that there is intra-clonal diversity and that a threshold of 7% is the most reliable and informative in terms of prognosis.[43] ZAP-70 encodes a tyrosine-kinase, which is expressed in normal T cells, NK cells, and a few B cells. Microarray studies in CLL have shown that the pattern of gene expression is very similar in cases with mutated or unmutated IgVH genes with only minor differences in a few genes. Among these, ZAP-70 is preferentially expressed in the cases with unmutated IgVH; thus it was suggested that ZAP-70 could be a surrogate marker for the mutational status. To this end, it is important to estimate its expression in purified B-CLL cells by RNA analysis or by a quadruple flow cytometry method that allows the assessment of ZAP-70 expression in T, NK, and CLL cells (Fig. 14.5).[44] At present, it is uncertain which is the best threshold (10% or 20%) for ZAP-70+ CLL cells to consider that this marker is positive.

McAb Against the Variable Regions of the β TCR

There is a set of McAb that identifies T-lymphocytes that bear the various variable regions of the TCR β and hence might be useful to demonstrate clonality of the T-cell population, particularly in cases with LGL lymphocytosis, when molecular studies (e.g., polymerase chain reaction) cannot easily be performed. There is also a potential role in identifying T-cell clones in patients with hypereosinophilia.

McAb Against CD20 and CD52 (Campath-1H)

The expression of the CD20 and CD52 antibodies should be assessed in patients in whom antibody therapy is contemplated.

Immunological Profiles of Chronic Lymphoproliferative Disorders

The most common immunophenotypes of the B- and T-cell disorders are shown in Tables 14.6 and 14.7. CLL has a phenotype that clearly distinguishes this disease from the other B-cell leukaemias. By contrast, there is overlap on the marker expression in the other B-cell malignancies; for this reason, in

Table 14.6   Membrane markers in mature B-cell disorders (CD2–)

Disease	SmIg	CD5	CD23	FMC7	CD22	CD79b
CLL	Weak	++	++	–/+	Weak/–	Weak/–
B-PLL	Strong	–/+	–	++	+	++
HCL	Strong	–	–	++	++	+
HCL-variant	Strong	–	–	++	++	+
SLVL	Strong	–/+	–/+	++	++	++
FL	Strong	–/+	–/+	++	++	++
Mantle	Strong	++	–	++	++	++
Large-cell	Strong	–/+	–/+	++	++	++
PCL*	Negative	–	–	–	–	–

*Express cytoplasmic immunoglobulin (light chain restricted), CD38, CD79a, and, with a variable frequency, other B-cell markers.
Scoring: (–): negative or positive in less than 10% of cases; (–/+): positive in 10–25% of cases; (+): positive in 25–75% of cases; and (++): positive in more than 75% of cases.
SmIg, surface immunoglobulin; CLL, chronic lymphocytic leukaemia; B-PLL, B-prolymphocytic leukaemia; HCL, hairy cell leukaemia; SLVL, splenic lymphoma with villous lymphocytes; FL, follicular lymphoma; PCL, plasma cell leukaemia.

Table 14.7   Immunological markers in mature T-cell disorders (CD2+)

Marker	T-PLL	LGL leukaemia*	ATLL	SS	T-NHL
CD3	++	++	++	++	+
CD7	++	+	–/+	+	+
CD4+, CD8–	+	–	++	++	+
CD4+, CD8+	–/+	–	–	–	+
CD4–, CD8+	–/+	++	–	–	+
CD4–, CD8–	–	–/+	–	–	+

*A proportion of cases are CD3 negative and have a natural killer phenotype: CD56+, CD16+.
Scoring: (–): negative or positive in less than 10% of cases; (–/+): positive in 10–25% of cases; (+): positive in 25–75% of cases; and (++): positive in more than 75% of cases.
T-PLL, T-prolymphocytic leukaemia; LGL, large granular lymphocyte; ATLL, adult T-cell leukaemia lymphoma; SS, Sézary syndrome; T-NHL, post-thymic T-cell lymphoma.

cases with a B-cell marker profile different from CLL, the immunophenotypic analysis needs to be interpreted in the light of morphology and other clinical and laboratory information to establish the precise diagnosis.

There is no specific immunological profile that distinguishes the various T-cell diseases (Table 14.7). However, expression of CD8, with or without that of NK-associated markers such as CD16 or CD56, is characteristic of T-cell large granular lymphocyte (LGL) leukaemia, whereas such expression is rarely seen in other conditions.[45] By contrast, coexpression of CD4 and CD8 is almost exclusively seen in a subgroup, approximately 25%, of T-cell prolymphocytic leukaemia (T-PLL) (Table 14.7).[46] Other markers may also be differentially expressed in various T-cell malignancies. Thus, for example, there is expression of CD25 in adult T-cell leukaemia lymphoma (ATLL); strong reactivity with CD7 in T-PLL[45,47]; and expression of granzyme B, TIA-1, or perforins in T-cell or NK cell LGL leukaemias and TCR γδ in hepatosplenic T-cell lymphoma.[45]

Immunological Markers for the Detection of Minimal Residual Disease

Immunophenotyping can be a useful tool to detect small numbers of residual leukaemic cells in peripheral blood or bone marrow specimens when such cells are not detected by standard morphology or histopathology. This can be carried out by double or triple colour immunofluorescent methods with a combination of McAbs aimed at identifying "aberrant" phenotypes not present in normal haemopoietic cells or by quantification of antigens that are expressed at a different density in normal and leukaemic cells.[48,49] For example, although normal bone marrows, particularly in infants or when regenerating after therapy, have a minor cell population with a B-cell precursor phenotype (e.g., TdT+, CD10+, CD19+), similar to that of ALL blasts, quantitative studies provide discrimination between the normal precursors (strong TdT and weak CD10 and CD19) and ALL blasts (weak TdT, strong CD10/CD19).[48,49] Similarly, there is a small B-cell population in normal blood and bone marrow that coexpresses CD5, a phenotype characteristic of CLL. However, by estimating the proportions of CD5+ cells within the whole B-cell population (CD19+), it is possible to

demonstrate whether cells represent residual leukaemia or normal B-lymphocytes (Fig. 14.6).[50] More recently quadruple flow cytometry using CD79b, CD20, CD5, and CD19 has been shown to be extremely sensitive in the detection of residual CLL cells.[51] In bone marrow tissue sections, occasional residual abnormal leukaemic cells can be highlighted and easily recognized using immunohistochemistry with markers known to react with the

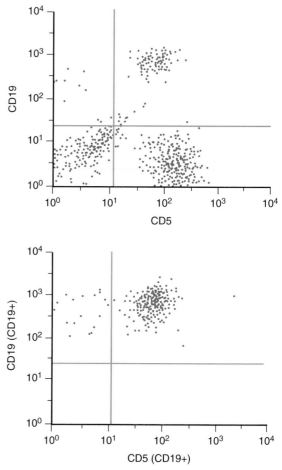

Figure 14.6   Minimal residual disease detection. **Upper:** Dot plot showing a small proportion of lymphocytes coexpressing CD5 and CD19 in a patient with chronic lymphocytic leukaemia following treatment; the majority of lymphocytes are T cells (CD5+, CD19–). **Lower:** Dot plot showing enrichment of the CD5+ CD19+ population acquired on a gate for the CD19+ cells in the above image.

leukaemic cells (e.g., DBA44 or CD103) in HCL.[52] Detection of MRD applies to both acute and chronic lymphoid leukaemias, and it is likely to have prognostic significance in terms of probability of relapse.

It is essential to identify any phenotypic aberrancy present at diagnosis in an individual patients so as to look for the same leukaemia-associated aberrancy during follow-up.

Abbreviations used specifically in this chapter:

ABC	antibody binding capacity
ALL	acute lymphoblastic leukaemia
APAAP	alkaline phosphatase anti-alkaline phosphatase
ATLL	adult T-cell leukaemia/lymphoma
B-PLL	B-cell prolymphocytic leukaemia
BSA	bovine serum albumin
CD	cluster of differentiation
CLL	chronic lymphocytic leukaemia
CLL/PL	chronic lymphocytic leukaemia with increased prolymphocytes
Cy	cytoplasmic
DAB	diaminobenzidine
EGIL	European Group for the Immunological Classification of Leukaemias
FITC	fluorescein isothiocyanate
FL	follicular lymphoma
FSC	forward light scatter
HCL	hairy cell leukaemia
Ig	immunoglobulin
IP	immunoperoxidase
LGL	large granular lymphocyte
McAb	monoclonal antibody
MESF	molecules equivalent soluble fluorochrome
MPO	myeloperoxidase
MRD	minimal residual disease
NHL	non-Hodgkin's lymphoma
PBS-azide-BSA	PBS containing sodium azide and bovine serum albumin
PCL	plasma cell leukaemia
PE	phycoerythrin
PML	protein encoded by the *PML* gene
QSC	quantum simply cellular
SSC	sideways light scatter
SLVL	splenic lymphoma with villous lymphocytes
SmIg	surface membrane immunoglobulin
SS	Sézary syndrome
TBS	Tris buffered saline
TCR	T-cell receptor
TdT	terminal deoxynucleotidyl transferase
T-PLL	T-cell prolymphocytic leukaemia

REFERENCES

1. Groeneveld K, Temarvelde JG, van den Beemd MWM, et al 1996 Flow cytometry detection of intracellular antigens for immunophenotyping of normal and malignant leukocytes. BTS Technical Report. Leukemia 10:1383–1389.
2. Pizzolo G, Vincenzi C, Nadali G, et al 1995 Detection of membrane and intracellular antigens by flow cytometry following ORTHO PermeaFix fixation. Leukemia 9:226–228.
3. Bikoue A, George F, Poncelet LW, et al 1996 Quantitative analysis of leukocyte membrane antigen expression: normal adult values. Cytometry 26:137–147.
4. Poncelet P, George F, Papa S, et al 1996 Quantitation of haemopoietic cell antigens in flow cytometry. European Journal of Histochemistry 40 (suppl 1):15–32.
5. Erber WN, Mynheer LC, Mason DY 1986 APAAP labelling of blood and bone-marrow samples for phenotyping leukaemia. Lancet i:761–765.
6. Mason DY, Erber WN 1991 Immunocytochemical labeling of leukemia samples with monoclonal antibodies by the APAAP procedure. In: Catovsky D (ed) The leukemic cell, p. 196. Churchill Livingstone, Edinburgh.
7. Bene MC, Castoldi G, Knapp W, et al 1995 Proposals for the immunological classification of acute leukemias. Leukemia 9:1783–1786.
8. Bain BJ, Barnett D, Linch D, et al 2002. Revised guideline on immunophenotyping in acute leukaemias and chronic lymphoproliferative disorders. Clinical and Laboratory Haematology 24:1–13.
9. Janossy G, Coustan-Smith E, Campana D 1989 The reliability of cytoplasmic CD3 and CD22 antigen expression in the immunodiagnosis of acute leukemia: a study of 500 cases. Leukemia 3:170–181.

10. Buccheri V, Shetty V, Yoshida N, et al 1992 The role of an anti-myeloperoxidase antibody in the diagnosis and classification of acute leukaemia: a comparison with light and electron microscopy cytochemistry. British Journal of Haematology 80:62–68.

11. Buccheri V, Milhaljevic B, Matutes E, et al 1993 mb-1: a new marker for B-lineage lymphoblastic leukemia. Blood 82:853–857.

12. Tetteroo PAT, Lansdorp PM, Leeksma OC, et al 1983 Monoclonal antibodies against human platelet glycoprotein IIIa. British Journal of Haematology 55:509–522.

13. O'Connor SJ, Forsyth PD, Dalal S, et al 1997 The rapid diagnosis of acute promyelocytic leukaemia using PML (5E10) monoclonal antibody. British Journal of Haematology 99:597–604.

14. Falini B, Flenghi L, Lo Coco F, et al 1997 Immunocytochemical diagnosis of acute promyelocytic leukemia (M3) with the monoclonal antibody PG-M3 (anti-PML). Blood 90:4046–4053.

15. Behm FG, Smith FO, Raimondi SC, et al 1996 Human homologue of the rat chondroitin sulfate proteoglycan, NG2, detected by monoclonal antibody 7.1 identifies childhood acute lymphoblastic leukemias with t(4;11)(q21;q23) or t(11;19)(q23;p13) and MLL rearrangements. Blood 87:1134–1139.

16. Wutchter C, Schnittger S, Schoch C, et al 1998 Detection of acute leukemia cells with 11q23 rearrangements by flow cytometry: sensitivity and specificity of monoclonal antibody 7.1. Blood 92 (suppl 1):228a.

17. Smith FO, Rauch C, Williams DE, et al 1996 The human homologue of rat NG2, a chondroitin sulfate proteoglycan is not expressed on the cell surface of normal hematopoietic cells but is expressed by acute myeloid leukemia blasts from poor prognosis patients with abnormalities of chromosome band 11q23. Blood 87:1123–1133.

18. Mauvieux L, Delabesse E, Bourquelot P, et al 1999 NG2 expression in MLL rearranged acute myeloid leukaemia is restricted to monoblastic cases. British Journal of Haematology 107:674–676.

19. Brunning RD, Borowitz M, Matutes E, et al 2001. Precursor B lymphoblastic leukaemia/lymphoblastic lymphoma. In: Jaffe ES, Harris NL, Stein H et al (eds) World Health Organization classification of tumours: tumours of haemopoietic and lymphoid tissues, pp. 111–114. IARC Press, Lyon.

20. Bene MC, Bernier M, Casasnovas RO, et al 1998 The reliability and specificity of c-kit for the diagnosis of acute myeloid leukemias and undifferentiated leukemias. Blood 92:596–599.

21. Bennett JM, Catovsky D, Daniel MT, et al 1985 Proposed revised criteria for the classification of acute myeloid leukemia. Annals of Internal Medicine 103:620–625.

22. Matutes E, de Oliveria MP, Foroni L, et al 1988 The role of ultrastructural cytochemistry and monoclonal antibodies in clarifying the nature of undifferentiated cells in acute leukaemia. British Journal of Haematology 69:205–211.

23. Bennett JM, Catovsky D, Daniel MT, et al 1991 Proposals for the recognition of minimally differentiated acute myeloid leukaemia (AML-MO). British Journal of Haematology 78:325–329.

24. Buccheri V, Matutes E, Dyer MJS, et al 1993 Lineage commitment in biphenotypic leukemia. Leukemia 7:919–927.

25. Matutes E, Morilla R, Farahat N, et al 1997 Definition of acute biphenotypic leukemia. Haematologica 82:64–66.

26. Brunning RD, Matutes E, Borowitz M, et al 2001 Acute leukaemias of ambiguous lineage. In: Jaffe ES, Harris NL, Stein H and Vardiman JW (eds) World Health Organization classification of tumours. Tumours of haemopoietic and lymphoid tissues, p. 27. IARC Press, Lyon.

27. Feulliard J, Jacob MC, Valensi F, et al 2002 Clinical and biological features of CD4+ CD56+ malignancies. Blood 99:1556–1563.

28. Chan JKC, Wong KF, Jaffe ES, et al 2001 Aggressive NK cell leukaemia. In: ES Jaffe, NL Harris, H Stein and JW Vardiman (ed) World Health Organization classification of tumours: tumours of haemopoietic and lymphoid tissues, pp. 198–2000. IARC Press, Lyon.

29. Matutes E, Owusu-Ankomah K, Morilla R, et al 1994 The immunological profile of B-cell disorders and proposal of a scoring system for the diagnosis of CLL. Leukemia 8:1640–1645.

30. Zomas AP, Matutes E, Morilla R, et al 1996 Expression of the immunoglobulin associated protein B29 in B-cell disorders with the monoclonal antibody SN8 (CD79b). Leukemia 10:1966–1970.

31. Moureau EJ, Matutes E, A'Hern RP, et al 1997 Improvement of the chronic lymphocytic leukemia scoring system with the monoclonal antibody SN8 (CD79b). American Journal of Clinical Pathology 108:378–382.

32. Cabezudo E, Morilla R, Carrara P, et al 1999 Quantitative analysis of CD79b, CD5 and CD19 in B-cell lymphoproliferative disorders. Haematologica 84:413–418.

33. Delgado J, Matutes E, Morilla A, et al 2003 Diagnostic significance of CD20 and FMC7

expression in B cell disorders. American Journal of Clinical Pathology 120:754–759

34. Matutes E, Morilla R, Owusu-Ankomah K, et al 1994 The immunophenotype of hairy cell leukemia (HCL): proposal for a scoring system to distinguish HCL from B-cell disorders with hairy or villous lymphocytes. Leukemia and Lymphoma 14 (suppl 1):57–61.

35. del Giudice I, Matutes E, Morilla R, et al 2004 The diagnostic value of CD123 in B-cell disorders with hairy or villous lymphocytes. Haematologica 89: 303-308

36. De Boer CJ, Schuuring E, Dreef E, et al 1995 Cyclin D1 protein analysis in the diagnosis of mantle-cell lymphoma. Blood 86:2715–2723.

37. Delmer A, Ajchenbaum-Cymbalista F, Tang R, et al 1995 Overexpression of cyclin D1 in chronic B-cell malignancies with abnormality of chromosome 11q13. British Journal of Haematology 89:798–804.

38. Elenaei MO, Jadayel DM, Matutes E, et al 2001 Cyclin D1 flow cytometry as a useful tool in the diagnosis of B-cell malignancies. Leukemia Research 25:115–123.

39. Thornton PD, Gruzka-Westwood AM, Hamoudi RA, et al 2004 Characterisation of TP53 abnormailities in chronic lymphocytic leukaemia. The Hematology Journal 5:47-54.

40. Lens D, Dyer MJS, Garcia Marco JA, et al 1997 p53 abnormalities in CLL are associated with excess of prolymphocytes and poor prognosis. British Journal of Haematology 99:848–857.

41. Dohner H, Fischer K, Bentz M, et al 1995 p53 gene deletion predicts for poor survival and non-response to therapy with purine analogs in chronic B-cell leukemias. Blood 85:1580–1589.

42. Damle RN, Walie T, Fais F, et al 1999 Immunoglobulin V gene mutation status and CD38 expression as novel prognostic indicators in chronic lymphocytic leukemia. Blood 94:1840–1847.

43. Thornton PD, Fernandez C, Giustolisi G, et al 2004 CD38 as a prognostic indicator in chronic lymphocytic leukaemia. The Hematology Journal 5:145–151.

44. Crespo M, Bosch F, Villamor N, et al 2003 ZAP-70 expression as a surrogate for Immunoglobulin variable gene region mutations in chronic lymphocytic leukemia. New England Journal of Medicine 348:1764–1775.

45. Matutes E 2003 Chronic T-cell lymphoproliferative disorders. Reviews in Clinical and Experimental Haematology 6:401–420.

46. Matutes E, Brito-Babapulle V, Swansbury J, et al 1991 Clinical and laboratory features of 78 cases of T-prolymphocytic leukemia. Blood 78:3269–3274.

47. Ginaldi L, Matutes E, Farahat N, et al 1996 Differential expression of CD3 and CD7 in T-cell malignancies: a quantitative study by flow cytometry. British Journal of Haematology 93:921–927.

48. Farahat N, Lens D, Zomas A, et al 1995 Quantitative flow cytometry can distinguish between normal and B-cell precursors. British Journal of Haematology 91:640–646.

49. Campana D, Counstan-Smith E 2002 Advances in the immunological monitoring of childhood acute lymphoblastic leukaemia. Best Practice Research on Clinical Haematology 15:1–19.

50. Cabezudo E, Matutes E, Ramrattan M, et al 1997 Analysis of residual disease in chronic lymphocytic leukemia by flow cytometry. Leukemia 11:1909–1914.

51. Rawstron AC, Kennedy B, Evans PA, et al 2001 Quantitation of minimal residual disease levels in chronic lymphocytic leukemia improves the prediction of outcome and can be used to optimize therapy. Blood 98:29–35.

52. Matutes E, Meeus P, McLennan K, et al 1997 The significance of minimal residual disease in hairy cell leukaemia treated with deoxycoformycin: a long term follow-up study. British Journal of Haematology 98:375–383.

15 Diagnostic radioisotopes in haematology

Inderjeet Dokal and S. Mitchell Lewis

Radioactive isotopes must be distinguished from nonradioactive isotopes of the same chemicals. The radioactive forms are usually referred to as radionuclides or radioisotopes. These terms are interchangeable, and in this chapter the latter term is used.

Methods using radioisotopes have an important place in haematological diagnosis. Tests that may be undertaken in haematology departments include blood volume (BV), red cell survival studies, vitamin B_{12} absorption (Schilling) tests, and occasionally ferrokinetic studies. Other investigations are more likely to be referred to a department of medical physics or nuclear medicine. Even when the tests are not carried out directly in the haematology department, it is essential for the haematologist to understand their principles and limitations and to be able to interpret the results in clinical terms. Various textbooks (e.g., Wagner et al,[1] Maisey et al[2]) provide more complete accounts of the theory and practice of nuclear medicine techniques, as does a monograph on radioisotopes in haematology by Lewis and Bayly[3] The main properties of the radioisotopes useful in diagnostic haematology are summarised in Table 15.1. The units used to express radioactivity and the effects of radiation on the body are given on page 697. As discussed in this chapter, anyone handling radioisotopes must be aware of the potential radiation hazard. It is also important to be aware of the potential biohazard of handling blood products and administering them to patients (see Chapter 25).

Table 15.1   Radioisotopes used for diagnostic investigations in haematology

Element	Half–life (T$_{1/2}$)	Energies (MeV)	Pharmaceutical	Application	Activities (MBq)	Radiation dose (mSv)	Chest X–ray equivalence*
^{57}Co	270 days	0.122 0.136	Vitamin B$_{12}$	Investigation of megaloblastic anaemias	0.02	0.05	3
^{58}Co	711.3 days	0.811 0.511			0.2	10	
^{51}Cr	27.8 days	0.320	Sodium chromate	Red cell volume Red cell lifespan Gastrointestinal bleeding Spleen scan Spleen pool	0.8 2 4 4 4	0.3 0.6 1 1 1	15 30 50 50 50
•^{59}Fe	45 days	1.09 1.29	Ferric chloride or citrate	Oral iron absorption Ferrokinetic studies	0.4 0.4	4 4	200 200
^{125}I	60 days	0.035	Iodinated human serum albumin	Plasma volume	0.2	0.06†	3
^{111}In	2.81 days	0.247 0.173	Indium chloride→ oxine/tropolone	Red cell volume Spleen scan Platelet lifespan	2 5 4	1 2 2	50 100 100
^{99m}Tc	6 hours	0.141	Pertechnetate	Red cell volume Spleen scan Spleen pool	2 100 100	0.02 1 1	1 50

MBq, megabecqueral; 1 MBq = 10^6 Bq = approximately 27 µCi; Sv, Sievert; 10^3 mSv = 1 Sv.
*The number of chest X-rays that would expose the subject to the same amount of radiation as the radioisotopes that are listed. A simple chest X-ray has a radiation dose of 0.02 mSv, but for some radiological investigations it is far greater. For example, for intravenous urography, computed tomography (CT) scan of the chest, and a large bowel barium study the effective radiation doses are 4.0, 8.0, and 9.0 mSv, respectively.
†Provided that thyroid is blocked and the label is excreted in the urine; if not blocked, about 20% will accumulate in the thyroid, resulting in a radiation dose of 1 mSv to the thyroid.

SOURCES OF RADIOISOTOPES

Radioisotopes that emit γ-rays are particularly useful because they have the advantage of emissions that penetrate tissues well, so they can be detected at the surface of the body when they have originated within organs. The radioisotope should have as short a half-life (T$_{1/2}$) as is compatible with the duration of the test. A radioisotope with a very short half-life can be administered in much higher amounts than those that are likely to remain active in the body for a considerably longer time.

The longer-lived radioisotopes that are used for haematological investigations are generally available from commercial suppliers. The usual way of obtaining certain short-lived radioisotopes is by means of a radioisotope generator, in which a moderately long-lived parent radioisotope decays to produce the required short-lived isotope. In this way ^{99m}Tc (T$_{1/2}$ = 6 h) can be derived from ^{99}Mo (T$_{1/2}$ = 66 h).

RADIATION PROTECTION

The quantity of radioactivity used in diagnostic work is usually small, and good laboratory practice is all that is necessary for safe working. However, before using radioisotopes, workers should familiarise themselves with the regulations concerning radiation protection for themselves, their fellow workers, and patients.[4]

The effect of radiation on the body depends on the amount of energy deposited and is expressed in grays (Gy). The unit that describes the overall effect of radiation on the body, or the "dose equivalent," is measured in sieverts (Sv) or millisieverts (mSv). The annual whole-body dose limit for somebody working with radioisotopes is in the order of 20 mSv, whereas 1 mSv is the annual limit for the general public. To put this into perspective, 1 mSv is produced by normal background radiation in 6 months and the radiation dose from a single chest X-ray is 0.02 mSv.[5] No statutory limit of total annual radiation dose has been set for patients, but it is an important requirement that radioisotopes should be handled only in approved laboratories under the direction of a trained person who holds a certificate from the appropriate authority specifying the radioisotopes that the individual is authorized to use and the dose limits that must not be exceeded. In the United Kingdom, this authority is the Administration of Radioactive Substances Advisory Committee (ARSAC).[5] Radioisotopes should not be given to pregnant women unless the investigation is considered imperative; if an investigation is necessary during lactation, breast-feeding should be discontinued until radioactivity is no longer detectable in the milk. When radioisotope investigations are necessary in children, the dose relative to that for an adult should be based on surface area rather than body weight (Table 15.2).

In general, the radioactive waste from radioisotopes used in haematological diagnostic procedures may be poured down a single designated laboratory sink. It should be washed down with a large quantity of running water. If the waste material exceeds the amount allowed for disposal in this way, it should be stored in a suitable place until its radioactivity has decayed sufficiently for it to be disposed of via the refuse system. All working and storage areas

Table 15.2   Radioisotope doses for children as Fraction of adult dose

Weight (kg)	Fraction of Adult Dose
10	0.3
15	0.4
20	0.5
30	0.6
40	0.75
50	0.9
60	0.95
70	1.0

and disposal sinks should be clearly labelled with the internationally recognised trefoil symbol.

Decontamination of working surfaces, walls, and floors can usually be achieved by washing with a detergent such as Decon 90 (Decon Laboratories, Ltd.). Glassware can be decontaminated by soaking in Decon 90, and plastic laboratory ware can be decontaminated by washing in dilute (e.g., 1%) nitric acid.

Protective gloves must always be worn when handling radioisotopes; any activity that does get on the hands can usually be removed by washing with soap and water or, if that fails, with a detergent solution. For each laboratory in which isotopes are used, a radiation protection officer should be nominated to supervise protection procedures and to ensure that a careful record is kept of all administered radioisotopes. This officer should work in association with the departmental safety officer (p. 647) and must ensure that all personnel working with radioactive materials wear dosimetry badges,* which must be checked at regular intervals.

Apparatus for Measuring Radioactivity in Vitro

The radioisotopes used for most haematological tests are measured in a scintillation counter with thallium-activated sodium iodide crystals. These are

---

*Available from ISO Pharma, Norway; Mallinckrodt Medical (Nuclear Medicine Division), Northampton.

available in various shapes and sizes. A "well-type" crystal contains a cavity into which is inserted a small container or test tube holding up to 5 ml of fluid. Because the sample is almost surrounded by the crystal, counting is achieved with high efficiency. Because the geometric efficiency of a well-type counter depends on the position of the sample in relation to the crystal, it is important to use the same volume for each sample in a series. Another form of crystal detector is a solid circular cylinder, 2.5–10 cm in diameter. In this form, it is used for *in vivo* measurements and occasionally for the measurement of bulky samples (e.g., samples of faeces or 24-hour urine specimens), thus avoiding the need to concentrate them to a smaller volume.

An alternative method for measuring bulky material is by using two opposed detectors in a single counting system. The sample is placed in a 450-ml waxed cardboard carton with a screw-top lid and positioned between two counters placed above and below it and with a plastic ring over the lower counter to ensure that the specimen in the carton is approximately equidistant from both crystals. The counting system is surrounded by lead, and the responses of both crystals are counted together. If a single detector system is used, it is essential to homogenise the samples.

Apparatus for Measuring Radioactivity *in Vitro*

Surface Counting

Surface counting depends on shielding the crystals by means of a lead collimator to exclude as far as possible the radiation from outside a well-defined area of the body. It is thus possible to measure the radioactivity in individual organs such as the spleen and liver.

Imaging

The most widely used method for imaging is by the scintillation camera. It consists of a lead shielding, a large thin sodium iodide detector, an array of photomultiplier tubes, a collimator with multiple parallel holes, and a system for pulse height analysis and for storage and display of the data. By scanning down the body, an image of the distribution of the label is built up and recorded. It can also be used to measure the quantity of the isotope in various organs. Positron emission tomography (PET) has augmented scintillation scanning, and a further refinement is single photon emission computed tomography (SPECT).[6,7]

Measurement of Radioactivity with a Scintillation Counter

Standardisation of Working Conditions

For each radioisotope, it is necessary to plot a spectrum of pulse height distribution and to identify a window corresponding to the energy at which the maximum number of pulses is emitted. Examples of spectra and selected settings are illustrated in Figure 15.1. The setting of the apparatus, once determined, should remain constant for many months.

Counting Technique

Measurement of Radioactivity

Measurements are usually carried out for a fixed time period, and the results are recorded as counts per second (cps) or counts per minute (cpm). Radioactivity is subject to random but statistically predictable variation similar to that in blood cell counts (see p. 683). The accuracy of the count depends on the total number of the counts recorded as the variance (σ) of a radioactive count = $\sqrt{\text{total count}}$.

Thus, on a count of 100 the inherent error is 10%; it is 1% on a count of 10,000. Any measured activity represents the difference between the sample count and the background count, in which the errors of both counts are cumulative. In practice, a net count of 2500 over background is adequate for the accuracy required for clinical studies.

Background counts should be measured alongside that of the radioactive material. If the count rate of the sample is not much above background, then the background should be counted for as long a time as the sample. If the sample-count rate is less than the background, accurate measurement requires extremely long counting times.

Correction for Physical Decay

Because physical decay is a continuous process that proceeds at an exponential rate, it is possible to correct mathematically for the loss of radioactivity and to convert any measurement back to the initial reference time. This is necessary when successive observations made at different times after the administration of a radionuclide to a patient are compared.

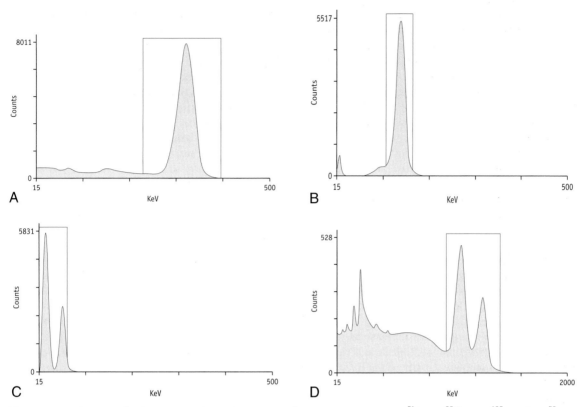

Figure 15.1   Spectra of radioisotopes obtained on a scintillation spectrometer. A: ^{51}Cr, B: ^{99m}Tc, C: ^{125}I, and D: ^{59}Fe. The radionuclides should be counted with the window set within the limits indicated by the vertical lines.

Double Radioisotope Measurements

If more than one radionuclide is present in a sample, it is possible to measure the radioactivity of each radioisotope separately by one of the following techniques.

Differential Decay

Differential decay is of value especially when one of the labels has a very short half-life (e.g., ^{99m}Tc, half-life 6 hours). The method is to count the activity in the mixture twice—the second count when the short-lived label has effectively disappeared.

Physical Separation

When the two radioisotopes produce γ-rays of different energies, they can be identified by their characteristic features and separated using an energy analyser. Correction for any "cross talk" is carried out by counting a standard of each radionuclide (A and B) at both channel settings. The proportion of A (P_A) spilling over into channel B = channel B counts ÷ channel A counts from the radionuclide A standard (both corrected for background), and the proportion of B (P_B) spilling over into channel A = channel A counts ÷ channel B counts from the radionuclide B standard. The total counts obtained for labels A and B in their correct channels can then be corrected for the proportion of "foreign" counts.

BLOOD VOLUME

The haemoglobin content, total red cell count, and packed cell volume (PCV) do not invariably reflect the total red cell volume (RCV). Whereas in most cases for practical purposes there is adequate correlation between peripheral blood values and (total) RCV,[8] there will be a discrepancy if the plasma volume is reduced or increased disproportionately. Fluctuation in plasma volume may result in haemodilution or conversely in haemoconcentration, giving rise to pseudoanaemia or pseudopolycythaemia, respectively.

An increase in plasma volume occurs in pregnancy, returning to normal soon after delivery. Increased plasma volume may also be found in patients with cirrhosis, nephritis, and congestive cardiac failure and when there is marked splenomegaly. Reduced plasma volume occurs in stress, with oedema, with dehydration, following the administration of diuretic drugs, and in smokers. It also occurs during prolonged bed rest.

In contrast to the fluctuations in plasma volume, RCV does not fluctuate to any extent if erythropoiesis is in a steady state.

Blood volume should thus be measured whenever the PCV is persistently higher than normal; demonstration of an absolute increase in RCV is necessary to diagnose polycythaemia and to assess its severity. The component parts of the BV (i.e., red cell and plasma volume) should also be measured separately in the elucidation of obscure anaemias when the possibility of an increase in plasma volume cannot be excluded.

Measurement of Blood Volume

Principle
The principle is that of dilution analysis. A small volume of a readily identifiable radioisotope is injected intravenously, either bound to the red cells or to a plasma component, and its dilution is measured after time has been allowed for the injected material to become thoroughly mixed in the circulation but before significant quantities have left the circulation or become unbound. The most practical method now available is to use a small volume of the patient's red cells labelled with radioactive chromium (^{51}Cr), technetium (pertechnetate) (^{99m}Tc), or indium (^{111}In). The labelled red cells are diluted in the whole blood of the patient, and from their dilution the total BV can be calculated; the RCV, too, can be deduced from knowledge of the PCV. The plasma volume can be measured directly by injecting human albumin labelled with radioactive iodine (^{125}I) that is diluted in the plasma compartment.

In contrast to measurement of RCV, plasma volume measurements are only approximations because the labelled albumin undergoes continuous slow interchange between the plasma and extravascular fluids, even during the mixing period. For this reason, it is undesirable to attempt to calculate RCV from plasma volume on the basis of the observed PCV. However, because the RCV is generally more stable, calculation of total BV from RCV is usually more reliable, provided that the difference between whole-body and venous PCV is appreciated and allowed for (see p. 364). Measurement of red cell and plasma volumes separately by direct methods is to be preferred.

Red Cell Volume

Radioactive Chromium Method
For the radioactive chromium method,[9] add approximately 10 ml of blood to 1.5 ml of sterile NIH-A acid–citrate–dextrose (ACD) solution (see p. 683) in a sterile bottle with a screw cap. Centrifuge at 1200–1500 g for 5 min. Discard the supernatant plasma and buffy coat and slowly, with continuous mixing, add to the cells 8×10^3 Bq of Na_2 $^{51}CrO_4$ per kg of body weight. The sodium chromate should be in a volume of at least 0.2 ml, being diluted in 9 g/l NaCl (saline). Allow the blood to stand for 15 min at 37°C for labelling to take place. Wash the red cells twice in 4–5 volumes of sterile saline.*

Finally, resuspend the cells in a volume of sterile saline sufficient for an injection of about 5 ml and the preparation of a standard. Take up the appropriate volume into a syringe that is weighed before and after the injection. The volume injected is calculated from the following formula:

Volume injected (ml)

$$= \frac{\text{Weight of suspension injected (g)}}{\text{Density of suspension (g/ml)}}$$

---

*For all procedures requiring sterile saline, this should be 9 g/l (0.9%) sodium chloride BP (nonpyrogenic); 12 g/l NaCl should be used when red cell osmotic fragility is greatly increased (e.g., in cases of hereditary spherocytosis).

The density of the suspension = 1.0 + Hb concentration of suspension (g/l) × 0.097/340, assuming that packed red cells have a mean cell haemoglobin concentration (MCHC) of 340 g/l and a density of 1.097.

Inject the suspension intravenously without delay and note the time; at 10, 20, and 30 min later, collect 5–10 ml of the patient's blood and add it to the appropriate amount of K_2 EDTA anticoagulant. This blood should preferably be drawn from a vein other than that used for the injection. However, it is often convenient to insert a self-retaining (e.g., butterfly) needle; in this case, care must be taken to ensure that the isotope is well-dispersed into the bloodstream when injected by flushing through with 10 ml of sterile saline. When the mixing time is likely to be prolonged, as in splenomegaly, cardiac failure, or shock, another sample should be taken 60 min after the injection.

Measure the PCV of each sample.* Deliver 1 ml volumes into counting tubes and lyse with saponin; a convenient method is to add 2 drops of 2% saponin. Measure their radioactivity in a scintillation counter. Then dilute an aliquot of the original suspension that was not injected 1 in 500 in water (for use as a standard) and determine the radioactivity of a 1 ml volume. Then:

Red cell volume (RCV) (ml) =

$$\frac{\text{Radioactivity of standard (cpm/ml)} \times \text{Dilution of standard} \times \text{Volume injected (ml)}}{\text{Radioactivity of post-injection sample (cpm/ml)}} \times \text{PCV (on blood sample)}$$

Total Blood Volume

The total blood volume (TBV) can be calculated by multiplying the value for RCV by 1/(whole-body PCV) (see p. 31). Plasma volume can be calculated by subtracting RCV from TBV.

If a sample has been taken at 60 min in cases in which delayed mixing is suspected, and there is a significant difference between the measurements at 10–30 min and 60 min, then the 60 min measurement should be used for calculating the RCV.

Technetium Method

^{99m}Tc is available as sodium pertechnetate. This passes freely through the red cell membrane and will become attached to the cells only if it is present in a reduced form as it enters the cells when it binds firmly to β-chains of haemoglobin. For this to occur, the red cells must be treated with a stannous (tin) compound by the following *in vivo* procedure.

Dissolve a vial of Stannous Reagent[†] in 6 ml of sterile saline and inject intravenously 0.03 ml/kg body weight.

After 15 min, collect 5 ml of blood into a sterile container to which has been added 200 iu of liquid heparin. Add 2 MBq of freshly generated ^{99m}Tc in approximately 0.2 ml of saline or 100 MBq if measurement of splenic red cell pool and scanning are also required. Allow to stand at room temperature for 5 min. Centrifuge; wash twice in cold sterile saline, and resuspend in a sufficient volume of cold sterile saline for an injection of 5–10 ml. Draw 5 ml into a syringe that is weighed before and after injection, and carry out subsequent procedures as for the chromium method. Because of the short half-life of ^{99m}Tc, radioactivity must be measured on the day of the test. Because 5–10% of the radioactivity is eluted from the red cells within an hour, the method is less suitable than the chromium and indium methods when delayed mixing is suspected (e.g., in splenomegaly).

Indium is available as ^{111}In chloride. The labelling procedure is simpler than with ^{99m}Tc, and because there is less elution than with technetium during the first hour,[10] it is particularly suitable for delayed sampling. For labelling blood cells, the indium is complexed with oxine[11] or tropolone.[12]

---

*PCV should be obtained by microhaematocrit centrifugation for 5 min, or for 10 min if the PCV is more than 0.50, and correcting for trapped plasma by deducting 2% from the measurement. A more accurate measurement of the PCV can be obtained by the International Council for Standardization in Haematology (ICSH) surrogate reference method (p. 32).

†Stannous fluoride and sodium medronate (Amerscan, Amersham International).

Plasma Volume

^{125}I–Human Serum Albumin Method

Human serum albumin (HSA) labelled with ^{125}I or ^{131}I is available commercially.* The albumin concentration should not be less than 20 g/l. The user must be reassured that only donors who are negative for human immunodeficiency virus (HIV) and hepatitis B and C have been used as the source of albumin. ^{125}I is readily distinguishable from ^{51}Cr, ^{99m}Tc, and ^{111}In, and this makes possible the simultaneous direct determination of RCV and plasma volume (see below). If further doses of the radioisotope are to be administered for repeat tests, it is advisable to block the thyroid by administering 30 mg of potassium iodide by mouth on the day before the test and daily for 2–3 weeks thereafter.

Withdraw approximately 20 ml of blood into a syringe containing a few drops of sterile heparin solution and transfer to a 30 ml sterile bottle with a screw cap. After centrifuging at 1200–1500 g for 5–10 min, transfer approximately 7 ml of plasma to a second sterile bottle and add 2.5×10^{3} Bq of the radionuclide-labelled HSA per kg body weight (approximately 0.2 MBq in total). Inject a measured amount (e.g., 5 ml) and retain the residue for preparation of a standard.

After 10, 20, and 30 min, withdraw blood samples from a vein other than that used for the original injection (or after flushing through with 10 ml of sterile 9 g/l NaCl [saline] if a butterfly needle has been used) and deliver into bottles containing EDTA or heparin.

Measure the PCV (see footnote, p. 363), centrifuge the sample, and separate the plasma. Prepare a standard by diluting part of the residue of the uninjected HSA 1 in 100 in saline.

Measure the radioactivity of the plasma samples in a scintillation counter, and by extrapolation on semilogarithmic graph paper, calculate the radioactivity of the plasma at zero time. If only a single sample is collected 10 min after the injection, the radioactivity at zero time may be approximated by multiplying by 1.015 to allow for early loss of the radioisotope from the circulation. Reliance on a single 10 min sample will lead to error if the mixing of the albumin in the plasma is delayed. After measuring the radioactivity of the standard, the plasma volume (ml) is calculated as follows:

$$\frac{\text{Radioactivity of standard (cpm/ml)} \times \text{Dilution of standard} \times \text{Volume injected (ml)}}{\text{Radioactivity of postinjection sample (cpm/ml, adjusted to zero time)}}$$

Total Blood Volume

As has already been indicated, the TBV is frequently calculated from the RCV and PCV. Before this can be done, however, the observed PCV has to be corrected for the difference between the whole-body and venous PCV.

Whole-Body and Venous Packed Cell Volume Ratio

PCV measured on venous blood is not identical with the average PCV of all the blood in the body. This is mainly because the red cell:plasma ratio is less in small blood vessels (capillaries, arterioles, and venules) than in large vessels. The ratio between the whole body PCV and venous blood PCV is normally about 0.9,[9] and it is thus necessary in the calculation of TBV from measurements of RCV to multiply the observed PCV by 0.9. Thus, TBV is given by the following:

$$\text{Red cell volume} \times \frac{1}{\text{PCV} \times 0.9}$$

However, the ratio varies in individuals, especially in splenomegaly, and it is better to estimate RCV and plasma volume by separate measurements rather than to attempt to calculate one of these from an estimate of the other.

Simultaneous Measurement of Red Cell Volume and Plasma Volume

Collect blood and label the red cells by one of the methods described earlier. If ^{99m}Tc is used, it is necessary first to inject stannous reagent (p. 363). Then add ^{125}I HSA (see above) and mix it with the labelled red cell suspension. Inject an accurately measured amount and dilute the remainder 1 in 500 in water for use as a standard. Collect three blood samples at 10, 20, and 30 min, respectively, after the administration of the labelled blood and estimate the radioactivity of a measured volume of each sample and a similar volume of the standard.

When ^{99m}Tc has been used in combination with ^{125}I, count on the same day; then leave for 2 days to

---

*Available from ISO Pharma, Norway; Mallinckrodt Medical (Nuclear Medicine Division), Northampton.

allow the ^{99m}Tc to decay and count again for ^{125}I activity. Because the radioactivity in the preparation from ^{125}I is much smaller than that from ^{99m}Tc, the count from the red cells is not likely to be significantly affected by interference from ^{125}I in the initial count. However, if necessary, a correction can be made by subtracting the ^{125}I counts on day 2 (corrected for decay) from the original counts to obtain a measurement of the counts owing only to the ^{99m}Tc.

When ^{51}Cr has been used in combination with ^{125}I, and a multichannel counter is available, measure the radioactivity owing to the ^{51}Cr and ^{125}I at the appropriate settings for ^{51}Cr and ^{125}I.

Calculate the radioactivity owing to the red cell label in the blood from the mean of the 10-, 20-, and 30-min samples, and obtain that owing to ^{125}I from the value extrapolated to zero time. Calculate RCV as described on page 363.

Plasma volume is calculated from the formula:

$$\frac{\text{Radioactivity of standard (cpm/ml)} \times \text{Dilution of standard} \times \text{volume injected (ml)} \times (1-\text{PCV})}{\text{Radioactivity of postinjection sample (cpm/ml, corrected to zero time)}}$$

Total blood volume = RCV + plasma volume

Expression of Results of Blood Volume Estimation

RCV, plasma volume, and total BV are usually expressed in ml/kg of body weight. Because fat is relatively avascular, low values are obtained in obese subjects and the relation between BV and body weight varies according to body composition. Blood volume is more closely correlated with lean body mass (LBM).[13] Earlier methods for determination of LBM were not practical as a routine procedure, and discounting excess fat by using an estimate of so-called "ideal weight" is arbitrary and tends to overcorrect for the avascularity of fat. The International Council for Standardisation in Haematology (ICSH) developed two formulae, based on body surface area, which provide normal reference values in men and women, respectively.[14] They are as follows.

Mean Normal Red Cell Mass (ml)

Men: [1486 × S] – 825; ± 25% includes 98% limits
Women: [1.06 × age (yr)] + [822 × S]; ± 25% includes 99% limits

Mean Normal Plasma Volume (ml)

Men: 1578 × S; ± 25% includes 99% limits
Women: 1395 × S; ± 25% includes 99% limits

$$S = [W^{0.425} \times H^{0.725} \times 0.007184],$$

where S = surface area (m²), W = weight (kg), H = height (cm)

However, the problem of establishing the LBM has been overcome to some extent because there are now instruments that are simple to use for estimating body composition by the different response of fat and other tissues to electrical impedance.*[13,15]

Thus, RCV can now be obtained by a direct measurement that discounts the effect of fat. The graph in Figure 15.2 shows the normalisation of the RCV in ml/kg LBM.[13] It is obtained as follows: On arithmetic graph paper with % Fat on the horizontal (x) axis and RCV in ml/kg total body weight on the vertical (y) axis, plot the intercepts of the following:

Fat 20% with RCV 29 ml; Fat 50% with RCV 19 ml

Join these two points and extend the line to the right and left.

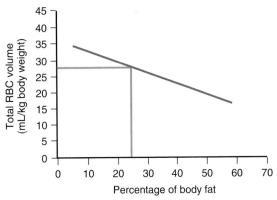

Figure 15.2 Normalisation of red cell volume in ml/kg lean body mass (see text). The example shows a patient with 25% body fat; from the slope of the graph the normalised red cell volume for that person should be 28 ml/kg body weight. A measurement more than 120% of this value (i.e., 33.6 ml) would indicate polycythaemia.

---

*Body composition analyser, Holtain Ltd, Crosswell, Dyfed, Wales; Body fat monitor, Tanita Corporation.

When the % fat is known in any individual (male or female), draw a line vertically from this reading on the x axis to the slope, and where this line intersects the slope draw a horizontal line to the y axis. The reading of this line on the y axis is the normalised RCV for that individual. When the measured RCV is >120% of this figure, it is equivalent to 43 ml/kg LBM, and a diagnosis of polycythaemia can be made with confidence in men or women.

Range in Health

The TBV is 250–350 ml at birth. After infancy, the volume increases gradually until adult life when the RCV in men is 30 ± 5 ml (2SD)/kg, and in women it is 25 ± 5 ml (2SD)/kg. Plasma volume (for men and women) is 40–50 ml/kg; total BV is 60–80 ml/kg.

As a rule, the BV remains remarkably constant in an individual, and rapid adjustments take place within a few hours after blood transfusion or intravenous infusion. In pregnancy, both the plasma volume and total BV increase. The plasma volume increases especially in the first trimester, and the total volume increases later; by full term the plasma volume will have increased by about 40%, and total BV will have increased by 32% or even more. The BV returns to normal within a week postpartum.[16]

Bed rest causes a reduction in plasma volume, and muscular exercise and changes in posture cause transient fluctuations. In practice, the patient should always be allowed to rest in a recumbent position for 15 min before measuring the blood volume.

Splenic Red Cell Volume

The red cell content of the normal spleen (the red cell "pool") is less than 5% of the total RCV (i.e., <100–120 ml in an adult). In splenomegaly, the pool is increased (e.g., by perhaps as much as 5–10 times in myelofibrosis, polycythaemia, hairy cell leukaemia, and lymphoproliferative disorders).[17] An increase in the volume of the splenic red cell pool may itself be a cause of anaemia; measurement of the pool may be useful in investigating the anaemia in these conditions. It is also useful in determining the cause of erythrocytosis because the expanded pool in polycythaemia vera contrasts with that in secondary polycythaemia, in which it is normal.[18]

An approximate estimate of the splenic RCV can be obtained from the difference between the RCV calculated from the measurement of the blood sample that has been collected 2–3 min after the injection of labelled cells and that measured after mixing has been completed (i.e., after a delay of 20 min). The splenic RCV can be estimated more accurately by quantitative scanning, after injecting viable red cells labelled with ^{99m}Tc.[19] The blood volume is measured in the usual way using 100 MBq of ^{99m}Tc. The splenic area is scanned 20 min after the injection or after 60 min when there is splenomegaly. To delineate the spleen more precisely, it may be necessary to carry out a second scan after an injection of heat-damaged labelled red cells (see p. 374). From the radioactivity in the spleen, relative to that in a standard, and knowledge of the total RCV, the proportion of the total RCV contained in the spleen can be calculated. This technique has also been used for demonstrating localised accumulation of blood in haemangiomas in the liver,[20] telangiectasia, and other vascular abnormalities.[21]

FERROKINETICS

Whereas much can be learned about the rate and efficiency of erythropoiesis from the red cell count and reticulocyte counts, studies of iron metabolism and measurement of red cell lifespan with radioactive isotopes may provide useful additional information.

Radioactive iron (^{59}Fe)* has a moderately short half-life, 45 days, and labels haemoglobin after injection. It also labels the plasma iron pool, and this allows the measurement of iron clearance and calculation of plasma iron turnover. Its subsequent appearance in haemoglobin permits the assessment of the rate of haemoglobin synthesis and the completeness of the utilisation of iron. Because it is a γ-ray emitter, radioactivity can be measured *in vivo* and the sites of distribution of the administered iron and the probable sites of erythropoiesis can thus be determined.

---

*^{59}Fe is not available at present from the former supplier, Amersham plc, but it may be available from POLATOM, www.polatom.pl.

Iron Distribution

Principle

Iron is transported to the bone marrow bound to transferrin. At the surface of the erythroblasts, the complex releases its iron, which enters the cell to be incorporated into haem, leaving the transferrin free for recycling. Iron not bound to transferrin finds its way to the liver and to other organs rather than to the bone marrow, whereas colloidal particles of iron are rapidly removed by phagocytic cells.

The ferrokinetic studies with ^{59}Fe that provide information on erythropoiesis include the rate of clearance of the radioiron from the plasma and iron incorporation into circulating red cells (iron utilisation). These are relatively simple procedures but they do not take account of the recirculation of iron that returns to the plasma from tissues, nor of iron turnover resulting from dyserythropoiesis or haemolysis. To take account of these factors requires much more complex and time-consuming procedures with multiple sampling over an extended period,[22] but the simpler tests provide sufficiently reliable and useful measurements for clinical purposes.

In ferrokinetic studies, it is important to ensure that any iron administered is bound to transferrin. In most cases, plasma has an adequate amount of transferrin. However, the unsaturated iron-binding capacity (UIBC) or transferrin concentration of the patient's plasma should be measured before the test is carried out, and, if the UIBC is <1 mg/l (20 μmol/l) or the transferrin concentration is <0.6 g/l, normal donor plasma (HIV and hepatitis B and C negative) should be used instead of that of the patient for the subsequent labelling procedure.

Method

Under sterile conditions, obtain 5–10 ml of plasma from freshly collected heparinised blood. Add 0.4 MBq of ^{59}Fe ferric citrate (specific activity >0.2 MBq/μg). Incubate at room temperature for 15 min. Fill a syringe with all but 1 ml of the mixture. Weigh the syringe to the nearest 10 mg. Inject its content intravenously into the patient, starting a stopwatch at the midpoint of the injection. Reweigh the empty syringe and calculate the volume injected:

$$\text{Volume of plasma (ml)} = \frac{\text{Weight of plasma (g)}}{1.015}$$

Dilute the residual portion of the dose (1 ml) 1 in 100 in water and use as a measure of the total amount of radioactivity and as a standard in subsequent measurements.

Plasma Iron Clearance

Take a sample at 3 min and 4 or 5 further samples over a period of 1–2 hours, collecting them into heparin or EDTA. Retain a portion of one sample for measurement of plasma iron. Measure the radioactivity in unit volumes of plasma from the samples and plot the values obtained on log linear graph paper. A straight line will usually be obtained for the initial slope. The radioactivity at the moment of injection is inferred by extrapolation back to zero time, and the time taken for the plasma radioactivity to decrease to half its initial value ($T_{1/2}$-plasma clearance) is read off the graph (Fig. 15.3).

Range of $T^1/_2$-Plasma Clearance in Health

60–140 min.

The clearance rate is influenced by the intensity of erythropoiesis and also by the activity of the macrophages of the reticuloendothelial (RE) system, especially in the liver, spleen, and bone marrow, where the iron is retained as storage iron. Also, to a lesser extent, circulating reticulocytes may take up some of the iron. A rapid clearance indicates hyperactivity of one or more of these mechanisms, as for

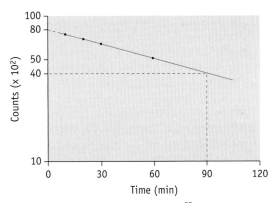

Figure 15.3   Plasma iron clearance. [59]Fe activity in plasma at 10, 20, 30, and 60 min extrapolated to the vertical axis to obtain activity at zero time. The $T_{1/2}$ was 90 min.

instance in iron deficiency anaemias, haemorrhagical anaemias, haemolytic anaemias, and polycythaemia vera. The clearance rate is decreased in aplastic anaemia. In leukaemia and in myelofibrosis, the results are variable, depending on the amount of erythropoietic marrow and the extent of extra-medullary erythropoiesis; in myelofibrosis, however, rapid clearance is by far the more common finding. In dyserythropoiesis, the clearance may be normal or accelerated.

Iron Utilisation

Collect blood samples daily, or at least on alternate days, for a period of about 2 weeks after the administration of the ^{59}Fe. Measure the radioactivity per ml of whole blood and calculate the percentage utilization on each day from the formula:

$$\frac{\text{cpm/ml daily whole blood sample} \times 100 \times f}{\text{cpm/ml whole blood sample at zero time}}$$

where f is a PCV correction factor

$$\text{i.e.,} \quad \frac{0.9 \text{ PCV}}{1 - 0.9 \text{ PCV}}$$

When there is reason to suspect that the body:venous PCV ratio is not 0.9, measure the RCV by a direct method (p. 364). Note, however, that because calculation of plasma volume from extrapolation of the ^{59}Fe disappearance curve is often unreliable, it should not be used as the basis for calculation of RCV.

Calculate the percentage utilisation on each day from the formula:

Percentage utilization =
$$\frac{\text{Red cell volume (ml)} \times \text{cpm/ml red cells} \times 100}{\text{Total radioactivity injected (cpm)}^\ddagger}$$

Plot the daily measured percentages against time on arithmetic graph paper. Record the maximum utilization (Fig. 15.4).

The calculation gives a measure of effective erythropoiesis. In normal subjects, red cell radioactivity increases steadily from 24 hours and reaches a maximum of 70–80% utilisation on the 10th to 14th day.

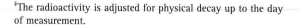

‡The radioactivity is adjusted for physical decay up to the day of measurement.

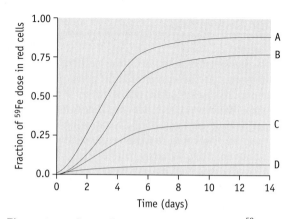

Figure 15.4   Iron utilization. Red-cell uptake of ^{59}Fe in A: iron deficiency and polycythaemia, B: a normal subject, C: dyserythropoiesis, and D: severe aplastic anaemia.

A rapid plasma clearance is usually associated with early and relatively complete utilisation, and the converse also applies. The results are inconsistent in megaloblastic anaemias and in haemoglobinopathies in which there is ineffective erythropoiesis; they also are inconsistent in myelofibrosis, depending on the extent of extramedullary erythropoiesis and whether the red cell lifespan is reduced. If there is rapid haemolysis, the utilisation curve will be distorted by destruction of some of the labelled red cells; this may be recognized if frequent (daily) samples are measured. In aplastic anaemia, the utilisation is usually 10–15%; in ineffective erythropoiesis, it is as a rule 30–50%.

The ferrokinetic patterns in various diseases are shown in Table 15.3 and Fig. 15.4.

Body Iron Distribution

An overall picture of ferrokinetics can be constructed from surface counting with a scintillation probe positioned over the liver, spleen, sacrum (for bone marrow), and heart (for blood pool) after an intravenous injection of ^{59}Fe. By counting over several days, it is possible to identify sites of erythropoiesis from early counts and sites of red cell destruction from later counts. This test is rarely performed nowadays, although it has some clinical value for determining the extent of extramedullary erythropoiesis in the spleen before splenectomy.

Table 15.3   Ferrokinetic patterns in various diseases

	Plasma clearance $T_{1/2}$	Red cell utilisation*
Normal	60–140 min	80%
Iron deficiency	Shortened	Increased (90%)
Aplastic anaemia	Prolonged	Decreased (10%)
Chronic infection	Slightly shortened	Normal
Dyserythropoiesis	Slightly shortened	Decreased (30%)
Myelofibrosis	Shortened	Decreased (50%)
Haemolytic anaemia	Shortened	Increased (85%)

*Average figures are shown, but there is a wide range, depending on the stage and severity of the disease.

Where there are facilities for using cyclotron-produced [52]Fe and positron emission tomography (PET), high-resolution images of the intramedullary and extramedullary distribution of erythropoietic tissue can be obtained. This is especially helpful in the myeloproliferative disorders for diagnosing transition of polycythaemia to myelofibrosis and for differentiating essential thrombocythaemia from reactive thrombocytosis.[23] It is also useful in identifying residual skeletal erythropoiesis in aplastic anaemia.

ESTIMATION OF THE LIFESPAN OF RED CELLS IN VIVO

There is extensive literature on the survival of red cells in haemolytic anaemias using radioisotope labelling of red cells (see review by Bentley and Miller[24]). Although now undertaken less frequently than in the past, measurement of red cell survival can still provide important data in cases of anaemia in which increased haemolysis is suspected but not clearly demonstrated by other tests. In the usual procedure, a population of circulating red cells of all ages is labelled ("random labelling"). By contrast, in "cohort labelling" a radionuclide (e.g., ^{59}Fe) is incorporated into haemoglobin during its synthesis by erythroblasts, and radioactivity is measured in red cells that appear in the circulation as a cohort of closely similar age. Red cell lifespan can be calculated from measurements of red cell iron turnover,[25] but the results have to be interpreted with caution because of the reutilisation for haem synthesis of iron derived from red cells at the end of their lifespan. Random labelling is a much more practical method than cohort labelling.

Radioactive Chromium (^{51}Cr) Method

Radioactive chromium (^{51}Cr) is a γ-ray emitter with a half-life of 27.8 days. As a red cell label, it is used in the form of hexavalent sodium chromate. After passing through the surface membrane of the red cells, it is reduced to the trivalent form that binds to protein, preferentially to the β-polypeptide chains of haemoglobin.[26] In this form, it is not reutilised nor transferred to other cells in the circulation.

The main disadvantage of ^{51}Cr is that it gradually elutes from red cells as they circulate; there may be, too, an increased loss over the first 1–3 days, and uncertainty as to how much has been lost makes it impossible to measure red cell lifespan accurately. Chromium, whether radioactive or nonradioactive, is toxic to red cells, probably by its oxidising actions; it inhibits glycolysis in red cells when present at a concentration of 10 μg/ml or more[27] and blocks glutathione reductase activity at a concentration exceeding 5 μg/ml.[28] Blood should thus not be exposed to more than 2 μg of chromium per ml of packed red cells.

$Na_2{}^{51}CrO_4$ is available commercially at a specific activity of about 15–20 GBq/mg Cr. For administration, the stock solution usually must be dissolved in 9 g/l NaCl (saline) (see below). ACD must not be used as a diluent because this reduces the chromate to the cationic chromic form.

Care must be taken to avoid lysis when the red cells are washed; it may be necessary, especially if the blood contains spherocytes, to use a slightly hypertonic solution (e.g., 12 g/l NaCl). This should certainly be used if an osmotic fragility test has demonstrated lysis in 9 g/l NaCl. In patients whose plasma contains high-titre, high-thermal-amplitude cold agglutinins, the blood must be collected in a warmed syringe, and delivered into ACD solution previously warmed to 37°C; the labelling and washing in saline should be carried out in a "warm room" at 37°C.

Method

The technique of labelling red cells is the same as for TBV measurement (see p. 362).[29] To ensure as little damage to red cells as possible, with subsequent minimal early loss and later elution, it is important to maintain the blood at an optimal pH. This can be achieved by adding 10 volumes of blood to 1.5 volumes of NIH-A ACD solution (see p. 689).

For a red cell survival study, 0.02 MBq per kg body weight (an average total dose of $2c$ MBq) is recommended. If this is to be combined with a spleen scan or pool measurement, a higher dose (4 MBq) should be used, bearing in mind that <2 µg of chromium should be added per ml of packed red cells.

After injection, allow the labelled cells to circulate in the recipient for 10 min (or for 60 min in patients with cardiac failure or splenomegaly, in whom mixing may be delayed). Then collect a sample of blood from a vein other than that used for the injection (or after washing the needle through with saline if a butterfly needle is used) and mix with EDTA as anticoagulant. The radioactivity in this sample provides a baseline for subsequent observations. Retain part of the labelled cell suspension that was not injected into the patient to serve as a standard. This enables the blood volume to be calculated if required.

Take further 4–5 ml blood samples from the patient 24 hours later (day 1) and subsequently at intervals, the frequency of the samples depending on the rate of red cell destruction: in general, three specimens between day 2 and day 7, and then two specimens per week for the duration of the study. Measurements should be continued until at least half the radioactivity has disappeared from the circulation.

Measure the haemoglobin or PCV in a part of each sample; then lyse the samples with saponin, mix well, and deliver 1 ml into counting tubes, if possible in duplicate.

Measurement of Radioactivity

Estimate the percentage survival (of ^{51}Cr) on any day (t) by comparing the radioactivity of the sample taken on that day with that of the day 0 sample (i.e., the sample withdrawn 10 [or 60] min after the injection of the labelled cells). Thus ^{51}Cr survival on day t (%) is given by the following:

$$\frac{\text{cpm/ml of blood on Day t}}{\text{cpm/ml of blood on Day 0}} \times 100$$

No adjustment is necessary for the physical decay of the isotope, provided that the standard is counted within a few minutes of the day t sample.

Carry out the measurements in any high-quality scintillation counter, at least 2500 counts being recorded to achieve a precision within ±2%.

Processing of Radioactivity Measurements

Before the data can be analysed and interpreted, factors, other than physical decay, that are involved in the disappearance of radioactivity from the circulation have to be considered. There are two processes: ^{51}Cr-labelled cells are lost from the circulation by lysis, phagocytosis, or haemorrhage and, in addition, ^{51}Cr is eluted from intact red cells that still circulate.

Elution

The rate of elution differs to a small extent from one individual to another. It is thought to vary to a greater extent between different diseases, especially when the red cell lifespan is considerably reduced. However, in such cases, elution and variation in the rate of elution become unimportant. The rate of elution is also influenced by technique, especially by the anticoagulant solution into which the blood is collected prior to labelling. With the NIH-A ACD solution, the rate of elution is about 1% per day.[29]

Early Loss

Sometimes, in addition to the elution that occurs continuously and at a relatively low and constant rate, up to 10% of the ^{51}Cr may be lost within the first 24 hours. The cause of this major early loss is obscure, and several components may be involved. If this major loss does not continue beyond the first 2 days, it is often looked on as an artefact, in the sense that it does not denote an increased rate of lysis *in vivo,* and it can be, and typically is ignored by replotting the figures as described on page 373. This procedure is acceptable, at least for clinical studies, but it does not take into account the possibility that a small proportion of red cells are present that lyse rapidly. It is common practice to calculate the T_{50}Cr,* (i.e., the time taken for the concentration of ^{51}Cr in the blood to fall to 50% of its initial value) after correcting the data for physical decay but not for elution. The chief objection to the use of T_{50}Cr is that it may be misleading without additional information on the pattern of the survival curve. Moreover, the mean red cell lifespan cannot be directly derived from it. With the technique described earlier, the mean value of T_{50} in normal subjects is 30 days, with a range of 25–33 days (Table 15.4).

Correction for Elution

When haemolysis is marked, elution is of minor importance and can be ignored. When haemolysis is not greatly increased, it is essential to correct for elution. This can be done by multiplying the measured survival by the factors given in Table 15.4.

Survival Curves

Normal red cell survival (corrected for elution) will be in the range shown in Figure 15.5. When survival is reduced, a survival curve should be drawn, and from this the mean red cell lifespan can be derived.

Plot the % radioactivity figures or count rates per ml of whole blood (corrected for physical decay and for elution) on arithmetic and semilogarithmic graph paper and attempt to fit straight lines passing through the data points.

*t_{50} is used rather than $T^1/_2$ because the elimination of the label is not a constant exponential fraction of the original amount.

Table 15.4   Normal range for ^{51}Cr survival curves with correction for elution

Day	% ^{51}Cr (corrected for decay; not corrected for elution)	Elution correction factors*
1	93–98	1.03
2	89–97	1.05
3	86–95	1.06
4	83–93	1.07
5	80–92	1.08
6	78–90	1.10
7	77–88	1.11
8	76–86	1.12
9	74–84	1.13
10	72–83	1.14
11	70–81	1.16
12	68–79	1.17
13	67–78	1.18
14	65–77	1.19
15	64–75	1.20
16	62–74	1.22
17	59–73	1.23
18	58–71	1.25
19	57–69	1.26
20	56–67	1.27
21	55–66	1.29
22	53–65	1.31
23	52–63	1.32
24	51–60	1.34
25	50–59	1.36
30	44–52	1.47
35	39–47	1.53
40	34–42	1.60

*To correct for elution, multiply the % ^{51}Cr by the elution factor for the particular day.

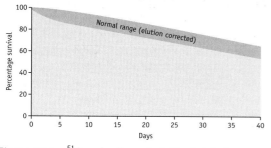

Figure 15.5 ^{51}Cr red cell survival. The hatched area shows the normal range.

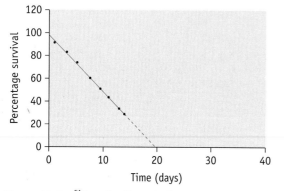

Figure 15.6 ^{51}Cr red cell survival curve. Patient with hereditary spherocytosis. The results give a straight line when plotted on arithmetic graph paper. The mean cell lifespan is indicated by the point at which its extension cuts the abscissa (20 days).

1. If a straight line can be fitted to the arithmetic plot, the mean red cell lifespan is given by the point in time at which the line or its extension cuts the abscissa (Fig. 15.6).
2. As a rule, however, a straight line is better fitted to the semilogarithmic plot; the mean red cell lifespan can be read as the exponential e^{-1} that is, the time when 37% of the cells are still surviving, (Fig. 15.7) or calculated by multiplying the half-time of the fitted line by the reciprocal of the natural log of 2 (0.693) (i.e., multiplying by 1.44).

A computer programmed curve-fitting procedure is more precise but is not likely to improve overall accuracy of the results for clinical purposes.

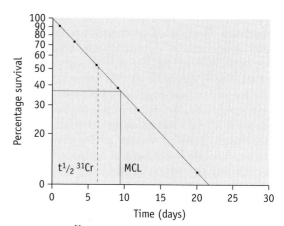

Figure 15.7 ^{51}Cr red cell survival curve. Patient with autoimmune haemolytic anaemia. The results have been plotted on semilogarithmic graph paper, and the mean cell lifespan was read as the time when 37% of the cells were still surviving (9–10 days). The T_{50}Cr was 6–7 days. MCL, mean cell lifespan.

Interpretation of Survival Curves

In the autoimmune haemolytic anaemias, the slope of elimination is usually markedly curvilinear when the data are plotted on arithmetic graph paper. Red cell destruction is typically random and the curve of elimination is thus exponential, and the data give a straight line when plotted on semilogarithmic graph paper.

In some cases of haemolytic anaemia (possibly only when there are intracorpuscular defects), the survival curve appears to consist of two components, an initial steep slope followed by a much less steeply falling slope. This suggests the presence of cells of widely varying lifespan. This type of "double population" curve is seen in paroxysmal nocturnal haemoglobinuria, in sickle cell anaemia, in some cases of hereditary enzyme-deficiency haemolytic anaemia, and when the labelled cells consist of a mixture of transfused normal cells and short-lived patient's cells. The mean cell lifespan of the entire cell population can be deduced by plotting the points on semilogarithmic graph paper, as described earlier. The proportion of cells belonging to the longer-lived population can be estimated by plotting the data on arithmetic graph paper and extrapolating the less steep slope back to the ordinate; the lifespan of this population can be

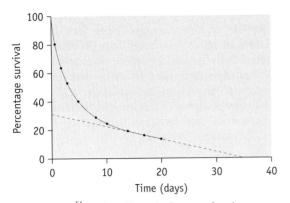

Figure 15.8 ^{51}Cr red cell survival curve showing a "double population." By plotting the data on semilogarithmic graph paper as described in Figure 15.6, the mean cell lifespan (MCL) of the entire cell population was deduced as 5 days. When plotted on arithmetic graph paper, by extrapolation of the less steep slope to the ordinate it was deduced that approximately 30% of the red cells belonged to one population, and by extrapolation of the same slope to the abscissa the MCL of this population was deduced as 35 days. The lifespan of the remaining 70% of cells was calculated to be 3.6 days (see formula). The T_{50}Cr was 3–4 days.

estimated by extending the same slope to the abscissa (Fig. 15.8). The lifespan of the short-lived cells can be deduced from the formula:

$$MCLs = \frac{\frac{\%S}{100}}{\frac{1}{MCL_T} - \frac{\%L}{MCL_L}}$$

where S = short-lived population, L = longer-lived population, T = entire cell population, and MCL = mean cell lifespan.

Correction for Early Loss

The simplest method is to ignore the early loss by taking as 100% the radioactivity still present at the end of 24–48 hours. Alternatively, the following method can be used; it has the advantage that the slope of the survival curve is not altered. Plot the data on arithmetic graph paper, extrapolate the line of the slope beyond the initial steep part back to the ordinate, and take the point of intersection as 100%; then calibrate the ordinate scale accordingly.

Blood Volume Changes

There is no need to correct the measurements of radioactivity per ml of whole blood for alterations in PCV provided that the total blood volume remains constant throughout the study. However, if it is suspected that the BV may be changing (e.g., in patients suffering from haemorrhage or being transfused), serial determinations of BV should be carried out and the observed radioactivity should be multiplied by the observed BV and divided by the initial BV. In practice, if a patient receives a blood transfusion during a survival study, it can, as a general rule, be assumed that the BV will have returned to its pretransfusion level within 24–48 hours.

Correction of Survival Data for Blood Loss

When there is a relatively constant loss of blood during a red cell survival study, the true mean red cell lifespan can be obtained by the following equation:

$$True\ MCL = \frac{Ta \times RCV}{RCV - (Ta \times L)}$$

where Ta = apparent time of MCL (days), RCV = red cell volume (ml), and L = mean rate of loss of red cells (ml/day).

Normal Red Cell Lifespan

The mean red cell lifespan in health is usually taken as 120 days.

COMPATIBILITY TEST

The behaviour of labelled donor cells in a recipient will provide important information on the compatibility or otherwise of the donor blood:

1. When serological tests suggest that all normal donors are incompatible
2. When in the presence of an alloantibody no nonreacting donor can be found
3. When the recipient has had an unexplained haemolytic transfusion reaction

Method

Remove 1–2 ml of blood from the donor bag using a sterile technique. Label 0.5 ml of the red cells with 0.8 MBq of ^{51}Cr, 2 MBq of ^{111}In, or 2 MBq of ^{99m}Tc in the standard way (p. 362) and administer to the recipient. Collect 5–10 ml of blood into EDTA or heparin at 3, 10, and 60 min after the injection from a vein other than that used for the injection. Prepare 1 ml samples in counting vials. Centrifuge the remainder of the specimens and pipette 1 ml of the plasma into counting vials. Measure the radio-activity in the usual way. Calculate the activity in the blood and plasma samples as a percentage of the 3 min blood sample.[29]

Interpretation

With compatible blood, the radioactivity in the 60 min sample is, on average, 99% of that of the 3 min sample, but it may vary between 94% and 104%. If the blood radioactivity at 60 min is not less than 70% and the plasma activity is not more than 3%, the donor cells may be transfused with minimal hazard.[29]

Determination of Sites of Red Cell Destruction Using ^{51}Cr

Because ^{51}Cr is a γ-ray emitter, the sites of destruc-tion of red cells, with special reference to the spleen and liver, can be determined by *in vivo* surface counting using a shielded scintillation counter placed, respectively, over the heart, spleen, and liver. This procedure is laborious, but occasionally it may provide clinically useful information on the role of the spleen in various types of haemolytic anaemia, especially by predicting response to splenectomy.[30]

VISUALIZATION OF THE SPLEEN BY SCINTILLATION SCANNING

Anatomical features of organs, including the spleen, are usually studied in radiology or nuclear medicine departments by means of magnetic resonance imaging (MRI), computed tomography imaging (CT scans), or ultrasound. Imaging of radioisotope-labelled red cells provides an alternative functional method. If red blood cells labelled with ^{99m}Tc are heat damaged, they will be selectively removed by the spleen. ^{99m}Tc-labelled colloid is also removed from circulation by the spleen, but this is not as specific because it is also taken up by reticuloen-dothelial cells in the liver and elsewhere. The rate of uptake of the isotope by the spleen is a measure of its function (see below). Imaging by scintillation

scanning is usually started about 1 hour after the injection of the damaged cells, but it can be performed up to 3–4 hours later. Accumulation of radioactivity within the spleen after administration of heat-damaged labelled cells thus provides a means of demonstrating its size and position, whether it is absent or has reduced function, and the presence of splenuncules. Satisfactory scans can also be obtained with ^{51}Cr or ^{111}In.

Method

With ^{99m}Tc as the label, carry out pre-tinning *in vivo* by an injection of a stannous compound as described on page 363. Then collect 5–10 ml of blood into a sterile bottle containing 100 iu of heparin. Wash twice in sterile 9 g/l NaCl (saline), centrifuging at 1200–1500 g for 5–10 min. Transfer 2 ml of the packed red cells to a 30 ml glass bottle with a screw cap; heat the bottle in a waterbath at a constant temperature of 49.5–50°C for exactly 20 min with occasional gentle mixing. Wash the cells in saline until the supernatant is free from haemoglobin and discard the final supernatant. Label with 40 MBq of ^{99m}Tc by the method described on page 363. After it has stood for 5 min, wash twice in saline. Resuspend in about 10 ml of saline and inject as soon as possible. After about 1 hour carry out a gamma camera scan.[31]

Spleen Function

Information on splenic activity may be obtained by measuring the rate of clearance of heat-damaged labelled red cells from the circulation. A blood sample is taken exactly 3 min after the midpoint of the injection, and further samples are collected at 5 min intervals for 30 min, at 45 min, and a final sample at 60 min. The radioactivity in each sample is measured and expressed as a percentage of the radioactivity in the 3-min sample. The results are plotted on semilogarithmic graph paper, the 3-min sample being taken as 100% radioactivity. For constant results, a carefully standardised technique is necessary to ensure that the red cells are damaged to the same extent.

The disappearance curve is, as a rule, exponential (Fig. 15.9). The initial slope reflects the splenic blood flow; the rate of blood flow is calculated as the reciprocal of the time taken for the radioactivity

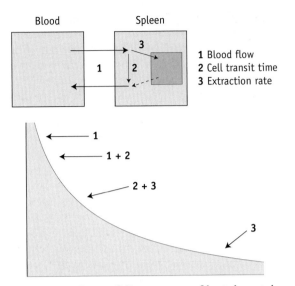

Blood	Spleen	
	3	**1** Blood flow
1	**2**	**2** Cell transit time
		3 Extraction rate

1
1 + 2
2 + 3
3

Figure 15.9   Curve of disappearance of heat-damaged red cells from circulation. The curve shows the sequence of blood flow, transient pooling, sequestration, and irreversible trapping of cells.

to fall to half the 3-min value (i.e., $\dfrac{0.693}{t^{1}/_{2}}$)

where 0.693 is the natural log of 2.

When the spleen is functioning normally, the $t_{1/2}$ is 5–15 min, and fractional splenic blood flow is 0.05–0.14 ml/min (i.e., 5–14% of the circulating blood per min). The clearance rate is considerably prolonged in thrombocythaemia and in conditions associated with splenic atrophy such as sickle cell anaemia, coeliac disease, and dermatitis herpetiformis.[17] It thus provides some indication of spleen function. However, the disappearance curve is a complex of at least two components. The first (mentioned earlier) reflects the splenic blood flow, and the second component mainly measures cell trapping, the consequence of both transient sequestration and phagocytosis with irreversible extraction of the cells from circulation.[32,33] Measurement of phagocytosis alone is obtained more reliably with immunoglobulin G (IgG) (anti-D)-coated red cells.[34]

Leucocyte Imaging

The main diagnostic value of ^{111}In-labelled granulocyte scintigraphy is to localise specific sites of infection and abscesses and, in investigation of patients with fever of unknown origin, to rule out an infectious cause for the fever.[35] For this it is necessary to prepare a granulocyte concentrate separated from other leucocytes (see p. 67). This is then labelled with ^{111}In in a procedure similar to that for labelling platelets (p. 376)[36] and administered. The sites of granulocyte accumulation are shown by gamma camera scan.

Miscellaneous Imaging

In addition to the radioisotopes discussed earlier, there are other radioisotopes that can be used to provide information in haematological disorders. For example, 18F-FDG (fluorine-18 fluorodeoxyglucose), a tracer of glucose metabolism, with position emission tomography (PE) can be useful in the assessment of tumour metabolism.[37,38] The information generated can assist in clinical staging of patients with malignancies, including lymphoma. Malignant tissue shows enhanced uptake of this tracer, and this information can be used to monitor progress of patients receiving chemotherapy.

Similarly, other more mainstream radiological investigations can be useful in the management of haematological diseases. For example, MRI can assist in monitoring the progress of patients with lymphoma and myeloma. In the management of patients with iron overload, MRI scans (by specified imaging method T2) can provide important information on liver and cardiac iron that can be used to optimize iron chelation regimens.[39]

MEASUREMENT OF BLOOD LOSS FROM THE GASTROINTESTINAL TRACT

The ^{51}Cr method of red cell labelling can be used to measure quantitatively blood lost into the gastrointestinal tract because ^{51}Cr is neither excreted nor more than minimally reabsorbed. Accordingly, when the blood contains ^{51}Cr-labelled red cells faecal radioactivity is at a very low level unless bleeding has taken place somewhere within the gastrointestinal tract. Measurement of the faecal radioactivity then gives a reliable indication of the extent of the blood loss.

Method

Label the patient's own blood with approximately 4 MBq of ^{51}Cr, as described on p. 362. On each day of the test, collect the faeces in plastic or waxed cardboard cartons. Prepare a standard by adding a measured volume (3–5 ml) of the patient's blood, collected on each day, to approximately 100 ml of water in a similar carton. Compare the radioactivity of the faecal samples and the corresponding daily standard in a large-volume counting system (see p. 360). Then:

$$\text{Volume of blood in faeces (in ml)} = \frac{\text{cpm/24 hour faeces collection}}{\text{cpm/ml standard}}$$

Blood loss from any other source (e.g., surgicalal operation or menstruation) can be measured in a similar way by counting swabs, dressings, and so on placed in a carton. It is not, however, possible to measure blood or haemoglobin loss in the urine (haematuria or haemoglobinuria) by this method because free ^{51}Cr is normally excreted in the urine.

An imaging procedure has also been described in which blood is labelled with ^{99m}Tc and a large-field scintillation scan is performed after 60–90 min and, if necessary, again at intervals for 24 hours.[40]

MEASUREMENT OF PLATELET LIFESPAN

Principle

The procedure for measuring platelet lifespan is broadly similar to that for red cell survival (see p. 367). A method using ^{111}In-labelled platelets was recommended by ICSH.[41] A modification of this method especially for use with low platelet counts[42] is described in the following.

Method

Collect 51 ml of blood into 9 ml of NIH-A ACD (p. 689); a proportionately lower amount is required if the platelet count is normal or high. Distribute the blood equally into three 30-ml polystyrene tubes, each containing 2 ml of 60 g/l hydroxyethyl starch (Hespan, Bristol Myers Squibb). Mix and immediately centrifuge at 150 g for 10 min. Transfer the supernatant platelet-rich plasma into clean centrifuge tubes and add ACD, 1 volume to 10 volumes of the platelet-rich plasma. If necessary,

centrifuge again at 150 g for 5 min to remove residual red cells.[42]

Centrifuge the platelet-rich plasma at 640 g for 10 min to obtain platelet pellets. Carefully remove the supernatant plasma but do not discard. Add 1 ml of this platelet-poor plasma to the platelet pellets, gently tap the tubes to resuspend, and pool the contents.

Prepare a solution of tropolone, 4.4 mmol/l (0.54 mg/ml) in HEPES-saline buffer, pH 7.6 (p. 691). Mix 0.1 ml with 8 MBq (250 µCi) of ^{111}InCl in less than 50 µl of 40 mmol/l HCl. Add the platelet suspension with gentle mixing and leave at room temperature for 5 min. Then add 5 ml of platelet-poor plasma. Centrifuge at 640 g for 10 min. Remove the supernatant and resuspend the platelet pellet in 5 ml of platelet-poor plasma. Take up the platelet suspension into a 10-ml plastic syringe.

Add 0.5 ml of the platelet suspension to 100 ml of water in a volumetric flask as a standard. Weigh the syringe, inject the platelets into the patient through a butterfly needle, and reweigh.

$$\text{Volume injected} = \text{Wt (g)} \times 1/1.015,$$

where 1.015 is the specific gravity of plasma.

Collect 5-ml blood samples in EDTA at 45 min, at 2, 3, and 4 hours after injection, and then daily for up to 10 days.

Measure the packed cell volume (p. 31) and centrifuge part of each sample at 1500 g for 10 min to obtain cell-free plasma.

Lyse part of the whole blood sample with 2% saponin and measure the radioactivity in 1 ml sample of whole blood, plasma, and diluted standard.

From radioactivity in 1 ml of whole blood sample subtract the radioactivity in 1 ml of plasma, corrected for the true volume of plasma in 1 ml of whole blood (i.e., 1-PCV).

Calculation of Platelet Recovery at Each Sampling Time:

$$\frac{\text{cpm/ml blood sample (corrected for plasma activity)} \times \text{Total BV (ml)}^*}{\text{cpm/ml standard} \times \text{dilution of standard} \times \text{volume injected}}$$

---

*If total blood volume is not measured, an approximate estimate can be obtained from the subject's height and weight.[43]

Analysis of Data

Plot the percent survival against time on arithmetic graph paper and estimate the survival time as for red cell survival (p. 367).

By this method, normal platelet lifespan is 8–10 days, but the validity of the analysis is based on the assumption that the blood volume is constant and the pattern of disappearance of platelets from the circulation remains constant during the course of the study.

Platelet Survival in Disease

In idiopathic thrombocytopenia purpura, platelet lifespan is considerably reduced. It is also shortened in consumption coagulopathies and in thrombotic thrombocytopenic purpura. In thrombocytopenia, because of defective production of platelets, the lifespan should be normal, provided that platelets are not being lost by bleeding during the course of the study. In thrombocytopenia associated with splenomegaly, the recovery of injected labelled platelets is low, but their survival is usually almost normal. By quantitative scanning with ^{111}In, it is possible to measure the splenic platelet pool and to distinguish the relative importance of pooling and destruction of platelets in the spleen.[44-46] The splenic platelet pool is normally about 30% of the total platelet population, and it is thought that each platelet spends one third of its lifespan in the spleen. The size of the pool is increased in splenomegaly, resulting in thrombocytopenia but not necessarily in a reduced mean platelet lifespan.

REFERENCES

1. Wagner HN, Szabo Z, Buchanan JW 1995 Principles of nuclear medicine. Saunders, Philadelphia.
2. Maisey MN, Britton KE, Collier BD 1998 Clinical nuclear medicine, 3rd ed. Chapman and Hall, London.
3. Lewis SM, Bayly RJ (eds) 1986 Methods in hematology 14: radionuclides in haematology. Churchill Livingstone, Edinburgh.
4. National Radiation Protection Board 2000 The ionizing radiation (medical exposure) regulations 2000. HSE Book, London.
5. ARSAC 1993 Notes for guidance on the administration of radiopharmaceuticals and use of sealed radioactive sources. National Radiation Protection Board, Chilton, Didcot Oxon OX11 0RQ. See also website *www. ARSAC>NRPB.*
6. Alavi A (ed) 2002 Impact of FDG-PET imaging on the practice of medicine. Seminars in Nuclear Medicine 32:1–76.
7. Jamar F Lonneux M 2003 Positron emission tomography in haematology. In Peters AM (ed) Nuclear medicine in radiological diagnosis, p 519–529, Martin Dinitz, London.
8. Bentley SA, Lewis SM 1976 The relationship between total red cell volume, plasma volume and venous haematocrit. British Journal of Haematology 33:301–307.
9. International Committee for Standardization in Haematology 1980 Recommended methods for measurements of red-cell and plasma volume. Journal of Nuclear Medicine 21:793–800.
10. Ferrant A, Lewis SM, Szur L 1974 The elution of 99mTc from red cells and its effect on red cell volume measurement. Journal of Clinical Pathology 27:983–985.
11. Goodwin DA 1978 Cell labelling with oxine chelates of radioactive metal ions: techniques and clinical implications. Journal of Nuclear Medicine 19:557–559.
12. Osman S, Danpure HJ 1987 A simple in vitro method of radiolabelling human erythrocytes in whole blood with 113mIn-tropolonate. European Journal of Haematology 39:125–127.
13. Berlin NI, Lewis SM 2000 Measurement of total red-cell volume relative to lean body mass for diagnosis of polycythaemia. American Journal of Clinical Pathology. 114:922–926.
14. International Council for Standardization in Haematology (Expert Panel on Radionuclides) 1995 Interpretation of measured red cell mass and plasma volume in adults. British Journal of Haematology 89:747–756.
15. Lukaski HC, Johnson PE, Bolunchuk WW, et al 1985 Assessment of fat-free mass using bioelectrical impedance measurements of the human body. American Journal of Clinical Nutrition 41:810–817.
16. Lund CJ, Sisson TRC 1958 Blood volume and anemia of mother and baby. American Journal of Obstetrics and Gynecology 76:1013–1023.
17. Pettit JE 1977 Spleen function. Clinics in Haematology 6:639–656.
18. Bateman S, Lewis SM, Nicholas A, et al 1978 Splenic red cell pooling: a diagnostic feature in polycythaemia. British Journal of Haematology 40:389–396.
19. Hegde UM, Williams ED, Lewis SM, et al 1973 Measurement of splenic red cell volume and

visualization of the spleen with 99mTc. Journal of Nuclear Medicine 14:769–771.

20. Miller JH 1987 Technetium-99m-labelled red blood cells in the evaluation of the liver in infants and children. Journal of Nuclear Medicine 28:1412–1418.

21. Front D, Israel O 1981 Tc-99m-labelled red blood cells in the evaluation of vascular abnormalities. Journal of Nuclear Medicine 22:149–151.

22. Cavill I 1986 Plasma clearance studies. Methods in Hematology 14:214–244.

23. Peters AM, Swirsky DM 1998 Blood disorders. In: Maisey MN, Britton KE, Collier BD (eds) Clinical nuclear medicine, 3rd ed. Chapman and Hall, London.

24. Bentley SA, Miller DT 1986 Radionuclide blood cell survival studies. Methods in Hematology 14:245–262.

25. Ricketts C, Cavill I, Napier JAF 1977 The measurement of red cell lifespan using 59Fe. British Journal of Haematology 37:403–408.

26. Pearson HA 1963 The binding of 51Cr to hemoglobin. I. In vitro studies. Blood 22:218–230.

27. Jandl JH, Greenberg MS, Yonemoto RH, et al 1956 Clinical determination of the sites of red cell sequestration in hemolytic anemias. Journal of Clinical Investigation 35:842–867.

28. Koutras GA, Schneider AS, Hattori M, et al 1965 Studies of chromated erythrocytes: mechanisms of chromate inhibition of glutathione reductase. British Journal of Haematology 11:360–369.

29. International Committee for Standardization in Haematology 1980 Recommended methods for radioisotope red-cell survival studies. British Journal of Haematology 45:659–666.

30. International Committee for Standardization in Haematology 1975 Recommended methods for surface counting to determine sites of red-cell destruction. British Journal of Haematology 30:249–254.

31. Royal HD, Brown ML, Drum DE, et al 1998 Procedure guideline for hepatic and splenic imaging. Journal of Nuclear Medicine 39:1114–1116.

32. Peters AM, Ryan PFJ, Klonizakis I, et al 1981 Analysis of heat-damaged erythrocyte clearance curves. British Journal of Haematology 49:581–586.

33. Peters AM, Ryan PFJ, Klonizakis I, et al 1982 Kinetics of heat damaged autologous red blood cells. Scandinavian Journal of Haematology 28:5–14.

34. Peters AM, Walport MJ, Elkon KB, et al 1984 The comparative blood clearance kinetics of modified radiolabelled erythrocytes. Clinical Science 66:55–62.

35. Kjaer A, Lebech A-M 2002 Diagnostic value of ^{111}In-granulocyte scintigraphy in patients with fever of unknown origin. Journal of Nuclear Medicine 43:140–144.

36. Buscombe J 1998 Infection. In: Maisey MN, Britton KE, Collier BD (eds) Clinical nuclear medicine, 3rd ed. Chapman and Hall, London.

37. Weber WA, Schwaiger M, Avril N 2000 Quantitative assessment of tumour metabolism using FDG-PET imaging. Nuclear Medicine and Biology 27:683–687.

38. Schöder H, Larson SM, Yeung HW 2004 PET/CT in oncology: Integration into clinical management of lymphoma, melanoma, and gastrointestinal malignancies. Journal of Nuclear Medicine 45:72S–81S.

39. Anderson LJ, Wonke B, Prescott E et al 2002 Comparison of effects of oral deferiprone and subcutaneous desferrioxamine on myocardial iron concentrations and ventricular function in beta-thalassaemia. Lancet 360:516–520.

40. Ford PV, Bartold SP, Fink-Bennett DM, et al 1999 Procedure guideline for gastrointestinal bleeding and Meckel's diverticulum scintigraphy. Journal of Nuclear Medicine 40:1226–1232.

41. International Committee for Standardization in Haematology 1988 Recommended methods for ^{111}In platelet survival studies. Journal of Nuclear Medicine 29:564–566.

42. Danpure HJ, Osman S, Peters AM 1990 Labelling autologous platelets with ^{111}In tropolonate for platelet kinetic studies: limitations imposed by thombocytopenia European Journal of Haematology 45:223–230.

43. Hurley PJ 1975 Red cell and plasma volumes in normal adults. Journal of Nuclear Medicine 16:46–52.

44. Peters AM, Swirsky DM 1998 Blood disorders In: Maisey MN, Britton KE, Collier BD (ed) Clinical nuclear medicine, 3rd ed. pp. 525–539, Chapman and Hall, London.

45. Peters AM, Saverymuttu SH, Bell RN, et al 1985 The kinetics of short-lived indium-111 radiolabelled platelets. Scandinavian Journal of Haematology 34:137–145.

46. Peters AM, Saverymuttu SH, Wonke B, et al 1984 The interpretation of platelet kinetic studies for the identification of site of abnormal platelet destruction. British Journal of Haematology 57:637–649.

16 Investigation of haemostasis

Mike Laffan and Richard Manning

COMPONENTS OF NORMAL HAEMOSTASIS

The haemostatic mechanisms have several important functions: (a) to maintain blood in a fluid state while it remains circulating within the vascular system; (b) to arrest bleeding at the site of injury or blood loss by formation of a haemostatic plug; and (c) to ensure the eventual removal of the plug when healing is complete. Normal physiology thus constitutes a delicate balance between these conflicting tendencies, and a deficiency or exaggeration of any one may lead to either thrombosis or haemorrhage. There are at least five different components involved: blood vessels, platelets, plasma coagulation factors, their inhibitors, and the fibrinolytic system. In this chapter a brief review of normal haemostasis is presented followed by a discussion on the general principles of basic tests used to investigate haemostasis and bleeding disorders.

The Blood Vessel

General Structure of the Blood Vessel

The blood vessel wall has three layers: intima, media, and adventitia. The intima consists of endothelium and subendothelial connective tissue and is separated from the media by the elastic lamina interna. Endothelial cells form a continuous monolayer lining all blood vessels. The structure and the function of the endothelial cells vary according to their location in the vascular tree, but in their resting state they all share three important characteristics: they are "non-thrombogenic" (i.e., they promote maintenance of blood in its fluid state), they play an active role in supplying nutrients to the subendothelial structures, and they act as a barrier to macromolecules and particulate matter circulating in the bloodstream. The permeability of the endothelium may vary under different conditions to allow various molecules and cells to pass.

Endothelial Cell Function[1]

The luminal surface of the endothelial cell is covered by the glycocalyx, a proteoglycan coat. It contains heparan sulphate and other glycosamino-glycans, which are capable of activating antithrombin, an important inhibitor of coagulation enzymes. Tissue factor pathway inhibitor (TFPI) is present on endothelial cell surfaces bound to these heparans but also tethered to a GPI (glycophosphoinositol) anchor. The relative importance of these two TFPI pools is not known. Endothelial cells express a number of coagulation active proteins that play an important regulatory role such as thrombomodulin and the endothelial protein C (PC) receptor. Thrombin generated at the site of injury is rapidly bound to a specific product of the endothelial cell, thrombomodulin. When bound to this protein, thrombin can activate PC (which degrades factors Va and VIIIa) and a carboxypeptidase (which inhibits fibrinolysis; discussed later). Thrombin also stimulates the endothelial cell to produce plasminogen activator. The endothelium can also synthesize protein S, the cofactor for PC. Finally, endothelium produces von Willebrand factor (VWF), essential for platelet adhesion to the subendothelium. This is both stored in specific granules called Weibel Palade bodies and secreted constitutively, partly into the circulation and partly toward the subendothelium. The expression of these and other important molecules such as adhesion molecules and their receptors are modulated by inflammatory cytokines. The lipid bilayer membrane also contains ADPase (adenosine diphosphatase), an enzyme that degrades ADP (adenosine diphosphate), which is a potent platelet agonist (see p. 430). Many of the surface proteins are found localised in the specialized lipid raft invaginations called caveolae.[2]

The endothelial cell participates in vasoregulation by producing and metabolising numerous vasoactive substances. On one hand it metabolises and inactivates vasoactive peptides such as bradykinin; on the other hand, it can also generate angiotensin II, a local vasoconstrictor, from circulating angiotensin I. Under appropriate stimulation the endothelial cell can produce vasodilators such as nitric oxide (NO) and prostacyclin or vasoconstrictors such as endothelin and thromboxane. These substances have their principal vasoregulatory effect via the smooth muscle but also have some effect on platelets.

The subendothelium consists of connective tissues composed of collagen (principally types I, III, and VI), elastic tissues, proteoglycans, and non-collagenous glycoproteins, including fibronectin and VWF. After vessel wall damage has occurred, these components are exposed and are then responsible for platelet adherence. This appears to be mediated by VWF binding to collagen, particularly under high shear rate, and also to the microfibrils, which have a greater affinity for VWF under some conditions. VWF then undergoes a conformational change, and platelets are captured via their surface membrane glycoprotein Ib binding to VWF. Platelet activation follows, and a conformational change in glycoprotein IIbIIIa allows further, more secure, binding to VWF via this receptor as well as to fibrinogen. At low shear rates platelet binding directly to collagen appears to dominate.[3]

Vasoconstriction[1,4]

Vessels with muscular coats contract following injury thus helping to arrest blood loss. Although not all coagulation reactions are enhanced by reduced flow, this probably assists in the formation of a stable fibrin plug. Vasoconstriction also occurs in the microcirculation in vessels without smooth muscle cells. Endothelial cells themselves can produce vasoconstrictors such as angiotensin II. In addition, activated platelets produce thromboxane A_2 (TXA$_2$), which is a potent vasoconstrictor.

Platelets[5,6]

Platelets are small fragments of cytoplasm derived from megakaryocytes. On average they are 1.5–3.5 μm in diameter but may be larger in some disease states. They do not contain a nucleus and are bounded by a typical lipid bilayer membrane. Beneath the outer membrane lies the marginal band of microtubules, which maintain the shape of the platelet and depolymerise when aggregation begins. The central cytoplasm is dominated by the three types of platelet granules: the δ granules, α granules, and lysosomal granules. The contents of these various granules are detailed in Table 16.1. Finally there exists the dense tubular system and the canalicular membrane system; the latter communicates with the exterior. It is not clear how all these elements act together to perform such functions as contraction and secretion, which are characteristic of platelet activation.

The platelet membrane is the site of interaction with the plasma environment and with the damaged vessel wall. It consists of phospholipids cholesterol; glycolipids; and at least nine glycoproteins, named GpI–GpIX. The membrane phospholipids are asym-

---

Table 16.1 Some contents of platelet granules

Dense (δ) granules	α Granules	Lysosomal vesicles
ATP	PF4	Galactosidases
ADP	β-Thromboglobulin	Fucosidases
Calcium	Fibrinogen	Hexosaminidase
Serotonin	Factor V	Glucuronidase
Pyrophosphate	Thrombospondin	Cathepsin
P selectin (CD62)	Fibronectin	Glycohydrolases
Transforming growth factor-beta (1)	PDGF	+ others
Catecholamines (noradrenaline/adrenaline)	PAI-1	
GDP/GTP	Histidine-rich glycoprotein α$_2$ Macroglobulin Plasmin inhibitor P selectin (CD62)	

ADP, adenosine 5′-diphosphate; ATP, adenosine 5′-triphosphate; GDP, guanosine 5′-diphosphate; GTP, guanosine 5′-triphosphate; PAI-1, plasminogen activator inhibitor-1; PDGF, platelet-derived growth factor.

metrically distributed, with sphingomyelin and phosphatidylcholine predominating in the outer leaflet, and phosphatidyl-ethanolamine, -inositol and -serine in the inner leaflet. After platelet activation the membrane also expresses binding sites for several coagulation proteins such as factor XI and factor VIII.

The contractile system of the platelet consists of the dense microtubular system and the circumferential microfilaments, which maintain the disc shape. Actin is the main constituent of the contractile system, but myosin and a regulatory calcium-binding protein, calmodulin, are also present.

Platelet Function in the Haemostatic Process[7]

The main steps in platelet functions are adhesion, activation with shape change, and aggregation. When the vessel wall is damaged, the subendothelial structures, including basement membrane, collagen, and microfibrils, are exposed. Surface-bound VWF binds to GpIb on circulating platelets, resulting in an initial monolayer of adhering platelets. Binding via GpIb initiates activation of the platelet via a G-protein mechanism. Once activated, platelets immediately change shape from a disc to a tiny sphere with numerous projecting pseudopods. After adhesion of a single layer of platelets to the exposed subendothelium, platelets stick to one another to form aggregates. Fibrinogen, fibronectin, and the glycoprotein Ib–IX and IIbIIIa complexes are essential at this stage to increase the cell-to-cell contact and facilitate aggregation. Certain substances (agonists) react with specific platelet membrane receptors to promote platelet aggregation and further activation. The agonists include exposed collagen fibres, ADP, thrombin, adrenaline, serotonin, and certain arachidonic acid metabolites including TXA_2. In areas of nonlinear blood flow, such as may occur at the site of an injury, locally damaged red cells release ADP, which further activates platelets.

Platelet Aggregation

Platelet aggregation may occur by at least two independent but closely linked pathways. The first pathway involves arachidonic acid metabolism. Activation of phospholipase enzymes (PLA_2) releases free arachidonic acid from membrane phospholipids (phosphatidyl choline). About 50% of free arachidonic acid is converted by a lipo-oxygenase enzyme

to a series of products including leucotrienes, which are important chemoattractants of white cells. The remaining 50% of arachidonic acid is converted by the enzyme cyclooxygenase into labile cyclic endoperoxides, most of which are in turn converted by thromboxane synthetase into TXA_2. TXA_2 has profound biological effects, causing secondary platelet granule release and local vasoconstriction, as well as further local platelet aggregation via the second pathway below. It exerts these effects by raising intracellular cytoplasmic free calcium concentration and binding to specific granule receptors. TXA_2 is very labile with a half-life of less than 1 min before it is degraded into the inactive thromboxane B_2 (TXB_2) and malonyldialdehyde.

The second pathway of activation and aggregation can proceed completely independently from the first one: various platelet agonists, including thrombin, TXA_2, and collagen, bind to receptors and, via a G-protein mechanism, activate phospholipase C. This generates diacylglycerol and inositol triphosphate, which in turn activate protein kinase C and elevate intracellular calcium, respectively. Calcium is released from the dense tubular system to form complexes with calmodulin; this complex and the free calcium act as coenzymes for the release reaction, for the activation of different regulatory proteins and of actin and myosin and the contractile system, and also for the liberation of arachidonic acid from membrane phospholipids and the generation of TXA_2.

The aggregating platelets join together into loose reversible aggregates, but after the release reaction of the platelet granules, a larger, firmer aggregate forms. Changes in the platelet membrane configuration now occur; "flip-flop" rearrangement of the surface brings the negatively charged phosphatidyl-serine and -inositol on to the outer leaflet, thus generating platelet factor 3 (procoagulant) activity. At the same time specific receptors for various coagulation factors are exposed on the platelet surface and help coordinate the assembly of the enzymatic complexes of the coagulation system. Local generation of thrombin will then further activate platelets.

Platelets are not activated if in contact with healthy endothelial cells. The "nonthrombogenicity" of the endothelium is the result of a combination of control mechanisms exerted by the endothelial cell:

synthesis of prostacyclin, capacity to bind thrombin and activate the PC system, ability to inactivate vasoactive substances, and so on. Prostacyclin released locally binds to specific platelet membrane receptors and then activates the membrane-bound adenylate cyclase (producing cyclic adenosine monophosphate, or cAMP). cAMP inhibits platelet aggregation by inhibiting arachidonic acid metabolism and the release of free cytoplasmic calcium ions.

Thus platelets have at least three roles in haemostasis:

1. Adhesion and aggregation forming the primary haemostatic plug
2. Release of platelet activating and procoagulant molecules
3. Provision of a procoagulant surface for the reactions of the coagulation system.

Blood Coagulation[8]

The central event in the coagulation pathways is the production of thrombin, which acts upon fibrinogen to produce fibrin and thus the fibrin clot. This clot is further strengthened by the crosslinking action of factor XIII, which itself is activated by thrombin. The two commonly used coagulation tests, the activated partial thromboplastin time (APTT) and the prothrombin time (PT) have been used historically to define two pathways of coagulation activation: the intrinsic and extrinsic paths, respectively. However, this bears only a limited relationship to the way coagulation is activated *in vivo*. For example, deficiencies of factor XII or of factor VIII both produce marked prolongation of the APTT, but only deficiency of the latter is associated with a haemorrhagic tendency. Moreover, there is considerable evidence that activation of factor IX (intrinsic pathway) by factor VIIa (extrinsic pathway) is crucial to establishing coagulation after an initial stimulus has been provided by factor VIIa-tissue factor (TF) activation of factor X.[8] See Figure 16.1.

Investigation of the coagulation system centres on the coagulation factors, but the activity of these proteins is also greatly dependent on specific surface receptors and phospholipids largely presented on the surface of platelets but also by activated

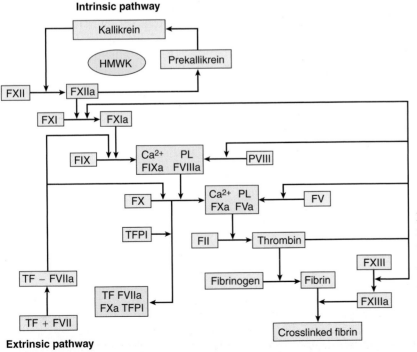

Figure 16.1   Schematic representation of the coagulation network. The major interactions are shown by the bold arrows. Inhibitory factors and clot limiting mechanisms are not shown. HMWK, high molecular weight kininogen; PL, phospholipid; TFPI, tissue factor pathway inhibitor.

endothelium. The necessity for calcium in many of these reactions is frequently used to control their activity *in vitro*. The various factors are described in the following sections, as far as possible in their functional groups; their properties are detailed in Table 16.2.

The Contact Activation System[9]

The contact activation system comprises factor XII (Hageman factor), high molecular weight kininogen (HMWK) (Fitzgerald factor), and prekallikrein/kallikrein (Fletcher factor). As mentioned earlier, these factors do not appear to be essential for haemostasis *in vivo*. There is evidence that their ability to activate the fibrinolytic system may be functionally more important as may their ability to generate vasoactive peptides; in particular, bradykinin is released from HMWK by prekallikrein or FXIIa cleavage. Kallikrein and factor XIIa also function as chemoattractants for neutrophils.

When bound to a negatively charged surface *in vitro*, factor XII and prekallikrein are able to reciprocally activate one another by limited proteo-lysis, but the initiating event is not clear. It may be that a conformational change in factor XII on binding results in limited autoactivation that triggers the process. HMWK acts as a (zinc-dependent) cofactor by facilitating the attachment of prekallikrein and factor XI, with which it circulates in a complex, to the negatively charged surface. It has been shown in *in vitro* studies that platelets or endothelial cells can provide the necessary negatively charged surface for this mechanism and also possess specific receptors for factor XI. The contact system can activate fibrinolysis by a number of mechanisms: plasminogen cleavage, urokinase plasminogen activator (uPA) activation, and tissue plasminogen activator (tPA) release. Most importantly from the laboratory point of view, the contact activation system results in the generation of factor XIIa, which is able to activate factor XI, thus initiating the coagulation cascade of the intrinsic pathway.

Tissue Factor

TF is the cofactor for the extrinsic pathway and the physiological initiator of coagulation. It is a lipo-

Table 16.2   The coagulation factors

No.	Factor	RMM (Daltons)	Half–life	Concentration in plasma	
				μg/ml	nmol/l
I	Fibrinogen	340 000	90 h	1.5–4 × 10	–
II	Prothrombin	70 000	60 h	100–150	1400
V	–	330 000	12–36 h	5–10	20
VII	–	48 000	6 h	0.5	10
VIII	–	200 000	12 h	0.2	0.7
vWF	–	800 000–140 000 000	24 h	10	–
IX	–	57 000	24 h	4	90
X	–	58 000	40 h	10	170
XI	–	158 000	60 h	6	30
XII	–	80 000	48–52 h	30	375
Pre-kallikrein	–	85 000	48 h	40	450
HMWK	–	120 000	6.5 days	80	700
XIII	–	32 000	3–5 days	30 (A+B)	900 (tetramer)

RMM, Relative molecular mass (molecular weight); h, hours; HMWK, high molecular weight kininogen; vWF, von Willebrand factor.

protein that is membrane bound and constitutively present in many tissues outside the vasculature and on the surface of stimulated inflammatory cells such as monocytes and, under some conditions, endothelial cells. Factor VIIa binds to TF in the presence of calcium ions and then becomes enzymatically active. Small amounts of factor VIIa are present in the circulation but have virtually no enzymic activity unless bound to TF. The factor VIIa–TF complex can activate both factor X and factor IX, and therefore two routes to thrombin production are stimulated. Factor Xa subsequently binds to TFPI and then to factor VIIa to form a quaternary (Xa–TF–VIIa–TFPI) complex. This mechanism therefore functions to shut off the extrinsic pathway after an initial stimulus to coagulation has been provided.

The Vitamin K–Dependent Factors

The vitamin K–dependent factors group includes coagulation factors II, VII, IX, and X. However, it is important to remember that the anticoagulant proteins S, C, and Z are also vitamin K-dependent. Each of these proteins contains a number of glutamic acid residues at its amino terminus that are γ-carboxylated by a vitamin K–dependent mechanism. This results in a novel amino acid, γ-carboxyglutamic acid, which is important in promoting a conformational change in the protein that promotes binding of the factor to phospholipid. Because this binding is crucial for coordinating the interaction of the various factors, the proteins produced in the absence of vitamin K (PIVKAs) that are not γ-carboxylated are essentially functionless. The vitamin K–dependent factors are proenzymes or zymogens, which require cleavage sometimes with release of a small peptide (activation peptide) to become functional. Measurement of these activation peptides has been used as a means of assessing coagulation activation.

Cofactors

Factors VIII and V are the two most labile of the coagulation factors, and they are rapidly lost from stored blood or heated plasma. They share considerable structural homology and are cofactors for the serine proteases FIX and FX, respectively; they both require proteolytic activation by factor IIa or Xa to function. Factor VIII circulates in combina-tion with VWF, which is present in the form of large multimers of a basic 200 kD monomer. One function of VWF is to stabilize factor VIII and protect it from degradation. In the absence of VWF the survival of factor VIII in the circulation is extremely short (i.e., <2 hours instead of the normal 8–12 hours). VWF may also serve to deliver factor VIII to platelets adherent to a site of vascular injury. Once factor VIII has been cleaved and activated by thrombin it no longer binds to VWF.

Fibrinogen[10,11]

Fibrinogen is a large dimeric protein, each half consisting of three polypeptides named Aα, Bβ, and γ held together by 12 disulphide bonds. The two monomers are joined together by a further three disulphide bonds. A variant γ chain denoted γ' is produced by a variation in messenger RNA splicing. In the process a platelet binding site is lost and high-affinity binding sites for FXIII and thrombin are gained. The γ' variant constitutes approximately 10% of plasma fibrinogen. A less common (<2%) a chain variant "γE" is also produced by splice variation. Fibrinogen is also found in platelets, but the bulk of this is derived from glycoprotein IIbIIIa–mediated endocytosis of plasma fibrinogen, which is then stored in alpha granules, rather than synthesis by megakaryocytes. Fibrin is formed from fibrinogen by thrombin cleavage of the A and B peptides from fibrinogen. This results in fibrin monomers that associate to form a polymer that is the visible clot. The central E domain exposed by thrombin cleavage binds with a complementary region on the outer or D domain of another monomer. The monomers thus assemble into a staggered overlapping two-stranded fibril. More complex interactions subsequently lead to branched and thickened fibre formation

Factor XIII

The initial fibrin clot is held together by non-covalent interactions and can be deformed and resolubilized. Factor XIII, which is also activated by thrombin, is able to covalently crosslink these fibrin monomers. Factor XIII is a transglutaminase that joins a glutamine residue on one chain to a lysine on an adjacent chain. This loss of resolubility is the basis of the screening test for factor XIII deficiency.

Inhibitors of Coagulation[12,13]

A number of mechanisms exist to ensure that the production of the fibrin clot is limited to the site of injury and is not allowed to propagate indefinitely. First there are a number of proteins that bind to and inactivate the enzymes of the coagulation cascade. Probably the first of these to become active is TFPI, which rapidly quenches the factor VIIa–TF complex that initiates coagulation. It does this by combining first with factor Xa so that coagulation is thereafter dependent on the small amount of thrombin that has been generated activating the intrinsic pathway.

The principal physiological inactivator of thrombin is antithrombin (AT, formerly ATIII), which belongs to the serpin group of proteins. This binds to factor IIa forming an inactive thrombin–antithrombin complex (TAT), which is subsequently cleared from the circulation by the liver. This process is greatly enhanced by the presence of heparin or vessel wall heparan. AT is responsible for approximately 60% of thrombin-inactivating capacity in the plasma; the remainder is provided by heparin cofactor II and less specific inhibitors such as α2 macroglobulin. AT is also capable of inactivating factors X, IX, XI, and XII but to lesser degrees than thrombin.

As thrombin spreads away from the area of damage it is also bound by thrombomodulin on the surface of endothelial cells. In this way it is changed from a primarily procoagulant protein to an anticoagulant one. Although remaining available for binding to AT, thrombin bound to thrombomodulin no longer cleaves fibrinogen. It now has a greatly enhanced preference for PC as a substrate. PC activated by thrombin cleavage acts to limit and arrest coagulation by inactivating factors Va and VIIIa. This action is further enhanced by its cofactor protein S, which does not require prior activation. In larger vessels, where the effective concentration of thrombomodulin is low, the binding of PC is enhanced by the endothelial PC receptor (EPCR). PC is subsequently inactivated by its own specific inhibitor.

The Fibrinolytic System

The deposition of fibrin and its removal are regulated by the fibrinolytic system.[14] Although this is a complex multicomponent system with many activators and inhibitors, it centres around the fibrinogen- and fibrin-cleaving enzyme plasmin. Plasmin circulates in its inactive precursor form, plasminogen, which is activated by proteolytic cleavage. The principal plasminogen activator (PA) in humans is tissue plasminogen activator (t-PA) which is another serine protease. tPA and plasminogen are both able to bind to fibrin via the amino acid lysine. When they are both bound, the rate of plasminogen activation is markedly increased, and thus plasmin is generated preferentially at its site of action and not free in plasma. The second important physiological PA in humans is called urokinase (u-PA). This single chain molecule (scu-PA) is activated by plasmin or kallikrein to a two-chain derivative (tcu-PA), which is not fibrin-specific in its action. However, the extent to which this is important *in vivo* is not clear, and the identification of cell surface receptors for uPA suggests that its primary role may be extravascular. The contact activation system also appears to generate some plasminogen activation via factor XIIa, and bradykinin stimulates release of tPA. The degradation products released by the action of plasmin on fibrin are of diagnostic use and are discussed later in this chapter. The activation of plasmin on fibrin is restricted by the action of a carboxypeptidase, which removes the amino terminal lysine residues for plasminogen and tPA binding. This carboxypeptidase is activated by thrombomodulin-bound thrombin and is referred to as thrombin-activated fibrinolysis inhibitor (TAFI).

PAI-1 (plasminogen activator inhibitor-1) is a potent inhibitor of tPA, produced by endothelial cells, hepatocytes, platelets, and placenta. Levels in plasma are highly variable. It is a member of the serpin family and is active against tPA and tcu-PA but not scu-PA. A second inhibitor PAI-2 has also been identified, originally from human placenta, but its role and importance are not yet established.

The main physiological inhibitor of plasmin in plasma is plasmin inhibitor (α2-antiplasmin), which inhibits plasmin function by forming a 1:1 complex (plasmin–antiplasmin complex, PAP). This reaction in free solution is extremely rapid but depends on the availability of free lysine-binding sites on the plasmin. Thus, fibrin-bound plasmin in the clot is not accessible to the inhibitor. Deficiencies of the fibrinolytic system are rare but have sometimes been associated with a tendency to thrombosis or haemorrhage.

GENERAL APPROACH TO INVESTIGATION OF HAEMOSTASIS

This section begins with some general points regarding the clinical and laboratory approach to the investigation of haemostasis. Following this, the basic or first-line screening tests of haemostasis are described. These tests are generally used as the first step in investigation of an acutely bleeding patient, a person with a suspected bleeding tendency or as a precaution before an invasive procedure is carried out. They have the virtue that they are easily performed and the patterns of abnormalities obtained point clearly to the appropriate next set of investigations. It should be remembered, however, that these tests may be normal in the presence of a mild but significant bleeding diathesis such as VWD or disorders of platelets or vessels. Hence a normal "clotting screen" should not be taken to mean that haemostasis is normal.

Clinical Approach

The investigation of a suspected bleeding tendency may begin from three different points:

1. *Investigating a clinically suspected bleeding tendency.* The investigation properly begins with the bleeding history, which may suggest an acquired or congenital disorder of primary or secondary haemostasis. If the bleeding history or family history is significant, appropriate specific tests and assays should be performed, notwithstanding the results of screening tests such as the PT, APTT, and so on.
2. *Following up an abnormal first-line test.* The abnormalities already detected will determine the appropriate further investigations (discussed later).
3. *Investigation of acute haemostatic failure.* This is often required in the context of an acutely ill or postoperative patient. Investigations are therefore directed toward detecting disseminated intravascular coagulation (DIC) or a previously undetected coagulation defect (congenital or acquired). The availability of a normal premorbid coagulation screen and further questioning to determine a bleeding history can be extremely useful in this respect.

In all cases comprehensive clinical evaluation, including the patient's history, the family history, and the family tree, as well as the details of the site, frequency, and the character of haemorrhagic manifestations (purpura, bruising, large haematomata, haemarthroses, etc.), is required to establish a definitive diagnosis. If considered in conjunction with laboratory results, they will help avoid misinterpretation. It is also desirable to undertake a series of screening tests before proceeding to more specific tests. The results of the screening investigations, taken in conjunction with clinical information, usually point to the appropriate additional procedure.

Despite their simplicity it is clearly important that the results obtained from the first-line tests are reproducible and accurate. This requires attention to blood sample collection and processing, selection, preparation and storage of reagents, and the use of appropriate controls and standards. Laboratories should participate in local or national quality assessment schemes.

Principles of Laboratory Analysis

It is worth remembering that the tests of coagulation performed in the laboratory are attempts to mimic *in vitro* processes that normally occur *in vivo*. Not surprisingly, this may give rise to misleading results. One of the most striking is the gross prolongation of the APTT in complete factor XII deficiency in the absence of any bleeding tendency. Similarly, the amount of factor VII required to produce a normal PT is greatly in excess of the amount required for normal haemostasis. Conversely, normal screening tests do not necessarily imply that the patient has entirely normal haemostasis. The only *in vivo* test of coagulation that is commonly performed is the bleeding time, and even with this test there are notable discrepancies between the results and the clinical bleeding propensity.

The more detailed investigations of coagulation proteins also require caution in their interpretation depending on the type of assay performed. These can be divided into three principal categories, as described in the following sections.

Immunological

The immunological tests include immuno-diffusion, immuno-electrophoresis, radioimmunometric assays, latex agglutination tests, and tests using enzyme-linked immunosorbent assays (ELISA). Fundamentally, all these tests rely on the recognition of the protein in question by polyclonal or monoclonal antibodies. Polyclonal antibodies lack specificity but provide relatively high sensitivity, whereas monoclonal antibodies are highly specific but produce relatively low levels of antigen binding. Immunological assays are often easy to perform, particularly convenient for large batches, and can be bought as kits with standardised controls. The obvious drawback of these assays is that they may tell you nothing about the functional capacity of the antigen detected. If possible they should always be carried out in parallel with a functional assay.

With advances in automation, latex agglutination kits are becoming more popular and replacing the more established ELISA assays. Latex microparticles are coated with antibodies specific for the antigen to be determined. When the latex suspension is mixed with plasma an antigen–antibody reaction takes place, leading to the agglutination of the latex microparticles. Agglutination leads to an increase in turbidity of the reaction medium, and this increase in turbidity is measured photometrically as an increase in absorbance. Usually the wavelength used for latex assays is 405 nm, although for some assays a wavelength of 540 or 800 nm is used. Instrument-specific application sheets should be followed for each kit. This type of assay is referred to as immuno-turbidimetric. Do not freeze latex particles because this will lead to irreversible clumping. An occasional problem with latex agglutination assays is interference from rheumatoid factor or para-proteins. These may cause agglutination and overestimation of the protein under assay. It is then preferable to resort to an ELISA assay. Applications of latex particles include the following:

Calibration standards
Filter challenges
Agglutination assays
Phagocytosis studies

Flow cytometry standards
Laser Doppler velocimetry
Light scattering studies

Assays Using Chromogenic Peptide Substrates (Amidolytic Assays)

The serine proteases of the coagulation cascade have narrow substrate specificities. It is possible to synthesise a short peptide specific for each enzyme that has a dye (*p*-nitroaniline, *p*-NA) attached to the terminal amino acid. When the synthetic peptide reacts with the specific enzyme, the dye is released and the rate of its release or the total amount released can be measured photometrically. This gives a measure of the enzyme activity present. Chromogenic substrate assays can be classified into direct and indirect assays. Direct assays can be further subclassified into primary assays, in which a substrate specific for the enzyme to be measured is used, and secondary assays, in which the enzyme or proenzyme measured is used to activate a second protease for which a specific substrate is available. Specific substrates are available for many coagulation enzymes. However, the substrate specificity is not absolute and most kits include inhibitors of other enzymes capable of cleaving the substrate to improve specificity. Indirect assays are used to measure naturally occurring inhibitors and some platelet factors.[15]

It should be remembered that the measurement of amidolytic activity is not the same as the measurement of biological activity in a coagulation assay and in some cases may not accurately reflect this. This is particularly important when dealing with the molecular variants of various coagulation factors. Nevertheless, the continuing development of more specific substrates with good solubility and high affinity for individual enzymes, together with rapid advances in automation, make chromogenic substrate assays increasingly popular. The assays can be carried out in a microtitre plate or in a tube when a spectrophotometer is used to measure the intensity of the colour development.

Coagulation Assays

Coagulation assays are functional bioassays and rely on comparison with a control or standard preparation with a known level of activity. In the one-stage system optimal amounts of all the clotting factors are present except the one to be determined, which should be as near to nil as possible. The best one-stage system is provided by a substrate plasma obtained either from a patient with severe congenital deficiency or artificially depleted by immuno-adsorption. The principles of bioassay, its standardisation, and its limitations are considered in detail on page 407.

Coagulation techniques are also used in mixing tests to identify a missing factor in an emergency or to identify and estimate quantitatively an inhibitor or anticoagulant. The advantage of this type of assay is that it most closely approximates the activity *in vivo* of the factor in question. However, they can be technically more difficult to perform than the other types described earlier.

Other Assays

Other assays include measurement of coagulation factors using snake venoms, assay of ristocetin cofactor, and the clot solubility test for factor XIII. DNA analysis is becoming more useful and more prevalent in coagulation. However, this requires entirely different equipment and techniques (see Chapter 21).

NOTES ON EQUIPMENT

Waterbaths

A 37°C water bath is required for manual coagulation tests, incubation steps, and the rapid thawing of frozen specimens. Waterbaths set at 37°C should vary by no more than ± 0.5°C because slight variation in temperature will markedly affect the speed of clotting reactions. A waterbath with plastic or glass sides is preferable, and some type of cross-illumination helps to determine the exact time and appearance of fibrin clot formation. Check that the temperature is 37°C before and during use. Distilled water should be used to fill and maintain the water level.

Refrigerators and Freezers

Check that the temperature has not been out of the acceptable range of 4° ± 2°C for refrigerators and −20° ± 2°C for freezers, rechecking during the day. Records must be kept.

Centrifuges

Check to ensure each machine is clean before and after use. Also do a visual inspection of rotors, buckets, and liners for corrosion and cracks. Thorough maintenance records should be kept.

Reagents and Buffers

Attention must be paid to the age and condition of solutions. This is particularly important with the calcium chloride solution. Whenever a solution is prepared it should be correctly labeled and dated. Buffers should be inspected for bacterial growth before use. Contamination with microorganisms can cause errors and assay failures as a result of the release of enzymes and other active biological substances into solution. Azide may be added as a preservative to some buffers but should not be used in reagents for platelet studies or ELISA substrates. Chromogenic substrates should be reconstituted with sterile distilled water; contamination with bacterial enzymes may cause para nitro-aniline (pNA) release and yellow discolouration of the reagent. Records of batch numbers and expiry dates should be kept.

Plastic and Glass Tubes

For clotting tests, 75 × 10 mm glass rimless test tubes should be used. Plastic tubes should be used for sample dilutions, storage, and reagent preparation.

Pipettes

A range of graduated glass (certified Class A) and automatic pipettes must be obtained. The latter should be accurate and durable. Fluids should not be drawn into the pipette barrels and acids should not be pipetted with instruments containing metal piston assemblies, which may become pitted or corroded. Attention to technique is vital because contamination of reagents with used pipette tips may occur, there may be errors of volume as a result of fluid on the exterior of the pipette tip, or the manner of addition of a reagent may alter the results obtained. The amount of fluid drawn into the tip should be inspected visually with each pipetting procedure. Records of pipette accuracy and precision should be kept.

Stopwatches and Clocks

Stopclocks are useful for timing incubation periods of several minutes or more, but stopwatches that may be held in the hand, and controlled rapidly, should be used for measuring clotting times and for short incubations. At least four stopwatches are needed unless an automatic coagulometer is used.

Automated Coagulation Analysers

A wide variety of automated and semiautomated coagulation analysers are available. The choice of analyser depends on predicted workload, repertoire, and cost implications. A thorough evaluation of the current range of analysers is recommended. This is aided by reports of instrument evaluation, e.g., from the National Health Services Medical Devices Agency* (see p. 631).

If coagulation analysers are used, it is important to ensure that their temperature control and the mechanism for detecting the end-point are functioning properly. Although such instruments reduce observer error when a large number of samples are tested, it is important to apply stringent quality control at all times to ensure accuracy and precision.

Evaluating and Choosing an Automated Analyser

The purchasing or leasing of new equipment is a complicated process, and the most important factors to be considered will vary from one laboratory to another.

Specification standards can be classified into MANDATORY and DESIRABLE.

Mandatory requirements:

Performance of clotting, chromogenic, and immunological assays
Reliable test results with acceptable levels of accuracy and precision
Closed vial, cap piercing
Positive barcode identification
Effective flagging of abnormal results
Storage of quality control data
Stability of reagents
Sample throughput time appropriate for workload
Rapid analysis of urgent samples
Bidirectional interface

Continual sample loading
Conformity to national health and safety legislation

Desirable additional requirements:

Good reputation of supplier and satisfaction of other users
Acceptable level of service, telephone support, and availability of engineer support
Availability of independent evaluation report
Satisfactory performance of analyser and reagent combinations in an external quality assessment scheme
Satisfactory results on an on-site evaluation
Ease of implementation in laboratory with necessary changes to existing practice
Ease of implementation of future requirements and increase in workload
Guaranteed supply of reagents and consumables
Post-sales support, training, and education
Establishment of new reference range

The final decision is usually made after competitive tenders are submitted to ensure fairness to all relevant commercial firms and after achieving the lowest appropriate cost. The selection process should take into account the following cost implications:

Capital bid cost or leasing/rental cost
Cost of reagents and consumables per year
Cost of maintenance contracts per year
Cost of computer interfacing

The extent to which each analyser fulfills the *essential* and *desirable* attributes can be scored according to their relative importance. Thus, for example, the specification standard should be *weighted,* 10 for the most important, 1 for the least important criterion; compliance with the specification standard should be given a *mark,* 5 as the best and 1 as the worst score.

A total score is then calculated as Weighting × Mark and summed for each analyser.

Safety

Each laboratory should have its own safety recommendations and procedures to follow in case of accident or contamination (see Chapter 25).

---

*Now Medicines and Healthcare Products Regulatory Agency.

PREANALYTICAL VARIABLES INCLUDING SAMPLE COLLECTION

Many misleading results in blood coagulation arise not from errors in testing but from carelessness in the preanalytical phase. Ideally the results of blood tests should accurately reflect the values *in vivo*.

When blood is withdrawn from a vessel, changes begin to take place in the components of blood coagulation. Some occur almost immediately, such as platelet activation and the initiation of the clotting mechanism dependent on surface contact.

It is essential to take precautions at this early stage to prevent, or at least minimize, *in vitro* changes by conforming to recommended criteria during collection and storage. These criteria, as described below, have been established by the National Committee for Clinical Laboratory Standards (NCCLS).*

Collection of Venous Blood

Venous blood samples should be obtained whenever possible, even from the neonate. Capillary blood tests require modification of techniques, experienced operators, and locally established normal ranges; they are not an easy alternative to tests on venous blood. All blood samples must be collected by personnel who are trained and experienced in the technique. Patients requiring venipuncture should be relaxed and in warm surroundings. Excessive stress and vigorous exercise cause changes in blood clotting and fibrinolysis. Stress and exercise will increase factor VIII, VWF antigen, and fibrinolysis.

Whenever possible, venous samples should be collected without a pressure cuff, allowing the blood to enter the syringe by continuous free flow or by the negative pressure from an evacuated tube (see p. 3). Venous occlusion causes haemoconcentration, increase of fibrinolytic activity, platelet release, and activation of some clotting factors. In the majority of patients, however, light pressure using a tourniquet is required; this should be applied for the shortest possible time (i.e., less than 1 min). The venepuncture must be "clean"; blood sample from an indwelling line or catheter should not be used for tests of haemostasis because they are prone to dilution or heparin contamination.

*Now Clinical and Laboratory Standards Institute (CLSI).

To minimise the effects of contact activation, good-quality plastic or polypropylene syringes should be used. If glass blood containers are used, they should be evenly and adequately coated with silicon.

The blood is thoroughly mixed with the anticoagulant by inverting the container several times. The samples should be brought to the laboratory as soon as possible. If urgent fibrinolysis tests are contemplated, the blood samples should be kept on crushed ice until delivered to the laboratory. Assays of tPA and of PA1-1 antigen are preferably performed on samples taken into trisodium citrate to prevent continued tPA–PA1-1 binding (see p. 457).

If an evacuated tube system is used for collecting samples for different tests, the coagulation sample should be the second or third tube obtained.

Patient identification is of utmost importance. Care must be taken in labelling the patient sample both at the bedside and within the laboratory.

Blood Sample Anticoagulation

The most commonly used anticoagulant for coagulation samples is trisodium citrate. A 32 g/l (0.109 M) solution (p. 7) is recommended. Other anticoagulants, including oxalate, heparin, and EDTA, are unacceptable. The labile factors (factors V and VIII) are unstable in oxalate, whereas heparin and EDTA directly inhibit the coagulation process and interfere with end-point determinations. Additional benefits of trisodium citrate are that the calcium ion is neutralised more rapidly in citrate, and APTT tests are more sensitive to the presence of heparin.

For routine blood coagulation testing, 9 volumes of blood are added to 1 volume of anticoagulant (i.e., 0.55 ml of anticoagulant for a 5 ml specimen). When the haematocrit is abnormal with either severe anaemia or polycythaemia, the blood:citrate ratio should be adjusted.[75] For a 5 ml specimen, the amount of citrate should be as follows:

Haematocrit	Citrate (ml)
0.20	0.70
0.25	0.65
0.30	0.61
0.55	0.39
0.60	0.36
0.65	0.31
0.70	0.27

Time of Sample Collection

The time of day when the sample is collected can be an important factor in the interpretation of results. Fibrinolytic activity follows a definite circadian pattern with a trough at around 6 a.m.

The timing of the collection of the blood sample in relation to drug administration should also be taken into consideration (e.g., the APTT for monitoring heparin therapy).

The timing following administration of factor concentrate samples is very important. The following times are recommended.

Factor VIII: at 15 minutes
Factor IX: at 30 minutes
DDAVP: at 45 minutes

Transportation to the Laboratory

An efficient and regular collection service is necessary. It is important that samples are delivered as quickly as possible to prevent deterioration of the labile clotting factors such as factors V and VIII. For certain investigations it is necessary for the samples to be placed on ice once taken and delivered immediately to the laboratory.

Centrifugation: Preparation of Platelet Poor Plasma

Most routine coagulation investigations are performed on platelet poor plasma (PPP), which is prepared by centrifugation at 2000 g for 15 min at 4°C (approximately 4000 rev/min in a standard bench cooling centrifuge). The sample should be kept at room temperature if it is to be used for PT tests, lupus anticoagulant (LAC), or factor VII assays, and it should be kept at 4°C for other assays; the testing should preferably be completed within 2 hours of collection. Care must be taken not to disturb the buffy coat layer when removing the PPP.

Samples for platelet function testing, LAC, and the activated PC resistance (APCR) test should not be centrifuged at 4°C. These samples should be prepared by centrifugation at room temperature to prevent activation of platelets and release of platelet contents such as phospholipid and factor V. For LAC testing and APCR it is very important that the number of platelets and platelet debris in the samples is minimised. The platelet count should be below $10^4/\mu l$. This is best achieved by double centrifugation or filtration of the plasma through a 0.2 μm filter.

Storage of Plasma and Sample Thawing

Some tests such as the PT and APTT are carried out on fresh samples. Certain coagulation assays, unless urgently required, can be performed in batches at a later date on deep frozen plasma. Storage of small aliquots of samples in liquid nitrogen (–196°C) is the optimum, although samples may be frozen at –40°C or –80°C for several weeks without significant loss of most haemostatic activities. Gentle but thorough mixing of samples is essential after thawing and before testing. Once thawed the sample should never be refrozen.

Some Common "Technical" Errors

A false abnormality of the clotting time may occur in the following situations:

1. Faulty collection of the sample, resulting in it undergoing partial clotting (can lead to a shortening of the clotting times)
2. Underfilling or overfilling of the bottle or high or low haematocrit (can cause the volume of citrate in relation to the plasma volume to be incorrect; see above).
3. An unsuitable anticoagulant, such as EDTA, used in collecting the sample
4. Collection of blood through a line that has at some stage been in contact with heparin (leads to a marked prolongation of the APTT and thrombin time, or TT).
5. Contamination of the kaolin/platelet substitute reagent with a trace of thromboplastin (can shorten the APTT).
6. Undue delay in sample analysis.
7. Use of inaccurate pipettes. (Documented proof of pipette calibration is essential.)
8. Machine malfunction.
9. Incorrect waterbath temperature.
10. Calcium chloride at incorrect concentration or not freshly prepared.

Calibration and Quality Control

Reference Standard (Calibrator)

International (World Health Organization, or WHO) and national standards are available for a number of coagulation factors (see p. 694). For diagnostic tests it is necessary to have a calibrated normal reference preparation tested alongside the patients' plasmas.

Because the concentration of some coagulation factors may vary as much as fourfold in different normal plasma samples, it is inadvisable to use plasma from any one person as representing 100% clotting activity. The larger the number of donors in the pool, the more likely the pool clotting activity will be 100% or 1.0 u/ml. A suggested minimum for the normal pool is 20 donors. It is preferable to use a calibrated reference plasma for routine use with each assay. If this is not possible, then a locally prepared normal pool can be used provided it is itself calibrated against a reference preparation.

Calibration of Standard Pools and Suggested Calibration Procedure

Whenever possible, the normal pool should be calibrated as described in the following against a freeze-dried reference material already calibrated against the international standard. The reference material may be a national standard (e.g., National Institute for Biological Standards and Control) or a commercial standard. In the absence of reference materials the laboratory should obtain as large a normal pool as possible and assign it a value of 100 u/dl (1.0 u/ml).

The most important principle of calibration is repetition to minimise possible errors at each stage of calibration. It is necessary to carry out at least four independent assays, and preferably six. An independent assay is an assay for which a new ampoule of standard is opened, or if a freeze-dried standard is not available, for which a new set of dilutions are prepared from frozen previous reference plasma. Each plasma must be tested in duplicate; two replicate assays should be carried out each day, and the procedure should be repeated on at least 4 days (four independent assays). Whenever possible more than one operator should be involved.

Comparison should always be made with the previous normal pool. The potency of the new normal pool is calculated for each replicate assay on each day and an overall mean value is calculated. This calibration also enables an assessment of the precision of the method used.

Control Plasma

Controls are included alongside patient samples in a batch of tests. Inclusion of both normal and abnormal controls will enable detection of nonlinearity in the standard curve. Whereas a reference standard (calibrator) is used for accuracy, controls are used for precision. Precision control, the recording of the day-to-day variation in control values, is an important procedure in laboratory coagulation. Participation in an external assessment scheme (see p. 657) is also important to ensure interlaboratory harmonization. The use of lyophilised reference standard and control plasmas has become widespread, whereas locally calibrated standard pools are used especially in underresourced countries. The results of participation in external quality-control schemes require careful attention. The large number of different reagents, substrate plasmas, reference preparations, and analysers available makes comparison of like with like difficult. Ideally all combinations should give similar results, but this is often not the case and the results should be used to carefully choose the combination used.

A control must be stable and homogeneous; the exact potency is not important, although the approximate value should be known to select a preparation at the upper or lower limit of the normal reference range.

Fresh control blood is required for procedures such as platelet aggregation and should be obtained from "normal" healthy subjects. Fresh controls should be prepared in exactly the same way as the patient sample. Normal and abnormal controls are usually obtained from commercial companies.

Variability of Coagulation Assays

Within a laboratory, variability is most commonly the result of a dilution error, differences in the composition of reagents, failure to take the time-trend into account, and differences in experience and technique between operators. A coefficient of variation of 15–20% is not uncommon for factor VIII:C assays. Furthermore, the variability increases if like is not compared with like (e.g., if concentrate preparations are assayed against plasma).

Variability between laboratories is much higher. Apart from the factors described for the within-laboratory variability, there is the major effect of differences in methods and in the composition of reagents. Comparability between laboratories improves if standardized reagents are used.

The unavoidable variability associated with coagulation assays makes the use of reliable reference materials imperative.

Performance of Coagulation Tests

Handling of Samples and Reagents

All plasma samples should be kept in plastic or siliconized glass tubes and placed on melting ice or at 4°C until used, except when cold activation of factor VII and platelets is to be avoided, in which case the plasma is kept at room temperature. All pipetting should be performed using disposable plastic pipettes or autodiluter pipette tips. The actual clotting tests are performed at 37°C in new round-bottom glass tubes of standard size (10 or 12 mm external diameter). Ideally, all glassware should be disposable. If the tubes have to be reused, scrupulous cleaning using chromic acid and a detergent such as 2% Decon 90 is essential.

Eliminating a Time Trend

The potential instability of biological reagents used in tests of haemostasis makes it desirable to arrange results so as to reduce time-related errors. Thus, if there is a significant length of time between the results with the patient's plasma and the results with the control sample, the difference may be the result of the deterioration of one or more of the reagents or of the plasma itself rather than to a true defect or deficiency. In the simplest case, if there are two samples A and B, the readings should be carried out in the order A_1, B_1, B_2, A_2. Additional specimens are allowed for by inserting further letters into the design.

Assay Monitoring and End-Point Detection

Detecting clot formation as the end-point depends to some extent on the rate of its formation: the shorter the clotting time the more opaque is the clot and the easier it is to detect. A slowly forming clot may appear as mere fibrin wisps, which are difficult to detect by eye or machine. In manual work, the observer must try to adopt a uniform convention in selecting the moment in clot formation that will be accepted as the end-point. It is also important to ensure that the tube can be watched with its lower part under the water or while being quickly dipped in and out so as to avoid cooling and a slowing down of the clot formation. Bubbles also make the determination of the end-point difficult.

Manual clotting techniques are still used in WHO calibration schemes and therefore should be viewed as an essential skill despite the ever-increasing reliance on automation. It is worth remembering that not all results produced by an automated analyser are correct and sometimes they may be spurious; dubious or inconsistent results should be checked manually.

In instrumental work the coagulometer must be shown to detect long clotting times reliably and reproducibly. The various coagulometers available have different means of detecting the end-point, which may make comparison of results difficult. Some commonly used techniques are as follows.

Electromechanical

Impedance, Steel Ball (e.g., Amelung KC10)
The sample cuvette rotates and a steel ball remains stationary in a magnetic field until the formation of fibrin strands around the ball produces movement. This is detected by a change in the magnetic field, and the coagulation time is recorded.

Impedance, Steel Ball (Nycomed Thrombotrack)
A steel ball rotates under the influence of a magnet until the formation of fibrin strands around the ball stops it rotating. This is detected by a sensor, and the coagulation time is recorded.

Photo Optical

Scattered Light Detection for Clotting Assays (660 nm)
The turbidity during the formation of a fibrin clot is measured as an increase in scattered light intensity when exposed to light at a wavelength of 660 nm.

Transmitted Light Detection for Chromogenic Assays (405 nm, 575 nm, 800 nm)
Colour production leads to a change in light absorbance, which is detected as a change in transmitted light. Over time the change in absorbance per minute is calculated (Δ OD/min). Various wavelengths can be used such as 405 nm, 575 nm, and 800 nm.

Transmitted Light Detection for Immunoassays (405 nm, 575 nm, 800 nm)

The change in light absorbance caused by the antigen antibody reaction is detected as the change in transmitted light. Over time the change in absorbance per minute is calculated (Δ OD/min).

Waveform Analysis (Biomerieux)

Detection of light transmittance with Tungsten-Halogen light is performed at 35 wavelengths between 395 and 710 nm. Waveform analysis provides additional information from routine clotting assays. For example, the biphasic waveform A2 Flag is associated with sepsis and disseminated intravascular coagulation.

Nephelometry (IL ACL Analysers)

Nephelometry is the determination of the intensity of light scatter using a detector placed at right angles to the incident light path but of the same wavelength as the incident light. The procedure is particularly useful in measuring complexes of antigen and antibody produced by immunoprecipitation.

Electrochemical

INRatio Meter (Hemosense) Near Patient Testing Devices

The INRatio single-use test strip is made of laminated layers of transparent plastic. Each test strip has a sample well where blood is applied, three channels through which the blood sample flows to reach the testing areas, reagents to start the coagulation process, and electrodes that interface with the INRatio meter. The device detects a change in electrical resistance when blood clots.

Assay Analysis

The changes recorded by the methods described earlier may be analysed in a number of ways to derive an end-point. Some of these methods are described in the following.

Percentage Detection Method (Fig 16.2)

After the start of the clotting reaction the scattered light intensity is monitored and the baseline (bH) and maximum values are determined. In the percent detection method bH is referred to as 0% and change in scatter (dH) is taken as 100%. An arbitrarily chosen

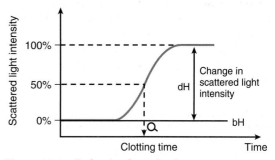

Figure 16.2   End-point determination: percentage detection method.

% change is then set as the end-point and the time taken to reach this is the clotting time. This percent detection value can be optionally set between 2% and 80%. Usually, the 50% point is used, at which point the rate of change of light scatter is greatest and the fibrin monomer polymerisation reaction rate (for example) is high.

Rate Method (Fig 16.3)

At a predefined point after the start of the kinetic reaction, the increase in absorbance per minute is monitored. At the predetermined end time the final increase in absorbance per minute measurement will be made. The program then calculates the rate of absorbance increase per minute between these two time point measurements. The calculated absorbance value is expressed as the raw data. The dOD/min may be calculated and used to construct a standard curve.

VLin Integral (Fig 16.4)

The VLin Integral method evaluates the time point at which the reaction reaches its steepest increase. At a predefined point after the start of the kinetic reaction the algorithm will monitor the reaction and determine when an increasing absorbance measurement starts. The algorithm then monitors the slope of the increasing curve signal using polynomial regression. Then linear regression is used to find the point of maximum velocity. The limit of the linear range around this point is defined, and the integral area between these points is used to calculate the reaction in absorbance per minute at the peak. It is a dynamic algorithm based on the strength of the reaction. Using this method allows for increase in analytical sensitivity, extended measuring range,

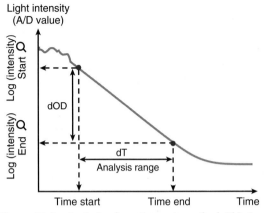

Figure 16.3   Analysis of reaction: rate method. This is used for chromogenic assays. (Reproduced by permission of Sysmex UK Ltd.)

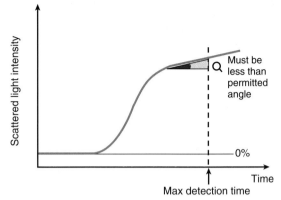

Figure 16.5   Examples of Error flags that may require manual clotting: "Analysis Time Over." (Reproduced by permission of Sysmex UK Ltd.)

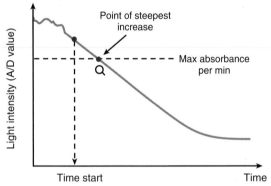

Figure 16.4   Analysis of reaction: VLin Integral (e.g., immunological assays). (Reproduced by permission of Sysmex UK Ltd.)

reduced measurement time, and improved reliability in monitoring an immunological reaction when there is excess antigen. The VLin Integral evaluation method can be used for immunological assays.

Analysis Time Over (Fig 16.5)

The "Analysis Time Over" check is able to detect whether the reaction end-point is correct. If the sample reaction end angle is greater than the permitted angle at maximum detection time, the result will be flagged with an "Analysis Time Over" error. The situation occurs when testing samples with prolonged clotting times.

Action steps for "Analysis Time Over" are as follows:

1. Check the sample for possible anticoagulant contamination, haemolysis, lipaemia, etc.
2. Verify delivery of sample and reagent.
3. Set the "Maximum Reading Time" to a longer time and reanalysis the sample.
4. If reanalysis of the sample results in a numeric value without an error flag, the result can be reported.
5. If reanalysis gives an "Analysis Time Over" message again, the sample may not be capable of forming a firm clot. In these situations the clotting time must be checked manually.

Turbidity Level Over (Fig 16.6)

If the dH exceeds the detection capacity of the A/D converter, the result will not be reported and it is suspected that sample plasma is turbid or lipaemic

Action steps for "Turbidity Level Over" are as follows:

1. Check the sample for turbidity, lipaemia, etc.
2. Verify delivery of sample and reagent.
3. For a fibrinogen level dilute the sample with Owren's veronal buffer and reanalyse.
4. If reanalysis of the sample results in a numeric value without an error flag, the result can be reported.

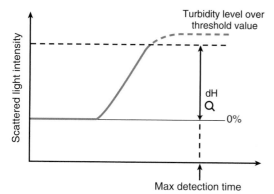

Figure 16.6 Examples of error flags that may require manual tests: "Turbidity Level Over." (Reproduced by permission of Sysmex UK Ltd.)

5. Clotting tests such as PT, APTT, and TT must be performed manually.

Waveform Analysis

It is important to realize that coagulation is a *dynamic* process and that the measurement of static end-points does not necessarily provide information on the quality of the clot or the kinetics of its formation.

Clot Signatures: Normal and Abnormal APTT Clot Waveforms (Fig 16.7)

Information on the dynamics of clot formation may also be extracted from the optical profiles generated when performing PT or APTT assays. It has been demonstrated that such profiles (clot waveforms) show a different pattern in certain clinical conditions compared to normal. Furthermore, the shape of this pattern is predictable for the particular abnormality and the term "clot signature" has been used in this context.

The A2 Flag on the MDA System identifies the presence of a biphasic APTT waveform often seen in patients with DIC, and a high sensitivity (98%), specificity (98%), and positive predictive value (74%) have been reported(16).

It is important to note that the biphasic aPTT waveform has also been observed in samples from patients not diagnosed as having DIC by standard criteria. In this respect it may indicate an emerging or occult and potentially serious clinical condition

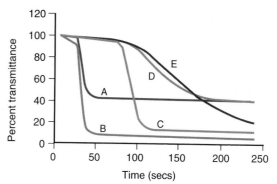

Figure 16.7 Clot signatures: normal and abnormal activated partial thromboplastin time (APTT) clot waveforms. A: Normal specimen; APTT = 29 sec, fibrinogen = 2.89 g/l. B: Biphasic response in a suspected disseminated intravascular coagulation (DIC) specimen with normal APTT (28.5 sec) and elevated fibrinogen (6.74 g/l). C: Patient treated with heparin (0.52 a-Xa U/ml); prolonged APTT (81.2 sec), and elevated fibrinogen (5.54 g/l). D: Factor VIII-deficient specimen (<1%), with prolonged APTT (84.1 sec) and reduced fibrinogen (1.56 g/l). E: Factor IX-deficient specimen (<1%) with prolonged APTT (83.4 sec) and normal fibrinogen (2.94 g/l). (Reproduced by permission of Biomerieux.)

associated with the activation of coagulation. Further clinical and laboratory investigation is then warranted.

Molecular Mechanism of the Biphasic Waveform: LC-CRP

The development of the biphasic waveform is a consequence of the formation of a divalent metal ion-dependent complex of C-reactive protein (CRP) and very low density lipoprotein (VLDL) and, to a lesser extent, intermediate density lipoprotein (IDL).[17]

This lipoprotein-complexed CRP has been designated LC-CRP. In the APTT assay, when the citrated plasma is recalcified, the formation of this complex results in a reduction in light transmission, detected by the first slope of the biphasic waveform.

Commonly Used Reagents

Some reagents are common to the majority of first-line tests. They are described here, whereas the reagents specific for one particular test or assay only are described with the details of the relevant test.

CaCl$_2$

The working solution is best prepared from a commercial molar solution. Small volumes of 0.025 mol/l concentration should be prepared frequently and stored for short periods to avoid proliferation of microorganisms. Prewarmed CaCl$_2$ should always be discarded at the end of the working day.

Barbitone buffered saline

pH 7.3–7.4 is recommended for most clotting tests. See p. 691 for preparation of barbitone buffered saline, pH 7.4.

Glyoxaline buffer.

Dissolve 2.72 g of glyoxaline (imidazole) and 4.68 g of NaCl in 650 ml of water. Add 148.8 ml of 0.1 mol/l HCl and adjust the pH to 7.4. Adjust the volume to 1 l with water.

Owren's veronal buffer

Sodium acetate: 3.89 g
Barbitone sodium: 5.89 g
Sodium chloride: 6.8 g
Dissolve the salts in 800 ml of water.
Add 21.5 ml of 1 mol/l HCl, then make up to 1 l with water, mix, and check that the pH is 7.4.

Factor-Deficient Plasmas

Plasmas deficient in specific factors are required for many bioassays. They may be obtained from individuals with congenital deficiency of the factor, but frequently these patients will have been treated with plasma concentrates and there is a danger of infection. Many laboratories now use commercial plasmas rendered deficient in the factor by immuno-depletion and then lyophilised. However, it is important to establish that these are completely deficient. Once reconstituted, lyophilised plasmas should be gently mixed and left to stand for 20 min before use. If an automated coagulation analyser is used, the factor deficient plasma should be placed in position 10 min prior to testing.

THE "CLOTTING SCREEN"

Basic tests of coagulation are often performed with no specific diagnosis in mind and in the absence of any clinical indication of a haemostatic disorder.

There may be numerous reasons for this, and the tests performed may give clues to diagnosis or may detect an unsuspected hazard that increases the risk of postoperative bleeding. The choice and extent of tests performed in this screening process will vary between hospitals. Our current practice is to perform PT, APTT, TT, and fibrinogen assay.

Prothrombin Time

Principle

The PT test measures the clotting time of plasma in the presence of an optimal concentration of tissue extract (thromboplastin) and indicates the overall efficiency of the extrinsic clotting system. Although originally thought to measure prothrombin, the test is now known to depend also on reactions with factors V, VII, and X and on the fibrinogen concentration of the plasma.[18]

Reagents

Patient and Control Plasma Samples

Platelet poor plasma (PPP) from the patient and control is obtained as described on p. 392. Note that plasma stored at 4°C may have a shortened PT as a result of factor VII activation in the cold.[19]

Thromboplastin

Thromboplastins were originally tissue extracts obtained from different species and different organs containing tissue factor and phospholipid. Because of the potential hazard of viral and other infections from handling human brain, it should no longer be used as a source of thromboplastin. The majority of animal thromboplastins now in use are extracts of rabbit brain or lung. A laboratory method for a rabbit brain preparation is described on p. 692.

The introduction of recombinant thromboplastins has resulted in a move away from rabbit brain thromboplastin. They are manufactured using recombinant human tissue factor produced in *Escherichia coli* and synthetic phospholipids, which do not contain any other clotting factors such as prothrombin, factor VII, and factor X. Therefore they are highly sensitive to factor deficiencies and oral anticoagulant–treated patient plasma samples and have an International Sensitivity Index (ISI) close to 1.

Each preparation has a different sensitivity to clotting factor deficiencies and defects, in particular the defect induced by oral anticoagulants (see Chapter 18). For control of oral anticoagulation a preparation calibrated against the International Reference Thromboplastin should be used; calibrated commercially available thromboplastin has its ISI determined and clearly labelled. It is important to remember that some thromboplastins are not sensitive to an isolated factor VII deficiency and that use of animal thromboplastin for analysis of human samples may produce abnormalities solely as a result of species differences. If the manufacturer does not state in the accompanying literature that the reagent is sensitive to factor VII deficiency, it is advisable to check whether it is capable of detecting this deficiency by performing a PT on a known factor VII deficient plasma.

CaCl$_2$.
  0.025 mol/l.

Method

Deliver 0.1 ml of plasma into a glass tube placed in a waterbath and add 0.1 ml of thromboplastin. Wait 1–3 min to allow the mixture to warm. Then add 0.1 ml of warmed CaCl$_2$ and start the stopwatch. Mix the contents of the tube and record the end-point. Carry out the test in duplicate on the patient's plasma and the control plasma. When a number of samples are to be tested as a batch, the samples and controls must be suitably staggered to eliminate the time bias. Some thromboplastins contain calcium chloride, in which case 0.2 ml of thromboplastin is added to 0.1 ml plasma and timing is started immediately.

Expression of Results

The results are expressed as the mean of the duplicate readings in seconds or as the ratio of the mean patient's plasma time to the mean normal control plasma time. The control plasma is obtained from 20 normal men and women (not pregnant and not taking oral contraceptives), and the logarithmic mean normal PT (LMNPT) is calculated. For further details and a discussion of the importance of the one-stage PTT test in oral anticoagulant control, when results may be reported as an International Normalized Ratio (INR), see Chapter 18.

Normal Values

Normal values depend on the thromboplastin used, the exact technique, and whether visual or instrumental end-point reading is used. With most rabbit thromboplastins the normal range of the PTT is between 11 and 16 sec; for recombinant human thromboplastin it is somewhat shorter (10–12 sec). Each laboratory should establish its own normal range.

Interpretation

The common causes of prolonged one-stage PTs are as follows:

1. Administration of oral anticoagulant drugs (vitamin K antagonists)
2. Liver disease, particularly obstructive
3. Vitamin K deficiency
4. Disseminated intravascular coagulation
5. Rarely, a previously undiagnosed factor VII, X, V, or prothrombin deficiency or defect (see p. 409). *Note:* With prothrombin, factor X, or factor V deficiency the APTT will also be prolonged.

Activated Partial Thromboplastin Time

Other forms of the APTT test are known as the partial thromboplastin time with kaolin (PTTK) and the kaolin cephalin clotting time (KCCT), reflecting the methods used to perform the test.

Principle

The test measures the clotting time of plasma after the activation of contact factors but without added tissue thromboplastin and so indicates the overall efficiency of the intrinsic pathway. To standardize the activation of contact factors, the plasma is first preincubated for a set period with a contact activator such as kaolin, silica, or ellagic acid. During this phase of the test factor XIIa is produced, which cleaves factor XI to factor XIa, but coagulation does not proceed beyond this in the absence of calcium. After recalcification, factor XIa activates factor IX and coagulation follows. A standardised phospholipid is provided to allow the test to be performed on PPP. The test depends not only on the contact factors and on factors VIII and IX, but also on the reactions with factors X, V, prothrombin, and fibrinogen. It is also sensitive to the presence of circulating anticoagulants (inhibitors) and heparin.

Reagents

PPP.

From the patient and a control, stored as described on p. 392.

Kaolin.

5 g/l (laboratory grade) in barbitone buffered saline, pH 7.4 (p. 690). Add a few glass beads to aid resuspension. The suspension is stable at room temperature. Other insoluble surface active substances such as silica, celite, or ellagic acid can also be used.

Phospholipid.

Many reagents are available; these contain different phospholipids.

When choosing a reagent for the APTT, it is important to establish that the activator–phospholipid combination is sensitive to deficiencies of factors VIII:C, IX, and XI at concentrations of 0.35 to 0.4 iu/ml. Reagents that fail to detect reductions of this degree are too insensitive for routine use. The system should also be responsive to unfractionated heparin over the therapeutic range of approximately 0.3–0.7 u/ml. In addition, some laboratories will wish the system to be sensitive to the presence of lupus-like anticoagulants.

$CaCl_2$.

0.025 mol/l.

Method

Mix equal volumes of the phospholipid reagent and the kaolin suspension and leave in a glass tube in the waterbath at 37°C. Place 0.1 ml of plasma into a new glass tube. Add 0.2 ml of the kaolin–phospholipid solution, mix the contents, and start the stopwatch simultaneously. Leave at 37°C for 10 min with occasional shaking. At exactly 10 min add 0.1 ml of prewarmed $CaCl_2$ and start a second stopwatch. Record the time taken for the mixture to clot. Repeat the test at least once on both the patient's plasma and the control plasma. It is possible to do four tests at 2-min intervals if sufficient stopwatches are available.

Expression of Results

Express the results as the mean of the paired clotting times.

Normal Range

The normal range is typically within 26–40 sec. The actual times depend on the reagents used and the duration of the preincubation period, which varies in manufacturer's recommendations for different reagents. These variables also greatly alter the sensitivity of the test to minor or moderate deficiencies of the contact activation system. Laboratories can choose appropriate conditions to achieve the sensitivity they require. Each laboratory should calculate its own normal range.

Interpretation

The common causes of a prolonged APTT are as follows:

1. Disseminated intravascular coagulation
2. Liver disease
3. Massive transfusion with plasma-depleted red blood cells
4. Administration of or contamination with heparin or other anticoagulants
5. A circulating anticoagulant (inhibitor)
6. Deficiency of a coagulation factor other than factor VII

The APTT is also moderately prolonged in patients taking oral anticoagulant drugs and in the presence of vitamin K deficiency. Occasionally, a patient with previously undiagnosed haemophilia or another congenital coagulation disorder presents with an isolated prolonged APTT. If the patient's APTT is abnormally long, the equal mixture test must be set up (see below).

Deficiency or Circulating Anticoagulant?

In cases with a long APTT, a 50:50 mixture of normal and test plasma should be tested to distinguish between factor deficiency and the effect of an inhibitor (see p. 413).

Thrombin Time

Principle

Thrombin is added to plasma and the clotting time is measured. The TT is affected by the concentration and reaction of fibrinogen and by the presence of inhibitory substances, including fibrinogen/fibrin degradation products (FDP) and heparin. The clotting time and the appearance of the clot are equally informative.

Reagents

PPP.
From the patient and a control.

Thrombin solution.
A commercial bovine thrombin is used. It is stored frozen as a 50 NIH unit solution, and it is freshly diluted in barbitone buffered saline in a plastic tube so as to give a clotting time of normal plasma of 15 sec (usually approximately 7–8 NIH thrombin units per ml). Shorter times with normal plasma may fail to detect mild abnormalities.

Method

Add 100 μl thrombin solution to 200 μl of control plasma in a glass tube at 37°C and start the stopwatch. Measure the clotting time and observe the nature of the clot (e.g., whether transparent or opaque, firm or wispy, etc.). Repeat the procedure with two tubes containing patient's plasma in duplicate and then with a second sample of control plasma.

Expression of Results

The results are expressed as the mean of the duplicate clotting times in seconds for the control and the test plasma.

Normal Range

A patient's TT should be within 2 sec of the control (i.e., 15–19 sec). Times of 20 sec and longer are definitely abnormal.

Interpretation of Results

The common causes of prolonged TT are as follows:

1. Hypofibrinogenaemia as found in DIC and, more rarely, in a congenital defect or deficiency.
2. Raised concentrations of FDP, as encountered in DIC or liver disease.
3. Extreme prolongation of the TT is nearly always a result of the presence of heparin, which interferes with the thrombin–fibrinogen reaction. If the presence of heparin is suspected, a Reptilase time test should be carried out (see p. 407). Low molecular weight heparin (LMWH) produces only a slight prolongation at therapeutic levels.
4. Dysfibrinogenaemia, either inherited or acquired, in liver disease or in neonates.
5. Hypoalbuminaemia.

Shortening of the TT occurs in conditions of coagulation activation.

A transparent bulky clot is found if fibrin polymerization is abnormal, as is the case in liver disease and some congenital dysfibrinogenaemias.

A gross elevation of the plasma fibrinogen concentration may also prolong the TT. Correction can be obtained by diluting the patient's plasma with saline (see p. 406).

Measurement of Fibrinogen

Numerous methods of determining fibrinogen concentration have been devised including clotting, immunological, physical, and nephelometric techniques, and all tend to give slightly different results, presumably partly because of the heterogeneous nature of plasma fibrinogen.[20] Many automated analysers will now provide a fibrinogen concentration estimated from the coagulation changes during the PTT (PT-derived fibrinogen). This is simple, inexpensive, and widely used. However, it tends to give higher estimates of fibrinogen than the Clauss assay and is inaccurate in some disease states and in patients who are anticoagulated.[21,22] Guidelines on fibrinogen assays have been published and recommend the Clauss technique for routine laboratory use.[23]

Fibrinogen Assay (Clauss Technique)[24]

Principle

Diluted plasma is clotted with a strong thrombin solution; the plasma must be diluted to give a low level of any inhibitors (e.g., FDPs and heparin). A strong thrombin solution must be used so that the clotting time over a wide range is independent of the thrombin concentration.

Reagents

Calibration plasma. With a known level of fibrinogen calibrated against an International Reference Standard.

PPP. From the patient and a control.

Thrombin solution. Freshly reconstituted to 100 NIH u per ml in 9 g/l NaCl.

Owren's veronal buffer, pH 7.4. See p. 398.

Method

A calibration curve is prepared each time the batch of thrombin reagent is changed or there is a drift in control results; this is used to calculate the results of unknown plasma samples.

Make dilutions of the calibration plasma in veronal buffer to give a range of fibrinogen concentrations (i.e., 1 in 5, 1 in 10, 1 in 20, and 1 in 40). Part (0.2 ml) of each dilution is warmed to 37°C, 0.1 ml of thrombin solution is added, and the clotting time is measured. Each test should be performed in duplicate. Plot the clotting time in seconds against the fibrinogen concentration in g/l on log/log graph paper. The 1 in 10 concentration is considered to be 100%, and there should be a straight line connection between clotting times of 5 and 50 sec. Make a 1 in 10 dilution of each patient's sample and clot 0.2 ml of the dilution with 0.1 ml of thrombin.

The fibrinogen level can be read directly off the graph if the clotting time is between 5 and 50 sec. However, outside this time range a different assay dilution and mathematic correction of the result will be required (i.e., if the fibrinogen level is low and a 1 in 5 dilution is required, divide answer by 2 and for a 1 in 20 dilution multiply answer by 2).

The clot formed in this method may be "wispy" as a result of the plasma being diluted, and end-point detection may be easier with optical or mechanical automated equipment. These have been assessed with available substrates and give reasonably consistent results.[25] The high concentration of thrombin used raises the risk of carry over into subsequent tests.

Normal Range

The normal range is 1.8–3.6 g/l.

Interpretation

The Clauss fibrinogen assay is usually low in inherited dysfibrinogenaemia but is insensitive to heparin unless the level is very high (>0.8 u/ml). High levels of FDPs, >190 µg/ml, may also interfere with the assay.[26] Because the chronometric Clauss assay is a functional assay it will generally give a relevant indication of fibrinogen function in plasma. When an inherited disorder of fibrinogen is suspected, a physicochemical estimation should be obtained (e.g., clot weight estimate of fibrinogen or total clottable fibrinogen or an immunological measure; see page 398). If a dysfibrinogenaemia is present, it will reveal a discrepancy between the (functional) Clauss assay and the physical amount of fibrinogen present.

Platelet Count

Before considering further investigation of a suspected bleeding disorder always check the platelet count (see Chapter 3).

INTERPRETATION OF FIRST-LINE TESTS

The pattern of abnormalities obtained using the first-line tests described earlier often gives a reasonably clear indication of the underlying defect and determines the appropriate further tests required to define it. The patterns are outlined in Table 16.3. The further tests that include specific factor assays and tests for DIC are described in the following sections.

SECOND-LINE INVESTIGATIONS

Relevant second-line investigations are described with each of the patterns of abnormalities detected by the first-line tests.

1.

PT	Normal
APTT	Normal
Thrombin time	Normal
Fibrinogen	Normal
Platelet count	Normal

If all the first-line investigations are normal in a patient who continues to bleed from the site of an injury or after surgery (or has a history of such bleeding), there are several possible diagnoses:

1. A disorder of platelet function, either congenital or acquired.

Table 16.3   First-line tests used in investigating acute haemostatic failure

	PT	APTT	TT	Fibrinogen	Platelet count	Condition
1.	N	N	N	N	N	Normal haemostasis. Disorder of platelet function. Factor XIII deficiency. Disorder of vascular haemostasis. Mild/masked coagulation factor deficiency. Mild von Willebrand disease. Disorder of fibrinolysis.
2.	Long	N	N	N	N	Factor VII deficiency. Early oral anticoagulation. Lupus anticoagulant (with some reagents). Mild II, V, or X deficiency.
3.	N	Long	N	N	N	Factor VIII, IX, XI, XII, prekallikrein. HMWK deficiency. Von Willebrand's disease. Circulating anticoagulant, e.g. lupus. Mild II, V, or X deficiency.
4.	Long	Long	N	N	N	Vitamin K deficiency. Oral anticoagulants. Factor V, X, or II deficiency. Multiple factor deficiency, e.g. liver failure. Combined V + VIII deficiency.
5.	Long	Long	Long	N or Abnormal	N	Heparin (large amount). Liver disease. Fibrinogen deficiency/disorder. Inhibition of fibrin polymerization. Hyperfibrinolysis.
6.	N	N	N	N	Low	Thrombocytopenia.
7.	Long	Long	N	N or Abnormal	Low	Massive transfusion. Liver disease.
8.	Long	Long	Long	Low	Low	Disseminated intravascular coagulation. Acute liver disease.

HMWK, high molecular weight kininogen; N, normal.

2. von Willebrand disease (VWD) in which the factor VIII is not sufficiently low to cause prolongation of the APTT. This is quite common in mild cases.

3. A mild coagulation disorder that is below the sensitivity of the routine tests to detect or that has been masked by the administration of blood products. This will include mild factor VIII deficiency (e.g., 30% of normal).

4. Factor XIII deficiency.

5. A vascular disorder of haemostasis.

6. Bleeding from a severely damaged vessel or vessels with normal haemostasis.

7. A disorder of fibrinolysis such as antiplasmin or PAI-I deficiency.

8. Administration of LMWH.

Second-line investigations required in this situation are specific factor assays for the suspected deficiencies or appropriate screening tests such as the PFA-100 system (p. 418), bleeding time, or clot solubility test. Note that some LMWH may be present at therapeutic levels without abnormality of the coagulation screening tests; an anti-Xa assay will reveal their presence.

2.

PT	Long
APTT	Normal
Thrombin time	Normal
Fibrinogen	Normal
Platelet count	Normal

This combination of results is found in the following:

1. With factor VII deficiency, congenital or secondary to liver disease or vitamin K deficiency.
2. At the start of oral anticoagulant therapy.
3. Some thromboplastins are sensitive to lupus-like anticoagulants and some APTT reagents are insensitive, giving rise to this pattern of results.
4. Depending on reagents used, mild deficiencies of II, V, or X may cause prolongation of PT, whereas the APTT remains in the normal range.

A mixing test should be performed. Factor VII assay is described later. It is usually, but not always, possible to establish from the history whether the patient has received oral anticoagulant drugs. Specific tests for lupus and specific factor assays should be performed, as indicated by the mixing test results. Biochemical measures of liver function should be obtained.

3.

PT	Normal
APTT	Long
Thrombin time	Normal
Fibrinogen	Normal
Platelet count	Normal

An isolated prolonged APTT is found in the following:

1. Congenital deficiencies or defects of the intrinsic pathway (i.e., factor VIII, factor IX, factor XI, and factor XII deficiency), as well as in prekallikrein and HMWK deficiencies.
2. Depending on the reagents used, mild deficiencies of II, V, or X may cause prolongation of APTT, whereas the PT remains in the normal range.
3. VWD, owing to low levels of factor VIII and when it may be associated with a prolonged bleeding time.
4. In the presence of circulating anticoagulants (inhibitors).
5. Heparin (a common cause), either because the patient is undergoing treatment or because of sample contamination. However, the TT is extremely sensitive to unfractionated heparin and will then also be prolonged. A Reptilase time will confirm this if necessary. Detecting LMWH may require an anti-Xa assay as noted earlier.

The next diagnostic step is to establish whether the patient has a deficiency or an inhibitor by performing the 50:50 mixture test described on p. 412. Mixing tests should be done immediately, followed by the specific assay or tests, as described later.

4.

PT	Long
APTT	Long
Thrombin time	Normal
Fibrinogen	Normal
Platelet count	Normal

The main causes of a prolonged PT and APTT are as follows:

1. Lack of vitamin K. In this case the PTT is usually relatively more prolonged than is the APTT.
2. The administration of oral anticoagulant drugs. The PTT is usually more prolonged than is the APTT.
3. Liver disease giving rise to multiple factor deficiencies. (In some cases the fibrinogen may also be abnormal.)

4. Rare congenital or acquired defects of factors V, X, prothrombin, and combined V and VIII deficiency.

Mixing experiments using the PTT may be useful if there is no history of anticoagulant therapy and no obvious reason for failure of vitamin K absorption (e.g., parenteral feeding, long-term antibiotic treatment). If correction is obtained, specific factor assays should be performed.

5.

PT	Long
APTT	Long
Thrombin time	Long
Fibrinogen	Normal/abnormal
Platelet count	Normal

Abnormalities in all three screening coagulation tests are found in the following:

1. In the presence of unfractionated heparin (TT usually disproportionately long).
2. In hypofibrinogenaemias, afibrinogenaemias, and dysfibrinogenaemias.
3. In some cases of liver disease.
4. In systemic hyperfibrinolysis.

To distinguish between these conditions, perform a Reptilase or Ancrod time, measure the fibrinogen concentration, and measure the level of FDPs or D-dimers in plasma. The pattern may also appear in incipient DIC, but usually the platelet count will also fall in this case.

6.

PT	Normal
APTT	Normal
Thrombin time	Normal
Fibrinogen	Normal
Platelet count	Low

If the only abnormality is a low platelet count, possible causes must be investigated. Premorbid counts should be sought to establish whether the

thrombocytopenia is long standing and possibly constitutional. When it appears to be acquired, the usual approach is to perform a bone marrow aspirate to exclude marrow failure and establish whether megakaryocytes are present. If the number and morphology of megakaryocytes in the marrow is normal, further investigations are undertaken to establish the cause of the presumed peripheral destruction of platelets. Heparin and other drugs are common causes in hospital practice.

7.

PT	Long
APTT	Long
Thrombin time	Normal
Fibrinogen	Normal/abnormal
Platelet count	Low

This pattern of abnormalities of the screening tests is found:

1. After massive transfusion with stored/plasma reduced blood that is deficient in coagulation factors.
2. In some cases of chronic liver disease, especially cirrhosis.
3. In DIC. Although disseminated coagulation activation will eventually result in depletion of fibrinogen, this is often a relatively late event.

Specific factor assays may be useful if the situation persists. Consider the possibility that the low platelet count has a separate aetiology and that the situation is in fact the same as in 4.

8.

PT	Long
APTT	Long
Thrombin time	Long
Fibrinogen	Low
Platelet count	Low

All the first-line tests are abnormal in the following:

1. Acute DIC
2. Some cases of acute liver necrosis with DIC

It is only exceptionally necessary to confirm the diagnosis of DIC with additional tests (e.g., by estimating FDP or D-dimer concentration or by carrying out a screening test for the presence of fibrin monomers). Consider the possibility that more than one pathology is present.

Correction Tests Using the PT or APTT

Principle
Unexplained prolongation of the PT or APTT can be investigated with simple correction tests by mixing the patient's plasma with normal plasma. Correction indicates a possible factor deficiency, whereas failure to correct suggests the presence of an inhibitor, but interpretation should initially be cautious; see below.

Reagents

Plasmas for Correction
Normal plasma contains all the coagulation factors; therefore mixing tests with normal plasma will identify the presence of an inhibitor or a factor deficiency. In previous editions the use of aged and adsorbed plasma is described, but these correction reagents may give misleading results if not used with great care. It is better to proceed directly to specific factor assays if appropriate factor deficient plasmas are available.

PPP.
From the patient and a control.
Other reagents. As described on p. 401.

Method
Perform a PT and/or APTT on control, patient's, and a 50:50 (0.05 ml of each) mixture of the control and patient plasma. Perform all the tests in duplicate using a balanced order to avoid time bias. Note that mixing experiments to detect factor VIII inhibitors may require incubation for 2 hours (see p. 414).

Interpretation
If the prolongation is the result of a deficiency of a clotting factor, the PT or APTT of the mixture should return to within a few seconds of normal. It is then necessary to identify the specific factor(s) that are deficient.

If the APTT is prolonged, and normal plasma fails to correct the APTT, an inhibitor should be suspected. An inhibitor screen and tests for an LAC should be performed.

However, mixing tests may be misleading in two particular circumstances:

1. Some inhibitors (usually anti-factor VIII antibodies) are time dependent in their action and testing immediately after mixing may show correction, whereas testing after 2 hours of incubation reveals an inhibitory effect.
2. Some lupus-like anticoagulants are relatively weak and may only be apparent if 25:75 mixes of normal and test plasma are used. For details of testing for inhibitors, see p. 412.

Comment
Correction tests are sometimes not as clearcut as the literature and theory would suggest. Incomplete correction can be difficult to interpret. If the correction tests fall into the "grey" area, specific factor levels should be measured, and tests for the presence of an LAC should be performed, checking for time-dependent effects and nonlinearity.

Correction Tests Using the Thrombin Time

Principle
The tests use certain physicochemical properties of reagents to bind to inhibitors or abnormal molecules and normalise the prolonged TT. Protamine sulphate has a net electropositive charge and interacts with heparin, as well as binds to FDP, neutralising the inhibitory effects of both. Toluidine blue is also a charged reagent that will neutralise heparin but has no effect on FDP. It is interesting that toluidine blue normalises the TT in some dysfibrinogenaemias, probably by interacting with the excess of sialic acid attached to the fibrinogen molecules. Mixing with serum will correct the prolongation of the TT resulting from hypoalbuminaemia.

Reagents
Patient's and control plasma.
Protamine sulphate.
1% and 10% in 9 g/l NaCl.

Toluidine blue.
0.05 g in 100 ml of 9 g/l NaCl.

Bovine thrombin.
As described under thrombin time.

Method

Perform the test as described for TT, adding 0.1 ml of saline to the controls and replacing in the test with protamine sulphate or toluidine blue solution. Also perform a TT on a 50:50 mixture of control and test plasma.

Interpretation

See Table 16.4.

Comment

The end-point may be difficult to see in samples with a low fibrinogen content in the presence of toluidine blue owing to the dark colour of the reagent. Grossly elevated fibrinogen concentrations or the presence of a paraprotein can cause a prolonged time not corrected by either protamine or toluidine blue. Diluting the test plasma in saline will shorten the TT.

Reptilase or Ancrod Time[27]

Reptilase, a purified enzyme from the snake *Bothrops atrox,* and Ancrod (Arvin), a similar enzyme from the snake *Agkistrodon rhodostoma*, may be used to replace thrombin in the TT test.

The venoms are reconstituted as directed by the manufacturers, and the test is performed exactly as described for the TT. The snake venoms are not inhibited by heparin and will give normal times for the clotting of normal plasma in the presence of heparin. The clotting times will, however, remain prolonged in the presence of raised FDP or abnormal or reduced fibrinogen or hypoalbuminaemia.

INVESTIGATION OF A BLEEDING DISORDER RESULTING FROM A COAGULATION FACTOR DEFICIENCY OR DEFECT

When the screening tests indicate that an individual has a coagulation defect, the plasma concentration of the coagulation factors should be assayed. Such assays establish the diagnosis of the deficiency or defect, and they assess its severity; they also can be used to monitor replacement therapy and to detect the carrier state in families in which one or more members are affected by a congenital bleeding disorder.

An individual may have a congenital deficiency of a coagulation factor because of impaired synthesis or because a variant of the molecule that is deficient in clotting activity is synthesised. In both instances the results of assays based on coagulation tests will be subnormal, but when a variant molecule is being produced, the result of an immunological assay may be normal or near normal.

General Principles of Parallel Line Bioassays of Coagulation Factors

If two materials containing the same coagulation factor are assayed in a specific assay system in a range of dilutions, and the clotting times are plotted against the plasma concentration on linear graph paper, curved dose-response lines are obtained. If the plot is redrawn on double-log paper, a sigmoid

Table 16.4	Interpretation of correction tests using the thrombin time (TT)				
	TT of test plasma corrected with			Interpretation	
Saline	Normal plasma	Protamine sulphate	Toluidine blue		
No	Yes	No	No	Deficiency	
No	Var	No	Yes	Dysfibrinogenaemia of liver disease	
No	Var	Yes	No	High concentration of FDP	

FDP, fibrin degradation products; var, variable.
It is essential to exclude the possibility of heparin contamination.

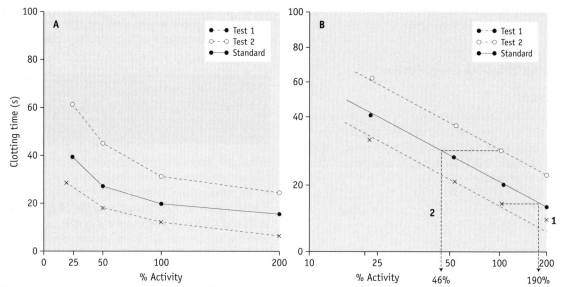

Figure 16.8   Parallel line bioassay of factor VII. A: Clotting times with 1 in 5, 1 in 10, 1 in 20, and 1 in 40 dilutions of test and standard plasma plotted on linear graph paper. B: The same data plotted on double log paper. Three parallel straight lines are obtained. The horizontal shift of the test line represents the difference in potency. In this case test 1 has a potency of 190% and test 2 has a potency of 46%. The 1 in 10 dilution of the standard plasma is assigned a potency of 100%.

curve with a straight middle section is obtained (Fig. 16.8), although in some cases (e.g., Factor VIII) semilog paper is required. If the dilutions of the test and standard materials are chosen carefully, it should be possible to draw two straight parallel lines. The horizontal distance between the two lines represents the difference in potency ("strength" or concentration) of the factor assayed. If the test line is to the right of the standard, it contains less of the factor than the standard; if it is to the left, it contains more. The assay is based on the assumption that both test and control behave like simple dilutions of each other. This assumption has caused some problems when assaying samples containing factor VIII or IX concentrates (see below).

When setting up and performing a parallel line assay, a number of measures must be taken to ensure that the assay is valid and reliable.

1. *Dilution range.* This should be chosen so that the coagulation times lie on the linear portion of the sigmoid curve. For example, when assaying factor VIII:C by one-stage assay, dilutions giving times between 60 and 100 sec are chosen if the blank clotting time is more than 120 sec. (The blank consists of a mixture of buffer and substrate or deficient plasma, which provides all factors except the one to be measured.)

2. *Number of dilutions.* At least three dilutions of the standard and the test are assayed to give the best graphic or mathematic solution.

3. *Responses.* Dilutions of the test sample should be chosen so that the clotting times fall within the range obtained for the standard. If it transpires that the test result falls outside this range, the standard curve should not be extrapolated but the dilutions of the test and/or the standard must be adjusted.

4. *Duplicates and replicates.* Duplicates are obtained from the same dilution of the sample and sometimes by subsampling from the same incubation mixture. Replicates are true repeats involving a fresh dilution and fresh reagents. Normally, coagulation times are measured on duplicates. Replicates are sometimes used for particularly difficult assays.

5. *Temporal drift.* This has already been discussed. Duplicates in a coagulation assay should always be tested in a balanced order (e.g., ABCCBA).

Note on Single Point Factor Assays

Factor assay results are dependent on obtaining parallel lines for the test and reference plasmas. Many automated coagulation analysers will give an assay result obtained from a single dilution assuming that this condition is met. However, this is not always true, and if an inhibitor is suspected, results from more than one dilution should be obtained for comparison and to determine parallelism. Similarly, if the result is above the linear part of the standard curve, further dilutions should be tested.

Assays Based on the Prothrombin Time

The investigation of an isolated prolonged one-stage PT (e.g., suspected factor VII deficiency or defect) in an individual with a lifelong history of bleeding includes a one-stage factor VII assay. If a reduced concentration of factor VII is found, further tests may include immunoassays of factor VII and, when possible, a family study.

One-Stage Assay of Factor VII

Principle
The assay of factor VII is based on the PT. The assay compares the ability of dilutions of the patient's plasma and of a standard plasma to correct the PT of a substrate plasma. It is easily adapted to assay of prothrombin, FV or FX.

Reagents
PPP from the patient.
Standard/reference plasma.
See page 392.

Factor VII deficient plasma.
Commercial or from a patient with known severe deficiency.

Barbitone buffered saline.
See page 690.

Thromboplastin.
It is recommended that a recombinant human thromboplastin is used for the assay of human FVII.

Rabbit brain thromboplastin known to be sensitive to factor VII deficiency has been used, but there is a danger of the interspecies differences giving misleading results. The thromboplastin should be reconstituted according to the manufacturer's instructions and may have sufficient Ca for the assay. Warm sufficient thromboplastin for the assay to 37°C.

$CaCl_2$.
0.025 mol/l (if not present in the thromboplastin preparation).

Method
Prepare 1 in 5, 1 in 10, 1 in 20, and 1 in 40 dilutions of the standard and test plasma in buffered saline. Transfer 0.1 ml of each dilution to a glass tube and add to it 0.1 ml of deficient (substrate) plasma. Mix and allow to warm to 37°C. Add 0.1 ml of dilute thromboplastin and start the stopwatch. Record the clotting time. If the thromboplastin does not contain calcium, start the stopwatch after adding 0.1 ml of $CaCl_2$. A blank must be included with every assay, and all tests must be carried out in duplicate and in balanced order.

Calculation of Results
Plot the clotting times of the test and standard against the concentration of factor VII on log–log graph paper. Read the concentration as shown in Fig. 16.8.

Normal Range
The normal range is 0.5–2.0 u/ml (for discussion of units see p. 413).

Interpretation
Patients with a congenital deficiency have factor VII levels of 0.30 u/ml and less. The concentration measured may vary according to the thromboplastin used in the assay, so human thromboplastin is preferable. A small proportion of patients have normal factor VII antigen despite abnormal functional activity.

Assays Based on the Activated Partial Thromboplastin Time

An APTT-based assay (e.g., factor VIII) may be indicated after obtaining correction of a prolonged APTT by mixing with another plasma. An assay for factor VIII is described, but this is easily adapted to FIX, FXI, or contact factor assay by substituting the relevant factor deficient plasma.

One-Stage Assay of Factor VIII:C[28,29]

Principle

The one-stage assay for factor VIII:C is based on the APTT according to the bioassay principle described earlier.

Reagents

PPP.
From the patient.

Standard/reference plasma.
See page 392.

Factor VIII deficient plasma (substrate plasma).
If using a commercial plasma, the reagent should be reconstituted according to the manufacturer's instructions. If a haemophiliac donor is used, his factor VIII:C concentration should be less than 1% and his plasma should be free of inhibitors. The plasma should be stored in suitable volumes (e.g., 2 ml) at $-20°C$ or lower until used. All samples obtained from patients must be considered potentially infective. Patient samples should be tested for antibodies to human immunodeficiency virus (HIV) and hepatitis C virus and for hepatitis B surface (HBs) antigen.

Barbitone buffered saline.
See page 690.

Reagents for APTT.
Plastic tubes.
To avoid contact activation while preparing samples.

Icebath.

Method

Place the APTT reagent and $CaCl_2$ at 37°C, and the patient's, standard, and substrate plasma in the icebath until used.

Make 1 in 10 dilutions of the test and standard plasma in buffered saline in plastic tubes in the icebath. Using 0.2 ml volumes, make doubling dilutions in buffered saline to obtain 1 in 20 and 1 in 40 dilutions. Place 0.1 ml of the three dilutions

(1 in 10, 1 in 20, and 1 in 40) in glass tubes. If the test plasma is suspected of having a very low factor VIII:C content, make 1 in 5, 10, and 20 dilutions of the test instead.

Add to each dilution 0.1 ml of freshly reconstituted or thawed substrate plasma and warm up at 37°C. Perform APTTs according to the laboratory protocol following a balanced order of duplicates.

The dilutions should be tested at 2-min intervals on the master watch. The assay must end with a blank consisting of 0.1 ml of buffered saline and 0.1 ml of substrate plasma.

Calculation of Results

Plot the clotting times of the test and standard against the concentration of factor VIII:C on semilog paper. Read the concentration as shown in Fig. 16.8. It is important to obtain straight and parallel lines if the result is to be accurate. The reasons for nonparallelism and curvature are as follows:

1. Technical error. Repeat the assay with fresh dilutions.
2. Activation of the plasma by poor collection. A new sample should be collected.
3. A low concentration of factor VIII:C in the test plasma giving rise to nonparallel lines. Stronger concentration of plasma should be prepared and tested.
4. The presence of an inhibitor. The tests described on p. 413 should be carried out.

Some automated coagulometers produce computed values using mathematic formulae. If the standard plasma is calibrated in terms of international units, the result can be expressed in iu. For example, if the standard plasma has a factor VIII:C concentration of 0.65 iu/ml and the test is shown to have 20% of the activity of the standard, the test plasma will have a factor VIII concentration of 0.13 iu/ml (20% of 65 iu/ml).

Normal Range

The normal range is 0.45–1.58 iu/ml. Each laboratory should determine its own normal range.

Interpretation

Some clinically normal people have factor VIII:C concentrations of 35–50 iu/dl. Values below 30 iu/dl are unequivocally abnormal; values below 50 iu/dl are significant in carriers of haemophilia (heterozygotes).

A reduced factor VIII:C concentration is found in the following:

1. Haemophilia A
2. Some carriers of haemophilia A (heterozygotes)
3. VWD, types I and III, and some cases of type II
4. Congenital combined deficiency of factors VIII and V (rare)
5. Disseminated intravascular coagulation
6. Acquired haemophilia (anti-factor VIII antibodies)

An elevated level of factor VIII has now been shown to have an association with thrombosis.[30]

Further Tests in Haemophilia A

Reduction in factor VIII secondary to VWD should be excluded. VWF:Ag and VWF:RCo (described later) should be measured, and the patient's family history should be investigated. A low factor VIII with normal VWF Ag and VWF:RCo may also result from the Normandy type VWD (Type 2N), which should be suspected when there is not a clear sex-linked, family history and which can be confirmed by a VWF-FVIII–binding assay.[31]

Two-Stage and Chromogenic Assays for Factor VIII

The one-stage factor VIII assay is sensitive to preactivation of coagulation factors in the patient sample. The two-stage and chromogenic assays circumvent this problem by preactivating all the available factor VIII and then assaying this in a separate system by its ability to generate Xa. In the chromogenic assay this is measured using a chromogenic Xa substrate; in the two-stage assay it is measured by a clotting end-point. In general these have proved too cumbersome or expensive for widespread use and preactivation is rarely a significant problem. However, a clinically significant discrepancy between the two types of assay has been reported in some cases of mild haemophilia. In these cases mutations destabilising the interaction between the A_1 and A_2 domains result in a one-stage assay result that is higher than that obtained by two stage. Most significantly, the patient's clinical problem is more in keeping with the two-stage assay result.[32,33] The chromogenic assay has also found utility in avoiding some of the problems encountered assaying factor VIII concentrates.

Tests Required for Monitoring Replacement Therapy in Coagulation Factor Defects and Deficiencies

Replacement therapy requires the following:
1. Calculation of the dose of the material to be administered and its frequency
2. Assessment of the response to the dose
3. Monitoring of any untoward effects

The *dose* to be administered is calculated from the patient's body weight and the rise in the plasma concentration of the defective coagulation factor that is desired. Thus the patient's plasma concentration of the factor and the potency or strength of the therapeutic material must be known. For the vast majority of patients in whom the defect is known and plasma concentration has been measured, and for whom a commercial freeze-dried factor concentrate is used, this means a calculation based on the following formulae:

For factor VIII the dose in iu per kg body weight = rise required in iu per dl divided by 1.5.
For plasma-derived factor IX, the dose in iu per kg body weight = rise required in iu per dl.
For recombinant factor IX, the dose in iu per kg body weight = rise required in iu per dl divided by 0.8

The rise required depends on the type of bleeding, the half-life and stability of the clotting factor used, and the concentration of the defective factor in the patient's plasma prior to treatment.

Assessment of the response to the therapy requires regular measurements of the plasma concentration of the coagulation factor infused by means of a functional assay. The response can be assessed from the following formula:

Rise in iu per dl divided by dose in iu per kg body weight = K, which is approximately 2 for haemophilia A and approximately 1 for haemophilia B (if plasma concentrates are used).

The response is usually measured immediately after the administration of the therapeutic material. If the response is inadequate, this may have been because of an error in calculating the dose, because the potency of the therapeutic material is less than expected, or because the patient is developing an inhibitor.

The main *untoward effects* are transmission of infection and the development of inhibitors. If the presence of an inhibitor is suspected, it must be confirmed using the tests described on p. 413 and later assessed quantitatively. Monitoring replacement and other types of therapy in patients with inhibitors are described by White and Roberts.[34]

Estimations of factor VIII in patients with haemophilia treated with factor VIII concentrates often yield discrepant results. This is primarily because the factor VIII concentrate (diluted in haemophilic plasma) is compared with a plasma standard. In general two-stage or chromogenic assays reveal greater potency than one-stage assays in this situation. This has been particularly noted in patients who have been treated with B domainless factor VIII (Refacto, Wyeth Pharmaceuticals). In this case a product-specific reference preparation is available from the company. It is recommended that this is used in conjunction with a chromogenic assay, but this may not be necessary.[35] In most other cases the clinical experience of using results from one-stage assays remains valid.

Assays of factor VIII concentrates are fraught with difficulty, and a detailed discussion is beyond the scope of this chapter.[36] The difficulties arise from several problems. First, the concentrate potency may be assigned using either a one-stage assay (as in the United States) or the chromogenic assay (as in Europe). Second, many concentrates, even when diluted in haemophilic plasma, behave differently in one-stage and chromogenic assays. As a result there are separate WHO standards for FVIII measurement: a plasma for measurement of FVIII in plasma samples and a concentrate is for measurement of FVIII in concentrates. This is based on the principle of assaying like against like, although there are so many different concentrates with different characteristics that this is difficult to truly achieve, and all must eventually be calibrated against a single plasma pool.[37]

Investigation of a Patient whose APTT and PT are Prolonged

A prolonged APTT and PT but a normal TT in a patient with a bleeding disorder may be the result of a defect or deficiency of one of the factors of the common pathway: factor X, factor V, or pro-thrombin. In addition, the patient could be suffering from the much rarer combined deficiency of factors V and VIII:C. Liver disease and vitamin K deficiency should always be excluded, even in the presence of a family history of bleeding. Mixing tests illustrated on p. 413 may help to pinpoint the defect; the missing factor or factors should be estimated quantitatively. Factor X, factor V, and prothrombin can all be assayed satisfactorily using a prothrombin-based assay as described for factor VII. The Taipan venom assay for prothrombin and the Russell's viper venom assay for factor X are described in the 8th edition.

INVESTIGATION OF A PATIENT WITH A CIRCULATING ANTICOAGULANT (INHIBITOR)[38]

Circulating anticoagulants or acquired inhibitors of coagulation factors are immunoglobulins arising either in congenitally deficient individuals as a result of the administration of the missing factor or in previously haemostatically normal subjects as a part of an autoimmune process. Usually, an inhibitor is suspected when a prolonged clotting test does not correct after mixing 50:50 with normal plasma or if an apparent factor deficiency does not fit with a patient's clinical history.

The most common anticoagulant in haemostatically normal people is the LAC, but despite the prolongation of clotting tests *in vitro,* this anticoagulant predisposes to thrombosis, and its diagnosis and investigation therefore are considered on p. 443. Of the anticoagulants that cause a bleeding tendency, antibodies to factor VIII:C are most common. They are present in 15% or more of haemophiliacs but also arise as autoantibodies in previously normal individuals. They fall into two general categories: those with simple kinetics and those with complex kinetics. Patients with haemophilia usually develop antibodies with simple kinetics;

this inhibitor reacts with factor VIII:C in a linear fashion and the antigen/antibody complex has no factor VIII:C activity. Antibodies in nonhaemophilic individuals or patients with mild/moderate haemophilia usually develop antibodies with complex kinetics: inactivation of factor VIII:C is at first rapid, but it then slows as the antigen/antibody complex either dissociates or displays some factor VIII:C activity. Addition of further factor VIII results to the same residual (equilibrium) factor VIII activity.

Inhibitors directed against other coagulation factors are very rare, but an acquired form of VWD commonly associated with a paraprotein has been increasingly recognised in recent years. Hypoprothrombinaemia owing to autoantibodies is a rare complication of systemic lupus erythematosus.[39] Only the factor VIII:C inhibitor assays are described in detail in this section.

Confusion may arise in the presence of inhibitor if different clotting factors are assayed. For instance, if a patient's plasma contains an inhibitor directed against factor VIII and the factor IX level in that plasma is assayed using factor IX deficient plasma, the clotting times in the factor IX assay will be prolonged. This may lead to the mistaken conclusion that the patient has factor IX deficiency, particularly if a single dilution of test plasma is used. Clotting factors should always be assayed at multiple dilutions. If the inhibitor is specifically directed against one clotting factor, that factor will appear to be equally deficient at all dilutions of the patient's plasma. The assayed level of other clotting factors will increase with increasing dilution as the inhibitor is diluted out.

Circulating Inhibitor (Anticoagulant) Screen Based on the APTT[38]

Principle

Circulating anticoagulants or inhibitors affecting the APTT may act immediately or be time dependent. Normal plasma mixed with a plasma containing an immediately acting inhibitor will have little or no effect on the prolonged clotting time. In contrast, if normal plasma is added to a plasma containing a time-dependent inhibitor, the clotting time of the latter will be substantially shortened. However, after 1–2 hours, correction will be abolished, and the clotting time will become long again. To detect both types of inhibition, normal plasma and test plasma samples are tested immediately after mixing and also after incubation together at 37°C for 120 min.

Reagents

Normal plasma.
Commercial lyophilised normal plasma or a plasma pool from 20 donors as described on p. 393.

PPP.
From the patient.

Reagents for the APTT.
(See p. 398.)

Method

Prepare 3 plastic tubes as follows: place 0.5 ml of normal plasma in a first tube, 0.5 ml of the patient's plasma in a second tube, and a mixture of 0.25 ml of normal and 0.25 ml of patient's plasma in a third tube. Incubate the tubes for 120 min at 37°C and then place all 3 tubes in an icebath or on crushed ice. Next, make a 50:50 mixture of the contents of tubes 1 and 2 into a 4th tube, which serves to check for the presence of an immediate inhibitor. Perform APTTs in duplicate on all 4 tubes.

Results and Interpretation

See Table 16.5. Note that the incubation period results in a prolongation of the normal plasma APTT.

Quantitative Measurement of Factor VIII:C Inhibitors

Principle

Factor VIII inhibitors are usually time dependent.[38] Thus if factor VIII:C is added to plasma containing an inhibitor and the mixture is incubated, factor VIII:C will be progressively neutralised. If the amount of factor VIII:C added and the duration of incubation are standardised, the strength of the inhibitor may be measured in units according to how much of the added factor VIII:C is destroyed.

In the Bethesda method, the unit is defined as the amount of inhibitor that will neutralise 50% of

Table 16.5 Interpretation of the inhibitor screen based on the activated partial thromboplastin time

Tube	Content	Clotting time		
1	Normal plasma	Normal	Normal	Normal
2	Patient's plasma	Long	Long	Long
3	50:50 mixture, patient: normal; incubated 2 h	Normal	Long	Long
4	50:50 mixture, patient: normal; no incubation	Normal	Long	Normal
Interpretation		Deficiency	Immediately acting inhibitor	Time-dependent inhibitor

1 unit of factor VIII:C in normal plasma after 2 hours of incubation at 37°C.

Dilutions of test plasma are incubated with an equal volume of the normal plasma pool at 37°C. The normal plasma pool is taken to represent 1 unit of factor VIII:C. Dilutions of a control normal plasma containing no inhibitor are treated in the same way. An equal volume of normal plasma mixed with buffer is taken to represent the 100% value.

At the end of the incubation period the residual factor VIII:C is assayed and the inhibitor strength is calculated from a standard graph of residual factor VIII:C activity versus inhibitor units.

Inhibitor Assay Modifications

The Bethesda assay and Nijmegen modification give similar results at high levels of factor VIII inhibition. However, at low levels (below 1.0) the Bethesda method can give false-positive levels of inhibition, whereas the Nijmegen method would give zero levels of inhibition. Reports have shown that shifts in pH and protein concentrations will lead to changes in factor VIII stability and inactivation. Factor VIII inactivation increases with pH, and reduced protein concentration leads to further inactivation of factor VIII activity. The Nijmegen modification prevents these discrep-ancies by buffering normal plasma with 0.1 M imidazole buffer at pH 7.4 and using immunodepleted factor VIII deficient plasma in the control mixture.[40] The assay can also be modified to use factor VIII concentrate (Oxford method) or by increasing the incubation time to 4 hours (New Oxford method).

Reagents

Glyoxaline buffer.
See p. 398.

Kaolin.
5 mg/ml and platelet substitute. Phospholipid or preferred APTT reagent.

Factor VIII C deficient plasma.

Standard plasma.
Normal plasma pool.

Method

Pipette into each of a series of plastic tubes 0.2 ml of normal pool plasma. Add 0.2 ml of glyoxaline buffer to the first tube (this tube serves as the 100% value); add 0.2 ml of test plasma dilutions in glyoxaline buffer to each of the other tubes. If the patient's inhibitor has been assayed previously, this can be used as a guide to the dilutions that should be used. If the patient has not been tested before, a range of dilutions should be set up ranging from undiluted plasma to a 1 in 50 dilution.

Cap, mix, and incubate all the tubes for 2 hours at 37°C. Then immerse all the tubes in an icebath. Perform factor VIII:C assays on all the incubation mixtures.

Calculation of Results

Record the residual factor VIII:C percentage for each mixture assuming the assay value of the control to be 100%. The dilution of test plasma that gives the residual factor VIII:C percentage nearest to 50% (between 30% and 60%) is chosen for calculating the strength of inhibitor. Results are calculated as shown in Table 16.6 and Fig. 16.9 for three different patients with a mild inhibitor only detected in undiluted plasma, a stronger inhibitor with simple kinetics, and an inhibitor with complex kinetics, respectively.

Interpretation

If the residual factor VIII:C activity is between 80% and 100%, the plasma sample does not contain an inhibitor. If the residual activity is less than 60%, the plasma unequivocally contains an inhibitor. Values between 60% and 80% are borderline, and repeated testing on additional samples is needed before the diagnosis can be established.

Tests for Other Inhibitors

Factor IX inhibitors can be measured in a system identical to that described earlier. Because factor IX inhibitors act immediately, there is no need for prolonged incubation; the mixtures can be assayed after 5 min at 37°C. The activity of the inhibitor against porcine factor VIII can be measured by substituting Hyate C (porcine factor VIII, concentrate,

appropriately diluted in factor VIII deficient plasma) for normal plasma.

INVESTIGATION OF A PATIENT SUSPECTED OF AFIBRINOGENAEMIA, HYPOFIBRINOGENAEMIA, OR DYSFIBRINOGENAEMIA

A patient suspected of afibrinogenaemia, hypofibrinogenaemia, or dysfibrinogenaemia usually has a prolonged APTT, PT, and TT. The prolongation of the PT is usually less marked than that of the APTT and TT. There may be either a history of bleeding or of recurrent thrombotic events, and many patients (c 50%) are asymptomatic. It is important that a physical estimation of fibrinogen (such as the clot weight) is obtained as well as a function-based assay (e.g., Clauss).

Fibrinogen Estimation (Dry Clot Weight)

Principle
Fibrinogen in plasma is converted into fibrin by clotting with thrombin and calcium. The resulting clot is weighed. The resulting clot may include other

Table 16.6	Example of the calculation of Bethesda units (u) in three plasma samples			
Patient	Plasma dilution	% residual VIII:C	Calculation u × dilution	Inhibitor in Bethesda u
A	Undiluted	61	0.70 × 1	= 0.07
B	1 in 5	33	1.60 × 5	= 8.0
	1 in 10	55	0.85 × 10	= 8.5
	1 in 15	68	0.55 × 15	= 8.3
C	1 in 5	40	1.30 × 5	= 6.5
	1 in 10	55	0.85 × 10	= 8.5
	1 in 15	61	0.70 × 15	= 10.5
	1 in 20	65	0.60 × 20	= 12

Patient A has a mild inhibitor, patient B an inhibitor with simple kinetics, and patient C an inhibitor with complex kinetics. All values are chosen for the percent residual factor VIII:C activity close to 50%. The units for the calculation are read from Figure 16.9 using the % residual VIII:C. (Modified from Kasper CK, Ewing NP. 1982 The haemophilias: measurement of inhibitor to factor VIII C (and IX C). Methods in Haematology 5:39)
Note that in patients B and C the results should be reported as 8.5 Bethesda units; in C, the calculated level of inhibitor may continue to rise with increasing dilution.

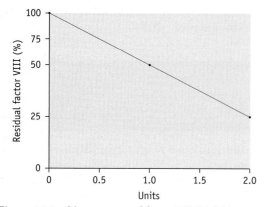

Figure 16.9 Measurement of factor VIII:C inhibitors Relationship between the residual factor VIII:C activity in normal plasma and the inhibitor activity of the test plasma can be read off this plot. At 50% inhibition the test plasma contains, by definition, 1 Bethesda inhibitor unit per ml. Note that the y axis is a logarithmic scale. See also Table 16.7.

proteins including some FDPs. It is, however, simpler than the total clottable protein method used for the international standard[41] and provides a useful comparison for the Clauss.

Reagents

Platelet poor plasma (PPP).

CaCl₂.
0.025 mol/l.

Bovine thrombin.
50 NIH u/ml.

Method

Pipette 1 ml of plasma into a 12×75 mm glass tube and warm to 37°C. Place a wooden applicator or swab stick in the tube, add 0.1 ml of $CaCl_2$ and 0.9 ml of thrombin, and mix. Incubate for 15 min at 37°C.

Gently wind the fibrin clot onto the stick, squeezing out the serum. Wash the clot in a tube containing at first 9 g/l NaCl, then water. Blot the clot carefully with filter paper, remove the fibrin from the stick, and put into acetone for 5–10 min. Dry the clot in a hot air oven or over a hot lamp for 30 min. Allow it to cool and then weigh it.

Results

The fibrinogen level is expressed as g/l (i.e., the weight of fibrin obtained from 1 ml of plasma $\times$ 1000).

Normal Range

Normal range is 1.5–4.0 g/l.

Further Investigations

Whenever a congenital fibrinogen abnormality is suspected, DIC and hyperfibrinolysis must be excluded; FDP should not be in excess and there should be no evidence of the consumption of other coagulation factors and platelets (see p. 434). Immunological or chemical determination of fibrinogen is the next step in investigation. In dysfibrinogenaemias there is often a normal or even raised plasma fibrinogen concentration using these methods, although the functional assays indicate a deficiency. Other tests that may be helpful are the Reptilase time, fibrinopeptide release, factor XIII crosslinking, tests of polymerisation, binding to thrombin, and lysis by plasmin. In some cases genomic DNA analysis can be performed.[42] Testing the parents or other family members is sometimes a useful means for establishing whether an hereditary fibrinogen abnormality is present.

DEFECTS OF PRIMARY HAEMOSTASIS

Investigation of the Vascular Disorders of Haemostasis

Vascular disorders of haemostasis are those that arise as a result of a defect or deficiency of the vessel wall. This may result from one of the inherited disorders of collagen or from an acquired disorder such as amyloid or scurvy.

In general the tests of coagulation available in the laboratory will be of little help in elucidating such defects. The only test of any use is the bleeding time. Tests of capillary resistance are of little value. A careful clinical history and physical examination are most likely to provide the basis for diagnosis. Particular attention should be paid to previous scars, associated signs of the inherited syndromes, and evidence of systemic disease. In some cases a tissue biopsy may be useful, but confirmation of the diagnosis requires analysis of collagen from cultured fibroblasts or DNA analysis of the relevant candidate genes.[43]

Bleeding Time

Principle
A standard incision is made on the volar surface of the forearm, and the time the incision bleeds is measured. Cessation of bleeding indicates the formation of haemostatic plugs, which are in turn dependent on an adequate number of platelets and on the ability of the platelets to adhere to the subendothelium and to form aggregates.[44]

Standardised Template Method[45]

Materials
Sphygmomanometer.

Cleansing swabs.

Template bleeding time device.
Such as "Simplate R" with a single retractable blade (Organon Teknika).

Filter paper.
1 mm thick.

Stopwatch.

Method
Place a sphygmomanometer cuff around the patient's arm above the elbow, inflate to 40 mm Hg, and keep it at this pressure throughout the test. Clean the area with 70% ethanol and allow to dry. Choose an area of skin on the volar surface of the forearm that is devoid of visible superficial veins. Use a commercial template device to make one or two standard longitudinal incisions. If not available then press a sterile metal template with a linear slit 7–8 mm long firmly against the skin aligned along the long axis of the arm and use a scalpel blade with a guard so arranged that the tip of the blade protrudes 1 mm through the template slit. In this way make an incision 6 mm long and 1 mm deep. Modifications of the template and blade making two simultaneous cuts with a spring mechanism are commercially available.

With the edge of a filter paper, at 15 sec intervals blot off the blood exuding from the cut. Avoid contact with the wound during this procedure because this may disturb the formation of the platelet plug. When bleeding has ceased, carefully oppose the edges of the incision and apply an adhesive strip to reduce the risk of keloid formation and an unsightly scar.

Normal Range
Normal range is 2-7 min. An upper limit of 4 min has been reported in one study on men and women who had not used aspirin or other relevant drugs in the ten days before the test.[46a] Ideally, every laboratory should determine its own normal range and if possible ensure that the test is performed by the same operator.

Ivy's Method[46]

Ivy's method is similar to the template method, but instead of a standardised incision, two separate punctures, 5–10 cm apart, are made in quick succession using a disposable lancet. Any microlance with a cutting depth of 2.5 mm and width of just more than 1 mm is suitable; it can be inserted to its maximum depth without fear of penetrating too deeply. A source of inaccuracy with Ivy's method is the tendency for the puncture wound to close before bleeding has ceased.

Normal Range
Normal range is 2–7 min. Ideally, every laboratory should determine its own normal range and if possible ensure that the test is performed by the same operator.

Interpretation of Results
A prolonged bleeding time may result from the following:

1. *Thrombocytopenia.* It is advisable to check the platelet count before carrying out the bleeding time test. Patients with a platelet count below 50×10^9/l may have a very long bleeding time and the bleeding may be difficult to arrest.
2. *Disorders of platelet function.* They may be congenital, such as thrombasthenia, storage pool defect, and the like (see below), or acquired, such as from drug use, uraemia, the presence of a paraprotein, or myelodysplastic/myeloproliferative syndromes.

3. *VWD.* This may occur as a result of defective platelet adherence to the subendothelium in the absence of a normal amount or of normally functioning VWF.
4. *Vascular abnormalities.* Examples of these abnormalities can be found in Ehler-Danlos's syndrome or in pseudoxanthoma elasticum.
5. *Occasionally, severe deficiency of factor V or XI, or afibrinogenaemia.*
6. *The bleeding time is subject to a large number of variables and confounding factors.* It is important to standardise the sphygmomanometer pressure, longitudinal orientation of the incision, volar aspect of arm, and the blotting technique. Attempting to repeat the test within a short period will usually give a shorter bleeding time. A normal bleeding time does not imply normal haemostasis, and the result of the test has been shown not to correlate with bleeding at other sites.

Laboratory Tests of Platelet–von Willebrand Factor Function

The PFA-100 System

The most widely used screening test for platelet disorders, the bleeding time, suffers from inherent variability and does not correlate well with the incidence of clinically significant bleeding.

An *in vitro* system for measuring platelet–VWF function PFA-100 (Dade Behring) is now available. The instrument aspirates a blood sample under constant vacuum from the sample reservoir through a capillary and a microscopic aperture cut into a membrane. The membrane is coated with collagen and/either epinephrine or adenosine 5'-diphosphate (ADP). It therefore attempts to reproduce under high shear rates VWF binding, platelet attachment, activation, and aggregation, which slowly build a stable platelet plug at the aperture. The time required to obtain full occlusion of the aperture is reported as the "closure time." Collagen/epinephrine is the primary screening cartridge, and the collagen/ADP is used to identify possible aspirin use.

Studies have shown this system to be sensitive to platelet adherence and aggregation abnormalities and to be dependent on normal VWF, glycoprotein Ib, and glycoprotein IIb/IIIa levels but not on plasma fibrinogen or fibrin generation.

The PFA-100 system may reflect VWF platelet function better than the bleeding time, but it is not sensitive to vascular-collagen disorders.[47,48] Studies have shown that many patients with minor platelet disorders such as secretion defects are not detected by the PFA-100.[49]

INVESTIGATION OF SUSPECTED VON WILLEBRAND'S DISEASE[50, 52]

A diagnosis of VWD should be considered in individuals with a relevant history or family history of bleeding, particularly of the mucosal type. Although a prolonged bleeding time and APTT in screening tests is suggestive, these are normal in many patients with VWD and specific assays must be performed. Preliminary screening with a test such as the PFA-100 may be useful in excluding borderline cases. All relevant activities (i.e., factor VIII:C concentration, VWF:Ag concentration, collagen binding activity [VWF:CB] and ristocetin cofactor activity [VWF:RCo]) should be measured. When interpreting the results, the very wide range of VWF levels in the normal population and the effect of ABO blood group should be borne in mind. It is apparent that many individuals with levels down to 30% of normal do not have any significant bleeding tendency and caution should be exercised in diagnosing VWD on the basis of moderately low VWF levels alone.[50-53]

If an abnormality is detected, the multimer analysis of the plasma should be performed. In normal plasma, each multimer of VWF (a large molecule consisting of 4 to more than 20 subunits of VWF) is seen to be composed of a "triplet," a dark central band sandwiched between two lighter bands; high molecular weight multimers predominate. In VWD, the multimer analysis may be superficially normal, there may be no VWF:Ag detectable, the high molecular weight forms necessary for normal platelet adhesion may be lacking, or the triplet pattern may be abnormal. On the basis of these results VWD can be classified as shown in Table 16.7.[50,52]

Enzyme-Linked Immunosorbent Assay for von Willebrand Factor Antigen[54]

Principle

ELISA involves coating a special microtitre plate with a primary antibody to VWF:Ag.[54] A suitable dilution of the test plasma is added to the wells,

Table 16.7   Classification of von Willebrand disease

Type	Inheritance	VIII:C	vWF:Ag	RiCoF	Mulimer analysis	Comments
1	Autos. dominant	L/N	L	L	Normal pattern	–
2A	Autos. dominant	L/N	L/N	L	Absent large and intermediate size multimers, some forms have abnormal triplets	–
2B	Autos. dominant	L/N	L	L/N	Large multimers absent normal triplets	Aggregation with low dose Ristocetin in platelet-rich plasma Thrombocytopenia
2M	Autos. dominant	N	N	L	Normal pattern	–
2N	Autos. recessive	L	N	N	Normal pattern	Abnormal FVIII binding
3	Autos. recessive	L	L	L	Virtually absent	–

Autos., autosomal; L, low; N, normal; RiCoF, ristocetin cofactor; vWF, von Willebrand factor.

allowing the VWF:Ag to bind to the primary antibody. After removal of excess antigen by washing the plate, a second antibody, conjugated to an enzyme, usually peroxidase, and called the "tag" antibody, is added and this binds to the VWF:Ag already bound to the plate. On addition of a specific substrate, a colour change occurs. After the reaction has been stopped with acid, the optical density (OD) of each well can be measured using an electronic plate reader; the OD is directly proportional to the amount of VWF:Ag present in the test plasma.

The primary antibody can be substituted by a monoclonal antibody specifically raised against the glycoprotein Ib binding site on the VWF (available from Porton, Cambridge). This modification was found to correlate with the functional activity of the VWF measured as ristocetin cofactor activity (VWF:RCo). However, because a number of exceptions to this relationship have been identified the ristocetin cofactor assay remains the gold standard for estimation of VWF functional activity.

Reagents

0.05 M Carbonate buffer.
1.59 g Na_2CO_3, 2.93 g $NaHCO_3$, 0.2 g NaN_3 in 1 litre of distilled water (pH 9.6).

0.01 M Phosphate buffered saline.
0.39 g $NaH_2PO_4.2H_2O$, 2.68 g $Na_2HPO_4.12H_2O$, 8.47 g NaCl in 1 litre distilled water (pH 7.2).

0.1 M Citrate phosphate buffer.
8.8 g citric acid, 24.0 g $Na_2HPO_4.12H_2O$ in 1 litre distilled water (pH 5.0).

Anti VWF:Ag antiserum.
Anti VWF:Ag conjugated with peroxidase.
Platelet poor (100%) calibration plasma.
PPP (tests and control).
1,2-o-Phenylenediamine dihydrochloride (ortho-phenylenediamine, OPD).
1 M Sulphuric acid.
Hydrogen peroxide 20 vol.
Tween 20.

Method

Dilute the antihuman VWF:Ag 1:500 in 0.05 M carbonate buffer (i.e., 40 µl antibody in 20 ml buffer) and add 100 µl to each well of the microtitre plate. Incubate for 1 hour at room temperature in a moist chamber. Discard antibody and wash 3 times by immersion in a trough of phosphate buffered saline (PBS) with 0.5 ml/l Tween for 2 min, followed by inversion onto absorbent paper.

Prepare dilutions of the 100% standard 1:10, 1:20, 1:40, and 1:60 in PBS with 1 ml/l Tween. Dilute patients' and control plasmas 1:10, 1:20, and 1:40 in the same way and add 100 µl of each dilution in duplicate to the wells of the microtitre plate. Incubate for 1 hour as before and repeat washing.

Dilute the antihuman VWF:Ag-peroxidase conjugate 1:500 in 1 ml/l PBS-Tween (i.e., 40 μl antibody in 20 ml buffer) and add 100 μl to each well. Incubate for 1 hour. Wash twice in 0.5 ml/l PBS Tween and once in 0.1 M citrate phosphate buffer.

Dissolve 40 mg of substrate (OPD) in 15 ml citrate phosphate buffer. Add 10 μl of 20 volume hydrogen peroxide to the substrate solution immediately before use, and then add 100 μl to each well.

When the yellow colour has reached an intensity at which a mid-yellow ring is clearly visible in the bottom of the wells, stop the reaction by the addition of 150 μl of 1 M sulphuric acid. Read the optical density across the plate at 492 nm using a microtitre plate reader. Plot the standard curve on log-linear graph paper. VWF:Ag levels are obtained by reading from the reference curve.

Normal Range

The normal range is 0.5–2.0 iu/ml.

Interpretation

The results must be interpreted in conjunction with the results of factor VIII:C assay and the ristocetin cofactor assay (Table 16.7). VWF:Ag can also be measured by an immunoelectrophoretic assay. The Laurell rocket method for this is described in the 7th edition of this book.

von Willebrand Factor Antigen Immunoturbidometric Assay

Latex microparticles, coated with antibodies specific for VWF, are incubated with plasma; an antigen-antibody reaction occurs resulting in agglutination of the latex microparticles. Agglutination of the microparticles leads to an increase in turbidity and hence absorbance, which is measured photometrically. Using a standard curve, the VWF concentration can be calculated (Instrumentation Laboratories and Stago).

Ristocetin Cofactor Assay[55]

Principle

Washed platelets do not "agglutinate" in the presence of ristocetin unless normal plasma is added as a source of VWF. "Agglutination" follows a dose-response curve dependent on the amount of plasma/VWF added. Freshly washed platelets or formalin-fixed platelets can be used in the assay. Fixed platelets take longer to prepare but are not susceptible to aggregation (as distinct from "agglutination") with ristocetin, and they can be stored so that they are available for emergency use. Freshly washed platelets are quicker to prepare and retain a functional platelet membrane, but they cannot be retained for later use.

Commercial lyophilised, fixed, washed platelet preparations are available. Once reconstituted these preparations are stable for several weeks and should enhance assay standardization.

Assay Using Fresh Platelets

Reagents

K_2EDTA. *0.134 mol/l.*

Citrate-saline.

One volume of 31.1 g/l trisodium citrate + 9 volumes of 9 g/l NaCl.

EDTA–citrate–saline.

One volume of 0.134 mol/l K_2EDTA + 9 volumes of citrate-saline.

Method

Collect 40–60 ml of normal blood into a one-tenth volume of EDTA-saline in flat-bottom plastic universal containers. Do not use conical bottom containers. Centrifuge at 150–200 g at room temperature (about 20°C) for 15 min.

Pipette, using a plastic pipette, the platelet-rich plasma (PRP) into a plastic container. Mark the level of plasma on the tube. Centrifuge at 1500–2000 g to obtain a platelet button.

Discard the PPP. Resuspend the platelet button in a 2 ml volume of EDTA–citrate–saline by gently squeezing the liquid up and down a pipette until a smooth suspension is formed. Add EDTA–citrate–saline to the 20 ml mark.

Centrifuge at 1500–2000 g for 15 min. Discard the supernatant. Resuspend in EDTA–citrate–saline and leave at room temperature for 20 min to elute the ristocetin cofactor off the platelets.

Centrifuge again, discard the supernatant, and resuspend in EDTA–citrate–saline two more times to a total of four washes.

Centrifuge at 1500–2000 g for 15 min. Discard the supernatant and resuspend in citrate–saline using a volume slightly under the original plasma volume (marked on the container). Centrifuge at 800 g for 5 min to remove platelet clumps, white cells, and red cells.

Remove the platelet-rich supernatant carefully. Perform a platelet count and dilute the platelet-rich suspension with citrate–saline until the platelet count is about $200 \times 10^9/l$.

Leave the platelets at room temperature for 30–45 min to allow the platelets to recover from the trauma of washing and centrifugation.

Reagents for Assay

Citrate–saline.
Ristocetin.
100 mg/ml. Stored frozen in 1 ml volumes.

Plasma standard.
PPP.
From the patient(s).

Assay Method

Confirm that the washed platelets do not "agglutinate" with ristocetin in the absence of added plasma. Deliver 0.5 ml of citrate–saline into an aggregometer cuvette and 0.4 ml of the platelet suspension + 0.1 ml of citrate–saline into another cuvette. Place in the warming block and leave it there for 3 min to warm. Add 5 µl of ristocetin and record at 1 cm/min for 2 min. The absorbance resulting from citrate–saline alone is taken to represent 100% agglutination, and that resulting from platelets alone represents zero (%) agglutination (blank). The absorbance resulting from the platelet suspension must not exceed 5 divisions on the chart paper. If it is greater, the platelets must be washed again and the procedure must be repeated. The reading of this blank must be repeated every hour.

All plasma samples and ristocetin should be kept in an icebath.

Standard Curve

A standard curve is obtained by making doubling dilutions, 1 in 2 to 1 in 32 in citrate–saline, of the standard plasma (donor pool, commercial reference plasma, or other reference materials). The absorbance resulting from a mixture of 0.4 ml of citrate–saline and 0.1 ml of plasma dilution is taken to represent 100% agglutination, and that resulting from the mixture of 0.4 ml of platelet suspension and 0.1 ml of plasma dilution represents zero (0%) agglutination.

Add 5 µl of ristocetin to the cuvette containing the mixture giving zero agglutination and record the agglutination for 2 min. Test each dilution of the standard plasma in a similar way.

The patient's plasma is tested at two dilutions, depending on the expected concentration of VWF in the plasma. Both dilutions should give agglutination within the range of that of the standard curve.

Reset 100% and zero aggregation for each patient.

A reading of the platelet blank should be repeated at hourly intervals. If the reading differs from the original, the difference must be subtracted from the results of subsequent tests.

Results

Measure "agglutination" at 1 or 2 min depending on the strength of "agglutination." All responses must be compared on the same time scale and not read at maximum "agglutination."

Plot the standard curve on semilog paper with "agglutination" on the linear scale and the concentration of VWF in u/dl on the log scale (Fig. 16.10). For assay purposes, assign the 1 in 2 dilution of standard plasma a value of 0.50 iu/ml. (Each batch of standard is precalibrated as described on p. 413 and may not necessarily be 1.0 iu/ml.)

Read the patient's VWF concentration directly off the standard curve, correct for the dilution factor, and average the two results from the different dilutions.

Normal Range

The normal range is 0.5–2.0 iu/ml.

Interpretation

The VWF concentration measured by ristocetin cofactor assay can only be interpreted in conjunction with other factor VIII:C and VWF:Ag assays, as shown in Table 16.7.

Assay Using Formalin-Fixed Platelets

Reagents

Sodium citrate solution.
32 g/l trisodium sodium citrate ($Na_3C_6H_5O_7.2H_2O$).

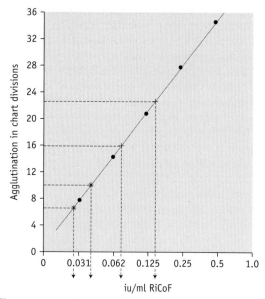

Figure 16.10 Ristocetin cofactor assay. The standard curve is plotted on semi-log paper. Each test plasma is assayed in two dilutions. Plasma 1 (+) produced the following readings: 1 in 4 dilution: 16 divisions of the chart paper = 7 iu (four times [dilution factor] = 28 iu/dl); 1 in 2 dilutions: 22 divisions = (13 iu/dl [twice dilution factor] = 26 iu/dl). The mean of the two readings is 27 iu/dl. Plasma 2 (*) gave the following results: 1 in 2 dilution: 7 divisions = (2.5 iu [twice dilution factor] = 5 iu/dl). 1 in 4 dilutions: 5 divisions (not shown). This result was similar to the blank and the plasma was next tested undiluted, giving a reading of 10 divisions = 4 iu/dl. The mean is 4.5 iu/dl (very low).

K_2EDTA.
0.134 mol/l.

2% formalin (40% formaldehyde).
In 9 g/l NaCl.

0.05% sodium azide.
In 9 g/l NaCl.

Method

Suitable preparations can be obtained from citrated blood in a blood donation bag, from a normal individual, or from a therapeutic venisection carried out on a patient with a normal platelet count. Acid–citrate–dextrose or citrate–phosphate–dextrose solution from the donor bag is ejected through the taking needle and replaced by the equivalent volume of sodium citrate. Collect c 500 ml of blood.

Centrifuge the blood at 300 g for 15 min at room temperature. Separate the PRP and add 9 volumes of PRP to 1 volume of EDTA solution. Incubate for 1 hour at 37°C to reverse the effect of ADP released during the preparation. Add an equal volume of 2% formalin and leave at 4°C for 1 hour. Centrifuge at 200 g for 10 min at 4°C. Decant the supernatant and recentrifuge it at 250 g for 20 min at 4°C. Discard the supernatant and resuspend the platelet sediment in chilled (4°C) 9 g/l NaCl. Wash the platelets twice more. After the final wash, resuspend the platelets in the sodium azide solution. Adjust the platelet count to 300–500 × 10^9/l. The suspension is stable for 1 month at 4°C.

Fixed platelets are also available commercially.

Reagents for Assay

Buffer for plasma dilutions.
Barbitone buffer, pH 7.4, containing 40 mg/ml of bovine serum albumin (p. 690).

Ristocetin, plasma standard, and patient's PPP.
As described in the previous assay.

Assay Method

Follow the method described for washed fresh platelets. Prepare all plasma dilutions in the albumin containing buffer.

Results, interpretation, and normal range are as described for the washed platelet assay.

Collagen Binding Assay (ELISA)

The ELISA-based VWF collagen binding assay (VWF:CB) was developed as an alternative to VWF:RCo as a measure of VWF functional activity. It has the advantage over VWF:RCo of using an ELISA-based system, giving a lower assay CV and greater precision. Clearly, because it measures a different ligand binding property to ristocetin, it should be seen as a complementary rather than alternative assay of VWF function. Indeed, some cases of VWD have reduced VWF:RCo but normal VWF:CB. The assay conditions have been adjusted to make the result sensitive to the presence of high molecular weight multimers of VWF and thus to its functional activity *in vivo*.[56]

The collagen binding assay ELISA method is based on the ability of VWF to bind collagen. The source of collagen is an important variable, and wells of the ELISA test strips are coated with human collagen type III.[57] After incubation with the test plasma, the amount of VWF bound is detected using an anti-VWF peroxidase-conjugated antibody. Antibody-peroxidase binding is quantified in the usual way, and the intensity of the colour generated is directly proportional to the VWF:CB concentration. Using a reference curve, the VWF:CB is quantified.

Collagen binding assay kits can be obtained through companies such as Technoclone and Gradipore. Assay details can be found in the manufacturer's instructions. They may vary with manufacturer and even from batch to batch of the same kit. Particular attention should be paid to the shelf life of the kits. Each laboratory should establish its own normal range.

Multimeric Analysis of von Willebrand Factor Antigen in Plasma Samples[58]

Nonradioactive Multimer Method

Multimeric analysis of von Willebrand factor antigen is important in the diagnosis and treatment of VWD. The gold standard method is the autoradiographic method described by Enayat and Hill.[58] This method uses radioactive iodine (I^{125}) and is performed in only a few specialised centres.

The nonradioactive method described here uses a peroxidase-conjugated antibody to VWF:Ag to replace the radioactive antibody described in previous editions.

Plasma samples are diluted in a buffer containing 8 M urea and sodium dodecyl-sulphate (SDS) and are heated to ensure mobility of protein is related to size and not molecular charge. Samples are electrophoresed through an agarose stacking gel at pH 6.8 and then through a running gel of higher agarose concentration at pH 8.8. After running overnight on a cooling plate, the protein is fixed in the gel, washed, and incubated with a peroxidase-conjugated antibody to VWF:Ag followed by extensive washing. The VWF:Ag multimers are revealed by adding a colour substrate reagent and scanning the gel. The scanned image is modified using photographic editing software (e.g., Microsoft Picture It or Corel Draw Graphics Suite) to produce a black-and-white image suitable for presentation.

The technique described here uses an agarose gel in a discontinuous buffer system. The method appears less prone to technical problems than an acrylamide/agarose system and yet can distinguish clearly the known patterns of VWD subtypes.

Reagents

Horseradish peroxidase-conjugated rabbit antihuman VWF:Ag.
DAKO Laboratories.

Agarose, ultra-pure DNA grade.
Seakem, code No. LE 49052-5.

SDS. BDH.

Glycine. BDH

Sodium EDTA. BDH

Hydrochloric acid. BDH

Propan-2-ol. BDH

Acetic acid. BDH

Tris base (T1503). BDH

Bromophenol blue. Sigma

Marvel or Baby Milk. Mothercare

Deionized water.

Preparation of Stock Solutions

2 M Tris 242.2 g per litre water (121.1 g/500 ml deionized water).
3 M HCl. 26.2 ml (1 N HCl, SG 1.18)/100 ml deionized water
0.01 M. Na2 EDTA. 3.3624 g/l or 0.336 g/100 ml deionized water.
These 3 reagents may be stored at 4°C for up to 3 months.

Preparation of Buffers

Stacking Buffer
25.0 ml 2 M Tris.

15.8 ml 3 M HCl.
Make up to 100 ml with deionized water.
Check pH is 6.8.
May be stored at 4°C for up to 2 weeks.

Running Buffer
75.0 ml 2 M Tris.
8.9 ml 3 M HCl.
Make up to 100 ml with deionized water.
Check pH is 8.8.
May be stored at 4°C for up to 2 weeks.

Sample Buffer
500 µl, 2 M Tris
10 ml stock EDTA
Make up to 100 ml with deionized water.
May be stored at 4°C for up to 4 weeks.

For use:
9.61 g urea
0.4 g SDS
Dissolve in sample buffer and make up to 20 ml.
May need to warm to dissolve.
Carefully adjust the pH to 8.0 with 1 M HCl
Use within 1 day of preparation.

10% SDS
1 g SDS dissolved in deionized water to a final volume of 10.0 ml. Store at 4°C to prevent bacterial growth; warm to room temperature just before use. Discard after 4 weeks of storage.

Electrophoresis Buffer
57.6 g glycine
12.0 g Tris base
2.0 g SDS
Dissolve and make up to 2 l with deionized water. Make up fresh on day of use. Cool to 4°C prior to electrophoresis.

Acid/Alcohol Fixative
100 ml propan-2-ol.
40 ml acetic acid.
Make up to 400 ml with deionized water.
Washing solutions (0.5 ml/l Tween 20 PBS).

0.01 M Phosphate Buffered Saline, pH 7.2
0.39 g $NaH_2PO_4.2H_2O$.
2.68 g $Na_2HPO_4.12H_2O$.

8.474 g NaCl.
Make up to 1 litre with deionized water.

The washing solution is prepared by adding 0.5 ml/l Tween 20.

Colour Buffer (0.1M Citrate Phosphate Buffer, pH 5.0)
8.8 g Citric acid.
24.0 g $Na_2HPO_4.12H_2O$.
Make up to 1 litre with deionized water.

Colour Reagent
60 mg ortho-phenylenediamine (OPD).
120 ml 0.1 M citrate phosphate buffer.
40 µl hydrogen peroxide (20 vol). Add just before use.

Preparation of Gels
Running gel (1.6% agarose, 0.1% SDS)
1.6 g agarose.
25.0 ml running buffer.
74.0 ml deionized water.
1.0 ml 10% SDS (add last to prevent frothing).

Dissolve the agarose by boiling in a conical flask using a microwave oven. Place a thick glass slide over the top of the conical flask to keep the loss of water to a minimum, thus maintaining the correct agarose concentration. Ensure that the agarose has fully dissolved. Add the SDS to the molten agarose last to prevent excessive frothing. Keep at 60°C in a waterbath.

Stick the hydrophilic side of standard gel bond (Pharmacia LKB) to a clean glass slide (10 × 205 mm) using a few drops of water. Cast the gel between the hydrophobic side and a clean glass plate separated by a 1 mm spacer, using Bulldog clips to clamp the mould together. Warm the mould prior to addition of molten agarose by standing it in a 37°C oven. Allow the resultant gel (183 × 100 mm) to set at 4°C in a refrigerator.

Stacking Gel (0.8% agarose, 0.1% SDS)
0.32 g agarose
10.0 ml stacking buffer four times.
29.6 ml deionized water.
0.4 ml 10% SDS.
Dissolve by boiling as explained earlier.

Addition of the Stacking Gel to the Running Gel
Carefully disassemble the running gel mould and remove the top 1.5 cm. of gel using a clean scalpel blade. After reassembly, pour the stacking gel to fill the mould. Allow gel to set at 4°C in a fridge for several hours.

Preparation of Samples
Dilute plasma samples in sample buffer as follows:
250 µl sample.
700 µl sample buffer.
15 µl 1% bromophenol blue dye.
Place diluted samples at 60°C for exactly 30 min, then keep them at 4°C for not more than 30 min prior to electrophoresis.

Electrophoresis (Day 1 Evening)

Set the cooling system used at 8°C to achieve a gel temperature of 13°C. Prepare wicks prepared from J-cloths (Johnson and Johnson) and Whatman No.1 24 cm filter papers. Fold a filter paper in half and mark the folded edge 27 mm from each end. From these marks draw lines at right angles and join the points where they cut the arc. Cut out the rectangle thus drawn, and it will act as part of one wick. Also cut two double-thickness J-cloth rectangles 183 × 120 mm. Place 500 ml of cold electrophoresis buffer in each reservoir of the electrophoresis tank.

Once again, carefully disassemble the mould; remove the gel bond, leaving the gel on the glass plate. Using a template, cut 10 wells 10 × 2 mm in the stacking gel 8 mm from the interface of running and stacking gels. Place the gel on the cooling platen. Soak two filter paper wicks in electrophoresis buffer and position over the gel by 5 mm at either end. Soak two J-cloth wicks in electrophoresis buffer, placing one completely over the paper wick at the running gel end and the other over the paper wick at the stacking gel end, leaving a small portion of the paper wick visible.

Pipette 35–40 µl of diluted sample into each well, taking care not to touch the wick. Electrophorese the gel at a constant current of 5 mA per gel (approximately 65V). Stop the electrophoresis when the blue dye has migrated 1 cm from each well. Carefully remove residual liquid from each well, and refill each well with molten stacking gel. Start electrophoresis at the same current. After a total of 18–20 hours, the dye will have run off the gel into the wick and electrophoresis is complete.

Gel Fixation (Day 2 Morning)

Remove the gel gently from the glass plate and fix for 1 hour using the acid/alcohol fixative solution in a suitable container.

Gel Washing (Day 2)

Once fixed, wash the gel in 3 changes of distilled water for a total of 3 hours. Transfer the gel to a small plastic tray and wash with 1% milk powder for 20 min followed by 10% milk powder for 20 min. Wash the gel extensively in 0.5 ml/l Tween 20 PBS for the remainder of the day.

Addition of the Peroxidase-Conjugated Rabbit Antihuman VWF:Ag (Day 2 Evening)

Dilute 400 µl of the peroxidase-conjugated rabbit antihuman VWF in 400 ml of 0.ml/l Tween 20 PBS. Then add this to the gel in the tray and mix gently overnight. Place a plastic sheet over the plastic tray to prevent evaporation.

Extensive Washing (Two Days and Nights)

Pour the peroxidase-conjugated rabbit antihuman VWF mixture to waste. Remove the gel from the plastic tray and place into another flat-bottomed tray. Then wash the gel extensively with frequent changes of 0.5 ml/l Tween 20 PBS for the next 2 days and 2 nights.

Addition of the Colour Substrate (Day 5)

Prepare the colour reagent by adding 6 × 10 mg OPD tablets to 120 ml 0.1 M citrate phosphate buffer. Add 40 µl of hydrogen peroxide just before use. Place the gel into a plastic tray, pour the colour reagent over the gel, and mix gently. Ensure the colour reagent gets underneath the gel. When the colour begins to develop, remove the gel from the plastic tray and place between two sheets of gel bond, draining off any excess substrate reagent.

Scanning the Developing Gel

When the multimer patterns become visible, the gel is ready to scan. The gel will continue to develop colour for several minutes and eventually the background gel will become too dark to see the multimer patterns clearly. Scan the gel several times

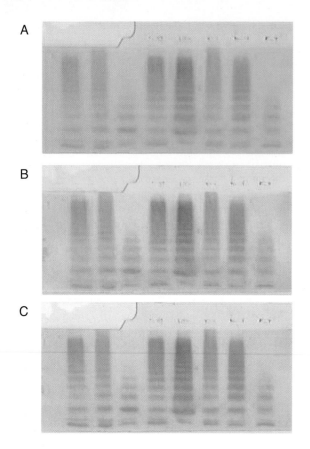

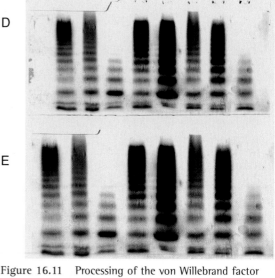

Figure 16.11   Processing of the von Willebrand factor multimer gel. See text for preparation. A: Scan of the original stained gel. B: Adjustment of image tint. C: Conversion to monochrome image. D: Adjustment of brightness and contrast. E: Final gel image.

as the colour develops to get the best image of the multimer patterns.

The scanned gel will appear shown as in Figure 16.11A. The top section is the stacking gel where the samples were added prior to electrophoresis; the main body of the gel is the running gel showing the multimer patterns. The scan is manipulated using photographic editing software such as Microsoft Picture It or Corel Draw Graphics Suite. The manipulations are shown in Figure 16.11A–E, during which the image tint is corrected, it is converted to a monochrome image, and adjustments to brightness and contrast are made.

Interpretation[51]

See Figure 16.12.

Investigation of a Suspected Disorder of Platelet Function, Inherited or Acquired

(For investigation assays of VWD, see p. 418; for diagnosis of thrombocytopenia, see pp. 20 and 681.)

Abnormalities of platelet function all lead to signs and symptoms characteristic of defects of primary haemostasis: bleeding into the mucous membranes, epistaxes, menorrhagia, and small skin ecchymoses. The patient may also suffer from abnormal intraoperative or postoperative bleeding and oozing from small cuts or wounds.

Laboratory Investigation of Platelets and Platelet Function[59]

The peripheral blood platelet count and the skin bleeding time or PFA-100 are first-line tests of platelet

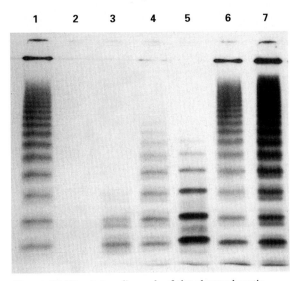

1 2 3 4 5 6 7

Figure 16.12   Autoradiograph of the electrophoretic analysis of von Willebrand factor (vWD) multimer patterns. The largest multimers appear at the top of the gel. The normal pattern with numerous large multimers and a triplet pattern visible in the smaller multimers are shown in lane 7. Lanes 1 and 6 are compatible with type 1 vWD in which there is a generalised decrease in multimer numbers but the normal triplet pattern is retained. In lane 2 there is virtually no vWF detected, indicating type 3 vWD. Lanes 3 and 5 show both abnormality of vWF amount and multimer pattern, indicating type 2A. In lane 4 there is a selective loss of the large multimers typical of type 2B vWD.

function. However, some disorders of platelet function are not detected by these tests.[49] Additional information may be obtained by inspecting a fresh blood film, which may show abnormalities of platelet size or morphology that may be of diagnostic importance.

If the screening procedures or clinical history suggest a disorder of primary haemostasis and VWF function is normal, further tests should be organized. Drugs and certain foods (Table 16.8) may affect platelet function tests, and the patient must be asked to refrain from taking such substances for at least 7 days before the test.

The usual sequence of investigation is shown in Figure 16.13. Platelet function tests can be divided into six main groups (Table 16.9): adhesion tests, aggregation tests, assessment of the granular content, assessment of the release reaction, investigation of the prostaglandin pathways, and tests of platelet coagulant activity. Expression of platelet glycoproteins can be assessed by flow cytometry, although this does not necessarily correlate with functional activity.

The *granular content* of the platelets can be assessed by electron microscopy or by measuring the substances released. Adenine nucleotide and serotonin release from the dense granules are probably best measured by a specialist laboratory. The release of β-thromboglobulin and platelet factor 4 can be measured using commercial radioimmunoassay kits, but there are problems with reproducibility and interpretation of the results. The release from the α granules is mostly investigated as a marker of *in vivo* platelet activation and thrombotic tendency. Platelet VWF is measured to diagnose some variants of VWD.

If the initial aggregation studies suggest a defect in the prostaglandin pathways, TXB_2 can be estimated quantitatively by radioimmune assay. Highly specific assays of various steps in arachidonic acid metabolism are also available but are outside the scope of a routine laboratory.

Platelet coagulant activity—the completion of the membrane "flip-flop"—can be indirectly measured using the prothrombin consumption index. This test is rarely performed now but is abnormal in Scott syndrome, a rare bleeding disorder; it was described in the 7th edition of this book. Alternatively, phosphatidyl serine exposure can be directly assessed by flow cytometry (see later).

Platelet Aggregation

Principle

The light absorbance of PRP plasma decreases as platelets aggregate. The amount and the rate of fall are dependent on platelet reactivity to the added agonist provided that other variables, such as temperature, platelet count, and mixing speed, are controlled. The absorbance changes are monitored on a chart recorder.

Reagents

Test and Control Platelet-Rich Plasma

The patient and control subject should not be ingesting any drugs, beverages, and foods that may

Table 16.8 Substances that commonly affect platelet function
Agents that affect prostanoids synthesis
Aspirin
Non-steroidal anti-inflammatory drugs
Corticosteroids
Agents that bind to platelet receptors and membranes
α-antagonists
β-blockers
Antihistamines
Tricyclic antidepressants
Local anaesthetics
Ticlopidine
Clopidogrel
IIb, IIIa blocking agents
Antibiotics
Penicillin
Cephalosporins
Agents that increase cyclic adenosine monophosphate (C-AMP) levels
Dipyridamole
Aminophylline
Prostanoids
Others
Herparin
Dextran
Ethanol
Clofibrate
Phenothiazine
Garlic

Table 16.9 Platelet function tests
Adhesion tests
Retention in a glass-bead column
Baumgartner's technique
PFA-100
Aggregation tests
Turbidometric technique using
ADP
Collagen
Ristocetin
Adrenaline
Thrombin
Arachidonic acid
Endoperoxide analogues
Calcium ionophore
Investigation of granular content and release
Dense bodies
Electron microscopy
ADP and ATP content (bioluminescence)
Serotonin release
Granules
β-Thromboglobulin
Platelet factor 4
vWF
Fluorescence by flow cytometry
Prostaglandin pathways
TXB_2 radio-immunoassay
Platelet coagulant activity
Prothrombin consumption index
Flow cytometry
Glycoprotein surface expression
Activation
P-selectin (CD62) surface expression
Fibrinogen binding
Annexin binding (to phosphatidyl serine)
Conformational changes in IIbIIIa
Platelet granule fluorescence

ADP, adenosine 5'-phosphatase; ATP, adenosine 5'-triphosphatase; vWF, von Willebrand factor.

affect aggregation for at least 10 days (see Table 16.8) and preferably should have fasted overnight because the presence of chylomicra may also disturb the aggregation patterns. Collect 20 ml of venous blood with minimal venous occlusion and add to a one-tenth volume of trisodium citrate (see p. 690) contained in a plastic or siliconised container. The blood should not be chilled because cold activates the platelets. PRP is obtained by centrifuging at room temperature (c 20°C) for 10–15 min at 150–200 g. Carefully remove the PRP, avoiding contamination with red cells or buffy coat, and place in a stoppered plastic tube. Store at room temperature until tested. This is stable for about 3 hours. It is important to test all samples after a similar interval of time (say 1 hour) and to store them at the same temperature to minimise variation.

Test and Control Platelet Poor Plasma
Centrifuge the remaining blood at 2000 g for 20 min to obtain PPP.

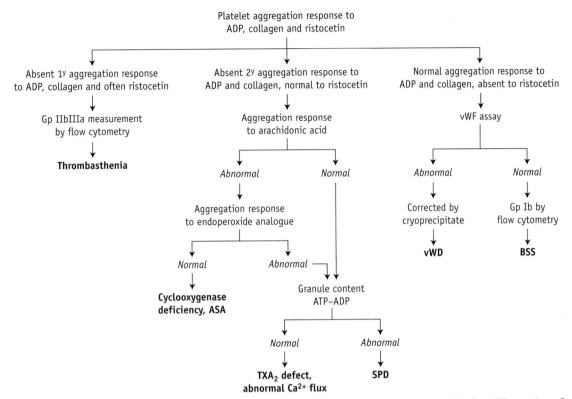

Figure 16.13   Flow chart for investigation of suspected platelet dysfunction. SPD, storage pool defect; ITP, coating of platelets by autoantibodies in idiopathic thrombocytopenic purpura; vWD, von Willebrand disease; B-SS, Bernard-Soulier syndrome; ASA, effect of aspirin ingestion.

Standardization of Platelet-Rich Plasma

A platelet count is performed on the PRP. The number of platelets will influence aggregation response if the count falls outside $200–400 \times 10^9/l$. For very high PRP counts, the count should be adjusted by diluting the PRP in the patient's PPP. Platelet counts of less than $200 \times 10^9/l$ give rise to diminished aggregation responses. Further centrifugation of PRP is not recommended because it induces platelet activation. The control PRP should be diluted to the same count and tested as a comparison.

PRP should always be stored in tightly stoppered tubes that are filled nearly to the top to avoid changes in pH, which also affect platelet aggregation and tests of nucleotide release.

Aggregating Agents

The five aggregating agents listed in the following should be sufficient for the diagnosis of most functional disorders. For research purposes and when investigating unusual kindreds, other agonists listed in Table 16.9 may also be used.

Adenosine 5-Diphosphate

The anhydrous sodium salt of ADP is used. Prepare a stock solution by dissolving 4.93 mg of the trisodium salt or 4.71 mg of the disodium salt in 10 ml of 9 g/l NaCl, pH 6.8. This makes a 1 mmol/l solution. Store in 0.5 ml volumes at $-40°C$ until use; they remain stable for up to 3 months at this temperature. Once thawed, the solution must be used within 3 hours and then discarded. For aggregation testing, prepare 100, 50, 25, 10, and 5 µmol/l solutions.

Collagen 1 mg/ml (Mascia Brunelli, Sigma, Helena)

This collagen is a 1 mg/ml stock solution. For use, dilute in the buffer supplied with the collagen or in

5% dextrose to obtain concentrations of 10 and 40 µg/l. When diluted 1:10 in PRP (see below), the final concentrations will be 1 and 4 µg/ml.

Ristocetin Sulphate (American Biochemical & Pharmaceutical Corporation)

Each vial of ristocetin sulphate contains 100 mg of ristocetin and should be stored at 4°C until dissolved; 8 ml of 9 g/l NaCl are added to each vial so as to obtain a 12.5 mg/ml solution. Store at −40°C in 0.5 ml volumes until used. Ristocetin may be refrozen after use. It should never be used in concentrations of greater than 1.4 mg/ml because protein precipitation may occur in plasma and give rise to false results.

Arachidonic Acid

Arachidonic acid is Na-salt, 99% pure. Dissolve the contents of a 10 mg vial in 1.5 ml of sterile water by gentle mixing to give a 20 mmol/l stock solution. This may be frozen in 0.5 ml volumes at −20°C for later use. Prepare a working solution by making doubling dilutions of the stock in saline to give 5 and 10 mmol/l solutions.

Adrenaline (Epinephrine)

Dissolve 1-epinephrine bitartrate, 3.33 mg, in 10 ml of water to prepare a 1 mmol/l stock solution. Store in 0.5 ml volumes at −40°C. Solutions of 20 and 200 µmol/l are prepared for use in barbitone buffered saline, pH 7.4.

Note.

All aggregation reagents should be kept on ice until used.

Method

Centrifugation may cause cellular release of ADP and platelet refractoriness to aggregation, and the actual aggregation test should not be started within 30 min of preparing the PRP. However, the tests should be completed within 3 hours and whenever possible within 2 hours of preparing the PRP. Platelets left standing at room temperature (c 20°C) become increasingly reactive to adrenaline and in some cases to collagen; the rate of change increases after 3 hours.

Switch the aggregometer on about 30 min before the tests are to be performed to allow the heating block to warm up to 37°C. Set the stirring speed to 900 rpm. Pipette the appropriate volume of PRP (this varies depending on the make of the aggregometer used) into a plastic tube or cuvette. Place the tube in the heating block. After 1 min insert the stirrer into the plasma. Set the transmission to 0 on the chart recorder. Replace with a cuvette containing PPP and set the transmission to 100%. Repeat this procedure until no further adjustments are needed and the pen traverses most of the width of the chart paper in response to the difference in absorbance between the PRP and PPP.

Allow the PRP to warm up to 37°C for 2 min and then add 1:10 vol of the agonist. Record the change in absorbance until the response reaches a plateau or for 3 min (whichever is sooner). Repeat this procedure for each agonist. The starting amount for each agonist is the lowest concentration prepared as described earlier. If no release is obtained, increase the concentration until a satisfactory response is obtained.

Interpretation

Normal and abnormal platelet aggregation curves are shown in Figures 16.14 and 16.15.

Adenosine 5-Diphosphate

Low concentrations of ADP (<0.5 to 2.5 µmol/l) cause primary or reversible aggregation. First, ADP binds to a membrane receptor and releases Ca^{2+} ions. A reversible complex with extracellular fibrinogen forms, and the platelets undergo a shape change reflected by a slight increase in absorbance. After this, the bound fibrinogen adds to the cell-to-cell contact and reversible aggregation occurs. At very low concentrations of ADP, platelets may disaggregate after the first phase. In the presence of higher concentrations of ADP an irreversible secondary wave aggregation is associated with the release of dense and α-granules as a result of activation of the arachidonic acid pathway. If only high doses of ADP are used, defects in the primary wave (measuring the second pathway as described on p. 382) will be missed.

Collagen

The aggregation response to collagen is preceded by a short "lag" phase lasting between 10 and 60 sec. The duration of the lag phase is inversely pro-

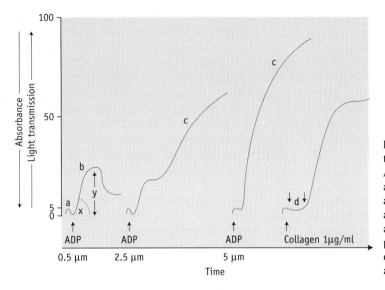

Figure 16.14. Traces obtained during the aggregation of platelet-rich plasma. A: Shape change. B: Primary wave aggregation. C: Secondary wave aggregation. X°, angle of the initial aggregation slope; Y, height of the aggregation trace; d, lag phase; μm = μmol/l. Reproduced with the permission of authors and publisher from Yardumian and colleagues.[60]

portional to the concentration of collagen used and to the responsiveness of the platelets tested. This phase is succeeded by a single wave of aggregation resulting from the activation of the arachidonic acid pathway and the release of the granules. Higher doses of collagen (>2 μg/ml) cause a sudden increase in intraplatelet calcium concentration, and this may bring about the release reaction without activating the prostaglandin pathway. Collagen responses should therefore always be measured using 1 and 4 μg/ml concentrations.

Ristocetin

Ristocetin reacts with VWF and the membrane receptor to induce platelets to clump together ("agglutination"). It does not activate any of the three aggregation pathways and does not initially cause granule release. The response is assessed on the basis of the angle of the initial slope. The platelet response to 1.2 mg/ml is initially studied. Concentrations above 1.4 mg/ml may cause nonspecific platelet "agglutination" as a result of an interaction between ristocetin and fibrinogen and protein precipitation.

Arachidonic Acid

Arachidonic acid induces TXA_2 generation and granule release even if there is a defect of agonist binding to the surface membrane or of the phospholipase-induced release of endogenous arachidonate. If

steps further along the pathway are impaired, such as absence or inhibition of cyclooxygenase (e.g., aspirin effect), arachidonic acid will not produce normal aggregation.

Adrenaline (Epinephrine)

No shape change precedes aggregation, but the response thereafter resembles the ADP response. Such a response is usually obtained with concentrations of 2–10 μmol/ml. Some clinically normal people have severely reduced responses to epinephrine.

Calculation of Results[59,60]

Results can be expressed in one of three ways:

1. As a percentage decrease in absorbance measured at 3 min after the addition of an agonist (see Fig. 16.14; y). This does not provide any information on the shape of the curve.
2. By the initial slope of the aggregation tracing (see Fig. 16.14; x^0). This indicates the rate of aggregation but does not show whether secondary aggregation has occurred.
3. By the minimum amount of agonist required to induce a secondary response.

Normal Range

The platelets of normal subjects usually produce a single reversible primary wave with 1 μmol/l ADP or less, biphasic aggregation with ADP at 2.5 μmol/l, and a single irreversible wave at 5 or 10 µmol/l. A single-phase response is observed after a lag phase lasting not more than 1 min with 1 and 4 µg/ml of collagen. A single phase or biphasic response is seen with 1.2 mg/ml of ristocetin and after 50 and 100 µmol/l of arachidonic acid. Biphasic aggregation is observed with 2–10 µmol/l of adrenaline. A response to a low concentration of ristocetin (0.5 mg/ml) is abnormal and is a feature of type 2B VWD (see below).

Interpretation and Technical Artifacts

The volumes of PRP used will depend on the aggregometer and cuvette used. The smaller the cuvette, the more responses can be tested with a given volume of PRP, but the poorer the optical quality (because of a shorter lightpath) and the more likely the influence of factors such as debris or air bubbles.

Care should be taken to exclude red cells and granulocytes from PRP because these will interfere with the light transmittance and cause reduced response heights, which can be mistaken for abnormal aggregation. In diseases such as thalassaemia, where there may be red cell fragments and membranes, these may be removed by further centrifugation of PRP at 150 g for 2 min or after settling has occurred.

If cryoglobulins are present, they may cause changes in transmittance such as spontaneous aggregation. Warming the PRP to 37°C for 5 min allows aggregation to be performed in the normal way.

Lipaemic plasma may cause problems in adjusting the aggregometer and the responses may be compressed owing to the small difference in transmitted light between PRP and PPP. Care should be taken in the interpretation of results from such samples.

The pattern of responses in various disorders of platelet function is shown in Table 16.10. For a discussion of hyperaggregability, see p. 458.

Some common technical problems associated with platelet aggregation are described in Table 16.11.

Further Investigation of Platelet Function

If an abnormal aggregation pattern is observed, it is advisable to check the assessment on at least one further occasion. If the aggregation tests are persistently abnormal, and the patient is not taking any drugs or substances known to interfere with

---

Table 16.10 Differential diagnosis of disorders of platelet function

Conditon	Platelet		Aggregation with					Comment/further tests
	Count	Size	ADP	Col	Ri	AA	A23187	
Thrombasthenia	N	N	0	0	1	0	0	IIbIIIa expression
Bernard-Soulier syndrome	Low	Large	N	N	0	N	N	GpIb expression
Storage pool defect (δ)	N	N	1	R	1	1/0	R	ATP:ADP pools
Cyclo-oxygenase deficiency	N	N	1/N	R	N	R	R	Responds to endoperoxide
Thromboxane synthetase deficiency	N	N	1/N	R	N	R/0	N	
Aspirin ingestion	N	N	1	R	N	R/0	N/R	Stop aspirin/NSAID and retest
Ehlers-Danlos syndrome	N	N	N	N	N	N	N	
von Willebrand disease	N	N	N	N	0/R	N	N	Assay vWF:Ag and RiCoF

N, normal; 0, absent; 1, primary wave only; R, reduced; Col, collagen; Ri, ristocetin; AA, arachidonic acid; A23187, calcium ionophore; ATP, adenosine 5′-triphosphatase; ADP, adenosine 5′-diphosphatase; NSAID, non-steroidal anti-inflammatory drug; RiCoF, ristocetin co-factor; vWF, von Willebrand factor.

Note that many other defects, such as found in oculocutaneous albinism, Chediak-Higashi syndrome and grey platelet syndrome, have also been described.

Table 16.11 Technical factors that may influence platelet aggregation tests

Centrifugation. At room temperature, *not* at 4°C. Should be sufficient to remove red cells and white cells but not the largest platelets. Residual red cells in the PRP may cause apparently incomplete aggregation.

Time. For 30 min after the preparation of the PRP, platelets are refractory to the effect of agonists. Progressive increase in reactiveness occurs thereafter; more marked from 2 h onward.

Platelet count. Slow and weak aggregation observed with platelet counts below 150 or over 400×10^9/l.

pH. <7.7 inhibits aggregation; pH >8.0 enhances aggregation.

Mixing speed. <800 rpm or >1200 rpm slows aggregation.

Haematocrit. >0.55 is associated with less aggregation, especially in the secondary phase owing to the increased concentration of citrate in PRP. It may also be difficult to obtain enough PPP. Centrifuging twice may help.

Temperature. <35°C causes decreased aggregation except to low dose ADP, which may be enhanced.

Dirty cuvette. May cause spontaneous platelet aggregation or interfere with the optics of the system.

Air bubbles in the cuvette. Cause large, irregular oscillations, even before the addition of agonists.

No stir bar. No response to any agonist obtained.

PPP, platelet-poor plasma; PRP, platelet-rich plasma.

platelet function, the following tests should be done (see also Fig. 16.13 and Table 16.10):

1. If thrombasthenia or the Bernard-Soulier syndrome is suspected, an analysis of membrane glycoproteins is necessary; most conveniently by flow cytometry.
2. If a release abnormality is suspected, additional agonists including synthetic endoperoxide analogues and calcium ionophores should be used in testing for aggregation. Release products can be measured directly or concurrently with aggregation in a lumoaggregometer.[61] In addition, the total adenine nucleotide content of the platelets and the amount released after maximal stimulation should be measured using a firefly bioluminescence technique.[59,62]
3. Whenever possible electron microscopic studies of platelet ultrastructure should be carried out.
4. Factor VIII:C, VWF:Ag, and ristocetin cofactor assay should be carried out on all patients investigated for an abnormality of platelet function who show abnormal ristocetin "agglutination" or in whom all platelet function tests are normal.

CLOT SOLUBILITY TEST FOR FACTOR XIII

Principle

Fibrin clots formed in the presence of factor XIII and thrombin are stable (as a result of crosslinking) for at least 1 hour in 5 mol/l urea, whereas clots formed in the absence of factor XIII dissolve rapidly. Quality assurance surveys in the United Kingdom have shown that the solubility test for XIII is more sensitive when the sample is clotted with thrombin rather than calcium. Thrombin preparations containing calcium should not be used. The use of 5 M urea as described here will detect factor XIII deficiency of up to 5 iu/dl. One study suggested that deficiency of up to 10% could be detected by using 2% acetic acid as the lysing solution.[63]

Reagents

PPP.
From the patient and a control subject

Thrombin.
10 NIH unit solution.

Urea.
5 mol/l in 9 g/l NaCl.

Method

In duplicate, 0.2 ml patient plasma is mixed with 0.2 ml 10 NIH unit thrombin solution in a glass test tube and incubated at 37°C for 20 min. Set up a normal plasma control in the same way; EDTA plasma can be included as a negative control. Each tube is filled with approximately 3 ml of urea solution, carefully dislodging the clot, and left undisturbed at 37°C for 24 hours. Inspect each tube for the presence of a clot at regular intervals.

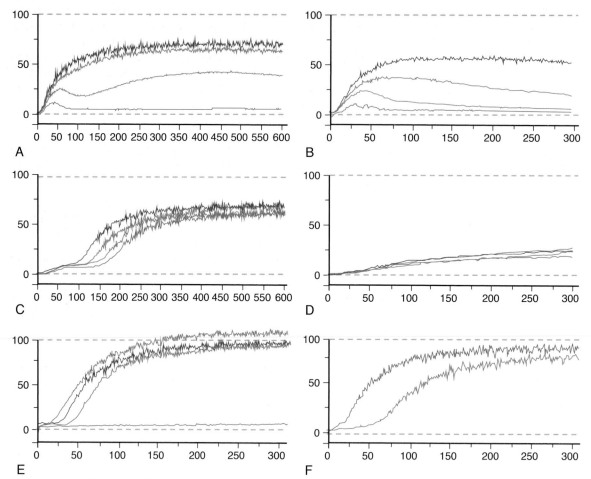

Figure 16.15.   Some examples of platelet aggregation analyses.
A Normal B Abnormal, responses to adenosine diphosphate
Black   0.5 µmol/l
Red   1.0 µmol/l
Green   2.0 µmol/l
Blue   5.0 µmol/l
C Normal and D Abnormal, responses to epinephrine
Black   0.5 µmol/ml
Red   1.0 µmol/ml
Green   2.0 µmol/ml
Blue   5.0 µmol/ml
E responses to collagen and ristocetin
Black   Low-dose ristocetin   0.75 mg/ml
Red   High-dose ristocetin   1.5 mg/ml
Green   Low-dose collagen   5 µg/ml
Blue   High-dose collagen   10 µg/ml
F responses to arachidonic acid
Black   High-dose arachidonic acid 0.5 mg/ml
Red   Low-dose arachidonic acid   0.25 mg/ml

Interpretation

The control clot, if normal, shows no sign of dissolving after 24 hours. However, in the absence of factor XIII, the clot will have dissolved. The test is reported as normal if the clot is present and abnormal if the clot is absent. The clot solubility test has poor sensitivity and may only detect levels below approximately 5 iu/dl. The relationship between factor XIII level and adequate haemostasis is uncertain, but there is some evidence that levels of 5–40 iu/dl may also be associated with bleeding. In suspected cases photometric and ELISA assays of factor XIII are available for quantitative measurements. However, these appear to have poor reproducibility so their role is not yet clear.[63]

DISSEMINATED INTRAVASCULAR COAGULATION

The term DIC encompasses a wide range of clinical phenomena of varying degrees of severity. It is also sometimes referred to as consumptive coagulopathy because its characteristic feature is excessive and widespread activation of the coagulation mechanism with consequent consumption of clotting factors and inhibitors with loss of the normal regulatory mechanisms. In acutely ill patients this usually results in defibrination and a haemorrhagic diathesis. In some situations, however, the activation may be less marked and partially compensated resulting in a tendency to thrombosis. This latter phenomenon is typical of the coagulation activation seen in association with malignancy and may be associated with slightly shortened clotting times.

The diagnosis of acute DIC can generally be made from abnormalities of the basic first-line screening tests described earlier in the presence of an appropriate clinical context. Characteristically, the PT, APTT, and TT are all prolonged and the fibrinogen level is markedly reduced. In association with the consumption of clotting factors responsible for these abnormalities there is also a fall in platelet count also resulting from consumption. As DIC develops, a decrease in platelet count is an early sign and hypofibrinogenemia may be relatively late. This distinguishes it from dilutional coagulopathy in which the reverse is usually the case. Concomitantly there is activation of the fibrinolytic system and an increase in circulating fibrin(ogen) degradation products. These abnormalities form the basis for the diagnosis of DIC. A diagnostic guideline is available but will be most useful in clinical trials rather than routine practice.[64] More elaborate tests are not usually performed but can demonstrate reductions in individual clotting factors, antithrombin, and antiplasmin and increased levels of thrombin–antithrombin and plasmin–antiplasmin complexes and of activation peptides such as prothrombin F1+2. Some analysers provide a waveform analysis that can detect early stages of DIC (see p. 434).[17]

Detection of Fibrinogen/Fibrin Degradation Products Using a Latex Agglutination Method[65]

Principle

A suspension of latex particles is sensitised with specific antibodies to the purified FDP fragments D and E. The suspension is mixed on a glass slide with a dilution of the serum to be tested. Aggregation indicates the presence of FDP in the sample. By testing different dilutions of the unknown sample, a semiquantitative assay can be performed.

Reagents

Venous blood.
Collected into a special tube (provided with the kit) containing the antifibrinolytic agent and thrombin.

Test Kit.
(Oxoid Ltd).

Positive and negative controls.
Provided by the manufacturer.

Glycine buffer.
Part of the kit.

Method

Allow the tube with blood to stand at 37°C until clot retraction commences. Then centrifuge the tube and withdraw the serum for testing. It is important that the fibrinogen in the sample is completely clotted or this will be detected by the test. This may be a problem in the presence of heparin or a dysfibrinogenaemia or high levels of FDPs. Addition of a few drops of 100 u (NIH)/ml thrombin will enhance clotting in these cases.

Make 1 in 5 and 1 in 20 dilutions of serum in glycine buffer. Mix 1 drop of each serum dilution with 1 drop of latex suspension on a glass slide. Rock the slide gently for 2 min while looking for macroscopic agglutination. If a positive reaction is observed in the higher dilution, make doubling dilutions from the 1 in 20 dilution until macroscopic agglutination can no longer be seen.

Interpretation

Agglutination with a 1 in 5 dilution of serum indicates a concentration of FDP in excess of 10 μg/ml; agglutination in a 1 in 20 dilution indicates FDP in excess of 40 μg/ml.

Normal Range

Healthy subjects have an FDP concentration of less than 10 μg/ml. Concentrations between 10 and 40 μg/ml are found in a variety of conditions including acute venous thromboembolism, acute myocardial infarction, and severe pneumonia and after major surgery. High levels are seen in systemic fibrinolysis associated with DIC and thrombolytic therapy with streptokinase.

Screening Tests for Fibrin Monomers[66–68]

Principle

When thrombin acts on fibrinogen, some of the monomers do not polymerise but give rise to soluble complexes with plasma fibrinogen and FDP. These complexes can be associated *in vitro* by ethanol or protamine sulphate.

Reagents

PPP.
From the patient and a control.

Positive control.
This is prepared by adding 0.1 ml of thrombin (0.2 NIH units/ml) to 0.9 ml of control plasma and incubating at 37°C for 30 min. Fibrin threads formed during the incubation are removed by centrifugation.

Protamine sulphate.
1% (10 g/l).

Ethanol.
50% (v/v) in water.

Method

1. Protamine sulphate test. Add 0.05 ml of protamine sulphate to 0.5 ml of patient's plasma and to 0.5 ml of positive control plasma. Incubate undisturbed at 37°C for 30 min. A positive result is indicated by the formation of a fine fibrin network or fibrin strands. The presence of amorphous material only is a negative result.
2. Ethanol gelation test. Add 0.15 ml of ethanol to 0.5 ml of patient's plasma and to 0.5 ml of the positive control plasma at room temperature (c 20°C). After gentle agitation inspect the tubes at 1 min intervals. A positive result is the formation of a definite gel within 3 min.

Interpretation

Positive gelation tests are found in the following scenarios:

1. The early stages of acute DIC
2. After major surgery
3. Severe inflammatory illness, in particular lobar pneumonia
4. Liver disease

Detection of Crosslinked Fibrin D-Dimers Using a Latex Agglutination Method

Principle

The latex agglutination method used to detect crosslinked fibrin D-dimers is identical to the test previously described for FDP, but in this case the latex beads are coated with a monoclonal antibody directed specifically against fibrin D-dimer in human plasma or serum. Because there is no reaction with fibrinogen, the need for serum is eliminated and measurements can be performed on plasma samples.

Reagents

Several manufacturers market kits for the measurement of D-dimers. These usually contain the latex suspension, dilution buffer, and positive and negative controls.

Method

The manufacturer's protocol should be followed. Undiluted plasma is mixed with one drop of latex suspension on a glass slide and the slide is gently rocked for the length of time recommended in the kit. If macroscopic agglutination is observed, dilutions of the plasma are made until agglutination can no longer be seen.

Interpretation

Agglutination with the undiluted plasma indicates a concentration of D-dimers in excess of 200 mg/l. The D-dimer level can be quantified by multiplying the reciprocal of the highest dilution showing a positive result by 200 to give a value in mg/l.

Normal Range

Plasma levels in normal subjects are <200 mg/l. There has been much study of D-dimer assays as a useful way of excluding thrombosis, but there is naturally a compromise between sensitivity and specificity, especially when a rapid turnaround time is required. The lack of an international standard and the poor correlation between kits mean that the use of kits for this purpose should be validated individually. A number of kits using ELISA methods for the detection of D-dimers are now available that have greater sensitivity but are more cumbersome to perform. Latex test using automated analysers may provide an acceptable compromise.[69] These tests have now been incorporated into clinical guidelines according to their sensitivity.[70,71]

INVESTIGATION OF CARRIERS OF A CONGENITAL COAGULATION DEFICIENCY OR DEFECT[72,73]

Carrier detection is important in genetic counselling, and antenatal diagnosis may enable heterozygotes to consider termination of pregnancy with a severely affected fetus and may optimise management of the pregnancy and delivery. The information of value in carrier detection is derived from family studies, phenotype investigations, and determination of genotype.

Family Studies

Haemophilia A and B (factor VIII and factor IX deficiency) are inherited by X-linked genes. This means that all the sons of a person with haemophilia will be normal and all of his daughters will be carriers. The children of a carrier have a 0.5 chance of being affected if they are sons and a 0.5 chance of being carriers if they are daughters. The other coagulation factor defects are inherited as autosomal traits. Heterozygotes possess approximately half the normal concentration of the coagulation factor and are generally not affected clinically; only homozygotes have a significant bleeding tendency. Factor XI is an exception to this where heterozygotes sometimes bleed excessively after trauma or surgery. The most common form of VWD (type 1) is inherited as an autosomal dominant trait.

A detailed family study is important in all coagulation factor defects to establish the true nature of the defect and its severity. Patients often describe any familial bleeding tendency as haemophilia, and it is therefore essential to prove the exact defect in every new patient and family. In inbred kindreds, the likelihood of homozygotes emerging is increased.

Phenotype Investigation

Theoretically one might expect the concentration of the affected coagulation factor in the heterozygote or carrier to be roughly half that of normal. However, in the case of factor VIII and factor IX, this is complicated by the phenomenon of X chromosome inactivation (XCI). Women possess two X chromosomes, but in each cell only one of these two is used and the other is largely inactivated. In each cell the choice of which X is active is essentially random and varies over a normal distribution. Thus, in carriers of haemophilia A or B, the level of factor VIII or IX also varies over roughly a normal distribution depending on the proportions of the normal and haemophiliac containing Xs that are used. As a result, some carriers may have an entirely normal level of factor VIII or factor IX and others may be significantly deficient. This chromosome inactivation is sometimes referred to as lyonisation after Mary Lyon, by whom it was first described.

In the case of factor VIII, the level of VWF has sometimes been found to be useful. The ratio of VIII:C to VWF:Ag is reduced in most carriers and can be used in conjunction with the family history to determine a probability that the subject is a carrier. These estimations are further complicated by the fact that factor VIII behaves as an acute-phase reactant and may be elevated by a number of intercurrent factors including pregnancy, stress, and exercise.

When a detailed family study has been carried out it may be possible to establish the statistical chance of inheriting a coagulation defect. For a review, see Graham et al.[72]

Genotype Assignment

The advent of molecular biology and the cloning of many of the genes for coagulation factors, especially factor VIII and factor IX, have revolutionised the approach to carrier determination. The discovery of genetic polymorphisms, some of which are multi-allelic, within the coagulation factor genes has meant that in most families the affected gene can be tracked and the carrier state can be determined with a high degree of probability. Increasingly, the genetic defect itself can be identified, resulting in unequivocal genotypic assignment in every member of a family. This must now be regarded as the standard of care, removing the ambiguity and uncertainty of preceding methods.

The techniques required for these analyses are described in Chapter 21. The problem of carrier determination and antenatal diagnosis has been dealt with in a comprehensive WHO/WFH review.[73] Although the options for affected families increase,[74] approximately one third of cases arise with no preceding family history.

REFERENCES

1. Cines DB, Pollak ES, Buck CA, et al 1998 Endothelial cells in physiology and in the pathophysiology of vascular disorders. Blood 91:3527–3561.
2. Frank PG, Woodman SE, Park DS, et al 2003 Caveolin, caveolae, and endothelial cell function. Arteriosclerosis, Thrombosis & Vascular Biology 23:1161–1168.
3. Ruggeri ZM 2003 Von Willebrand factor, platelets and endothelial cell interactions. Journal of Thrombosis & Haemostasis 1:1335–1342.
4. May AE, Neumann FJ, Preissner KT 1999 The relevance of blood cell-vessel wall adhesive interactions for vascular thrombotic disease. Thrombosis & Haemostasis 82:962–970.
5. Ruggeri ZM 1997 Mechanisms initiating platelet thrombus formation [published erratum appears in Thrombosis & Haemostasis 1997 Oct;78(4):1304] [see comments]. Thrombosis & Haemostasis 78:611–616.
6. Nurden AT 1999 Inherited abnormalities of platelets. Thrombosis & Haemostasis 82:468–480.
7. George J 2000 Platelets. Lancet 355:1531–1539.
8. Mann KG 1999 Biochemistry and physiology of blood coagulation. Thrombosis & Haemostasis 82:165–174.
9. Colman R, Schmaier A 1997 Contact system: a vascular biology modulator with anticoagulant, profibrinolytic, antiadhesive and proinflammatory attributes. Blood 90:3819–3843.
10. Mosesson MW 1998 Fibrinogen structure and fibrin clot assembly. Seminars in Thrombosis and Hemostasis 24:169–174.
11. Matsuda M, Sugo T, Yoshida N, et al 1999 Structure and function of fibrinogen: insights from dysfibrinogens. Thrombosis & Haemostasis 82:283–290.
12. van Boven HH, Lane DA. 1997 Antithrombin and its inherited deficiency states. Seminars in Hematology 34:188–204.
13. Dahlback B 1997 Factor V and protein S as cofactors to activated protein C. Haematologica 82:91–95.
14. Collen D 1999 The plasminogen (fibrinolytic) system. Thrombosis & Haemostasis 82:259–270.
15. Hutton RA 1987 Chromogenic substrates in haemostasis. Blood Reviews 1:201–206.
16. Toh CH 1999 APTT revisited: detecting dysfunction in the hemostatic system through waveform analysis. Thrombosis & Haemostasis:684–687.
17. Toh CH, Samis J, Downey C, et al 2002 Biphasic transmittance waveform in the APTT coagulation assay is due to the formation of a Ca(++)-dependent complex of C-reactive protein with very-low-density lipoprotein and is a novel marker of impending disseminated intravascular coagulation. Blood 100:2522–2529.
18. Quick AJ 1973 Quick on "Quick agglutination venostasis" bleeding time technique. Journal of Laboratory and Clinical Medicine 26:1812.
19. Miller GJ, Seghatchian MJ, Walter SJ, et al 1986 An association between the factor VII coagulant activity and thrombin activity induced by surface/cold exposure of normal human plasma. British Journal of Haematology 62:379–384.
20. Palareti G, Maccaferri M, Manotti C, et al 1991 Fibrinogen assays: a collaborative study of six different methods. C.I.S.M.E.L. Comitato Italiano per la Standardizzazione dei Metodi in Ematologia e Laboratorio. Clinical Chemistry 37:714–719.
21. Lawrie AS, McDonald SJ, Purdy G, et al 1998 Prothrombin time derived fibrinogen determination on Sysmex CA-6000. Journal of Clinical Pathology 51:462–466.
22. De Cristofaro R, Landolfi R 1998 Measurement of plasma fibrinogen concentration by the prothrombin-time-derived method: applicability

and limitations. Blood Coagulation & Fibrinolysis 9:251–259.

23. Mackie IJ, Kitchen S, Machin SJ, et al 2003 Guidelines on fibrinogen assays. British Journal of Haematology 121:396–404.

24. Clauss A.1957 Rapid physiological coagulation method in determination of fibrinogen. Acta Haematologica (Basel) 17:237.

25. Mackie J, Lawrie AS, Kitchen S, et al 2002 A performance evaluation of commercial fibrinogen reference preparations and assays for Clauss and PT-derived fibrinogen. Thrombosis & Haemostasis 87:997–1005.

26. Jespersen J, Sidelmann J 1982 A study of the conditions and accuracy of the thrombin time assay of plasma fibrinogen. Acta Haematologic 67:2–7.

27. Funk C, Gmur J, Herold R, et al 1971 Reptilase-R—a new reagent in blood coagulation. British Journal of Haematology 21:43–52.

28. Williams KN, Davidson JM, Ingram GI 1975 A computer program for the analysis of parallel-line bioassays of clotting factors. British Journal of Haematology 31:13–23.

29. Kirkwood TB, Snape TJ 1980 Biometric principles in clotting and clot lysis assays. Clin Laboratory Haematology 2:155–167.

30. Koster T, Blann A, Briet E, et al 1995 Role of clotting factor VIII in effect of von Willebrand factor on occurrence of deep vein thrombosis. Lancet 345:152–155.

31. Jorieux S, Tuley EA, Gaucher C, et al 1992 The mutation Arg (53)–Trp causes von Willebrand disease Normandy by abolishing binding to factor VIII: studies with recombinant von Willebrand factor. Blood 79:563–567.

32. Pipe SW, Eickhorst AN, McKinley SH, et al 1999 Mild hemophilia A caused by increased rate of factor VIII A2 subunit dissociation: evidence for nonproteolytic inactivation of factor VIIIa in vivo. Blood 93:176–183.

33. Keeling DM, Sukhu K, Kemball Cook G, et al 1999 Diagnostic importance of the two-stage factor VIII:C assay demonstrated by a case of mild haemophilia associated with His1954–>Leu substitution in the factor VIII A3 domain. British Journal of Haematology 105:1123–1126.

34. White GC, Roberts HR 1996 The treatment of factor VIII inhibitors: a general overview. Vox Sanguinis 70 (suppl 1):19–23.

35. Sukhu K, Harrison P, Keeling D 2003 Factor VIII assays in haemophilia a patients treated with ReFacto. British Journal of Haematology 121:379–380.

36. Barrowcliffe TW, Raut S, Hubbard AR 1998 Discrepancies in potency assessment of recombinant FVIII concentrates. Haemophilia 4:634–640.

37. Barrowcliffe TW 2003 Standardization of FVIII & FIX assays. Haemophilia 9:397–402.

38. Kasper CK 1984 Measurement of factor VIII inhibitors. Progress in Clinical Biological Research 150:87–98.

39. Galli M, Barbui T 1999 Antiprothrombin antibodies: detection and clinical significance in the antiphospholipid syndrome. Blood 93:2149–2157.

40. Verbruggen B, Novakova I, Wessels H, et al 1995 The Nijmegen modification of the Bethesda assay for factor VIII:C inhibitors: improved specificity and reliability. Thrombosis & Haemostasis 73:247–251.

41. Gaffney PJ, Wong MY 1992 Collaborative study of a proposed international standard for plasma fibrinogen measurement. Thrombosis & Haemostasis 68:428–432.

42. Haverkate F, Samama M 1995 Familial dysfibrinogenemia and thrombophilia: report on a study of the SSC Subcommittee on Fibrinogen. Thrombosis & Haemostasis 73:151–161.

43. Pepin M, Schwarze U, Superti Furga A, et al 2000 Clinical and genetic features of Ehlers-Danlos syndrome type IV, the vascular type [see comments]. New England Journal of Medicine 342:673–680.

44. Rodgers RP, Levin J 1990 A critical reappraisal of the bleeding time. Seminars in Thrombosis & Hemostasis 16:1–20.

45. Mielke CH, Jr, Kaneshiro MM, Maher IA, et al 1969 The standardized normal Ivy bleeding time and its prolongation by aspirin. Blood 34:204–215.

46. Ivy A, Nelson D, Bucher G 1940 The standardization of certain factors in the cutaneous 'venostasis' bleeding time technique. Journal of Laboratory and Clinical Medicine 26:1812.

46a.Bain BJ, Forster T 1980 A sex difference in the bleeding time. Thrombosis and Haemostasis 43:131–132.

47. Fressinaud E, Veyradier A, Truchaud F, et al 1998 Screening for von Willebrand disease with a new analyzer using high shear stress: a study of 60 cases. Blood 91:1325–1331.

48. Cattaneo M, Federici AB, Lecchi A, et al 1999 Evaluation of the PFA-100 system in the diagnosis and therapeutic monitoring of patients with von Willebrand disease. Thrombosis & Haemostasis 82:35–39.

49. Quiroga T, Goycoolea M, Munoz B, et al 2004 Template bleeding time and PFA-100 have low sensitivity to screen patients with hereditary mucocutaneous hemorrhages: comparative study in 148 patients. J Thrombosis & Haemostasis 2:892–898.

50. Sadler JE, Matsushita T, Dong Z, et al 1995 Molecular mechanism and classification of von

Willebrand disease. Thrombosis & Haemostasis 74:161–166.

51. Sadler JE 1994 A revised classification of von Willebrand disease: for the Subcommittee on von Willebrand Factor of the Scientific and Standardization Committee of the International Society on Thrombosis and Haemostasis. Thrombosis & Haemostasis 71:520–525.

52. Laffan M, Brown SA, Collins PW, et al 2004 The diagnosis of von Willebrand disease: a guideline from the UK Haemophilia Centre Doctors' Organization. Haemophilia:199–217.

53. Sadler JE 2003 Von Willebrand disease type 1: a diagnosis in search of a disease. Blood 101:2089–2093.

54. Bartlett A, Dormandy KM, Hawkey CM, et al 1976 Factor-VIII-related antigen: measurement by enzyme immunoassay. British Medical Journal 1:994–996.

55. Macfarlane DE, Stibbe J, Kirby EP, et al 1975 Letter: A method for assaying von Willebrand factor (ristocetin cofactor). Thrombosis Diatheses Haemorrhage 34:306–308.

56. Favaloro EJ 2002 A duplex issue: (i) time to re-appraise the diagnosis and classification of von Willebrand disorder, and (ii) clarification of the roles of von Willebrand factor collagen binding and ristocetin cofactor activity assays. Haemophilia 8:828–831.

57. Favaloro EJ 2000 Collagen binding assay for von Willebrand factor (VWF:CBA): detection of von Willebrands Disease (VWD), and discrimination of VWD subtypes, depends on collagen source. Thrombosis & Haemostasis 83:127–135.

58. Enayat MS, Hill FG 1983 Analysis of the complexity of the multimeric structure of factor VIII related antigen/von Willebrand protein using a modified electrophoretic technique. Journal of Clinical Pathology 36:915–919.

59. BCSH.1988 Guidelines on platelet function testing. The British Society for Haematology BCSH Haemostasis and Thrombosis Task Force. Journal of Clinical Pathology 41:1322–1330.

60. Yardumian DA, Mackie IJ, Machin SJ 1986 Laboratory investigation of platelet function: a review of methodology. Journal of Clinical Pathology 39:701–712.

61. Leon C, Vial C, Gachet C, et al 1999 The P2Y1 receptor is normal in a patient presenting a severe deficiency of ADP-induced platelet aggregation. Thrombosis & Haemostasis 81:775–781.

62. David JL, Herion F 1972 Assay of platelet ATP and ADP by the luciferase method: some theoretical and practical aspects. Adv Exp Med Biol 34:341–354.

63. Jennings I, Kitchen S, Woods TA, et al 2003 Problems relating to the laboratory diagnosis of factor XIII deficiency: a UK NEQAS study. Journal of Thrombosis & Haemostasis 1:2603–2608.

64. Taylor FB, Jr, Toh CH, Hoots WK, et al 2001 Towards definition, clinical and laboratory criteria, and a scoring system for disseminated intravascular coagulation. Thrombosis & Haemostasis 86:1327–1330.

65. Garvey MB, Black JM 1972 The detection of fibrinogen-fibrin degradation products by means of a new antibody-coated latex particle. Journal of Clinical Pathology 25:680–682.

66. Lipinski B, Worowski K.1968 Detection of soluble fibrin monomer complexes in blood by means of protamine sulphate test. Thrombosis Diatheses Haemorrhage 20:44–49.

67. Breen FA, Jr, Tullis JL 1968 Ethanol gelation: a rapid screening test for intravascular coagulation. Annals of Internal Medicine 69:1197–1206.

68. Breen FA, Jr, Tullis JL 1969 Ethanol gelation test improved. Annals of Internal Medicine 71:433–434.

69. Keeling DM, Wright M, Baker P, et al 1999 D-dimer for the exclusion of venous thromboembolism: comparison of a new automated latex particle immunoassay (MDA D-dimer) with an established enzyme-linked fluorescent assay (VIDAS D-dimer). Clinical Laboratory Haematology 21:359–362.

70. Keeling DM, Mackie IJ, Moody A, et al 2004 The diagnosis of deep vein thrombosis in symptomatic outpatients and the potential for clinical assessment and D-dimer assays to reduce the need for diagnostic imaging. British Journal of Haematology 124:15–25.

71. British Thoracic Society Standards of Care Committee Pulmonary Embolism Guideline Development G 2003 British Thoracic Society guidelines for the management of suspected acute pulmonary embolism. [See comment]. Thorax 58:470–483.

72. Graham J, Elston R, Barrrow E, et al 1982 The Hemophilias: statistical methods for carrier detection in hemophilias. Methods in Hematology 5:156.

73. Peake IR, Lillicrap DP, Boulyjenkov V, et al 1993 Report of a joint WHO/WFH meeting on the control of haemophilia: carrier detection and prenatal diagnosis [published erratum appears in Blood Coagulation & Fibrinolysis 1994] Blood Coagulation & Fibrinolysis 4:313–444.

74. Oyesiku JO, Turner CF 2002 Reproductive choices for couples with haemophilia. Haemophilia 8:348–352.

75. Ingram GIC, Hills M 1976 The prothrombin time test: effect of varying citrate concentration. Thrombosis and Haemostasis 36:230–232.

17 Investigation of a thrombotic tendency

Mike Laffan and Richard Manning

INTRODUCTION TO THROMBOPHILIA

Investigations to exclude an acquired or inherited thrombotic tendency are frequently carried out in neonates, children, and young adults who develop venous thrombosis; in those who have a strong family history of such events or have thrombosis at an unusual site; and in individuals of all ages with recurrent episodes of thromboembolism. These investigations are most commonly instituted in venous thrombosis, but some unexplained arterial events, especially in young people, are also studied. In general, the contribution of the inherited factors described here is less evident for arterial than venous thrombosis because their effect is then usually obscured by atherosclerosis. It should be remembered that many thromboses are almost entirely the result of circumstantial factors; these include trauma, fractures, operations, and acute-phase inflammatory response. Further investigation of coagulation is often unnecessary in these circumstances

In this chapter the investigations to diagnose or exclude an acquired thrombotic tendency are presented first, followed by a simplified battery of tests needed to establish the diagnosis of the more important inherited "thrombophilias." Although the number of coagulation factors known to contribute to a thrombotic tendency has increased greatly in the last few years, it remains clear that not all factors have been identified. Hence the failure to detect one of the traits described does not imply that the individual's risk of thrombosis is normal. An acquired thrombotic tendency is common and occurs in many conditions. The large number of traits identified, often with a small associated relative risk, makes their individual utility equally small. Until the interactions of these numerous factors are more completely understood, the clinical history remains a dominant factor in clinical management. The British Committee for Standards in Haematology has published guidelines on the investigation and management of thrombophilia.[1] An outline of appropriate investigations in different circumstances is described in this chapter and is shown in Figure 17.1.

TESTS FOR THE PRESENCE OF A LUPUS ANTICOAGULANT

The lupus anticoagulant (LAC) is an acquired autoantibody found in various autoimmune disorders and sometimes in otherwise healthy individuals.[2]

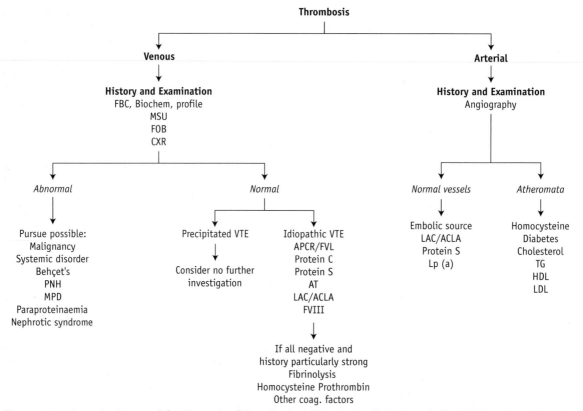

Figure 17.1 Investigations used for diagnosis of thrombosis. ACLA, Anticardiolipin antibody; APCR, activated protein C resistance; AT, antithrombin; CXR, chest X-ray; FBC, full blood count; FOB, faecal occult blood; FVL, factor V Leiden; HDL, high-density lipoprotein; LAC, lupus anticoagulant; LDL, low-density lipoprotein; Lp(a), lipoprotrein (a); MPD, myeloproliferative disorder; MSU, midstream specimen of urine; PNH, paroxysmal nocturnal haemoglobinuria; TG, triglyceride; VTE, venous tromboembolism.

LACs are immunoglobulins that bind to complexes of various proteins with phospholipids active in coagulation and thus prolong the clotting times of phospholipid-dependent tests such as the prothrombin time (PT) or activated partial thromboplastin time (APTT). The name "anticoagulant" is misleading because patients do not have a bleeding tendency. Instead, there is a clear association with recurrent venous thromboembolism, cerebrovascular accidents, and other arterial events and, in women, with recurrent abortions, fetal loss, and other complications of pregnancy.[3] Therefore tests for the presence of the LAC should be carried out in all young individuals with unexplained venous or arterial thrombosis and also in women with recurrent early or late pregnancy loss. The detection of an LAC should not preclude further investigation for other prothrombotic defects, such as coexistent antithrombin (AT), protein C (PC) and protein S (PS) deficiency, and factor V Leiden (FVL), although it may interfere with these tests.

The presence of an LAC may be detected by the clotting screen, depending on the reagents and methods used as well as on the potency and avidity of the antibody. However, the sensitivity of both APTT and PT to LAC varies considerably so that these tests may well be normal and, if clinically suspected, specific tests should always be performed.[4] The unmodified test for activated PC resistance (see below) is also sensitive to the presence of an LAC.

Patients with an LAC may show other abnormalities, including thrombocytopenia, a positive direct antiglobulin test, and a positive antinuclear factor test. In some rare cases, specific antibodies against coagulation factors are also found. Such patients may have a bleeding tendency. The specific tests most commonly used are as follows:

1. Dilute Russell's viper venom time (DRVVT) in conjunction with the platelet neutralisation test
2. Kaolin clotting time (KCT)
3. Tissue thromboplastin inhibition time

It is essential that all the samples of plasma tested for the LAC should be as free of platelets as possible. This is achieved by further centrifugation of plasma at 2000 g or by passing the test plasma through a 0.2-μm microfilter under pressure using a syringe. A platelet count of less than $10 \times 10^9/L$ should be achieved. The plasma is centrifuged at room temperature to avoid platelet activation because platelet microvesicles may also invalidate the test.

Guidelines for the investigation of antiphospholipid syndrome and detection of LACs have been published.[5]

Kaolin Clotting Time

Principle
When the APTT is performed in the absence of platelet substitute reagent, it is particularly sensitive to the LAC. If the test is performed on a range of mixtures of normal and patient's plasma, different patterns of response are obtained, indicating the presence of LAC, deficiency of one or more of the coagulation factors, or the "lupus cofactor" effect.

There are commercially available kits based on the KCT[6] such as Kaoclot (Gradipore Ltd.). This method uses a low-turbidity colloidal kaolin solution, making this reagent slow to settle and therefore suitable for use on automated coagulation analysers. Kaoclot shows high sensitivity to LACs but is not suitable for testing patients undergoing heparin therapy

Reagents
Kaolin. 20 mg/ml in Tris buffer, pH 7.4. This may need to be reduced to 5 mg/ml in some automated analysers (see p. 400).
Normal platelet poor plasma. Depleted of platelets by second centrifugation or microfiltration.
Patient's plasma. Also platelet depleted.
CaCl₂. 0.025 mol/l.

Method
Mix normal and patient plasma in plastic tubes in the following ratios of normal to patient's plasma: 10:0, 9:1, 8:2, 5:5, 2:8, 1:9, and 0:10. Pipette 0.2 ml of each mixture into a glass tube at 37°C. Add 0.1 ml of kaolin and incubate for 3 min, then add 0.2 ml of CaCl₂ and record the clotting time.

Results
Plot the clotting times against the proportion of normal to patient's plasma on linear graph paper as shown in Figure 17.2.

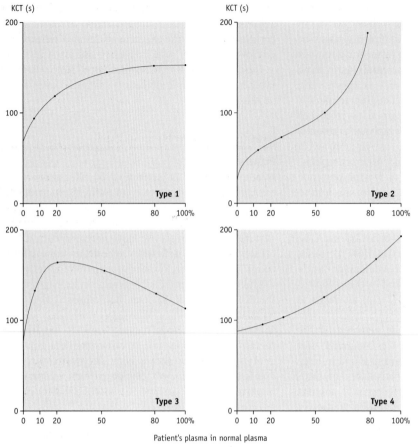

Figure 17.2 Curves obtained using the kaolin clotting time (KCT) to test for presence of lupus anticoagulant (see text).

Interpretation

The pattern obtained for each patient must be critically assessed. A convex pattern (Pattern 1) indicates a positive result, whereas a concave pattern (Pattern 4) indicates a negative result. Pattern 2 indicates a coagulation factor deficiency and LAC. Pattern 3 is found in plasma containing the anticoagulant and is also deficient in a cofactor necessary for the full inhibitory effect. The initial rate of slope is important because a steep slope indicates a positive result. This allows the test to be simplified so that only the tests of 100% normal and of 80% normal/20% test plasmas are performed. The slope can be calculated using the ratio of KCT at 20% test plasma and KCT at 100% normal control plasma (N). For a positive result the ratio at this point should be 1.2 or greater.

Thus,

$$\frac{\text{KCT (80\%N:20\%Test)}}{\text{KCT (100\% N)}} \geq 1.2$$

A control KCT of <60 s may indicate contamination of the control plasma with phospholipid.

Dilute Russell's Viper Venom Time

Principle

Russell's viper venom (RVV) activates factor X leading to a fibrin clot in the presence of factor V, prothrombin, phospholipid, and calcium ions. The LAC prolongs the clotting time by binding to the phospholipid and preventing the action of RVV. As the following test describes, dilution of the venom and phospholipid makes it particularly sensitive for detecting the LAC.[7] Because RVV activates factor X directly, defects of the contact system and factor VIII, IX, or XI deficiencies do not influence the test. The DRVVT[8] is usually combined with a platelet/phospholipid neutralisation procedure to add specificity, and this is incorporated into several commercial kits.

Reagents

Platelet poor plasma. From the patient and a control (p. 392).

Pooled normal plasma.

Glyoxaline buffer. 0.05 mol/l, pH 7.4 (p. 398).

RVV (American Diagnostica Inc.). Stock solution: 1 mg/ml in saline. For working solution dilute approximately 1 in 200 in buffer. The working solution is stable at 4°C for several hours.

Phospholipid. Platelet substitute; also available commercially.

CaCl₂. 0.025 mol/l (p. 398).

Reagent Preparation

The RVV concentration is adjusted to give a clotting time of 30–35 s when 0.1 ml of RVV is added to the mixture of 0.1 ml of normal plasma and 0.1 ml of undiluted phospholipid. The test is then repeated using doubling dilutions of phospholipid reagent. The last dilution of phospholipid before the clotting time is prolonged by 2 s or more is selected for the test (thus giving a clotting time of 35–37 s).

Method

Place 0.1 ml of pooled normal plasma and 0.1 ml of dilute phospholipid reagent in a glass tube at 37°C. Add 0.1 ml of dilute RVV and, after warming for 30 s, add 0.1 ml of CaCl₂. Record the clotting time. Repeat the sequence using the test plasma. Calculate the ratio of the clotting times of the test and control (normal pool) plasma.

Interpretation

The normal ratio should be determined in each laboratory; it is usually between 0.9 and 1.05. Ratios greater than 1.05 suggest the presence of the LAC but could also arise from an abnormality of factors II, V, or X; fibrinogen; or some other inhibitor. The presence of an inhibitor can be confirmed by testing a mixture of equal volumes of patient's and control plasma, whereas phospholipid dependence can be confirmed by using the platelet

neutralisation test described later. The addition of normal plasma corrects an abnormal dilute RVV test result as a result of factor deficiency or defect, but it does not do so in the presence of the LAC. The platelet neutralisation procedure shortens the clotting time in the dilute RVV test of plasma containing the LAC (see below).

Platelet Neutralisation Test

Principle

When platelets are used instead of phospholipid reagents in clotting tests, the tests become insensitive to the LAC. This appears to be a result of the ability of the platelets to adsorb the LAC. To utilise this property of platelets, they must be washed to remove contaminating plasma proteins and activated or "fractured" to expose their coagulation factor binding sites.

Reagents

Commercial Platelet Extract Reagent or Washed Normal Platelets

Acid–citrate–dextrose (ACD) anticoagulant solution (p. 689). pH 5.4, is required for washed platelets. For use, 6 parts of blood is added to 1 part of this anticoagulant.

Na₂EDTA 0.1 mol/l in saline.

Calcium-free Tyrode's buffer Dissolve 8 g NaCl, 0.2 g KCl, 0.625 g Na₂HPO₄, 0.415 g MgCl₂, and 1.0 g NaHCO₂ in 1 litre of water. Adjust pH if necessary to 6.5 with 1 mol/l HCl.

Method

Collect normal blood into ACD and centrifuge at 270 g for 10 min. Pipette the supernatant platelet rich plasma (PRP) into a plastic container, and centrifuge again to obtain more PRP, which is added to the first lot. Dilute the PRP with an equal volume of the calcium-free buffer, and add one-tenth volume of EDTA to give a final concentration of 0.01 mol/l. Centrifuge the mixture in a conical or round-bottom tube at 2000 g for 10 min, and discard the supernatant. Gently resuspend the platelet pellet in buffer and 0.01 mol/l EDTA. Centrifuge again, discard the supernatant, and resuspend the pellet in buffer alone. Then centrifuge the platelets a third time, and resuspend the pellet in buffer without EDTA to give a platelet count of at least 400 × 10⁹/l. The washed platelets may be stored below –20°C in volumes of 1–2 ml. Before use, they must be activated by repeatedly thawing and refreezing 3–4 times.

Use the washed platelets or the commercial reagent in the dilute RVV test or in the APTT in place of the usual phospholipid reagent. First, determine a suitable dilution by testing a range of doubling dilutions in the test system with control plasma. A suitable dilution gives a similar clotting time to that obtained using control plasma and the phospholipid reagent.

Interpretation

The addition of platelets or a commercial "confirm" phospholipid reagent to the DRVVT system shortens the clotting time when the LAC is present. It does not shorten the time when the prolongation is due to a factor deficiency or an inhibitor directed against a specific coagulation factor. However, the ability of different batches of platelets to perform this correction is variable and may vary further with storage. Accordingly, each time the test is performed a plasma sample known to contain an LAC should be tested in parallel to establish the efficacy of the platelets.

Many commercial kits are now available for performing the tests described earlier. As with all such tests, there is an inevitable tradeoff between sensitivity and specificity. This varies with different techniques, kits, and coagulometer. One survey of reagents found that the best discriminator of positivity was by using a normalised correction ratio (CR) of DRVVT clotting times as follows:

$$CR = \frac{\left(\dfrac{P_D}{N_D}\right) - \left(\dfrac{P_C}{N_C}\right)}{\dfrac{P_D}{N_D}}$$

where P is patient and N is normal plasma, and D represents the detection procedure and C represents the confirmation (platelet/phospholipid neutralisation) procedure.[7] A correction of >10% is regarded as positive, but care should be taken to establish a local normal range, and other calculations may also be used.[5]

False-positive results may be obtained in patients receiving intravenous heparin, and the interpretation may be difficult in patients receiving oral anticoagulants. The latter can sometimes be overcome by performing the test on a 50:50 mix with normal plasma.

Dilute Thromboplastin Inhibition Test

Principle

When the thromboplastin used for the PT is diluted, the PT becomes prolonged. At a certain point (usually 1:50–1:500 dilution) the concentration of phospholipid is low enough for the test to become sensitive to phospholipid binding antibodies, and when an LAC is present the ratio of the test plasma to normal plasma clotting time increases. This test is now considered more useful because some thromboplastin reagents (e.g., Innovin) are more sensitive to LAC. However, it should be noted that diluting thromboplastin makes the system sensitive to low levels of factor VIII as are encountered in mild haemophilia, acquired haemophilia, and low levels of factor V or factor VII. Care should be taken that these disorders are not confused. In one study, the test was determined to be positive when the dilute PT ratio (test/mean normal) using Innovin at 1:200 dilution was greater than 1.15.[9]

Textarin/Ecarin Ratio

Principle

The Textarin/Ecarin ratio is a sensitive and relatively specific test for the LAC based on fractions of two snake venoms. Textarin is a protein fraction of *Pseudonaja textilis* venom (Australian Eastern brown snake) that activates prothrombin in the presence of phospholipid, factor V, and calcium ions.[10] Ecarin is a protein fraction of *Echis carinatus* (Indian saw-scaled viper) venom that activates prothrombin in the absence of any cofactors. The activation of prothrombin by Textarin yields thrombin, whereas Ecarin yields meizothrombin (an intermediate of prothrombin activation). In the presence of an LAC, the Textarin time is prolonged, whereas the Ecarin time remains unaffected.

Results

The test results are reported as a ratio of Textarin/Ecarin times. A positive result is indicated by a ratio greater than 1.3.

Polybrene is incorporated with Textarin when testing heparinised samples for the LAC. False-positive results may be obtained in the presence of factor V deficiency and specific inhibitors of factor V. This test has been reported to be useful in identifying LACs in samples from patients who have received warfarin because the action of Ecarin is not affected by the lack of vitamin K.[11]

Interpretation of Tests for Lupus Anticoagulant

No single test detects all lupus-like anticoagulants, and if suspected clinically, then two or if possible three specific tests should be performed before concluding that one is not present.[4,12,13] Conversely, a single positive test should be repeated 6–8 weeks later because a transient positive may be the result of intercurrent illness or medication. It is crucial to distinguish them from specific anti-factor VIII antibodies, which are more typically time dependent but may have some immediate effect as well; specific factor assays may be of use. Similarly, some weak LAC are neutralised by 50:50 mixing with normal plasma and sometimes exhibit a time-dependent effect. Some transient nonspecific coagulation inhibitors are not detected by tests for LAC. Tests are frequently negative while taking warfarin.

Anticardiolipin Assay

The LAC effect is produced by members of the anti-phospholipid group of antibodies. These antibodies do not bind to phospholipid itself but to numerous different proteins to which binding is facilitated by the presence of phospholipid. The proteins that are bound in this way include $\beta2$ glycoprotein 1, prothrombin, annexin V, and cardiolipin. The most frequent of these are anticardiolipin antibodies.[14] These antibodies are detected using the relevant protein in immunoassay on microtitre plates or in coated polystyrene tubes. It is possible that the test for anticardiolipin that is currently most prevalent can be superseded by tests for anti-$\beta2$ glycoprotein 1 antibodies because these may have a closer relationship with thrombosis. However, this is not exclusively so and no standardisation is yet available. Commercial kits for these assays are available.

Care must be taken in the selection of control sera and in setting the cut-off point for normal values. It is also important to remember that anticardiolipin antibodies may be found after viral infections, including glandular fever, and after myocardial infarction.

There are numerous other disorders that are associated with an increased risk of thrombosis but are not usually diagnosed using coagulation-based tests. Their position in the investigation of thrombosis is illustrated in Figure 17.1, and appropriate tests for some of these such as myeloproliferative disorders and paroxysmal nocturnal haemoglobinuria are found elsewhere in this book. One of the most important factors precipitating thrombosis is malignancy. However, the value of extensive testing for possible malignancy in patients with thrombosis remains contentious; some studies have shown that a history and examination combined with a few simple tests as indicated in Figure 17.1 detect virtually all cases of malignancy and other systemic disorders. Other screening tests have been effective in detecting occult malignancy but without improvement in outcome.[16,17]

INVESTIGATION OF INHERITED THROMBOTIC STATES

Testing for thrombotic syndromes is becoming increasingly frequent despite doubts about its clinical utility.[1,18,19] Patients with disorders of pregnancy and those with thrombotic disorders are often referred for investigation. Screening must start by excluding the common causes of an acquired thrombotic tendency as described earlier. A careful family history must be taken next; however, a negative history does not exclude an inherited thrombotic tendency because the defects have variable penetration or a fresh mutation may have been responsible. As with a bleeding tendency, laboratory investigation is a stepwise procedure, starting with the simpler, first-line tests (as shown in Figure 17.1) The relevant tests are described below.

Antithrombin (AT)

AT[20,21] (previously known as antithrombin III) is the major physiological inhibitor of thrombin and factors IXa, Xa, and XIa. AT deficiency is found in approximately 2% of cases of thrombosis and may be acquired or congenital. Various methods are available for measuring either functional activity or antigenic quantity of AT. The functional methods are based on the reaction with thrombin or factor Xa and can be coagulation or chromogenic assays. A chromogenic assay is described below.

Antithrombin (AT) Measurement Using a Chromogenic Assay

Principle

In the presence of heparin, AT reacts rapidly to inactivate thrombin by forming a 1:1 complex. The chromogenic AT assay is a two-step procedure. In the first step the plasma sample is incubated with a fixed quantity of thrombin and heparin. In the second step the residual thrombin is measured spectrometrically by its action on a synthetic chromogenic substrate, which results in the release of para nitro-aniline (pNA) dye. The use of bovine thrombin avoids interference in the assay by heparin cofactor II; this can also be achieved by measuring the Xa neutralising capacity of the AT and an appropriate chromogenic substrate. The assay thus measures heparin cofactor activity rather than progressive AT activity and may therefore also detect AT variants with altered heparin binding.

Method

Carry out the procedure on dilutions of a standard plasma to construct a standard graph. Then test dilutions of the test plasma in an identical manner and read the results directly from the standard graph.

The reagents provided and details of the method vary among manufacturers and should be closely followed. There may also be variation between different batches of the same reagent.

Normal Range

The normal range is generally between 0.75 and 1.25 u/ml. Some manufacturers suggest a slightly narrower range (i.e., 0.8–1.20 u/ml), but it is preferable for each laboratory to establish its own normal range. Repeated freezing and thawing of samples, as well as storage at or above –20°C, result in a reduction in AT concentration.

Interpretation

In an inherited deficiency, the AT concentration is usually <0.7 iu/ml. Most cases are heterozygotes for null mutations and have levels of approximately 50% of normal. Be aware that numerous variants have been described, some of which give assay results that are close to normal. Further tests such as AT antigen or crossed immunoelectrophoresis may be required.[22] A low level of AT may be acquired during active thrombosis, liver disease, heparin therapy, nephrotic syndrome, or asparaginase therapy; very low values are sometimes encountered in fulminant disseminated intravascular coagulation (DIC) or liver failure. Normal newborns have a lower AT concentration (0.60–0.80 iu/ml) than adults. In neonates who are congenitally deficient, very low values (0.30 u/ml and lower) may be found. Very high values are encountered after myocardial infarction and in some forms of vascular disease. It is also important to remember that oral anticoagulant therapy may increase the AT concentration by approximately 0.1 u/ml in cases of congenital deficiency.

Antithrombin Antigen Determination

AT antigen can be assessed using various methods such as enzyme-linked immunosorbent assay (ELISA), immuno-electrophoresis assays, and latex agglutination (nephelometry).

Principle

Latex agglutination assays are based on the agglutination of a suspension of antibody-coated, micro-latex particles in the presence of plasma containing AT antigen, (The antibody is attached by covalent bonding.) The wavelength is such that light can pass through the latex suspension unabsorbed. However, in the presence of AT antigen, the antibody-coated latex particles agglutinate to form aggregates of diameter greater than the wavelength of the light; the latter is absorbed. There is a direct relationship between the observed absorbance value and the concentration of the antigen being measured. The convenience of this form of test is that it can be performed on automated analysers.

INVESTIGATION OF PROTEIN C (PC) DEFICIENCY

Protein C Assay

PC[23] is a vitamin K–dependent protein. After activation by thrombin, which is accelerated in the presence of thrombomodulin on the vascular endothelium, PC complexes with phospholipids and PS to degrade factors Va and VIIIa. Inherited heterozygous PC deficiency is found in 2–4% of first-episode thromboses and 5–7% of all recurrent thromboembolic episodes in young adults.[18,19] The importance of the

PC–PS system is evidenced by the catastrophic syndrome of purpura fulminans in neonates with homozygous PC or PS deficiency.[24] Acquired PC deficiency is found in all conditions associated with vitamin K deficiency or defect, including oral anticoagulant therapy. A low plasma concentration is also found in DIC, in liver disease, and in the early postoperative period.

PC can be measured using a chromogenic assay, a coagulation assay, or an antigenic method.

Measurement of Functional Protein C by the Protac Method

Principle

In the presence of a specific snake venom activator, PC is converted into its active form. This allows the activation to be carried out in whole plasma without separation of PC. Activated PC is measured by its action on one of the specific synthetic substrates (e.g., S-2366, CBS 65.25). The reaction is stopped by the addition of 50% acetic acid and the p-nitroalanine produced is measured in a spectrometer at 405 nm.

Reagents

Platelet poor plasma. Standard and test of samples are centrifuged at 1500–2000 g for 15 min. After centrifugation, plasma can be stored indefinitely at –40°C or below.

Protac. This is an activator derived from the venom of *Agkistrodon contortrix contortrix* (Southern copperhead). It is obtained commercially; each vial contains lyophilised powder, which is reconstituted and stored according to the manufacturer's instructions.

Specific chromogenic substrate. Reconstituted and stored according to the manufacturer's instructions.

Barbitone buffered saline. See p. 690.

Acetic acid. 50%.

Method

Construct the standard curve according to the instructions. Some manufacturers recommend the use of commercial calibrators or control plasma in preference to the normal pool.

The assay is carried out by a two-step method. In the first step plasma and activator are incubated for an exact period of time. In the second step the specific chromogenic substrate is added and the reaction is stopped with acetic acid again at a precise point in time. Read the amount of the dye produced at 405 nm against a blank obtained as follows: acetic acid, activator, and chromogenic substrate are first mixed; then standard or patient's plasma is added to the mixture and the absorbance is measured at 405 nm. The manufacturer's instructions must be closely followed. Plot the PC activity against the corresponding absorbance reading on linear graph paper.

Normal Range

The normal range is 0.70–1.40 u/ml. Preferably, each laboratory should establish its own normal range.

Further investigation for Protein C Deficiency

If inherited PC deficiency is suspected, an immunological assay should also be carried out with an ELISA-based kit. The amidolytic assay described here does not detect the rare type II PC deficiency due to mutations in the Gla domain, although they can be detected by a coagulation-based assay. A problem with the coagulation-based assay is its susceptibility to interference from FVL. Although the chromogenic substrate is said to be specific, this is not true. Specificity is conferred by the inclusion of substances that inhibit other enzymes capable of cleaving the substrate. In some circumstances this can fail and spuriously high PC activities can be obtained, which may obscure a PC deficiency.[25] PC activity and antigen are reduced in patients taking oral vitamin K antagonists, although it is sometimes possible to make a provisional diagnosis of PC deficiency by using a PC:VIIc ratio.[26] It is also important to exclude vitamin K deficiency by assaying other vitamin K-dependent factors that should be normal. Family studies should be carried out whenever possible.

Clotting-Based Protein C Assay

Principle

PC clotting assays use an APTT reagent incorporating a PC activator derived from the Southern copperhead snake venom (*Agkistrodon contortrix contortrix*), PC-deficient plasma, and calcium chloride. The APTT reagent activates both PC and the factors of the intrinsic pathway. The clotting time of normal plasma is long (>100 s), whereas that of PC-deficient plasma is normal (30 s). The degree of prolongation of the clotting time when patient plasma is mixed with PC-deficient plasma is proportional to the concentration of PC in the patient plasma.

Unlike chromogenic PC assays, PC clotting assays are sensitive to functional PC defects such as phospholipid binding (mutations in the Gla domain) and calcium binding. However, they are also sensitive to FVL, LACs, and raised factor VIII levels.

Protein C Antigen

PC antigen can be measured using a conventional ELISA. Commercial kits are available.

Protein S (PS) Assay

PS is also a vitamin K–dependent protein that acts as a cofactor for activated PC. It is similar to the serine proteases of the coagulation system in having a Gla domain and four EGF domains; however, instead of a protease domain it has a large terminal domain closely homologous to sex hormone-binding globulin (SHBG). In plasma, 60% of PS is bound to C4b-binding protein (C4bBP) via the SHBG[27] and does not possess any APC cofactor activity; the remaining 40% is free and available to interact with APC. The functional assays of PS are based on the capacity of PS to augment the prolongation of a clotting test time by APC. However, PS has some APC-independent anticoagulant activity that can also be measured in coagulation assays.[28] Measurement of the total and free PS antigen is possible using enzyme-linked immunoassays. Interpretation of PS assay results is frequently difficult, and the three measurements are considered together here.

Enzyme-Linked Immunosorbent Assay of Free and Total Protein S

Principle

The total PS in plasma is detected by a standard ELISA using polyclonal antibodies.[29] The analysis is then repeated using plasma in which C4bBP-bound PS has been removed by polyethylene glycol (PEG) precipitation. This gives a measure of free PS.

Reagents

Polytheneglycol (PEG) precipitation solution. Dissolve 100 g of PEG 8000 in 200 ml of sterile water. Prepare approximately 50 ml of working PEG by diluting the stock solution to exactly 18.75% with sterile water. Store in 2-ml aliquots at −20°C.

Coating buffer (phosphate buffered saline, pH 7.2). 0.39 g $Na_2HPO_4.2H_2O$, 2.68 g $Na_2HPO_4. 12H_2O$, 8.474 g NaCl. Make up to 1 litre and adjust to pH 7.2; store at 4°C.

Wash buffer. This is the same as the coating buffer, but it contains 0.5 M NaCl and 0.2% v/v Tween 20. Add 10.37 g of NaCl to 1 litre of coating buffer and 0.2% Tween 20. (Mix well.) Store at 4°C.

Dilution buffer. This is the washing buffer with 30 g/l PEG 8000. Store at 4°C.

Substrate buffer Na_2HPO_4 (citrate phosphate buffer, pH 5.0). 7.3 g citric acid, 23.87 g. $Na_2HPO_4.12H_2O$. Make up to 1 litre with water. Adjust pH to 5.0.

o-phenylenediamine.

Anti-PS and anti-PS peroxidase conjugated. (Dako Ltd.).

Sulphuric acid, 1 M.

Microtitre plates. (Greiner Labortechnick Ltd.).

Standards and controls.

Hydrogen peroxide. 30% w/v.

Methods

Dilute the antihuman PS immunoglobulin 1:1000 in coating buffer (i.e., 20 μl in 20 ml of buffer). Add 0.1 ml to each well of a microtitre plate, cover with parafilm, and leave overnight in a moist chamber at 4°C. On the day the assay is to be performed, warm an aliquot of working PEG solution to 30°C. Accurately pipette 200 μl of standard, patient's, and control plasma samples into conical Eppendorf tubes; warm for 5 min at 37°C. Add exactly 50 μl of warmed PEG, immediately cap, and vortex mix twice for exactly 5 s each. Place in water/crushed ice mixture. In turn treat all the samples identically. Leave for 30 min on the melted ice. Centrifuge for 30 s in the Eppendorf centrifuge. Then return to ice and remove 100 μl in a labelled tube (taking care not to remove any precipitate).

Prepare dilutions of control and patient's samples in PEG dilution buffer as follows. For total PS, dilute 0.05 ml of reference plasma in 8 ml of diluent. Use the PEG precipitated reference plasma for measuring free PS; add 0.1 ml to 4 ml of dilution buffer.

Prepare a range of standards from these stock solutions using the same dilution schedule for free and total PS.

A. Stock solution = 1.25 u/ml.
B. 0.8 ml stock + 0.2 ml buffer = 1.0 u/ml.
C. 0.6 ml stock + 0.4 ml buffer = 0.75 u/ml.
D. 0.4 ml stock + 0.6 ml buffer = 0.5 u/ml.
E. 0.2 ml stock + 0.8 ml buffer = 0.25 u/ml.
F. 0.1 ml stock + 0.9 ml buffer = 0.125 u/ml.
G. 0.05 ml stock + 0.95 ml buffer = 0.0625 u/ml.

Control and patient's samples are tested at two dilutions—total PS plasma: 1:200 and 1:400 and free PS PEG supernatants: 1:50 and 1:100. Shake out the contents of the previously prepared plate, and blot on tissue. Wash the plate three times in wash buffer by filling all the wells, leaving for 2 min, shaking out the contents, blotting, and repeating. Add 100 μl of each dilution of standard, control, or patient's plasma in duplicate across the plate. Cover and incubate for 3 hours in a wet box at room temperature. Wash the plate as described earlier. Dilute 2 μl of peroxidase-labelled antibody in 24 ml of dilution buffer. Add 100 μl of diluted tag (peroxidase-conjugated) antibody to each well and leave in a wet box for 2–3 hours at room temperature. Wash the plate as described earlier. Make up the substrate solution by adding 8 mg of o-phenylene diamine to 12 ml of citrate phosphate buffer. Immediately before use add 10 μl of hydrogen peroxide. Add 100 μl of substrate solution to each well. When the weakest standard has a visible yellow colour, add 150 μl of 1 M sulphuric acid to each well. Read the optical densities on a plate reader at 492 nm. Plot the optical densities against plasma dilutions on double-log graph paper and read the patient's values from the corresponding calibration curve (i.e., total against total and free against free).

The polyclonal antibody should have similar affinities for free and bound PS; high plasma dilutions and long incubation times help to avoid differential affinity leading to error. Alternatively, two monoclonal antibodies (capture and tag) with the same affinity for free and bound PS can be used (Asserchrom).

A new test using two separate antibodies to measure free and total PS is now available.[30]

Free Protein S Antigen by Immunoturbidometric Assay (Instrumentation Laboratories and Stago)

Free PS is assayed by measuring the increase of turbidity produced by the agglutination of two latex reagents. The first latex reagent is coated with purified C4BP, which has a high affinity for free PS in plasma in the presence of calcium ions. The free PS adsorbed on the C4BP latex initiates the agglutination reaction with a second latex reagent, which is coated with a monoclonal antibody directed against human PS. The amount of agglutination is directly proportional to the free PS concentration.

Protein S Functional Assay

Principle

Functional PS can be assessed using coagulation-based assays activated by different means. In one commercial assay (American Diagnostica) dilutions of normal and test plasmas are mixed with PS-deficient plasma. Activation of these mixtures is achieved by a reagent containing factor Xa, activated PC, and phospholipid. After a 5-min activation time, clot formation is initiated by the addition of calcium chloride. Under these conditions, the prolongation of the clotting time is directly proportional to the concentration of PS in the patient plasma. The use of factor Xa as the activator minimises the potential interference by high levels of factor VIII.

A PS function assay may also be based on the PT, in which case the effect of factor VIII is again bypassed. The PT-based PS assay uses PS-depleted plasma activated by Protac, thus providing activated PC. The PT is increased by the APC–PS mediated destruction of factor Va, which occurs in the presence of PS from the test and control plasmas. The PT is measured using bovine thromboplastin, and prolongation is proportional to PS activity.

The details of the tests are performed according to the manufacturer's instructions, and many tests can be automated.

Because the assays are subject to interference by other plasma factors, it is recommended that the test plasma is assayed at two different dilutions to ensure parallelism with the standard curve.

PS functional assays are designed to measure the PC cofactor activity of PS, but as discussed earlier, this is not its only anticoagulant activity. PS that is bound to C4bBP, is inadequately γ-carboxylated, or has been cleaved by thrombin has an indeterminate effect on these assays and does not contribute via PC cofactor activity.

Interpretation of Protein S Functional and Antigenic Assays

PS deficiency has been classified into three subtypes according to the pattern of results obtained in functional and antigenic assays.

Category	Total PS	Free PS	Functional PS
Type I	Low	Low	Low
Type II	Normal	Normal	Low
Type III	Normal	Low	Low

Studies have suggested that the type I and type III patterns are both the result of the same genetic defect and that the difference may be the result of an age-related increase in C4bBP.[31,32] Many examples of what were thought to be type II PS deficiency have subsequently been shown to be a result of the presence of FVL, which causes a spuriously low result in the functional PS assay.

Although an estimate of PS functional activity would be ideal for diagnosing PS deficiency, the functional PS assays available are problematic. Like other functional assays they are prone to external influences: FVL, LAC, and levels of other coagulation factors. Fortunately type II PS defects appear to be extremely rare; thus measurement of free PS is the preferred method for detecting PS deficiency.[33,34] An assay on free PS removed from plasma using a monoclonal antibody has been described and avoids these problems but is not in general use.[35]

Low levels of PS may be an acquired phenomenon during pregnancy and with oral anticoagulation, nephrotic syndrome, use of oral contraceptives, systemic lupus erythematosus, and liver disease. Catastrophically low levels have been reported in children after varicella infection owing to autoantibody production.[36] It is important to note that the normal range for women who are premenopausal is significantly lower than in other groups and local normal ranges should be determined to avoid misinterpretation, paying attention to the additional effects of hormonal therapy and artifactual reduction in PS as described earlier.[37,38] Although C4bBP is elevated during an acute-phase reaction, the PS-binding β chain does not increase, and as a result free PS does not decrease.[39]

Activated Protein C Resistance

In 1993 Dahlback et al[40] described an inherited tendency to thrombosis characterised by a defective plasma response to activated PC. This became known as activated PC resistance (APCR) and was subsequently shown in >90% of cases to result from a mutation Arg506Glu in factor V Leiden (FVL). This mutation destroys a cleavage site for APC, which greatly slows APC inactivation of Va. It also blocks the conversion by APC of factor V into factor Vi, which acts a cofactor for APC degradation of factor VIIIa. APCR is found in approximately 20% of patients with a first episode of venous thrombosis.

Principle[41]

When activated PC (APC) is added to plasma and an APTT is performed, there is normally a prolongation of the clotting time as a result of factor V and factor VIII degradation. The original detection of this phenomenon was by means of a modified APTT, but it can also be detected using modifications of the PT, RVV time, and Xa clotting time. These tests all vary somewhat in their sensitivity and specificity for the FVL mutation, which is generally improved by mixing the test plasma with factor V–deficient plasma. This reduces the effect of other factors such as factor VIII and prothrombin, which can alter estimation of APCR[42] and restores the sensitivity of the test in patients who are taking oral anticoagulants. However, the test remains sensitive to interference by LACs. Numerous commercial kits are available for these tests.

Expression of Results

APCR was originally reported as a simple ratio of clotting times with and without APC. The result can be normalised by expressing this as a ratio of the same result obtained with normal plasma, that is:

$$\text{Normalised APCR} = \frac{T + APC}{T - APC} \div \frac{N + APC}{N - APC}$$

The use of a normalised ratio improves day-to-day precision and may also improve accuracy. However, it is extremely important that the pooled normal plasma does not contain FVL because very small amounts (2.5%) markedly affect the response to APC. A normal range should be established locally, and its relationship to the presence of FVL should be investigated.

Interpretation

The Leiden thrombophilia survey estimated the relative risk of thrombosis for APCR to be approximately 7.[43] Studies using DNA analysis alone have generally found lower relative risks.[44] Most testing strategies have been directed toward producing tests that have a high sensitivity and specificity for FVL, but this may not be appropriate. It seems that "acquired APCR" or APCR resulting from other causes represents a prothrombotic state even in the absence of FVL[45] and also by the presence of acquired APCR in prothrombotic states such as pregnancy. These are not (except LACs) detected after mixing with factor V–deficient plasma. Many laboratories use a combination of plasma and DNA testing to assess patients' status.

Increased Prothrombin, Factor VIII, and Other Factors

A later finding from the Leiden thrombophilia survey was that elevated levels of prothrombin were significantly associated with thrombosis.[46] Most elevated levels were associated with a mutation in the 3′ untranslated region of the gene (G20210A). The mutation is detected by a simple polymerase chain reaction–based test. (See p. 557.) Subsequently, other factors, including factor VIII, factor IX, and factor XI, have been shown to have an association with thrombosis when elevated.[47-49]

Heparin Cofactor II Assay

Principle

Heparin cofactor II (HCII) present in test and standard plasma is activated by dermatan sulphate and incubated with human thrombin. The residual, uninhibited thrombin is then measured by cleavage of a chromogenic substrate.

Reagents

Reagents are commercially available in a kit form.

Buffer, pH 8.2. 0.05 mol/l Tris, 0.15 mol/l NaCl, 6.8 mmol/l Na_2EDTA, 2 mg/l Polybrene, 10 g/l bovine serum albumin, pH adjusted with HCl.
Dermatan sulphate (free of heparin).
Human thrombin.
Chromogenic substrate for thrombin.
50% Acetic acid.
Pooled normal plasma as standard.
Test plasma.

Method

It is important to follow the manufacturer's instructions that come with the kit. Prepare a range of dilutions of pooled normal plasma to construct a calibration curve. Prepare also a single dilution of each test plasma. Incubate the dilutions with dermatan sulphate at 37°C in a plastic tube or a microtitre plate. Then add thrombin, followed, after a further incubation, by the chromogenic substrate. After a suitable reaction time, in accordance with the manufacturer's instructions, add acetic acid to stop the reaction, and measure the absorbance at 405 nm in a spectrometer or a microtitre plate reader as appropriate.

Calculation

Read the absorbance of the test plasma from the calibration curve and express as percentage normal.

Normal Range

The normal range is generally 0.55–1.45 u/ml.

Interpretation

Plasma concentration of heparin cofactor II may be increased in healthy women taking oral contraceptive pills, in pregnancy, and as part of the acute-phase response. It is reduced in congenital deficiency, chronic haemolytic anaemias, liver disease, and DIC.[50] A deficiency is found in some individuals with recurrent thromboembolism. However, there is no clear evidence that HCII deficiency is more prevalent in this group than in the normal population; consequently, testing is not recommended as part of thrombophilia investigation.

FIBRINOLYTIC SYSTEM

Investigation of Suspected Dysfibrinogenaemia

Congenital dysfibrinogenaemia associated with thrombosis should be suspected in individuals with a prolonged thrombin time and a slightly or moderately reduced fibrinogen concentration in plasma. The presence of a dysfibrinogen is proved when a significant (usually twofold) discrepancy is found between the Clauss and clot weight assays. For details of investigation see p. 401.

Investigation of the Fibrinolytic System: General Considerations

The investigation of fibrinolysis has an uncertain place in haemostasis. It seems well-established that uncontrolled fibrinolytic capacity as a result of anti-plasmin or plasminogen activator inhibitor (PAI-1) deficiency can lead to a haemorrhagic tendency, although these are rare.[51,52] In contrast, there is no good evidence that an impaired fibrinolytic capacity results in a tendency to venous thrombosis. This may be attributed in part to the poor reproducibility of the global tests of euglobulin clot lysis or fibrin plate lysis, but the uncertainty has not been removed by use of either specific assays or genetic polymorphic markers.[53] Although reduced fibrino-lysis is a common finding in patients who have had a venous thrombosis, it appears to have no prospective value.[54] Similarly, high (sic) levels of tissue plasminogen activator (tPA) were shown to be predictive of myocardial infarction in the ECAT (European Concerted Action on Thrombosis and Disabilities) study, but it seems likely that in both cases the association can be best interpreted as demonstrating an abnormality of endothelial function rather than a problem with fibrinolysis *per se*.[55-58]

Fibrinolysis shows considerable diurnal variation as well as interference from plasma lipids and stress. It is therefore generally preferred to perform these tests in the morning after an overnight fast, after a period of no smoking, and after the subject has lain resting for ≥15 min (the plasma half-life of tPA is approximately 5 min). Great care is required in obtaining and handling samples for the assays described later.[59] Tests for fibrin and fibrinogen degradation products are described in Chapter 16.

Investigation of Suspected Plasminogen Defect or Deficiency

Inherited plasminogen deficiency or defect may be found in 2–3% of unexplained thromboses in young people.[60,61] However, the relationship between the deficiency and thrombosis is not clear. The laboratory screening should be carried out using a functional assay based on full transformation of plasminogen into plasmin by activators. Such assays can be caseinolytic, fibrin substrate, or chromogenic.

Chromogenic Assay for Plasminogen

Principle

In this two-step amidolytic assay, plasminogen is first complexed with excess streptokinase. In the second step, the plasmin-like activity of the strepto-kinase–plasminogen complex is measured by its effect on a plasmin-specific peptide. The amount of the dye released is proportional to the amount of plasminogen available in the sample for complexing with streptokinase. The streptokinase–plasminogen complex is not significantly inhibited by the plasma plasmin inhibitors.

Reagents and Method

Details can be found in the manufacturer's instructions. They vary among manufacturer's and even among batches of the same kit.

Normal Range

The normal range is 0.75–1.60 u/ml.

Interpretation

Plasminogen concentration is reduced in the newborn, in patients with cirrhosis, with DIC, and during and after thrombolytic therapy, but the assay is less reliable in these circumstances when fibrinogen/fibrin degradation products (or high levels of fibrinogen) may augment plasmin activity. Plasminogen is an acute-phase reactant, and an increased concentration is found in infection, trauma, myocardial infarction, and malignant disease. The diagnosis of inherited plasminogen deficiency must be confirmed by functional tests using other activators, immunological assays, and family studies.

Investigation of "Fibrinolytic Potential"

The "fibrinolytic potential" is measured as the combined effect of plasminogen activators and inhibitors. The concentration of activators may be increased by venous occlusion or by the administration of DDAVP (1-deamino-8-D-arginine vasopressin, also known as desmopressin). The tests used are, first, the assays of plasminogen activators, using a fibrin substrate (euglobulin lysis time, fibrin plate lysis, and many others) or a chromogenic substrate or ELISA techniques; and second, assays of inhibitors. The commonly used tests for inhibitors are the chromogenic assays of PAI and of α_2 antiplasmin (AP).[62,63] The finding of an increased or reduced fibrinolytic potential should be followed by assays of specific fibrinolytic factors.

Euglobulin Lysis Time

Principle

When plasma is diluted and acidified, the precipitate (euglobulin) that forms contains plasminogen activator (mostly tPA), plasminogen, and fibrinogen. Most of the plasmin inhibitors are left in the solution. The precipitate is redissolved, the fibrinogen is clotted with thrombin, and the time for clot lysis is measured.

Reagents

Acetic acid.
0.01%

Bovine thrombin.
10 NIH u/ml.

Fresh platelet poor plasma from the patient and control.
Because tPA is very labile, blood must be collected into cooled sample tubes, placed on ice, and processed immediately.

Glyoxaline buffer.
pH 7.4. (See p. 398).

Method

Place venous blood in a plastic tube containing citrate; after mixing, keep the tube in an icebath. Centrifuge the sample as soon as possible (never later than 30 min after collection) at 4°C at 1200–1500 g. Pipette 1.0 ml of plasma into 9 ml of acetic acid. Mix well and keep on ice for 15 min. Centrifuge at 4°C for 15 min, at 1500 g, to deposit the white euglobulin precipitate. Discard the supernatant, invert the tubes, then wipe the walls with cotton wool on an applicator stick until completely dry inside. Add 0.5 ml of glyoxaline buffer and dissolve the precipitate. Place duplicate 0.3 ml volumes of patient's and control plasma dissolved euglobulin fraction in glass tubes and obtain clotting with 0.1 ml of thrombin. Leave undisturbed at 37°C and inspect for clot lysis at 15-min intervals.

Normal Range

The normal range is 90–240 min.

Interpretation

A technical problem leading to an artifactually long lysis time is the failure to maintain a low temperature throughout all the stages of the test. Furthermore, the fact that a variable amount of PAI-1 precipitates in the euglobulin fraction makes it essential to analyse a normal control on each occasion the test is performed. Exercise and prolonged venous stasis shorten the lysis times. There is also a significant diurnal variation; lysis time is longer in the morning than at noon or in the afternoon. Prolonged fibrinolysis (as found during fibrinolytic therapy) may result in plasminogen depletion and give rise to a falsely long time. In DIC, a low fibrinogen concentration in the patient's plasma gives a wispy clot, which dissolves rapidly and results in a falsely short lysis time. Conversely, high levels of fibrinogen result in a prolonged lysis time.

Long lysis times are found in the last trimester of pregnancy, in the postoperative period, after myocardial infarction, in individuals who are obese, and in many cases of recurrent venous thrombosis. Very short lysis times are seen in some haematological or disseminated malignancies and in cirrhosis. A short lysis time is also seen in factor XIII deficiency.

Lysis of Fibrin Plates

Principle

Most commercially available fibrinogen preparations are contaminated with plasminogen. If a standard fibrinogen solution is poured into a petri dish and clotted with $CaCl_2$ and thrombin, a solid fibrin plate is obtained. If the euglobulin fraction under test is placed on the plate, the plasminogen in the plate converts into plasmin and a zone of lysis appears around the sample. The area of lysis is proportionate to the concentration of plasminogen activator in the euglobulin fraction.[64]

Reagents

Bovine fibrinogen.
Bovine thrombin.
50 NIH μ/ml.

Calcium.
0.025 mol/l.

Barbitone buffered saline.
(See p. 690.)

Platelet poor plasma.
From the patient and a control collected as described for euglobulin lysis time.

Equipment

Equipment includes plastic petri dishes.

Method

To prepare the fibrin plate, dilute the fibrinogen in buffered saline to obtain a final concentration of 1.5 g/l. Pipette 10 ml of diluted fibrinogen into a petri dish. Place it on a level tray. Add 0.5 ml of $CaCl_2$ and 0.2 ml of thrombin solution. Mix the contents by swirling quickly. The plate clots within 10 to 20 s; it must clot evenly to be suitable for the test. Leave the plate undisturbed for 20 min. The prepared plates can then be kept for 3–4 days at 4°C.

Carefully apply 30 μl of the euglobulin fraction, prepared as described in the previous test, to the surface of the plate. There is no need to cut a well. Place in an incubator at 37°C for 24 hours. This preparation time can be shortened by the addition of exogenous plasminogen.[64]

Perform all tests (patient and control) in duplicate.

Results

Calculate the zone of lysis by measuring two diameters in mm at right angles to each other. Multiply the two values to obtain the approximate area of lysis in mm^2.

Normal Range

The normal range is variable but is usually between 40 and 60 mm^2.

Interpretation

The area of lysis may be difficult to define because of incomplete lysis. Only areas of complete, clear lysis should be measured. In other respects the interpretation is as for the euglobulin clot lysis time except that the levels of plasminogen and fibrinogen in the test plasma do not affect the result. The same problems in preparing the euglobulin fraction apply as does the necessity for a normal control.

Venous Occlusion Test

Principle

Localised venous occlusion[65] of an arm for a standardised period is used as a stimulus for release of tPA from the vessel wall. The original intention was that this would be a better measure of functional defects in fibrinolysis than a resting sample. Preocclusion and postocclusion lysis times, using the previously described euglobulin lysis or the fibrin plate lysis tests, are measured. In normal subjects fibrinolysis is greatly enhanced by occlusion. However, given the problems associated with global assays of fibrinolysis, it seems preferable to perform specific measurements of tPA before and after occlusion.

Method

Withdraw blood from the arm to be tested without stasis, place it in a citrate-containing tube, and keep in an icebath. Inflate the sphygmomanometer cuff to a pressure midway between the systolic and diastolic pressure. Leave the inflated cuff on for 10 min. Take a sample of venous blood from below the cuff immediately before deflation and place on ice. Measure the lysis in both samples, as described previously. This test is uncomfortable and some patients may not be able to tolerate as much as 10 min of occlusion. Petechiae are commonly seen after the test is completed.

Results

The postocclusion lysis times should be shorter than the preocclusion times. Shortening by at least 30 min is found in most normal subjects.

Interpretation

Failure to enhance lysis is found in some cases of recurrent venous thrombosis; in people who are obese; after surgery, trauma, or severe illness; and in Behçet's syndrome.[63,65] It may also result from a failure to release the activator because insufficient pressure was applied or the occlusion time was too short. Normal people vary in the degree of response: "good" responders increase the concentration of tPA by threefold to fourfold, whereas "poor" responders may consistently show only a very slight enhancement of fibrinolysis even with longer occlusion times. When comparing plasma levels of proteins preocclusion and postocclusion, an adjustment for changes in haematocrit may be required.[66] The effect of the venous occlusion test and the levels of tPA are very variable over time.[67,68]

Tissue Plasminogen Activator (tPA) Amidolytic Assay

Principle

Different amidolytic assays for tPA have been described.[69,70] One relies on the activation of purified plasminogen to plasmin in the presence of fibrinogen fragments, which stimulate the tPA activity in the test plasma. The plasmin is measured using a specific chromogenic substrate. In the second method, tPA is captured on specific antibodies bound to a solid-phase matrix such as a microtitre plate; the various plasma inhibitors of tPA and plasmin are washed away, plasminogen is added together with a stimulator of tPA activity, and the plasmin produced is measured with chromogenic substrates. Alternatively, chromogenic substrates specific for tPA may be used, but there are specificity problems especially in the plasma assays.

Interpretation

tPA is secreted into plasma in its active form but rapidly complexes with its principal inhibitor PAI-1. The amount of active tPA in the plasma is a result of this equilibrium and represents only a small fraction of the total (antigenic) tPA. This process continues after blood sampling unless taken into appropriate acidic anticoagulant (see above).

tPA can also be measured by ELISA using monoclonal antibodies on microtitre plates. Although this closely parallels the PAI-1 concentration and says little about the proportion of free, active tPA, it has been found to have a predictive effect in patients with angina.[57] The tPA levels have a large number of disease associations.[71]

Plasminogen Activator Inhibitor Assay

Principle

A fixed amount of tPA is added in excess to undiluted plasma. Part of it rapidly complexes with the tPA inhibitor (PAI). Plasminogen in plasma is then activated into plasmin by the residual, uncomplexed tPA. The amount of plasmin formed is directly proportional to the residual tPA activity and inversely proportional to the PAI activity of the sample. The amount of plasmin generated is measured using a plasmin-specific substrate.

Reagents are available in kit form, and the manufacturer's instructions must be closely followed. The normal range is as yet poorly defined, and each laboratory should establish its own range until reliable normal values become available.

The time of sampling must be standardised. Early morning (7 a.m.) samples have much greater levels of activity than those done later in the day. Sample processing is extremely important because PAI leaks from platelets in sampled blood and PAI-1 in plasma rapidly converts to a latent (inactive) form. An ELISA assay is also available to measure the total PAI-1 present.

Plasminogen Activator Inhibitor Antigen Assay

Principle

Microplate wells coated with an anti-PAI-1 monoclonal antibody are incubated with samples and standards. PAI-1 present in the samples and standards is bound to the solid phase during this incubation. Unbound substances are then removed by washing. An enzyme-labelled anti-PAI-1 monoclonal antibody (conjugate) is added. The conjugate binds to the antibody–antigen complexes formed in the previous incubation. Unbound conjugate is then removed by washing. Finally enzyme substrate is added. The action of the bound enzyme on the substrate produces a blue colour, which turns yellow after stopping the reaction with acid. The absorbances are read in a microplate reader at 450 nm. The amount of colour is proportional to the concentration of PAI-1. The assay is specific for total PAI-1, including both free and complexed forms.

Specimen Collection

Blood should be collected into CTAD tubes or Diatube H (Stago) and immediately cooled on ice. Vacutainer coagulation tubes with CTAD (Becton-Dickinson) samples can be stored on ice for up to 7 hours in the collection tubes. If the sample is not tested immediately, it should be separated and frozen as soon as possible. (CTAD is a buffered tri-sodium citrate solution with theophylline, adenosine, and dipyridamole.)

Reagents and Method

This is available in a kit based on an ELISA (Chromogenix).

Normal Range

The normal range is usually 11–69 ng/ml. However, each laboratory should establish its own normal range.

Plasmin Inhibitor (α_2 Antiplasmin) Amidolytic Assay

Principle

Plasma dilutions are incubated with excess plasmin, a proportion of which are inhibited by antiplasmins. The residual, uninhibited plasmin is measured using a specific chromogenic substrate. α_2 Antiplasmin is the major circulating inhibitor of plasmin and forms complexes much faster than other inhibitors; if the reaction times are short, the assay effectively measures α_2 antiplasmin only.

Different commercial kits are available containing all the necessary reagents. The manufacturer's instructions should be carefully followed. Specificity is achieved by keeping the reaction times short. Care is required when aliquoting the plasmin solution, which has a high viscosity because of its glycerol content. Note that plasmin bound to α_2 macroglobulin may escape inhibition, thus underestimating inhibitor activity.

The usual normal range is between 0.80 and 1.20 u/ml. Congenital α_2 antiplasmin deficiency is associated with a severe bleeding tendency. A reduced concentration is also found in liver disease, in DIC, and during thrombolytic therapy. α_2 Antiplasmin increases with age and is higher in Caucasians than in Africans.

PLATELET "HYPERREACTIVITY" AND ACTIVATION

Platelets may be more reactive than normal as a consequence of in vivo activation by thrombin or nonendothelial surfaces, such as prosthetic valves or Dacron grafts. This can sometimes be detected by a lowered threshold (increased sensitivity) for aggregating agents. Because there is considerable variation in response to aggregating agents in normal people, the attempts to show platelet hyper-aggregability are rarely successful and the results are frequently inconsistent. Spontaneous aggregation of platelets in the blood can also be demonstrated.[72]

Platelets that have formed a part of a platelet thrombus and have been released into the circulation may show a measurable decrease in their ability to aggregate because of a loss of some granular content. The released contents can be measured in plasma; the α-granule proteins, β-thromboglobulin, and platelet factor 4 are the constituents most commonly measured. Overall the problems with these tests make them of doubtful utility;[56] they are described in previous editions of this book.

Several genetic polymorphisms have been reported to affect the reactivity of platelet glycoproteins and P selectin. Although they may be important in population studies, their clinical significance for individual patients remains unclear.[73-76]

Platelet Activation: Flow Cytometry

The problems associated with previous tests of platelet activation have been circumvented to some extent by the application of flow cytometric analysis of platelets in whole blood samples.

Principle

The activation of platelets is associated with the appearance of new antigenic determinants on the platelet surface. Some of these are molecules present in platelet granules brought to the surface during degranulation (e.g., CD62), and others are new conformations of existing molecules (e.g., GpIIbIIIa). These can by detected using fluorescein-conjugated antibodies, and the degree of expression can be quantified by flow cytometry. This gives a measure of platelet activation with a much greater degree of sensitivity than PF4 or β-TG estimation. Numerous alternative surface molecules are available (Table 17.1). These tests have not yet entered routine laboratory practice but are proving increasingly useful in research.[77,78]

An alternative approach is offered by the PFA-100 (see p. 478) in which short closure times may be indicative of platelet hyperreactivity and/or hyperreactive von Willebrand factor species.

HOMOCYSTEINE

Following the observation that patients with homocystinuria have venous and arterial thromboses with accelerated vascular damage, there has been considerable interest in patients with less marked elevation of plasma homocysteine (hyperhomocystinaemia).[79] This has been shown to have an association with arterial and venous thrombosis.

Until recently, homocysteine has been measured by high-performance liquid chromatography or mass spectroscopy, but an ELISA-based assay is now available that allows it to fit more easily into coagulation laboratory practice. To standardise study results, homocysteine is measured either while fasting or after a methionine load. Rapid processing of samples is required because homocysteine quickly leaches out of red blood cells.

MARKERS OF COAGULATION ACTIVATION

Numerous commercial kits are now available for measuring molecules produced by coagulation activation.

Principle

The activation of many proteins active in coagulation is mediated by proteolytic cleavage with the release of small peptides: activation peptides. The most frequently measured of these is prothrombin fragment 1 + 2, which is released when prothrombin is converted to thrombin. It has an appreciable half-life of approximately 45 min, which allows a measurable concentration to accumulate in plasma and provides an indication of the rate at which thrombin is being generated.

An alternative is to measure the concentration of thrombin–antithrombin complexes (TAT), which provides similar information. Plasmin–antiplasmin

Table 17.1   Indicators of platelet activation detectable by flow cytometry

Name	CD designation	Comment
GpIb, IX, V	CD42	Decreases
GpIIbIIIa	CD41	Increases
Phosphatidyl serine	–	Increases Detected by Annexin V binding
Lysosomal Integral membrane protein (gp53, granulophysin)	CD63	Indicates lysosomal degranulation
P-selection	CD62	Indicates α granule release
Fibrinogen	–	Surface bound fibrinogen increases
IIbIIIa activation	–	Conformation change in IIbIIIa produced by activation, detected by PAC-1 antibody

complexes provide corresponding information about fibrinolysis. These can all be measured using commercially available ELISA kits but are not used routinely and are not required for normal diagnostic work.[80] Other tests such as fibrinopeptide A require exceptional care and the use of specials anti-coagulants to prevent *in vitro* activation of the sample.

ACTIVATED FACTOR VIIa

As discussed in Chapter 16, factor VIIa is thought to be the physiological initiator of coagulation *in vivo;* therefore it is a potentially important thrombogenic factor. Most factor VII circulates in its inactive, zymogen form, but approximately 1% is activated (factor VIIa). Factor VIIa has an unusually long half-life in plasma of approximately 2.5 hours, which helps explain this level and makes its measurement possible.

Principle[81]

The assay is based on the availability of recom-binant soluble tissue factor, which functions as a cofactor for factor VIIa but does not support conversion of factor VII to factor VIIa. The clotting time after addition of soluble tissue factor thus depends on the amount of factor VIIa in the test sample. The test is performed on a dilution of the test plasma in factor VII–deficient plasma to improve specificity. A standard curve is produced using purified VIIa.

Interpretation

The clinical utility of factor VIIa assays is not established; however, elevated levels have been found in some thrombotic disorders such as diabetes and have been implicated as a predictor of ischaemic heart events. Reduced levels are found in patients with factor IX but not factor VIII deficiency.

GLOBAL TEST OF COAGULATION

As a response to the failure of reductive approaches to identify assays that reliably predict thrombosis or thrombotic risk, some workers have moved in the opposite direction and devised global assays that assess the overall coagulation potential of a blood or plasma sample. These tests include the endo-genous thrombin potential (ETP) and the thrombo-elastograph (TEG). Neither of these is in routine diagnostic use. Some manufacturers have developed kits for global assessment of the PC/PS pathway.

REFERENCES

1. Haemostasis, Thrombosis Task Force BCSH 2001 Investigation and management of heritable thrombophilia. British Journal of Haematology 114:512–528.
2. Greaves M 1999 Antiphospholipid antibodies and thrombosis [see comments]. Lancet 353:1348–1353.
3. Brenner B 2004 Clinical management of thrombophilia-related placental vascular complications. Blood 103:4003–4009.
4. Brandt JT, Barna LK, Triplett DA 1995 Laboratory identification of lupus anticoagulants: results of the Second International Workshop for Identification of Lupus Anticoagulants. On behalf of the Subcommittee on Lupus Anticoagulants/Antiphospholipid Antibodies of the ISTH. Thrombosis and Haemostasis 74:1597–1603.
5. British Committee for Standards in Haematology 2000 Guidelines on the investigation and management of the antiphospholipid syndrome. British Journal of Haematology 109:704–715.
6. Exner T, Rickard KA, Kronenberg H 1978 A sensitive test demonstrating lupus anticoagulant and its behavioural patterns. British Journal of Haematology 40:143–151.
7. Lawrie AS, Mackie IJ, Purdy G, et al 1999 The sensitivity and specificity of commercial reagents for the detection of lupus anticoagulant show marked differences in performance between photo-optical and mechanical coagulometers. Thrombosis and Haemostasis 81:758–762.
8. Thiagarajan P, Pengo V, Shapiro SS 1986 The use of the dilute Russell viper venom time for the diagnosis of lupus anticoagulants. Blood 68:869–874.
9. Arnout J, Vanrusselt M, Huybrechts E, et al 1994 Optimization of the dilute prothrombin time for the detection of the lupus anticoagulant by use of a recombinant tissue thromboplastin. British Journal of Haematology 87:94–99.
10. Hoagland LE, Triplett DA, Peng F, et al 1996 APC-resistance as measured by a Textarin time assay:

comparison to the APTT-based method. Thrombosis Research 83:363–373.

11. Moore GW, Smith MP, Savidge GF 2003 The Ecarin time is an improved confirmatory test for the Taipan snake venom time in warfarinized patients with lupus anticoagulants. Blood Coagulation and Fibrinolysis 14:307–312.

12. Jennings I, Kitchen S, Woods TA, et al 1997 Potentially clinically important inaccuracies in testing for the lupus anticoagulant: an analysis of results from three surveys of the UK National External Quality Assessment Scheme (NEQAS) for Blood Coagulation. Thrombosis and Haemostasis 77:934–937.

13. Triplett DA 1996 Antiphospholipid-protein antibodies: clinical use of laboratory test results (identification, predictive value, treatment). Haemostasis 26 (suppl 4):358–367.

14. Kandiah DA, Krilis SA 1996 Laboratory detection of antiphospholipid antibodies. Lupus 5:160–162.

15. Wright SD, Tuddenham EG 1994 Myeloproliferative and metabolic causes. Baillieres Clinical Haematology 7:591–635.

16. Lee AY 2003 Screening for occult cancer in patients with idiopathic venous thromboembolism: no. Journal of Thrombosis and Haemostasis 1:2273–2274.

17. Piccioli A, Prandoni P 2003 Screening for occult cancer in patients with idiopathic venous thromboembolism: yes. Journal of Thrombosis and Haemostasis 1:2271–2272.

18. Lane DA, Mannucci P, Bauer K, et al 1996 Inherited thrombophilia. I. Thrombosis and Haemostasis 76:651–662.

19. Lane DA, Mannucci P, Bauer K, et al 1996 Inherited thrombophilia. II. Thrombosis and Haemostasis 76:824–834.

20. Tollefsen DM 1990 Laboratory diagnosis of antithrombin and heparin cofactor II deficiency. Seminars in Thrombosis and Hemostasis 16:162–168.

21. van Boven HH, Lane DA 1997 Antithrombin and its inherited deficiency states. Seminars in Hematology 34:188–204.

22. Lane DA, Olds RJ, Conard J, et al 1992 Pleiotropic effects of antithrombin strand 1C substitution mutations. Journal of Clinical Investigation 90:2422–2433.

23. Bertina RM 1990 Specificity of protein C and protein S assays. Ricerca in Clinica E in Laboratorio 20:127–138.

24. Marlar RA, Neumann A 1990 Neonatal purpura fulminans due to homozygous protein C or protein S deficiencies. Seminars in Thrombosis and Hemostasis 16:299–309.

25. Mackie IJ, Gallimore M, Machin SJ 1992 Contact factor proteases and the complexes formed with alpha 2-macroglobulin can interfere in protein C assays by cleaving amidolytic substrates. Blood Coagulation and Fibrinolysis 3:589–595.

26. Jones DW, Mackie IJ, Winter M, et al 1991 Detection of protein C deficiency during oral anticoagulant therapy use of the protein C:factor VII ratio. Blood Coagulation and Fibrinolysis 2:407–411.

27. Van Wijnen M, Stam JG, Chang GT, et al 1998 Characterization of mini-protein S, a recombinant variant of protein S that lacks the sex hormone binding globulin-like domain. Biochemical Journal 330:389–396.

28. van Wijnen M, van't Veer C, Meijers JC, et al 1998 A plasma coagulation assay for an activated protein C-independent anticoagulant activity of protein S. Thrombosis and Haemostasis 80:930–935.

29. Comp PC, Doray D, Patton D, et al 1986 An abnormal plasma distribution of protein S occurs in functional protein S deficiency. Blood 67:504–508.

30. Aillaud MF, Pouymayou K, Brunet D, et al 1996 New direct assay of free protein S antigen applied to diagnosis of protein S deficiency. Thrombosis and Haemostasis 75:283–285.

31. Simmonds RE, Zoller BH, Ireland H, et al 1997 Genetic and phenotypic analysis of a large (122 member) protein S deficient kindred provides an explanation for the co-existence of type I and type III plasma phenotypes. Blood 89:4364–4370.

32. Zoller B, Garcia dFP, Dahlback B 1995 Evaluation of the relationship between protein S and C4b-binding protein isoforms in hereditary protein S deficiency demonstrating type I and type III deficiencies to be phenotypic variants of the same genetic disease. Blood 85:3524–3531.

33. Persson KE, Dahlback B, Hillarp A 2003 Diagnosing protein S deficiency: analytical considerations. Clinical Laboratory 49:103–110.

34. Lawrie AS, Lloyd ME, Mohamed F, et al 1995 Assay of protein S in systemic lupus erythematosus. Blood Coagulation and Fibrinolysis 6:322–324.

35. D'Angelo A, Vigano D'Angelo S, Esmon CT, et al 1988 Acquired deficiencies of protein S: protein S activity during oral anticoagulation, in liver disease, and in disseminated intravascular coagulation. Journal of Clinical Investigation 81:1445–1454.

36. Levin M, Eley BS, Louis J, et al 1995 Postinfectious purpura fulminans caused by an autoantibody

directed against protein S. Journal of Pediatrics 127:355–363.

37. Gari M, Falkon L, Urrutia T, et al 1994 The influence of low protein S plasma levels in young women, on the definition of normal range. Thrombosis Research 73:149–152.

38. Faioni EM, Valsecchi C, Palla A, et al 1997 Free protein S deficiency is a risk factor for venous thrombosis. Thrombosis and Haemostasis 78:1343–1346.

39. Garcia de Frutos P, Alim RI, Hardig Y, et al 1994 Differential regulation of alpha and beta chains of C4b-binding protein during acute-phase response resulting in stable plasma levels of free anticoagulant protein S. Blood 84:815–822.

40. Dahlback B, Carlsson M, Svensson PJ 1993 Familial thrombophilia due to a previously unrecognized mechanism characterized by poor anticoagulant response to activated protein C: prediction of a cofactor to activated protein C. Proceedings of the National Academy of Science U.S.A. 90:1004–1008.

41. Bertina RM 1997 Laboratory diagnosis of resistance to activated protein C (APC-resistance). Thrombosis and Haemostasis 78:478–482.

42. Laffan MA, Manning R 1996 The influence of factor VIII on measurement of activated protein C resistance. Blood Coagulation & Fibrinolysis 7:761–765.

43. Koster T, Rosendaal FR, de RH, et al 1993 Venous thrombosis due to poor anticoagulant response to activated protein C: Leiden Thrombophilia Study [see comments]. Lancet 342:1503–1506.

44. Ridker PM, Glynn RJ, Miletich JP, et al 1997 Age-specific incidence rates of venous thromboembolism among heterozygous carriers of factor V Leiden mutation. Annals of Internal Medicine 126:528–531.

45. de Visser MCH, Rosendaal FR, Bertina RM 1999 A reduced sensitivity for activated protein C in the absence of factor V Leiden increases the risk of venous thrombosis. Blood 93:1271–1276.

46. Poort S, Rosendaal F, Reitsma P, et al 1996 A common genetic variation in the 3′ untranslated region of the prothrombin gene is associated with elevated plasma prothrombin levels and an increase in venous thrombosis. Blood 88:3698–3703.

47. Koster T, Blann A, Briet E, et al 1995 Role of clotting factor VIII in effect of von Willebrand factor on occurrence of deep vein thrombosis. Lancet 345:152–155.

48. Meijers JC, Tekelenburg WL, Bouma BN, et al 2000 High levels of coagulation factor XI as a risk factor for venous thrombosis. New England Journal of Medicine 342:696–701.

49. O'Donnell J, Tuddenham EG, Manning R, et al 1997 High prevalence of elevated factor VIII levels in patients referred for thrombophilia screening: role of increased synthesis and relationship to the acute phase reaction. Thrombosis and Haemostasis 77:825–828.

50. Tollefsen DM 2002 Heparin cofactor II deficiency. Archives of Pathology and Laboratory Medicine 126:1394–1400.

51. Lind B, Thorsen S 1999 A novel missense mutation in the human plasmin inhibitor (alpha2-antiplasmin) gene associated with a bleeding tendency. British Journal of Haematology 107:317–322.

52. Fay WP, Parker AC, Condrey LR, et al 1997 Human plasminogen activator inhibitor-1 (PAI-1) deficiency: characterization of a large kindred with a null mutation in the PAI-1 gene. Blood 90:204–208.

53. Lane D, Grant P 2000 Role of hemostatic gene polymorphisms in venous and arterial thrombotic disease. Blood 95:1517–1532.

54. Crowther MA, Roberts J, Roberts R, et al 2001 Fibrinolytic variables in patients with recurrent venous thrombosis: a prospective cohort study. Thrombosis and Haemostasis 85:390–394.

55. Thompson SG, Kienast J, Pyke SD, et al 1995 Hemostatic factors and the risk of myocardial infarction or sudden death in patients with angina pectoris. European Concerted Action on Thrombosis and Disabilities Angina Pectoris Study Group. New England Journal of Medicine 332:635–641.

56. Pyke SD, Thompson SG, Buchwalsky R, et al 1993 Variability over time of haemostatic and other cardiovascular risk factors in patients suffering from angina pectoris. ECAT Angina Pectoris Study Group. Thrombosis and Haemostasis 70:743–746.

57. Juhan VI, Pyke SD, Alessi MC, et al 1996 Fibrinolytic factors and the risk of myocardial infarction or sudden death in patients with angina pectoris. ECAT Study Group. European Concerted Action on Thrombosis and Disabilities. Circulation 94:2057–2063.

58. Ridker PM, Vaughan DE, Stampfer MJ, et al 1993 Endogenous tissue-type plasminogen activator and risk of myocardial infarction. Lancet 341:1165–1168.

59. Kluft C, Meijer P 1996 Update 1996: Blood collection and handling procedures for assessment of plasminogen activators and inhibitors (Leiden fibrinolysis workshop). Fibrinolysis 10:171–179.

60. Dolan G, Greaves M, Cooper P, et al 1988 Thrombovascular disease and familial plasminogen

deficiency: a report of three kindreds. British Journal of Haematology 70:417–421.

61. Heijboer H, Brandjes DP, Buller HR, et al 1990 Deficiencies of coagulation-inhibiting and fibrinolytic proteins in outpatients with deep-vein thrombosis [see comments]. New England Journal of Medicine 323:1512–1516.

62. Wiman B, Chmielewska J 1985 A novel fast inhibitor to tissue plasminogen activator in plasma, which may be of great pathophysiological significance. Scandinavian Journal of Clinical Laboratory Investigation Suppl 177:43–47.

63. Nilsson IM, Ljungner H, Tengborn L 1985 Two different mechanisms in patients with venous thrombosis and defective fibrinolysis: low concentration of plasminogen activator or increased concentration of plasminogen activator inhibitor. British Medical Journal Clinical Research and Education 290:1453–1456.

64. Marsh NA, Gaffney PJ 1977 The rapid fibrin plate: a method for plasminogen activator assay. Thrombosis and Haemostasis 38:545–551.

65. Juhan VI, Valadier J, Alessi MC, et al 1987 Deficient t-PA release and elevated PA inhibitor levels in patients with spontaneous or recurrent deep venous thrombosis. Thrombosis and Haemostasis 57:67–72.

66. Wieczorek I, Ludlam CA, MacGregor I 1993 Venous occlusion does not release von Willebrand factor, factor VIII or PAI-1 from endothelial cells: the importance of consensus on the use of correction factors for haemoconcentration [letter] [see comments]. Thrombosis and Haemostasis 69:91, 93.

67. Marckmann P, Sandstrom B, Jespersen J 1992 The variability of and associations between measures of blood coagulation, fibrinolysis and blood lipids. Atherosclerosis 96:235–244.

68. Stegnar M, Mavri A 1995 Reproducibility of fibrinolytic response to venous occlusion in healthy subjects. Thrombosis and Haemostasis 73:453–457.

69. Mahmoud M, Gaffney PJ 1985 Bioimmunoassay (BIA) of tissue plasminogen activator (t-PA) and its specific inhibitor (t-PA/INH). Thrombosis and Haemostasis 53:356–359.

70. Holvoet P, Cleemput H, Collen D 1985 Assay of human tissue-type plasminogen activator (t-PA) with an enzyme-linked immunosorbent assay (ELISA) based on three murine monoclonal antibodies to t-PA. Thrombosis and Haemostasis 54:684–687.

71. Collen D 1999 The plasminogen (fibrinolytic) system. Thrombosis and Haemostasis 82:259–270.

72. Wu KK, Hoak JC 1976 Spontaneous platelet aggregation in arterial insufficiency: mechanisms and implications. Thrombosis and Haemostasis 35:702–711.

73. Lozano ML, Gonzalez-Conejero R, Corral J, et al 2001 Polymorphisms of P-selectin glycoprotein ligand-1 are associated with neutrophil-platelet adhesion and with ischaemic cerebrovascular disease. British Journal of Haematology 115:969–976.

74. Theodoropoulos I, Christopoulos C, Metcalfe P, et al 2001 The effect of human platelet alloantigen polymorphisms on the in vitro responsiveness to adrenaline and collagen. British Journal of Haematology 114:387–393.

75. Bennett JS, Catella-Lawson F, Rut AR, et al 2001 Effect of the Pl(A2) alloantigen on the function of beta(3)-integrins in platelets. Blood 97:3093–3099.

76. Afshar-Kharghan V, Li CQ, Khoshnevis-Asl M, et al 1999 Kozak sequence polymorphism of the glycoprotein (GP) Ib alpha gene is a major determinant of the plasma membrane levels of the platelet GP Ib-IX-V complex [see comment]. Blood 94:186–191.

77. Abrams CS, Ellison N, Budzynski AZ, et al 1990 Direct detection of activated platelets and platelet-derived microparticles in humans. Blood 75:128–138.

78. Michelson AD 1996 Flow cytometry: a clinical test of platelet function. Blood 87:4925–4936.

79. D'Angelo A, Selhub J 1997 Homocysteine and thrombotic disease. Blood 90:1–11.

80. Bauer KA, Rosenberg RD 1994 Activation markers of coagulation. Baillieres Clinical Haematology 7:523–540.

81. Morrissey JH, Macik BG, Neuenschwander PF, et al 1993 Quantitation of activated factor VII levels in plasma using a tissue factor mutant selectively deficient in promoting factor VII activation. Blood 81:734–744.

18 Laboratory control of anticoagulant, thrombolytic, and antiplatelet therapy

Mike Laffan and Richard Manning

Anticoagulant and antithrombotic therapy is given in various doses to prevent formation or propagation of thrombus. Apart from those that act via fibrinolysis, anticoagulant drugs have little if any effect on an already-formed thrombus. There are five main classes of drugs that require consideration:

1. Oral anticoagulants, coumarins, and indanediones, which act by interfering with the γ-carboxylation step in the synthesis of the vitamin K–dependent factors (see p. 385).
2. Heparin and heparinoids (low molecular weight and synthetic compounds), which have a complex action on haemostasis, the main effect being the potentiation and acceleration of the effect of antithrombin on thrombin and factor Xa.
3. Defibrinating agents such as ancrod (Arvin) and Reptilase, which induce hypocoagulability by the removal of fibrinogen from the blood.
4. Direct thrombin inhibitors, such as hirudin (natural or recombinant), which is a highly specific inhibitor of thrombin and thus a potent anticoagulant. New orally active thrombin inhibitors are now undergoing clinical trials.
5. Antiplatelet drugs such as aspirin, nonsteroidal anti-inflammatory drugs, dipyridamole and

clopidogrel, and inhibitors of IIb/IIIa function, some of which are antibodies.

ORAL ANTICOAGULANT TREATMENT

It is not possible to produce a therapeutic reduction in thrombotic tendency without increasing the risk of haemorrhage. The purpose of laboratory control is to maintain a level of hypocoagulability that effectively minimises the combined risks of haemorrhage and thrombosis: the therapeutic range. Individual responses to oral anticoagulant treatment[1] are extremely variable and so must be regularly and frequently controlled by laboratory tests to ensure that the anticoagulant effect remains within the therapeutic range.

Selection of Patients

Haemostasis is not usually investigated before starting oral anticoagulant treatment, but it is advisable to perform the first-line coagulation screen (prothrombin time [PT], activated partial thromboplastin time [APTT], thrombin time [TT], and platelet count). An abnormality of these tests must be investigated because a contraindication to the use of oral anticoagulants may be revealed and the tests may be used for controlling anticoagulant effect. History and clinical examination should be assessed to ensure that no local or general haemorrhagic diathesis exists.

Methods Used for the Laboratory Control of Oral Anticoagulant Treatment

The one-stage PT of Quick is the most commonly used test. Originally, lack of standardisation of the thromboplastin preparations and methods of expressing the PT results led to great discrepancies in the reported results and hence also in anticoagulant dosage. The use of ISI, the International Sensitivity Index, to assess the sensitivity of any given thromboplastin, and the use of INR, the International Normalized Ratio, to report the results, has minimised these difficulties and greatly improved uniformity of anticoagulation and interpretation throughout the world.

Chromogenic substrates have been used for the control of anticoagulant treatment in factor X, VII, or II assays. Although it is possible to use such a single factor measurement, it must be remembered that the one-stage PT measures the effect of three vitamin K–dependent factors (factors VII, X, and II) and is also affected by the presence of PIVKAs (proteins induced by vitamin K absence or antagonism) or the acarboxy forms of vitamin K–dependent factors. It thus gives a better assessment of the situation *in vivo*. Chromogenic substrate assays may be of use where the presence of an inhibitor invalidates the PT and coagulation-based assays.

The Thrombotest of Owren and the prothrombin and proconvertin (P&P) method of Owren and Aas were used in the past, but they are no longer recommended for oral anticoagulant control.

Standardisation of Oral Anticoagulant Treatment

Standardisation of oral anticoagulant therapy comprises the following steps:

1. A thromboplastin is chosen, and its ISI is determined by comparison with a reference thromboplastin.
2. The log mean normal PT is determined for that thromboplastin.
3. PTs are performed on patient samples, and the results are converted to an INR.

Reference thromboplastins (rabbit and bovine) are available as World Health Organization (WHO) Reference Preparations or certified reference materials from the European Union Bureau of Reference (BCR) (see p. 695). All the reference preparations have been calibrated in terms of a primary WHO reference of human brain thromboplastin, which was established in 1967.

The following terms are used in the calibration procedure described below:

International Sensitivity Index (ISI)[2] This is the slope of the calibration line obtained when the PTs obtained with the reference preparation are plotted on the vertical axis of log–log paper and the PTs obtained by the test thromboplastin are plotted on the horizontal axis. The same normal and anticoagulated patient's plasma samples are used for both sets of results.

International Normalized Ratio (INR) This is the PT ratio, which, by calculation, would have been obtained had the original primary, human reference thromboplastin been used to perform the PT.

Calibration of Thromboplastins

Principle

The test thromboplastin must be calibrated against a reference thromboplastin of the same species (rabbit vs. rabbit, bovine vs. bovine).[3] All reference preparations are calibrated in terms of the primary material of human origin and have an ISI, which is assigned after a collaborative trial involving many laboratories from different countries.

Reagents

Normal citrated plasma.
From 20 healthy donors.

Anticoagulated plasma.
From 60 patients stabilised on oral anticoagulant treatment for at least 6 weeks.

The tests need not all be done at the same time but may be carried out on freshly collected samples on successive days.

Reference and test thromboplastins.

CaCl₂.
0.025 mol/l.

Method

Carry out PT tests as described on p. 398. Allow the plasma and thromboplastin to warm up to 37°C for at least 2 min before mixing or adding $CaCl_2$. Test each plasma in duplicate with each of the two thromboplastins in the following order with minimum delay between tests:

	Reference Thromboplastin	Test Thromboplastin
Plasma 1	Test 1	Test 2
	Test 4	Test 3
Plasma 2	Test 5	Test 6
	Test 8	Test 7, etc.

Record the mean time for each plasma. If there is a discrepancy of more than 10% in the clotting times between duplicates, repeat the test on that plasma.

Calibration

Plot the PTs on log–log graph paper, with results using the reference preparation (y) on the vertical axis and results with the test thromboplastin (x) on the horizontal axis (Fig. 18.1). On arithmetic paper, it is necessary to plot the logarithms of the PTs (Fig. 18.2). The relationship between the two thromboplastins is determined by the slope of the line (b).

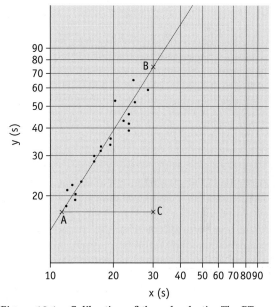

Figure 18.1 **Calibration of thromboplastin.** The PTs (in seconds) with the test thromboplastin are plotted on the horizontal axis (x) and with the reference thromboplastin on the vertical axis (y) on double log graph paper. The best-fit line is drawn by eye, and the slope is obtained as follows: Points (a) and (b) are marked on the line just below the lowest recorded PT and just above the longest recorded PT, respectively, (c) and a vertical through (b) meet. The distance between (b) and (c) is measured accurately in mm. The slope

$$b = \frac{[B \text{ to } C]}{[A \text{ to } C]}.$$ In this example B to C = 55 mm,

A to C = 35 mm, $b = 55/35 = 1.57$. The ISI of the reference thromboplastin was 1.11. Therefore, the ISI of the test thromboplastin = 1.11 × 1.57 = 1.74.

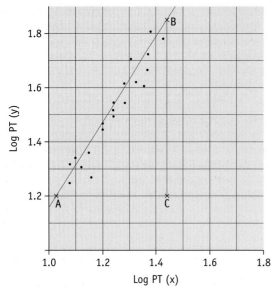

Figure 18.2   Calibration of thromboplastin. The PTs (in seconds) are converted to their logarithms which are plotted on arithmetic graph paper. The slope is calculated as in Figure 18.1. In this example, A to C = 42 mm, B to C = 65 mm, b = 65/42 = 1.54. Therefore, ISI = 1.11 × 1.54 = 1.71.

An estimate of the slope can be obtained as shown in Figures 18.1 and 18.2; this can then be used to obtain an approximation of the ISI of the test thromboplastin.

Whenever possible, however, to obtain a reliable measurement, the following more complicated calculation should be used instead.

Calculation of International Sensitivity Index

The natural logarithms of the PTs obtained using the reference thromboplastin and the test thromboplastin are called y_i and x_i, respectively, where $i=1,2,3....N$ for N pairs of results.

The following designations are then made:

x_0 and y_0 are the arithmetic means of the N values of x_i and y_i, respectively.

Q_1 and Q_2 are the sums of the squares of $(x_i - x_0)$ and $(y_i - y_0)$, respectively.
P is the sum of their products $\Sigma(x_i - x_0)(y_i - y_0)$

$$E = (Q_2 - Q_1)^2 + 4P^2$$

$$\text{And } b = \frac{Q_2 - Q_1 + E^{1/2}}{2P}$$

where b is the slope of the graph. The ISI of the preparation under test (ISI_t) is then given by the following:

$$ISI_t = ISI_{IRP} \times b$$

where IRP stands for International Reference Preparation.

Local Calibration of Thromboplastins

Although the ISI system has been very effective in standardising anticoagulant control and improving agreement between laboratories, it is not perfect. One reason is that the ISI of a thromboplastin may vary according to the coagulometer used and even with different models of the same instrument. To circumvent this, a system of local calibration has been suggested. In this system, a set of plasmas with an assigned INR are tested with the local thromboplastin–machine combination. These results are used to generate a standard curve from which the INRs of further test plasmas can be read by interpolation. In effect, the ISI of the system is determined in a reverse fashion.[3,4]

Mean Normal Prothrombin Time

The mean normal PT for each batch of thromboplastin should be determined by testing 20 normal samples or blood donors. An equal number of males and females should be tested.

Calibration Audits

External quality-assurance surveys (e.g., UKNEQAS, see p. 667) will reflect differences regarding thromboplastin–machine combinations but not differences in blood sampling techniques (i.e., capillary and venous blood sampling). This can be a problem when capillary blood sampling is used in an outpatient setting, whereas venous samples are taken for inpatient anticoagulant monitoring. Regular audits comparing results from a range of patients whose blood has been sampled by both capillary and venous techniques will provide information not provided by NEQAS surveys.[4,5]

Determination of the International Normalized Ratio

It is essential to use a thromboplastin whose ISI has been determined either by the commercial supplier or (preferably) according to a local, regional, or national procedure. The PT result can then be expressed as an INR. Using the INR/ISI system, the patients' INR should be the same in any laboratory in the world. To ensure safety and uniformity of anticoagulation, the results should be reported as an INR, either alone or in parallel with the locally accepted method of reporting.

INR = Prothrombin time ratio obtained using the test thromboplastin to the power of the ISI of the test reagent. The PT ratio is calculated using the patient's test result and the log mean normal prothrombin time (LMPT) from 20 normal donors:
$$INR = (PT\ patient/LMNPT)^{ISI}$$

For example, a ratio of 2.5 using a thromboplastin with ISI of 1.4 can be calculated from the formula to be $2.5^{1.4} = 3.61$, which is either read from a logarithmic table or calculated on an electronic calculator.

The LMNPT is the logarithmic mean normal PT (i.e., $e^{(\Sigma lnPT/N)}$). In this way the level of anticoagulation in all plasma samples can be compared and a meaningful therapeutic range can be established regardless of the thromboplastin used.

Capillary Reagent

Reagents are commercially available for monitoring the INR using samples of capillary blood. These are usually a mixture of thromboplastin, calcium, and adsorbed plasma so that when whole blood is added the reagent measures the overall clotting activity; it is sensitive to deficiency of factors II, VII, and X. The reagents have an ISI assigned to

them in the same way as individual thromboplastins, and the INR is calculated from the PT ratio. These reagents are frequently used in anticoagulant clinics when a large number of INRs need to be performed rapidly and in point-of-care testing (p. 637).

Therapeutic Range and Choice of Thromboplastin

Several authorities have now published recommended therapeutic ranges denoting the appropriate degree of anticoagulation in different clinical circumstances.[1,6,7] These are partly based on controlled clinical trials but to some extent also represent a consensus on practice that has emerged over many years.

The choice of thromboplastin largely determines the accuracy with which anticoagulant control can be maintained. If the ISI of the thromboplastin is high, then a small change in PT represents a large change in the degree of anticoagulation. This affects the precision of the analysis, and the coefficient of variation for the test increases with the ISI. Moreover, the prothrombin ratio range becomes very small for any given range of INR. This is illustrated in Figure 18.3 and Table 18.1. For these reasons it is strongly recommended that a thromboplastin with a low ISI (i.e., close to 1) is used.

Management of Overanticoagulation

The approach to management of a patient whose INR exceeds the therapeutic range with or without bleeding is shown in Table 18.2.[6]

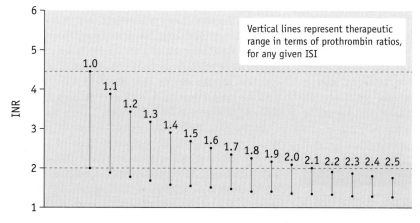

Vertical lines represent therapeutic range in terms of prothrombin ratios, for any given ISI

Figure 18.3 The ratios obtained with thromboplastins with given ISI values equivalent to INR therapeutic range of 2.0–4.5. (Slightly modified, from Poller L 1987 Oral anticoagulant therapy. In: Bloom AL, Thomas DP (eds) Haemostasis and thrombosis, 2nd edn. Churchill Livingstone, Edinburgh with the permission of the editors and the publisher.)

Table 18.1   Therapeutic ranges equivalent to an INR of 2.0–4.0 using different commercial thromboplastins. (Modified from Poller L 1987 Oral anticoagulant therapy. In: Bloom AL, Thomas DP (eds) Haemostasis and thrombosis, 2nd edn. Churchill Livingstone, Edinburgh, p. 870.)

Thromboplastin	ISI	Ratios equivalent to INR 2.0–4.0
Thrombotest	1.03	2.0–3.8
Thromborel	1.23	1.7–3.1
Dade FS	1.35	1.65–2.8
Simplastin	2.0	1.3–2.0
Boehringer	2.1	1.35–1.9
Ortho	2.3	1.3–1.8

ISI, International Sensitivity Index; INR, International Normalized Ratio

Table 18.2   Recommendations for management of bleeding and excessive anticoagulation

3.0 < INR < 6.0 (target INR 2.5)	1. Reduce warfarin dose or stop
4.0 < INR < 6.0 (target INR 3.5)	2. Restart warfarin when INR < 5.0
6.0 < INR < 8.0 No bleeding or minor bleeding	1. Stop warfarin 2. Restart when INR < 5.0
INR > 8.0 No bleeding or minor bleeding	1. Stop warfarin 2. Restart warfarin when INR < 5.0 3. If other risk factors for bleeding give 0.5–2.5 mg of vitamin K (oral or IV)
Major bleeding	1. Stop warfarin 2. Give prothrombin complex concentrate 50 u/kg of FFP 15 ml/kg 3. Give 5 mg of vitamin K (oral or IV)

FFP, fresh-frozen plasma; INR, International Normalized Ratio

Point-of-Care Testing

There are now schemes for monitoring INR at point of care outside the hospital clinic. These require selection and standardisation of appropriate analysers and a quality-control programme that includes participation in an external quality assessment scheme. It is essential to have liaison with the local laboratory for training of staff and supervision of the quality-control programme. There should be an established procedure for checking any problems of instrument performance and for referring to the specialist centre patients who are difficult to control.[8,9]

Self-management of warfarin treatment akin to home glucose monitoring may also be an effective point-of-care procedure for selected patients. They should first attend two or more training sessions on the use and quality control of the appropriate analyser, interpretation of INR in terms of adjustment of their warfarin dosage, and guidance on when it is necessary to be seen at the specialist clinic.[10] (See p. 634.)

HEPARIN TREATMENT

The anticoagulant action of heparin is primarily a result of its ability to bind to antithrombin (AT), thereby accelerating and enhancing the latter's rate of inhibition of the major coagulation enzymes (i.e., factors IIa and Xa and to lesser extents IXa, XIa, and XIIa). The two main effects of heparin, the AT and the anti-Xa effects, are differentially dependent on the size of the heparin molecule. The basic minimum sequence needed to obtain anticoagulant activity has been identified as a pentasaccharide unit. Of the molecules containing this pentasaccharide, those comprising less than 18 saccharide units and of molecular weight less than 5000 can only augment inhibitory activity of AT against Xa. In contrast, longer chains can augment AT activity as well by formation of a tertiary complex bridging both AT and thrombin molecules.

Hence low molecular weight heparins (LMWH), which have an average molecular mass of 5000 Da, have a ratio of anti-Xa to antithrombin effect of 2–5 compared to that of unfractionated heparin (UFH), which is defined as 1. However, all heparin preparations are heterogeneous mixtures of molecules with different molecular weight and many do not contain the crucial pentasaccharide sequence. Heparin also produces some anticoagulant effect by promoting the release of tissue factor pathway inhibitor (TFPI) from the surface endothelium (see p. 386).

Selection of Patients

It is advisable to perform the first-line tests of haemostasis as described in Chapter 16 before starting treatment. In the presence of a reduced platelet count or deranged coagulation, heparin may be contraindicated or, if used, the dose must be reduced.

Laboratory Control of Heparin Treatment[11]

The pharmacokinetics of heparins are extremely complicated, partly because of the variation in molecule size. Large molecules are cleared by a rapid saturable cellular mechanism and bind to numerous acute-phase proteins such as von Willebrand factor and fibronectin. Smaller molecules are cleared by a nonsaturable renal route and bind less to plasma proteins. As a result therapeutic doses of UFH result in a variable degree of anticoagulation and require close monitoring (Table 18.3). The dose-response relationship is much more predictable for the LMWHs, and most trials have not monitored therapy with these agents, which are simply given on a "units per kg" basis. Thus the approach to monitoring heparin therapy varies according to the type of heparin used and the clinical circumstance.

Prophylactic therapy with either UFH or LMWH is given by subcutaneous injection and is usually not monitored. However, LMWH may be monitored in some circumstances when it is expected that pharmacokinetics may be altered, such as during pregnancy and in renal failure. A blood sample is taken 2–4 hours after injection to detect the peak heparin level. Some authors have also measured trough levels prior to injection.

Therapeutic treatment with UFH is given by continuous intravenous infusion and is usually monitored using the APTT, which is repeated 6 hours after every dose change. Rarely, therapeutic UFH is given twice daily by subcutaneous injection, in which case samples for testing should be taken at the midpoint between injections. If heparin resistance is suspected, then an anti-Xa assay must be performed.

Therapeutic treatment with LMWH is not monitored except when the dose-response relationship is expected to be altered such as in the case of pregnancy, children, and renal failure. LMWHs produce relatively little effect on the APTT, and if monitoring is required, a specific heparin assay must be

Table 18.3 Tests used in the laboratory control of heparin treatment

Test	Advantages	Disadvantages
Whole blood clotting time	Simple, inexpensive, no equipment needed	Time consuming, can only be carried out at the bedside, one at a time, insensitive to <0.4 iu and to LMW heparins
APTT	Simple, many tests can be carried out in parallel	Not all reagents sensitive to heparin, insensitive to <0.2 iu and to LMW heparins, affected by variables other than heparin
TT	Simple, many tests can be carried out in parallel	Insensitive to <0.2 iu and to LMW heparins
Protamine neutralisation	Sensitive to all concentrations	Time consuming and insensitive to LMW heparins
Anti-Xa assays	Sensitive to all concentrations and to LMWT heparins	Expensive if commercial kits used; time consuming if home-made reagents used

APTT, activated partial thromboplastin time; LMW, low molecular weight; TT, thrombin time used. The result will then be reported as heparin activity in u/ml. In general, unless stated otherwise, this is measured as anti-Xa activity. An international standard for LMWH is now available.[12]

It is important to note that therapeutic levels of LMWH may be present without producing prolongation of PT, APTT, or TT. The dose-response curve of the TT is too steep to make it useful for monitoring heparin therapy. However, it is very sensitive to the presence of UFH and is a useful laboratory indicator of its presence.

Activated Partial Thromboplastin Time for Heparin Monitoring

Principle

The APTT is currently the most widely used test for monitoring unfractionated heparin therapy.[6] It is very sensitive to heparin but has a number of shortcomings that must be kept in mind. First, different APTT reagents have different sensitivities to heparin. It is important to establish that the reagent in use has a linear relationship between clotting times and heparin concentration in the therapeutic range (0.3–0.7 iu/ml). An example of different responses is shown in Fig. 18.4. The result is expressed as a ratio of the time obtained with that for the normal pool containing no heparin (often called "the heparin ratio").

The second shortcoming of the APTT in the control of heparin treatment is that the APTT is affected by a number of variables not related to heparin. The most important of these are fibrinogen and factor VIII:C concentration and the presence of fibrinogen/fibrin degradation products (FDP). When these factors are abnormal, there may be dissociation of the APTT and heparin level causing "apparent heparin resistance." In these circumstances a heparin assay must be performed. Last, the use of the APTT may be rendered invalid by the presence of inhibitors, factor deficiency (including liver disease), or other coagulation active drugs. In severely ill patients a significant prolongation of the APTT may arise from disseminated intravascular coagulation (DIC) or haemodilution, giving a misleading impression of heparin effect.

Reagents and Method

The reagents and method are described on p. 400.

Therapeutic Range

The therapeutic range for heparin is 0.3–0.7 iu/ml by anti-Xa assay and 0.2–0.4 units by protamine titration. The prolongation of the APTT achieved with these concentrations varies between reagents according to the reagents and coagulometer used. The results may be expressed as clotting time in seconds or as a ratio. For the majority of sensitive reagents, ratios of 1.5–3.0 cover the therapeutic range, but this must be determined for each reagent and, ideally, each batch of reagent. It is important that samples from patients treated with heparin are used for calibration because these give significantly

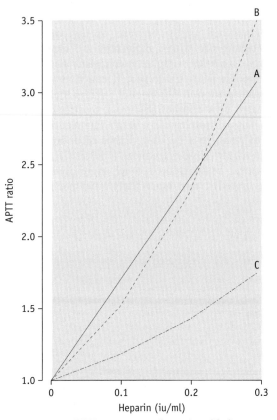

Figure 18.4   APTT response to heparin added to plasma in vitro. APTT response expressed as ratio (APTT of heparinized plasma/APTT of plasma without heparin). Three different reagents and methods shown. (Slightly modified, from Thomson JM (ed) 1985 Blood coagulation and haemostasis. A practical guide. Churchill Livingstone, Edinburgh, p 370, with the permission of the editor and the publisher.)

different results from those obtained when normal plasma is "spiked" with heparin. Regression analysis is used to determine the normal range, and a better fit may be obtained using logarithmically transformed APTT values.

Heparin Monitoring at the Bedside[13]

The whole blood activated clotting time (ACT) is routinely used to assess heparin effects during cardiac surgery. However, the ACT is not a specific assay for heparin and may be influenced by several other factors such as hypothermia, haemodilution, and platelet dysfunction. For these reasons the ACT may be misleading with regard to the proper administration of heparin and protamine.

Principle

The ACT is determined by using one of several different clotting cascade activators, such as kaolin or celite (diatomaceous earth activator), and a method of end-point detection such as optical or electro-magnetic. No additional phospholipid is added.

ACT monitors include the *Hemochron ACT monitors* (International Technidyne, Inc, Edison, NJ), and the *HemoTec Automated Coagulation Timer* (HemoTec, Inc., Englewood, CO). The Hemochron ACT monitor uses 2.0 ml of whole blood in glass tubes with celite. The HemoTec ACT monitor uses 0.8 ml of whole blood in dual-chamber, high-range kaolin cartridges. The ACT is thus primarily a system with little laboratory involvement.

Anti-Xa Assay for Heparin

Principle

Plasma anti-Xa activity as a result of antithrombin is enhanced by the addition of heparin, and either a coagulation or amidolytic (chromogenic) assay of anti-Xa activity can be adapted to measure this effect. A standard curve is constructed by adding varying amounts of heparin to a normal plasma pool, which provides the source of the antithrombin. A known amount of Xa is added and after incubation, the amount of Xa remaining is assayed by chromogenic or coagulation-based assay. A number of commercial kits such as Heptest and Hepaclot, as well as various kits based on chromogenic substrates, are in use and give linear and reproducible responses.

A standard curve should be constructed that is appropriate for the level of heparin expected. Some but not all assays add an exogenous source of antithrombin to the test sample, but it is not clear how important this is in patients with low antithrombin levels.

Chromogenic Method

The assay is performed as instructed with the kit. The concentration of heparin is read off a standard curve constructed according to the manufacturer's instructions.

Clotting Method

Principle

The anti-Xa activity of antithrombin III is enhanced by the addition of heparin. The inhibition of factor Xa by heparin is measured in a modified factor-X assay.

Reagents

Pooled normal plasma. From 20 normal donors.
Patient's plasma. Citrated platelet-poor plasma (PPP) should be collected between 2 and 4 hours after the injection of heparin; it should be tested as soon as possible after the collection and kept at 4°C or on crushed ice until tested.
Buffer. Trisodium citrate 30 vol, glyoxaline buffer (p. 398) 150 volumes, and 20% bovine albumin 1 volume.
Commercially prepared artificial factor X deficient plasma. Reconstitute according to instructions.
Platelet substitute. Mix equal volumes of factor X deficient plasma and platelet substitute. This is the working reagent and is kept at 37°C.
Factor Xa. Reconstitute as instructed by the manufacturer. Dilute further in the buffer to give a 1 in 100 dilution. Keep on crushed ice until used.
Heparin. 1000 iu/ml. Dilute in 9 g/l NaCl to 10 iu/ml. Ideally, the same batch of heparin as the patient is receiving should be used.
$CaCl_2$. 0.025 mol/l.

Method

A standard curve is constructed as shown in Table 18.4. Add 0.05 ml of each dilution to 0.45 ml of the normal plasma pool. This will give final concentra-

Table 18.4 Preparation of a standard curve for an anti–Xa assay

Reagent	Tube					
	1	2	3	4	5	6
Heparin (10 iu/ml)	0.05	0.10	0.15	0.20	0.25	0.30
Saline (ml)	0.95	0.90	0.85	0.80	0.75	0.70
Concentration of heparin (iu/ml)	0.5	1.0	1.5	2.0	2.5	3.0
Final conc. of heparin after addition to normal plasma pool	0.05	0.10	0.15	0.20	0.25	0.30

tions of heparin from 0.05 to 0.30 iu/ml in 0.05 iu steps.

Pipette 0.3 ml of diluted factor Xa into a large glass tube at 37°C.

Add 0.1 ml of the first standard dilution. Start the stopwatch. At 1 min and 30 s exactly transfer duplicate 0.1 ml volumes of the mixture into two tubes each containing 0.1 ml of prewarmed CaCl$_2$.

At 2 min after subsampling add 0.2 ml of the mixture of factor X deficient plasma and platelet substitute, start the stopwatch, mix, and record the clotting time.

Repeat for each dilution of standard. The patient's sample is tested undiluted in pooled normal plasma if the clotting time is longer than the times used to construct the standard curve.

Calculation

Plot the clotting times against the heparin concentration on log-linear graph paper, with the clotting times on the linear axis. The concentration of heparin in the patient's sample can be read directly from the standard curve. It is multiplied by the dilution factor if necessary.

Protamine Neutralization Test

Principle

This test is an extension of the TT, various amounts of protamine sulphate being added to the plasma before the addition of thrombin. When all the heparin present in plasma has been neutralised, the clotting time should become normal. The concentration of heparin in the plasma can be calculated from the amount of protamine sulphate required to produce this effect. The protamine neutralisation test is used mainly to calculate the dose of protamine sulphate needed to neutralise circulating heparin after cardiopulmonary surgery and haemodialysis, but it is also used to control treatment or to calculate the dose of protamine to be administered if the patient needs rapid reversal of heparinisation.

Reagents

Protamine sulphate.
Prepare dilutions (0–50 mg/ml) in barbitone buffer, pH 7.4. Dilute 5 ml of protamine sulphate (10 g/l) 1 in 20 with buffer to give 1 dl of a stock solution containing 500 µg/ml. Then make working solutions to cover the range of 0–500 µg/ml in 50 µg steps from the stock solution by dilution with buffer. The solutions keep indefinitely at 4°C.

Thrombin.
Dilute thrombin in barbitone buffer to a concentration of about 20 NIH u/ml. Adjust the concentration so that 0.1 ml of thrombin clots 0.2 ml of normal plasma at 37°C in 10 ± 1 s. Keep the thrombin in a plastic tube in melting ice during the assay.

Plasma.
Citrated PPP from the patient.

Method

Place 0.2 ml of test plasma and 20 µl of barbitone buffer in a glass tube kept in a waterbath at 37°C. Allow the mixture to warm and then add 0.1 ml of thrombin. Record the clotting time. If this is c 10 s, there is no demonstrable heparin in the plasma. If the TT is prolonged, repeat the test using 20 µl of the 500 µg/ml protamine solution instead of buffer. Repeat the test if necessary, until a concentration of protamine is found that gives a clotting time of c 10 s.

Calculation

If 20 µl of 150 µg/ml protamine sulphate produce a normal TT (whereas the clotting time is prolonged with 100 µg/ml protamine), then the concentration of 15 µg of protamine is sufficient to neutralise the heparin in 1 ml of plasma. Assuming weight-for-weight neutralisation, the patient's plasma contains 15 µg of heparin per ml or 1.5 iu, assuming that 1 mg of heparin is equivalent to 100 iu. This figure can be further converted to concentration of heparin per ml of whole blood by multiplying by 1 – PCV.

In the previous example, for *in vivo* neutralisation of heparin by protamine sulphate, assuming a total blood volume of 75 ml per kg body weight, the required dose of protamine would be as follows:

$$\frac{15 \times 75 \times \text{body weight} \times (1 - \text{PCV}) \text{ mg}}{1000 \text{ mg}}$$

Heparin-Induced Thrombocytopenia

Most patients receiving unfractionated heparin experience a small and immediate drop in their platelet count. This is referred to as type I HIT (heparin-induced thrombocytopenia) and is completely harmless. It is thought to arise as a result of heparin binding to platelets. A second more serious thrombocytopenia (type II HIT) is seen in approximately 5% of patients receiving UFH and is a result of development of antibodies against heparin-PF4 complexes. These bind to and activate platelets via the FCRγII, resulting in accelerated clearance. Type II HIT develops 5–12 days after starting heparin therapy and causes a profound decrease in platelets to <50% of preheparin value and usually <50 × 10^9/l. The process of activation sometimes results in arterial and venous platelet thrombus formation particularly in patients who are ill or septic, and skin necrosis has also been reported. This syndrome of heparin-induced thrombocytopenia and thrombosis (HITT) has a high mortality. Heparin must be stopped immediately, and alternative immediate-acting anticoagulation must be instituted.[14]

The diagnosis of HIT is primarily clinical, and there is no test that can be performed with sufficient speed, sensitivity, and specificity to be of use in making the primary decision to stop heparin. However, confirmatory information is useful and a number of tests can be performed to substantiate the diagnosis.[15] These may be either *functional* tests in which platelet activation is detected or *immunological* tests in which the presence of PF4-heparin dependent antibodies are detected. Examples of the former include what is regarded as the "gold standard" test, the serotonin release assay,[16] but this is too cumbersome and inconvenient for routine use. Alternatives are heparin-induced platelet aggregation and flow cytometry–based tests.[17,18] The simplest for routine use is a modified platelet aggregation test as described in the following section. Immunological tests, including enzyme-linked immunosorbent assay (ELISA), which is also a particle gel immunoassay.[19] Although the immunological tests appear to have greater sensitivity and are more easily reproducible, they do not demonstrate the functional significance of the antibodies.

Heparin-Induced Thrombocytopenia: Detection by Platelet Aggregation

Addition of heparin to the patient's PPP results in heparin/PF4 complexes that are bound by the pathological antibody. The antibody–heparin/PF4 complexes then bind to and activate the platelets. Platelet activation is detected as aggregation.

Principle

Blood is centrifuged gently to obtain platelet rich plasma (PRP), which is stirred in a cuvette at 37°C, between a light source and a photocell.

Reagents

Normal Control Platelet Rich Plasma (PRP)
Preferably blood group O or the same group as the patient should be used. For method see page 427. A platelet count is performed on the PRP. The number of platelets will influence aggregation response if the count falls outside a range of 200–400 × 10^9/l. If necessary the PRP is adjusted to give a platelet count of 300 × 10^9/l by diluting with control platelet poor plasma (PPP).

Patient and normal control PPP is obtained by centrifuging at 2000 g for 20 min. Check that the platelet count is zero.

Heparin
A sample of the type (batch identical) of heparin previously given to the patient is required. The heparin is diluted to give working concentrations of 10 and 20 u/ml (final concentration of 1.0 and 2.0 u/ml).

Method

Following the scheme shown in Table 18.5, four aggregation cuvettes are set up. Add 300 µl of normal PRP to each cuvette. Then add 200 µl of the appropriate patient or control PPP, along with a magnetic stir bar. Set the 100% baselines with the normal control PPP and the 0% baselines with PRP and PPP. Set the stir rate at 1200 rev/min. Observe the baselines for 1 min. Initiate aggregation by the addition of 50 µl of either heparin or saline. Observe aggregation for a minimum of 15 min (Fig. 18.5).

Interpretation

1. If aggregation is observed in cuvette 4 with a final heparin concentration of 1.0 and 2.0 u/ml, the test is repeated using normal platelets, patient plasma, and a final heparin concentration of 0.2 u/ml.
2. Aggregation observed in cuvette 4 only, with subsequent demonstration of heparin at a final concentration of 0.2 u/ml, is considered positive for heparin-induced platelet aggregation.
   Alternatively, aggregation can be repeated with a much higher final concentration of heparin (10 u/ml). Inhibition of aggregation is suggestive of heparin-induced platelet aggregation.
3. Aggregation observed in cuvette 4 without demonstration of aggregation with the lower concentration of heparin is considered questionable.
4. Aggregation observed in cuvettes 1, 2, or 3 indicates that the reaction may be a result of some-

thing other than heparin-induced platelet aggregation and the test is repeated using different normal donor platelets and control PPP.

With experience subjective assessment of aggregation responses is usually sufficient for clinical interpretation. A positive test result is shown in Figure 18.5. The total amount of aggregation seen may be reported.

Technical Problems

See platelet aggregation (p. 427).

The literature suggests that test sensitivity can be improved by the use of the patient's own platelets, platelets from selected donors known to be reactive in the assay, or washed platelets. The reactivity of the donor platelets can be established by using a known positive serum. Test specificity may be enhanced by the use of two point assays that include neutralisation of the reaction by a high dose of heparin.

Detection by Diamed Heparin-PF4 Antibody Test

The Diamed Heparin-PF4 antibody test is a particle gel immunoassay consisting of red-coloured polymer particles coated with Heparin-PF4 complex. When the patient's serum is mixed with the polymer

Table 18.5 The combinations of platelets, plasma, and heparin required to test for heparin-induced thrombocytopenia

	Cuvette 1	Cuvette 2	Cuvette 3	Cuvette 4
Normal control PRP	300 µl	300 µl	300 µl	300 µl
Patient PPP	None	200 µl	None	200 µl
Normal control PPP	200 µl	None	200 µl	None
Heparin (10 or 20 iu/ml)	None	None	50 µl	50 µl
Saline (0.85%)	50 µl	50 µl	None	None

PRP, platelet-rich plasma; PPP, platelet-poor plasma.

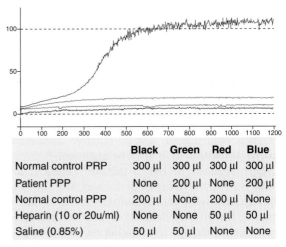

	Black	Green	Red	Blue
Normal control PRP	300 µl	300 µl	300 µl	300 µl
Patient PPP	None	200 µl	None	200 µl
Normal control PPP	200 µl	None	200 µl	None
Heparin (10 or 20u/ml)	None	None	50 µl	50 µl
Saline (0.85%)	50 µl	50 µl	None	None

Figure 18.5 The combinations of platelets, plasma, and heparin required to test for heparin-induced thrombocytopenia shown in Table 18-5. The aggregation traces show that platelet aggregation occurs only when the patient plasma is exposed to heparin (blue trace).

particles, specific antibodies react with the Heparin-PF4 complex on the particle surface, resulting in particle agglutination. The particles are centrifuged through a gel filtration matrix, agglutinated particles are trapped on top of the gel or within the gel, and nonagglutinated particles form a button at the bottom of the tube. The result can be read visually.

Hirudin

Recombinant manufactured hirudin is now available and licensed for both prophylactic and therapeutic use in some indications. It is a direct thrombin inhibitor and is given intravenously or subcutaneously. It is most easily monitored using the APTT with the same target range as for heparin. The TT may be prolonged and will be corrected using Reptilase. An alternative measure is the Ecarin clotting time. This is thought to be more accurate at high doses of hirudin but may give falsely high results when the amount of prothrombin in the sample is reduced below 50%. It is also useful when other factors such as antiphospholipid antibodies are causing prolongation of the APTT.

After 5 days therapy 45% of patients will develop antihirudin antibodies, which may enhance or reduce the therapeutic effect. Hirudin is excreted via the kidneys, and close monitoring is necessary, with dose reduction if renal impairment is present.

THROMBOLYTIC THERAPY

The thrombolytic agents currently in use are principally streptokinase and recombinant tissue type plasminogen activator (rtPA). Tenectplase and Reteplase are genetically modified forms of tPA.

Streptokinase

Streptokinase is a purified fraction of the filtrate from cultures of *Streptokinase haemolyticus*. Streptokinase interacts with plasminogen or plasmin to form a plasminogen activator in plasma. The activator complex in turn cleaves a bond in the plasminogen molecule to give rise to free plasmin. Streptokinase therefore results in systemic fibrinogenolysis as well as lysis of fibrin clot. Streptokinase is a foreign protein and induces antibody production in humans, limiting a course of treatment to 3–5 days.

It is recommended that 2 years should elapse before repeated administrations of streptokinase. It also crossreacts with antistreptococcal antibodies, which may cause resistance to therapy, although this is usually overcome with large doses.

Tissue-Type Plasminogen Activator

The tissue-type plasminogen activator is a single- or double-chain polypeptide obtained by recombinant techniques or from tissue cultures. It is a potent activator of plasminogen when the two molecules are bound to fibrin for which it has a strong affinity. It thus causes less systemic fibrinogenolysis than any of the previously mentioned agents, although some decrease in circulating fibrinogen does occur, particularly with prolonged administration. It induces a thrombolytic state of longer duration than either streptokinase or urokinase infusion.

Selection of Patients

Thrombolytic treatment carries a serious risk of bleeding, and thrombolytic agents should not be given to individuals suffering from a variety of illnesses where there is a high risk of bleeding. In addition, each patient should have haemostatic function and platelet count measured before treatment is started.

Laboratory Control of Thrombolytic Therapy[20]

Many laboratory tests are abnormal during thrombolytic therapy, but a perfect and specific procedure for monitoring is not available. In practice, thrombolytic therapy is given rapidly according to protocol, with no time or need for adjustment of dosage. During thrombolytic therapy all screening tests of coagulation are prolonged, reflecting the hyperplasminaemic state with the reduction in the fibrinogen concentration and the presence of FDP. The prolongation is most marked with streptokinase and streptokinase–plasminogen complex; it is less marked with urokinase and least with tPA. The fibrinogen concentration commonly decreases to below 0.05 g/l, and the FDP concentration may increase to more than 1000 ng/l.

Monitoring of therapy is only recommended for treatment lasting longer than 24 hours. If possible, a sample should be obtained prior to treatment. Samples taken after fibrinolysis has begun should be taken into citrate plus an inhibitor of fibrinolysis such as aprotinin (250 u/ml) or ε-aminocaproic acid (EACA: 0.07 mol/l). The fibrinolytic state will affect several tests.

Activated Partial Thromboplastin Time

With effective fibrinolysis the APTT is likely to be prolonged >1.5 times control. This is a result of fibrinogen, FV and FVIII depletion, and interference from FDPs. There are, however, no data to correlate APTT with therapeutic effect.

Thrombin Time

The TT can be used to monitor therapy. A few hours after the start of the infusion, the TT is prolonged to 40 s or more (control 15 ± 1 s); it then settles to approximately 20–30 s. Very long TTs carry a high risk of bleeding and are indicative of severe hyperplasminaemia.

Plasma Fibrinogen

Depending on duration of therapy and the specific plasminogen activator used, there is a variable decrease in fibrinogen. The fibrinogen should be measured by a method dependent on clottable fibrinogen (e.g., Clauss technique, p. 401). The PT-derived fibrinogen is likely to be unreliable. Fibrin(ogen) degradation products will be elevated, but this is unlikely to be helpful.

Investigation of a Patient Who Bleeds While Taking Thrombolytic Agents or Immediately Afterward

Haemorrhage is an inevitable risk associated with fibrinolytic therapy and may occur despite normal coagulation tests. When severe, bleeding will necessitate cessation of fibrinolysis and administration of aprotinin or tranexamic acid to inhibit its activity. Coagulation tests may guide replacement therapy with plasma or cryoprecipitate. The tests, the timing, and the likely mechanism of bleeding are shown in Table 18.5.

ANTIPLATELET THERAPY

Many drugs inhibit platelet function *in vitro*, but only a few have antiplatelet activity in acceptable doses. Each category of drugs has a different pharmacological action and requires different methods to demonstrate its effect on platelets. Antiplatelet agents are used in primary and secondary prevention of coronary heart disease, in unstable angina, in certain forms of cerebrovascular disease, to prevent thrombo-embolism associated with valvular disease and prosthetic heart valves, and to prevent thrombosis in arteriovenous shunts. Haematologists are only rarely asked to monitor these aspects of antiplatelet therapy. Indeed, it is said that the advantage of these agents is that monitoring is unnecessary.

Interest has been revived in the observation that some patients do not respond to aspirin. "Aspirin resistance" is poorly defined and may refer either to a failure to inhibit platelet function or a failure to suppress thromboxane A_2 production. The former may be detected by platelet function analysers such as the PFA100 or by platelet aggregation responses; the latter may be detected by serum thromboxane B2 levels. However, the clinical utility of this assessment and the appropriate responses are not established.[21]

A proportion of patients with thrombocytosis or thrombocythaemia experience episodes of arterial thrombosis. Such patients are often prescribed antiplatelet drugs, and the effect of these drugs is sometimes monitored. Three techniques are available for monitoring: prolongation of the bleeding time or PFA (p. 417), inhibition of platelet aggregation response to standard agonists (p. 427), and normalization of platelet survival using [111]indium-labelled platelets (p. 376).

REFERENCES

1. Hirsh J, Dalen JE, Anderson DR, et al 1998 Oral anticoagulants: mechanism of action, clinical effectiveness, and optimal therapeutic range. Chest 114:445s–469s.
2. World Health Organization 1999 Guidelines for thromboplastins and plasma used to control oral anticoagulant therapy. WHO Technical Report Series 889:64–93.
3. World Health Organization 1999 Guidelines for thromboplastins and plasma used to control oral anticoagulant therapy. WHO Technical Report Series 889:Annex 3.

4. Kitchen S, Preston FE 1999 Standardization of prothrombin time for laboratory control of oral anticoagulant therapy. Seminars Thrombosis Hemostasis 25:17–25.

5. Poller L, Barrowcliffe TW, van den Besselaar AM, et al 1997 A simplified statistical method for local INR using linear regression. European Concerted Action on Anticoagulation [see comments]. British Journal of Haematology 98:640–647.

6. Guidelines on oral anticoagulation, 3rd ed 1998. British Journal of Haematology 101:374–387.

7. Hirsh J, Dalen J, Anderson DR, et al 2001 Oral anticoagulants: mechanism of action, clinical effectiveness, and optimal therapeutic range. Chest 119:8S–21S.

8. Shiach CR, Campbell B, Poller L, et al 2002 Reliability of point-of-care prothrombin time testing in a community clinic: a randomized crossover comparison with hospital laboratory testing. British Journal of Haematology 119:370–375.

9. Murray ET, Fitzmaurice DA, McCahon D 2004 Point pf care testing for INR monitoring: where are we now? British Journal of Haematology 127:373–378.

10. Fitzmaurice D, Murray ET, Gee KM, et al 2002 Training of patients in a randomised controlled trial of self management of warfarin treatment. British Medical Journal 328:437–438.

11. Hirsh J, Warkentin TE, Raschke R, et al 1998 Heparin and low-molecular-weight heparin: mechanisms of action, pharmacokinetics, dosing considerations, monitoring, efficacy, and safety [published erratum in Chest 1999 Jun;115(6):1760]. Chest 114:489s–510s.

12. Gray E, Heath AB, Mulloy B, et al 1995 A collaborative study of proposed European Pharmacopoeia reference preparations of low molecular mass heparin. Thrombosis and Haemostasis 74:893–899.

13. Popma JJ, Prpic R, Lansky AJ, et al 1998 Heparin dosing in patients undergoing coronary intervention. American Journal of Cardiology 82:19–24.

14. Warkentin TE 2003 Heparin-induced thrombocytopenia: pathogenesis and management [see comment]. British Journal of Haematology 121:535–555.

15. Chong BH 2003 Heparin-induced thrombocytopenia. Journal of Thrombosis & Haemostasis 1:1471–1478.

16. Sheridan D, Carter C, Kelton JG 1986 A diagnostic test for heparin-induced thrombocytopenia. Blood 67:27–30.

17. Warkentin TE 1999 Heparin-induced thrombocytopenia: a clinicopathologic syndrome. Thrombosis and Haemostasis 82:439–447.

18. Amiral J, Meyer D 1998 Heparin-induced thrombocytopenia: diagnostic tests and biological mechanisms. Baillieres Clinical Haematology 11:447–460.

19. Meyer O, Salama A, Pittet N, et al 1999 Rapid detection of heparin-induced platelet antibodies with particle gel immunoassay (ID-HPF4). Lancet 354:1525–1526.

20. Ludlam CA, Bennett B, Fox KA, et al 1995 Guidelines for the use of thrombolytic therapy. Haemostasis and Thrombosis Task Force of the British Committee for Standards in Haematology. Blood Coagulation & Fibrinolysis 6:273–285.

21. Patrono C 2003 Aspirin resistance: definition, mechanisms and clinical read-outs [see comment]. Journal of Thrombosis & Haemostasis 1:1710–13.

19 Blood cell antigens and antibodies: erythrocytes, platelets, and granulocytes

Sue Knowles and Fiona Regan

ERYTHROCYTES

Red Cell Antigens

Since Landsteiner's discovery in 1901 that human blood groups existed, a vast body of serological, genetic, and biochemical data on red cell (blood group) antigens has been accumulated. More recently, the biological functions of some of these antigens have been appreciated.

Twenty-five blood group systems have been described (Table 19.1). Each system is a series of red cell antigens, determined either by a single genetic locus or very closely linked loci. In addition to the blood group systems, there are five "collections" of antigens (e.g., Cost), which bring together other genetically, biochemically, or serologically related sets of antigens, and a separate series of low-frequency (e.g., Rd) and high-frequency (e.g., Vel) antigens, which do not fit into any system or collection. A numeric catalogue of red cell antigens is being maintained by an International Society of Blood Transfusion (ISBT) Working Party.[1,2]

Apart from those of the ABO system, most of these antigens were detected by antibodies stimulated by transfusion or pregnancy.

Alternative forms of gene coding for red cell antigens at a particular locus are called alleles, and individuals may inherit identical or nonidentical alleles. Most blood group genes have been assigned to specific chromosomes (e.g., ABO system on chromosome 9, Rh system on chromosome 1). The term genotype is used for the sum of the inherited alleles of a particular gene (e.g., AA, AO), and most red cell genes are expressed as codominant antigens (i.e., both genes are expressed in the heterozygote).

Table 19.1   Blood group systems recognized by the ISBT working party

System number	System name conventional	System symbol ISBT	Chromosomal location	Gene(s)
001	ABO	ABO	9q34.1-q34.2	ABO
002	MNS	MNS	4q28-q31	GYPA GYPB
003	P	PI	22q11.2-qter	P
004	Rh	RH	1p36.2-p34	RHD RHCE
005	Lutheran	LU	19q12-q13	LU
006	Kell	KEL	7q33	KEL
007	Lewis	LE	19p13.3	FUT3
008	Duffy	FY	1q22-q23	FY
009	Kidd	JK	18q11-q12	HUT11
010	Diego	DI	17q12-q21	SLC4A1
011	Yt	YT	7q22	ACHE
012	Xg	XG	Xp22.32	XG
013	Scianna	SC	1p36.2-p22.1	SC
014	Dombrock	DO	12p13.2-p12.1	DO
015	Colton	CO	7p14	AQP1
016	LW	LW	19p13.2-cen	LW
017	Chido/Rogers	CH/RG	6p21.3	C4A,C4B
018	H	H	19q13	FUT1
019	Kx	XK	Xp21.1	XK
020	Gerbich	GE	2q14-q21	GYPC
021	Cromer	CROM	1q32	DAF
022	Knops	KN	1q32	CR1
023	Indian	IN	11p13	CD44
024	Ok	OK	19pter-p13.2	OK
025	MER2	RAPH	11p15	MER2

ISBT, International Society of Blood Transfusion.

The phenotype refers to the recognizable product of the alleles, and there are many racial differences in the frequencies of red cell phenotypes, as shown in Table 19.2.

Red cell antigens are determined either by carbohydrate structures or protein structures. Carbohydrate-defined antigens are indirect gene products (e.g., ABO, Lewis, P). The genes code for an

Table 19.2   Frequencies of red cell phenotypes in U.S. Black and White populations

System	Phenotype	U.S. Black population (%)	U.S. White population (%)
ABO	O	49	43.7
	A	26	41.7
	B	20.5	10.6
	AB	4.5	4
Lewis	Le (a–b–)	28.5	6
Rh	Dce	47.8	2.1
	DCcEe	4.2	13.4
	dce	5.6	14.6
	DCe	2.6	18.9
MNSs	S–s+	68.1	45
	S+s+	24.5	44
	S+s–	5.9	11
	S–s–	1.5	Rare
Duffy	Fy (a–,b–)	63.7	Rare
	Fy (a–, b+)	18.8	34
	Fy (a+,b+)	2	44
	Fy (a+,b–)	15.5	17
Kidd	Jk (a+,b–)	50	27.5
	Jk (a+b+)	41.4	49.4
	Jk (a–b+)	8.6	23.1

intermediate product, usually an enzyme that creates the antigenic specificity by transferring sugar molecules onto the protein or lipid. Protein-defined antigens are direct gene products, and the specificity is determined by the inherited amino acid sequence and/or the conformation of the protein. Proteins carrying red cell antigens are inserted into the membrane in one of three ways: single pass, multipass, or linked to phosphotidylinositol (GPI-linked). Only a few red cell antigens are erythroid-specific (Rh, LW, Kell, and MNSs), the remainder being expressed in many other tissues. The structure and functions of the membrane proteins and glycoproteins carrying blood group antigens have been reviewed by Cartron et al[3] and Daniels.[4] An illustration of the putative functions of molecules containing blood group antigens is provided in Table 19.3.

However, the main clinical importance of a blood group system depends on the capacity of alloan-tibodies (directed against the antigens not possessed by the individual) to cause destruction of transfused red cells or to cross the placenta and give rise to haemolytic disease in the fetus or newborn. This in turn depends on the frequency of the antigens and the alloantibodies and the characteristics of the latter—thermal range, immunoglobulin class, and ability to fix complement. On these criteria, the ABO and Rh systems are of major clinical importance. Anti-A and anti-B are naturally occurring and are capable of causing severe intravascular haemolysis after an incompatible transfusion. The RhD antigen is the most immunogenic red cell antigen after A and B, being capable of stimulating anti-D produc-tion after transfusion or pregnancy in the majority of RhD-negative individuals.

ABO System

Discovery of the ABO system by Landsteiner marked the beginning of safe blood transfusion. The ABO antigens, although most important in relation to transfusion, are also expressed on most endothelial and epithelial membranes and are important histo-compatibility antigens.[5] Transplantation of ABO-incompatible solid organs increases the potential for hyperacute graft rejection. Major ABO-incompatible stem cell transplants (e.g., group A stem cells into a group O recipient) will provoke haemolysis, unless the donation is depleted of red cells.

ABO Antigens and Encoding Genes

There are four main blood groups: A, B, AB and O (Table 19.4). In the British Caucasian population, the frequency of group A is 42%, B 9%, AB 3%, and O 46%, but there is racial variation in these frequencies.[6] The epitopes of ABO antigens are determined by carbohydrates (sugars), which are linked either to polypeptides (forming glyco-proteins) or to lipids (glycolipids).

The expression of ABO antigens is controlled by three separate genetic loci: *ABO* located on chromosome 9 and *FUT1* (*H*) and *FUT2* (*Se*), both of which are located on chromosome 19. The genes from each locus are inherited in pairs as Mendelian dominants. Each gene codes for a different enzyme (glycosyltransferase), which attaches specific mono-saccharides onto precursor disaccharide chains

Table 19.3   Putative functions of molecules containing blood group antigens

Class	Blood group system	Structure	Function
Transporter/channel	Kidd	Multipass GP	Urea transporter
	Colton	Aquaporin 1	
		Multipass CP	Water channel
	Diego	Band 3, multipass GP	Anion exchanger
Receptors	Duffy	DARC, multipass GP	Chemokine (*Plasmodium vivax* receptor)
	Indian	Single-pass GP	Hyaluronate receptor
Complement pathway	Chido/Rogers	Complement absorbed onto red cells	Complement component Complement regulator
	Cromer	DAF	Complement regulator
	Knops	Complement receptor 1	
Adhesion	LW	IgSF	Binds CD11/CD18 Integrins
Molecule	Lutheran	IgSF	? Laminin receptor
Enzyme	Yt	GPI-linked GP Acetylcholinesterase	Unknown on red cells
	Kell	Single-pass GP	? Endopeptidase
Structural protein	Gerbich	Glycophorins C and D Single-pass GP	Attachment to membrane skeleton

Table 19.4   ABO blood group system

Blood group	Subgroup	Antigens on red cells	Antibodies in plasma
A	A₁	A + A₁	Anti-B
	A₂	A	(Anti-A₁)*
B	–	B	Anti-A, Anti-A₁
AB	A₁B	A + A₁ + B	None
	A₂B	A + B	(Anti-A₁)*
O	–	(H)†	Anti-A
			Anti-A₁
			Anti-B
			Anti-A,B†

*Anti-A₁ found in 1–2% of A₂ subjects and 25–30% of A₂B subjects.
†The amount of H antigen is influenced by the ABO group; O cells contain most H and A₁B cells least. Anti-H may be found in occasional A₁ and A₁B subject (see text).
†Crossreactivity with both A and B cells.

(Table 19.5). There are four types of disaccharide chains known to occur on red cells, on other tissues, and in secretions. The Type 1 disaccharide chain is found in plasma and secretions and is the substrate for the *FUT2* (*Se*) gene, whereas Types 2, 3, and 4 chains are only found on red cells and are the substrate for the *FUT1* (*H*) gene. It is likely that the *O* and *B* genes arose by mutation of the *A* gene. The *O* gene does not encode for the production of a functional enzyme; group O individuals commonly have a deletion at nucleotide 261 (the *O1* allele), which results in a frame-shift and premature termination of the translated polypeptide and the production of an enzyme with no catalytic activity. The *B* gene differs from *A* by consistent nucleotide substitutions.[7] The expression of A and B antigens is determined by the *H* and *Se* genes, which both give rise to glycosyltransferases that add L-fucose, producing the H antigen. The presence of an *A* or *B* gene (or both) results in the production of further glycosyltransferases, which convert H substance into A and B antigens by the terminal addition of

Table 19.5 Glycosyltransfereases produced by genes encoding for antigens within the ABO, H, and Lewis blood group systems

Gene	Allele	Transferase
FUT1	H	α-2-L-fucosyltransferase
	H	None
A	A	α-3-N-acetyl-D-galactosaminyltransferase
B	B	α-3-D-galactosyltransferase
0	0	None
FUT2	Se	α-2-L-fucosyltransferase
	se	None
FUT3	Le	α-3/4-L-fucosyltranferase
	le	None

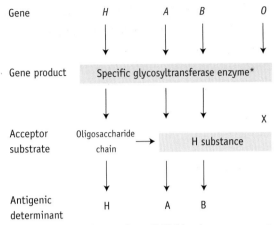

Figure 19.1 Pathways from HAB blood group genes to antigens. *Glycosyltransferase H transfers L-fucose; A transfers N-acetyl-D-galactosamine; B transfers D-galactose; 0 is inactive.

N-acetyl-D-galactosamine and D-galactose respectively (Fig. 19.1). Because the O gene produces an inactive transferase, H substance persists unchanged as group O. In the extremely rare Oh Bombay phenotype, the individual is homozygous for the h allele of FUT1 and hence cannot form the H precursor of the A and B antigen. Their red cells type as group O, but their plasma contains anti-H, in addition to anti-A, anti-B, and anti-A,B, which are all active at 37°C. As a consequence, individuals with an Oh Bombay phenotype can only be safely transfused with other Oh red cells.

Serologists have defined two common subgroups of the A antigen. Approximately 20% of group A and group AB individuals belong to group A_2 and group A_2B, respectively, the remainder belonging to group A_1 and group A_1B. These subgroups arise as a result of inheritance of either the A^1 or A^2 alleles. The A_2 transferase is less efficient in transferring N-acetyl-D-galactosamine to available H antigen sites and cannot utilize Types 3 and 4 disaccharide chains. As a consequence, A_2 red cells have fewer A antigen sites than A_1 cells and the plasma of group A_2 and group A_2B individuals may also contain anti-A_1. The distinction between these subgroups can be made using the lectin Dolichos biflorus, which only reacts with A_1 cells. The H antigen content of red cells depends on the ABO group and when assessed by agglutination reactions with anti-H, the strength of reaction tends to be graded O >

$A_2 > A_2B > B > A_1 > A_1B$. Other subgroups of A are occasionally found (e.g., A_3, A_x) that result from mutant forms of the glycosyltransferases produced by the A gene and are less efficient at transferring N-acetyl-D-galactosamine onto H substance.[7]

The A, B, and H antigens are detectable early in fetal life but are not fully developed on the red cells at birth. The number of antigen sites reaches "adult" level at around 1 year of age and remains constant until old age, when a slight reduction may occur.

Secretors and Nonsecretors

The ability to secrete A, B, and H substances in water-soluble form is controlled by FUT2 (dominant allele Se). In a Caucasian population, about 80% are secretors (genotype SeSe or Sese) and 20% are nonsecretors (genotype sese) (Table 19.6). Secretors have H substance in the saliva and other body fluids together with A substances, B substances, or both, depending on their blood group. Only traces of these substances are present in the secretions of nonsecretors, although the antigens are expressed normally on their red cells and other tissues.

An individual's secretor status can be determined by testing for ABH substance in saliva (p. 506).

ABO Antigens and Disease

Group A individuals rarely may acquire a B antigen from a bacterial infection that results in the release of a deacetylase enzyme. This converts N-acetyl-D-

Table 19.6 Secretor status in the caucasian population

Genes	Blood group of red cells	ABH substance present in saliva	Incidence (%)
Secretor			
SeSe	A	A + H or B	B + H
Sese	AB	A + B + H	80
		O	H
Nonsecretors			
sese	A, B, AB, or O	None	20

galactosamine into α-galactosamine, which is similar to galactose, the immunodominant sugar of group B, thereby sometimes causing the red cells to appear to be group AB. In the original reported cases, five out of seven of the patients had carcinoma of the gastrointestinal tract. Case reports attest to the danger of individuals with an acquired B antigen being transfused with AB red cells, resulting in a fatal haemolytic transfusion reaction following the production of hyperimmune anti-B.[8]

The inheritance of ABH antigens is also known to be weakly associated with predisposition to certain diseases. Group A individuals have 1.2 times the risk of developing carcinoma of the stomach than group O or B; group O individuals have 1.4 times more risk of developing peptic ulcer than non-group O individuals; and nonsecretors of ABH have 1.5 times the risk of developing peptic ulcer than secretors.[9] The ABO group also affects plasma von Willebrand factor (vWF) and factor VIII levels; group O healthy individuals have levels around 25% lower than those of other ABO groups.[10] It has been shown that it is H antigen expression (which is highest in group O individuals) that mediates this effect—and may result from accelerated clearance of vWF via a fucose-mediated mechanism.[11] ABH antigens are also frequently more weakly expressed on the red cells of persons with leukaemia.

ABO Antibodies

Anti-A and Anti-B

ABO antibodies, in the absence of the corresponding antigens, appear during the first few months after birth, probably as a result of exposure to ABH antigen-like substances in the diet or the environment (i.e., they are "naturally occurring") (Table 19.4). This allows for reverse (serum/plasma) grouping as a means of confirming the red cell phenotype. The antibodies are a potential cause of dangerous haemolytic transfusion reactions if transfusions are given without regard to ABO compatibility. Anti-A and anti-B are always, to some extent, immunoglobulin M (IgM). Although they react best at low temperatures, they are nevertheless potentially lytic at 37°C. Hyperimmune anti-A and anti-B occur less frequently, usually in response to transfusion or pregnancy, but they may also be formed following the injection of some toxoids and vaccines. They are predominantly of IgG class and are usually produced by group O and sometimes by group A_2 individuals. Hyperimmune IgG anti-A and/or anti-B from group O or group A_2 mothers may cross the placenta and cause haemolytic disease of the newborn (HDN). These antibodies react over a wide thermal range and are more effective haemolysins than the naturally occurring antibodies. Group O donors should always be screened for hyperimmune anti-A and anti-B antibodies, which may cause haemolysis when group O platelets or whole blood are transfused to recipients with A and B phenotypes.

Plasma-containing blood components from these "dangerous" (high titre) universal donors should be reserved for group O recipients.

Anti-A_1 and Anti-H

Anti-A_1 reacts only with A_1 and A_1B cells and is occasionally found in the serum of group A_2 individuals (1–8%) and not uncommonly in the serum of group A_2B subjects (25–50%). However, anti-A_1 normally acts as a cold agglutinin and is very rarely reactive at 37°C, when it is only capable of limited red cell destruction. There have been a few reports of red cell haemolysis ascribed to anti-A_1, which some authors have questioned because, although the antibodies reacted only with A_1 red cells, no attempts were made to absorb them with A_2 cells, which would have revealed their anti-A specificity.

Anti-H reacts most strongly with group O and A_2 red cells and also normally acts as a cold agglutinin. A notable, but rare, exception is the anti-H that occurs in the Oh Bombay phenotype, which is an IgM antibody and causes lysis at 37°C (Table 19.4) so that Oh Bombay phenotype blood would be required for transfusion.

Lewis System

Lewis Antigens and Encoding Genes

The Lewis antigens (Le^a and Le^b) are located on soluble glycosphingolipids found in saliva and plasma and are secondarily absorbed into the red cell membranes from the plasma.

The Le gene at the *FUT3 (LE)* locus is located on chromosome 19 and codes for a fucosyltransferase, which acts on an adjacent sugar molecule to that acted on by the *Se* gene. Where *Se* and *Le* are present, the Le^b antigen is produced; where *Le* but not *Se* is present, Le^a is produced; and where *Le* is not present, neither Le^a nor Le^b is produced. After transfusion of red cells, donor red cells convert to the Lewis type of the recipient owing to the continuous exchange of glycosphingolipids between the plasma and red cell membrane.

Neonates have the phenotype Le(a–b–) because low levels of the fucosyltransferase are produced in the first 2 months of life.

Lewis Antibodies

Lewis antibodies are naturally occurring and are usually IgM and complement binding. *In vitro*, their reactivity is enhanced with the use of enzyme-treated red cells, when lysis may occur. However, only rare examples of anti-Le^a, strictly reactive at 37°C, have given rise to haemolytic transfusion reactions and there is no good evidence that anti-Le^b has ever caused a haemolytic episode. Explanations for the relative lack of clinical significance include their thermal range, neutralisation by Lewis antigens in the plasma of transfused blood, and the gradual elution of Lewis antigens from the donor red cells. Consequently, it is acceptable to provide red cells for transfusion that have not been typed as negative for the relevant Lewis antigen but are compatible with the recipient plasma when the compatibility test is performed strictly at 37°C.

Lewis antibodies have not been implicated in haemolytic disease of the fetus or newborn. The role of Lewis in influencing the outcome of renal transplants is unclear.

The P System and Globoside Collection

Antigens

The P_1 antigen of the P system and the P and P^k antigens of the globoside collection are related. Little is known of the genes involved or their products, but all are derived from the precursor, lactosyl ceramide dehexoside. Carbohydrate products related to the P system are widely distributed in nature.

Expression of P_1 varies considerably between individuals. One in 100,000 individuals is p (negative for P) and is resistant to parvovirus B19 infection.

Antibodies

Anti-P_1 is a common naturally occurring antibody of no clinical significance, and red cells for transfusion can be provided that are crossmatch compatible at 37°C. Allo anti-P is also a naturally occurring antibody found in individuals with the rare P^k phenotype. Auto-anti-P is the specificity attributed to the Donath–Landsteiner antibody; it is a potent biphasic haemolysin, responsible for paroxysmal cold haemoglobinuria.

Anti-PP$_1$P^k is a naturally occurring high-titre IgM or IgG antibody, and it is found only in individuals with the rare p phenotype. It is reactive at 37°C and is capable of causing intravascular haemolysis and HDN. It is also associated with spontaneous abortion in early pregnancy.

Rh System

The Rh system, formerly known as the Rhesus system, was so named because the original antibody that was raised by injecting red cells of rhesus monkeys into rabbits and guinea pigs reacted with most human red cells. Although the original antibody (now called anti-LW) was subsequently shown to be different from anti-D, the Rh terminology has been retained for the human blood group system. The clinical importance of this system is that individuals who are D negative are often stimulated to make anti-D if transfused with D positive blood or, in the case of pregnant women, if exposed to D positive fetal red cells that have crossed the placenta.

Rh Antigens and Encoding Genes

This is a very complex system. At its simplest, it is convenient to classify individuals as D positive or D negative, depending on the presence of the D antigen. This is largely a preventive measure, to avoid transfusing a D-negative recipient with the cells expressing the D antigen, which is the most immunogenic red cell antigen after A and B. At a more comprehensive level, it is convenient to consider the Rh system as a gene complex that gives rise to various combinations of three alternative antigens—C or c, D or d, and E or e—as originally suggested by Fisher. The d gene was thought to be amorphic without any corresponding antigen on the red cell. More recently it has been confirmed that the *RH* locus is on chromosome 1 and comprises two highly homologous, very closely linked genes, *RHD* and *RHCE*, each with 10 exons. Each gene codes for a separate transmembrane protein with 417 residues and 12 putative transmembrane domains. The D and CE proteins differ at 35 residues. The *RHCE* gene has four main alleles; *CE, Ce, ce,* and *cE.* Positions 103 and 226 on the CE polypeptide, situated in the external loops, determine the C/c (serine/proline) and E/e (proline/alanine) polymorphisms, respectively. This concept of D and CcEe genes linked closely and transmitted together is consistent with the Fisher nomenclature.

In Caucasian, D negative individuals, the *RHD* gene is deleted, whereas in Black races and other populations, single-point mutations, partial deletions, or recombinations have been described. In individuals with a weak D antigen (D^u), there is a quantitative reduction in D antigen sites, believed to arise from an uncharacterised transcriptional defect. These individuals do not make anti-D antibodies following a D antigen challenge. Partial D individuals lack one or more epitopes of the D antigen, defined using panels of monoclonal reagents. D^{VI} is perhaps the most important partial D phenotype because such individuals not infrequently make anti-D. Partial D phenotypes arise from DNA exchanges between *RHD* and *RHCE* genes and from other rearrangements. Comprehensive reviews of this system have been provided by Cartron and Agre,[12] Huang,[13] and Avent and Reid.[14]

The Rh haplotypes are named either by the component antigens (e.g., CDe, cde) or by a single shorthand symbol (e.g., R^1 = CDe, r = cde). Thus, a person may inherit *CDe* (R^1) from one parent and *cde* (r) from the other and have the genotype *Cde/cde* (R^{1}r). The haplotypes in order of frequency and the corresponding shorthand notation are given in Table 19.7. Although two other nomenclatures are also used to describe the Rh system, namely, Wiener's Rh-Hr terminology and Rosenfeld's numeric notation, the CDE nomenclature, derived from Fisher's original theory, is recommended by a World Health

Table 19.7 The Rh haplotypes in order of frequency (Fisher nomenclature) in caucasians and the corresponding short notations

Fisher	Short notations	Approximate frequency (%)
CDe	R^1	41
cde	r	39
cDE	R^2	14
cDe	R^0	3
C^{w}De	R^{1w}	1
cdE	r$''$	1
Cde	r$'$	1
CDE	R^Z	Rare
CdE	r^y	Rare

Organization Expert Committee[15] in the interest of simplicity and uniformity. The Rh antigens are defined by corresponding antisera, with the exception of "anti-d," which does not exist. Consequently, the distinction between homozygous DD and the heterozygous Dd cannot be made by direct serological testing but may be resolved by informative family studies. It is still routine practice to predict the genotype from the phenotype on the basis of probability tables for the various Rh genotypes in the population (Table 20.3, p. 532). However, in women with anti-D and a history of an infant affected by HDN, *RH* DNA typing is used in prenatal testing for the fetal D status to decide on the clinical management of the pregnancy. DNA typing requires less fetal tissue and can be performed earlier in pregnancy before the Rh proteins are expressed on red cells. Suitable sources include amniotic fluid (amniocytes) and trophoblastic cells (chorionic villi), and it has also been established that maternal blood can be used because it contains fetal DNA.[16,115] In practice, multiplex polymerase chain reaction (PCR) is used, with more than two primer sets, to detect the different molecular bases for D-negative phenotypes in non-Caucasians. *RH* DNA typing also has applications in paternity testing and forensic medicine. There are racial differences in the distribution of Rh antigens—for example, D negativity is more common in Caucasians (approximately 15%), whereas R^0 (cDe) is found in approximately 48% of Black Americans but is uncommon (approximately 2%) in Caucasians. The Rh antigens are present only on red cells and are a structural part of the cell membrane. Complete absence of Rh antigens (Rh null phenotype) may be associated with a congenital haemolytic anaemia with spherocytes and stomatocytes in the blood film, increased osmotic fragility, and increased cation transport. This phenotype arises either as a result of homozygosity for a silent allele at the *RH* locus (the amorph type) or more commonly by homozygosity for an autosomal suppressor gene (X^0r), genetically independent of the *RH* locus (the regulator type). Rh antigens are well-developed before birth and can be demonstrated on the red cells of very early fetuses.

Antibodies

Fisher's nomenclature is convenient when applied to Rh antibodies, and antibodies directed against all Rh antigens, except d, have been described: anti-D, anti-C, anti-c, anti-E, and anti-e. Rh antigens are restricted to red cells and Rh antibodies result from previous alloimmunization by previous pregnancy or transfusion, except for some naturally occurring forms of anti-E and anti-C^W. Immune Rh antibodies are predominantly IgG (IgG1 and/or IgG3), but may have an IgM component. They react optimally at 37°C, they do not bind complement, and their detection is often enhanced by the use of enzyme-treated red cells. Haemolysis, when it occurs, is therefore extravascular and predominantly in the spleen.

Anti-D is clinically the most important antibody; it may cause haemolytic transfusion reactions and was a common cause of fetal death resulting from haemolytic disease of the newborn before the introduction of anti-D prophylaxis. Anti-D is accompanied by anti-C in 30% of cases and anti-E in 2% cases. Primary immunization following a transfusion of D positive cells becomes apparent within 2–5 months, but it may not be detectable following exposure to a small dose of D positive cells in pregnancy. However, a second exposure to RhD-positive cells in a subsequent pregnancy will provoke a prompt anamnestic or secondary immune response.

Of the non-D Rh antibodies, anti-c is most commonly found and can also give rise to severe haemolytic disease of the fetus and newborn. Anti-E is less common, whereas anti-C is rare in the absence of anti-D.

Kell and Kx Systems

Antigens and Encoding Genes

Twenty-five antigens have been identified (K1–K25), but three very closely linked sets of alleles are clinically important: *K* (KEL1) and *k* (KEL2); *Kp^a* (KEL3), *Kp^b* (KEL4), and *Kp^c* (KEL21); and *Js^a* (KEL6) and *Js^b* (KEL7). These antigens are encoded by alleles at the *KEL* locus on chromosome 7, but their production also depends on genes at the *KX* locus on the X chromosome. The K antigen is present in 9% of the English population. The Kp^b antigen has a high frequency in Caucasians; the Js^b antigen is universal in Caucasians and almost universal in black races.

The Kell protein is a single-pass glycoprotein and is believed to be complexed by a disulphide bridge to the Kx protein, which is multipass with 10 putative transmembrane domains. It has considerable sequence homology to other neutral endopeptidases.

In the McLeod phenotype, red cells lack Kx, and there is a marked decrease in all Kell antigens, an acanthocytic morphology, and a compensated haemolytic anaemia. The McLeod syndrome is X-linked with slow progression to cardiomyopathy, skeletal muscle wasting, and neurological defects.

Kell Antibodies

Immune anti-K is the most common antibody found outside the ABO and Rh systems. It is commonly IgG1 and occasionally complement binding. Other immune antibodies directed against Kell antigens are less common. The presence of some of these antibodies, such as anti-k, anti-Kp^b, and anti-Js^b, may cause extensive difficulties in the selection of antigen-negative units for transfusion.

Duffy System

Duffy Antigens and Encoding Genes

The Duffy (Fy) locus is on chromosome 1 and encodes a multipass protein with seven or nine putative transmembrane domains.

The locus has the following alleles: Fy^a, Fy^b, which code for the co-dominant Fy^a and Fy^b antigens, respectively; Fy^x, which is responsible for a weak Fy^b antigen; and Fy, which is responsible when homozygous for the Fy(a−b−) phenotype in black races. This Fy gene is identical to the Fy^b gene in its structural region but has a mutation in the promoter region, resulting in the lack of production of red cell Duffy glycoprotein.

The Fy glycoprotein (also known as Duffy antigen receptor for chemokines, DARC) is a receptor for the CC and CXC classes of proinflammatory chemokines and is expressed on vascular endothelial cells and Purkinje cells in the cerebellum, but its precise role as a potential scavenger of excess chemokines is unknown. The Fy glycoprotein is also a receptor for *Plasmodium vivax*.

Duffy Antibodies

Anti-Fy^a is much more common than anti-Fy^b, and all other Duffy antibodies are rare. They are predominantly IgG1 and are sometimes complement binding.

Kidd (JK) System

Kidd Antigens and Encoding Genes

Genes at the *HUT11 (JK)* locus on chromosome 18 encode for a multipass protein, which carries both the Kidd antigens and the human erythroid urea transporter. The codominant alleles, Jk^a and Jk^b, produce a polymorphism on *HUT11,* which differs by a single amino acid substitution at position 280 (Asp/Asn).

The Jk(a−b−) phenotype is very rare and is caused by homozygous inheritance of the silent allele, Jk, at the *JK* locus or by inheritance of the dominant inhibitor gene *In (Jk)* unlinked to the *JK* locus. These Jk(a−b−) cells are resistant to lysis by solutions of urea and have a selective defect in urea transport.

Kidd Antibodies

Anti-Jk^a is more common than anti-Jk^b; both are usually IgG. Kidd antibodies are usually complement binding, which is thought to be because most of them contain an IgG3 fraction. Anti-Jk3 is produced by individuals of the Jk(a−b−) phenotype.

Kidd antibodies can be difficult to detect because they often show dosage (may only react with cells showing homozygous expressions of Jk^a or Jk^b), they fall to undetectable levels in plasma, and they are often present in mixtures of alloantibodies.

MNSs System

MNSs Antigens and Encoding Genes

GYPA and *GYPB* are closely linked genes on chromosome 4 and encode glycophorin A (GPA) and glycophorin B (GPB), respectively. Both GPA and GPB are single-pass membrane sialoglycoproteins. *M* and *N* are alleles of *GYPA* (encoding the M and N antigens on GPA), and *S* and *s* are alleles of *GPYB* (encoding the S and s antigens on GPB). Many rare variants have been described owing to gene deletions, mutations, and segmental exchanges.

The U antigen is found on the red cells of Caucasians and 99% of black races. U-negative individuals are, with rare exceptions, S−s− and lack GPB or have an altered form of GPB.

MNSs Antibodies

Anti-M is a relatively common antibody that may be IgM or IgG. Rare examples are reactive at 37°C when they can give rise to haemolytic transfusion reactions. Anti-M very rarely gives rise to HDN.

Anti-N is uncommon and of no clinical significance.

Anti-S and anti-s are usually IgG; both rarely have been implicated in haemolytic transfusion reactions and HDN.

Anti-U is a rare immune antibody, usually containing an IgG1 component. It has been known to cause fatal haemolytic transfusion reactions and severe HDN.

Other Blood Group Systems

Lutheran System

The antigens in the Lutheran system are not well-developed at birth, and as a consequence there are no documented cases of clinically significant haemolytic disease owing to Lutheran antibodies.

Anti-Lu^a is uncommon and rarely of clinical significance. Anti-Lu^b has caused extravascular haemolysis.

Yt (Cartwright) System

The antigens Yt^a and Yt^b are found on GPI-linked acetylcholinesterase. Some examples of anti-Yt^a have caused accelerated red cell destruction.

Colton System

The antigens in the Colton system, Co^a and Co^b, are carried on the water-transport protein, channel-forming integral protein (CHIP-1). Anti-Co^a and the rarer anti-Co^b are both sometimes clinically significant.

Dombrock System

The antigens in the Dombrock system include Do^a and Do^b and also include the high-incidence antigens Gy^a, Hy, and Jo^a. Antibodies of this system are usually weak, but all should be considered as potentially significant.

Clinical Significance of Red Cell Alloantibodies

The significance of the alloantibodies described, with respect to the nature of the haemolytic transfusion reaction they produce, is provided in Table 19.8. The majority of haemolytic transfusion reactions, however, are the result of ABO incompatibility,[17] as shown in Table 19.9.

Mollison et al[18] analysed the significance of blood group antigens other than those of the ABO system and D by looking at the prevalence of transfusion-induced red cell alloantibodies, excluding anti-D, -CD, and -DE (Table 19.10). Rh antibodies, mainly anti-c or anti-E, accounted for 53% of the total, and anti-K and anti-Fy^a accounted for a further 38%, leaving only about 9% for all other specificities. A similar distribution of the different red cell antibodies was found in a smaller group of patients who experienced immediate haemolytic transfusion reactions (HTR). However, the figures for delayed HTR showed a striking increase in the relative frequency of Jk antibodies, which reflects the outlined characteristics of Jk antibodies.

Haemolytic disease of the fetus and newborn has not been associated with antibodies directed against Lewis antigens, and only very mild disease is produced by anti-Lu^a and anti-Lu^b. With these exceptions, all other IgG antibodies directed against antigens in the systems mentioned should be

Table 19.8   Antibody specificities related to the mechanism of immune haemolytic destruction

Blood group system	Intravascular haemolysis	Extravascular haemolysis
ABO,H	A, B, H	
Rh		All
Kell	K	K, k, Kp^a, Kp^b, Js^a, Js^b
Kidd	Jk^a	Jk^a, Jk^b, Jk^3
Duffy		Fy^a, Fy^b
MNS		M, S, s, U
Lutheran		Lu^b
Lewis	Le^a	
Cartwright		Yt^a
Colton		Co^a, Co^b
Dombrock		Do^a, Do^b

Table 19.9   Fatal acute haemolytic transfusion reactions reported in the United States to the FDA between 1976 and 1985

Incompatibility	No. of deaths
O recipient and A red cells	80
O recipient and B/AB red cells	26
B recipient and A/AB red cells	12
A recipient and B red cells	6
O plasma to A/AB recipient	6
B plasma to AB recipient	1
Total ABO incompatibilities	131
Anti-K	5
Anti-E+K+P_1	1
Anti-Jk^b	1
Anti-Jk^a+Jk^b+Jk^3	1
Anti-Fy^a	1
Total non–ABO incompatibilities	9

Table 19.10 Relative frequency of immune red cell alloantibodies*

Patient group	No. studied	Blood group alloantibodies (% of total)				
		Rh[+]	K	Fy	Jk	Other
Transfused (some pregnant)	5228	53.1	28.1	10.2	4.0	4.7
Immediate HTR[+]	142	42.2	30.3	18.3	8.5	0.7
Delayed HTR[+]	82	34.2	14.6	15.9	32.9	2.4

*Excluding antibodies of ABO, Lewis, P systems, and anti-M and anti-N.
[+]Excluding anti-D (or –CD or –DE); almost all were anti-c or anti-E.
[+]Haemolytic transfusion reaction.
Adapted from Mollison PL, Engelfriet CP, Contreras M 1997 Blood transfusion in clinical medicine, 9th ed. Blackwell Scientific, Oxford, p. 112, based on published data from several sources.

considered capable of causing haemolysis in this setting.

The significance of the many other blood group antigens not referred to in the text is summarised in Table 19.11. However, it should be noted that the antibodies listed are usually wholly or predominantly IgG and would be detectable in routine pretransfusion testing using the indirect antiglobulin test (IAT).

It is difficult to find suitable blood for transfusion to a patient whose serum contains an antibody, such as anti-Vel, which has a specificity for a high-frequency antigen and which can cause severe haemolytic transfusion reactions. In addition to using blood from a frozen blood bank, autologous blood should be considered, and if necessary, the compatibility of red cells from close relatives (particularly siblings) should be investigated. Antibodies such as anti-Kn[a] are commonly found and not clinically important, but their presence may cause delay in the provision of blood until their specificity has been determined.

Mechanisms of Immune Destruction of Red Cells

Immune-mediated haemolysis of red cells depends on the following[19]:

1. The immunoglobulin class of the antibody (for all practical purposes, antibodies directed against red cell antigens are either IgM or IgG or both).
2. The ability of the antibody to bind complement.

3. Interaction with the reticuloendothelial system (mononuclear phagocytic system). The most important phagocyte participating in immune haemolysis is the macrophage, predominantly in the spleen.

The mechanism of immune haemolysis also determines the site of haemolysis:

a. *Intravascular haemolysis* owing to sequential binding of complement components (C1 to C9) cascade and the formation of the membrane attack complex (MAC; $C5b678(9)_n$). This is characteristic of IgM antibodies, but some IgG antibodies can also act as haemolysins. Red cells are usually destroyed by intravascular complement lysis in ABO incompatible transfusion reactions (p. 549). Most other alloimmune red cell destruction is extravascular and mediated by the mononuclear-phagocytic system.

Red cell autoantibodies may also cause intravascular lysis, especially the IgG autoantibody of PCH (p. 255) and some autoantibodies of the cold haemagglutinin disease (CHAD) (p. 254). Complement-mediated intravascular lysis may also occur in drug-induced immune haemolysis (p. 258).

b. *Extravascular haemolysis* by the mononuclear phagocytic system is characteristic of IgG antibodies and occurs predominantly in the spleen. This is caused by noncomplement–binding IgG antibodies or those that bind sublytic amounts of complement. Macrophages have Fcγ receptors for cell-bound IgG, and

Table 19.11   "Minor" blood group antigens

Antigen	Antigen frequency (%)caucasians	Associated HTR	Associated HDN	Comments
Diª	0	Yes	Yes	Part of DI system. Diª
Diᵇ	100	Yes	Yes	More common in American Indians and Orientals
Wrª	<0.1	Yes	Yes	
Xgª	65 (males) 88 (females)	Rarely	Rarely	Xgª only antigen in system
Sc1	>99.9	No	No	3 antigens in SC system
Sc2	<0.1	No	Mild	
Ge2	100	Some	No	7 antigens in GE system
Ge3	>99.9	Some	No	
Crª	100	Some	No	10 antigens in CR system
Ch1	96	No	No	9 antigens in CH/RG systems, reside on C4
Rg1	98	No	No	
Knª	98	No	No	Belong to KN system of 5 antigens
McCª	98	No	No	
Ykª	92	No	No	
Inª	0.1	Yes	No	Inª has incidence of 4% in Asian Indians
Inᵇ	99	Yes	No	
LWª	100	Some	Mild	—
JMH	>99.9	No	No	One of 901 series of high-incidence antigens
Vel	>99.9	Yes	No	One of 901 series; complement binding
Bgª	approx 15	No	No	Corresponds to HLA-B7, detectable on red cells

HTR, haemolytic transfusion reactions; HDN, haemolytic disease of the newborn.

sensitised red cells may be wholly phago-cytosed or lose part of the membrane and return to the circulation as microspherocytes. Spherocytes are less deformable and more readily trapped in the spleen than normal red cells; this shortens their lifespan. In addition to Fc receptor–mediated phagocytosis, anti-body-dependent cell-mediatedcytotoxicity (ADCC) may also contribute to cell damage during the close contact with splenic macro-phages. Red cells are destroyed external to the monocyte membrane by lysosomal enzymes secreted by the monocyte.[20]

Complement components may enhance red cell destruction. Complement activation by some IgM and most IgG antibodies is not always complete, and the red cell escapes intravascular lysis. The activation of complement stops at the C3 stage, and, in these circumstances, complement can be detected on the red cell by the antiglobulin test using appropriate anticomplement reagents. The first activation product of C3 is membrane-bound C3b, which is constantly being broken down to C3bi. Red cells with these components on their surface adhere to phagocytes (monocytes, macrophages, and granulocytes), which have complement receptors, CR1 (CD35) and CR3 (CD11b/CD18). These sensitised cells are rapidly sequestered in the liver because of its bulk of phagocytic cells (Küpffer) cells and large blood flow, but no engulfment occurs. When C3bi is cleaved, leaving only C3dg on the cell surface, the cells tagged with "inactive" C3dg return to the circulation, as in chronic haemagglutinin disease. However, when IgG is also present on the cell surface, C3b enhances phagocytosis, and under these circumstances both liver and spleen are important sites of extravascular haemolysis. Hence, C3b and C3bi augment macrophage-mediated clearance of IgG-coated cells, and antibodies binding sublytic amounts of complement (e.g., Duffy and Kidd antibodies), often cause more rapid destruction and more marked symptoms than noncomplement binding antibodies (e.g., Rh antibodies).

Macrophage activity is an important component of cell destruction, and further study of cellular interactions at this stage of immune haemolysis may provide an explanation for the differing severity of haemolysis in patients with apparently similar antibodies. *In vitro* macrophage (monocyte) assays have been introduced to supplement conventional serological techniques to assess this aspect of immune haemolysis.[21]

Factors that may affect the interaction between sensitised cells and macrophages include the following:

1. *IgG subclass.* IgG1 and IgG3 antibodies have a higher binding affinity to mononuclear Fcγ receptors than IgG2 and IgG4 antibodies.
2. *Antigen density.* This affects the number of antibody molecules bound to the cell surface.
3. *Fluid-phase IgG.* Serum IgG concentration is a determinant of Fc-dependent mononuclear-phagocytic function. Normal levels of IgG block the adherence of sensitized red cells to monocyte Fc receptors (particularly FcγR1) *in vitro*. Haemoconcentration within the splenic sinusoids is probably a major factor in minimising this effect *in vivo,* which may explain why the spleen is about 100 times more efficient at removing IgG-sensitised cells than the liver despite the greater macrophage mass and higher blood flow of the latter organ.

The initial effect of high-dose intravenous IgG is to cause blockade of macrophage FcγR. This reduces the immune clearance of antibody-coated cells and has particular application in the management of autoimmune thrombocytopenia and post-transfusion purpura.

4. *Regulation of macrophage activity.* Cytokines are now known to be important in the upregulation of macrophage receptors. Interferon gamma enhances macrophage phagocytic activity by increasing the expression of FcγRI *in vitro* and *in vivo* and also activates FcγII without increasing the number of these receptors.[22]

Interleukin-6 also enhances FcγRII activation, and increased activity of the CR1 receptor occurs through the action of T-cell cytokines and through chemotactic agents released in the inflammatory response.[23] The increased levels of proinflammatory cytokines and other biological mediators and their effects on the activity of the monocyte phagocytic system have been monitored in patients with systemic inflammatory response syndrome.[24] It is therefore possible that release of cytokines during viral and bacterial infections could, at least in part, trigger some episodes of autoimmune cell destruction.

The rate of immune destruction is therefore determined by antigen and antibody characteristics and the level of activation of the monocyte phagocytic system.

Antigen–Antibody Reactions

The red cell is a convenient marker for serological reactions. Agglutination or lysis (owing to complement action) is a visible indication (end-point) of an antigen–antibody reaction. The reaction occurs in two stages: in the first stage the antibody binds to the red cell antigen (sensitisation) and the second stage involves agglutination (or lysis) of the sensitised cells.

The *first stage* (i.e., association of antibody with antigen [sensitisation]) is reversible and the strength of binding (equilibrium constant) depends on the "exactness of fit" between antigen and antibody. This is influenced by the following:

1. *Temperature.* Cold antibodies (usually IgM) generally bind best to the red cell at a low temperature (e.g., 4°C), whereas warm antibodies (usually IgG) bind most efficiently at body temperature (i.e., 37°C).
2. *pH.* There is relatively little change in antibody binding over the pH range 5.5–8.5, but to ensure comparable results, it is preferable to buffer the saline in which serum or cells are diluted to a fixed pH, usually 7.0. Some antibody elution techniques depend on altering the pH to less than 4 or more than 10.
3. *Ionic strength of the medium.* Low ionic strength increases the rate of antibody binding. This is the basis of antibody detection tests using low ionic strength saline (LISS).

The *second stage* depends on various laboratory manipulations to promote agglutination or lysis of sensitised cells. The cell surface is negatively charged (mainly owing to sialic acid residues), which keeps individual cells apart; the minimum distance between red cells suspended in saline is about 18 nm. Agglutination is brought about by antibody crosslinking between cells. The span between antigen-binding sites on IgM molecules (30 nm) is sufficient to allow IgM antibodies to bridge between saline-suspended red cells (after settling) and so cause agglutination. IgG molecules have a shorter span (15 nm) and are usually unable to agglutinate sensitised red cells suspended in saline; notwithstanding this, heavy IgG sensitisation owing to high-antigen density lowers intercellular repulsive forces and is able to promote agglutination in saline (e.g., IgG anti-A, anti-B). The agglutination of red cells coated by either IgM or IgG antibodies is enhanced by centrifugation. However, it is standard procedure to promote agglutination of IgG-sensitised red cells by the following:

1. Reducing intercellular distance by pretreatment of red cells with protease enzymes (e.g., papain or bromelin), which reduce the surface charge of red cells (p. 497).
2. Adding polymers (e.g., albumin), although the mechanism by which albumin or other water-soluble polymers enhance agglutination is uncertain.

3. Bridging between sensitised cells with an anti-globulin reagent in the antiglobulin test (p. 501).

Some complement-binding antibodies (especially IgM) may cause lysis *in vitro* (without noticeable agglutination), which can be enhanced by the addition of fresh serum as a source of complement. However, complement activation may only proceed to the C3 stage; in these circumstances cell-bound C3 can be detected by the antiglobulin test using an appropriate anticomplement reagent (p. 501).

Quality Assurance within the Laboratory

It has long been appreciated that the test systems used for routine pretransfusion testing are of the utmost importance because errors can and do lead to patient morbidity and mortality. It is therefore of little surprise that within the European Union all reagents, calibrators, and control materials for red cell typing and for determining the presence of "irregular anti-erythrocytic antibodies" have been included under the In-vitro Diagnostics (IVD) Medical Devices Directive.[25] (See also p. 658). This means that all reagents sold within the European Union must display the CE mark to show that they conform to the agreed Common Technical Specifications (CTS). In each European country, a Competent Authority will be able to withdraw or suspend certification of any reagent, depending on the information received from its Notified Body, which will perform batch release approval and monitor the performance of the manufacturer and the product.

The arrival of this Directive further reinforces the potential liabilities of an individual laboratory, which takes on the product liability of a manufacturer if reagents are made "in-house" or if the manufacturer's recommended method is not strictly adhered to.

The majority of the following points are taken from the British Committee for Standards in Haematology (BCSH) guidelines[26,27] for pretransfusion compatibility testing:

1. General Aspects
a. The laboratory should document its Quality System, appropriate to its requirements.

b. Attention should be given to the sensible inclusion of internal controls in all the tests undertaken.

c. The laboratory should participate in External Quality Assessment exercises.

d. The laboratory should only make use of systems that have been validated against its documented requirements.

e. The laboratory should ensure that they have procedures to cover the failure of automated equipment and computer(s). The laboratory should develop procedures to build in checks for all critical points in transfusion testing (e.g., preserving the identity of patient samples, transcribing results).

2. Reagents

a. The head of the laboratory should refer to available specifications for reagents given by, for example, the International Society of Blood Transfusion (ISBT), the American Association of Blood Banks (AABB), or the Guidelines for the Blood Transfusion Services.[28,29]

b. All reagents or systems should be used in accordance with the manufacturer's instructions. Where this is not possible, the procedure should be validated in accordance with the BCSH Guidelines on evaluation, validation, and implementation of new techniques for blood grouping, antibody screening, and crossmatching.[30]

c. There should be a record of all batch numbers and expiry dates of all reagents used in the laboratory.

3. Techniques

a. All procedures used should be in accordance with recommended practice as outlined here.

b. It is essential that the antiglobulin technique chosen has been validated against the documented requirements of the laboratory and has been subjected to a thorough field trial before being introduced into the laboratory.[31]

c. All changes in techniques must be thoroughly validated in accordance with the BCSH Guidelines on evaluation, validation and implementation of new techniques before being introduced into routine use.

d. Written authorised standard operating procedures (SOPs) which cover all aspects of the laboratory work must be available and reviewed regularly.

e. The regular checking and maintenance of all laboratory equipment must be documented. In particular, there should be a documented quality-assurance procedure for cell washers (e.g., using the National Institute of Biological Standards and Control [NIBSC] anti-D standard)[32] (See p. 694.)

4. Staff Training and Proficiency

a. There should be a documented programme for training laboratory staff, which covers all SOPs in use and which fulfils the documented requirements of the laboratory.

b. Laboratory tasks should only be undertaken by appropriately trained staff.

c. There must be a documented programme for assessing staff proficiency (e.g., replicate testing for the IAT), which should include details of the action limits for retraining.[33]

5. Auditing and Reviewing Practice

a. There should be a system in place for documenting and reviewing all incidents of noncompliance with procedures.

b. The systems should enable a full audit trail of laboratory steps, including the original results, interpretations, authorisations, and all staff responsible for conducting each step.

c. A programme of independent audits should be conducted to assess compliance with documented "in-house" procedures.

6. Health and Safety

When appropriate, reagents should have been screened for human immunodeficiency virus and hepatitis B and C virus. All high-risk samples must be handled in accordance with the laboratory safety code (see Chapter 25).

General Points of Serological Technique

Serum versus Plasma

Serum is preferred to plasma for the detection of red cell alloantibodies. Nevertheless, plasma is being used increasingly for convenience in microplate technology and in automated systems.

When plasma is used, complement is inactivated by the ethylenediaminetetra-acetic acid (EDTA) anticoagulant. This is relevant for the detection of some complement-binding antibodies (e.g., of Kidd specificity) that may be missed or give only weak reactions with anti-IgG in the routine antiglobulin test but can be readily detected by anticomplement (p. 501). It is therefore essential, before using plasma, to optimise the sensitivity of techniques for detecting weak IgG antibodies and to validate the procedure (p. 502). For example, in antibody screening, increased sensitivity can be achieved by using panel cells with homozygous expression of selected antigens (p. 532).

Collection and Storage of Blood Samples

Positive identification of the patient and careful labelling of blood samples are essential to avoid misidentification errors. Venous blood is desirable for blood-grouping purposes, and 5–10 ml of blood should be taken and either allowed to clot at room temperature or anticoagulated with EDTA in a sterile glass tube. This will provide serum or plasma and red cells. If serum is required urgently, the specimen may be placed in a 37°C waterbath and centrifuged as soon as the clot can be seen to have started to retract.

Storage of Sera or Plasma

Great care must be taken to identify and label correctly any serum or plasma separated from the patient's original sample.

Whole blood samples will deteriorate over time. Problems associated with storage include red cell lysis; loss of complement in the serum; decrease in potency of red cell antibodies, particularly IgM antibodies; and bacterial contamination. However, in the absence of evidence, it has been suggested that whole blood can be stored at room temperature for up to 48 hours and up to 7 days at 4°C. It has also been recommended that laboratories evaluate the stability of weak antibodies before making local decisions for storage conditions. Patient's serum or plasma is best stored frozen at –20°C or below in 1–2 ml volumes in plastic vials. Repeated thawing of a sample is harmful. If the sera are stored at –20°C or below, no precautions are necessary with respect to sterility. Complement deteriorates rapidly on storage, but sera separated from blood as quickly as possible and stored at –20°C retain most of their complement activity for 1–2 weeks. For compatibility tests, samples of serum should be separated from the red cells as soon as possible and stored at –20°C until used because the content of complement may be important for the detection of some antibodies.

Red Cell Suspensions

Normal Ionic Strength Saline

A 2–3% suspension of washed red cells in phosphate buffered saline (PBS), pH 7.0, is generally recommended. Cells suspended in normal ionic strength saline (NISS) are routinely used for antibody titrations, but their use in routine pretransfusion testing has declined over the last decade as observations from external quality assessment exercises have demonstrated that laboratories using NISS have a significantly lower detection rate of antibodies than those using other technologies.[34]

Low Ionic Strength Saline

It is known that the rate of association of antibodies with red cell antigens is enhanced by lowering the ionic strength of the medium in which the reactions take place. Hence, a major advantage of low ionic strength saline (LISS) is that the incubation period in the IAT (p. 502) can be shortened while maintaining or increasing sensitivity to the majority of red cell antibodies. The LISS solution can be made up in the laboratory (p. 690) or purchased commercially.

There was historical reluctance to use low ionic strength media in routine laboratory work for two reasons: first, nonspecific agglutination may occur when NaCl concentrations <2 g/l (0.03 mol/l) are used, and second, complement components are bound to the red cells at low ionic strengths.

To avoid false-positive results, the following rules should be followed:

a. Red cells resuspended in LISS and serum or plasma should be incubated together in equal volumes: 2 volumes of cells to 2 volumes of serum are recommended to ensure the optimal molarity in the test of the order of 0.09 mol. Doubling the serum to cell ratio (by halving the cell concentration from 3% to 1.5%) will enhance the detection of some antibodies (e.g., anti-K) that might otherwise be missed.[35]

b. The red cells should be washed in saline twice and then once in LISS before suspending in LISS at 1.5–2% cell suspension.

c. The working solution of LISS should be freshly made and kept at room temperature.
d. Centrifugation force and time should be optimal to give maximum sensitivity with freedom from false-positive or false-negative reactions (p. 503).

False-positive reactions may still infrequently occur with some sera/plasma. If plasma is used, subsequent serological work may be performed using NISS; if serum is used, anti-IgG should replace the polyspecific antiglobulin reagent.

Reagent Red Cells

Red cells of selected phenotypes are required for ABO and RhD grouping, Rh phenotyping, and antibody screening and identification (see Chapter 20). Such cells are available commercially or from blood transfusion centres.

Use of Enzyme-Treated Cells

Enzyme-treated red cells are useful reagents in the detection and investigation of autoantibodies and alloantibodies. Papain and bromelin are currently used for this purpose. Enzyme treatment is known to increase the avidity of both IgM and IgG antibodies. The receptors of some red cell antigens, however, may be inactivated by enzyme treatment (e.g., M, N, S, Fy^b).

The most sensitive techniques are those using washed enzyme-pretreated red cells (two-stage), which should match the performance of the spin tube LISS antiglobulin test (p. 502) One-stage mixtures and papain inhibitor techniques are relatively insensitive and are now not recommended. An ISBT/International Council for Standardization in Haematology (ICSH) protease enzyme standard and an agreed method for its use are available from listed centres.[36]

Preparation of Papain Solution (Low's Method)

A 1% solution of papain is made as follows: Grind 2 g of papain in a mortar in 100 ml of Sorenson's phosphate buffer, pH 5.4 (p. 692). Centrifuge for 10 min and add 10 ml of 0.5 mol/l cysteine hydrochloride to the supernatant to activate the enzyme. Dilute the solution to 200 ml with the phosphate buffer and incubate for 1 hour at 37°C. Dispense the enzyme in small volumes (e.g.,

0.1–0.2 ml); it will keep satisfactorily for many months at –20°C, but once a tube is unfrozen any of the solution not immediately used should be discarded.

The enzyme activity should be standardised using an azoalbumin assay[37] because this will determine the incubation time for enzyme treatment of the cells. The enzyme preparation should also be compared with the ISBT/ICSH papain standard using the same batch of azoalbumin, and so serve as an "in house" standard.[36]

Two-Stage Papain Method

For the two-stage papain method,[38] add 1 volume of 1% papain (activated as described earlier) to 9 volumes of Sorenson's phosphate buffer, pH 7.0 (p. 692) in a 10 × 75 mm plastic tube. Incubate at 37°C equal volumes of the freshly diluted papain and packed washed red cells for a time that must be determined for each batch of papain depending on the azoalbumin activity; this is normally 15–30 min. After incubation, wash the cells in two changes of saline, pH 7.0, then dilute as required to 3% in NISS or 1.5% in LISS. For NISS tests, add 1 drop of NISS–suspended cells to 1 drop of serum. For LISS tests, add 2 drops of LISS–suspended cells to 2 drops of serum. Incubate for 15 min in a 37°C waterbath.

Preparation of Bromelin Solution[39]

Prepare a 0.5% solution by dissolving the bromelin powder in a mixture of 9 volumes of saline and 1 volume of Sorensen's phosphate buffer, pH 5.4 (p. 692). Store the solution in 0.5–1.0 ml volumes at –20°C, at which temperature it will keep for months. As preservatives, add 0.1% sodium azide and 0.5% Actidione (a fungicide). Add the bromelin, in the same way as papain is added in Low's technique, to the serum just before the addition of the red cells. There is no need to pretreat the red cells with the enzyme. Bromelin activity can be standardised by an azoalbumin assay as for papain.

Controls are particularly important when enzyme-treated cells are being used, and it must be established without question that the altered cells are reacting appropriately with sera of known antibody content. Only in this way can the potency of the enzyme and the method of enzyme treatment be checked. Enzyme-treated cells are compared with untreated cells in reactions with a positive control (0.25 iu/ml anti-D) and a negative control (AB serum or fresh compatible serum).

Agglutination of Red Cells by Antibody: A Basic Method

Agglutination tests are usually carried out in tubes or microtitre plates, using centrifugation or sedimentation. Slide tests are sometimes used for emergency ABO and RhD grouping (p. 528 and 529). For microplate tests, see page 529.

Tube Tests

Add 1 volume of a 2% red cell suspension to 1 volume of serum or serum dilution in a disposable plastic or glass tube. Mix well and leave undisturbed for the appropriate time (see later).

Tubes

For agglutination tests, use medium-sized (75 × 10 or 12 mm) disposable plastic or glass tubes. Similar tubes should be used for lysis tests when it is essential to have a relatively deep layer of serum to look through, if small amounts of lysis are to be detected. The level of the fluid must rise much higher than the concave bottom of the tubes.

Glass tubes should always be used if the contents are to be heated to 50°C or higher or if organic solvents are being used. Glass tubes, however, are difficult to clean satisfactorily, particularly small bore tubes, and cleaning methods such as those given on page 695 should be followed carefully.

Temperature and Time of Exposure of Red Cells to Antibody

In blood group serology, tube tests are generally done at 37°C, room temperature, or both. There is some advantage in using a 20°C waterbath rather than relying on "room temperature," which in different countries and seasons may vary from 15°C (or less) to 30°C (or more).

Sedimentation tube tests are usually read after 1–2 hours have elapsed. Strong agglutination will, however, be obvious much sooner than this. In spin tube tests, agglutination can be read after only 5–10 min incubation if the cell–serum mixture is centrifuged.

Slide Tests

Because of evaporation, slide tests must be read within about 5 min. Reagents that produce strong agglutination within 1–2 min are normally used for rapid ABO and RhD grouping. Because the results are read macroscopically, strong cell suspensions should be used (35–45% cells in their own serum or plasma)

Reading Results of Tube Tests

Only the strongest complete (C) grade of agglutination seems to be able to withstand a shake procedure without some degree of disruption, which may downgrade the strength of reaction. The BCSH Blood Transfusion Task Force has therefore recommended the following reading procedure.[40]

Microscopic Reading

It is essential that a careful and standardised technique be followed. Lift the tube carefully from its rack without disturbing the button of sedimented cells. Holding the tube vertically, introduce a Pasteur pipette, with its tip cut at 90 degrees. Carefully draw up a column of supernatant about 1 cm in length and then, without introducing an air bubble, draw up a 1–2 mm column of red cells by placing the tip of the pipette in the button of red cells. Gently expel the supernatant and cells onto a slide over an area of about 2 × 1 cm. It is important not to overload the suspension with cells, and the method described earlier achieves this.

A scheme of scoring the results is given in Table 19.12.

Macroscopic Reading

A gentle agitation tip-and-roll "macroscopic" method is recommended. It is possible to read agglutination tests macroscopically with the aid of a hand reading glass or concave mirror, but it is then difficult to distinguish reactions weaker than + (microscopic reading) from the normal slight granular appearance of unagglutinated red cells in suspension. Macroscopic reading thus gives lower titration values than does microscopic reading, but the former is recommended. Follow the system of scoring in Table 19.12.

A good idea of the presence or absence of agglutination can often be obtained by inspection

Table 19.12   Scoring of results in red cell agglutination tests

Symbol	Agglutination score*	Description
4+ or C (complete)	12	Cell button remains in one clump, macroscopically visible
3+	10	Cell button dislodges into several large clumps, macroscopically visible
2+	8	Cell button dislodges into many small clumps, macroscopically visible
1+	5	Cell button dislodges into finely granular clumps, macroscopically just visible
(+) or w (weak)	3	Cell button dislodges into fine granules, only visible microscopically[†]
–	0	Negative result—all cells free and evenly distributed

*Titration scores are the summation of the agglutination scores at each dilution.
[†]May be further classified depending on the number of cells in the clumps (e.g., clumps of 12–20 cells [score 3]; 8–10 cells [score 2]; 4–6 cells [score 1]. This is the minimum agglutination that should be considered positive.

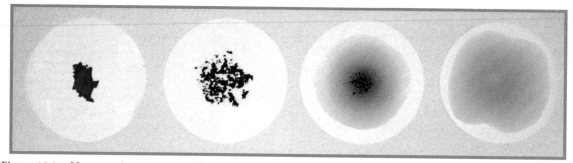

Figure 19.2   Macroscopic appearances of agglutination in round-bottom tubes or hollow tiles. Agglutination is shown by various degrees of "graininess"; in the absence of agglutination, the sedimented cells appear as a smooth round button, as on the extreme right.

of the deposit of sedimented cells: a perfectly smooth round button suggests no agglutination, whereas agglutination is shown by varying degrees of irregularity, "graininess," or dispersion of the deposit (Fig. 19.2).

Demonstration of Lysis

Many blood-group antibodies lyse red cells under suitable conditions in the presence of complement. This is particularly true of anti-A and anti-B, anti-P, anti-Le^a and Le^b, anti-PP$_1$P^k (anti-Tj^a), and certain autoantibodies (p. 253). If it is necessary to add fresh complement, this should be mixed with the serum being tested before the addition of red cells.

Otherwise, agglutination occurs and could block complement access. Lysis should be looked for at the end of the incubation period before the tubes are centrifuged, if the cells have sedimented sufficiently; lysis may be scored semiquantitatively after centrifuging the suspensions and comparing the colour of the supernatant with that of the control.

If the occurrence of lysis is of interest, then the final volume of the cell-serum suspension has to be greater than is required for the reading of agglutination. Tubes (75 × 10 or 12 mm) should be used, and the level of the cell–serum suspension must rise much higher than the concave bottom of the tubes.

In testing for lytic activity, a high concentration of complement may be required. Therefore, in contrast to tests for agglutination, it is advantageous to use a stronger red cell suspension (c 5%).

Lysis tests are usually carried out at 37°C, but with cold antibodies a lower temperature (e.g., 20°C or 30°C) would be appropriate, depending on the upper thermal range of activity of the antibody or, in the case of the Donath–Landsteiner antibody, 0°C followed by 37°C (p. 255).

With certain antibodies the pH of the cell–serum suspension affects the occurrence of lysis. In these, optimal pH is 6.5–6.8.

Controls

It is necessary to be sure that any lysis observed is not artefactual (i.e., that lysis is brought about by the serum under test and not by the serum added as complement) and that the added complement is potent. A complement control (no test serum) is thus necessary, as is a control using a serum known to contain a lytic antibody.

In lysis tests, great care should be taken to deliver the cell suspension directly into the serum. If the cell suspension comes into contact with the side of the tube and starts to dry, this in itself will lead to lysis.

Antiglobulin Test

The antiglobulin test (Coombs test) was introduced by Coombs, Mourant, and Race in 1945[41] as a method for detecting "incomplete" Rh antibodies (i.e., IgG antibodies capable of sensitising red cells but incapable of causing agglutination of the same cells suspended in saline) as opposed to "complete" IgM antibodies, which do agglutinate saline-suspended red cells.

Direct and indirect antiglobulin tests can be carried out. In the *direct* antiglobulin test (DAT), the patient's cells, after careful washing, are tested for sensitisation that has occurred *in vivo*; in the *indirect* antiglobulin test (IAT), normal red cells are incubated with a serum suspected of containing an antibody and subsequently tested, after washing, for *in vitro*-bound antibody.

The antiglobulin test is probably the most important test in the serologist's repertoire. The DAT is used to demonstrate *in vivo* attachment of antibodies to red cells, as in autoimmune haemolytic anaemia (p. 246), alloimmune HDN (p. 540), and

alloimmune haemolysis following an incompatible transfusion (p. 549). The IAT has wide application in blood transfusion serology, including antibody screening and identification and crossmatching.

Antiglobulin Reagents

Polyspecific (Broad-Spectrum) Reagents

The majority of red cell antibodies are noncomplement-binding IgG; anti-IgG is therefore an essential component of any polyspecific reagent. Anti-IgA is not required because IgG antibodies of the same specificity always occur in the presence of IgA antibodies. Anti-IgM is also not required because clinically significant IgM alloantibodies that do not cause agglutination in saline are much more easily detected by the complement they bind.

Anticomplement has also traditionally been considered essential—namely, anti-C3c and anti-C3d. However, if plasma is used, only anti-IgG is necessary because EDTA prevents complement activation. In addition, it seems that most, if not all, antibodies detected by the C3-anti-C3 reaction in normal ionic strength tests can be detected with anti-IgG in polybrene, polyethylene glycol (PEG), and LISS. Laboratories using techniques other than NISS have adopted the use of anti-IgG alone, supported by changes to guidelines from the AABB in 1990 and from the BCSH in 1996. Nevertheless, the BCSH guidelines stress the importance of having screening cells with homozygous expression of Jk[a] before deciding to use anti-IgG rather than a polyspecific antiglobulin reagent. Anti-C3 will certainly be required for DATs for the diagnosis of autoimmune haemolytic anaemia.

Monospecific Reagents

Monospecific reagents can be prepared against the heavy chains of IgG, IgM, and IgA and are referred to as anti-γ, anti-μ, and anti-α; antibodies against IgG subclasses are also available. Specific antibodies against the complement components C4 and C3 and C3 breakdown products can be prepared as mentioned earlier.

The main clinical application of these monospecific reagents is to define the immunochemical characteristics of antibodies. This is relevant to the mechanisms of *in vivo* cell destruction and, in the case of IgG, the subclasses have different biological properties (p. 494).

Quality Control of Antiglobulin Reagents

The quality control of antiglobulin reagents must always be carried out by the exact technique by which they are to be used. All reagents should be used according to the manufacturer's instructions, unless appropriately standardised for other methods.

An ISBT/ICSH freeze-dried reference reagent is available for evaluating either polyspecific anti-human globulin reagents or those containing their separate monospecific components.[28] The validation of a new antiglobulin reagent should assess the following qualities of the reagent:

1. *Specificity.* The reagent should only agglutinate red cells sensitised with antibodies and/or coated with significant levels of complement components.
2. *Potency of anti-IgG by serological titration.*
3. *Specificity and potency of anticomplement antibodies.* A polyspecific reagent should contain anti-C3c and anti-C3d at controlled levels to avoid false-positive reactions or a suitable potent monoclonal anti-C3d (e.g., BRIC-8). It should contain little or no anti-C4. The assessment of these qualities requires red cells specifically coated with C3b, Cb3i, C3d, and C4. Details of the procedures recommended for the preparation of such cells have been published by an ISBT/ICSH Working Party.[42]

It is appreciated that some hospital blood banks will be unable to evaluate an antiglobulin reagent as comprehensively as outlined earlier. They should, however, carry out the following minimal assessment of all new antiglobulin reagents:

1. Test the antiglobulin reagent for freedom from false-positive results by simulated crossmatch tests:
    a. Test for excess anti-C3d by incubating fresh serum at 37°C by NISS and LISS tests with 6 ABO-compatible cells from CPD-A1 donor unit segments (10–30 days old). This is a critical test for false-positive results owing to C3d uptake by stored blood, which is further augmented by incubation with fresh serum.
    b. Tests for contaminating red cell antibodies (against washed A₁, B, and O cells) must be negative.

Only proceed further if the antiglobulin reagent passes the previously listed tests.

2. Compare the antiglobulin reagent with the current reagent using a selection of weak antibodies. These antibodies may be selected from those encountered in routine work or can be obtained from a transfusion centre or reference laboratory. Store such antibodies in small volumes at 4°C for repeated tests.
3. Dilute a weak IgG anti-D (0.8 iu/ml), as used for routine antiglobulin test controls, from undiluted (neat) to 1 in 16 and sensitise R₁r red cells with each dilution of anti-D. These sensitised cells (washed four times) should then be tested with neat to 1 in 8 dilutions of the antiglobulin reagents. The antiglobulin reagent should not show prozones by immediate spin tests using 2 volumes of antiglobulin per test. The potency of the test antiglobulin should at least match the current antiglobulin reagent.

The ISBT/ICSH antiglobulin reference reagent can be used to calibrate an "in-house" antiglobulin reagent for use as a routine standard.

The quality control of Ig class and subclass specific antiglobulin reagents, although following the previously listed general principles, is more complex. Details of the appropriate techniques are beyond the scope of this chapter; the reader should consult the review by Engelfriet et al.[43]

Recommended Antiglobulin Test Procedure

A spin tube technique is recommended for the routine antiglobulin test; the procedure described here is based on BCSH *Guidelines for Compatibility Testing in Hospital Blood Banks.*[26,40] Reliable performance depends on the correct procedure at each stage of the test and appropriate quality-control measures.

The test should be carried out in glass tubes (75 × 10 or 12 mm). Plastic tubes are not recommended because they may adsorb IgG, which could neutralize anti-IgG of the antiglobulin reagent.

1. *Sensitise red cells* (not relevant to the direct test) by using the following serum:cell ratios:
    a. For NISS, use at least 2 volumes of serum (preferably 4) and 1 volume of a 3% suspen-

sion of red cells washed (3 times) and suspended in PB) or 0.15 mol/l NaCl (p. 690).

b. For LISS, use 2 volumes of serum and 2 volumes of a 1.5% suspension of red cells washed twice in PBS or 0.15 mol/l NaCl and washed once in LISS and then suspended in LISS (p. 690).

c. For commercial low ionic strength additive solutions, the manufacturer's instructions must be followed.

Because the volume of "a drop" varies according to the type of pipette or dropper bottle, a measured or known drop volume should be used to ensure that appropriate serum:cell ratios are maintained.

Mix the reactants by shaking, then incubate at 37°C, preferably in a waterbath, for a minimum period of 15 min for LISS tests and 45 min for NISS tests.

2. *Wash the test cells* 4 times with a minimum of 3 ml of saline per wash. Vigorous injection of saline is necessary to resuspend the cells and achieve adequate mixing. As much of the supernatant as possible should be removed after each wash to achieve maximum dilution of residual serum.

3. *Add 2 volumes of a suitable antiglobulin reagent* to each test tube and centrifuge without delay after thorough mixing. The combinations of centrifugal force (RCF) and time for spin-tube tests are as follows:

RCF (g)	100	200–220	500	1000
Time (s)	60	25–30	15	8–10

4. *Read agglutination* as previously described (p. 499).

5. *Quality control of the test* should be monitored by the following:

a. An IgG anti-D diluted to give 1+ or 2+ reactions with RhD-positive (R_1r) cells as a *positive control*.

b. An inert group AB serum with the same RhD-positive cells as a *negative control*; this is not essential because most tests are negative.

c. The addition of sensitised cells to all negative tests. This is widely used to detect neutralisation of the antiglobulin reagent owing to incomplete removal of serum by the wash step. The value of this test as a control depends on the strength of reaction of the sensitised cells. Appropriate control cells sensitised with IgG anti-D should give a 3+ reaction when tested directly with the antiglobulin reagent and should still be positive (if the reagent is potent) when added to negative tests but downgraded (1+ or 2+) owing to the "pooled-cell" effect of the nonsensitised cells. The reaction will, of course, be negative if the antiglobulin has been neutralised by residual serum.

The production of satisfactory antiglobulin control cells can be achieved by limiting the level of anti-D sensitisation to that which gives a negative test in the presence of 1 in 1000 parts serum in saline.[40]

The suitability of the antiglobulin control cells can be checked as follows:

i. Prepare two tubes (10 × 75 mm) with 1 volume of 3% unsensitised cells; wash four times.

ii. Add 2 volumes of antiglobulin to each of the tubes, mix well, spin, and read the tubes to confirm the tests are negative.

iii. Add 1 volume of 1 in 1000 serum in saline to 1 tube and 1 volume of saline as a control to the other tube. Mix and incubate for 1 min at room temperature.

iv. Add 1 volume of control cells to each tube, mix, spin, and read the tests.

The test containing 1 in 1000 serum in saline should be negative, and the control tube should give at least 2+ reaction. A negative reaction with the control tube suggests a washing deficiency and demands corrective action. If an automated cell-washing centrifuge is used, the washing efficiency should be checked; see *Quality Control of Cell Washing Centrifuges.*[32,40]

Alternative Technology for Antibody Detection by the Antiglobulin Test

Alternative techniques have emerged that have a simpler reading phase than the manually read spin-tube IAT. These are of two main types: solid-phase red cell adherence methods[44] and column agglutination techniques. A well-performed spin-tube IAT, as described earlier, is the standard against which any new system should be compared.

Solid-phase red cell adherence methods involve systems in which known red cells, which may also be sensitised, are immobilised on a solid matrix. In the method referenced, ABO and RhD typing plates are prepared by immobilising A_1, B, and RhD-positive red cells to chemically modified U-bottom strips. The cells are then exposed to the appropriate antibody, and the sensitised red cell monolayers are then dried. The unknown test cells are added, and the plates are centrifuged after incubation. In a positive reaction, the cells spread over the surface of the well because they have adhered to the bound antibody. In a negative reaction, there is no adherence and the cells form a small button in the centre of the well when the plates are centrifuged.

For reverse typing and antibody screening, A_1, B, and O screening cell monolayers are prepared and dried. The test serum is added and, if antibodies to any of the immobilised antigens are present, they attach to the monolayer. The tests are read by the addition of A_1B cells that are coated with anti-IgG.

Solid-phase methods are highly suited for automated reading by passing a light beam through the well at a point at which it will not be interrupted by the button of cells in a negative test but will be dispersed by the layer of red cells spread across the well in a positive test.

With *column agglutination techniques* very small volumes of serum and cells are mixed in a reservoir at the top of a narrow column that contains either a Dextran gel* or glass beads.** The columns with the integral reservoirs are supplied in card or cassette form, respectively. After a suitable incubation period, the cards/cassettes containing the tests are spun in a centrifuge in which the axis of the column is strictly in line with the centrifugal force. The red cells, but not the medium in which they are suspended, enter the column. Agglutinated red cells are trapped at the top of the column, and unagglutinated red cells form a pellet at the bottom of the column (see Fig. 20.5, p. 528).

The columns can also contain an antiglobulin reagent for performing DATs or IATs. Because, during centrifugation, the red cells but not the suspending fluid pass through the gel, the red cells do not have to be washed before coming into contact with the antiglobulin reagent. The columns can also include an antibody (e.g., anti-D) for cell typing. Antigen positive cells are agglutinated and trapped in the upper portion of the column.

The advantages of column agglutination technology are as follows:

1. Ease of use and reading and can theoretically be performed by relatively unskilled staff.
2. Less chance of aerosol contamination from infected samples because no cell washing before IATs.
3. The cards can be kept for up to 24 hours, enabling the results to be reviewed by experienced staff.
4. Ease of automation and positive sample identification.

However, the technology is expensive and its performance does not always compare favourably with the standard LISS–IAT in experienced hands.

Assessment of Individual Worker Performance

It is recommended that all staff (including "on-call" staff who do not routinely work in the blood bank) should be assessed at regular intervals. A procedure based on "blind" replicate antiglobulin tests may be used for this purpose.[33,40]

The procedure is as follows:

1. A low-titre (8–16) IgG anti-D, as used for the control of the antiglobulin test, should be titrated against OR^1r or pooled O RhD-positive cells to find the dilution of anti-D that gives 1+ or 2+ sensitised cells (most workers use around 0.3 iu/ml). A standard BCSH–NIBSC anti-D reference reagent (95/784)[46] is available for this purpose (available from NIBSC (p. 694).
2. A batch of sensitised cells is prepared (e.g., by incubating 16 ml of the selected anti-D dilution with 8 ml of 3% washed OR^1 red cells at 37°C for 45 min).
3. Twelve tubes are labelled for blind tests by another person. One volume of 3% 1+ or 2+ sensitised cells and 2 volumes of group AB inert serum (to simulate the volumes of serum used in routine tests) are placed in 9 random tubes, and then 1 volume of unsensitised cells + 2 volumes of group-AB inert serum are placed in the

---

*DiaMed, AG, Switzerland.
**Bio Vue, Ortho-Clinical Diagnostics, New Jersey.

remaining tubes. The position of the various tests is recorded.

4. The cells are washed thoroughly four times, antiglobulin is added, and the tubes are spun and read.

5. The number of false-negative (and false-positive) results are recorded for each worker and analysed in relation to reading and/or washing technique. It is advisable to give immediate tuition to any workers with washing or reading test faults, followed by further blind replicate trials to demonstrate improvement in procedure and to restore confidence.

Titration of Antibodies

A method for preparing primary dilutions of serum and subsequent antibody titration is illustrated in Figure 19.3.

External quality assessment exercises have demonstrated the wide range of titres reported for a single sample, reflecting the differing sensitivities of technologies in use, and have also highlighted the lack of reproducibility.[47] The following points are taken from an addendum to the BCSH guidelines.[48]

Preparation of serial dilutions of patient's or other sera

1. All dilutions and titrations should be made using calibrated pipettes and a separate tip for each step.

2. The diluent should be buffered saline, pH 7.0, for agglutination tests; for lysis tests undiluted ABO-compatible fresh normal human serum should be acidified so that the pH of the cell–serum mixture is c 6.8. The normal serum serves as a source of complement.

3. Tube sizes and assay volumes should be chosen to permit thorough mixing of the dilutions.

4. When assaying high-titre samples, an initial dilution should be made to reduce the number of doubling serial transfers to less than 10. A sufficient range of dilutions should be chosen to ensure that two negative results can be observed.

5. The end-point should be macroscopic and well-defined. The use of visual comparator aids should be considered where possible.

6. Wherever possible, each sample should be tested in parallel with the previous sample.

7. Titrations should be repeated if there is more than a one-tube difference in the titres obtained from sequential samples.

Addition of red cell suspensions to dilutions of serum

It is conventional to add 1 volume of red cell suspension to 1 volume of serum or serum dilution. This means that each antibody dilution, and hence the "final" titre, will be twice that of the original serum dilution. Because red cell antigen expression

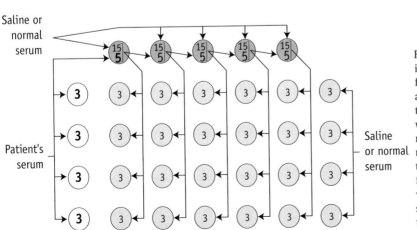

Serum dilution	1 in 1	1 in 4	1 in 16	1 in 64	1 in 256	1 in 1024	Control

Figure 19.3 Diagram illustrating method of preparing four sets of fourfold dilutions of a serum. The large circles at the top represent the large tubes in which the primary dilutions are made; the smaller circles represent the tubes in which the titrations are carried out. The figures represent drops or volumes. The patient's neat serum is indicated by the bold type.

varies with the source and age of the sample, wherever possible, the same cell sample should be used.

Test for ABH Substance Secretion

In the majority of the population, substances with the appropriate A, B, and H antigenic activity are distributed widely in saliva and all body fluids, controlled by a regulator secretor gene (Se), which is inherited independently of ABH genes. Only about 20% of people are nonsecretors. An individual's secretor status can be determined by testing saliva.

Method

Dilute an anti-A or anti-B serum so that it gives good visible agglutination with A_2 or B cells at the end of 1 hour at room temperature (e.g., if the titre of the serum is 128, use it at a dilution of 1 in 16).

Collect several milliliters of saliva in a centrifuge tube. Place the tube in boiling water for 10 min and then centrifuge. Serially dilute the clear supernatant in saline so as to give dilutions ranging from 1 in 2 to 1 in 32. Use a tube containing saliva alone as a control. Add an equal volume of the diluted anti-A (or anti-B) serum to each tube and, after shaking the rack of tubes, allow them to stand at room temperature for 10–15 min. Then add an equal volume of a 2% suspension of A_2 (or B) red cells in saline to each tube. Mix the contents and allow to stand at room temperature for 1–2 hours; then inspect for agglutination. If the saliva contains A or B substances, agglutination is usually inhibited in all the tubes except the saline control tube.

H substance can be demonstrated in a similar way using an extract of Ulex, eel serum, or the naturally occurring "incomplete" cold antibody as the source of anti-H.

PLATELET AND GRANULOCYTES

Platelet and Granulocyte Alloantigen Systems

Platelet and granulocyte alloantigens may be exclusive to each cell type (cell-specific) or shared with other cells. The currently recognised human platelet antigens (HPA) and human neutrophil antigens (HNA) are shown in Tables 19.13–19.15.[49-51]

The historical nomenclature for granulocyte antigens used the letter N to indicate neutrophil specificity, and this has been retained, although it is recognised that many studies used granulocytes rather than pure neutrophils and many "neutrophil-specific" antibodies can also target granulocyte precursors. In the HPA nomenclature, HPA-1, -2, -3, -4, and -5 were designated as separate diallelic alloantigen systems. The high-frequency allele of a system was designated with the letter a, and the low-frequency allele was designated with the letter b. However, this system is difficult to reconcile with recent molecular genetic knowledge, which suggests that each new base exchange does not constitute a new diallelic alloantigen system but rather defines a single allele that expresses a single new epitope. Currently, eight different GPIIIa alleles have been found in the human gene pool, three allelic variants have been described for GPIa and GPIIb, and two allelic variants have been found for the GPIbα and GPIbβ subunits. A database of human platelet antigens is available at the NIBSC website (www.nibsc.ac.uk). Of the shared antigens, the HLA system is the most important clinically; only class 1 antigens (HLA-A, -B, and to a lesser extent -C) are expressed on platelets and granulocytes. ABH antigens are also expressed on platelets (in part absorbed from the plasma) but cannot be demonstrated on granulocytes.

Clinical Significance of Platelet and Granulocyte Antibodies

Platelet and granulocyte antibodies may be classified on the basis of the antigenic stimulus (e.g., allo-, iso-, auto- and drug-induced antibodies).

Alloantibodies

Alloimmunization to platelet and granulocyte antigens is most commonly a result of transfusion or pregnancy. The associated clinical problems depend on the specificity of the antibody, which determines the target cell involved. Cell-specific alloantibodies are associated with well-defined clinical conditions, which are summarised in Tables 19.16 and 19.17.

Alloimmune fetal and neonatal thrombocytopenia are commonly caused by anti-HPA-1a and less frequently by anti-HPA-5b. The chance of HPA-1a alloimmunisation is strongly associated with

Table 19.13   Molecular genetics of human platelet antigens (HPA)

Antigen	Synonym location	Glycoprotein substitution	Nucleotide substitution	Amino acid
HPA-1a	Zw^a, Pl^{A1}	GPIIIa	T_{196}	Leu_{33}
HPA-1b	Zw^b, Pl^{A2}		C_{196}	Pro_{33}
HPA-2a	Ko^b	GPIbα	C_{524}	Thr_{145}
HPA-2b	Ko^a Sib^a		T_{524}	Met_{145}
HPA-3a	Bak^a, Lek^a	GPIIb	T_{2622}	Ile_{843}
HPA-3b	Bak^b		G_{2622}	Ser_{843}
HPA-4a	Yuk^b, Pen^a	GPIIIa	G_{526}	Arg_{143}
HPA-4b	Yuk^a, Pen^b		A_{526}	Gln_{143}
HPA-5a	Br^b, Zav^b	GPIa	G_{1648}	Glu_{505}
HPA-5b	Br^a, Zav^a, Hc^a		A_{1648}	Lys_{505}
HPA-6bW	Ca^a, Tu^a	GPIIIa	A_{1564}	Gln_{489}
			G_{1564}	Arg_{489}
HPA-7bW	Mo^a	GPIIIa	G_{1317}	Ala_{407}
			C_{1317}	Pro_{407}
HPA-8bW	Sr^a	GPIIIa	T_{2004}	Cys_{636}
			C_{2004}	Arg_{636}
HPA-9bW	Max^a	GPIIb	A_{2603}	Met_{837}
			G_{2603}	Val_{837}
HPA-10bW	La^a	GPIIIa	A_{281}	Gln_{62}
			G_{281}	Arg_{62}
HPA-11bW	Gro^a	GPIIIa	A_{1996}	His_{633}
			G_{1996}	Arg_{633}
HPA-12bW	Iy^a	GPIbβ	A_{141}	Glu_{15}
			G_{141}	Gly_{15}
HPA-13bW	Sit^a	GPIa	T_{2531}	Met_{799}
			C_{2531}	Thr_{799}
HPA-15a	Gov^b	CD109	C_{2108}	Ser^{703}
HPA-15b	Gov^a	CD109	A_{2108}	Tyr^{703}
HPA-	Oe^a	GPIIIa		
HPA-	Va^a	GPIIIa		
HPA-	Pe^a	GPIbα		

HPA, human platelet antigens; GP, glycoprotein location of epitopes.

Table 19.14   Human platelet antigen frequencies (%) in different populations

Antigen	Dutch	Finns	American caucasian	Japanese	Korean
HPA-1a	97.9	99.0	98.0	100.0	99.5
HPA-1b	28.8	26.5	20.0	0.3	2.0
HPA-2a	100.0	99.0	97.0	99.2	99.0
HPA-2b	13.5	16.5	15.0	19.7	14.0
HPA-3a	81.0	83.5	88.0	85.1	82.5
HPA-3b	69.8	66.5	54.0	66.2	71.5
HPA-4a	100.0		100.0	100.0	100.0
HPA-4b	0.0		0.0	2.0	2.0
HPA-5a	100.0	99.5	98.0	99.0	100.0
HPA-5b	19.7	10.0	21.0	7.0	4.5
HPA-6a		100.0		99.7	100.0
HPA-6b		2.4		4.8	4.0

Table 19.15   The human neutrophil antigen systems

Antigen system	Antigen phenotype	Location	Acronym	Caucasian frequency (%)
HNA-1	HNA-1a	FcγRIIIb	NA1	58
	HNA-1b	FcγRIIIb	NA2	88
	HNA-1c	FcγRIIIb	SH	5
HNA-2	HNA-2a	gp50–64	NB1	97
HNA-3	HNA-3a	gp70–95	5b	97
HNA-4	HNA-4a	CD11b	MART	99
HNA-5	HNA-5a	CD11a	OND	96

HNA, human neutrophil antigen.

maternal HLA class–II DRB3*0101 (DR52a) type.[52] Partners should be offered HPA genotyping, and if heterozygous, with a severely affected previous child, fetal HPA grouping should be considered in the first trimester of the next pregnancy using amniocyte DNA. There is some evidence that severe thrombocytopenia is associated with a third trimester anti-HPA-1a titre >32, using monoclonal antibody immobilisation of platelet antigens (MAIPA)[53] (see later). Potential strategies for routine antenatal screening and the acceptability and cost effectiveness of such a programme are discussed in several publications.[53,54]

Posttransfusion purpura is most commonly caused by anti-HPA-1a but can be associated with HPA antibodies with other specificities against HPA-1b, HPA-2b, HPA-3a, HPA-3b, HPA-4a, and HPA-5b.[55]

Immunological refractoriness to platelet transfusions is usually the result of anti-HLA antibodies. However, in multitransfused patients with HLA immunization, up to 25% may also have anti-HPA antibodies.[56,57]

Table 19.16   Clinical significance of platelet-specific alloantibodies[80]
1. Neonatal alloimmune thrombocytopenia
2. Posttransfusion purpura
3. Refractoriness to platelet transfusion Usually as a result of human leukocyte antigen antibodies.

Table 19.17   Clinical significance of granulocyte-specific alloantibodies[112–114]
1. Neonatal alloimmune neutropenia
2. Febrile reactions following transfusion (HLA antibodies also involved)
3. Transfusion-related acute lung injury (TRALI) (transfusion of high-titre antibody)
4. Poor survival and function of transfused granulocytes (HLA antibodies also involved)
5. Autoimmune neutropenia—some autoantibodies have allospecificity for HNA system antigens.
HLA, human leukocyte antigen; HNA, human neutrophil antigen.

Isoantibodies

Rarely, after blood transfusion or pregnancy, patients with type I Glanzmann's disease make antibodies that react with platelet glycoprotein (GP) IIb/IIIa not present on their own platelets but present on normal platelets (i.e., isotypic determinants).[58–61] Similarly, patients with Bernard–Soulier syndrome may make antibodies against isotypic determinants on GP Ib/V/IX not present on their own platelets.[62] This may present a serious clinical problem because no compatible donor platelets can be found to treat severe bleeding episodes.

Autoantibodies

Autoimmune thrombocytopenia may be idiopathic or secondary in association with other conditions. Demonstration of a platelet autoantibody is not required; even with the most suitable techniques now available, platelet autoantibodies remain elusive in a variable proportion (10–20%) of patients. The autoreactive antibodies target epitopes on certain glycoproteins. In 30–40% of patients these are directed against epitopes on the αIIbβ3 integrin heterodimer, platelet glycoprotein (GP) IIb/IIIa (CD41) and in 30–40% against the von Willebrand receptor or complex GpIbα/GPIbβ/IX (CD42).[63–66]

In the diagnosis of autoimmune thrombocytopenia it is important to consider and exclude three other immunological conditions:

1. *Post-transfusion purpura (PTP).* A blood transfusion within 2 weeks will suggest this possibility.[55]
2. *Drug-induced immune thrombocytopenia.* A drug history is essential. Heparin-induced thrombocytopenia (HIT) is the most frequent drug-induced thrombocytopenia and can be confirmed by the demonstration of antibodies to the heparin/platelet factor 4 (PF4) complex by ELISA (enzyme-linked immunosorbent assay).[67]
3. *Pseudothrombocytopenia.* The patient has an EDTA-dependent platelet antibody that is active only *in vitro*. The antibody (IgG and/or IgM) reacts with hidden (cryptic) antigens on platelet GP IIb/IIIa, which are exposed owing to confirmational changes in the complex caused by the removal of Ca^{2+} by EDTA.[68] The antibody causes platelet agglutination in the EDTA blood sample associated with large platelet clumps on the blood film or platelet satellitism around neutrophils, both of which lead to a falsely low platelet count. To overcome this, blood should be taken into a tube containing citrate instead.

Autoimmune neutropenia may be idiopathic or secondary. Idiopathic autoimmune neutropenia is more common in infants than in adults, in whom it is usually associated with other disorders that have in common a postulated imbalance of the immune system.[69] However, it is the least well-studied of the autoimmune cytopenias because it is rare and performing granulocyte assays is difficult, lengthy, labour-intensive, and expensive.

Granulocyte autoantibodies (which are usually IgG) are unusual in that they often have well-defined specificity for alloantigens, especially NA1 or NA2.[70] These autoantibodies may suppress granulocyte precursors in the bone marrow and cause more severe neutropenia. The investigation of suspected autoimmune neutropenia should, when possible, include granulocyte immunology and clonal assays (e.g., CFU-GM) on bone marrow precursors as target cells.

Drug-Induced Antibodies

Drug-induced antibodies may cause selective haemolytic anaemia (p. 257), thrombocytopenia or neutropenia, or various combinations of these in the same patient.[71,72]

A drug may cause an immune cytopenia by stimulating production of either an *autoantibody* (which reacts directly with the target cell independently of the drug itself) or a *drug-dependent antibody* (which destroys the target cell by reacting with a drug-membrane complex on the target cell).[73] Laboratory tests may demonstrate both types of antibody in some patients.[74]

Demonstration of Platelet and Granulocyte Antibodies

No single method will detect all types of platelet and granulocyte antibodies equally well. In practice, it is useful to have a basic screening method that will detect most commonly occurring antibodies, both cell-bound (direct test) and in serum (indirect test), and to supplement this with other selected methods for demonstrating particular properties of an antibody and for measuring the amount of cell-bound antibody.

The various techniques used over the last decade by participants in Australasian Platelet Workshops are shown in Table 19.18.[75]

Alloantibodies

Reports of national and international workshops make it possible to formulate guidelines for *platelet immunological tests*. The basic procedure for demonstrating platelet alloantibodies should include the following:

1. *A platelet test for platelet-reactive antibodies.* The ISBT/ICSH Working Party on Platelet Serology[76] recommended the platelet suspension immunofluorescence test[77] as the standard for assessment of other platelet antibody techniques.

    It is important to combine a sensitive binding assay, such as the platelet immunofluorescence

Table 19.18 Changing patterns shown in number of workshop participants using various platelet immunology techniques in the Australasian platelet workshops between 1989 and 1998[75]

Technique	1989	1992	1995	1998
PIFT microscopic	5	4	1	2
PIFT flow cytometric	3	5	5	7
ELISA	5	2	0	0
SPRCA	3	5	10	8
Chloroquine or acid HLA removal	3	12	11	9
Western immunoblot	3	1	0	0
MAIPA or MACE	0	4	4	6
DNA-based genotype of panel	0	0	7	8
No. of participants	14	17	15	14

PIFT, platelet immunofluorescence test; ELISA, enzyme-linked immunosorbent assay; SPRCA, solid-phase red cell adherence; MAIPA, monoclonal antibody immobilization of platelet antigens; MACE, modified antigen capture.

test (PIFT), with an antigen-capture method, such as the MAIPA,[78] to increase the chance of detecting weak antibodies or those that react with relatively few antigen sites.

2. *A lymphocyte test for detecting HLA antibodies.* Because HLA antibodies also react with platelets, a lymphocyte cytotoxicity and/or ELISA assay should be included in the basic antibody screening procedure.

3. *Tests to differentiate platelet-specific from HLA antibodies.* The MAIPA technique using appropriate monoclonal antibodies is particularly useful for resolving mixtures of platelet-reactive antibodies (p. 517). The chloroquine-"stripping" technique to inactivate HLA Class I molecules on platelets[79] is also helpful in this respect (p. 516). Conventional serological techniques (e.g., differential reactions with a panel of normal lymphocytes and platelets; differential absorption of HLA antibodies) can also be used to differentiate

cell-specific and HLA antibodies, but these are less suitable for rapid screening than the chloroquine-"stripping" technique.

Further characterisation of platelet-specific antibodies will require referral to a reference laboratory. Identification of allospecificity should be carried out as for red cell antibodies by reaction with a selected genotyped panel of group O platelets, preferably with reference to the patient's platelet genotype.

An important consideration in platelet serology is the occasional occurrence of antibodies against hidden (cryptic) antigens of the GP IIb/IIIa complex, which are exposed by EDTA and paraformaldehyde (PFA) fixation.[80] These antibodies, which are only active *in vitro,* are unpredictable but when suspected can be avoided by using unfixed test platelets from citrated blood.

The detection and identification of granulocyte alloantibodies should be left to experienced reference laboratories, but should follow a similar schedule with the use of monoclonal antibody immobilisation of granulocyte antigens (MAIGA)[81,82] or adsorption of the sera with pooled platelets to differentiate between granulocyte-specific and HLA antibodies.

Autoantibodies

The detection of autoantibodies and drug-induced antibodies requires special consideration.

It can be misleading, when looking for platelet (or granulocyte) autoantibodies, only to test the patient's serum against normal platelets (granulocytes) because positive reactions may result from the presence of alloantibodies (e.g., HLA or cell-specific) induced by previous transfusion or pregnancy. It is important to show that an autoantibody in the patient's serum reacts with the patient's own cells. Ideally a DAT (e.g., PIFT) should be performed, before treatment is given, to detect antibody bound *in vivo.* Where a severe cytopenia exists, it may not be possible to harvest enough cells for the test; nevertheless, serum samples should be stored at −20°C and tested retrospectively against the patient's cells when the peripheral platelet (or neutrophil) count has increased in response to treatment.

A major interest in platelet autoimmunity has been the quantitative measurement of platelet-associated immunoglobulins as an indication of *in vivo* sensitisation. A criticism of these quantitative methods is that they detect not only platelet autoantibody but also Ig nonspecifically trapped or bound to platelets and platelet fragments[83] and are therefore generally nonspecific in the diagnosis of autoimmune thrombocytopenia.[84] It is now more customary to use the direct PIFT,[85,86] using flow cytometry. The patient's platelets are incubated with isotype-specific fluorescein-isothiocyanate (FITC)-labelled conjugates (anti-IgG, anti-IgM, and anti-IgA) and the test is reported as positive when the fluorescence intensity is > mean + 2SD when compared with the results obtained with pooled (10 or more) normal donor platelet suspensions. In a study of 75 patients with idiopathic thrombocytopenic purpura, using microscopy rather than flow cytometry, von dem Borne and colleagues[87] found a weak positive (± to +) direct PIFT in 60% of patients and strong reactions (++ to ++++) in only 26% of patients. In the same study, the indirect PIFT was positive with the patient's serum in 66% of cases who had a positive direct PIFT, and it was positive with an ether eluate of the patient's platelets in 94% of the same cases. Although these results may be a reflection of the relative insensitivity of the method, they may result from a low-affinity antibody that is easily eluted during the assay procedure[83] or indicate an alternative immune mechanism for thrombocytopenia in some cases.

The Ig class of platelet autoantibodies is similar in idiopathic and secondary autoimmune thrombocytopenia; mostly it is IgG (92%), but often (also) it is IgM (42%) and sometimes (also) IgA (9%).[87] All IgG subclasses occur, but IgG1 and/or IgG3 are the most frequent.

A combination of the granulocyte immunofluorescence test (GIFT)[88] and the granulocyte agglutination test (GAT)[89] provides the most effective means of granulocyte antibody detection. However, immune complexes and aggregates in a patient's serum can still cause false-positive results. This can cause a problem for sera from adult patients with secondary autoimmune neutropenia, which should also be investigated for immune complexes (e.g., Clq-enzyme-linked immunosorbent assay). The granulocyte chemiluminescence test (GLCT)[90] is relatively insensitive to the presence of immune complexes when inactivated serum is used, but it is unable to detect antibodies of the IgM. Several reviews provide an appraisal of the techniques available for detecting granulocyte-specific antibodies and antigens.[91,92]

Drug-Induced Antibodies

The serological investigation of drug-induced immune thrombocytopenia (neutropenia) follows the same pattern as for haemolytic anaemia (p. 257), with the exception that it is not always possible to collect enough cells to test at the nadir of thrombocytopenia or neutropenia. The following blood samples are therefore necessary:

1. *Acute phase blood sample when the cell count is at the nadir.* If there are too few cells to test for cell-bound antibody and complement at this time, it is necessary to test the acute-phase serum against the patient's cells during remission. These tests will demonstrate the immune basis of the cytopenia.

   If the patient's acute-phase serum is tested against *normal* donor cells, it is essential to take account of positive reactions owing to HLA or cell-specific alloantibody in the patient's serum. Furthermore, negative results with normal donor cells may be the result of absence of the antigen for the particular drug-dependent antibody (e.g., owing to genetic restriction of the antigen concerned).[93]

2. *Subsequent samples after stopping the drug.* Ideally, sampling should be done when the drug has been eliminated and the antibody is still detectable. Tests using this sample with and without the drug in the assay system are necessary to demonstrate the part played by the drug in causing the immune cytopenia. The drug may be added directly to the assay system (and included in the wash solution) or the cells may be pretreated with the drug. For some drugs, a metabolite and not the native drug is the appropriate antigen for testing; in these cases an "*ex vivo*" drug antigen from urine or plasma may be used.[94]

Methods of Demonstrating Antibodies

The basic immunofluorescent antiglobulin method and the MAIPA assay will be described in detail. Only brief mention will be made of other methods.

The Immunofluorescent Antiglobulin Methods

The immunofluorescent antiglobulin methods are based on the conventional antiglobulin technique (p. 501) and are suitable for platelet,[77] granulocyte,[88] and lymphocyte[95] serology. The PIFT and GIFT* are described in detail in this chapter.

These tests can either be read by direct examination of a cell suspension using fluorescence microscopy or by flow cytometry. These tests can detect allo-, auto-, and drug-induced antibodies and by using appropriate monospecific antiglobulin reagents can determine the Ig class and subclass of the antibody and cell-bound complement components. Both tests can be used with chloroquine-treated cells to differentiate cell-specific from HLA antibodies.[96]

Patient's and Screening Panel Cells

Platelets and granulocytes are prepared from venous blood taken into 5% (w/v) Na_2EDTA in water (9 volumes blood:1 volume anticoagulant).

Screening panel cells should be obtained from group O donors for platelet serology to avoid positive reactions owing to anti-A and anti-B, but this is not necessary for granulocyte serology because A and B antigens cannot be demonstrated on granulocytes. If a patient's serum must be tested with ABO-incompatible platelets, anti-A and/or anti-B can be absorbed with corresponding red cells or A or B substance.

The best results are obtained with the freshest cell preparations, but some delay is tolerable (see later). Neutrophils are more susceptible to storage damage than platelets; cells should be fixed (see later) on the day of collection, but serology may be delayed to the following day. Platelets are more resilient, and an anticoagulated blood sample may be satisfactory for testing for up to 2 days at ambient temperature (c 20°C). Once fixed, platelets may be kept for 3–4 days at 4°C before serological testing. For longer storage, platelet-rich plasma may be kept at –40°C for at least 2 months; however, there is some membrane damage after recovery of frozen platelets, which causes increased background fluorescence that may limit the sensitivity of the test.[97,98] For

---

*Fison Ltd., Loughborough, UK.

longer-term storage a cryoprotectant (e.g., DMSO), may be used.[98]

Patient's Serum

Serum from clotted venous blood should be heated at 56°C for 30 min to inactivate complement and stored in 1–2 ml volumes at –40°C (to avoid repeated thawing of a stock).

Control Sera

Negative control serum is prepared from a pool of 10 sera from normal group AB male donors who have never been transfused. *Positive control* sera containing platelet-specific antibodies (e.g., anti-HPA-1a), granulocyte-specific antibodies, or multi-specific HLA antibodies should be obtained from reference centres.

Eluate from Patient's Sensitised Cells

Elution is important to confirm the antibody nature of cell-bound immunoglobulin and to determine the specificity of antibodies. This applies especially when no antibody is demonstrable in the patient's serum, which often occurs in patients with auto-immune thrombocytopenia and neutropenia.

Elution by lowering the pH of the medium, by ether (or DMSO) and by heating to 56°C, has been used.[99] For routine platelet serology, ether elution for platelet autoantibodies or heating to 56°C for platelet-specific alloantibodies is most convenient.

Heat Eluate

Incubate platelets or granulocytes suspended in 0.5 ml of 0.2% bovine serum albumin (BSA) in PBS for 60 min at 56°C. Centrifuge and remove the supernatant that contains the eluted antibody.

Ether Eluate

Using glass or plastic tubes, mix washed packed platelets from 50 ml of EDTA blood with 1 part of PBS/BSA (0.2%) and 2 parts of ether, by vigorous shaking for 2 min. Incubate the mixture for 30 min at 37°C in a waterbath with repeated shaking. After centrifugation (2800 g, 10 min), 3 layers are present, consisting of ether, stroma, and the eluate. Pipette off the eluate with a Pasteur pipette and test it in the indirect PIFT with normal donor platelets as described for serum.

Platelet Preparation

1. Prepare platelet rich plasma (PRP) by centrifugation of anticoagulated blood (200 g, 10 min).
2. Wash the platelets three times (2500 g, 5 min) in PBS/EDTA buffer (8.37 g of Na_2 EDTA dissolved in 2.5 l of PBS, pH 7.2); resuspend the platelets thoroughly each time.
3. Fix the platelets in 3 ml of 1% paraformaldehyde solution for 5 min at room temperature. A stock solution of PFA is prepared by dissolving 4 g of PFA (BDH) in 100 ml of PBS by heating to 70°C with occasional mixing. Add 1 mol/l NaOH dropwise with continuous mixing until the solution clears. This 4% stock solution may be stored at 4°C protected from light for several months. Prepare a 1% PFA working solution by adding 1 volume of the 4% PFA stock solution to 3 volumes of PBS and by correcting the pH if necessary to 7.2–7.4 with 1 mol/l HCl.)

Wash the platelets twice as before and resuspend in PBS/EDTA buffer at a concentration of 250–500 $\times 10^9$/l for use in the PIFT.

Granulocyte Preparation

1. Mix anticoagulated blood or blood retained from platelet preparation after removal of PRP (and made up to its original volume with PBS) with 2 ml of Dextran solution per 10 ml of blood (Dextran 150 injection BP in 5% dextrose). Incubate this mixture at 37°C for 30 min at an angle of about 45 degrees to accelerate red cell sedimentation, and then remove the leucocyte-rich supernatant (LRS).
2. Granulocytes can be separated by double-density sedimentation (Fig. 19.4). The LRS is under-layered with 2 ml of lymphocyte separating medium (LSM) (LSM = Ficoll-hypaque sp gr 1.077), which is then underlayered with 2 ml of mono-poly resolving medium (MPRM) (MPRM = Ficoll-hypaque sp gr 1.114).* The density gradient tube is then centrifuged at 2500 g for 5 min. Granulocytes form an opaque layer at the LSM/MPRM interface from which they are harvested by careful pipetting (microscopic

---

*LSM and MPRM supplied by Flow Laboratories Ltd.

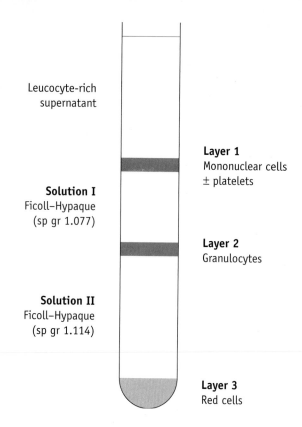

Leucocyte-rich
supernatant

Solution I
Ficoll–Hypaque
(sp gr 1.077)

Solution II
Ficoll–Hypaque
(sp gr 1.114)

Layer 1
Mononuclear cells
± platelets

Layer 2
Granulocytes

Layer 3
Red cells

Figure 19.4 Double-density separation of lymphocytes and granulocytes. A leucocyte-rich supernatant is underlayered with Ficoll–Hypaque with a specific gravity of 1.077 (Solution 1) and 1.114 (Solution 2) and then centrifuged at 2500 g for 5 min. Lymphocytes concentrate in layer 1; granulocytes concentrate in layer 2.

examination shows that the cells from this layer are predominantly neutrophil polymorphs). Lymphocytes can similarly be harvested from the plasma/LSM interface (e.g., for use in the lymphocyte immunofluorescence test, or LIFT).[95]

3. Wash the granulocytes three times at 400 g for 5 min) in PBS/BSA buffer (PBS pH 7.2 with 0.2% BSA).

4. Fix the granulocytes in 3 ml of 1% PFA for 5 min at room temperature.

5. Wash the granulocytes twice as before, and resuspend in PBS/BSA buffer at a concentration

of about $10 \times 10^9/l$ for use in the GIFT.

Platelet and Granulocyte Immunofluorescence Tests

The serological methods for testing platelets and granulocytes in the suspension immunofluorescence test are similar, except that platelets are washed throughout in PBS/EDTA buffer and granulocytes are washed in PBS/BSA buffer. A flow diagram of the PIFT is shown in Figure 19.5.

FITC-labelled antiglobulin reagents are used as follows: anti-Ig (polyspecific), anti-IgG, anti-IgM, and anti-C3. F(ab)$_2$ fragments of these reagents should be used to minimise nonspecific membrane fluorescence owing to Fc receptor binding, which is a particular problem with granulocytes. The optimal dilution for each reagent should be determined by chequerboard titration. Centrifuge the FITC conjugates at 2500 g for 10 min before use to remove fluorescent debris and reduce background fluorescence.

Positive and negative controls (as described earlier) should be included with each batch of tests.

Indirect Test

1. In plastic precipitin tubes (7 × 50 mm), mix 0.1 ml of serum and 0.1 ml of the appropriate cell suspension, as prepared earlier. (The method can also be adapted for use with microtitre plates, which has the advantage of using smaller volumes.)

2. Incubate for 30 min at 37°C (for IgG and C3 tests) and at room temperature (for IgM tests). For C3 tests *only*, sediment cells (1000 g, 5 min), remove the supernatant, and resuspend the cell button in 0.1 ml of freshly thawed human serum as a source of complement. Incubate for 30 min at 37°C.

3. Wash the cells three times at 1000 g, for 5 min with appropriate buffer—PBS/EDTA for platelets, PBS/BSA for granulocytes; decant the final supernatant. This and subsequent steps are common for both the *indirect* test (i.e., patient's serum with donor cells) and the *direct* test (i.e., patient's own cells to detect *in vivo* sensitisation).

4. Add the fluorescent antiglobulin reagent (0.1 ml of the appropriate dilution determined by che-querboard-titration), mix with the cell button,

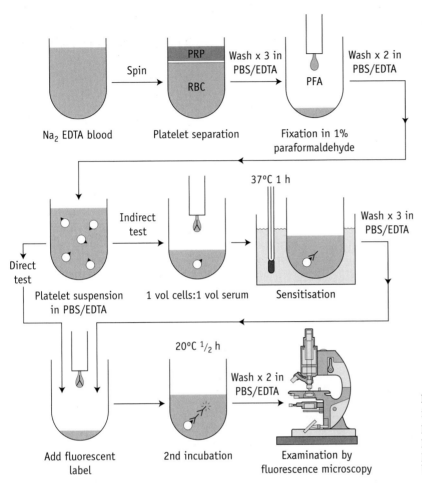

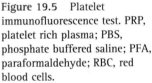

Figure 19.5   Platelet immunofluorescence test. PRP, platelet rich plasma; PBS, phosphate buffered saline; PFA, paraformaldehyde; RBC, red blood cells.

and leave at room temperature for 30 min in the dark.

5. Wash twice as before, and remove the supernatant.

6. Mix 0.5 ml of glycerol–PBS (3 volumes glycerol:1 volume PBS) with the cell button and mount on a glass slide under a coverslip.

7. Examine microscopically using ×40 objective and epifluorescent ultraviolet illumination.

Scoring Results

Reactions in the PIFT and GIFT may be scored on a scale from negative (–) through graded positives + to + + + +. Although subjective, this method of scoring in experienced hands can produce semiquantitative results in the PIFT.[100]

In general, normal platelets and granulocytes incubated with AB serum do not fluoresce after incubation with an appropriately diluted FITC antiglobulin reagent. Sometimes the negative control may show weak fluorescence (up to two fluorescing points on some cells); in these cases, the test result is classified as positive only if it is clearly stronger than the negative control (AB serum). Stronger fluorescence in the negative control should raise doubts about the performance of the test.

Use of Flow Cytometry

With simplification of flow cytometers and improved software, more platelet reference laboratories are using them for primary analysis in PIFT because sensitivity is improved. Nevertheless, platelets are more difficult to work with flow cytometrically than other cells, and particular attention has to be paid to prevent aggregation and to ensure single cell suspensions. Presence of platelet particles and debris may also cause confusion. The technical considerations of applying flow cytometry to platelet work are the subject of several reviews.[85,86]

Chloroquine Treatment of Platelets and Granulocytes

Platelets for chloroquine treatment should be prepared from fresh blood or blood stored overnight at 4°C; granulocytes are suitable only if freshly prepared.[79,101] An important consideration is the extent of chloroquine-induced cell membrane damage, which is minimal with fresh cells.

1. Cells are prepared as already described. Two-thirds of the cells are treated with chloroquine; the remaining one-third is not treated. After washing, and before PFA fixation, the cell button is incubated with 4–5 ml of chloroquine diphosphate in PBS (200 mg/ml, pH adjusted to 5.0 with 1 mol/l NaOH) for 2 hours at room temperature with occasional mixing, or overnight at 4°C without mixing, if this is more convenient for the laboratory routine.
2. Wash three times in the appropriate buffer and fix in 1% PFA as previously described. Cell clumping during washing may be a problem after chloroquine treatment, especially with granulocytes; cell clumps should be dispersed by repeated gentle aspiration with a Pasteur pipette. The final cell suspension for serological testing should be prepared as previously described.

When reading the test under fluorescence microscopy, it is important to recognise and allow for any fluorescence owing to chloroquine-induced cell damage, which is more likely to occur with granulocytes than platelets. Damaged cells are easily recognised by bright homogeneous fluorescence. Such cells should be excluded from assessment; only cells showing obvious punctuate fluorescence should be considered positive.

Chloroquine-treated cells were tested initially in the fluorescent antiglobulin method, but they may also be used in enzyme and radionuclide-labelled antigen methods.

Interpretation of Results with Chloroquine-Treated Cells

Typical results with HLA- and cell-specific antibodies are shown in Table 19.19. If a serum that has been shown to contain HLA antibodies by LCT and/or LIFT gives equal or stronger reactions with chloroquine-treated cells than with untreated cells, then a cell-specific antibody is also present. The Second Canadian Workshop on Platelet Serology[97] concluded that a weaker reaction with chloroquine-treated platelets should be interpreted with caution; this could indicate residual HLA reactivity, especially in the presence of high-titre multispecific HLA antibodies. If a platelet-specific antibody is nevertheless still suspected, other methods should be used to confirm this (e.g., MAIPA using appropriate monoclonal antibodies for capture; see later).

Similar caution should be observed in interpreting the GIFT results with chloroquine-treated cells.

Table 19.19 Platelet and granulocyte antibody reactions using cells prepared with and without treatment with chloroquine

Sera	Untreated cells		Chloroquine–treated cells	
	Platelets	Granulocytes	Platelets	Granulocytes
Negative	–	–	–	–
Multispecific HLA antibodies	+++	++	–	–
Granulocyte-specific antibody	–	++	–	+++
Platelet-specific antibody	+++	–	+++	–
HLA, human leucocyte antigen.				

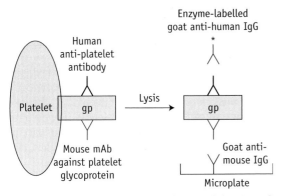

Figure 19.6 Monoclonal antibody immobilisation of platelet antigens (MAIPA): principle of the method. gp, platelet membrane glycoprotein; mAb, monoclonal antibody.

MAIPA Assay

The principle of the MAIPA assay is shown in Figure 19.6. The test is based on the use of monoclonal antibodies, such as anti-IIb/IIIa, anti-Ib/IX, anti-Ia/IIa, and anti-HLA class I, to "capture" specific platelet membrane glycoproteins. The availability of appropriate monoclonal antibodies has led to the wider clinical application of this method.[78] The same principle can be used with granulocytes, depending on the availability of appropriate monoclonal antibodies.[78,102]

The following assay protocol was developed from the original method described by Kiefel.[78,103]

1. Prepare platelets as for the PIFT (p. 513) except that paraformaldehyde fixation is omitted.
2. Resuspend a pellet of $50-100 \times 10^6$ platelets in 30 µl of human serum or plasma to be tested and incubate at 37°C for 30 min in a U-well microplate.
3. Wash platelets twice in PBS/EDTA buffer (8.37 g of Na_2EDTA in 2.5 l of phosphate buffered saline [p. 691]). Resuspend the platelets in 30 µl of mouse monoclonal antibody (anti-Gp IIb/IIIa, Ia/IIa, Ib/IX, or HLA at 20 µg/ml), and incubate at 37°C for 30 min.
4. Wash platelets twice in PBS/EDTA buffer, lyse by the addition of 100 µl of Tris buffered saline (TBS) containing 0.5% Nonidet P-40, and leave at 4°C for 30 min.

5. Transfer the platelet lysate to a 2 ml conical tube and centrifuge at 11,600 g for 30 min at 4°C to remove particulate matter.
6. Dilute 60 µl of the resulting supernatant with 180 µl of TBS wash buffer (0.5% Nonidet P-40, 0.05% Tween 20, and 0.5 mmol $CaCl_2$). Transfer 100 µl of diluted platelet lysate, in duplicate, to a flat-well microplate previously coated with goat anti-mouse IgG.* Leave at 4°C for 90 min.
7. Wash the microplate well four times with 200 µl of TBS wash buffer and then add 100 µl of alkaline phosphatase-labelled anti-human IgG (Jackson, code 109–055–008) diluted 1:4000 in TBS wash buffer.

   Leave at 4°C for a further 90 min, then wash the wells four times with TBS wash buffer and add 100 µl of substrate solution (1 mg/ml p-nitrophenyl phosphate in diethanolamine buffer, pH 9.8) to each well.
8. Measure the resulting colour change at 30 min using a dual-wavelength spectrometer (e.g., Bio-Rad model 450).

Express results as the mean absorbance at 405 nm of duplicate tests minus the mean of eight blanks containing TBS wash buffer instead of platelet lysate.

Use pooled AB serum as a negative control.

Other Methods

Several other methods have been developed for the detection of platelet antibodies.

Solid-phase red cell adherence (SPRCA) techniques (some commercially available) evolved as alternatives to the microscopic reading initially required for the PIFT. These assays combine traditional red cell serology technology with platelet serology. Platelets are captured on microtitre wells; test antibodies are applied; and, after washing and addition of antihuman globulin, platelet or HLA alloantibody binding is detected using tanned sheep

---

*The microplate is prepared by adding to each well 100 µl of goat antimouse IgG (Sera-Lab, code SBA 1030-01) at 3 µg/ml in carbonate coating buffer, pH 9.6. Leave the plate to stand overnight at 4°C. Next morning, wash the plate four times with TBS wash buffer. Leave the last wash supernatant for 30 min to "block" nonspecific protein adsorption to the plastic and then decant.

red cells[104] or anti-D sensitised RhD positive red cells.[105] SPRCA are robust, sensitive tests that lend themselves to automation, and the chloroquine treatment of platelets can be used effectively to screen out HLA antibodies.

GTI PakPlus is a platelet antibody kit based on an ELISA principle.** Microwells coated with platelet glycoproteins or HLA class I antigens are incubated with test serum. After incubation, followed by washing to remove unbound proteins, any antibody bound to the microwell is detected using an alkaline-phosphatase–conjugated antihuman globulin reagent (anti-GAM or anti-IgG) and the appropriate substrate. Results are considered positive when the ratio of the mean absorbance of the test sample to that of the normal control sera is 2.0 or more.[106]

With respect to testing for granulocyte antibodies when working with the GIFT or GAT, elucidation of the alloantibody requires panels of typed granulocytes, which cannot be preserved for more than a few hours. A technique has been reported that uses extracted granulocyte antigens coated onto U-well Terasaki plates and a micromixed passive haemagglutination test. Patient's serum and appropriate controls (sera known to contain granulocyte-specific antibodies, monoclonal antibodies, such as anti-CD16 and anti-NA1, and sera from normal donors) are added to the wells, and, following incubation and washing, indicator blood cells are added (sheep red blood cells coated with antihuman IgG and antimouse IgG). If successful on a large scale, such a technique, together with molecular characterisation of the antigens, could make granulocyte immunology more readily available in reference laboratories.[107]

Molecular Genotyping of Platelet Alloantigens

The application of DNA technology for platelet genotyping is based on the knowledge that the platelet antigen systems are the result of single DNA base changes, which lead to single amino acid polymorphisms in the platelet membrane glycoproteins (see Table 19.13).

Molecular genotyping involves amplification of the relevant segments of genomic DNA from any nucleated cell by the PCR in combination with sequence-specific primers[108] or by allele-specific restriction enzyme analysis[109] or by allele-specific oligonucleotide dot blot hybridisation.[110]

Of the variety of PCR-based techniques available, the PCR with sequence-specific primers (PCR–SSP) is the most widely used in the UK[111] for the determination of HPA 1 to 5. Molecular genotyping has now been accepted to be an essential part of confirming the specificity assigned to platelet alloantibodies, as well as allowing the investigation of patients with severe thrombocytopenia and making possible the determination of the fetal platelet genotype in early pregnancy to assess the risk of alloimmune thrombocytopenia.

REFERENCES

1. Daniels GL, Anstee DJ, Cartron JP 1995 Blood group terminology 1995: From the ISBT Working Party on Terminology for Red Cell Surface Antigens. Vox Sanguinis 69:265–279.
2. Daniels GL, Anstee DJ, Cartron JP 1999 Terminology for red cell surface antigens. Vox Sanguinis 77:52–57.
3. Cartron JP, Bailly P, Le Van Kim C 1998 Insights into the structure and function of membrane polypeptides carrying blood group antigens. Vox Sanguinis 74 (Suppl. 2):29–64.
4. Daniels G 1999 Functional aspects of red cell antigens. Blood Reviews 13:14–35.
5. Eastlund T 1998 The histo-blood group ABO system and tissue transplantation. Transfusion 38:975–988.
6. Mourant AE, Kopec AC, Domaniewska-Sobczak K 1976 The distribution of the human blood groups and other biochemical polymorphisms, 2nd ed. Oxford University Press, Oxford.
7. Yamamoto F 1995 Molecular genetics of the ABO histo-blood group system. Vox Sanguinis 69:1–7.
8. Garratty G, Arndt P, Co S 1993 Fatal ABO haemolytic transfusion reaction resulting from acquired B antigen only detectable by some monoclonal grouping reagents. Transfusion 33 (Suppl. 47S).
9. Garratty G 1996 Association of blood groups and disease: do blood group antigens and antibodies have a biological role? History and Philosophy of the Life Sciences 18:321–344.

**Quest Biomedical, Solihull B90 2EL (UK).

10. O'Donnell J, Laffan M 2001 The relationship between ABO histo-blood group, factor VIII and von Willebrand factor. Transfusion Medicine 11:343–351

11. O'Donnell J, Boulton FE, Manning RA, et al 2002 The amount of H antigen expressed on circulating vWF is modified by ABO blood group genotype and is a major determinant of plasma vWF:Ag levels. Arteriosclerosis Thrombosis and Vascular Biology 22:335–341

12. Cartron JP, Agre P 1993 Rh blood group antigens: protein and gene structure. Seminars in Hematology 30:193–208.

13. Huang CH 1997 Molecular insights into the Rh protein family and associated antigens. Current Opinion in Haematology 4:94–103.

14. Avent ND, Reid ME 2000 The Rh blood group system: a review. Blood 95:375–387.

15. World Health Organization (WHO) 1977 Twenty-eighth Report of WHO Expert Committee on Biological Standardization. Technical Report Series 610. WHO, Geneva.

16. Lo YM, Bowell PJ, Selinger M et al 1994 Prenatal determination of fetal rhesus D status by DNA amplification of peripheral blood of rhesus–negative mothers. Annals of the New York Academy of Sciences 731:229–236.

17. Sazama K 1990 Reports of 355 transfusion-associated deaths: 1976 through 1985. Transfusion 30:583–590.

18. Mollison PL, Engelfriet CP, Contreras M 1997 Blood transfusion in clinical medicine, 10th ed. Blackwell Scientific, Oxford, p. 89.

19. Engelfriet CP 1992 The immune destruction of red cells. Transfusion Medicine 2:1–6.

20. Horsewood P, Kelton JG 1994 Macrophage-mediated cell destruction. In: Garratty G (ed) Immunobiology of transfusion medicine. Marcel Dekker, New York, p. 434–464.

21. Zupanska BA 1994 Cellular bioassays and their use in predicting the clinical significance of antibodies. In: Garratty G (ed) Immunobiology of transfusion medicine. Marcel Dekker, New York, p. 465–492.

22. Guyre PM, Miller R 1983 Recombinant immune interferon increases immunoglobulin G Fc receptors on cultured human mononuclear phagocytes. Journal of Clinical Investigation 72:393–397.

23. Griffin JA, Griffin FM 1979 Augmentation of macrophage complement receptor function in vitro. Journal of Experimental Medicine 150:653–675.

24. Volk HD, Reinke P, Krausch D 1996 Monocyte deactivation–rationale for a new therapeutic strategy in sepsis. Intensive Care Medicine 22:S474–S481.

25. In-vitro diagnostics IVD Medical Devices Directive 1998 Official Journal of the European Communities (7.12.98) 1331.

26. British Committee for Standards in Haematology 1996 Guidelines for pre-transfusion compatibility testing in blood transfusion laboratories. Transfusion Medicine 6:273–283.

27. British Committee for Standards in Haematology 2004 Guidelines for compatibility procedures in blood transfusion laboratories. Transfusion Medicine 14:59–73

28. Case J, Ford DS, Chung A 1999 International reference reagents: antihuman globulin. Vox Sanguinis 77:121–127.

29. Department of Health 1998 Guidelines for the blood transfusion services in the United Kingdom, 4th ed. HMSO, London.

30. British Committee for Standards in Haematology 1995 Recommendations for the evaluation, validation and implementation of new techniques for blood grouping antibody screening and crossmatching. Transfusion Medicine 5:145–150.

31. Voak D 1992 Validation of new technology for antibody detection by antiglobulin tests. Transfusion Medicine 2:177–179.

32. Phillips PK, Voak D, Whitton CM, et al 1993 BCSH–NIBSC anti-D reference reagent for antiglobulin tests: the in-house assessment of red cell washing centrifuges and of operator variability in the detection of weak macroscopic agglutination. Transfusion Medicine 3:143–148.

33. Voak D, Downie DM, Moore BPL 1988 Replicate tests for the detection and correction of errors in anti-human globulin AHG tests: optimum conditions and quality control. Haematologia 2:3–16.

34. Knowles SM, Milkins CE, Chapman JF, Scott M 2002 The United kingdom National External Quality Assessment Scheme (Blood Transfusion Laboratory practice): trends in proficiency and practice between 1985 and 2000 Transfusion Medicine 12:11–23.

35. Voak D, Downie DM, Haigh T, Cook N 1982 Improved antiglobulin tests to detect difficult antibodies: detection of anti-Kell by LISS. Medical Laboratory Sciences 39:363–370.

36. Scott ML, Voak D, Phillips P 1994 Review of the problems involved in using enzymes in blood group serology – provision of freeze-dried

ICSH/ISBT protease enzyme and anti-D reference standards. Vox Sanguinis 67:89–98.

37. Scott ML, Voak D, Downie DM 1988 Optimum enzyme activity in blood grouping and a new technique for antibody detection: an explanation for the poor performance of the one-stage mix technique. Medical Laboratory Sciences 45:7–18.

38. Scott ML, Phillips PK 1987 A sensitive two-stage papain technique without cell washing. Vox Sanguinis 52:67–70.

39. Pirofsky B 1959 The use of bromelin in establishing a standard cross–match. American Journal of Clinical Pathology 32:350–356.

40. British Committee for Standards in Haematology 1991 Standard haematology practice (Roberts B, ed.) Blackwell Scientific, Oxford, p. 150–163.

41. Coombs RRA, Mourant AE, Race RR 1945 A new test of the detection of weak and "incomplete" Rh agglutinins. British Journal of Experimental Pathology 26:255–266.

42. Voak D, Downie DM, Moore PBL, et al 1986 Anti-human globulin reagent specification: the European and ISBT/ICSH view. Biotest Bulletin 1:7.

43. Engelfriet CP, Overbeeke MAM, Voak D 1987 The antiglobulin test, Coombs test and the red cell. In: Cash JD (ed) Progress in transfusion medicine. Churchill Livingstone, Edinburgh, vol 2, p. 74–98.

44. Sinor LT 1992 Advances in solid-phase red cell adherence methods and transfusion serology. Transfusion Medicine Reviews 6:26–31.

45. Lapierre Y, Rigel D, Adams J, et al 1990 The gel test: a new way to detect red cell antigen–antibody reactions. Transfusion 30:109–113.

46. Phillips P, Voak D, Downie M 1998 New reference reagent for the quality assurance of anti-D antibody detection. Transfusion Medicine 8:225–230.

47. O'Hagan J, Milkins CE, Chapman JF, et al 1997 Antibody titres – results of a UK NEQAS BGS exercise and accompanying questionnaire. Transfusion Medicine 7:Suppl. 1.

48. British Committee for Standards in Haematology 1999 Addendum for guidelines for blood grouping and red cell antibody testing during pregnancy. Transfusion Medicine 9:99.

49. Santoso S 1998 Human platelet-specific alloantigens: update. Vox Sanguinis 74 (Suppl. 2):249–253.

50. Bux J, von dem Borne AEG, de Haas L 1999 ISBT Working Party on Platelet and Granulocyte Serology, Granulocyte Antigen Working Party: Nomenclature of granulocyte alloantigens. Vox Sanguinis 77:251.

51. Lucas GF, Metcalfe P 2000 Platelet and granulocyte polymorphisms. Transfusion Medicine 10:157–174.

52. Decary F, L'Abbe D, Tremblay L, et al 1991 The immune response to the HPA-1a antigen: association with HLA-DRw52a. Transfusion Medicine 1:55–62.

53. Williamson LW, Hackett G, Rennie J, et al 1998 The natural history of fetomaternal alloimmunization to the platelet-specific antigen HPA-1a PI^{A1} Zw^a as determined by antenatal screening. Blood 92:2280–2287.

54. Flug F, Karpatkin M, Karpatkin S 1994 Should all pregnant women be tested for their platelet PLA Zw HPA-1 phenotype? British Journal of Haematology 86:1–5.

55. Mueller-Eckhardt C, Kroll H, Kiefel V, et al 1991 European PTP Study Group: Post-transfusion purpura. Platelet immunology: fundamental and clinical aspects. (Kaplan-Gouet C, Schlegel N, Salmon C, McGregor J, eds.) INSERM/John Libbey Eurotext.

56. Schnaidt M, Northoff H, Wernet D 1996 Frequency and specificity of platelet-specific allo-antibodies in HLA-immunised haematologic-oncologic patients. Transfusion Medicine 6:111–114.

57. Kurz M, Hildegard G, Hocker P, et al 1996 Specificities of anti-platelet antibodies in multitransfused patients with haemato-oncological disorders. British Journal of Haematology 95:564–569.

58. Bierling P, Fromont P, Elbez A, et al 1988 Early immunization against platelet glycoprotein IIIa in a new born Glanzmann type I patient. Vox Sanguinis 55:109–113.

59. Brown CH 3rd, Weisberg RJ, Natelson EA, et al 1975 Glanzmann's thrombasthenia: assessment of the response to platelet transfusion. Transfusion 15:124–131.

60. Ribera A, Martin-Vega C, Pico M, et al 1988 Sensitization against platelet antigens in Glanzmann disease. Abstract XX, Congress of the International Society of Blood Transfusion in Association with British Blood Transfusion Society (BBTS), Manchester, p. 240.

61. Van Leeuwen EF, von dem Borne AEGKr, Von Riesz LE, et al 1981 Absence of platelet specific alloantigens in Glanzmann's thrombasthenia. Blood 57:49–54.

62. Degos L, Tobelem G, Lethielliux P, et al 1977 A molecular defect in platelets of patients with Bernard–Soulier syndrome. Blood 50:899–903.

63. Van Leeuwen EF, Helmerhorst FM, Engelfriet CP, et al 1982 Specificity of auto-antibodies in

autoimmune thrombocytopenia. Blood 59:23–26.

64. Fujisawa K, Tani P, O'Toole TE, et al 1992 Different specificities of platelet-associated and plasma auto-antibodies to platelet GPIIb–IIIa in patients with chronic immune thrombocytopenic purpura. Blood 79:1441–1446.

65. Fujisawa K, Tani P, McMillan R 1993 Platelet-associated antibody to glycoprotein IIb/IIIa from chronic immune thrombocytopenic purpura patients often binds to divalent cation-dependent antigens. Blood 81:1284–1289.

66. Hou M, Stockelberg D, Kutti J, et al 1995 Glycoprotein IIb/IIIa autoantigenic repertoire in chronic idiopathic thrombocytopenic purpura. British Journal of Haematology 91:971–975.

67. Kelton JG, Sheridan DP, Santos AV, et al 1988 Heparin-induced thrombocytopenia: laboratory studies. Blood 72:925–930.

68. Pegels JG, Bruynes ECE, Engelfriet CP, et al 1982 Pseudothrombocytopenia: an immunologic study on platelet antibodies dependent on ethylene diamine tetra-acetate. Blood 59:157–161.

69. Shastri KA, Logue GL 1993 Autoimmune neutropenia. Blood 81:1984–1995.

70. McCullough J, Clay ME, Thompson HW 1987 Autoimmune granulocytopenia. Baillière's Clinical Immunology and Allergy 1:303.

71. Bux J, Mueller-Eckhardt C 1992 Autoimmune neutropenia. Seminars in Hematology 29:45–53.

72. Mueller-Eckhardt C 1987 Drug-induced immune thrombocytopenia. Baillière's Clinical Immunology and Allergy 1:369.

73. Mueller-Eckhardt C, Salama A 1990 Drug-induced immune cytopenias: a unifying pathogenetic concept with special emphasis on the role of drug metabolites. Transfusion Medicine Reviews 4:69–77.

74. Salama A, Schutz B, Kiefel V, et al 1989 Immune-mediated agranulocytosis related to drugs and their metabolites: mode of sensitization and heterogeneity of antibodies. British Journal of Haematology 72:127–132.

75. Minchinton RM 2000 What can we learn from National and International Platelet Serology Workshops? Transfusion Medicine Reviews 14:74–83.

76. Metcalfe P, Waters AH 1990 Report on the fourth ISBT/ICSH platelet serology workshop. Vox Sanguinis 58:170–175.

77. Von dem Borne AE, Verheught FW, Oosterhof F, et al 1978 A simple immunofluorescence test for the detection of platelet antibodies. British Journal of Haematology 39:195–207.

78. Kiefel V 1992 The MAIPA assay and its applications in immunohaematology. Transfusion Medicine 2:181–188.

79. Nordhagen R, Flaathen ST 1985 Chloroquine removal of HLA antigens from platelets for the platelet immunofluorescence test. Vox Sanguinis 48:156–159.

80. von dem Borne AEGKr, van der Lelie J, Vos JJE, et al 1986 Antibodies against crypt antigens of platelets. Characterisation and significance for the serologist. Current Studies in Hematology and Blood Transfusion 52:33. Karger, Basel.

81. Bux J, Kober B, Kiefel V, et al 1993 Analysis of granulocyte-reactive antibodies using an immunoassay based upon monoclonal-antibody-specific immobilization of granulocyte antigens. Transfusion Medicine 3:157–162.

82. Minchinton RM, Noonan K, Johnson TJ 1997 Examining technical aspects of the monoclonal antibody immobilization of granulocyte antigen assay. Vox Sanguinis 73:87–92.

83. Shulman NR, Leissinger CA, Hotchkiss AJ, et al 1982 The non-specific nature of platelet associated IgG. Transactions of the Association of American Physicians 95:213–220.

84. Von dem Borne AEGKr 1987 Autoimmune thrombocytopenia. Baillière's Clinical Immunology and Allergy 1:269.

85. Goodall AH, Macey MG 1994 Platelet-associated molecules and immunoglobulins. In: Macey MR (ed) Flow cytometry–clinical applications. Blackwell Scientific, London, p. 148–191.

86. Ault KA 1988 Flow cytometric measurement of platelet-associated immunoglobulin. Pathology and Immunopathology Research 7:395–408.

87. Von dem Borne AE, Vos JJ, van der Lelie J, et al 1986 Clinical significance of positive platelet immunofluorescence test in thrombocytopenia. British Journal of Haematology 64:767–776.

88. Verheugt FWA, von dem Borne AEGKr, Decary F, et al 1977 The detection of granulocyte allo-antibodies with an indirect immunofluorescence test. British Journal of Haematology 36:533–544.

89. McCullough J, Clay ME, Press C, et al 1988 Granulocyte serology. A clinical and laboratory guide. ACSP, Chicago.

90. Lucas GF 1994 Prospective evaluation of the chemiluminescence test for the detection of granulocyte antibodies: comparison with the immunofluorescence test. Vox Sanguinis 66:141–147.

91. Bux J 1996 Challenges in the determination of clinically significant granulocyte antibodies and

antigens. Transfusion Medicine Reviews 10:222–232.

92. Stroncek DF 1997 Granulocyte immunology: is there a need to know? Transfusion 37:886–888.

93. Claas FHJ, Langerak J, de Beer LL, et al 1981 Drug-induced antibodies: interaction of the drug with a polymorphic platelet antigen. Tissue Antigens 17:64–66.

94. Salama A, Mueller-Eckhardt C, Kissel K, et al 1984 Ex vivo antigen preparation for the serological detection of drug-dependent antibodies in immune haemolytic anaemias. British Journal of Haematology 58:525–531.

95. Decary F, Vermeulen A, Engelfriet CP 1975 A look at HLA antisera in the indirect immunofluorescence technique LIFT. In: Histocompatibility testing. Munksgaard, Copenhagen, p. 380.

96. Metcalfe P, Minchinton RM, Murphy MF, et al 1985 Use of chloroquine-treated granulocytes and platelets in the diagnosis of immune cytopenias. Vox Sanguinis 49:340–345.

97. Decary F 1988 Report on the second Canadian workshop on platelet serology. Current Studies in Hematology and Blood Transfusion 54:1. Karger, Basel.

98. Helmerhorst FM, Ten Boerge ML, van der Plas–van Dalen C, et al 1984 Platelet freezing for serological purposes with and without a cryopreservative. Vox Sanguinis 46:318–322.

99. Helmerhorst FM, van Oss CJ, Bruynes ECE, et al 1982 Elution of granulocyte and platelet antibodies. Vox Sanguinis 43:196–204.

100. Vos JJE, Huisman JG, Winkel IN, et al 1987 Quantification of platelet-bound allo-antibodies by radioimmunoassay: a study on some variables. Vox Sanguinis 53:108–116.

101. Minchinton RM, Waters AH 1984 Chloroquine stripping of HLA antigens from neutrophils without removal of neutrophil specific antigens. British Journal of Haematology 57:703–706.

102. Metcalfe P, Waters AH 1992 Location of the granulocyte-specific antigen LAN on the Fc-receptor III. Transfusion Medicine 2:283–287.

103. Kiefel V, Santoso S, Weisheit M, et al 1987 Monoclonal antibody specific immobilization of platelet antigens MAIPA: a new tool for the identification of platelet-reactive antibodies. Blood 70:1722–1726.

104. Shibata Y, Juji T, Nishizawa Y, et al 1981 Detection of platelet antibodies by a newly developed mixed agglutination with platelets. Vox Sanguinis 41:25–31.

105. Lown JA, Ivey JG 1991 Evaluation of solid phase red cell adherence technique for platelet antibody screening. Transfusion Medicine 1:163–167.

106. Lucas GF, Rogers SE 1999 Evaluation of an enzyme-linked immunosorbent assay kit GTI PakPlus® for the detection of antibodies against human platelet antigens. Transfusion Medicine 9:63–67.

107. Araki N, Nose Y, Kohsaki M, et al 1999 Anti-granulocyte antibody screening with extracted granulocyte antigens by a micro-mixed passive haemagglutination method. Vox Sanguinis 77:44–51.

108. Metcalfe P, Waters AH 1993 HPA-1 typing by PCR amplification with sequence-specific primers PCR-SSP: a rapid and simple technique. British Journal of Haematology 85:227–229.

109. Simsek S, Faber NM, Bleeker PM, et al 1993 Determination of human platelet antigen frequencies in the Dutch population by immunophenotyping and DNA allele-specific restriction enzyme analysis. Blood 81:835–840.

110. McFarland JG, Aster RH, Bussel JB, et al 1991 Prenatal diagnosis of neonatal alloimmune thrombocytopenia using allele-specific oligonucleotide probes. Blood 78:2276–2282.

111. Cavanagh G, Dunn A, Chapman CE, et al 1997 HPA genotyping by PCR sequence specific priming PCR-SSP: a streamlined method for rapid routine investigations. Transfusion Medicine 7:41–45.

112. Engelfriet CP, Tetteroo PAT, van der Veen JPW et al 1984 Granulocyte-specific antigens and methods for their detection. In: McCullough J, Sandler SG, Sweeney GE (eds) Advances in Immunobiology: blood cell antigens and bone marrow transplantation. Liss, New York, p. 121.

113. McCullough J 1985 The clinical significance of granulocyte antibodies and in vivo studies of the fate of granulocytes. In: Garraty G (ed) Current Concepts in Transfusion Therapy. American Association of Blood Banks, Arlington, VA, p. 125.

114. Minchinton RM, Waters AH 1984 The occurrence and significance of neutrophil antibodies. British Journal of Haematology 56:521–528.

115. Lo YM, Tein MS, Lau TK, et al 1998 Quantitative analysis of fetal DNA in maternal plasma and serum: implications for noninvasive prenatal diagnosis. American Journal of Human Genetics 62:768–775.

20 Laboratory aspects of blood transfusion

Megan Rowley and Clare Milkins

Safe and effective blood transfusion requires the combined efforts of blood transfusion services, scientists, and clinicians to ensure the highest standards are applied to all the systems in a complex process from "vein to vein." This chapter provides a description of the laboratory framework required to provide the right blood products to the right patients at the right time. The increased awareness of what can go wrong comes from a number of sources including the Serious Hazards of Transfusion UK haemovigilance scheme, which was started in 1996.[1,2]

This confidential reporting scheme, using detailed analysis of errors, has provided data that have enabled both national bodies and local transfusion services to introduce measures to reduce risk. It is clear that multiple errors can occur and that many of these are outside the control of the transfusion laboratory (Figs. 20.1 and 20.2). Within the laboratory setting, the application of strict protocols for sample labelling and testing, robust laboratory procedures, reliable documentation, and frequent staff training should be used.

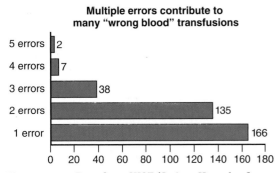

Multiple errors contribute to many "wrong blood" transfusions

Errors	Count
5 errors	2
4 errors	7
3 errors	38
2 errors	135
1 error	166

Figure 20.1   Data from SHOT (Serious Hazards of Transfusion) 2003[1,2] showing that in 348 analysed cases where wrong blood was transfused, multiple errors occurred in 52% of cases.

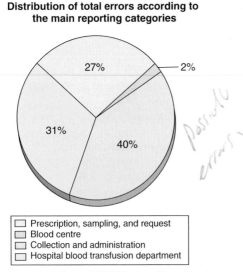

Distribution of total errors according to the main reporting categories

27%   2%
31%
40%

☐ Prescription, sampling, and request
☐ Blood centre
☐ Collection and administration
☐ Hospital blood transfusion department

Figure 20.2   Data from SHOT (Serious Hazards of Transfusion) 2003[1,2] showing distribution of errors, according to the main reporting categories, of a total of 588 errors from the analysis of 348 completed reports.

This chapter is concerned with the testing of patient samples prior to the provision of appropriate compatible blood products including identification of red cell antibodies. It also covers compatibility testing and investigation of transfusion reactions and the testing required in other special situations including the antenatal and postnatal settings. National professional bodies such as the British Committee for Standards in Haematology (BCSH)[3]

and the AABB[4] (formerly American Association of Blood Banks) issue guidance to transfusion laboratories and this has been referenced where appropriate. The European Blood Directive (Directive 2002/98/EC) became law in member countries in 2005; this has important implications for hospital transfusion practice, particularly in terms of the "vein to vein" traceability of blood products, the need to store transfusion records for 30 years, and the requirement for a quality management system.[5] The UK government continues to promote the safe and effective transfusion of blood products through its two Health Service Circulars.[6,7] These documents aim to ensure that a corporate approach to blood transfusion safety is taken via the local clinical governance arrangements and to promote good transfusion practice via the Hospital Transfusion Committees and Teams.

RECENT DEVELOPMENTS IN BLOOD TRANSFUSION

Since the previous edition of this book, a number of important changes have taken place in the blood transfusion laboratory. Bar-coded labels on blood products, reagents, patient samples, and equipment are now commonplace, and these result in safer transfer of information, free from the transcription errors associated with manual methods.

Column agglutination and solid-phase technology (Chapter 19) can be used both on automated machines and by manual techniques, and in 80% of UK hospital laboratories these technologies have partly or wholly replaced tube techniques and liquid-phase microplates for antibody screening.[8] Although there are many advantages, there are some restrictions imposed by having six columns on most of the column agglutination technology cards/cassettes in common use.

Individual laboratories need to make decisions about the selection of profiles and reagents when using this technology for blood grouping, and it is vital that any abbreviated testing in an automated or semiautomated system is carefully evaluated for the risks that could ensue if important controls were omitted.[9] Computer systems store patient details and results of laboratory tests, allowing timely and accurate access to important information. Many are interfaced to automated blood grouping analysers, and some use programmes for interpretation of test results. Computer algorithms support the "electronic issue" of blood to patients with a negative antibody screen without the need to use an antiglobulin crossmatch and, in the UK, 19% of laboratories are using this system for some or all of their patients.[8] The application and use of automation for all aspects of compatibility testing continues to increase. Automation brings several or all of the discrete activities of compatibility testing into a single platform process. It provides various levels of increased security over manual testing and may provide justification for abbreviated pretransfusion testing (e.g., abandoning duplicate D [previously termed "RhD] grouping or reverse ABO grouping). A risk assessment must be made and documented prior to any abbreviation of an established procedure, with consideration being given to the presence or absence of key functions in the automated equipment. The BCSH guidelines for compatibility procedures[9] give a list of factors to be taken into consideration, and the reader is advised to consult these prior to implementing automated or semiautomated systems.

PRETRANSFUSION COMPATIBILITY SYSTEMS

The process of providing blood for transfusion involves many steps, all of which have to be reliably completed. These include the following:

Blood samples have to be taken from the correct patient and labelled at the bedside in a single uninterrupted procedure. The sample must be identified by a minimum of the correctly spelled forename and surname, the exact date of birth, and an accurate unique patient number. The sample should be dated and signed by the person taking the sample.[9] Some guidelines recommend that addressograph labels should not be accepted on blood samples for compatibility testing. The laboratory should have a policy for rejecting badly labelled samples,[10] although a recent survey of hospitals in England and North Wales showed considerable variation in the content and application of these policies.[11] A request for services should include the previously outlined patient identifiers as well as clear information about the source of the request and the location of the patient and clinical details including a detailed justification for the request. Previous transfusion history and any special considerations for the selection of blood (e.g., cytomegalovirus [CMV] tested or irradiated) are also needed.

An ABO and D group of the patient sample must be accurately performed.

An antibody screen of the patient's plasma/serum (or mother's plasma/serum in the case of a neonate) should be able to detect any clinically significant red cell antibodies. In the event of a positive red cell antibody screen, antibody identification should be undertaken to assist the selection of compatible blood.

There should be a check of existing transfusion records to compare current and historical results.

The appropriate blood component should be selected and issued as suitable for transfusion to a named patient using a serological crossmatch or electronic issue

Traceable documentation should exist to ensure that the results of laboratory compatibility procedures are available at the patient's bedside to allow a check before transfusing the blood product. This may include a blood bag compatibility label (Fig. 20.3) and a compatibility form. The patient must be identified with a wristband, and the blood product must be prescribed on a drug or fluid administration chart.[10] In some countries, an additional bedside check of the patient's blood group is undertaken prior to commencing the transfusion.

Identification and Storage of Blood Samples

Depending on laboratory practice, blood transfusion tests may require a clotted sample or EDTA-anticoagulated blood. Clotted samples should be taken into a plain tube **but not a tube with a separating gel** (see Chapter 19, p. 497). On being received in the laboratory, the details on the request form must be checked against the blood sample. Each blood sample must be labelled with a unique sample number. Bar code labels offer the advantage of positive sample identification and reduce the number of transcription errors. Samples inadequately

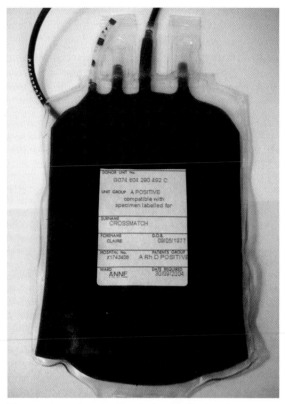

Figure 20.3 A unit of packed red cells showing a compatibility label.

or inaccurately labelled should NOT be used for pretransfusion testing.[9] Great care must be taken to select and identify the sample prior to any testing. Transposition of samples in the laboratory can lead to an incorrect blood group being assigned to a patient, with serious consequences, including ABO incompatible transfusions. Where possible, the primary sample should be used for testing. If samples are separated, the plasma/serum must be clearly and accurately identified and special precautions must be taken (Fig. 20.4). If repeated testing on this sample is anticipated, storing separate small aliquots reduces the risk of sample deterioration, which occurs with repeated thawing/freezing of larger samples.

Whole blood samples should be tested as soon as possible because they will deteriorate over time. Problems associated with storage include lysis of the red cells, loss of complement in the serum, and decrease in potency of antibodies. The BCSH

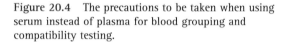

When using **serum** for blood grouping and compatibility testing, any **red cells** in the test system should be washed and suspended in EDTA-containing saline. The presence of complement in serum can cause lysis and hence may lead to misinterpretation of tests based on agglutination. In addition, false negative reactions may occur in immediate spin crossmatching with potent ABO antibodies, where rapid complement fixation causes a prozone effect (bound C1 inhibits agglutination). EDTA saline is not necessary when using **plasma**.

Figure 20.4 The precautions to be taken when using serum instead of plasma for blood grouping and compatibility testing.

guidelines[9] indicate working limits as outlined in Table 20.1. If separated plasma or serum samples are stored for later serological crossmatch, care must be taken to ensure that the patient has not been transfused in the interim. It has been recommended that samples should be stored for 7 days on all patients who have been transfused to allow investigation of any subsequent transfusion reactions.[12,13]

Documentation of Transfusion Process

All stages of the transfusion process must be clearly documented, and European Union regulations now require that the records must be accessible for 30 years.[5] This allows any blood product to be traced from the donor to the recipient should information come to light about any potential infective risks to the recipient. This system has been tested in the hepatitis C look-back exercise undertaken by the UK National Blood Service.[14]

Computer records are easier to search than paper records, but computer systems are likely to become obsolete and be replaced several times within this mandatory 30-year period so provision must be made to store historical data in an accessible format when procuring a replacement computer system.[15] Patient-held records are useful for patients who are treated in more than one institution, particularly if they have red cell antibodies and require phenotyped blood or if they have special requirements because of their underlying disease or its treatment. Credit card–sized records are issued by some transfusion centres to patients with red cell antibodies, and similar cards exist for patients who require irradiated cellular blood products.[16] In

Table 20.1 Recommended limits for storage of samples used for compatibility testing[9]

Sample	18–25°C	4°C	–20°C
EDTA-anticoagulated whole blood	Up to 48 hours	Up to 7 days	Not applicable
Separated plasma/serum	Not applicable	Up to 7 days	6 months

Hong Kong, a system has been proposed to phenotype red cells of all citizens, making this information available as part of an identity card.[17]

ABO AND D GROUPING

ABO and D grouping must be performed by an approved technique with appropriate controls. Before use, all new batches of grouping reagents should be checked for reliability by the techniques used in the laboratory. Grouping reagents should be stored according to manufacturer's instructions.

ABO Grouping

ABO grouping is the single most important serological test performed in compatibility testing; consequently it is imperative that the sensitivity and security of the test system are not compromised. The fact that anti-A and anti-B are naturally occurring antibodies allows the patient's plasma/serum to be tested against known A and B cells in a "reverse" group.

This is an excellent built-in check for the "forward" or cell group and has always been considered to be an integral part of ABO grouping, allowing the reading and recording of test results to be split into two discrete tasks. However, with the advent of secure, fully automated systems, linked to secure information technology systems that, in combination, have the ability to prevent procedural ABO grouping errors, some laboratories now omit the reverse group when testing samples for which a historical group is available. This should only be considered following a careful risk assessment and taking into account that the first sample taken may have been from the wrong patient.[9,11] This may be in the order of 1:2000 samples.[18] Any discrepancy between the forward and reverse groups should be investigated further, and any repeat tests should be undertaken using cells taken from the original sample rather than from a prepared cell suspension.

Reagents for ABO Grouping

Prior to the introduction of monoclonal reagents, polyclonal anti-A, anti-B, and anti-A,B were traditionally used for red cell grouping tests. The anti-A,B reagent (from group O serum) acted as an additional check on cells that were agglutinated by anti-A and/or anti-B but was also capable of detecting weak A antigens (e.g., A_x). Superior monoclonal anti-A and anti-B reagents have replaced polyclonal reagents), and although anti-A,B and anti-A+B monoclonal reagents are available, there is no requirement to include them in routine grouping tests. A_1 and B cells are used for reverse grouping; group O cells or an auto-control may be included to ensure that reactions with anti-A and anti-B are not a result of the presence of cold autoantibodies.

D Grouping

D grouping is usually undertaken at the same time as ABO grouping for convenience and to minimise clerical errors that may arise through repeated handling of patients' samples. In the absence of secure automation, testing should be undertaken in duplicate because there is no counterpart of the "reverse" grouping of ABO testing.

Reagents for D Grouping

Monoclonal reagents do not have the problem of possible contamination with antibodies of unwanted specificities, as was the case with polyclonal reagents. Therefore, the duplicate testing may be undertaken using the same anti-D reagent, although this should be dispensed as though it were two separate reagents. D^{VI} is the partial D with the fewest epitopes; therefore D^{VI} individuals are those most likely to form anti-D.[9,19] For this reason, anti-D monoclonal

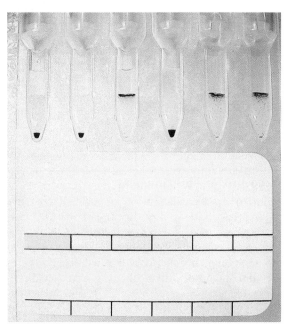

Figure 20.5 Column agglutination technology: blood group O D positive.

reagents that do not detect D^{VI} should be selected for testing patients' samples.[20] The use of anti-CDE reagents has lead to the misinterpretation of r′ and r″ cells in UK National External Quality Assessment Scheme (NEQAS) exercises and, because they are of no value in routine patient typing, their use is not recommended.[9] Selection of high-avidity monoclonal anti-D reagents will allow detection of all but the weakest examples of weak D, negating the need to use more sensitive techniques to check the D status of apparent D negatives.

Some anti-D reagents have high levels of potentiator (e.g., polyethylene glycol) and should be used with caution; a diluent control is essential to demonstrate that the diluent does not promote agglutination of the test red cells as may happen if the patient's cells are coated *in vivo* with immunoglobulin G (IgG); any positive seen with the control, however weak, invalidates the test result. Anti-D reagents are provided in many different kits, and those responsible for selection and purchase should make themselves aware of the content, specificity, and potentiation of the chosen reagent.

Methods

There are several techniques available for ABO and D grouping including tube, slide, microplates, and columns. Other techniques for blood grouping have been described (e.g., flow cytometry),[21] but they are not in routine use. Care should be taken to use the appropriate reagent because not all reagents have been validated by the manufacturer for all techniques.

Tube and Slide Tests

Spin-tube tests are commonly used, particularly for urgent testing, where small numbers of tests are performed at once. Slide or tile techniques are widely used in under-resourced countries for ABO and D grouping. Spin-tube tests should be performed in 75 × 10 or 75 × 12 mm plastic tubes. Immediate spin tests may be used in an emergency, whereas routine tests are usually left for 15 min at room temperature (about 20°C) before centrifugation for 1 min at 150 g. Equal volumes (1 or 2 drops from either a commercial reagent dropper or a Pasteur pipette) of liquid reagents or serum/plasma and 2% cell suspensions are used. The patient's red cells (diluted in phosphate buffered saline [PBS]) should be tested against monoclonal anti-A and anti-B grouping reagents. The patient's serum or plasma should be tested against A_1 and B reagent red cells (reverse grouping). In addition, the serum or plasma should be tested against either the patient's own cells or group O cells (i.e., a negative control) to exclude reactions with A and B cells as a result of cold agglutinins, other than anti-A or anti-B, in the patient's sample. To prevent misinterpretation of results resulting from haemolysis when serum is used, it is recommended that the diluent for resuspension of reverse grouping cells contains EDTA (see later). Mix the suspensions by tapping the tubes, and leave them undisturbed for 15 min. Agglutination should be read as described on p. 499. Any discrepancy between the results of the red cell grouping and the reverse grouping should be investigated further, and any repeat tests should involve cells taken from the original sample rather than the prepared suspension. Reverse grouping is not carried out for infants younger than 4 months of age because the corresponding antibodies are normally absent.

EDTA for Diluents

Stock solution. Prepare a 0.1 mol/l solution of EDTA (dipotassium salt) in distilled water. Adjust the pH to 7.0 using 5 mol/l NaOH.

Working solution. Mix 1 volume of stock solution with 9 volumes of saline or low ionic strength saline (LISS). Check the pH and adjust to 7.0 if necessary.

Slide Method

In an emergency, rapid ABO grouping may be carried out on slides or tiles. The method is satisfactory if potent grouping reagents are used (see p. 499). An immediate spin-tube test is preferable.

Liquid-Phase Microplate Methods

Liquid-phase microplate technology provides a cheap and secure method for batch testing when semiautomation is utilised for dispensing and reading; it is the grouping technique most commonly used in the United Kingdom. ABO and D grouping may be performed in a single microplate if monoclonal reagents are used. A resuspension technique, using untreated U-well rigid polystyrene microplates, is recommended for grouping. If microplates are to be reused they should be cleaned in mild detergent, rinsed thoroughly in distilled water, and left to dry face down; alternatively, an ultrasonic bath may be used. Scored or otherwise damaged plates should be discarded.

The plate is usually laid out as 12 × 8 (12 tests and 8 reagents) but may be used in the opposite orientation (8 × 12), depending on the number of reagents and controls required. The anti-D reagents should be kept away from the anti-A and anti-B reagents because splashing between wells can happen when dispensing reagents and handling the plates during testing if insufficient care is taken. The following method is recommended[22]:

1. Add 1 drop of antiserum and diluent control (if required) to each appropriate well.
2. Add 1 or 2 drops of test plasma/serum to the appropriate wells for reverse grouping and auto controls (if required).
3. Make a visual check to ensure that there are no empty wells.
4. Add 1 drop of a 3% cell suspension of test cells to the appropriate wells containing antiserum, diluent control, and auto control.
5. Add 1 drop of 3% reagent red cells to the appropriate wells containing test plasma/serum.
6. Agitate carefully to mix, preferably using a microplate shaker.
7. Leave the plate to incubate at ambient temperature for 15 min and then centrifuge at 100 g for 40 s.
8. Resuspend the red cells using a microplate shaker. Excessive agitation will reduce the strength of agglutination. It should be remembered that agglutinates formed by some weaker examples of weak D may be disrupted and interpreted as D negative in microplate methods.
9. Results may be read visually or using an automated plate reader.

Column Agglutination Techniques

Agglutination techniques (see Chapter 19, p. 499) using either a sephadex gel (DiaMed ID) or a glass microbead matrix (Ortho BioVue) are increasingly being used for grouping, especially where automated systems are in place; these should always be performed in accordance with the manufacturer's instructions. The number of reagents and controls is limited to six, making the inclusion of two anti-D reagents, a control, and a reverse group, in addition to a cell group, impossible. There are several different profiles to choose from, and some cards/cassettes include monoclonal antibodies to other blood group antigens (e.g., K) in addition to ABO or D. Forward and reverse grouping may be undertaken in separate cards/cassettes.

Solid-Phase Techniques

ABO/D grouping using solid-phase techniques would usually be used as part of a fully automated system, and testing should be undertaken in accordance with the manufacturer's instructions.

Controls

Positive and negative controls should be included with every test or batch of tests. The anti-A reagent should be tested against group A (positive control) and B (negative control) cells, and the anti-B reagent should be tested against group B (positive control) and group A (negative control) cells. In fully automated systems, the controls should be set up at least twice daily. The timings should coincide with machine startup and changing of reagents, taking account of the length of time that reagents have been kept at room temperature on the machine. The control samples should be loaded in the same way as the test samples. The required controls are shown in Table 20.2. Where controls do not give the expected reactions, investigations should be undertaken to determine the validity of all tests undertaken subsequent to the most recent valid control results.

Table 20.2	Control cells for blood grouping	
Reagent	Positive control	Negative control
Anti-A	A cells	B cells
Anti-B	B cells	A cells
Anti-D	D positive cells	D negative cells
A₁ cells	Anti-A	Anti-B
B cells	Anti-B	Anti-A

Causes of Discrepancies in ABO/D Grouping

False-Positive Reactions

Rouleaux

Rouleaux may occur in various clinical conditions, where the ratio of normal albumin to globulin is altered in plasma (e.g., multiple myeloma), and in the presence of plasma substitutes such as dextrans. The stacking of red cells on top of one another in columns may be misinterpreted as weak agglutination by inexperienced workers (see Fig. 20.6). Rouleaux will usually disperse on a slide if a drop of saline is added; alternatively, the reverse grouping can be repeated using plasma/serum diluted 1 in 2 or 1 in 4 with saline.

Cold Autoagglutination and Cold Reacting Alloantibodies

Cold autoantibodies that are reactive at room temperature may lead to autoagglutination in the cell group (ABO and D) and panagglutination in the reverse group, causing a grouping anomaly (see p. 254). The tests should be repeated using cells washed in warm saline and plasma/serum prewarmed to 37°C, and an autocontrol should be included. Cold reacting alloantibodies (e.g., anti-P₁) may cause agglutination of reverse grouping cells, and, if

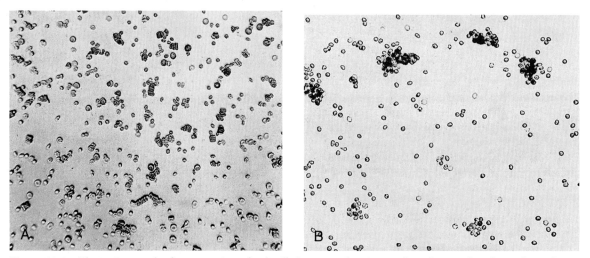

Figure 20.6   Photomicrograph of a suspension of red cells in serum showing a minor degree of rouleaux formation (A) and weak agglutination (B).

this is suspected, reverse grouping should be repeated using prewarmed plasma/serum or grouping cells that lack the implicated antigen.

T-Activation/Polyagglutination

Polyagglutination[23] describes agglutination of red cells by all or most normal adult sera as the result of IgM antibodies reacting with a cryptantigen on the red cells. The most common form is T-activation, which occurs when neuraminidase, produced by bacteria, cleaves N-acetyl neuraminic acid from the red cell membrane, exposing the T antigen.

This can be a problem when grouping with polyclonal reagents, which contain anti-T, and clinically most often occurs in sick infants and young children (e.g., infants with necrotising enterocolitis). Tests using monoclonal reagents are not affected by this phenomenon. Special tests may need to be undertaken to confirm T activation where necrotising enterocolitis has been diagnosed or is suspected.

Acquired B

The acquired B antigen is usually caused by deacetylation of A_1 red cells by bacterial red cell enzymes. Some anti-B reagents react strongly with the acquired B antigen (e.g., those derived from the ES4 clone).[24] This usually results in a discrepancy between forward and reverse grouping, which may be overlooked if the patient's own anti-B is weak or if the reverse group is omitted. Such anti-B reagents should be avoided.

Potentiators

Red cells may be coated with IgG as a result of *in vivo* sensitisation. The use of potentiated techniques, such as the antiglobulin test for D typing, or of potentiated reagents for ABO or D typing may result in a false-positive reaction; the latter would also result in a positive reaction with the diluent control, but UK NEQAS data[25] have shown that some laboratories fail to include an appropriate control or fail to understand the significance of a positive control. For this reason, use of potentiated techniques or reagents for blood grouping is not advised.

Contaminating Antibodies

Polyclonal anti-D reagents were susceptible to contamination by antibodies of other specificities that had not been adequately absorbed (e.g., it was not uncommon for an anti-D reagent to be contaminated with anti-A, anti-B, or anti-C, leading to false-positive reactions with A, B, or r' red cells, respectively).

In vitro Bacterial Contamination

In vitro bacterial contamination of antisera, patients' red cells, or reverse grouping cells may cause false-positive agglutination.

False-Negative Reactions

Failure to Add Reagents

The most likely cause of a false-negative grouping result is failure to add the reagent or test plasma/serum. For this reason, in liquid phase tests, the serum or plasma should always be added first to the reaction chamber, and a visual check should be made before red cells are added. The use of colour-coded reagents for ABO grouping is helpful in this respect.

Loss of Potency

Inappropriate storage or freezing and thawing may cause a loss of potency of blood grouping reagents. The use of regular controls will alert the user to this problem.

Failure to Identify Lysis

In the presence of complement, anti-A and anti-B may cause *in vitro* lysis of reagent red cells. If lysis is not recognised as a positive reaction, falsely negative results may be recorded in reverse grouping tests. To avoid this, reverse grouping cells should be resuspended in EDTA saline, where serum rather than plasma is used (see Fig. 20.4).

Mixed Field Appearance

A dual population of red cells may be present in both ABO and D grouping. It is important to recognise this as a mixed-field picture and not to confuse it with weak agglutination. The most likely cause of a mixed-field picture is the transfusion (either deliberate or accidental) of non-identical ABO or D red cells. Investigation will be required to determine the actual blood group of the patient, who may have been transfused in a different establishment or may have received an intrauterine transfusion. A mixed-field ABO group may be the first indication of a previous ABO-incompatible transfusion.

An ABO or D incompatible bone marrow transplant will result in a mixed-field picture until total engraftment has occurred; the mixed-field picture may subsequently reappear when a graft is failing. Rarely, a dual population of cells is permanent and results from a weak subgroup of A (A_3) or a blood group chimerism. Interpretation of a dual population of red cells will depend on the technique used. In a tube, microscopic reading will reveal strong agglutinates in a sea of free cells; in column agglutination techniques there will be a line of agglutinated cells at the top of the column, with the negative cells travelling through to the bottom of the column. Automated systems should be set up to detect mixed-field pictures.

D Variant Phenotypes

Discrepant results between different anti-D reagents or weak results are usually the result of weak or partial D phenotypes. In weak D, the entire D antigen is present but there are fewer D antigen sites per cell. Patients who are weak D are unable to make anti-D and may be treated as D positive*. However, a weak reaction with a single anti-D reagent should be investigated with a second anti-D before assigning a result of D positive. It is essential to be able to distinguish between a weak reaction and a mixed-field reaction because the latter may be the result of a patient who is D negative being transfused with D positive blood. If in doubt, it is safer to call the patient D negative, at least until investigations have been undertaken by a reference centre. This will be of no clinical consequence because it is safe to transfuse D negative blood to a patient who is D positive, and a pregnant woman who is D positive would be unlikely to be harmed by the injection of prophylactic anti-D. Most weak D types group as D positive with the currently available high-avidity commercial monoclonal anti-D reagents.

Where differing reactions are obtained with two reagents the patient may be a partial D (i.e., one or more of the epitopes of the D antigen is missing). These individuals are capable of making anti-D following sensitisation with the missing epitope. Category D^{VI} lacks the most epitopes, and such individuals are likely to make anti-D when challenged

by transfusion or pregnancy. For this reason, anti-D reagents for routine grouping of patients' samples should not detect D^{VI}. There is little evidence to suggest that a D^{VI} donor would elicit an immune response in a recipient who is D negative; however, weak D positive donors, including D^{VI} donors, should be classified as D positive. There are some important ethnic differences in the frequency of different Rh haplotypes, as shown in Table 20.3.

ANTIBODY SCREENING

Antibody screening is usually undertaken at the same time as blood grouping and in advance of selecting blood for transfusion. Antibody screening may be more reliable and sensitive than cross-matching against donor cells because some antibodies react more strongly with red cells with homozygous expression (double dose) of the relevant antigen than with those with heterozygous expression (single dose)—most notably anti-Jk^a/Jk^b but also anti-Fy^a, -Fy^b, -S, and –s. Screening cells can be selected to reflect this, whereas donor cells are usually of unknown zygosity. In addition, reagent red cells are easier to standardise than donor cells, and there is potentially less opportunity for procedural error, particularly in automated systems.

Clinically significant antibodies are those that are capable of causing patient morbidity as a result of accelerated destruction of a significant proportion of transfused red cells. With few exceptions, clinically significant antibodies are those that are reactive in the indirect antiglobulin test at 37°C;

*DNA red cell genotyping may change our definition of weak and partial D.

Table 20.3 Approximate frequencies of common haplotypes in selected populations[26]

Haplotype	Approximate frequencies		
	English	Nigerian	Chinese
DCe R^1	0.421	0.060	0.730
dce r	0.389	0.203	0.023
DcE R^2	0.141	0.115	0.187
Dce R^0	0.026	0.591	0.033
dcE r″	0.012	0	0
dCe r′	0.010	0.031	0.019

however, it is not possible to predict serologically which of these antibodies will definitely be of clinical significance, so the term "of potential clinical significance" is often used.

Red Cell Reagents

The patient's serum or plasma should be tested against at least two individual screening cells, used individually, not pooled. The screening cells should be group O and encompass the common antigens of the indigenous population.

In the United Kingdom, the following antigens should be expressed as a minimum: C, c, D, E, e, K, k, Fy^a, Fy^b, Jk^a, Jk^b, S, s, M, N, and Le^a; one cell should be R_2R_2 and another R_1R_1 or $R_1^WR_1$. The following phenotypes should also be represented in the screening set: Jk(a+b−), Jk(a−b+), S+s−, S−s+, Fy(a+b−), and Fy(a−b+) (see Table 20.4). These recommendations for homozygosity are based on UK data regarding the incidence of delayed haemolytic transfusion reactions, the need for high sensitivity in the detection of Kidd antibodies, and the poorer performance of column agglutination techniques in the detection of some examples of Kidd antibodies using heterozygous cells.[2,26] The requirement for the expression of C^w and Kp^a antigens on screening cells has been the cause of much debate, and there is no real international consensus. In the United Kingdom and the United States a detection of anti-C^w or anti-Kp^a is not a requirement even in the absence of an antiglobulin crossmatch.[9,27] This is because these are low-frequency antigens and the antibodies are rarely causes of delayed haemolytic transfusion reactions or severe haemolytic disease of the newborn.

Methods

Antibody screening should always be carried out by an indirect antiglobulin test as the primary method. Additional methods (e.g., two-stage enzyme or Polybrene) may also be used but are inferior for the detection of some clinically significant antibodies and should not be used alone. A large retrospective study showed that the vast majority of antibodies reactive only by enzyme technique are of no clinical significance.[28] In Issitt's study of 10,000 recently transfused patients, only one anti-c, initially unreactive by indirect antiglobulin test, caused a

Table 20.4 Expression of red cell antigens on screening cells[9]

Blood group system	Antigen	Homozygous cells recommended
Rh	C	Yes (R_1R_1 or $R_1^WR_1$)
	c	Yes (R_2R_2)
	D	Yes (R_1R_1 and R_2R_2)
	E	Yes (R_2R_2)
	e	Yes (R_1R_1 or $R_1^WR_1$)
Kell	K	No*
	k	No (always likely)
Duffy	Fy^a	Yes
	Fy^b	Yes
Kidd	Jk^a	Yes
	Jk^b	Yes
MNSs	M	No
	N	No
	S	Yes
	s	Yes
Lewis	Le^a	No

*Although desirable, KK cells are unlikely to be available

delayed haemolytic transfusion reaction. There has been one report of an anti-E that was only detectable by indirect antiglobulin test posttransfusion, causing a fatal delayed haemolytic transfusion reaction.[1] For liquid-phase techniques, BCSH guidelines recommend the use of red cells suspended in LISS, rather than in standard normal ionic strength saline (NISS), because LISS increases the sensitivity of detection of many potentially clinically significant antibodies.[9,25] There are conflicting reports about whether sensitivity can also be improved by adding polyethylene glycol.[29,30]

Indirect Antiglobulin Techniques

Column Agglutination

In many countries column agglutination is now more commonly used than traditional tube or liquid-phase microplate techniques because it has been shown to be at least as sensitive as a standard LISS spin-tube technique,[30,31] it is simpler to perform because it requires no washing phase, it uses small volumes of plasma/serum and reagents, it has a more objective reading phase, and it is easy to automate. The antihuman globulin (AHG) incorporated in the matrix is available as either a polyspecific or anti-IgG reagent. Red cell concentrations and volumes can be critical, and it is important to follow manufacturers' instructions at all times. Similarly, microcolumns are also available that use an affinity gel matrix, where protein G and protein A, rather than anti-IgG, are incorporated into the gel.

Column agglutination crossmatching tests have been shown to be less sensitive than standard tube techniques in detection of weak ABO antibodies such as anti-A with A_2B cells[25,32,33] and Kidd antibodies with heterozygous red cells.[25] It has been suggested that these failures may be the result of shear forces occurring during centrifugation, which cause weak agglutinates to be disrupted, especially when the antigen site density is low.[32]

Solid-Phase Systems

Solid-phase techniques (e.g., Capture-R [Immucor] and Solid Screen II [Biotest]) are also becoming more popular because they have been shown to have a high level of sensitivity and they also lend themselves to full automation.[30]

Liquid-Phase Techniques—Tubes and Microplates

Tube techniques are still used for antibody screening in some parts of the world. With LISS-suspension techniques it is important to keep a high serum:cell ratio, without affecting the ionic strength. Equal volumes of serum and 1.5–2% cells suspended in LISS[34] will result in a serum:cell ratio of >60:1, ensuring optimal sensitivity. Reagents should be incubated for 15–20 min at 37°C, and the cells then should be washed in PBS. After adding AHG, the red cells should be examined using a careful "tip and roll" procedure to prevent disruption of weak agglutinates. Reading aids such a light box or concave mirror may also be used with this technique.

Liquid-phase microplate technology has never achieved a huge popularity for antibody screening because it is relatively difficult to introduce and standardise and it cannot be automated. Because it is becoming increasingly difficult to obtain AHG reagents standardised for use in microplates, no method is detailed here. However, further information is available in the BCSH guidelines, including a recommended method for screening in V-well plates, using a streaming technique.[9]

Controls

A weak anti-D should be used on a regular basis to ensure the efficacy of the whole procedure, although the exact frequency will depend on work patterns as described in the blood grouping section. Additional weak controls are also recommended to confirm the sensitivity of the procedure and the integrity of the red cell antigens throughout their shelf life; anti-Fy^a and/or anti-S are good examples because Duffy and S antigens are protease labile and may deteriorate more quickly on reagent cells than the D antigen and their use will also ensure that enzyme-treated cells have not been used by mistake. Consideration should also be given to selecting controls that demonstrate that the correct screening cell has been added to the batch of tests.

The use of red cells weakly sensitised with anti-D is essential to control the washing phase of every negative liquid-phase test because inadequate washing may result in complete or partial neutralisation of AHG by unbound globulin. Any test that does not give a positive reaction at the expected strength, following addition of these cells (and subsequent centrifugation), indicates insufficient free anti-IgG and should be repeated. The washing phase of solid-phase systems is difficult to control, and it may be necessary to add a weak control to every column to ensure that every probe has dispensed wash solution during each wash cycle.

ANTIBODY IDENTIFICATION

When an antibody is detected in the antibody screen, its specificity should be determined and its likely clinical significance should be assessed before blood is selected for transfusion or relevant advice is given during pregnancy. It is essential to use a systematic approach to antibody identification to ensure that all specificities of potential clinical significance are identified. It may be tempting to match a reaction pattern immediately and look no further, but this is likely to result in additional specificities being missed.

Principles

As a starting point, the test plasma/serum should be tested against an identification panel of reagent red cells by the technique with which it was detected in the screen. The next section on reagents outlines the minimum requirements for the panel. Inclusion of an autoantibody test is helpful in distinguishing between an autoantibody, an antibody directed against a high-frequency antigen, and a complex mixture of alloantibodies. The positive and negative reactions should be compared with the panel profile in conjunction with the screening results.

Each antibody specificity should be taken in turn, and its presence should be systematically excluded, by identifying antigen positive cells that have given negative reactions; wherever possible a negative reaction should be obtained with a red cell with homozygous expression of the relevant antigen—for example, if a negative reaction has been recorded against a Jk(a+b−) cell, then the presence of anti-Jk^a can be excluded, but if the only negative reactions are against Jk(a+b+) cells, then anti-Jk^a cannot immediately be safely excluded. This will leave a list of potential specificities, which should be considered by matching the positive reactions to the antigen-positive cells to determine if any are definitely present. Once this process is complete with the initial screen and identification panel, further cells and techniques may need to be used to complete the exclusion process (e.g., where anti-S has been identified as being present, an enzyme-treated panel may be required to exclude the presence of anti-E, where all of the E positive cells were also S positive, or a K+S− cell may need to be selected to exclude the presence of anti-K). The more specificities present, the more complicated the process, and where resources are limited, samples may need to be sent to a reference centre to elucidate all specificities. If the antisera are available, phenotyping the patient's red cells early on in the process will allow exclusion of specificities for which the patient is antigen positive.

The specificity of an antibody should only be assigned when it is reactive with at least two examples of reagent red cells carrying the antigen and nonreactive with at least two examples of reagent red cells lacking the antigen. This is because a single positive reaction could occur if the panel cell unexpectedly expressed a low-frequency antigen, and a single negative reaction could occur if the panel cell lacked a high-frequency antigen.

Phenotyping

When an antibody has been identified, the patient's own red cells should be phenotyped for the relevant antigen. If the patient's red cells are negative for the antigen, this confirms that the patient is capable of making an antibody of that particular specificity. If the patient's red cells are positive for the antibody this suggests one of the following:

1. The antibody is an autoantibody, in which case the direct antiglobulin test should be positive.
2. The patient's red cells are antibody-coated and a potentiated method has been used for phenotyping, thus negating the result.
3. The initial identification result is incorrect.

Extended phenotyping can be helpful where a mixture of antibodies is present because it will allow the exclusion of antibodies specific for antigens for which the patient is positive, reducing the number of additional reagent cells required.

Additional Panels/Techniques

The chances of identifying antibodies, where two specificities are present, are significantly improved by using a two-stage enzyme technique, where at least one of the relevant antigens is affected by enzymes[25] (e.g., Rh antibodies are enhanced by proteolytic enzymes, whereas M, N, S, Fy^a and Fy^b antigens are destroyed by proteolytic enzymes). Similarly, two different panels of reagent cells provide an increased chance of excluding further specificities where a mixture of two antibodies has been identified.

Direct agglutination at room temperature or 4°C may be helpful to distinguish between an antibody of potential clinical significance and a cold reacting antibody; again this is particularly useful where a mixture of antibodies is present. Weak examples of

Kidd antibodies are often enhanced by the use of an indirect antiglobulin test using enzyme-treated cells, and this can be particularly helpful where the antibody is only reacting against homozygous cells by indirect antiglobulin test.

Reagents

An identification panel should consist of red cells from at least eight group O donors, although ten is more common in commercial panels and allows easier elucidation of antibody mixtures. To be functional, the panel must permit confident identification of the most commonly encountered, clinically significant antibodies. The UK guidelines[9] can be summarised as follows:

1. For each of the commonly encountered clinically significant red cells antibodies, there should be at least two examples of phenotypes lacking, and at least two examples of phenotypes carrying, the corresponding antigen.
2. There should be at least one example of each of the phenotypes R_1R_1 and $R_1{}^wR_1$. Between them, these two samples should express the antigens K, k, Fy^a, Fy^b, Jk^a, Jk^b, M, N, S, and s.
3. There should be at least one example of each of the phenotypes R_2R_2, r′r, and r″r and at least two examples of the phenotype rr.
4. The following phenotypes should be expressed in those samples lacking both D and C antigens: K+, K−, Jk(a+b−), Jk(a−b+), S+s−, S−s+, Fy(a+b−) and Fy(a−b+). The panel should be able to resolve as many likely antibody mixtures as possible.

Antibody Cards

Delayed haemolytic transfusion reactions can occur when antibodies have not been detected or have been *incorrectly* identified, often by a different establishment.[1,2] It has been suggested that antibody cards, produced either by the hospital or the reference centre, could be carried by the patient for presentation on admission to hospital. To be effective, such cards would have to be accompanied by patient information leaflets, explaining the significance of the antibodies, and preferably handed personally to the patient by someone with a clear understanding of blood transfusion practice. There are potential pitfalls with this suggestion, not least that the level of proficiency in identifying anti-bodies and appreciating clinical significance varies between establishments. A better long-term approach may be to have a national database that includes the presence of clinically significant antibodies.

SELECTION AND TRANSFUSION OF RED CELLS

Once the blood group of a patient has been established and any antibodies have been identified, a set of procedures is required to select units of red cells that are appropriate for transfusion. These include selecting ABO/D compatible units, which will also need to be negative for antigens to which the recipient has a clinically significant red cell alloantibody (see Table 20.5); however, it is important that they include selection based on certain clinical criteria (e.g., the requirement for CMV negative, irradiated, or washed red cells). Selection according to these criteria depends on good clinical information, accurate ABO and D typing, and a sensitive antibody screen.

Some patients are identified as definitely needing transfusion of blood, but others may be undergoing surgery where blood is crossmatched to "stand by." Audits have shown that blood is often crossmatched but not transfused. The transfusion ratio, or cross-match index, can be used to assess how well blood stocks are managed. One option is to perform a blood group and antibody screen on a patient and then save the sample, only crossmatching blood if certain pre-agreed transfusion triggers are met. Local policy should define a maximum surgical blood ordering schedule, indicating which surgical procedures can be "group and screen/group and save" and how many units of blood need to be crossmatched for procedures with a high likelihood of intraoperative transfusion.[35] The decision as to which category is chosen may relate to local factors including the proximity of the blood transfusion laboratory to the operating theatre (or other location where blood is to be transfused) and the time it takes to provide compatible blood following a request. Once the appropriate red cells have been selected, compatibility needs to be ensured. This is usually referred to as crossmatching, which may include an indirect antiglobulin test to check for incompatibility as a result of IgG antibodies and

Table 20.5   Recommendations for the selection of blood for a patient with red cell antibodies[9]

System	Antibody	Recommendation
ABO	Anti-A$_1$	IAT crossmatch compatible at 37°C
Rh	Anti-D, -C, -c, -E, -e	Antigen negative*
Rh	Anti-C^w	IAT crossmatch compatible[†]
Kell	Anti-K, -k	Antigen negative*
Kell	Anti-Kp^a	IAT crossmatch compatible[†]
Kidd	Anti-Jk^a, -Jk^b	Antigen negative*
MNS	Anti-M (active at 37°C)	Antigen negative*
MNS	Anti-M (not active at 37°C)	IAT crossmatch compatible at 37°C
MNS	Anti-N	IAT crossmatch compatible at 37°C
MNS	Anti-S, -s, -U	Antigen negative*
Duffy	Anti-Fy^a, -Fy^b	Antigen negative*
P	Anti-P$_1$	IAT crossmatch compatible at 37°
Lewis	Anti-Le^a, -Le^b, Le^{a+b}	IAT crossmatch compatible at 37°C
Lutheran	Anti-Lu^a	IAT crossmatch compatible at 37°C
Diego	Anti-Wr^a (anti-Di3)	IAT crossmatch compatible[†]
H	Anti-HI (in A$_1$ and A$_1$B patients)	IAT crossmatch compatible at 37°C
All	Other active by IAT at 37°C	Seek advice from blood centre

This guidance is suitable for patients undergoing hypothermia during surgery[26].
IAT indirect antiglobulin test.
*Antigen negative and crossmatch compatible.
[†]These recommendations apply when the antibody is present as a sole specificity. If present in combination, antigen-negative blood may be provided by the blood centre to prevent wastage of phenotyped units.
Mollison et al, 1993. Blood Transfusion in Clinical Practice. Blackwell, Oxford.

ABO antibodies or an immediate spin test to check for ABO incompatibility only. Instead of a serological test, an assessment of ABO compatibility may be based on a "computer check," usually referred to as "electronic issue." Some transfusion laboratories, where surgery takes place in a different hospital, have extended electronic issue to the selection of compatible units—as dictated by the transfusion laboratory—from a remote issue refrigerator.

The process of crossmatching blood is to prevent the transfusion of incompatible red cells and a subsequent haemolytic transfusion reaction. The different types of crossmatch are outlined in the following paragraphs. Whatever crossmatch technique is chosen, it should be clear that all patients with known red cell antibodies, even if currently undetectable, should have an antiglobulin crossmatch and are not suitable for group and screen/save or electronic issue.[9,15]

CROSSMATCHING

Choice of Technique

Indirect Antiglobulin Crossmatch
The arguments for retaining an indirect antiglobulin crossmatch are based on the failure to identify

antibodies against low-frequency antigens in the antibody screen. However, there is evidence summarised by Garratty[27] that the likelihood of missing a clinically significant antibody is about 1 in 10,615 crossmatches if the indirect antiglobulin test component is omitted and antibody detection relies on a sensitive antibody screen alone. Moreover, the usual outcome of transfusion if an antibody is present but undetected by the antibody screen is limited to shortened red cell survival.

An indirect antiglobulin crossmatch should always be performed if the patient has red cell antibodies of likely clinical significance, even if currently undetectable. The reasons for this are as follows:

1. It acts as a double check that the donation has been correctly phenotyped and labelled as negative for the corresponding antigen(s).
2. It ensures serological compatibility even if the identification of the antibody(ies) is incorrect or incomplete.
3. It allows detection of antibodies to low-frequency antigens not present on the screening cells, which may be more likely to be present in a patient who is clearly a "responder" and which may be masked by other alloantibodies.

Other circumstances in which an indirect antiglobulin crossmatch should be performed include the following:

1. The patient has had an ABO-incompatible solid organ transplant and is being transfused within 3 months of the transplant—this is necessary to detect IgG anti-A or anti-B that may be produced by passenger lymphocytes in the transplanted organ.[36]
2. The patient has an alloantibody of low clinical significance detectable in the routine antibody screen; in this case blood may be issued if compatible in the antiglobulin crossmatch performed strictly at 37°C, without the need for antigen-negative blood (see Table 20.5).

Methods for indirect antiglobulin crossmatching are the same as those used for antibody screening. Crossmatching may be less effective than antibody screening at detecting incompatibility as a result of IgG antibodies. This is partly because the cells may only show heterozygous expression of an antigen to which the patient has an antibody, potentially leading to weaker or negative reactions, and also because the cell suspensions and other techniques (e.g., cutting pigtails from donations, labelling tubes, washing cells) are less likely to be standardised and present more opportunity for transposition errors than the screening processes.

Immediate Spin Crossmatch

The sole purpose of this technique is to detect ABO incompatibility. It can be used in order to issue blood for transfusion when the patient has a full blood group and negative antibody screen. It may be used to convert a group and save/screen when blood is required and is often used in addition to an antiglobulin crossmatch. The immediate spin crossmatch will ensure that the correct units have been selected and that the correct ABO group has been assigned to the unit of donor red cells. Clearly it is not a suitable test to use for detection of ABO incompatibility if the reverse blood group reveals a very weak anti-A or anti-B, or if the patient falls into one of the categories described in the previous section.

There is evidence of poor standardisation of this technique,[37] but its sensitivity can be optimised by selecting the appropriate cell suspension, incubation time, and serum:cell ratio. The following tube method is recommended:

Mix 2 volumes of plasma/serum with 1 volume of 2–3% cells suspended in PBS or LISS (or EDTA saline if serum is used; see Fig. 20.4).
Incubate at room temperature for 2–5 min to enhance the detection of weak ABO antibodies.
Centrifuge at 100 g for 1 min.
Read the reaction carefully using a "tip and roll" technique.

False-Negative Results

Incompatibilities between A_2B donor cells and group B patient sera are not consistently detected with this technique.[38] Of more concern is the potential failure of agglutination with potent ABO antibodies[39,40] on account of rapid complement fixation with bound C1 interfering with agglutination—if using serum, red blood cells must be suspended in saline containing EDTA (Fig. 20.4).

False-Positive Results

Cold reacting antibodies other than anti-A and anti-B may cause agglutination in an immediate spin crossmatch. This has the potential to cause delays to transfusion while further procedures are used to rule out ABO incompatibility.

Electronic Issue

In many countries electronic issue is a commonly used alternative to the immediate spin crossmatch for issuing blood for transfusion when the patient has had a full blood group and no history of clinically significant antibodies. ABO and D compatible units are selected and issued through a computer system, which contains logic rules to prevent the issue of ABO and D incompatible blood.

Both BCSH guidelines[15] and AABB standards[41] require that there be concordant determinations of the patients ABO and D type on at least two separate samples, at least one of which must be a current sample. In addition, there must be no clinically significant antibodies detected and no record of any having been detected previously. The AABB recommends that the group of donor units is rechecked, but the BCSH accepts written verification by the supplying transfusion service of the accuracy of the donor unit label. It is strongly recommended by the BCSH that ABO and D grouping procedures are automated with positive sample identification (e.g., bar codes) and electronic transfer of results from the analyser to the transfusion laboratory computer, whereas the AABB does not have such a requirement. Ideally, computer algorithms should direct the procedure, only allowing issue if all the criteria are fulfilled—for example, issue of red cells for transfusion will be prevented if only one ABO and D group is on file or if the previous and current group do not agree. Any manually controlled part of this process increases the risk of error. Electronic issue, based on fully validated systems, has been in place in several countries for some time and has proved to be clinically safe, providing the recommendations are rigidly adhered to.[42–44]

EMERGENCY BLOOD ISSUE

In clinical emergencies in which immediate red cell support is required, there may not be time for full compatibility testing. Either abbreviated testing is employed and rapid techniques are used, or group O red cells are issued. There must be a documented procedure for dealing with emergencies. Local policies on this should be formally assessed for risk, and adequate training should be given to staff, particularly those providing the service out of routine laboratory hours. Out-of-hours staff should be included in internal proficiency testing as well as external quality assessment exercises designed to test emergency tests and techniques.

The transfusion laboratory should be involved in the development of emergency procedures within the hospital, including the Major Accident Plan. All staff should receive regular training and should take part in emergency practice drills. Communication is key to the success of provision of blood products in an emergency, and the transfusion laboratory needs to be fully informed about the current status of the patient or patients so as to provide an efficient and timely service.

Rapid ABO and D Typing

In an emergency, a sample *must* be obtained prior to transfusion and the patient's ABO and D type should be determined as rapidly as possible using the techniques already described. Tube and slide tests are most convenient.

Confirmation

A reverse group, a repeat cell group, or an immediate spin crossmatch should be carried out on the sample before issuing blood of an appropriate ABO group. The ABO and D group must always be confirmed by a further test on a second aliquot from the sample. If an inadequately labelled sample is provided, group O units should be issued until a further sample can be tested.

Selection of Units

Some hospitals provide one or two units of O D negative red cells for use by clinicians pending the availability of ABO and D specific compatible red cells. Because of the relatively short supply of O D negative red cells (only 8% of Caucasian blood donors are O D negative) in the United Kingdom the National Blood Service has issued guidance to hospitals[45] about the restrictions on the use of O

D negative red cells in patients of another blood group.

Compatibility Testing

Group-specific red cells can be issued following an immediate spin crossmatch to check for ABO incompatibility, or a LISS antiglobulin crossmatch and antibody screen can be done if more time is available. If no matching procedure is performed, the red cell units must be group-checked unless the supplier has indicated confidence in the validity of the donor unit labelling. Units issued following abbreviated testing must be labelled as such (i.e., "Selected for patient . . . but not crossmatched"). Cells from the donor units should be removed before issuing the units to enable retrospective crossmatch. A retrospective crossmatch can be performed but is only necessary if the antibody screen is positive.

Antibody Screening

Good practice requires a simultaneous antibody screen and crossmatch, and antibody identification if the antibody screen is positive. If group-specific units have been issued without an indirect antibody test crossmatch (or antiglobulin crossmatch), an antibody screen must be performed as soon as possible. If the antibody screen is negative, it is not necessary to carry out a retrospective crossmatch. It is not acceptable to perform a crossmatch and not carry out an antibody screen. Any untransfused incompatible units must be withdrawn from issue as soon as possible.

Massive Transfusion

Massive transfusion is defined as more than one blood volume within 24 hours and is usually taken to mean 8 or 10 units for an adult.[46] After this volume of transfusion, it is no longer necessary to undertake an antiglobulin crossmatch, but immediate spin crossmatch or electronic issue is recommended to check for ABO compatibility. If ABO nonidentical blood is given initially, blood of the same group as the patient should be used as soon as possible after the first transfusion. In some situations the recipient's need for red cell transfusion may necessitate the use of incompatible units, but this is a clinical decision based on the need for blood balanced against the known clinical significance of the red cell antibody detected.

Selection of Platelets and Plasma

Other blood products may be required in massive transfusion situations, and the use of platelets, fresh frozen plasma, and cryoprecipitate should be determined by clinical evaluation of the patient's haemostatic state as well as frequent full blood counts and coagulation screen tests. These will help determine the need for and response to blood products.

Potential Errors

Errors leading to transfusion of incorrect blood components are more likely to occur out of routine laboratory hours; therefore it has been recommended that only genuine emergency transfusions should take place out of hours.[1,2]

ANTENATAL SEROLOGY AND HAEMOLYTIC DISEASE OF THE NEWBORN

Maternal ABO and D grouping and red cell antibody screening must be done early in pregnancy as a routine. This is the basis for the prevention, detection, and, with antibody titration or quantification, the management of haemolytic disease of the newborn.

Haemolytic Disease of the Newborn

Haemolytic disease of the newborn is a haemolytic anaemia of the fetus and newborn infant that occurs when maternal alloantibody to fetal antigens crosses the placenta and causes haemolysis of fetal red cells or suppression of fetal red cell progenitors, the latter occurring with antibodies within the Kell system.[47]

As IgG is the only immunoglobulin that crosses the placenta, only red cell antibodies of this class are a potential cause of haemolytic disease of the newborn. Anti-D causes the most severe form of haemolytic disease of the newborn, but the success of postnatal prophylaxis with anti-D immuno-globulin has reduced the number of cases and routine antenatal anti-D prophylaxis will reduce it even further. The relative proportion of other IgG red cell antibodies has increased. Although haemolytic disease of the newborn resulting from anti-D is the most severe form of the disease, anti-c can give rise to significant haemolysis *in utero*—sufficient to cause intrauterine death and to warrant investigation in pregnancy. Anti-K has a different mode of action[47] but can also result in a severely affected fetus. Other IgG antibodies (e.g., anti-E, anti-Ce, anti-Fy[a], and anti –Jk[a]) uncommonly give rise to fetal haemolysis of sufficient severity to merit antenatal intervention. Haemolytic disease of the newborn as a result of ABO antibodies can also occur and is described later. For a detailed discussion of the investigation and management of haemolytic disease of the newborn, the reader is referred to the review by Bowman[48] and the textbook by Mollison et al.[26]

Antenatal Serology

ABO and D Grouping and Antibody Screening

Maternal ABO and D grouping as well as antibody screening and identification are performed early in pregnancy (i.e., when first seen and "booked in") and then at 28 weeks gestation. All pregnant women, whether D positive or D negative, should be screened for red cell antibodies.[49,50] Further testing depends on the specificity of any antibodies detected, whether they are capable of causing haemolytic disease of the newborn, and the obstetric history.

Follow-Up Antibody Screening

Protocols for antenatal screening and follow-up vary from country to country. In the United Kingdom, the following is recommended by the BCSH[49,50]:

1. All pregnant women have ABO, D, and antibody screen when booked in and at 28 weeks gestation. Repeat testing is no longer required at 36 weeks if the antibody screen at 28 weeks is negative.
2. Pregnant women with anti-D, antibodies to Kell-related antigens, and anti-c should be tested monthly to 28 weeks and then every 2 weeks to delivery. These women should have antibody titration or quantification as well as testing for additional red cell antibodies.
3. Pregnant women with other red cell antibodies have a titration done when booked in and again at 28 weeks.
4. All pregnant women with a previous history of haemolytic disease of the newborn or those who have a significant increase in anti-D, antibodies to Kell-related antigens, or anti-c should be referred to a specialist unit for further assessment of the need for antenatal intervention.
5. Pregnant women who have red cell antibodies of other specificities, capable of giving rise to haemolytic disease of the newborn and which demonstrate a significant increase in titre over the course of the pregnancy, should have their condition discussed with their obstetrician. It is now appreciated that an increasing titre rather than an individual level is more predictive of an affected fetus.[51]

Prediction of Fetal Blood Group

Partner Testing

The paternal blood group phenotype should be determined in all cases in which the mother has a clinically significant red cell alloantibody. If the paternal red cells lack the corresponding antigen, the baby is not at risk. However, caution is advised because the assumed parent may not be the biological father of the fetus. It is useful to predict whether the partner of a woman who is D negative and who has anti-D is homozygous or heterozygous for the D antigen. This helps to forecast the chances of having children affected by anti-D haemolytic disease of the newborn.

No antisera against the "d" antigen are available because the "d" allele does not exist. Because of the lack of anti-"d" serum, the zygosity of the D antigen is usually predicted from the results of tests with anti-c, anti-C, anti-e, and anti-E and from the likelihood of the homozygous or heterozygous association with these antigens (see Tables 20.3 and 20.6). These data have been compiled for different racial groups. It is important, therefore, to tell the specialist laboratory the racial origin of the patient. Because the genetic basis for the common D types is now known, DNA typing provides a better alternative for predicting the potential for haemolytic disease of the newborn.[52]

Fetal Blood Sampling

Using ultrasound guidance, it is possible to take a sample of fetal blood for blood grouping, but this carries some risks. Contamination by maternal blood can hinder analysis of the sample obtained, leading to false-negative results. In addition, the procedure itself can lead to fetomaternal haemorrhage and hence further sensitisation to fetal antigens. There is also a risk of miscarriage.[53]

Testing Fetal DNA in the Maternal Circulation

It is now possible to detect fetal DNA in the maternal circulation and, using DNA amplification techniques (see Chapter 21), to obtain D and K types on these cells. This has proved to be accurate at predicting the D type and, in the United Kingdom it is now offered as a clinical service at the beginning of the second trimester.[54] This may replace more invasive tests and supplement partner typing. It can be especially helpful if the partner is absent or unknown.

Antenatal Assessment of the Severity of Haemolytic Disease of the Newborn

There has been considerable change in antenatal assessment of the severity of haemolytic disease of the newborn in recent years. Many new non-invasive techniques have been developed to assess the degree of fetal anaemia and, if necessary, to proceed to intrauterine transfusion in severely affected cases.

Antibody Titrations during Pregnancy

Techniques for antibody titration are described in Chapter 19), but these have variable reproducibility and sensitivity. In some laboratories tube techniques have been replaced by column agglutination technology or solid-phase microplates. The role of the serologist is to carry out serial antibody measurements to determine changes in the titre or concentration of the antibody. It is recommended that the technique chosen for titration should be validated against the National Institute for Biological Standards and Control anti-D standard (p. 694).[49] Hence, laboratories should ensure that titres obtained with the anti-D standard are always within one doubling dilution when it is used as an internal control. In addition, antibody titrations performed in pregnancy should always be performed in parallel with the previous sample. Increases in titres of more than one doubling dilution should always be monitored in conjunction with obstetricians.

Antibody Quantitation

Individual laboratories should work closely with reference laboratories and obstetricians. Automated quantification is considered to be a more accurate predictor of when to proceed to more active investigation of the fetus but is usually only available for anti-D and sometimes anti-c. Results in iu or μg/ml are used as part of clinical algorithms to proceed to the next step of fetal investigation.[48,55,56] Other methods of predicting fetal risk include cellular assays such as the monocyte monolayer assay and the antibody-dependent cytotoxicity assay as models of *in vivo* haemolysis in the fetus. The place of cellular assays in *in vitro* testing to predict severity of haemolytic disease of the newborn has been reviewed by Hadley.[57]

Assessment of Fetal Anaemia

In a mother with increasing antibody levels and a fetus suspected or known to carry the red cell antigen against which the antibody is directed, an assessment of the severity of haemolysis is required. Traditionally this was done using amniocentesis to measure the optical density of the amniotic fluid (Lilley's lines) using spectrophotometry.

This, however, is an indirect measurement, whereas direct fetal blood sampling by ultrasound-guided cordocentesis provides not only direct diagnostic information but also a new approach to fetal therapy by direct fetal intravascular transfusion. However, both of these procedures carry the risk of miscarriage and further fetomaternal haemorrhage.[53] More recently, specialist units have been able to offer noninvasive tests to determine fetal anaemia; cerebral artery Doppler studies have been very useful in this regard.[58] The incidence and severity of anti-D haemolytic disease of the newborn is declining, and the increasingly specialised management of severely affected pregnancies has meant that these women are now being referred to specialist centres dealing with this condition early in pregnancy, thus decreasing the involvement of the routine transfusion laboratory in any but the early stages.

Tests on Maternal and Cord Blood at Delivery

In all pregnancies with red cell antibodies, blood samples should be collected at delivery for the following tests. There should be a local protocol for these procedures, especially noting the importance of labelling these samples to avoid misidentification errors.

(a). *Cord blood* (this is preferable to a sample from the baby because of the quantity of blood required)
1. ABO and D group and phenotype for the red cell antigen against which the antibody is directed
2. Direct antiglobulin test
3. Haemoglobin
4. Bilirubin

(b). *Maternal blood*
1. Repeat ABO and D group
2. Repeat antibody screen
3. Test to determine degree of fetomaternal haemorrhage by acid elution (Chapter 13) or by flow cytometry.

Prevention of Haemolytic Disease of the Newborn as a Result of Anti-D

Correct identification of women in early pregnancy who are D negative offers the chance to give intramuscular anti-D immunoglobulin to prevent sensitisation to the D antigen at times during the pregnancy when significant fetomaternal haemorrhage is likely to occur.[59] Accuracy in D grouping is particularly important because women who are D negative erroneously grouped as D positive risk not receiving prophylactic anti-D immunoglobulin (or being transfused with D positive cells). Sensitisation to the D antigen could result in severe haemolytic disease of the newborn as a result of development of anti-D in subsequent pregnancies.

Anti-D Prophylaxis

Anti-D immunoglobulin should be given routinely as soon as possible after delivery (but always within 72 hours) to women who are D negative who deliver babies that are D positive. It should also be given at times during pregnancy when sensitisation could occur, such as during termination of pregnancy, chorionic villus sampling and amniocentesis, and following any abdominal trauma. It should also be given for episodes of vaginal bleeding where the pregnancy remains viable.[59] At delivery and for sensitising events after 20 weeks of gestation, it is necessary to quantitate the fetomaternal haemorrhage using an acid elution or flow cytometry method so that extra anti-D immunoglobulin can be given if the standard dose in use does not cover the

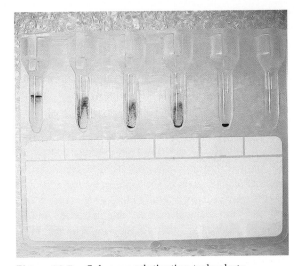

Figure 20.7   Column agglutination technology antibody screening showing reaction grades 4+ to 0.

estimated bleed. It takes 125 iu of anti-D immunoglobulin to cover a bleed of 1.0 ml fetal cells, and preparations containing 500 iu, 1000 iu, 1250 iu, and 1500 iu are in routine prophylactic use.

Because of the risk of silent fetomaternal haemorrhage in pregnancy, routine antenatal anti-D prophylaxis is being offered to women in some countries. In the United Kingdom this has been the subject of an appraisal by the National Institute of Clinical Excellence.[60] This can be given as two doses at 28 and 34 weeks or a single larger dose at 28 weeks in addition to the postnatal dose. Women can decline this if they know the father is D negative or if they do not want any further pregnancies. The typing of fetal DNA in the maternal circulation may be used in the future to select women with fetuses that are D positive who would benefit from this additional prophylaxis, but, at the moment, it is not universally offered.

The administration of prophylactic anti-D results in a positive maternal antibody screen. It is difficult to distinguish between passive anti-D and low-level acquired anti-D antibodies, particularly in the absence of a history of anti-D administration (this may have taken place at another institution). It is therefore important to take the 28-week sample for blood group and antibody screen *before* the administration of the anti-D injection. Although further antibody screens are not routinely required,[50] events in the third trimester may result in a sample being sent to the transfusion laboratory. Laboratories need to have a strategy for dealing with these samples—some implement screening against rr screening cells, whereas others proceed to full antibody identification on all samples.

Measurement of Fetomaternal Haemorrhage

The following tests are performed to determine the quantity of fetal cells in the maternal circulation by the difference between fetal and maternal cells. Most commonly used is acid elution, which depends on the Hb F in fetal cells resisting the acid elution to a greater extent than the Hb A in maternal cells. The calculation of the volume of fetal cells is based on the work by Mollison,[26] which assumed that the maternal red cell volume is 1800 ml, fetal red cells are 22% larger than maternal cells, and only 92% of fetal cells stain darkly (p. 317). Mollison's formula for calculating volume of fetomaternal haemorrhage is as follows:

Uncorrected volume of bleed =

$$\frac{1800 \times \text{fetal cells counted (F)}}{\text{Adult cells counted (A)}}$$

Corrected for fetal volume (1.22) =

$$\left(1800 \times \frac{F}{A}\right) \times 1.22 = J$$

Corrected for staining efficiency (1.09) = $J \times 1.09$ = volume of fetomaternal haemorrhage (ml fetal cells)

Occasionally the Kleihauer test is used to investigate intrauterine deaths or stillbirths where a large but silent fetomaternal haemorrhage is suspected as the cause of death. Often the D group of the mother is known but not that of the fetus. In these circumstances, acid elution is by far the better test. Anti-D prophylaxis should be given to women who are D negative in these circumstances if the fetus is D positive or the D type of the fetus is unknown. Flow cytometry uses anti D to measure a minority of D positive cells in the maternal D negative blood, but flow cytometry may not always be possible. Techniques using anti-Hb F have also been developed. The BCSH guidelines[61] give full details on performance and use of all these tests.

Recommended Action at Delivery (or Sensitising Event)

All women who are D negative should be given a standard intramuscular dose (into the deltoid muscle) of anti-D within 72 hours of delivery (or sensitising event) unless the baby (or fetus) is known to be D negative.

On the basis of a Kleihauer test (or equivalent), further anti-D should be given if the volume of fetomaternal haemorrhage exceeds the volume covered by the standard anti-D (Fig. 20.8).

If the fetomaternal haemorrhage is more than 4 ml, the maternal sample, if possible, should be retested by a second technique such as flow cytometry; alternatively, the test should repeated on the same sample by a different operator.

A repeat sample for Kleihauer and red cell antibody screen should be tested at 48 hours to check for clearance of fetal cells and for the presence of free anti-D. Further anti-D may be required if fetal cells are present.

Women with a large fetomaternal haemorrhage should be tested 6 months postpartum to see if sensitisation to the D antigen has occurred.

ABO Haemolytic Disease of the Newborn

ABO incompatibility as a result of high-titre maternal IgG anti-A and anti-B antibodies can cause prolonged neonatal jaundice and anaemia with spherocytosis in babies that are group A or B born to mothers that are group O. It should be distinguished from nonspherocytic haemolysis and from haemolytic disease of the newborn resulting from other red cell antibodies. Although confirmatory tests are best carried out on cord blood samples, it is often the case that babies have been

---

125 iu anti-D immunoglobulin is sufficient for a fetomaternal haemorrhage of 1 ml cells

500 iu will cover a FMH of less than 4 ml

1250 iu will cover a FMH of less than 10 ml

Additional doses should be calculated using 125 iu for each 1.0 ml fetal cells and rounded to the nearest vial size. Special preparations e.g., 2500 iu, are available for large bleeds.

Figure 20.8   Dosage of anti-D immunoglobulin to cover calculated fetomaternal haemorrhage.[59]

discharged from hospital before the problem is detected. In Caucasian populations, about 15% of births are susceptible, but only about 1% are affected; even then the condition is mild and very rarely severe enough to need exchange transfusion. The condition is more common in Asian populations. A number of special factors combine to protect the fetus from the effects of ABO incompatibility. These include the relative weakness of A and B antigens on the fetal red cells and the widespread distribution of A and B glycoproteins in fetal fluids and tissues, which diverts much of the maternal IgG antibody away from the fetal red cell "target." ABO haemolytic disease of the newborn may occur in the first incompatible pregnancy, unlike haemolytic disease of the newborn resulting from the D antigen, where sensitisation takes place at the end of the first pregnancy, the first child thus being unaffected. Antenatal prediction of ABO haemolytic disease of the newborn is not essential for medical management because there is time to observe the baby after birth and treat according to the severity of the condition. Nevertheless, a baby is more likely to be affected if the maternal IgG anti-A (or B) antibody titre is greater than 1 in 128.

Serological Investigation

ABO haemolytic disease is difficult to diagnose, especially in Caucasians, because the direct antiglobulin test may be negative or weak even in a case of severe haemolytic disease. Furthermore, anti-A or anti-B is present in the mother's serum and special tests may be required to demonstrate high-titre IgG antibodies in the presence of IgM

Table 20.6 The most common Rh phenotypes with possible genotypes and frequencies in an English population (accounting for >99% of all Rh genotypes in this population)[53]

D	C	c	E	e	Phenotype/most probable genotype	Possible genotypes	Frequency
+	+	+	−	+	DCe/dce R_1r	DCe/dce R^1r	32.68
						DCe/Dce R^1R^0	2.16
						Dce/dCe R^0r'	0.05
+	+	−	−	+	DCe/DCe R_1R_1	DCe/DCe R^1R^1	17.68
						DCe/dCe R^1r'	0.82
−	−	+	−	+	dce/dce rr	dce/dce rr	15.10
−	+	+	−	+	Cde/cde r'r	Cde/cde r'r	0.76
−	−	+	+	+	cdE/cde r''r	cdE/cde r''r	0.92
+	+	+	+	+	DCe/DcE R_1R_2	DCe/DcE R^1R^2	11.87
						DCe/dcE R^1r''	1.00
						DcE/dCe R^2r'	0.28
						DCE/cde R^2r	0.19
						Dce /DCE R^0R^z	0.01
						Dce/dCE R^0R^y	<0.01
+	−	+	+	+	DcE/dce R_2r	DcE/dce R^2r	10.97
						DcE/Dce R^2R^0	0.73
						Dce/dcE R^0r''	0.06
+	−	+	−	+	Dce/cde R_0r	Dce/cde R^0r	2.00
						Dce/Dce R^0R^0	0.07
+	−	+	+	−	DcE/DcE R_2R_2	DcE/DcE R^2R^2	1.99
						DcE/dcE R^2r''	0.34

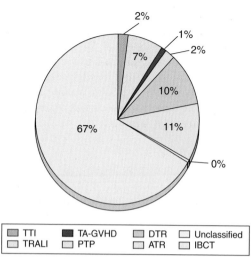

2%

1%

2%

7%

10%

67%

11%

0%

TTI   TA-GVHD   DTR   Unclassified
TRALI   PTP   ATR   IBCT

Figure 20.9   Cumulative data from SHOT (Serious Hazards of Transfusion) 1996–2003[1,2] (n = 2191) showing the different types of adverse event IBCT, incorrect blood component transfused; TTI, transfusion transmitted infection; TRALI, transfusion associated acute lung injury; TA-GVHD, transfusion-associated graft versus host disease; PTP, posttransfusion purpura; DTR, delayed transfusion reaction; ATR, acute transfusion reaction.

antibodies with the same specificity. The following are helpful pointers to diagnosis when ABO haemolytic disease of the newborn is suspected:

1. It is almost always confined to mothers who are group O because there are higher titres of IgG anti-A and anti-B in group O than in group A or B.
2. Because anti-A and anti-B are always present in mothers who are group O, evidence for ABO haemolytic disease of the newborn depends on demonstrating a high titre of IgG anti-A or anti-B by treating the mother's plasma/serum to remove the IgM antibodies (see p. 257) and then testing by the antiglobulin technique against adult A_1, B, and O cells.
3. The direct antiglobulin test on the cord blood or baby's sample may be weak or negative; the latter at least excludes any other serological incompatibility.
4. The simplest evidence for the occurrence of ABO haemolytic disease of the newborn is obtained by testing plasma/serum from the cord blood or baby's

sample for anti-A or anti-B by the antiglobulin technique against adult A_1, B, and O cells. The sooner after birth these tests are done, the better. Delays will lead to absorption of the antibody and the destruction of the red cells.

5. The best diagnostic test of ABO haemolytic disease of the newborn is to prepare an eluate from the baby's red cells and test it (together with the last wash supernatant as a control) by the antiglobulin test against adult A_1, B, and O cells. In some cases reactions occur with both A_1 and B cells because of the presence of anti-A,B crossreacting antibodies, although most severe cases of ABO haemolytic disease of the newborn contain separate specific anti-A and anti-B antibodies. The test with cells and the last wash control should be negative.

COMPATIBILITY TESTING IN SPECIAL TRANSFUSION SITUATIONS

Neonates and Infants within First Four Months of Life

Infants younger than 4 months of age do not generally make alloantibodies but may have passively acquired maternal antibodies (see sections on haemolytic disease of the newborn and ABO and other red cell antigens).

Investigations on the Maternal Sample
ABO and D group
Antibody screen

Investigations on the Infant Sample
ABO and D group (cell group only), repeated on the same sample if no historical group
Antibody screen if mother's sample not available
Direct antiglobulin test

If the direct antiglobulin test is positive or any red cell antibodies are detected in the maternal or infant serum, the diagnosis of haemolytic disease of the newborn should be considered (see earlier).

Selection of Blood and Other Components
Where possible the *cellular* product chosen should be ABO and D identical or an alternative compatible

ABO group (see Table 20.7). Care should be taken when giving group O products containing anti-A and anti-B to infants that are not group O. Despite high-titre anti-A and anti-B donors being excluded from donating products for this group, there have been reports of haemolysis of group A infants' red cells when given group O platelets.[1,2] Current production methods for fresh frozen plasma remove any red cell stroma; therefore plasma products do not need to be D compatible. If the maternal and infant antibody screens are negative (including absent maternal IgG anti-A in the infant), ABO- and D-typed blood can be given with no serological crossmatch, even after repeated small volume transfusions, because formation of red cell antibodies is rare in infants younger than 4 months old. Repeat antibody screen is not necessary if repeat transfusions are required within the first 4 months of life.[62] In the case of haemolytic disease of the newborn (ABO or non-ABO) or maternal red cell antibodies, a crossmatch is required against maternal plasma/serum using group O blood (which has been tested and shown to have low titres of anti-A and anti-B) or other group compatible with red cell antibodies in the maternal serum. If there is no suitable alternative, group O cells can be reconstituted in AB plasma. For neonates and infants, the product for transfusion should be <5 days old for exchange transfusion, negative for CMV antibodies, plasma reduced (or washed), Hb S negative, leucodepleted, and K negative. There is no need to irradiate the product unless the baby has previously been given an intrauterine transfusion.[62]

Intrauterine (Fetal) Transfusion

Intrauterine (fetal) transfusion is usually carried out in specialist fetal medicine units where local protocols should be in place. It is important for maternity units and associated neonatal units to have information about previous intrauterine transfusion because it may influence the selection of appropriate blood products (see above). This is particularly important when the units are in different institutions and therefore serviced by different transfusion departments. Shared-care protocols are one way of ensuring effective communication. When providing red cells for intrauterine transfusion, an antiglobulin crossmatch should be performed using maternal plasma/serum, and this must be repeated with a fresh maternal sample with every transfusion. Intrauterine transfusion can result in fetomaternal haemorrhage and hence sensitisation to new antigens, so antibody identification must be performed on all maternal samples. Red cells selected should be group O D negative (except where mother has made anti-c, when it will be necessary to give D positive, c negative blood) and K negative. Further selection of phenotyped blood will depend on the maternal red cell antibody profile. In addition to the stipulations listed earlier for selection of blood for infants and neonates, blood for intrauterine transfusions should also be irradiated to a minimum of 25 Gy to prevent transfusion-associated graft versus host disease and should be transfused within 24 hours of irradiation.[62]

Patients Receiving Transfusions at Close Intervals

Patients who are acutely ill, particularly those on intensive care units and those undergoing intensive chemotherapy for haematological malignancy, may

Table 20.7 Choice of ABO group for blood products for administration to neonates and infants younger than age 4 months[62]

Infants ABO	ABO group of blood product to be transfused		
Group	Red cells	Platelets	FFP*
O	O	O	O
A	A or O[†]	A	A or AB
B	B or O[†]	B[†] or A or O	B or AB
AB	AB or A or B or O[†]	AB[†] or A	AB

FFP, fresh frozen plasma.
*Only babies and infants who are blood group O should receive group O FFP because of anti-A and anti-B antibodies, whereas group AB FFP contains no naturally occurring antibodies.
[†]Group O products must be checked for high-titre anti-A and anti-B before being given to recipients that are not group O. This is particularly important for platelets because of the relatively large volumes of plasma.
[†]Group B or AB platelets may not be available.

require frequent blood transfusions. This section does not include transfusions to neonates and infants within the first 4 months of life (see earlier) and other special considerations are necessary for recipients of stem cell transplant (see below).

Alloantibodies can develop quickly following a transfusion. Therefore, a sample should be obtained for compatibility testing before each transfusion if they are separated by an interval of 3 days or more. There is no need for daily samples, but an antibody screen at least every 72 hours is recommended as being practical and safe.

Chronic Transfusion Programmes

Examples of patients in whom a decision has been made that regular transfusions are required include those with β thalassaemia major and congenital or acquired bone marrow failure. It is important to establish a treatment plan for each patient with clear triggers for transfusion and regular checks for the adverse effects of transfusion including iron overload. The risk of developing alloantibodies to red cell antigens on transfused blood influences the timing of blood samples (see Table 20.8). If a less rigorous approach is taken for patients in whom repeated transfusions have not led to alloantibody formation, a mutual decision should be made by the clinician and the transfusion department after careful consideration of the risks.

A pretransfusion Rh phenotype allows matching for D, C, c, E, and e. Some ethnic groups commonly have the phenotype cDe (R_0), and D positive blood negative for C and E may be difficult to find, particularly if there are other red cell antibodies. In this situation D negative blood is selected. Additionally, patients with haemoglobinopathies should have an extended red cell phenotype before they are first transfused to include the antigens K, Jk^a, Jk^b, Fy^a, Fy^b, M, N, S, and s.[63] This may be used to select blood but is also helpful when investigating antibodies formed as a result of repeated transfusions. Although provision of red cells with a matched extended phenotype is undertaken by some units treating haemoglobinopathies,[64] the degree of matching depends on local resources and should not impede the delivery of effective transfusion support. There is insufficient evidence to make this recommendation for other patients who have been chronically transfused.

Table 20.8 Timing of pretransfusion compatibility samples in patients having repeated transfusions*

Patient transfused within	Sample to be taken
3–14 days	Within 24 hours of transfusion
15–28 days	Within 72 hours of transfusion
29 days to 3 months	Within 1 week of transfusion

*From British Committee for Standards in Haematology compatibility guidelines[9] and based on Serious Hazards of Transfusion delayed haemolytic transfusion reaction data.

Allogeneic Haemopoietic Stem Cell Transplantation

An allogeneic haemopoietic stem cell transplant may introduce a new blood group—an ABO antigen (major mismatch), ABO antibody (minor mismatch), or both. The recipient/donor pairs have different ABO and D groups in about 15–20% of sibling stem cell transplants, and this is more common in unrelated donor stem cell transplants. If there is a major ABO mismatch and alloagglutinins persist in the recipient's plasma, engraftment may result in a positive direct antiglobulin test when substantial numbers of donor red cells start to enter the circulation and some haemolysis may occur.

A *minor ABO mismatch* is when the donor has antibodies to the recipient's red cells (e.g., donor O, recipient A). Transfuse plasma-depleted red cells of the donor ABO group until the recipient's own red cells are no longer detectable.

A *major ABO mismatch* is when the recipient has antibodies to the donor red cells (e.g., donor A, recipient O). Transfuse red cells of the patient's own type until red cells antibodies are no longer detectable by the indirect antiglobulin test and the direct antiglobulin test is negative, then transfer to donor type.

A *major plus minor mismatch* is when there are antibodies to recipient and donor red cells (e.g., donor A, recipient B). Transfuse group O red cells until the recipient's red cell antibodies are no longer detectable by the indirect antiglobulin test and the direct antiglobulin test is negative.

Prior to the transplant, recipient type red cells, platelets, and fresh frozen plasma are given, but following engraftment, the choice of blood products depends on the ABO and D mismatch between the donor/recipient pairs.[9] For a recipient who is D positive with a donor who is D negative, D negative components should be used.

From the time of conditioning therapy, throughout the period of prophylaxis for graft versus host disease, all cellular blood products should be irradiated. The stem cells to be reinfused are purged of red cells to prevent an acute haemolytic transfusion reaction.

INVESTIGATION OF A TRANSFUSION REACTION

Adverse events related to transfusion can be acute (within 24 hours) or delayed (see Table 20.9). Transfusion laboratories should immediately be informed of a suspected transfusion reaction, being ideally placed to coordinate investigation, to communicate with clinicians and transfusion services, and to advise about appropriate choice of blood products for subsequent transfusions. Serious adverse events should be reported confidentially to the national haemovigilance scheme, the local blood centre, and the Hospital Transfusion Committee. Acute transfusion reactions are easier to attribute to the transfusion than delayed reactions, although, in patients who are already very ill, they can go undiagnosed. The symptoms and signs of acute transfusion reactions are similar regardless of the cause; treatment, and investigation of causes is simultaneous. It is easier to distinguish between the causes of delayed transfusion reactions, but it may be more difficult to recognise their relationship to the transfusion episode because of the delay in onset. The following scheme outlines the role of the laboratory in investigation and management of transfusion reactions, and a very useful algorithm can be found in the *Handbook of Transfusion Medicine*.[64]

Acute Transfusion Reactions

Acute life-threatening transfusion reactions can result from the following:

1. Acute intravascular haemolysis as a result of ABO incompatibility

2. Acute intravascular haemolysis can occur, although rarely as a result of other red cell antibodies that activate complement through to the membrane attack complex (e.g., anti-Vel and anti-PP_1P^k)

3. Severe extravascular haemolysis—this may happen where a strong antibody, which does not bind complement or only binds it to the C3 stage, is missed in pretransfusion testing and causes rapid extravascular clearance of incompatible transfused red cells. These reactions are usually less severe than those caused by ABO incompatibilities.

4. Anaphylaxis and severe acute allergic reactions—these are more commonly associated with blood products containing large amounts of plasma where the recipient has been presensitised to an allergen in the donor plasma. Recipients with IgA deficiency can develop antibodies to IgA.

5. Transfusion of an infected blood product—this is more common with platelets because they are stored at room temperature. If contamination is proven, the blood centre must be informed so that other components from the same donor can be traced.

6. Transfusion-associated acute lung injury is an acute respiratory disorder, with one mechanism being passive transfer of antibodies in the donor

Table 20.9 Types of transfusion reaction	
Acute transfusion reactions	**Delayed transfusion reactions**
Acute haemolytic reaction	Delayed haemolytic reaction
Anaphylaxis	Transfusion transmitted infection
Bacterial contamination of blood product	Transfusion-associated graft versus host disease
Transfusion-associated acute lung injury	Posttransfusion purpura
Acute fluid overload	Iron overload
Allergic reaction	Immunosuppression
Febrile nonhaemolytic transfusion reaction	–

unit that react with the recipient's own white blood cells, resulting in noncardiogenic interstitial pulmonary oedema.

Although rare, the onset of acute transfusion reactions is usually very dramatic and the patient is acutely ill. Treatment is aimed at resuscitating the patient and elucidating the cause to try and prevent any further incidents (Table 20.10). In addition, there are unpleasant but not life-threatening reactions that may occur during transfusion. They include the following:

Allergic reactions—a mild urticaria or itching caused by a reaction to plasma proteins in the donor unit

Febrile non-haemolytic transfusion reactions—recipient's antibodies that react to donor white cells and cause an increase in temperature of no more that 1°C; alternatively, cytokines released from white cells in the donor units can cause a similar reaction. These conditions usually settle on slowing the transfusion and administration of antipyretics and antihistamines. They do not require detailed investigation.

Acute Intravascular Haemolysis

Transfused red cells react with the patient's own anti-A or anti-B, and the red cells are destroyed in the circulation, causing collapse, renal failure, and disseminated intravascular coagulation. Transfusion of ABO-incompatible cells usually results from an identification error. This can occur at point of blood sampling and labelling (wrong blood in tube), laboratory testing (technical error), blood unit labelling (administrative error), and collection from the blood refrigerator or inadequate bedside checking. If red cells are mistakenly transfused to the wrong patient, there is approximately a 1 in 3 chance that ABO incompatibility will occur. The reaction is most severe if group A blood is transfused to a patient who is group O, and only a few millilitres of red cells are required to cause this reaction. Prompt action in recognising this acute emergency and stopping the transfusion may lead to a better outcome because the severity depends on the volume of blood transfused. If an acute transfusion reaction is suspected, the laboratory must be informed immediately and the unit of blood and giving set must be returned to the laboratory

---

Table 20.10   Immediate investigations in the case of an acute transfusion reaction

Check for haemolysis
Perform visual examination of patient's plasma and urine (plasma and urine haemoglobin can be checked but this is not essential).
Blood film will show spherocytosis, red cell fragmentation.
Bilirubin and lactate dehydrogenase (LDH) levels will be raised.

Check for incompatibility
Check the documentation and the patient's identity.
Repeat ABO group of patient pretransfusion and posttransfusion and of the donor unit(s).
Screen the patient for red cell antibodies pretransfusion and posttransfusion.
Repeat crossmatch with pretransfusion and posttransfusion samples.
Direct antiglobulin test (DAT) on patient.
Eluate from patient's red cells if DAT is positive.

Check for disseminated intravascular coagulation
Perform blood count and film, coagulation screen, and fibrin degradation products (or D-dimers).

Check for renal function
Check blood urea, creatinine, and electrolytes.

Check for bacterial infections
Take blood cultures from the patient and donor unit including immediate gram stain.

Immunological investigations
Check immunoglobulin A (IgA) levels and anti-IgA antibodies.

with blood and urine samples from the patient (Table 20.10).

Documentation Check

Patient identification, the compatibility form, and the compatibility label of the blood unit should be checked again at the bedside. Any discrepancies must be notified to the transfusion laboratory immediately. If the wrong blood has been administered, the units intended for that patient must be withdrawn from issue to prevent another parallel error occurring with another patient who may have the same or a similar name.

Serological Investigations

Serological investigations have a twofold purpose: (a) to check for any laboratory errors in the pretransfusion sample group and compatibility check and (b) to repeat the group and compatibility tests with the posttransfusion sample to see if the pretransfusion sample was from the correct patient. Reactions in liquid-phase tests should be read microscopically to detect any mixed-field reaction.

Tests for Haemolysis

Because not all acute transfusion reactions are the result of haemolysis, haematological and biochemical tests as well as visual inspection of the plasma/serum and urine are required (see Chapter 9). Further tests may be required to manage the resuscitation of the patient and direct the use of blood products to treat disseminated intravascular coagulation.

Microbiological Tests

If the cause of the acute transfusion reaction is still unclear, blood cultures should be taken from the unit and the patient. Blood centres issue guidance for the investigation of potentially contaminated units.

Delayed Haemolytic Transfusion Reaction

A delayed haemolytic transfusion reaction occurs when the recipient has been immunised to a red cell antigen by a previous transfusion or during pregnancy but the antibody is present at low or undetectable levels. A secondary immune response is mounted to the incompatible antigen that has been transfused. The IgG- and/or complement-coated red cells are destroyed in the spleen and liver. Kidd antibodies are often implicated in delayed transfusion reactions because they are difficult to detect, often displaying a dosage effect, fall rapidly to undetectable levels, and are frequently present in combinations of antibodies.

Haematological Investigation

The following suggest a delayed haemolytic transfusion reaction:

Haemoglobin concentration falls more rapidly than would be expected after a red cell transfusion
Increase in haemoglobin concentration is less than expected for the number of units transfused
Blood film shows spherocytosis
Positive direct antiglobulin test
Unconjugated bilirubin raised

Serological Investigation

It is desirable to have the pretransfusion sample available to test in addition to a post-transfusion sample, but this is not always possible because of the delay between the time of the transfusion and the investigation. It has been recommended by some that plasma/serum samples are saved on all patients who are transfused, but this is not always practical. Unless the reaction is acute, the units transfused will not be available for retesting. In the United Kingdom, the phenotype of each unit is provided by the National Blood Service, and this information can help in the investigation of a delayed transfusion reaction. The following tests should be carried out, preferably using different or more sensitive techniques:

1. Confirm the ABO and D group of the patient on a pretransfusion and posttransfusion sample.
2. Perform a direct antiglobulin test on the patient's pretransfusion and posttransfusion washed red cells. In the event of a positive direct antiglobulin test, elution of the antibody may aid identification or confirm specificities in cases of non-ABO incompatibility.
3. Repeat the crossmatch, if possible, using pretransfusion and posttransfusion samples.
4. Screen the pretransfusion and posttransfusion samples for red cell antibodies and identify any antibodies. The immediate posttransfusion sample

may have no detectable red cell antibodies, although they may be eluted from the patient's red cells if the direct antiglobulin test is positive. It is also possible to have a delayed haemolytic transfusion reaction with a negative direct antiglobulin test because the antibody-coated red cells have been removed from the circulation. If the immediate posttransfusion investigation is inconclusive, repeat the tests 10 days later to allow antibody levels to increase.

REFERENCES

1. Serious Hazards of Transfusion (SHOT). Annual reports 1996–2003: www.shot-uk.org.
2. Serious Hazards of Transfusion Annual Report 2003 ISBN 0-9532-789-6-4.
3. British Committee for Standards in Haematology (BCSH). Guidelines available at www.bcshguidelines.com/.
4. AABB (previously American Association of Blood Banks): www.aabb.org.
5. Faber J-C 2004 The European Blood Directive: a new era of blood regulation has begun. Transfusion Medicine 14:257–273.
6. Department of Health. Better blood transfusion. Health Service Circular 1998/224.
7. Department of Health. Better blood transfusion 2. Health Service Circular 2002/009.
8. Annual Reports of UK National External Quality Assessment Scheme (Blood Transfusion Laboratory Practice); contact scheme via www.ukneqas.org.uk/Directory/HAEM/bgs.htm.
9. British Committee for Standards in Haematology 2004 Guidelines for compatibility procedures in blood transfusion laboratories. Transfusion Medicine 14:59–73.
10. British Committee for Standards in Haematology 1999 The administration of blood and blood components and the management of transfused patients. Transfusion Medicine 9:227–238.
11. Murphy MF, Stearn BE, Dzik WH 2004 Current performance of patient sample collection in the UK. Transfusion Medicine 14:113–121.
12. Brecher ME 2002. AABB Technical manual. 14th ed. AABB, Bethesda MD20814-2749.
13. Report of the Working Party of the Royal College of Pathologists and the Institute of Biomedical Science 1999 The retention and storage of pathological records and archives. 2nd ed. (corrected 2003); available at www.rcpath.org.
14. Transfusion transmission of HCV infection before anti-HCV testing of blood donations in England: results of the national HCV lookback program. 2002 Transfusion 42:1146–1153.
15. British Committee for Standards in Haematology 2000 Guidelines for blood bank computing. Transfusion Medicine 10:307–314.
16. Information for patients needing irradiated blood products. NHS INF/PCS/MS/001/03 or available at www.blood.co.uk/hospitals/library/pi/index.htm.
17. Lau FY, Cheng G 2001 To err is human nature: can transfusion errors due to human factors ever be eliminated? Clinical Chimica Acta 313:59–67.
18. Biomedical Excellence for Safer Transfusion (BEST) Working Party of the ISBT 2003 An international study of the performance of sample collection from patients. Vox Sanguinis 85:40–47.
19. Scott ML, Voak D 2000 Monoclonal antibodies to Rh D: development and uses. Vox Sanguinis 78(suppl 2):79–82.
20. Jones J, Scott ML, Voak D 1995 Monoclonal anti-D specificity and Rh D structure: criteria for selection of monoclonal anti-D reagents for routine typing of donors. Transfusion Medicine 5:171–184.
21. Roback JD, Barclay S, Hillyer CD 2003 An automatable format for accurate immunohematology testing by flow cytometry. Transfusion 43:918–927.
22. BCSH Blood Transfusion Task Force 1990 Guidelines for microplate techniques in liquid-phase blood grouping and antibody screening: a joint publication of the British Society for Haematology and the British Blood Transfusion Society. Clinical and Laboratory Haematology 12:437–460.
23. Horn KD 1999 The classification, recognition and significance of polyagglutination in transfusion medicine. Blood Reviews 13:36–44.
24. Garratty G, Arndt P, Co A, et al 1996 Fatal haemolytic transfusion reaction resulting from ABO mistyping of a patient with acquired B antigen detectable only by some monoclonal anti-B reagents. Transfusion 36:351–357.
25. Knowles SM, Milkins CE, Chapman JF, et al 2002 The United Kingdom National External Quality Assessment Scheme (Blood Transfusion Laboratory Practice): trends in proficiency and practice between 1985 and 2000. Transfusion Medicine 12:11–23.
26. Mollison PL, Engelfriet CP, Contreras M 1997 Blood transfusion in clinical medicine. 10th ed. Blackwell Science Ltd, Oxford.
27. Garratty G 2002 Screening for RBC antibodies—what should we expect from antibody detection RBCs. Immunohaematology 18:71–77.

28. Issitt PD, Combs MR, Bredehoeft SJ et al 1993 Lack of clinical significance of "enzyme-only" red cell alloantibodies. Transfusion 33:284–293.

29. Shirey RS, Boyd JS, Ness PM 1994 Polyethylene glycol versus low-ionic-strength solution in pre-transfusion testing: a blinded comparison study. Transfusion 34:368–370.

30. MDA Evaluation report MDA/96/14. Six systems for the detection of red cell antibodies. MHRA, Hannibal House, London SE1 6TQ.

31. Bromilow IM, Eggington JA, Owen GA, et al 1993 Red cell antibody screening and identification: a comparison of two column technology methods. British Journal of Biomedical Science 50:329–333.

32. Phillips P, Voak D, Knowles S et al 1997 An explanation and the clinical significance of the failure of microcolumn tests to detect weak ABO and other antibodies. Transfusion Medicine 7:47–53.

33. Cummins D, Downham B 1994 Failure of DiaMed-ID microtyping system to detect major ABO incompatibility. Lancet 343:1649–1650.

34. Voak D, Downie DM, Haigh T, et al 1982 Improved antiglobulin tests to detect difficult antibodies: detection of anti-K by LISS. Medical Laboratory Science 39:363–370.

35. British Committee for Standards in Haematology 1990 Guidelines for implementation of a maximum surgical blood order schedule. Cinical and Laboratory Haematology 12:321–327.

36. Contreras M, Hazlehurst GR, Armitage SE 1983 Development of "auto-anti-A1antibodies" following alloimmunisation in an A2 recipient. British Journal of Haematology 55:657–663

37. O'Hagan J, White J, Milkins CE, et al 1999 Direct agglutination crossmatch at room temperature (DRT): the results of a NEQAS (BTLP) questionnaire. Transfusion Medicine 9 (Suppl 1):42.

38. Lamberson RD, Boral LI, Berry-Dortch S 1986 Limitations of the crossmatch for detection of incompatibility between A_2B red blood cells and B patient sera. American Journal of Clinical Pathology 86:511–513.

39. Shulman IA, Odono V 1994 The risk of overt acute hemolytic transfusion reaction following the use of an immediate-spin crossmatch. Transfusion 34:87–88.

40. Berry-Dortch S, Woodside CH, Boral LI 1985 Limitations of the immediate spin crossmatch when used for detecting ABO incompatibility. Transfusion 25:176–178.

41. AABB 2003 Guidelines for implementing the electronic crossmatch.

42. Säfwenberg J, Högman CF, Cassemar B 1997 Computerized delivery control—a useful and safe complement to the type and screen compatibility testing. Vox Sanguinis 72:162–168.

43. Chapman JF, Milkins C, Voak D 2000 The computer crossmatch: a safe alternative to the serological crossmatch. Transfusion Medicine 10:251–256.

44. Judd WJ 1998 Requirements for the electronic crossmatch. Vox Sanguinis 74(suppl 2):409–417.

45. Stainsby D, Murphy MF [for the National Blood Service Transfusion Medicine Clinical Policies Group] 2003 Guidelines for the use of group O D negative red cells including contingency planning for large scale emergencies. www.blood.co.uk/hospitals/guidelines/index.htm.

46. Stainsby D, MacLennan S, Hamilton PJ 2000 Management of massive blood loss: a template guideline. British Journal of Anaesthetics 85:487–491.

47. Daniels G, Hadley A, Green CA 2003 Causes of fetal anemia in haemolytic disease due to anti-K. Transfusion 43:115–116.

48. Bowman J 1997 The management of hemolytic disease in the fetus and newborn. Seminars in Perinatology 21:39–44.

49. British Committee for Standards in Haematology 1996 Guidelines for blood grouping and red cell antibody testing during pregnancy. Transfusion Medicine 6:71–74.

50. British Committee for Standards in Haematology 1999 Addendum for guidelines for blood grouping and red cell antibody testing during pregnancy. Transfusion Medicine 9: 99.

51. Van Dijk BA, Dooren MC, Overbeeke MA 1995 Red cell antibodies in pregnancy: there is no "critical titre." Transfusion Medicine 5:199–202.

52. Daniels G 2004 Molecular blood grouping. Vox Sanguinis 87(suppl 1):S63–S66.

53. Daniels G 2002 Human blood groups. 2nd ed., Blackwell Publishing, Oxford.

53. Kumar S, O'Brien A 2004 Recent developments in fetal medicine. British Medical Journal 328:1002–1006.

54. Finning K, Martin P, Daniels G 2004 A clinical service in the UK to predict fetal Rh (Rhesus) D blood group using free fetal DNA in maternal plasma. Annals of the New York Academy of Science 1022:119–123.

55. Urbaniak SJ, Greiss MA 2000 RhD haemolytic disease of the fetus and the newborn. Blood Reviews 14:44–61.

56. Moise KJ 2002 Management of Rhesus alloimmunisation in pregnancy. Obstetrics and Gynecology 100:600–611.

57. Hadley AG 1998 A comparison of in vitro tests for predicting the severity of haemolytic disease of the fetus and newborn. Vox Sanguinis 74(suppl 2):375–383.

58. Abdel-Fattah SA, Soothill PW, Carroll SG, et al 2002 Middle cerebral artery Doppler for the prediction of fetal anaemia in cases without hydrops: a practical approach. British Journal of Radiology 75:726–730.

59. Lee D, Contreras M, Robson SC et al 1999 Joint Working Group of the British Blood Transfusion Society and the Royal College of Obstetricians and Gynaecologists. Use of anti-D immunoglobulin for Rh prophylaxis (Green top Guideline No 22—revised 2002) Transfusion Medicine 9:93–97. Also available at www.rcog.org.uk.

60. National Institute for Clinical Excellence 2002 Pregnancy - routine anti-D prophylaxis for rhesus negative women. Technology Appraisal No. 41. April 2002 www.nice.org.uk.

61. British Committee for Standards in Haematology1999 The estimation of fetomaternal hemorrhage. Transfusion Medicine 9:87–92.

62. British Committee for Standards in Haematology 2004 Transfusion guidelines for neonates and older children. British Journal of Haematology 124:433–453.

63. British Committee for Standards in Haematology 2003 Management of acute painful crisis in sickle cell disease. British Journal of Haematology 120:744–752.

64. Vichinsky EP, Luban NLC, Wright E et al Stroke prevention trial in sickle cell anaemia. Transfusion 41:1086–1092.

65. McClelland DBL2001 Handbook of transfusion medicine, 3rd ed. Blood Transfusion Services of the United Kingdom, London: The Stationery Office.

21 Molecular and cytogenetic analysis

Tom Vulliamy and Jaspal Kaeda
With contributions from Barbara Bain

INTRODUCTION TO THE ANALYSIS OF DNA

DNA analysis is playing an increasingly important role in refining haematological diagnosis and determining treatment. Over recent years our understanding of the molecular basis of both inherited and acquired haematological disorders has improved considerably. There are several ways in which this knowledge is now being applied in diagnostic haematology. These include the identification of families at risk for haemoglobinopathies allowing the provision of early prenatal diagnosis, the assessment of genetic risk factors in thrombophilia, the diagnosis and characterisation of leukaemias, the monitoring of minimal residual disease, and the study of host–donor chimerism following bone marrow transplantation.

In this chapter we will describe some of the methods that can be applied in these situations, although this cannot be exhaustive and will reflect the interests of our laboratory. The following points should help in the understanding of the methods described:

1. Information for the construction of proteins is encoded by four bases—adenine (A), cytosine (C), guanine (G), and thymine (T)—that lie along the sugar-phosphate backbone of the DNA molecule.
2. The DNA found in the nucleus of all eukaryotic cells is a double-stranded molecule.
3. The two strands are held together by hydrogen bonds that form specifically between A and T residues and between G and C residues.
4. Because of this, the sequence of bases on one strand of the DNA molecule (say, TAGGCTAG) has only one possible partner on the other strand (ATCCGATC). These sequences are called complementary.
5. The strands have a polarity; one end is called the 5′ end, and the other is the 3′ end. The two strands run in opposite directions (i.e., they are antiparallel).

The ability to manipulate DNA as recombinant molecules followed from the discovery of bacterial DNA modifying enzymes, specifically restriction enzymes. These are endonucleases that cut DNA molecules wherever there is a short, specific sequence of bases. More than 100 different restriction enzymes are now commercially available. Using these enzymes it is possible to cut the genetic material found in human nuclei—the human genome—into specific fragments of a manageable size. With the necessary DNA-modifying enzymes, these restriction fragments can be inserted into cloning vectors such as plasmids or cosmids. Bacteria that host these vectors can be isolated as colonies and subsequently propagated indefinitely.

In this way, genes can be isolated as cloned recombinant DNA molecules, and their DNA sequence can be established. The cloning and sequencing of the human genome is now virtually complete.[1,2] Expressed sequences, cloned as complementary DNAs (cDNAs), are known for almost all human genes. This dramatic increase in sequence information over recent years has been made accessible through parallel developments in computing technology. The ability to amplify specific DNA fragments from small amounts of starting material by the polymerase chain reaction (PCR)[3] has become the basis of most DNA analysis. Because this technique is relatively simple, rapid, and inexpensive and requires only some basic pieces of laboratory equipment, it has opened up molecular genetics, permitting access to molecular diagnosis away from specialist centres.

Many alternative protocols for the manipulation of DNA have become available; a comprehensive laboratory manual describing the techniques of molecular biology runs to three volumes.[4] Guidelines from the American Association for Molecular Pathology address the choice and development of appropriate diagnostic assays, quality control, and validation and implementation of molecular diagnostic tests.[5] In the United Kingdom, a national external quality assessment scheme has been approved for the molecular genetics of thrombophilia, and a pilot study for DNA diagnostics for haemoglobinopathies is under way. It is true, however, that the development and implementation of quality control methods and assurance standards still lag behind the rapid rate of expansion of molecular techniques.[6,7] In this chapter, some of the applications of the PCR in a diagnostic haematology laboratory are described. For the reasons just mentioned, PCR analysis has largely superseded other techniques, including Southern blot analysis. There are situations in which the latter is still appropriate, and for information about these, the reader is referred to previous editions of this book.

EXTRACTION OF DNA

DNA can be extracted from any blood or tissue sample. The quality and quantity of the DNA obtained will vary depending on the size, age, and cell count of the sample. As a rule, 3 ml of blood in EDTA will suffice (see p. 6). The DNA is extracted from all nucleated cells and is called genomic DNA.

In the nucleus, the DNA is tightly associated with many different proteins as chromatin. It is important to remove these as well as other cellular proteins to extract the DNA. This is achieved through the use of organic solvents or salt precipitation. An aqueous solution of DNA is obtained, from which the DNA is further purified by ethanol precipitation. The method described in Appendix A on p. 580 yields DNA that is of sufficiently high quality for all routine analysis.[8]

A number of DNA extraction kits are now commercially available. These can significantly reduce the amount of time required for DNA extraction, bypass the use of organic solvents, and provide good quality control of the reagents used. However, the use of kits in all aspects of molecular biology may inhibit the development of improvements.[4]

POLYMERASE CHAIN REACTION

Development of the PCR[3] has had a dramatic impact on the study and analysis of nucleic acids. Through the use of a thermostable DNA polymerase, Taq polymerase extracted from the bacterium *Thermus aquaticus,* the PCR results in the amplification of a specific DNA fragment such that it can be visualised by ethidium bromide staining on an agarose gel. The procedure takes only a few hours, does not require the use of radionucleotides, and requires only a very small amount of starting material.

Principle

A DNA polymerase will synthesise the complementary strand of a DNA template *in vitro.* A stretch of double-stranded DNA is required for the synthesis to be initiated. This double-stranded sequence can be generated by annealing an oligonucleotide (oligo), which is a short, single-stranded DNA molecule usually between 17 and 22 bases in length, to a single-stranded DNA template. These oligos, which are synthesised *in vitro,* will prime the DNA synthesis and are therefore referred to as primers.

In the PCR, at least two oligos are used. One primes the synthesis of DNA in the forward direction, or along the coding strand of the DNA, whereas the other primes DNA synthesis in the reverse direction, or along the noncoding strand. The other components of the reaction are the DNA template from which the DNA fragment will be amplified, the four deoxynucleotide triphosphates (dATP, dTTP, dCTP, and dGTP) required as the building blocks of the DNA that is to be synthesised, the necessary buffer, and the thermostable DNA polymerase (Taq polymerase).

The first step of the reaction is to denature the template DNA by heating the reaction mixture to 95°C. The reaction is then cooled to a temperature, usually between 50°C and 65°C, that permits the annealing of the oligos to the DNA template but only at their specific complementary sequences. The temperature is then raised to 72°C, at which temperature the Taq polymerase efficiently synthesises DNA, extending from the oligo in a 5′ to 3′ direction. Cyclical repetition of the denaturing, annealing, and extension steps, by simply changing

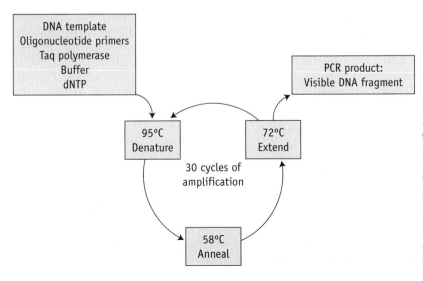

Figure 21.1   The polymerase chain reaction. Cyclical repetition of three temperatures for denaturing, annealing, and extending DNA, respectively, gives rise to an exponential amplification of a DNA fragment between two primer sequences directing DNA synthesis on opposite strands of the DNA template.

the temperature of the reaction in an automated heating block, results in exponential amplification of the DNA that lies between the two oligos (Fig. 21.1).

The specificity of the DNA fragment that is amplified is therefore determined by the sequences of the oligos used. A sequence of 17 base pairs (bp) is theoretically unique in the human genome, and so oligos of this length and longer will anneal at only one specific place on a template of genomic DNA. One general requirement of the PCR is therefore some knowledge of the DNA sequence of the gene that is to be amplified. The relative positioning of the two oligos is another important consideration. They must prime DNA synthesis in opposite directions but pointing toward one another. There is also an upper limit to the distance apart that the oligos can be placed; fragments of several kilobase pairs (kb) in length can be amplified, but the process is most efficient for fragments of several hundred bp.

Reagents and Methods

See Appendix B, p. 582.

Problems and Interpretation

If the amplification has been successful, a discrete fragment of the expected size is seen in an ethidium-bromide–stained agarose gel in all samples, except where a blank control is loaded. If a product is seen in the blank control, then one of the solutions has been contaminated. In this case, the experiment and all the working solutions must be discarded and the micropipettes must be cleaned.

The absence of a fragment in all tracks indicates that the PCR has failed. This could occur for a number of reasons, the most obvious being the poor quality or omission of one of the essential reagents. The reaction may also fail if the magnesium concentration is too low or if the annealing temperature is too high. DNA quality is often one of the major reasons for failure. If one particular DNA sample repeatedly fails to amplify, then the sample should be reextracted with phenol and chloroform and reprecipitated in one-tenth volume of 5 mol/l ammonium acetate and 2.5 volumes of ethanol (see DNA extraction protocol, p. 580). Another problem is the presence of nonspecific fragments or just a smear of amplified product. This can occur if the magnesium concentration is too high or if the annealing temperature is too low.

ANALYSIS OF POLYMERASE CHAIN REACTION PRODUCTS

Presence or Absence of a Polymerase Chain Reaction Product

PCR products are most commonly and conveniently visualised by agarose gel electrophoresis. If appropriate primers and controls are included in an experiment, the actual presence of a product can be highly informative.

Amplification Refractory Mutation System

Principle

Point mutations and small insertions or deletions can be identified directly by the presence or absence of a PCR product using allele-specific primers.[9,10] Two different oligos are used that differ only at the site of the mutation (the amplification refractory mutation system, or ARMS, primers) with the mismatch distinguishing the normal and mutant base located at the 3′ end of the oligo. In a PCR, an oligo with a mismatch at its 3′ end will fail to prime the extension step of the reaction. Each test sample is amplified in two separate reactions containing either a mutant ARMS primer or a normal ARMS primer. The mutant primer will prime amplification together with one common primer from DNA with this mutation but not from a normal DNA. A normal primer will do the opposite. To increase the instability of the 3′ end mismatch, and so ensure the failure of the amplification, it is sometimes necessary to introduce a second nucleotide mismatch three or four bases from the 3′ end of both oligos. A second pair of unrelated primers at distance from the ARMS primers is included in each reaction as internal control to demonstrate that efficient amplification has occurred. This is essential because a failure of the ARMS primer to amplify is interpreted as a significant result and must not be the result of suboptimal reaction conditions.

Interpretation

In all the samples, apart from the blank control, the fragment produced by amplification with the internal control primers must be seen. If this is the case, then the presence or absence of a mutation is simply determined by the presence or absence of the expected fragment produced by amplification with the mutant ARMS primer and the common primer. The presence or absence of the normal allele is determined in the same way in the reaction that includes the normal ARMS primer. In this way, heterozygous, homozygous normal, and homozygous mutant genes can be distinguished. An example of this analysis in the diagnosis of a β thalassaemia mutation is given on p. 561.

Gap-PCR

Large deletions can be detected by Gap-PCR. Primers located 5′ and 3′ to the breakpoints of a deletion will be too far apart on the normal chromosome to generate a fragment in a standard PCR. When the deletion is present, these primers will be brought together, enabling them to give rise to a product. An example of this is given for the detection of deletions in α° thalassaemia on p. 562.

By the same principle, primers can be brought together by chromosomal translocation, giving rise to a diagnostic product. Breakpoints may be clustered over too large a region for genomic DNA to be used in these instances. However, leukaemic translocations can also give rise to transcribed fusion genes. Primers from different genes are then juxtaposed in a hybrid messenger RNA (mRNA) molecule and can give rise to a reverse transcription-PCR (RT-PCR) product. An example of this is given in the analysis of minimal residual disease in chronic myeloid leukaemia (CML) on p. 565.

Size of the PCR Product

Principle

Deletions and insertions can be identified simply, after agarose gel electrophoresis, when their size significantly alters that of the PCR product. An example of this analysis is given for a β thalassaemia mutation on p. 561.

A higher resolution of fragment sizes is obtained after polyacrylamide gel electrophoresis. This is particularly appropriate in the analysis of short tandem repeat (STR) sequences that can be highly variable in length and, therefore, useful as genetic markers of different individuals. High resolution of DNA fragments is now often performed on the acrylamide gels or capillaries of the *Advanced Appliedbiosystems (ABI)* 370 or 3700 DNA analysers. These read fluorescently labelled DNA fragments as they exit the gel and enable single base resolution from around 50–800 bp. PCR reactions can be easily converted by using fluorescently labelled primers, and these analysers are therefore commonly used in genotyping STRs and in deriving DNA sequence data. An example of the use of STR genotyping in chimerism studies is given on p. 576.

A high-resolution gel is also used in PCR analysis of immunoglobulin and T-cell receptor (TCR) gene rearrangement in the diagnosis of lymphoproliferative disorders described on p. 576. A modification of this technique, running the denatured PCR products in a nondenaturing gel, enables the migration of single-stranded fragments to be determined. In these gels, the migration of the products depends not only on their size but also on their sequence because fragments with different sequences fold in different ways and the secondary structure formed affects their mobility. This is the basis of the single-strand conformation polymorphism (SSCP) technique, which is commonly used to locate point mutations and can also be used in gene rearrangement studies.

Reagents and Methods

See Appendix C, p. 584.

Restriction Enzyme Digestion

Principle

Restriction enzymes (RE) cleave DNA at short specific sequences. Because many RE are available, it is not uncommon for a single point mutation to coincidentally create or destroy an RE recognition sequence. If this is the case, digestion of the appropriate PCR product prior to agarose gel electrophoresis enables the mutation to be identified. A difference in the size of the restriction fragments seen in normal and mutant samples can be predicted from a restriction map of the amplified fragment and the site of the mutation that changes a restriction site.

The observed fragments should be consistent with either the mutant or the normal pattern. An example is shown on p. 561 in the diagnosis of the sickle cell mutation.

Even when a mutation does not itself create or destroy an RE site, this method can be applied if one of the primer sequences is modified. In this technique, which has been called the amplification created restriction enzyme site (ACRES), one or two deliberate mismatches are introduced into one primer, 2 to 5 bases from its 3′ end, which is then located immediately adjacent to the site of the mutation. These mismatches will be incorporated into the PCR product and can be designed such that an RE site is created in the presence of either the normal or the mutant base at the appropriate site. Cleavage with that enzyme will then distinguish mutant from normal sequences. An example of this analysis is shown for factor V Leiden (FVL) and prothrombin 3′ untranslated region (UTR) mutations on p. 564.

Method

See Appendix D, p. 585.

Allele-Specific Oligonucleotide Hybridization

Principle

Under appropriate conditions, short oligonucleotide probes will hybridize to their exact complementary sequence but not to a sequence where there is even a single base mismatch.[11] A pair of oligos is therefore used to test for the presence of a point mutation: a mutant oligo complementary to the mutant sequence and a normal oligo complementary to the normal sequence, with the sequence difference placed near the centre of each oligo.

The stability of the duplex formed between the oligo and the target DNA being tested (the product of a PCR reaction) depends on the temperature, the base composition and length of the oligo, and the ionic strength of the washing solution. For allele-specific oligonucleotide hybridization (ASOH) studies, an empirical formula has been derived for the dissociation temperature (Td), the temperature at which half of the duplexes are dissociated. This value is used as a guideline; the exact temperature at which

only perfect base pairing is maintained is usually determined by trial and error. The method is described in specialised laboratory manuals.[4]

Interpretation

The oligos should hybridise to their exact DNA sequence, such that the mutant oligo gives a signal with a homozygous mutant control but not with a normal control. When this is the case, the interpretation of the result is straightforward; a positive signal from a particular oligo indicates the presence of that allele in the test sample. Heterozygotes and homozygotes are distinguished by using the mutant and normal oligos in tandem. If there is no significant difference in the intensity of the radioactive signal seen in the control samples, a further wash of the filters at a higher temperature (e.g., Td + 2°C) may be necessary. A problem with the method is that it is relatively time consuming and care has to be taken in establishing the correct washing condition for each oligo. Nonradioactive probes, with detection systems involving horseradish peroxidase, are now quite widely used in this procedure.[12] This technique has been modified such that the allele-specific oligonucleotides are immobilised on the nylon membrane and the patient-specific PCR product is used as the probe—the reverse dot blot procedure.[13] This allows for several different mutations to be analysed simultaneously and has proved particularly useful in the diagnosis of β thalassaemia mutations.[14]

INVESTIGATION OF HAEMOGLOBINOPATHIES

Sickle Cell Disease

The presence of a sickle cell gene can be determined by haemoglobin cellulose acetate electrophoresis or a sickling test. However, there are occasions when it is beneficial to make this diagnosis by DNA analysis (e.g., in prenatal diagnosis, which can be performed at 10 weeks of pregnancy, in distinguishing HbS/S from HbS/β thalassaemia, or in confirming the diagnosis of sickle cell anaemia in a neonate). For the type of specimens collected for prenatal diagnosis, refer to p. 312.

The sickle cell mutation in codon 6 of the β globin gene (GAG → GTG) results in the loss of a Bsu36 I (or Mst II, Sau I, OxaN I, or Dde I) restriction enzyme site that is present in the normal gene. It is therefore possible to detect the mutation directly by restriction enzyme analysis of a DNA fragment generated by the PCR. A pair of primers are used to amplify exons 1 and 2 of the β globin gene, and the products of the PCR are digested with Bsu36 I. The loss of a Bsu36 I site in the sickle cell gene gives rise to an abnormally large restriction fragment that is not seen in normal individuals (Fig. 21.2).

β Thalassaemia

The ethnic groups with the highest incidence of β thalassaemia are the Mediterranean populations, Asian Indians, Chinese, and Africans. Although more than 100 β thalassaemia mutations are known, each of these groups has its own subset of mutations, so that as few as 5 different mutations may account for more than 90% of the affected individuals in a population. This makes the direct detection of β thalassaemia mutations a reasonable possibility, and it has become the method of choice where it is most important—in prenatal diagnosis.[14,15]

The majority of mutations causing β thalassaemia are point mutations affecting the coding sequence,

splice sites, or promoter of the β globin gene. Favoured methods for their detection are either ARMS or reverse dot blot analysis. Larger deletions can be identified directly from the size of the amplified product. If the mutation is not known, it may be identified by sequence analysis.

Example 1: The 619bp Deletion

Using primers that flank this common deletion mutation, the size of the product of the PCR is directly informative (Fig. 21.3). A small fragment of 224 bp is seen when the deletion is present, compared to the 843 bp fragment derived from the normal chromosome. This pair of primers can also be used as internal controls for the PCR when using ARMS primers.

Example 2: The 41/42 Frameshift Mutation

In this diagnosis, the presence or absence of the product generated by the ARMS oligos and the common primer determine the genotype of the test individual. An example of this is shown in Fig. 21.4. All individuals have amplified with the control primers (*upper band*) and the normal primer (*lower band*, lanes 6–9). Two have also amplified with the mutant primer (*lanes 3 and 4*); these two individuals are therefore heterozygous for the 41/42 frameshift mutation.

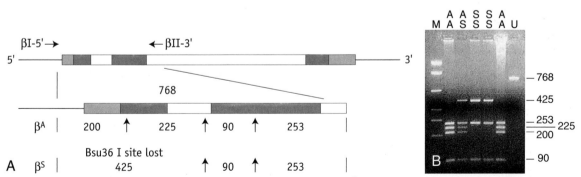

Figure 21.2 Detection of the sickle cell mutation. A: A sketch of the β globin gene shows the position of the primers used to amplify a 768 bp fragment in a polymerase chain reaction (PCR). The sequence of β I-5′ is 5′TAAGCCAGTGCCAGAAAGAGCC3′ and that of β II-3′ is 5′CATTCGTCTGTTTCCATTCTA3′. Maps of the Bsu36 I restriction sites and the fragment sizes from βA and βS genes are shown below. B: An ethidium–bromide–stained mini-gel illustrates the fragment sizes generated by Bsu36 I digestion of the PCR product from normal (A/A), sickle cell trait (A/S), and sickle cell anaemia (S/S) individuals, along with the undigested amplified fragment (U) and the molecular size marker (M).

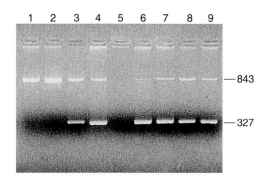

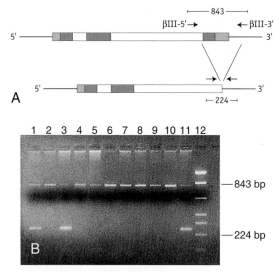

Figure 21.3 Detection of a 619 bp deletion using the polymerase chain reaction (PCR). A: A sketch of the normal β globin gene and the deleted gene shows the location of the primers (*arrows*) used to amplify across this deletion. The sequence of β III-5′ is 5′ACAGTGATAATTTCTGGGTT 3′ and that of β III-3′ is 5′TAAGCAAGAGAACTGAGTGG3′. B: A mini-gel shows the expected 843 bp fragment yielded by the two primers from a normal β globin gene in all lanes and the 224 bp fragment derived from a deleted gene in individuals who are heterozygous for the mutation in lanes 1, 3, and 11.

Figure 21.4 Diagnosis of the 41/42 (–TTCT) frameshift mutation using amplification refractory mutation system (ARMS). The gel shows the 843 bp fragment generated by the internal control primers (β III-5′ and β III-3′) in all lanes, except lane 5, which is the blank control. Four DNA samples are tested with the mutant ARMS primer (5′GTCTACCCTTGGACCCAGAGGTTGA3′) in combination with the common primer (5′CATTCGTCTGTTTCCCATTCTA3′) in lanes 1–4 and with the normal ARMS primer (5′GTCTACCCTTGGACCCAGAGGTTCTT3′) in combination with the common primer in lanes 6–9. The presence of a 327 bp product in lanes 3 and 4 and lanes 6–9 indicates that the individuals in lanes 3 and 4 are heterozygous for the 41/42 frameshift mutation, whereas individuals 1 and 2 are normal with respect to this mutation.

α Thalassaemia

In contrast to the β thalassaemias, the most common α thalassaemia mutations are deletions. Two categories exist: those that remove only one of the two alpha globin genes on any one chromosome (α+ thalassaemia) and those that remove both of the alpha genes from one chromosome (α0 thalassaemia). Although PCR amplification around the alpha globin locus has proved to be rather difficult, the common deletions can now be identified by a reasonably robust Gap-PCR.[16] In these reactions dimethylsulphoxide (DMSO) and betaine are added (see Appendix B, p. 582). Two different multiplex PCR reactions are set up, one for the common α+ thalassaemias (α-3.7 and α-4.2) and one for the common α0 thalassaemias (--SEA, --MED, --FIL, and α-20.5) The fragment generated by these primers across the deletion breakpoint is different in size to the fragment generated from the normal chromosome. The primers that flank the deletion breakpoint are too far apart to generate a fragment from the normal chromosome in the PCR. Only when these are brought closer together as a result of the deletion can a fragment be produced. Primer sequences used in this analysis are given in Table 21.1, and an example of their application in the detection of α0 thalassaemias is shown in Figure 21.5. More than 30 nondeletional forms of α thalassaemia have been described. Of these, Hb Constant Spring and the α^HphI α mutation are relatively common in Southeast Asian and Mediterranean populations, respectively. These can be detected by ASOH, ARMS, restriction enzyme digestion, or direct sequencing of the appropriate PCR product. Unlike the β thalassaemias, α thalassaemias are not easily diagnosed using routine haematological techniques. The diagnosis of α thalassaemia is often made following exclusion of β thalassaemia and iron deficiency. Because the vast

Table 21.1   Primers used in Gap-PCR analysis of α-thalassaemia

Primer name	Sequence, 5′→3′	Concentration (μmol/l)
α°	Multiplex PCR	From ref 15
20.5(F)	GGGCAAGCTGGTGGTGTTACACAGCAACTC	0.1
20.5(R)	CCACGCCCATGCCTGGCACGTTTGCTGAGG	0.1
α/SEA(F)	CTCTGTGTTCTCAGTATTGGAGGGAAGGAG	0.3
α(R)	TGAAGAGCCTGCAGGACCAGGTCAGTGACCG	0.15
MED(F)	CGATGAGAACATAGTGAGCAGAATTGCAGG	0.15
MED(R)	ACGCCGACGTTGCTGCCCAGCTTCTTCCAC	0.15
SEA(R)	ATATATGGGTCTGGAAGTGTATCCCTCCCA	0.15
FIL(F)	AAGAGAATAAACCACCCAATTTTTAAATGGGCA	1.6
FIL(R)	GAGATAATAACCTTTATCTGCCACATGTAGCAA	1.6
α+	Multiplex PCR	From J Old, personal communication
3.7F	CCCCTCGCCAAGTCCACCC	0.4
3.7/20.5R	AAAGCACTCTAGGGTCCAGCG	0.4
4.2F	GGTTTACCCATGTGGTGCCTC	0.6
4.2R	CCCGTTGGATCTTCTCATTTCCC	0.8
α2R	AGACCAGGAAGGGCCGGTG	0.1

PCR, polymerase chain reaction.

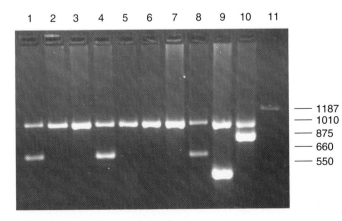

Figure 21.5   Detection of α^0 thalassaemia by multiplex Gap-PCR. The sequences of the primers used are shown in Table 21.1. A normal fragment of 1010 bp is generated by the primers α/SEA(F) and α/(R)in all lanes (although this is very faint in lane 11). In addition, a fragment of 660 bp is generated by the primer pair α/SEA(F) and SEA(R) in lanes 1, 4, and 8 in individuals who are heterozygous for the – –SEA deletion; a fragment of 550 bp is generated by the primer pair FIL(F) and FIL(R) in lane 9 in an individual who is heterozygous for the – –FIL deletion; a fragment of 875 bp is generated by the primer pair MED(F) and MED(R) in lane 10 in an individual who is heterozygous for the – –MED deletion; and a fragment of 1187 bp is generated by the primer pair 20.5(F) and 20.5(R) in lane 10 in an individual who is heterozygous for the $-\alpha^{20.5}$ deletion.

majority of cases of α thalassaemia are of the clinically benign type (i.e., α^+ thalassaemia), it is debatable whether molecular analysis is justified to reach a diagnosis in these individuals. However, it is important that individuals with α^0 thalassaemia are identified, and the only definitive diagnostic test is DNA analysis. The α^0 thalassaemias are almost entirely restricted to at-risk ethnic groups, namely those of southeast Asian or Mediterranean origin, and so it is most efficient to target these groups specifically. The diagnosis of α^0 thalassaemia is particularly relevant if prenatal diagnosis is to be offered to a couple who are at risk of having a fetus with hydrops, where there is an increased risk of maternal death at delivery. Guidelines derived from the UK experience as to how and when DNA analysis should be implemented have been proposed,[17] but these remain under review.

DISORDERS OF COAGULATION

Thrombophilia

Considerable advances have been made in our understanding of the genetic risk factors found in patients with venous thromboembolism (VTE).[18] Among these are the diverse mutations causing protein C, protein S, and antithrombin deficiency. An increased factor VIII level is also a risk factor for VTE, but the genetic determinants of this are unclear. Homozygosity for the common C677T mutation of the methylenetetrahydrofolate reductase gene, which gives rise to a thermolabile variant of this protein, has been reported to be a risk factor for VTE, although other studies have not supported this claim. A point mutation in the 3′ UTR of the prothrombin gene associated with elevated protein levels has been identified as a genetic risk factor for VTE.[19] The most common of the known genetic risk factors for VTE is a resistance to the anticoagulant effect of activated protein C caused by the Arg506Gln substitution in factor V (FVL)[20]; around 20% of subjects of north European origin presenting for the first time with thromboembolism are heterozygous for this mutation. Because of their prevalence, and because the tests have become relatively simple, there is a tendency toward indiscriminate testing for these genetic risk factors in thrombophilia, but

without careful and informed counselling this may often be inappropriate.[21] (See also Chapter 17.)

Method

A variety of different methods have been used to detect these mutations. The method described here is a multiplex that simultaneously detects the prothrombin and factor V mutations. We have adapted primer sequences to create Taq I sites in both genes—an example of the ACRES technique—which are lost when a mutation is present.

PCR is performed as described in Appendix B, using buffer III with an $MgCl_2$ concentration of 2.0 mmol/l. The forward primer in the factor V gene is 5′GTAAGAGCAGATCCCTGGACAGtC3′, with the deliberate mismatch shown in lowercase. The reverse primer is 5′TGTTATCACACTGGTGCTAA3′. The normal sequence of the gene at the position of the mutation is AGGCGA, altered to AGGCAA in FVL. The last 4 bases of the mutagenic oligo (AGtC) will create a Taq I site (TCGA) in the normal gene (AGtCGA), which will not be present in the FVL gene (AGtCAA). A similar principle applies for the prothrombin gene for which the forward and reverse primers are 5′CAATAAAAGTGACTCTCAtC3′ and 5′AGGTGGTGGATTCTTAAGTC3′, respectively. The PCR products are digested with Taq I at 65°C as described on p. 585.

Interpretation

The factor V primer pair gives rise to a fragment of 181 bp; after Taq I cleavage, the normal gene (1691G) gives rise to fragments of 157 bp and 24 bp, whereas the mutant gene (1691A) remains uncut at 181 bp. Although the 24 bp fragment is not easily detected, the 157 bp and 181 bp fragments are clearly resolved on a 3% agarose gel (Fig. 21.6). When only the smaller fragment is seen, the sample is normal (1691 G/G); when both the smaller and larger fragments are seen, the sample is heterozygous for FVL (1691 A/G); when only the larger fragment is seen, the sample is homozygous for FVL (1691 A/A). The same principle applies for the prothrombin fragment, with the normal gene (20210G) being cut by Taq I to 98 bp and the mutant gene (20210A) remaining uncut at 118 bp (Fig. 21.6). The Taq I enzyme is relatively robust, and partial digestion—the only potential pitfall in this analysis—

is avoided by using a significant excess of enzyme. The presence of both the factor V and prothrombin fragments in the same tube controls for the efficacy of the restriction enzyme because one of these is usually normal and therefore shows complete digestion. The analysis only requires confirmation when an individual appears to have both the prothrombin and factor V mutations.

Clotting Disorders

Diverse mutations underlie haemophilia A and haemophilia B, and these are usually identified by screening exons for mutation by SSCP, denaturing high-performance liquid chromatography, or direct DNA sequence analysis in specialised laboratories.[22] It may still be relevant to determine carrier status and offer prenatal diagnosis through genetic linkage analysis. Problems with this include the number of sporadic cases, lack of informative markers, unavailable family members, and the possibility of recombination.

Of particular diagnostic significance is the fact that from between one third and one half of all patients with severe haemophilia A have a large genomic inversion mutation involving recombination between a region in intron 22 of the factor VIII gene and telomeric homologous sequences.[23] These inversions are readily detected by Southern blot analysis using the p482.6 probe[24] to Bcl I digests of genomic DNA. A method has also recently been described using long-distance PCR, enabling identification of these deletion mutations in a single tube reaction.[25]

(See Chapter 16 for more information on bleeding disorders.)

LEUKAEMIA AND LYMPHOMA

Cytogenetic Principles and Terminology

Cytogenetic analysis is usually carried out by specially trained cytogeneticists in a separate laboratory that often has no specific relationship to the haematology laboratory. For this reason no details of techniques will be given. However, cytogenetic analysis is so crucial to the diagnosis and management of haematological neoplasms that it is necessary for haematologists to understand the principles and be able to understand the reports that are received. In addition, haematologists are often involved in collection of appropriate samples.

Classical cytogenetic analysis is carried out on cells that have entered mitosis and have been arrested in metaphase so that individual chromosomes can be recognised by their size and their banding pattern following staining (e.g., Giemsa staining [G-banding] or staining with a fluorescent dye). Alternating dark and light bands are numbered from the centromere toward the telomere to facilitate description of any abnormalities detected. An example showing the balanced translocation t(9;22) (q34;q11) in CML is shown in Fig 21.7. The standard terminology applied to chromosomes is shown in Table 21.2.

The results of cytogenetic analysis may be displayed visually (a karyogram) or written according to standard conventions (a karyotype). Thus 46,XY, t(3;3)(q21;q26)[20] indicates a pseudodiploid karyotype in a male; a reciprocal translocation has occurred between the paired chromosomes 3 following a break at 3q21 on one chromosome (i.e., involving

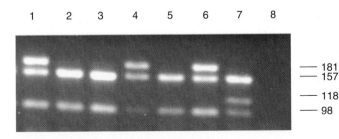

1 2 3 4 5 6 7 8

— 181
— 157

— 118

— 98

Figure 21.6   Detection of the factor V Leiden (FVL) and prothrombin 3′UTR mutations using amplification created restriction enzyme site (ACRES). Polymerase chain reaction products are digested with Taq I prior to agarose gel electrophoresis, as described in the text. Heterozygotes for the FVL mutation are identified in lanes 1, 4 (where the prothrombin fragment is weak), and 6, whereas a heterozygote for the prothrombin mutation is identified in lane 7. The other subjects are normal. Lane 8 is the blank control.

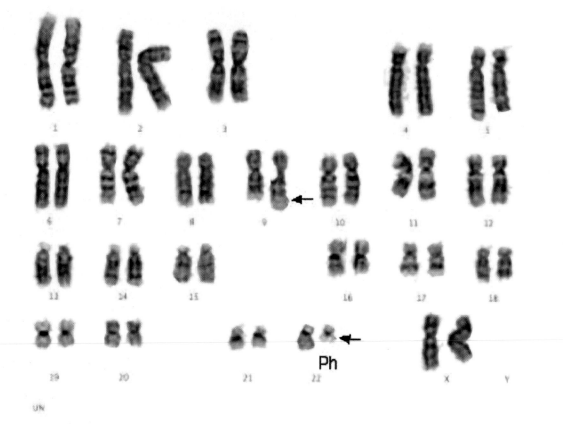

Figure 21.7 G-Banded karyotype. Female karyotype with a balanced reciprocal translocation between chromosomes 9 and 22 (arrowed) giving rise to the Philadelphia chromosome (Ph). Courtesy of J. Howard.

the long arm of chromosome 3, band 2, sub-band 1) and at 3q26 on the other. 46,XY,inv(3)(q21q26) indicates a pseudodiploid karyotype with a paracentric inversion of the long arm of a single chromosome 3; the breakpoints are the same as in the first instance but are on a single chromosome. Note the use of semicolons in describing a translocation, whereas these are absent from the notation of an inversion. Numbers shown within square brackets in a karyotype indicate the number of cells showing the specified normal or abnormal finding. Cytogenetic analysis can be carried out on the following:

1. Skin fibroblasts or phytohaemagglutinin (PHA)-stimulated lymphocytes (to study constitutional abnormalities)
2. Bone marrow cells
3. Blood cells
4. Cells isolated from lymph nodes or other organs suspected of being infiltrated by a lymphoid or other neoplasm
5. Cells isolated from serous effusions

In studying suspected haematological neoplasms, there are two reasons for seeking to detect constitutional abnormalities. First, there may be a constitutional abnormality underlying a haematological neoplasm as when megakaryoblastic leukaemia occurs in Down's syndrome. Second, there may be an irrelevant and previously undetected constitutional chromosomal abnormality that has to be recognised so that it can be distinguished from an acquired chromosomal abnormality associated with a neoplastic process.

Table 21.2   Terminology and abbreviations used in classical cytogenetic analysis

Term	Abbreviation	Explanation
Centromere	Cen	The junction of the short and long arms of a chromosome
Telomere	Ter	The termination of the short or long arm of a chromosome, pter or qter
Long arm	Q	The longer of the two arms of the chromosome that are joined at the centromere
Short arm	P	The shorter of the two arms of the chromosome that are joined at the centromere
Diploid		Having the full complement of 46 chromosomes, 44 paired autosomes, and two sex chromosomes in a cell or clone
Haploid		Having 23 chromosomes, a single copy of each autosome, and either an X or a Y chromosomes in a cell or clone
Tetraploid		Having a total of 92 chromosomes, four of each autosome and four sex chromosomes in a cell or clone
Aneuploid		Having a chromosome number that is neither diploid nor a fraction or a multiple of the diploid number, in a cell or clone
Pseudodiploid		Having 46 chromosomes in a cell or clone but with either structural abnormalities or with loss and gain of different chromosomes so that not all chromosomes are paired
Hyperdiploid		The presence of more than 46 chromosomes in a cell or clone
Hypodiploid		The presence of fewer than 46 chromosomes in a cell or clone
Monosomy	− (a minus sign before the chromosome number, e.g., −7)	Loss of one of a pair of chromosomes
Trisomy	+ (a plus sign before the chromosome number, e.g., +13)	Gain of a chromosome so that there are three rather than two copies
Deletion	del or a minus sign after the number and the designation of the arm of a chromosome, e.g., del(20q) or 20q−	Loss of part of the long or the short arm of a chromosome
Translocation	T	Movement of a chromosomal segment or segments between two or more chromosomes; a translocation can be reciprocal or nonreciprocal
Reciprocal translocation		Exchange of segments between two or more chromosomes
Nonreciprocal translocation		Movement of a segment of a chromosome from one chromosome to another but without reciprocity

Table 21.2   Terminology and abbreviations used in classical cytogenetic analysis—cont'd

Term	Abbreviation	Explanation
Centromere	Cen	The junction of the short and long arms of a chromosome
Balanced translocation		A translocation that occurs without loss of chromosomal material, or at least without loss of sufficient chromosomal material to be detectable by microscopic examination of chromosomes
Unbalanced translocation		A translocation that is associated with gain or loss of part of a chromosome
Inversion	inv	The inversion of a part of a chromosome, either pericentric or paracentric
Pericentric inversion		An inversion that follows breaking of both the long and short arms so that the part of the chromosome that is inverted includes the centromere
Paracentric inversion		An inversion that follows the occurrence of two breaks in either the long or the short arm of a chromosome so that the part of the chromosome that is inverted does not include the centromere
Insertion	ins	The insertion of a segment of one chromosome into another chromosome or into a different position on the same chromosomes. Can be direct or inverted
Isochromosome	i	A chromosome with two long arms or two short arms joined at the centromere, e.g., i(17q)
Derivative	der	A chromosome that is derived from another; a derivative chromosome derived from two or more chromosomes carries the number of the chromosome that contributed the centromere
Duplication	dup	The duplication of part of a chromosome
Clone		A population of cells derived from a single cell; in cytogenetic analysis a clone is considered to be present if two cells share the same structural abnormality or extra chromosome or if three cells have lost the same chromosome
Marker	mar	An abnormal chromosome of uncertain origin that "marks" a clone
Constitutional	c	A chromosomal abnormality that is part of the constitution of an individual rather than being acquired, e.g. 21c in Down's syndrome

The indications for cytogenetic analysis in a definite or suspected haematological neoplasm are as follows:

To provide evidence of clonality and permit a diagnosis of a neoplastic condition when this is not otherwise demonstrated (e.g., in some patients with eosinophilia or an increase in natural killer lymphocytes)

To confirm a specific diagnosis (e.g., acute promyelocytic leukaemia, Burkitt's lymphoma)

To permit classification (e.g., to apply the World Health Organization classification of acute myeloid leukaemia and the myelodysplastic syndromes)

To give prognostic information (e.g., the detection of hyperdiploidy [prognostically good] in acute lymphoblastic leukaemia [ALL])

To indicate which fusion genes are likely to be present and thus give information permitting detection of minimal residual disease by molecular analysis

To distinguish a phenotypic switch occurring within a single clone from a therapy-related secondary leukaemia

To distinguish therapy-related acute leukaemia following alkylating agents from that following topoisomerase II-interactive drugs.

For investigation of haematological neoplasms, a bone marrow aspirate is usually the preferred tissue. It is also possible to disaggregate bone marrow cells from a trephine biopsy specimen into tissue culture medium. Peripheral blood may yield metaphases when large numbers of immature cells are present, but it is generally less reliable than the bone marrow in yielding dividing cells. In theory, any infiltrated tissue can provide cells that can be disaggregated and analysed. In haematological practice it is mainly lymph node cells that are studied, but clinically relevant information is sometimes obtained from other infiltrated tissues.

A bone marrow aspirate for cytogenetic analysis should be anticoagulated by the addition of preservative-free heparin or tissue culture medium containing heparin. It can be stored at room temperature for some hours or at 4°C if delay in analysis is expected. If it is being sent to a central laboratory, detailed clinical and haematological information must accompany the sample so that the central laboratory is aware if there is clinical urgency in obtaining results and so that appropriate techniques are used.

Fluorescence *in situ* Hybridization

Fluorescence *in situ* hybridization (FISH) bridges classical cytogenetic analysis and molecular diagnostic techniques. Chromosomes can be stained and visualised but the technique is also dependent on the recognition of specific DNA sequences by means of a fluorescent probe that can anneal to a specific DNA sequence. FISH can be carried out of metaphase preparations or on cells in interphase. FISH probes may identify the following:

Centromeres of a specific chromosome (useful for detecting trisomy or monosomy and chimerism following sex-mismatched bone marrow transplantation; Fig. 21.8A)

Specific oncogenes (locus-specific probe, useful for detecting translocations; Fig. 21.8B and C)

Specific tumour-suppressor genes (locus-specific probe, loss is relevant to tumour progression)

Other diagnostically useful genes (locus-specific probe, for example, for the *CHIC2* gene, which is lost when an interstitial deletion leads to formation of a *FIP1L1-PDGFRA* fusion gene)

Whole chromosomes (whole chromosome painting, useful in identifying complex chromosomal rearrangements).

Advantages of FISH analysis in comparison with conventional chromosomal analysis include the following:

Many more cells can be examined (useful for detecting residual disease)

Metaphases are not essential, so abnormalities can be detected in nondividing cells (useful in chronic lymphocytic leukaemia)

FISH can be performed in a shorter period of time (may be critical in confirming a diagnosis of acute promyelocytic leukaemia)

Abnormalities that cannot be detected by conventional cytogenetic analysis may be detected (e.g., *SIL-TAL* fusion in T-lineage ALL or t(12;21) (p12;q22) in B-lineage ALL)

The main disadvantage is that only those abnormalities that are specifically sought will be found, whereas conventional cytogenetic analysis permits all chromosomes to be evaluated.

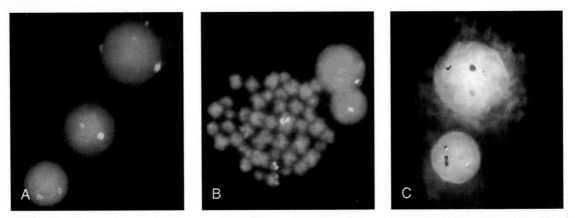

Figure 21.8   Fluorescent in situ hybridisation (FISH). A: Use of the X/Y dual-label probe (Abbott Diagnostics, Vysis) in a sex-mismatched bone marrow transplant patient. Two interphases show 1 red signal (X chromosome) and 1 green signal (Y chromosome) indicating male cells, whereas one interphase shows 2 red signals (X chromosomes) indicating a female cell. B: Use of the *BCR/ABL* dual-colour, dual-fusion translocation probe (Abbott Diagnostics, Vysis). One metaphase and one interphase cell show 2 red signals (from the *ABL* gene locus on chromosome 9) and 2 green signals (from the *BCR* gene locus on chromosome 22). These cells are therefore negative for the *BCR–ABL* gene fusion at the molecular cytogenetic level. C: Use of the *BCR-ABL* dual-colour, dual-fusion translocation probe (Abbott Diagnostics, Vysis). Interphase cells show 2 red/green fusion signals (from the *BCR–ABL* fusion on chromosome 22 and the *ABL-BCR* fusion on chromosome 9), 1 red signal (*ABL* gene locus on chromosome 9), and 1 green signal (*BCR* gene locus on chromosome 22). This sample is therefore positive for the *BCR–ABL* gene fusion at the molecular cytogenetic level. (Courtesy of J. Howard.)

Translocations, Molecular Analysis, and Minimal Residual Disease

The accurate characterization of haematological malignancies at the chromosomal and molecular level has advanced greatly in recent years and now makes an important contribution to initial treatment decisions. For example, many patients with acute leukaemia, CML, and lymphomas have specific chromosomal lesions known to be associated with particularly favourable or unfavourable prognoses, and the proportion of such patients with defined chromosomal lesions is increasing. Usually the presence of these cytogenetic abnormalities can be confirmed by molecular biology techniques, and in some cases the latter may be more informative than cytogenetics.

The Philadelphia (Ph) chromosome (22q-) present in 95% of cases of CML may be identified by routine cytogenetic studies; its presence can be confirmed by demonstrating the presence of the *BCR–ABL* fusion gene by RT-PCR. The Ph chromosome may

also be found in 25% and 5% of adult and childhood ALL respectively,[26] where it is associated with relatively poorer prognosis and indicates the need for a more aggressive therapy. Patients suspected of having CML or a myeloproliferative disorder should be tested for *BCR–ABL* for definitive diagnosis.

To optimize clinical management, patients with ALL should also be tested for *BCR–ABL*.

Small cleaved lymphoid cells are observed in a number of conditions with different treatments and prognoses. In such cases, detection of a translocation involving *BCL-1* is commonly associated with mantle cell lymphoma, t(11;14), whereas identification of *BCL-2* involvement implies a follicular lymphoma, t(14;18).[27] The former is much more aggressive with poor prognosis, thus requiring a more intensive treatment. Translocations associated with lymphomas usually lead to the deregulation of a normal gene—for example, t(14;18) places the *BCL-2* gene adjacent to the IgH gene, leading to deregulation of the former. In contrast, the leukaemia-associated translocations often give rise to a chimeric gene that is transcribed—for example, t(15;17), which yields a novel *PML/RARA* fusion gene.[28]

Frequently, the breakpoints within the translocation are too widely distributed to allow direct amplification of DNA by PCR. In such cases, the mRNA from the fusion gene can be reverse transcribed using RT to yield cDNA, which can than be amplified by PCR. In addition, RT-PCR is an exquisitely sensitive tool that has been exploited in the detection of residual disease. It is beyond the scope of this chapter to describe the extensive range of applications of these techniques, and they have been reviewed elsewhere.[29] We will illustrate their application in the analysis of the *BCR–ABL* fusion gene.

BCR–ABL Reverse Transcriptase-Polymerase Chain Reaction

Principle and Interpretation

The *BCR–ABL* analysis is performed by two-stage RT-PCR. The RNA extracted from nucleated cells is reverse transcribed by RT to generate coding or cDNA using random primers 6 bp long, or hexamers. Following the RT step, the samples are subjected to multiplex PCR, to test for the presence or absence of *BCR–ABL*.[30] Multiplex PCR is similar to conventional PCR but includes more than one pair of primers in a single PCR test. This strategy enables the detection of the vast majority of the *BCR–ABL* transcripts. The most commonly observed transcripts are b3a2, b2a2, and e1a2, giving rise to 385, 310, and 481 bp amplicons, respectively (Fig. 21.9).

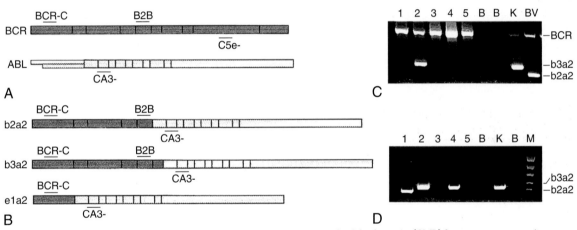

Figure 21.9   Detection of minimal residual disease in chronic myeloid leukaemia (CML) by reverse transcriptase-polymerase chain reaction (RT-PCR). A: Diagrammatic representation of the processed exons of the *BCR* and *ABL* genes together with the relative position of the B2B and C5e–primers used to coamplify *BCR* in the multiplex PCR. B: Commonly observed *BCR-ABL* derivatives, b2a2 and b3a2 which give rise to p210 *BCR-ABL*, and e1a2, which gives rise to p190 *BCR-ABL*. The relative positions of the primers used to amplify the chimeric transcripts by multiplex PCR are shown. C: A 2.0% agarose gel containing ethidium bromide through which amplicons generated by multiplex PCR using complementary DNA (cDNA) from 5 patients (lanes 1 to 5) were electrophoresed. The coamplified normal *BCR* fragment, 808 bp in length, is seen in all samples except for the lanes containing the blank controls (*B*). The diagnostic sample from a patient with suspected CML, in lane 2, revealed a fragment corresponding to the b3a2 *BCR-ABL* transcript, 385 bp in length, in addition to the *BCR* amplicon. *BCR-ABL* is not detectable in lanes 1, 3, 4, and 5 containing follow-up samples from patients following stem cell transplant (SCT). D: The cDNA of these individuals was subjected to nested PCR to exclude residual disease. This reveals *BCR-ABL* transcripts, b3a2 (385 bp) and b2a2 (310 bp) in lanes 1 and 4, previously undetectable by the less sensitive multiplex PCR. However, *BCR-ABL* is not detectable in lanes 3 and 5, implying these samples are from patients in molecular remission post-SCT. B, blank controls; K (K562-b3a2) and BV (BV173-b2a2), positive controls; M, molecular size marker.

In addition to *BCR–ABL*, the normal *BCR* gene is coamplified, yielding a 808 bp amplicon. The coamplification of *BCR* is an indication of the quality of RNA and the efficiency of cDNA synthesis. Absence of any fragments indicates failure of the procedure. The latter is often the result of an aged sample (i.e., more than 72 hours old). For RT-PCR analysis, the sample should be processed to lysate stage (see nuclear lysate preparation, p. 586) within 48 hours of collection. In addition, the *BCR* fragment is often not observed in diagnostic samples where the *BCR–ABL* is preferentially amplified.

If *BCR–ABL* is undetectable by multiplex PCR in follow-up samples from patients undergoing therapy, the cDNA is tested at higher level of sensitivity by nested PCR.[31] Nested PCR enables the detection of one leukaemic cell in a background of 10^5 to 10^6 normal cells. The choice of primers for nested PCR is dependent on the type of transcript detected by multiplex PCR at presentation. The primers for b3a2 and b2a2 are the same; however, for e1a2 transcript a different set of primers is used. The nested PCR yields fragments of 385bp (b3a2), 310bp (b2a2), or 481bp (e1a2) in length. Nested PCR is not indicated for testing cDNA from a patient suspected of having CML. Diagnosis is made by expression of BCR-ABL by multiplex PCR. Furthermore, in post-therapy samples this will indicate molecular relapse.

Reagents and Methods

See Appendix E, p. 586.

Monitoring Minimal Residual Disease

Effective clinical management of haematological malignancies depends on accurate and precise measurement of a patient's response to therapeutic agents. This includes examination of cellular morphology in peripheral blood and marrow specimens. Although these studies are essential, they lack sensitivity; therefore the malignant clone has frequently advanced to levels at which it is refractory to further treatment before relapse is recognised. The last 3 decades have seen a remarkable advance in the development of technology to monitor patients' response to therapy to a sensitivity of 1×10^{-5} (i.e., the detection of one malignant cell in a background of 100,000 normal cells). To enable this, a disease-specific marker is essential, as illustrated

by targeting the novel fusion gene *BCR–ABL*, which maps to the Philadelphia chromosome associated with CML. The principle aim is to detect and measure minimal residual disease (MRD) using the most sensitive techniques available to a clinical laboratory with accuracy and precision and thus recognise early signs of relapse. The clinical utility of such studies has been amply confirmed by close and regular measurement of MRD in patients with CML. This is increasingly being shown to apply to other adult and childhood leukaemias using disease-specific markers.

For purposes of clarity and because of space limitation, the principle and aims of MRD studies will be confined to CML. Although qualitative PCR (i.e., multiplex and nested PCR; see p. 571) is very useful, it provides no information about the kinetics of the disease. The latter can only be obtained by measuring the tumour load; this is achieved by quantification of *BCR–ABL* mRNA molecules. Several groups developed a semi-quantitative competitive RT-PCR strategy to measure quantification of *BCR–ABL* and an endogenous control gene to circumvent this difficulty. A detailed description of competitive PCR is beyond the scope of this book. In brief, competitive PCR involves coamplification of the target gene and a competitor at varying concentrations of copy number. The number of *BCR–ABL* transcripts is estimated by determining the concentration at which equivalence is obtained between the target and the competitor.[32]

Because the amount of total RNA added to each reverse transcription reaction and its quality (i.e., the degree of degradation) are variable, the transcripts of a housekeeping gene are quantified as an endogenous control. Furthermore, amplification of an endogenous control gene also allows for the intersample PCR dynamics variation. There are a number of control genes that can be used as endogenous control genes (e.g., *GAPDH*, β_2-microglobulin, and *ABL)*. An endogenous control gene should not be too highly expressed and should show no intersample variation in levels of expression; also, there should be no related pseudogenes nor alternative splicing.[33] However, the complexity and the expanse of competitive PCR assays limited their use to specialised centres. The introduction of quantitative real-time PCR (QR-PCR) at the end of the last millennium made quantification of MRD more widely accessible. QR-PCR is linear over five orders of magnitude in contrast to the short range of linearity of competitive PCR.

Principle

QR-PCR permits quantification of number of transcripts of gene of interest at high levels of sensitivity. This is achieved by developing the technology that permits the detection of PCR products as they accumulate. Furthermore, the rate of accumulation is proportional to the number of mRNA molecules of the target gene in the starting material during the exponential phase of the PCR. The accumulation of amplicons is detected by including a sequence-specific specific probe labelled with fluorochromes in addition to the primers as in conventional PCR (Fig. 21.10). Since the advent of QR-PCR several types of probes have been developed, although all are dependent on the fluorescence resonance energy transfer (FRET) principle. The two commonly used systems involve hybridisation or hydrolysis of the probe. A widely used methodology is TaqMan, which involves hydrolysis of the probe.[34] This technology is based on the 5′exonuclease assay, which exploits the inherent 5′ to 3′ exonuclease activity of the *Taq* DNA polymerase.[35] The *Taq* DNA polymerase cleaves a dual-labelled probe annealed to the target sequence during PCR amplification (Fig. 21.11A). Briefly, the cDNA synthesised from total RNA is added to the PCR reaction containing standard PCR components plus a probe that anneals to the template between the two primers as per conventional PCR. The probe has a fluorescent reporter dye, FAM, at the 5′-end (6′carboxyfluorescein; emission λ_{max} = 518 nm) and quencher dye, TAMRA, at the 3′-end (6-carboxytetramethylrhodamine; emission λ_{max} = 582 nm). While the probe is intact, the proximity of the quencher greatly reduces the fluorescence emitted by the reporter dye by Forster resonance energy transfer (FRET)[36] through space. Adequate quenching is observed for probes with the reporter dye at the 5′ end and the quencher at the 3′ end.

Thus, while although TAMRA and FAM are closely attached to the probe, fluorescent from the reporter dye is quenched by TAMRA. During PCR, as the *Taq* DNA polymerase replicates the DNA strand to which the TaqMan probe is annealed, the probe is degraded by the intrinsic 5′–3′ exonuclease activity of the polymerase. The effect is to dissociate FAM from TAMRA; therefore FRET is no longer applicable and fluorescence from FAM can be detected by a laser integrated in the sequence detector (TaqMan ABI 7700 Sequence Detection system, *Applied Biosystems, Foster City, CA*). Fluorescence increases, in each cycle, proportional to the rate of probe degradation. The number of cycles taken for the fluorescence to cross a threshold value of ×10

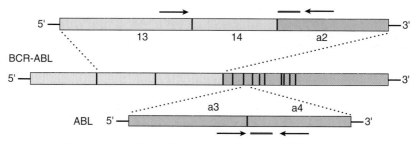

Figure 21.10   **Probes and primers.** The position of probes and primers used for quantification of *BCR–ABL* and ABL transcripts are shown. The *BCR–ABL* fusion gene is shown in yellow- and purple-filled boxes, with the yellow representing the exons derived from the *BCR* gene and purple those originating from the *ABL* gene. The dual-labelled probes are shown as red lines, and primers are shown as arrows. Probes and primers were designed using the Primer Express software to detect e13a2 and e14a2 junctions in a single reaction by QR-PCR. The *BCR–ABL* (FAM-cccttcagcggccagtagcatctga-TAMRA) and ABL (FAM-tgcttctgatggcaagctctacgtctcct-TAMRA) probes are dual labelled with 6-carboxyfluorescein (FAM) and 6-carboxy-tetramethyl-rhodamine (TAMRA). *BCR–ABL* forward primer: 5′-tccgctgaccatcaayaagga-3′; *BCR–ABL* reverse primer: 5′-cactcagaccctgaggctcaa-3′; ABL forward primer: 5′-gatacgaagggagggtgttacca-3′; ABL reverse primer: 5′ctcggccagggtgttgaa-3′. The *BCR–ABL* probe and primer set was designed in association with Europe Against Cancer Collaborative study.

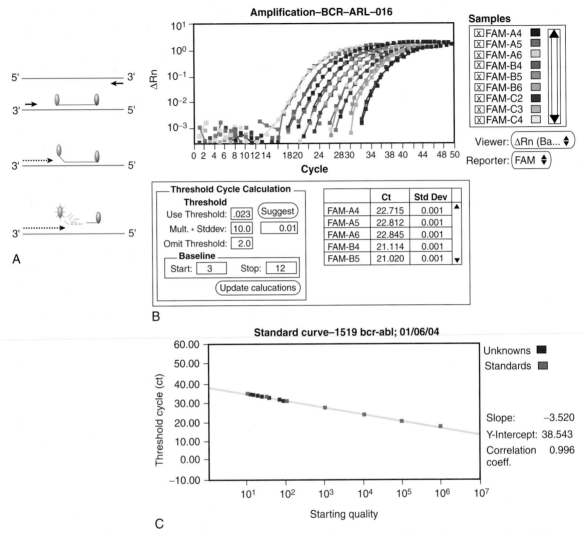

Figure 21.11   Quantitative real-time polymerase chain reaction (QR-PCR). A: Schematic representation of the principle of real-time PCR. The forward and reverse primers (*blue lines*) are extended by the *Taq* DNA polymerase as per conventional PCR. The quencher (*red symbol*) suppresses the fluorescence from the reporter (*green symbol*) dye while the two are attached to the probe. As the forward primer is extended, the probe is displaced and is cleaved by the *Taq* DNA polymerase 5′–3′ exonuclease activity. Fluorescence is detected once the reporter dissociates from the quencher on probe being degraded and the synthesis of the new DNA continues to completion. Therefore the fluorescence increases with increment in number of amplicons. **B: Amplification plot.** The real-time PCR amplification plot of the standards in log increments is shown. A 0.5 log standard between 10 and 100 *BCR–ABL* copies is included. The number of cycles for the fluorescence to cross the threshold is reported as Ct (cycle threshold). The greater the number of copies, the lower the Ct value (i.e., it is inversely proportional). **C: A standard curve.** A standard curve drawn from Q-PCR data from serial dilutions of plasmid containing *BCR–ABL* (*black symbols*) is shown. The *BCR–ABL* transcripts for the unknown samples (*red symbols*) are read off the standard curve.

the standard deviation of baseline emission is used for quantitative measurement. The threshold is set significantly above the baseline and can be adjusted manually. A significant increase in fluorescence above the baseline value during the 3–15 cycles indicates the detection of accumulated PCR product The upper baseline limit can be altered by the operator. The fluorescence is plotted as δRN against number of cycles (i.e., time; Fig. 21.11B. The δRN is $\delta RN = (Rn^+)-(Rn^-)$. The Passive reference, ROX (6-carboxy-X-rhodamine), is included in the Q-PCR Universal Master Mix. The formulae used to calculate the Rn^+ and Rn^- follow:

From PCR with template:

$$Rn^+ = \frac{\text{Emission intensity of reporter}}{\text{Emission intensity of passive reference (ROX)}}$$

and from PCR without template or early cycles of PCR:

$$Rn^- = \frac{\text{Emission intensity of reporter}}{\text{Emission intensity of passive reference (ROX)}}$$

The number of cycles taken to achieve this is called the cycle threshold (Ct), and it is inversely proportional to the starting material of the target. The number of transcripts of the target is read off a standard curve. The target gene and endogenous control gene transcripts are measured off the respective standard curves. The level of expression of the target gene is reported as a percentage ratio to obtain a normalised value for the gene of interest independent of the integrity of the RNA and efficiency of the reverse transcription reaction.

Interpretation

Patients who achieve complete cytogenetic remission may harbour up to 1×10^{10} leukaemic cells. The kinetics of the leukaemic load in these patients and their response to therapeutic agents can only be monitored by measuring MRD.[37] Although it should be noted that patients in whom QR-PCR fails to detect BCR–ABL may still harbour up to 1×10^6 leukaemic cells. Of those who are in complete cytogenetic remission, the BCR–ABL:ABL ratio is invariably <2.0%. Investigators have also reported that patients who achieve BCR–ABL:ABL ratio <0.045%

while receiving α-interferon therapy have a considerably reduced risk of cytogenetic relapse, and therefore it might be possible to reduce or withdraw chemotherapy from these individuals.[38] Thus with close regular monitoring of MRD it is possible to reduce or avoid exposing patients to toxic drugs unnecessarily. More recently, Q-PCR has been used to monitor patients being treated with imatinib mesylate. Early results from an international multicentre study indicate that a 3 log reduction in BCR–ABL copies is consistent with a good prognosis.[39] Quantification of BCR–ABL also helps to identify patients at risk of relapse, and therefore provides a window for early clinical intervention with the aim of reversing disease progression. For patients who have undergone stem cell transplantation (SCT) this invariably means infusion of lymphocytes isolated from the original donor (i.e., adoptive immunotherapy). Although there is some debate as to the precise criteria for molecular relapse, there is little doubt that a confirmed 1 log increase in BCR–ABL transcripts is clinically significant (i.e., from 0.002% to 0.02%). Patients who achieve a 0.02% BCR–ABL:ABL ratio on three consecutive occasions are said to be in molecular relapse.

Advantages of QR-PCR

The major advantage of QR-PCR is the ability to detect accumulation of amplicons during the exponential phase of PCR. This permits quantification of the DNA of interest in the starting material. This is not possible with conventional PCR because samples are analysed at the end of the PCR run and therefore any differences in the copy number between samples in the starting material are generally not discernable. This is illustrated by the amplification plot shown in Fig. 21.11B where all the samples at the end of 50 cycles have the same level of fluorescence, despite having varying target copy numbers in the starting material as seen in the exponential phase of the PCR. Post-PCR handling is eliminated, on completion of an assay, the sealed micro-titre plate is discarded and thereby minimising risk of contamination. This also eliminates the need to handle carcinogenic ethidium–bromide–stained gel on completion of QR-PCR assay. The QR-PCR offers higher level of specificity because, in addition to primers annealing to DNA sequence of interest, a third oligonucleotide (the probe) anneals to the region between the primers at a higher temperature. To achieve a level of sensitivity that is similar to QR-PCR, nested conventional PCR is required, but this is associated with a greater risk of contamination. Conventional PCR is also less amenable to automation. More importantly, because QR-PCR can be automated, interlaboratory standardisation becomes feasible when measuring patients' response to therapy. This permits rapid evaluation of new therapeutic modalities because methodology and protocols can be standardised, permitting international interlaboratory studies.

Reagents and Methods

See Appendix F, p. 588.

The Lymphoproliferative Disorders

The majority of lymphoproliferative disorders can be readily diagnosed using cytochemical and immunological techniques as described in Chapters 13 and 14. However, in monitoring residual disease, and in certain cases in which the diagnosis is ambiguous, genetic techniques may be useful.[29,40] Examples include cases of controversial lineage, lymphomas in which the histology is ambiguous, and occult lymphomas. DNA analysis may also help in determining whether a lymphocytosis is monoclonal, oligoclonal, or polyclonal. Translocations do occur in these disorders and may be used in monitoring disease, as described for CML earlier. However, the most commonly used markers, because they are more universally applicable, are the rearranged immunoglobulin (Ig) and *TCR* genes.

Principle

This analysis is possible because the Ig and *TCR* genes undergo a rearrangement during the normal differentiation of B and T lymphocytes, respectively, but not during differentiation of other cells. This rearrangement results in a unique fusion of variable diversity and joining (VDJ) segments, interdigitated by random nucleotide (N region) insertion or deletion. The sequence and length of the DNA at these sites of recombination are therefore characteristic of any particular lymphocyte clone.

For many years, Southern blot analysis has been the gold standard for the detection of rearranged Ig and *TCR* genes. Rearranged restriction enzyme fragments are detected as different in size to germline fragments seen at the joining regions of these loci. However, the rearranged fragments from any one clone are only detected when it represents an abnormally large proportion of the cells in the population being studied, as it will in a clonal lymphoproliferative disorder. In a polyclonal population, each of the many different rearranged fragments that are present, which are derived from the large number of different clones, will be below the level of detection by this method. In this situation only the germline fragments will be seen. The most informative probes used in gene rearrangement studies are the JH probe, for the joining region of the Ig heavy-chain gene, and the Cβ probe, for the constant region of the *TCR* α chain gene. For details on how these are performed and interpreted, we refer the reader to previous editions of this book.

More recently, because of its simplicity, the small amount of DNA required, and potential sensitivity, PCR has been used to detect rearrangement of the Ig and *TCR* genes. Because of the N region diversity, a polyclonal population of cells will give rise to a ladder of various fragment sizes; however, if one clone becomes abnormally large, a discrete fragment size will begin to dominate the products of the PCR—the basis of the so-called "fingerprinting" method for the diagnosis of lymphoproliferative disorders.[41] This analysis can be refined using heteroduplex analysis or SSCP gels in which the sequence as well as the size of the amplified product determines its mobility. To gain further sensitivity in following disease, the product of a "clonal" amplification can be sequenced to derive a clone-specific sequence at the site of rearrangement. This sequence can then be used for the design of clone-specific oligonucleotide probes or primers that can be used in ASOH, ARMS, or real-time PCR. This methodology has been used to monitor MRD in lymphoproliferative disorders.[42,43]

A comprehensive report has been published on the design and standardisation of PCR primers and protocols for the detection of Ig and *TCR* gene rearrangements.[40] The detection rate of clonal rearrangements is very high, but the comprehensive nature of the test requires 107 primer pairs in 18 multiplex PCR tubes, which are now commercially available. The methods described here are more restricted but more widely applicable.

Method: Immunoglobulin Gene Rearrangement

To study Ig gene rearrangement, the locus of choice is the heavy chain gene. A single primer can be used, which will anneal to a consensus sequence shared by all joining (JH) segments. The choice of variable (VH) segment primers is more difficult, and for the more comprehensive analysis, primers from all three framework regions for each of the six or seven VH families are used.[40] A reasonable starting point, however, is to use the JH primer in conjunction with a different primer derived from a consensus sequence of the framework 1 region for each VH family. These primers are as follows:

JH 5′ ACCTGAGGAGACGGTGACCAGGGT 3′
VH1 5′ CCTCAGTGAAGGTCTCCTGCAAGG 3′
VH2 5′ GAGTCTGGTCCTGCGCTGGTGAAA 3′
VH3 5′ GGTCCCTGAGACTCTCCTGTGCA 3′
VH4 5′ TTCGGA(GC)ACCCTGTCCCTCACCT 3′
VH5 5′ AGGTGAAAAAGCCCGGGGAGTCT 3′
VH6 5′ CCTGTGCCATCTCCGGGGACAGTG 3′

PCR buffer I is used in these reactions, with an annealing temperature of 60°C. The products of the reactions are in the order of 320 bp and can be visualised as either a smear or discrete band in thick agarose gels. However, a better resolution is obtained when the products are resolved on a 6% denaturing polyacrylamide gel (see Appendix C, p. 584). They can be visualised by ethidium–bromide staining, autoradiography (if a trace of [α^{32}P] dCTP is included in the PCR reaction), or silver staining.[44] With access to an automated fragment analyser (e.g., the ABI 3700 DNA Analyser), this method is easily converted by attaching a fluorescent label to the JH primer and reading the peaks of fluorescence as a "GeneScan." Alternatively, the PCR products can be subjected to heteroduplex or SSCP analysis, denaturing them at 95°C for 5 min and annealing on ice for 1 hour, prior to electrophoresis in a nondenaturing 6% polyacrylamide gel (see Appendix C, p. 584).

Interpretation

Because of the variable number of nucleotides either removed or added at the point of joining of VDJ segments of the immunoglobulin heavy-chain gene, the distance between V segment and J segment primers will alter accordingly. For the gene to be functional, the reading frame must be maintained, and therefore variations in length must be in multiples of 3 bp. The polyclonal population of B cells therefore gives rise to a characteristic "ladder" or Gaussian size distribution, with peak intensity observed at the median length at its centre. If one B-cell clone is abnormally large, it will give rise to a disproportionately intense band at the size (and using a V primer from the appropriate family) corresponding to its VDJ length. At presentation of a B-cell malignancy, this band may be the only one visible, confirming the presence of an abnormal B-cell clone. Subsequently, an abnormal intensity of this fragment size in the background of a ladder can be used to monitor the disease.

In heteroduplex or SSCP analysis, the polyclonal population of B cells will give rise to fragments with many different sequences, which, on denaturing and reannealing, will generate heteroduplexes that will appear as a smear spreading across the gel. If one large B-cell clone is present, however, homoduplexes will form and these will migrate as a discrete fragment with a migration consistent with its size alone.

There are two main problems that can be encountered in this analysis. The first is that the consensus V primers may not amplify all V segments because of variations in sequence. This is particularly true for diffuse large B-cell lymphomas and myelomas that may harbour many somatic mutations. Second, the evolution of a B-cell clone or the emergence of other subclones during the course of the disease may result in a change in the fragment size and family.

Method: T-Cell Receptor Gene Rearrangement

The choice of locus for PCR analysis of the *TCR* gene rearrangement is the TCR gamma locus as it is rearranged in the vast majority of T-cell clones and does not have the complexity of the TCR beta locus, which has 24 different V segment families. Amplification of DNA around the joining region of the TCR gamma gene is performed in a similar way to that described above earlier for the IgH locus, using a consensus primer for the joining segment (JγC) and one for each of the four variable segment families (Vγ1–4). The primer sequences are as follows:

JγC: 5′ CAACAAGTGTTGTTCCAC 3′
Vγ1: 5′ TGCAGCCAGTCAGAAATCTTCC 3′
Vγ2: 5′ TGCAGGTCACCTAGAGCAACCT 3′
Vγ3: 5′ AGCAGTTCCAGCTATCCATTTCC 3′
Vγ4: 5′ TGCAATTGCACTTGGGCAGTTG 3′

Standard PCR amplification conditions can be employed using these primer combinations, and analysis is again performed on acrylamide gels (Appendix C, p. 584) or an automated fluorescence analyser.

Interpretation

As in the analysis of the immunoglobulin heavy chain gene, discrete bands of amplified product are obtained from clonal T-cell populations, while whereas smears are obtained from polyclonal populations. A greater resolution can be obtained in SSCP gels in which fragment mobility is determined by sequence as well as by size. Products from a polyclonal population have a great variety of sequences, and after denaturing, they do not easily re-anneal to give the double-stranded product, but migrate as a long smear of single-stranded products. If a large T-cell clone is present, many copies of the same product are present that will re-anneal to give a double-stranded fragment, and also show up as discrete single-stranded fragments (Fig. 21.12).

The main problem with the interpretation of this kind of data is that it does not distinguish reactive T-cell clones from malignant T-cell clones. Three different patterns are clearly distinguished: a large malignant clonal population, an oligoclonal population, and a polyclonal population. However, because of the sensitivity of this method, problems can arise in trying to detect a small malignant clone against a polyclonal population compared to a clonal population stimulated by antigen, particularly when a patient is lymphopenic.

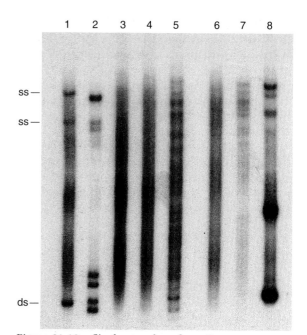

Figure 21.12   Single-strand conformation polymorphism (SSCP) analysis of T-cell receptor (TCR) γ-chain gene rearrangement. Electrophoresis of denatured radiolabelled polymerase chain reaction products in a native 6% polyacrylamide gel, visualised by autoradiography. Discrete single- (ss) and double- (ds) stranded fragments, indicating the presence of abnormal T-cell clones, are seen in lanes 1, 2, and 8 from patients with hypereosinophilia, cutaneous T-cell lymphoma, and a γδ lymphoma, respectively. Polyclonal smears of single-stranded fragments are seen in lanes 3, 4, and 6 and multiple single-stranded fragments against a background smear are seen in lanes 5 and 7 indicating an oligoclonal expansion of T-cell clones.

HOST-DONOR CHIMERISM STUDIES

Following allogeneic stem cell transplantation it is important to monitor the engraftment of donor cells in the host. This can be achieved in a number of ways, one of which is the use of DNA markers. The method of choice is the PCR amplification of STR loci, which, because of their highly polymorphic nature, are likely to give informative differences between any host-donor pair.[45]

Principle

Provided the amplification cycle number is kept reasonably low (25 cycles) the PCR reaction is semi-quantitative, and the amount of product will reflect the amount of starting material. Therefore, once an informative difference is established, the amount of PCR product of the different host and donor alleles will reflect the proportion host and donor DNA in a sample. Fluorescent-labelled primers are used in multiplex PCR reactions that are run on a capillary-based genetic analyser.

Method

This method has been modified from Mann et al[46] by Griffiths and Mason (personal communication). Five primer pairs are used, as listed in Table 21.3. PCR reactions are carried out using buffer III with 1.5 mM $MgCl_2$. Amplification conditions are 94°C for 5 min, then 25 cycles of 94°C for 30 s, 57°C for 1 min, and 72°C for 2 min followed by an extension at 72°C for 5 min. No oil is used when products are to be run on the DNA analyser. One µl of the PCR product, which may need to be diluted from 1:4 to 1:10 in water, is added to 10 µl of formamide containing the size marker Rox 500 (diluted 7.5 µl per 500 µl of formamide), aliquoted into an optical 96-well reaction plate, and run on the ABI 3700 DNA analyser (or equivalent). Peaks representing the DNA fragments are visualised with the Genotyper software (ABI).

Interpretation

Comparing the host (pretransplant) and donor DNA samples, an informative difference is sought at one or more of the STR loci such that host- and/or donor-specific alleles are identified. Correction factors are established by comparing the relative peak heights of the two host or donor alleles at these STRs. Posttransplant, the area under each informative peak is recorded and used to assess the relative proportion of host and donor DNA. Examples of full-engraftment and mixed chimerism are given in Figure 21.13.

Table 21.3   PCR primers used for multiplex STR amplification

Marker	Label	Primer sequence (5'–3')	Concentration (µmol/l)
D13S634F	6-FAM	GGCAGATTCAAT CGGATAAATAGA	0.12
D13S634R	–	GTAACCCCTCAG GTTCTCAAGTCT	0.12
D18S386F	HEX	TGAGTCAGGAG AATCACTTGGAAC	0.2
D18S386R	–	CTCTTCCATGAA GTAGCTAAGCAG	0.2
D18S391F	HEX	TAGACTTCACTA TTCCCATCTGAG	0.12
D18S391R	–	TAGACTTCACTA TTCCCATCTGAG	0.12
FGAF	6FAM	CCATAGGTTTTG AACTCACAG	0.2
FGAR	–	CTTCTCAGATCC TCTGACAC	0.2
MBPF	6FAM	GGACCTCGTGAA TTACAATC	0.6
MBPR	–	ATTTACCTACCT GTTCATCC	0.6

PCR, polymerase chain reaction; STR, short tandem repeat.

GLUCOSE-6-PHOSPHATE DEHYDROGENASE DEFICIENCY

Most of the polymorphic variants of glucose-6-phosphate dehydrogenase (G6PD) that are associated with acute haemolysis have been defined at the molecular level, and it may be important to distinguish these from a G6PD-deficient variant that is the cause of chronic haemolysis. Because it is an X-linked disorder, it may be difficult to identify heterozygous females, in whom levels of enzyme activity may vary from reduced to normal. This is particularly important in female relatives of men with chronic haemolytic anaemia caused by G6PD deficiency. Furthermore, G6PD deficiency can be masked by reticulocytosis in individuals with acute haemolysis (particularly in individuals with an A-variant) and in neonates.

In such cases, it may be beneficial to test for a G6PD-deficient variant by DNA analysis. Although more than 100 G6PD mutations have now been described,[47] some of the most common deficient variants are readily diagnosed by restriction enzyme digestion of the appropriate PCR products. For example, the G6PD Mediterranean mutation creates an Mbo II site in exon 6, and the two mutations found in G6PD A create an Nla III site in exon 4 and a Fok I site in exon 5 of the G6PD gene. (See also Chapter 10, p. 217.)

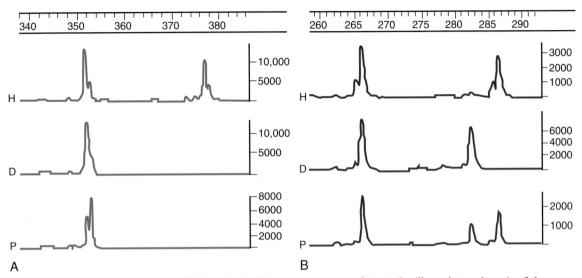

Figure 21.13   Short tandem repeat (STR) analysis of bone marrow engraftment. Capillary electrophoresis of the polymerase chain reaction (PCR) products of STR amplification as viewed by the Genotyper software. H, host DNA; D, donor DNA; P, posttransplant DNA. **Panel a:** the host and donor share an allele at 352 bp, whereas a host-specific allele is seen at 376 bp with the marker D18S386; the latter is not detected in the posttransplant sample. **Panel b:** the host and donor share an allele at 266 bp but have specific alleles at 286 and 282 bp, respectively. All three alleles are seen in the posttransplant DNA, indicating that the sample is chimeric. From the relative area under the host- and donor-specific peaks, the proportion of donor DNA is estimated at 39%.

APPENDICES: TECHNICAL METHODS

Appendix A: Extraction of Genomic DNA

Reagents

General note. For all the buffers and solutions described in this chapter, it is recommended that reagents of the highest grade available and double distilled deionised water are used throughout.

Stock Solutions

NaCl 5 mol/l. Weigh 146.1 g of NaCl into a beaker and make up the volume to 500 ml with water; stir until dissolved.

Tris-HCl, 1 mol/l, pH 8.5. Dissolve 60.5 g of Trizma base (tris[hydroxy]methylaminomethane) in 350 ml water; add concentrated HCl until the pH falls to 8.5; make up to 500 ml with water.

Tris-HCl, 1 mol/l, pH 7.4. Prepare as for the above, but reduce the pH to 7.4 with HCl.

NaOH, 5 mol/l. Add 200 g of NaOH to 800 ml water and stir until dissolved; make up to 1 litre with water.

EDTA, 0.5 mol/l, pH 8.0. Weigh 93 g of EDTA disodium salt (dihydrate) and add to 400 ml of water; stir until most of it has dissolved. Add 0.5 mol/l NaOH until the pH rises to 8.0, when the rest of the solid should go into solution. Make up to 500 ml with water.

Phosphate buffered saline (PBS), pH 7.3. See p. 690 for preparation.

Nonidet P-40 (NP40), 10%. Add 10 ml of NP40 to 90 ml water and mix well.

Sodium dodecyl sulphate (SDS, lauryl sulphate), 20%. Weigh 100 g of SDS and add to 350 ml of water. Stir and heat to 65°C until it is in solution and top up to 500 ml with water. **Caution: SDS is a respiratory irritant. Wear a face mask and weigh out in a fume hood.**

Working Solutions

PBS + 0.1% NP40. Add 5 ml of 10% NP40 to 495 ml of PBS.

Ten times concentrated (×10) lysis buffer). Mix 60 ml of 5 mol/l NaCl, 20 ml of 0.5 mol/l EDTA, 10 ml of 1 mol/l Tris pH 7.4, and 10 ml of water to give 100 ml of 3 mol/l NaCl, 100 mmol/l EDTA, and 100 mmol/l Tris.

Lysis solution. Prepare an appropriate amount of this solution fresh every time; for 50 ml weigh 21 g of urea (7 mol/l), add 5 ml of ×10 lysis buffer, and make up to a final volume of 50 ml with water.

Chloroform/isoamyl alcohol (24:1). Add 20 ml of isoamyl alcohol to 480 ml of chloroform.

Ethanol 70%. Add 30 ml of water to 70 ml of absolute ethanol.

Tris EDTA (TE) (10 mmol/l Tris, 1 mmol/l EDTA). Add 5 ml of 1 mol/l Tris pH 7.4 and 1 ml of 0.5 mol/l Na_2 EDTA to 494 ml water.

TE equilibrated phenol. The condition of the phenol is crucial to the quality of the DNA obtained. DNA is soluble in acidic water-saturated phenol, and so it is necessary to equilibrate it to a neutral pH.

1. Take 500 ml of water-saturated phenol. Prepare 500 ml of 0.5 mol/l Tris pH 8.5, add 150 ml of this to the phenol, and mix by inversion for 2–3 min. Leave to stand until the aqueous and organic phases have separated.

2. Remove and discard the upper aqueous layer. Add another 125 ml of 0.5 mol/l Tris, mix, stand, remove the aqueous layer as before, and then repeat.

3. To the remaining 100 ml of 0.5 mol/l Tris, add 400 ml of water to give 500 ml of 0.1 mol/l Tris. Add 150 ml of this to the phenol, and then mix, stand, and remove. Repeat two more times.

4. To the remaining 50 ml of 0.1 mol/l Tris add 449 ml of water and 1 ml of 0.5 mol/l EDTA to give 500 ml of TE. Add, mix, stand, and remove this in three stages as before. The phenol will have reduced in volume during this procedure but is now TE equilibrated and ready for use.

Method

1. Freeze an anticoagulated blood sample at −20°C. EDTA is the preferred anticoagulant. It is convenient to collect the blood in a tube that can be centrifuged, such as a disposable plastic 25 ml universal container. Any sample size from 2 to 20 ml will be satisfactory. Blood can be shipped at room temperature to a reference laboratory, preferably within a few days of taking it. The sample can be stored at −20°C for several weeks; storage for longer periods is better at −80°C.

2. Thaw the blood and centrifuge at 700 g for 15 min. Carefully pour off the supernatant. The pellet is hard to see at this stage and may be quite loose.

3. Resuspend the pellet in 1–2 ml of PBS + 0.1% NP40 by mixing up and down in a wide-bore standard plastic transfer pipette. Top up the suspension to the original volume with PBS + 0.1% NP40.

4. Centrifuge again at 700 g for 15 min and pour off the supernatant. If necessary, repeat until the pellet has lost most of its red colour.

5. Add 2–3 drops of lysis solution. Break up the pellet into this solution using a nonwettable sterile stick (e.g., a plastic disposable bacterial inoculating loop) or a clean siliconised glass rod. The solution will become viscous. Make it as homogeneous as possible.

6. Add successive 0.5 ml volumes of the lysis solution, mixing each time, until the viscosity is such that the solution can be pipetted up and down without difficulty. The final volume will depend on the size, nature, and quality of the blood sample. For 10 ml of freshly frozen normal blood, use 2–3 ml of lysis solution.

7. Add 1/10 volume of 20% SDS. Mix gently with a transfer pipette and incubate at 37°C for a minimum of 15 min. The samples can be left overnight at this stage.

8. Transfer the sample to a capped polypropylene tube. Add an equal volume of chloroform/isoamyl alcohol and an equal volume of phenol. Mix gently by inversion for 5 min. Centrifuge at 1300 g for 15 min.

9. Transfer the upper aqueous phase to a new polypropylene tube. Leave behind the white protein interface and the organic phase. This may be difficult if the solution is too viscous, in which case further dilution with lysis solution is necessary.

10. Repeat steps 8 and 9 at least once more and continue until the interface is clear. Add an equal volume of chloroform/isoamyl alcohol and mix gently by inversion for 5 min. Centrifuge as before and again transfer the aqueous phase to a universal or capped 10 ml tube.

11. Add 2.5 volumes of absolute ethanol. Mix the solution by inverting the tube several times. The DNA should precipitate as a "cotton wool"

ball. Using a micropipette tip, transfer the DNA to a microcentrifuge tube containing 1 ml of 70% ethanol.

12. Centrifuge in a microcentrifuge at 12,000 g for 5 min. Pour off the residual ethanol, and remove all of this with a micropipette.

13. Leave to dry on the bench for 10 min.

14. Add 50–500 μl of TE depending on the size of the pellet. Aim to have a DNA concentration of approximately 0.5 mg/ml. Leave to resuspend for at least one night. Mix gently by flicking the tube; never vortex. The DNA can be stored for long periods at 4°C or frozen at −20° C.

Extraction of DNA from Other Sources

For the analysis of Ig and TCR gene rearrangements, it is necessary to enrich a peripheral blood sample for lymphocytes prior to DNA extraction. This is achieved through the separation of mononuclear cells on Ficoll/Hypaque (or Lymphoprep). After washing the cell pellet in PBS, lysis and DNA extraction can proceed as from step 5.

DNA is extracted from bone marrow aspirates in the same way as from peripheral blood, except that before freezing they are diluted in at least 5 volumes of PBS.

Tissue biopsies vary greatly in nature, size, and cell content and, as a result, so does the quality and quantity of DNA obtained from them. To obtain sufficient quantities of high molecular weight DNA for Southern blot analysis, the biopsy must be several mm^3 in size and fresh frozen. If such a biopsy is available, sufficient cells can be obtained by mechanically disrupting it into PBS first by chopping it finely with a clean blade and then breaking it up with the blunt end of a 5 ml syringe plunger. The suspension is centrifuged to obtain a pellet, from which DNA is extracted as before (from step 5). For smaller biopsies, it is better to treat the sample with proteinase K prior to extraction, as follows:

1. Place the tissue in 700 μl of 50 mmol/l Tris-HCl, pH 8.0, 100 mmol/l NaCl, 1% (w/v) SDS containing 100 μg/ml proteinase K.

2. Cut up the tissue with a fine pair of scissors, and incubate at 50°C overnight.

3. Proceed with phenol/chloroform extraction and DNA precipitation as from step 8 earlier.

Determining the DNA Concentration

Take 5 μl of the DNA solution and dilute into 245 μl of water. Mix well by vortexing. (This DNA is to be discarded and can therefore be treated in this way.) Read the absorbance (A) in a spectrometer at 260 nm against a water blank. An A of 1.0 is obtained from a solution of DNA at a concentration of 50 μg/ml. Therefore, multiply the A reading obtained by 2500 to get the concentration of the original DNA solution in μg/ml. The ratio of the A_{260} to the A_{280} gives an indication as to the purity of the DNA solution. This ratio should be in the range of 1.7–2.0.

Appendix B: Polymerase Chain Reaction

Reagents

Taq polymerase and oligonucleotide primers. These can be purchased from a variety of different companies. The oligos are usually 18–22 bases in length.

PCR buffers. These are usually supplied along with the Taq polymerase. Three different buffers can be prepared as follows:

- *×10 PCR buffer I:* 100 mmol/l Tris-HCl, pH 8.3, 500 mmol/l KCl, 15 mmol/l $MgCl_2$, 0.1% (w/v) gelatin, 0.5% (v/v) NP40, and 0.5% (v/v) Tween 20.
- *×10 PCR buffer II:* 670 mmol/l Tris, pH 8.8, 166 mmol/l $(NH_4)_2SO_4$, 25 mmol/l $MgCl_2$, 670 μmol/l Na_2 EDTA, 1.6 mg/ml bovine serum albumin (BSA), and 100 mmol/l β-mercapto-ethanol. This buffer is used in conjunction with 10% dimethyl sulphoxide (DMSO) in the final reaction mixture.
- *×10 PCR buffer III:* 750 mmol/l Tris, pH 8.8, 200 mmol/l $(NH_4)_2SO_4$, 0.1% (v/v) Tween 20. A solution of 25 mmol/l $MgCl_2$ is also prepared and added separately to the PCR reaction.

dNTP, 10 mmol/l. Take 10 μl of 100 mmol/l dATP, 10 μl of 100 mmol/l dTTP, 10 μl of 100 mmol/l dCTP, 10 μl of 100 mmol/l dGTP, and 60 μl of water to make a 100 μl of 10 mmol/l dNTP.

DMSO.

Agarose, Type II medium electroendosmosis.

×10 Tris-borate-EDTA (TBE) buffer. Add 216 g of Trizma base, 18.6 g of EDTA, and 110 g of orthoboric acid to 1600 ml water. Dissolve and top up to 2l; dilute 1 in 20 for use as ×0.5 TBE buffer.

Ethidium bromide, 10 mg/ml. Dissolve 1 g of ethidium bromide in 100 ml of water, and keep in brown or foil-wrapped bottle. **Caution: Ethidium bromide is a known teratogen. Wear a face mask and handle with double gloves.**

Tracking dye. Weigh 15 g of Ficoll (type 400), 0.25 g of bromophenol blue, and 0.25 g of xylene cyanol. Make up to 100 ml with water, cover, and mix by inversion; it will take a considerable amount of mixing to get the solution homogeneous. Dispense into aliquots.

Method

Optimal conditions for the reaction have to be derived empirically, with the magnesium concentration and annealing temperature being the most important parameters.[48] The choice of buffer depends on the enzyme being used, and the company will usually supply the most appropriate one. For genes with a high GC content, buffer II (explained earlier) in combination with 10% DMSO may give better amplification. In most cases, a 25 μl reaction volume suffices, although 50 μl should be used if it is necessary to check whether the amplification has been successful prior to one subsequent manipulation. A blank control should always be included (i.e., a reaction without any template) to control for contamination. If the blank control yields a product, the analysis is invalidated. A DNA sample that is known to amplify can also be included, and this sample may then be used as a normal or positive control.

The risk of contamination cannot be over-emphasised. It can be minimised by using plugged tips and having dedicated micropipettes and areas for each step of the analysis. The optimum cycling conditions need to be determined for each thermocycler. Specificity is often improved by "hot start" PCR. This is achieved by setting up all the PCR tests on wet ice and transferring the tubes to the thermocycler once it reaches 95°C or by using an enzyme that only becomes activated when heated at 95°C for several minutes. In preparing a group of reactions, pipetting errors can be minimised by making a premix solution that can be dispensed into microcentrifuge tubes containing the DNA template. When a particular PCR is to be performed repetitively over a period of time, it is helpful to prepare a large volume (e.g., 10 ml) of the reaction mixture (without DNA or Taq polymerase), aliquot it, and store it at –20°C.

1. Prepare a PCR mixture for 10 reactions (with a final volume of 50 μl for each DNA sample) as follows:

Stock Solution	Vol (μl)	Final Concentration
×10 PCR buffer	50	×1
10 mmol/l dNTP	5	0.2 mmol/l
Primer (1) 10 μmol/l	10	0.2 μmol/l
Primer (2) 10 μmol/l	10	0.2 μmol/l
Taq polymerase 5 u/ml	2	0.02 u/ml
Water	–	410
Final volume	–	490

Add the Taq polymerase last, mix well, and pulse-spin in a microcentrifuge to bring down the contents of the tube.

Note. For some PCR reactions and in using PCR buffer III as explained earlier, appropriate volumes of 25 mmol/l $MgCl_2$ should be added; the correct final concentration, usually between 1.5 mmol/l and 3.0 mmol/l, should be determined empirically for each primer pair. Adjust the volume of water to compensate for this.

2. Put 1 μl of template DNA at approximately 0.5 mg/ml into each of nine 0.5 ml microcentrifuge tubes and 1 μl of double distilled water into the tenth tube. Aliquot 49 μl of the mix prepared as explained earlier into each tube.

3. Overlay the mixture with 50 μl of light paraffin oil and place the tubes in a PCR machine, programmed for the following conditions: an initial step of 5 min at 94°C and then 30 cycles of 58°C for 1 min, 72°C for 1 min, and 94°C for 1 min in sequence followed by a final extension step at 72°C for 10 min. These conditions are suitable for many primer pairs, although some will require different annealing temperatures or longer extension times.

4. While the PCR program is running, a 1.5% agarose mini-gel is prepared: add 0.75 g of agarose to 50 ml of ×0.5 TBE buffer and heat

until completely dissolved. Add 2 µl of ethidium bromide (10 mg/ml), allow the agarose to cool slightly, and pour with the appropriate comb in position.

5. To check if the amplification has been successful, add 1 µl of tracking dye to a 10 µl aliquot of the PCR reaction mixture, being careful not to pipette the mineral oil overlaying the PCR reaction.

6. Load the gel and run at a constant voltage of 100 V for 1 hour in ×0.5 TBE buffer. A molecular size marker should be included to establish the size of the amplified fragment; these are commercially available. The marker used in this chapter is the plasmid pEMBL 8 digested with Taq I and Pvu II to yield fragments of 1443, 1008, 613, 357, 278, 193, and 108 bp.

7. Visualise the DNA on an ultraviolet (UV) trans-illuminator and, if required, take a photograph.

Modifications and Developments

The procedure described earlier is a guideline for setting up and checking a standard PCR amplification. As the test dictates, modifications can be used, such as the following:

Radiolabelling. A PCR can be labelled with ^{32}P by adding 0.1 µl of $[\alpha^{32}P]dCTP$ per tube to the reaction mixture.

Multiplex. More than one fragment can be amplified in the same tube simply by adding in further primer pairs. It is important that the different pairs all work equally well under the same conditions.

Nested PCR. This involves successive rounds of amplification using two pairs of primers; the second pair, located within the sequence amplified by the first, allows products to be generated from as little as a single cell.

Long-range amplification. Fragments upward of 10 kb can now be generated by PCR using modified polymerases.

Automation. High-throughput PCR amplification is being achieved through the use of robots and 96-well plate technology.

Automated fragment analysis. The method of gel electrophoresis is modified for the detection of fluorescently labelled PCR products on DNA fragment analysers (e.g., the ABI 3700 DNA analyser).

Appendix C: Polyacrylamide Gel Electrophoresis

Equipment and Reagents

A vertical gel electrophoresis tank with appropriate plates, combs, and spacers.
A slab gel dryer with vacuum pump.
40% (w/v) acrylamide solution.
Caution: Acrylamide is a potent neurotoxin.
2% (w/v) bis-acrylamide solution.
Glycerol.
Urea (ultrapure).
10% (w/v) ammonium persulphate.
TEMED.
×10 TBE buffer (see Appendix B).
Formamide dye. To 10 ml deionised formamide, add 10 mg xylene cyanol FF, 10 mg bromophenol blue, and 200 µl of 0.5 mol/l EDTA.

Method

The following procedure describes the preparation of a large, thin (34 cm × 40 cm × 0.4 mm) 6% denaturing polyacrylamide gel.

1. Clean the glass plates thoroughly with detergent and a scourer. Rinse well and dry. Swab the larger plate with 100% ethanol. Treat one surface of the smaller plate with a siliconising solution or a nontoxic gel coating solution (e.g., Gel Slick from FMC) by applying a few ml and buffing dry with a paper towel. Assemble the gel using spacers, bulldog clips, and electrical tape around the bottom of the gel. Ensure that the gaskets closely abut the smaller plate.

2. Mix 12 ml of 40% acrylamide, 12 ml 2% bis-acrylamide, 8 ml ×10 TBE, and 36.8 g urea, and adjust the volume to 80 ml with double distilled water. Add 500 µl of 10% ammonium persulphate and 50 µl of TEMED; mix and pour the solution slowly between the glass plates using a 50 ml syringe. When full, insert an inverted shark's tooth comb (smooth surface downward) no more than 6 mm into the gel. Leave to polymerise.

3. Remove the electrical tape and bulldog clips and place the gel in the electrophoresis tank. Fill the top and bottom chambers with ×1 TBE. Remove the comb, and flush the surface of the gel with TBE buffer using a syringe and bent needle. Clean and invert the comb and insert it between

the plates until the teeth just indent the surface of the gel.

4. Mix 1–4 µl of the radiolabelled PCR product with 6 µl of formamide dye. Heat at 95°C for 5 min. Snap chill on wet ice. Flush out each well using TBE buffer and load 5 µl of each sample between the teeth. Run the gel at 40–60 V until the appropriate resolution has been obtained. (As a guide, the bromophenol blue and xylene cyanol will comigrate with 25 bp and 105 bp DNA fragments, respectively, in a 6% denaturing polyacrylamide gel).

5. Disconnect the power supply, remove the plates, and place them on a flat surface. Pull one of the spacers out from between the plates. Insert a metal spatula or a fine plastic wedge horizontally into the gap between the plates at the bottom corner where the spacer was. Lift the smaller siliconised plate off the gel. Cut a piece of 3 MM Whatman paper so that it is slightly larger than the gel area, and lay it down onto the gel. Return the smaller plate over the Whatman paper, apply gentle pressure, and invert the plates. Carefully pull up the larger plate, ensuring that the gel sticks to the Whatman paper. Cover the gel with cling film (e.g., Saran Wrap) and trim all the edges.

6. Dry the gel under vacuum at 80°C for about 1 hour. Peel off the cling film and expose the gel to X-ray film overnight at –80°C to obtain an autoradiograph.

For SSCP analysis, a nondenaturing gel is used. The procedure is the same as described earlier, but the composition of the gel is different. The following gel mix can be used for a large gel run overnight at 8–12 mA in a cool (20–22°C) laboratory: 12 ml of 40% acrylamide, 2.4 ml of 2% bis-acrylamide, 4 ml glycerol, 8 ml of ×10 TBE, and 53.6 ml water. Variations are often introduced to increase the chances of observing aberrant mobilities (or shifts) of mutant DNA strands. These include altering the content of the gel such as the % of glycerol and the % of the acrylamide and the acrylamide:bis-acrylamide ratio used as well as applying variations in the temperature and speed of electrophoresis.

As an alternative to using ^{32}P-labelled PCR reactions, it is possible to visualise the DNA products in these polyacrylamide gels by silver staining using a method such as that described as follows.

Silver Staining of DNA in Polyacrylamide Gels (Courtesy of Dr. P. Goncalves)

1. Dismantle the gel and fix it by soaking it in 100 ml of 10% acetic acid for 20 min at room temperature, preferably on a shaking platform.

2. Pour off the acetic acid and keep it. Wash the gel with water, ×3 for 2 min.

3. Incubate for 30 min at room temperature with a silver nitrate reagent composed of 0.1 g silver nitrate, 150 µl of 37% (v/v) formaldehyde, and water to a final volume of 100 ml.

4. Pour off and wash for 30 s with water.

5. Add 100 ml of a sodium carbonate reagent: make 200 ml 3% (w/v) Na_2CO_3 and just prior to use add 300 µl 37% (v/v) formaldehyde and 40 µl of 10 mg/ml sodium thiosulphate. Incubate with agitation until the bands begin to appear.

6. Pour off, and add the remaining 100 ml of the sodium carbonate solution. When the bands are clearly visible, pour off this solution and stop the reaction by adding back the 100 ml 10% acetic acid that was kept from step 2.

Appendix D: Restriction Enzyme Digestion of Polymerase Chain Reaction Products

Reagents

A number of companies now supply a comprehensive list of restriction enzymes (RE), but they may vary greatly in their cost. Those that are in regular use are generally quite inexpensive compared with the more specialised enzymes that are used only occasionally and that may be 10–100 times more expensive. RE buffers are now almost always supplied with each RE. Buffer compositions are always given and will vary from enzyme to enzyme. Many commonly used REs cut perfectly well in a single "universal" buffer. This is prepared using the following stock solutions:

Tris-acetate, 2 mol/l, pH 7.5. Dissolve 24.2 g of Trizma base in 60 ml of water, adjust the pH to 7.5 with glacial acetic acid and make up to 100 ml.

Potassium acetate, 2 mol/l. Weigh out 19.62 g, make up to 100 ml with water and dissolve.

Magnesium acetate, 2 mol/l. Weigh out 42.89 g, make up to 100 ml with water and dissolve.

BSA fraction V (molecular biology grade). 20 mg/ml.

Dithiothreitol (DTT), 0.5 mol/l. Weigh out 0.771 g,

make up to 10 ml with water, dissolve, and store at −20°C.

Spermidine (N-(3-aminopropyl)-1, 4-butane-diamine), 1 mol/l. Weigh out 1.273 g, make up to 10 ml with water, dissolve, and store at −20°C.

×10 RE buffer. For a ×10 concentrated buffer, prepare a solution that is 300 mmol/l Tris-acetate, pH 7.5, 660 mmol/l potassium acetate, 100 mmol/l magnesium acetate, 1 mg/ml BSA, 10 mmol/l DTT, and 30 mmol/l spermidine; aliquot into micro-centrifuge tubes and store at −20°C.

Method

1. Transfer 30 µl of the amplified product to another microcentrifuge tube, being careful not to transfer any of the mineral oil. Add 4 µl of ×10 restriction enzyme buffer, 4.5 µl of double-distilled water, and 2–5 units of the appropriate restriction enzyme (usually 0.5 µl), giving a final volume of 40 µl.

2. Incubate at 37°C (or other temperature as specified by the manufacturer) for a minimum of 4 hours. In preparing more than one digestion with the same restriction enzyme, sufficient buffer, enzyme, and water can be premixed and dispensed into microcentrifuge tubes before adding 30 ml of the PCR product.

3. Pour a 3.0% agarose mini gel in a taped casting tray with the appropriate comb. The gel is made up of 1:1 mixture of type II medium electroen-dosmosis agarose and Nusieve agarose (from FMC Bioproducts)—that is, 0.75 g of agarose and 0.75 g of Nusieve agarose in 50 ml of half-strength (×0.5) TBE buffer (see Appendix B).

4. After the incubation period, add 3 µl of tracking dye to the digests and load the samples on to the gel. The electrophoresis is continued until a clear separation of all the expected fragments is achieved, which may be checked at intervals by placing the gel on a UV transilluminator.

Appendix E: Reverse Transcriptase Polymerase Chain Reaction

Reagents

×10 concentrated red cell lysis buffer (RCLB). For 3 l, weigh 248.7 g of NH$_4$Cl (1.55 mol/l), 30.03 g of KHCO$_3$ (0.1 mol/l). Add 6 ml of 0.5 mol/l EDTA (0.1 mmol/l), pH 7.4, and make up to 3 l with sterile water and store at 4°C.

RCLB. Make 500 ml of ×10 RCLB up to 5 l with sterile water and cool to 4°C. Adjust the working solution pH to 7.4 with HCl, and store at 4°C.

1 mol/l citrate, pH 7.0. Neutralize 1 mol/l trisodium citrate with 1 mol/l citric acid.

Sodium acetate. 3 mol/l sodium acetate is adjusted to pH 5.2 with glacial acetic acid.

Guanidinium thiocynate (GTC). Because GTC is highly toxic, it is advisable to use the entire amount as purchased from the manufacturer, rather than weighing a required amount. Thus, with 1 kg of GTC add 21.15 ml of 0.5 mol/l EDTA (5.0 mmol/l), pH 8.0, 52.87 ml of 1 mol/l citrate, pH 7.0, 35.25 ml of 30% sarcosyl (0.5%) and make up to 2.115 l with sterile water. Store this solution in 50 ml aliquots. Add 7.1 µl of β-mercapto-ethanol per ml of GTC immediately before use.

Solutions for the complementary DNA Mix

5 mg/ml random hexamer primers: reconstitute 50 U pdN$_6$ (Pharmacia) with 539 µl of sterile water and add 21 µl of 0.5 mol/l KCl.

5′ RT-buffer (usually supplied) with M-MLV reverse transcriptase (RT): 0.25 mol/l Tris-HCl, pH 8.3, 0.375 mmol/l KCl, 15 mmol/l MgCl$_2$.

25 mM dNTP stock: Mix an equal volume of ultrapure 100 mmol/l dATP, dCTP, dGTP, and dTTP 0.1 M dithiothreitol (DTT), which is usually supplied with M-MLV RT.

cDNA mix: To 428 µl of 5′ RT-buffer, add 21.5 µl of DTT, 85.5 µl of 25 mmol/l dNTPs, and 45 µl of 5 mg/ml random hexamers; make up to 1000 µl with sterile water.

The composition for the multiplex and nested PCR mixes are given in Table 21.4, including the optimum MgCl$_2$ concentration for each mix as well as the primers used in the different PCR reactions.

Methods

Nuclear Lysate Preparation

1. Either blood or bone marrow aspirate can be analysed for MRD in CML, although bone marrow aspirates are preferred for ALL MRD studies. Centrifuge the anticoagulated peripheral blood sample at 700 g for 15 min. Bone marrow

aspirates can be dealt with in the same way as buffy coats by proceeding directly to step 4.

2. Carefully remove and discard the plasma, taking care not to disturb the buffy coat.

3. Using a sterile plastic Pasteur pipette, collect the buffy coat and transfer it to a 50 ml polypropylene tube. It is not necessary to collect all of the buffy coat layer if the white cell count is >50 × 10^9/l.

4. To lyse the contaminating red cells, resuspend the buffy coat in ice-cold RCLB to a final volume of 50 ml, and vortex for a few seconds. The suspension is then incubated on wet ice for 10 min, inverting the tube occasionally.

5. Centrifuge again at 700 g for 10 min and discard the supernatant by inverting the tube, taking care not to lose the nuclear pellet.

6. Repeat steps 4 and 5 until the nuclear pellet is void of pink-red colour. Usually two washes with RCLB are sufficient.

7. Wash the nuclear pellet once with 20–30 ml PBS by centrifuging at 700 g for 10 min.

8. Resuspend the nuclear-pellet in 1–2 ml GTC containing β-mercaptoethanol. Homogenize the suspension by passing it through a 2 ml syringe and 21G needle repeatedly until it loses its viscosity (i.e., the DNA is degraded). In some cases, it may be necessary to add more GTC.

9. The lysate can now be stored at –20°C or –70°C for several years.

RNA Extraction

There are several protocols, including commercially available kits, yielding RNA of varying qualities. The protocol described in the following, originally described by Chomczynski and Sacchi,[49] can easily be applied in a clinical laboratory.

1. Add 50 μl of 2 M NaOAc pH 4.0 to 500 μl of GTC lysate in a 1.5 ml microcentrifuge tube and vortex briefly.

2. Add 500 μl of un-neutralised water saturated phenol and 100 μl of chloroform. Vortex the mixture for 10 s and transfer to wet ice for 20 min.

3. Centrifuge at 12,000 g for 30 min at 4°C.

4. After centrifugation, two distinct layers should be clearly discernible; if not, add a further 50 ml of chloroform. Vortex for 10 s and centrifuge again for 30 min at 4°C. Transfer the upper aqueous layer to another 1.5 ml microcentrifuge tube, taking care not to disturb the interface.

5. Add an equal volume of propan-2-ol (isopropanol), cap the tube, mix by inverting, and incubate at –20°C for 2 hours or overnight.

6. Microcentrifuge for 30 min at 4°C and discard the supernatant, taking care not to lose the pellet, which may be hard to see.

7. Wash the pellet in 1 ml of 80% ethanol. Do not mix. Centrifuge directly for 30 min at 4°C, and discard the supernatant. Recentrifuge briefly to collect the residual ethanol and discard using a micropipette.

8. Air dry the pellet for 10 min and reconstitute in 20–40 μl of sterile water. The RNA must be stored at –70°C. However, immediate reverse transcription is the preferred option.

cDNA Synthesis

1. Incubate 19 μl of RNA in a 1.5 ml microcentrifuge tube (approximately 20 μg) at 65°C for 10 min. This is to denature the RNA, which readily forms secondary structures reducing the efficiency of the reverse transcriptase. Centrifuge at 12,000 g briefly to collect the condensation to the bottom of the tube. Transfer the tube to wet ice.

2. On the wet ice, add 21 μl of cDNA mix containing 300 U M-MLV RT and 30 U of RNasin.

3. Incubate the mixture at 37°C for 2 hours. When using gene-specific primers in this reaction, the temperature should be increased to 42°C.

4. Terminate the reaction by incubating the mixture at 65°C for 10 min. cDNA can be stored at –20°C.

Multiplex PCR

Add 2 μl of cDNA to 20 μl of multiplex PCR mix (see Table 21.4); add 0.5 U of Taq polymerase. Overlay with 1 drop of mineral oil and amplify using conditions as described in Appendix B. Carry out electrophoresis on the PCR products through 2.0% agarose gel containing ethidium bromide.

Nested PCR

1. Add 5 μl cDNA to 20 μl first-step PCR mix (see Table 21.4) and add 0.75 U Taq polymerase. Overlay with mineral oil and amplify. The PCR cycling conditions used are as in Appendix B except that the annealing temperature is set at 68°C for 25 s.

2. Transfer 1 μl of the PCR products from the first step to 19 μl of the second step PCR mix (see Table 21.4). Overlay with 1 drop of mineral oil and amplify using an annealing temperature of 64°C for 50 s. Then electrophorese the PCR products through 2.0% agarose gel containing ethidium bromide. The procedure for nested PCR is the same as for p210 (b3a2 and b2a2) and p190 (e1a2).

Appendix F: Real-Time Quantitative PCR

Reagents

×2 *Universal master mix.* The ×2 Universal Master mix contains dATP, dCTP, dGTP, and dTTP at 200 μmol/l each, 5.5 mmol/l MgCl$_2$, and 0.025 μmol/l AmpliTaq-Gold. It also contains the passive background reference dye, ROX. The Universal master mix can be purchased with or without uracil DNA glycosylase, which degrades any PCR contaminating products prior to starting the PCR by heating the plate to 95°C for 10 min (see later). It is possible to assemble master mixes by purchasing various components, such as dNTP, Buffer, MgCl$_2$, and hot start *Taq* DNA polymerase. However, in-house preparation of master mixes is not recommended to minimise intraassay and interassay variation and contamination, essential for monitoring patients response to therapy.

Probe-Primer mix. For convenience and to minimise interassay variation a bulk preparation of the QR-PCR assay mix, containing the probes and

Table 21.4 Composition of PCR mixes used in the amplification of BCR–ABL to create restriction enzyme recognition sites

	Multiplex PCR	Nested PCR			
		p210		p190	
		1st step	2nd Step	1st step	2nd Step
PCR buffer (×10)	1.2×	1.25×	1.0×	1.25×	1.0×
MgCl$_2$ (mmol/l)	1.8	3.125	1.75	2.25	1.75
dNTP (μmol/l)	240	250	200	250	200
Primer 1 (μmol/l)	C5e– (0.6)	NB1 + (0.625)	CA3– (0.5)	BCR 1+ (0.625)	CA3– (0.5)
Primer 2 (μmol/l)	CA3– (0.6)	Abl3– (0.625)	B2A (0.5)	Ab13– (0.625)	E1N+ (0.5)
Primer 3 (μmol/l)	B2B (0.6)				
Primer 4 (μmol/l)	BCR-C (0.6)				
Primer sequences are as follows:					
BCR1+: 5′ GAACTCGCAACAGTCCTTCGAC 3′					
BCR-C: 5′ ACCGCATGTTCCGGGACAAAAG 3′					
*C5e–: 5′ ataggaTCCTTTGCAACCGGGTCTGAA 3′					
NB1+: 5′ GAGCGTGCAGAGTGGAGGGAGAACA 3′					
Ab13–: 5′ GGTACCAGGAGTGTTTCTCCAGACTG 3′					
B2A: 5′ TTCAGAAGCTTCTCCCTGACAT 3′					
CA3–: 5′ TGTTGACTGGCGTGATGTAGTTGCTTGG 3′					
E1N+: 5′ AGATCTGGCCCAACGATGACGA 3′					

PCR, polymerase chain reaction.
*Lowercase letters represent changes introduced to create restriction enzyme site.

primers at required concentration, minus the Master Mix, is recommended. The mixture is stored at −20°C or −70°C. This also avoids repeated freezing and thawing of probes and primers because this may affect the probe-primer integrity. Furthermore, the probe should not be left exposed for prolonged periods to direct sunlight because this leads to degradation. In general 300 nmol/l of each primer and 200 nmol/l of probe permits optimum QR-PCR sensitivity; however, this should be determined for each assay by titrating one primer against the other. The optimum concentration of the primers is one that gives the lowest Ct. Similarly; the optimum probe concentration is determined by varying the quantity of the probe. The quantity yielding the lowest Ct is the optimum probe concentration. The probe-primer mixture is then prepared using the determined optimum concentrations. The mixture can then be aliquoted into micro-centrifuge tubes for a required number of samples, allowing for standards and positive and negative controls. Furthermore, for MRD studies it is advisable to measure the target gene in replicates of three to minimise sampling error at low copy number values. Because the endogenous control gene copy number is expected, assays in duplicate will suffice. However, standards for the endogenous control should be performed in triplicate.

Designing probe and primers. The probe and primers are designed using Primer Express Software (Applied Biosystems, Foster City, CA). Optimum design of probes and primers is critical to sensitivity of QR-PCR. The probe is designed such that it has higher T_m than the primers and works optimally at default PCR conditions settings using the universal master mix. The probe should not have a guanine base at the 3′ end, and the number of guanine bases should be fewer than cytosine bases. Furthermore, there should not be more than 4 guanine bases in tandem. Similar rules apply to design of primers. The annealing temperature of the probe should be 10°C greater than that of the primers. It is essential to design probes and primers such that the assay is RNA specific. This is achieved by positioning the forward and reverse primers in separate exons or by placing either of the primers or the probe across a splice site.

Standard Curve. It is acceptable to report data as Ct, with an increase of 3.3 being clinically significant, because this represents 1 log increase in *BCR–ABL* copies; it takes 3.3 cycles for every log increase in amplicons. For clinical samples, however, it is essential to generate a standard curve from which unknowns can be calculated. The standard curve can be generated using serially diluted cDNA derived from a cell line expressing the target gene at high levels (e.g., K562 for *BCR–ABL).* As an alternative to using cDNA, a plasmid can be used to create this curve, which provides stability over time. The method of preparation of the plasmid is beyond the scope of this book. Serially diluted plasmids for commonly occurring fusion genes and endogenous control genes are commercially available. In the absence of a standard curve the MRD values are reported as a delta-delta Ct ($\Delta\Delta$Ct). This is calculated by first normalising the fusion gene Ct (CtFG) to the control gene (CtCG) to obtain a ΔCt for the follow-up samples—that is, the ΔCt(follow-up) = Ct_{FG} − Ct_{CG}. The same calculation is performed for the Ct value for the sample taken at diagnosis to obtain a ΔCt(diagnosis). The ΔCt(diagnosis) is then subtracted from the ΔCt(follow-up) to obtain a $\Delta\Delta$Ct. From this the MRD value is calculated as $10^{\Delta\Delta Ct/3.3}$. To apply the $\Delta\Delta$Ct method of reporting the slope and intercept values for the control and fusion genes must be similar. More precisely it is recommended that the slope values for the fusion and control gene should not differ by more than 0.01 (i.e., the PCR efficiency for CG and FG are similar). The major advantage of using $\Delta\Delta$Ct is it obviates the need for a standard curve. Therefore, eliminating the need for a plasmid- or RNA-based standard curve reduces the risk of contamination further and frees microtitre plate wells for patient samples.

PCR cycling conditions. It is convenient to design the probes and primers so that they are able to work efficiently using standard QR-PCR conditions to amplify the cDNA, which are 2 min at 50°C (to allow uracil DNA glycosylase-mediated elimination of exogenous PCR product contamination), an enzyme heat-activation step of 10 min at 95°C, followed by 50 cycles of 15 s at 95°C for denaturation and 1 min at 60°C for annealing and extension.

Method

The QR-PCR assay is normally performed in 96-well microtitre plates in a 25 μl final reaction volume containing universal master mix. The composition of a 25 μl Q-PCR reaction is shown in Table 21.5.

1. Dispense 20 μl of QR-PCR mixture into the required number of microtitre wells. To minimise intersample differences an 8 channel automatic pipette is recommended to dispense the Q-PCR assay mix. Note the location of each sample, including the standards and controls, on a grid map in which each of the 96 wells is represented.
2. Using the grid map, add 5 μl of the appropriate cDNA or standard to each well.
3. To the No Template Control wells genomic DNA is included in mRNA-based studies. Add HL60 cell line derived cDNA to the No Amplification Control wells for *BCR–ABL* QR-PCR assays because this cell line does not express this fusion gene.
4. Also included are cDNA derived from K562 and BV173 cell lines diluted to give a known number of copies.
5. On dispensing all the samples, secure the wells with optical caps or a film adhesive.
6. Centrifuge the plate for 2–3 seconds at 1000 rpm to collect all the contents to the bottom of the wells and expel any trapped bubbles prior to placing it in the instrument.
7. Initiate the run as per manufacturer's instructions, adjusting the sample volume and number of cycles accordingly. The plate is normally subjected to between 40 and 50 cycles.
8. On completion, assign the microtitre wells as per Grid map and analyse the assay as per the manufacturer's instructions.

The instrument sets the threshold at ×10 the standard deviation of baseline emission; however this can be reset manually within the exponential phase of the PCR to avoid any background fluorescent interference. Alternatively, the threshold can be set at the same value for each assay, for instance, at 0.05, assuming this is within the exponential phase of PCR, thus avoiding operator variation. The data for any samples with a Ct greater than 38 are considered unreliable.

The baseline limits are set by the instrument; however, this should be adjusted so that the upper limit of the baseline is 4 cycles less than the lowest Ct value for a sample. For example, if the lowest Ct is 20, then the upper baseline limit is set at 16, thus giving a clear margin between the baseline and the samples. The lower limit set by instrument rarely requires adjusting.

The standard curve is generated and accepted if the slope value is between –3.3 and –3.6. A slope value of –3.3 represents 100% PCR efficiency because it takes 3.3 cycles for every log increase

Table 21.5	25 μl Q-PCR assay			
Stock solution	**Concentration**	**Volume (μl)**	**Volume (μl, 110 reactions)**	**Working concentration**
Universal Master Mix	×2	12.5	1375	×1
Forward primer	80 μmol/l	0.094	10.31	300 nmol/l
Reverse primer	189 μmol/l	0.04	4.37	300 nmol/l
Dual-labelled probe	20 μmol/l	0.125	13.75	100 nmol/l
Complementary DNA	–	5.0	–	–
Sterile water	–	7.24	796.6	–

Q-PCR, quantitative polymerase chain reaction.
The volumes for bulk preparation of probe-primer mix are indicated; these are sufficient for 96 samples (i.e., 96 well microtitre plate) and allow for pipetting. The Universal Master Mix is added just prior to setting up the Q-PCR.

in PCR products. Ideally the curve correlation coefficient should not be less than 0.98. If the standard curve is acceptable, then the copy number for the samples can be recorded. The QR-PCR for the endogenous control gene is performed similarly using the appropriate probes and primers. On completion of QR-PCR for target and endogenous control, the data are reported as a percentage ratio (i.e., *BCR–ABL:ABL* × 100).

Notes

To minimise sampling error, the target gene and the standards are assayed in triplicate. It is essential to include positive controls with a known number of transcripts. To minimise risk of contamination the patients' samples and standards should be handled in geographically separate locations. Because QR-PCR assays are *BCR–ABL* transcript-type specific it is essential to perform a multiplex PCR on presentation sample to assign the transcript type expressed by the patient (see Appendix E). This ensures that correct QR-PCR assay is used. A QR-PCR assay designed for b2a2 or b3a2, now referred to as e13a2 and e14a2, respectively, would give rise to false-negative data in patients expressing e13a3 and/or e14a3. A single QR-PCR for e13a2 and e14a2 is recommended rather than two separate assays for e13a2 and e14a2. This is achieved by designing the assay such that the probe and reverse primer map to the second exon (i.e., a2) of the ABL gene and the forward primer maps to the e13 exon (i.e., b2) of the BCR gene (see Fig. 21.10). Apart from being cost effective and efficient, it increases the accuracy of the assay because a significant minority of patients with single nucleotide polymorphism in exon 13 of the BCR gene have the potential to express both e13a2 and e14a2.

GLOSSARY

Alleles. Alternate forms of a gene found at a particular locus (e.g., β^A, β^S and β^{thal}). There may be many different alleles in a population but two at the most in one individual.

Base pair (bp). A single pairing of the nucleotides A with T or G with C in a DNA double helix (in RNA, A pairs with U).

complementary DNA (cDNA). A DNA molecule complementary to an RNA molecule, usually synthesised *in vitro* by the enzyme reverse transcriptase (RT).

Clone, cellular. The progeny of a single cell. Cells belonging to the same clone are referred to as a monoclonal cell population.

Clone, molecular. A large number of identical DNA molecules, usually obtained by propagation of a single plasmid or bacteriophage molecule in bacteria.

Codon. A triplet of nucleotides that codes for an amino acid or a termination signal.

Deletion. A mutation caused by the removal of a sequence of DNA, with the regions on either side being joined together.

Exon. A segment of a gene that codes for protein.

Gene. The unit of inheritance. In biochemical terms, a gene specifies the structure of a protein, which is the gene product. In molecular terms, a gene is a stretch of DNA that is transcribed in one block, a transcription unit.

Genomic clone. A molecular clone consisting of a portion of cellular DNA.

Genotype. The genetic constitution of an individual.

Heterozygote. An individual with two different alleles at a particular locus.

Hybridization. The pairing of complementary RNA or DNA strands to give an RNA–DNA hybrid or a DNA duplex.

Intron. A segment of a gene that is transcribed but is removed in the mature messenger RNA (mRNA) and therefore does not code for protein.

Linkage. The coinheritance of genes as a result of their neighbouring location on the same chromosome.

Locus. The position on a chromosome where a particular gene is located.

Mutation. A change in the sequence of genomic DNA.

Northern blotting. A technique for transferring RNA from an agarose gel to a nitrocellulose or nylon filter on which it can be recognised by a suitable probe.

Oligonucleotide (Oligo). A short, single-stranded DNA molecule, usually synthesised *in vitro*.

Phenotype. The appearance of an individual person or cell. In relation to a particular genetic character, the phenotype reflects the genotype conferring that character plus the effects of the environment.

Plasmid. An autonomously replicating extrachromosomal circular DNA molecule (e.g., pBR322 and pUC19).

Point mutation. A change of a single base pair in DNA.

Polymerase chain reaction (PCR). A technique for amplifying an individual DNA sequence *in vitro*. The reaction is primed by using specific oligonucleotides.

Primers. Oligonucleotides used to initiate DNA synthesis *in vitro* by the enzyme DNA polymerase.

Probe. A fragment of DNA that can be used to hybridize to a specific DNA sequence or RNA molecule.

Recombinant DNA. Any DNA molecule constructed artificially by bringing together DNA segments of different origin.

Restriction enzymes. Enzymes that recognize short DNA sequences (usually 4 or 6 bp) and cut the DNA wherever those sequences are found (e.g., BamH I, Bgl II, EcoR I, Hind III, Pst I and Sac I). These sequences are called restriction sites.

Southern blotting. The procedure for transferring denatured DNA from an agarose gel to a nitrocellulose or nylon filter, where it can be recognised by an appropriate probe.

Vector. A DNA molecule capable of replication and specifically engineered to facilitate the cloning of another DNA molecule of interest.

REFERENCES

1. International Human Genome Sequencing Consortium 2001 Initial sequencing and analysis of the human genome. Nature 409:860–921.
2. Venter JC, Adams MD, Myers EW, et al 2001 The sequence of the human genome. Science 291:1304–1351.
3. Saiki RK, Gelfand DH, Stoffel S, et al 1988 Primer-directed enzymatic amplification of DNA with a thermostable DNA polymerase. Science 239:487–491.
4. Sambrook J, Russell DW 2001 Molecular cloning. A laboratory manual, 3rd ed. Cold Spring Harbor Laboratory Press, Cold Spring Harbor, New York.
5. Association for Molecular Pathology statement. 1999 Recommendations for in-house development and operation of molecular diagnostic tests. American Journal of Clinical Pathology 111:449–463.
6. Schwartz MK 1999 Genetic testing and the clinical laboratory improvement amendments of 1988: present and future. Clinical Chemistry 45:739–745.
7. Williams LO, Cole EC, Lubin IM, et al 2003 Quality assurance in human molecular genetics testing: status and recommendations. Archives of Pathology and Laboratory Medicine 127:1353–1358.
8. Sykes BC 1983 DNA in heritable disease. Lancet ii:787–788.
9. Newton CR, Graham A, Heptinstall LE, et al 1989 Analysis of any point mutation in DNA. The amplification refractory mutation system (ARMS). Nucleic Acids Research 17:2503–2516.
10. Old JM, Varawalla NY, Weatherall DJ 1990 Rapid detection and prenatal diagnosis of β-thalassaemia: studies in Indian and Cypriot populations in the U.K. Lancet 336:834–837.
11. Wallace RB, Shaffer J, Murphy RF, et al 1979 Hybridization of synthetic oligodeoxyribonucleotides to PhiX174 DNA: the effect of single base pair mismatch. Nucleic Acids Research 6:3543–3547.
12. Saiki RK, Chang CA, Levenson CH, et al 1988 Diagnosis of sickle cell anemia and beta-thalassemia with enzymatically amplified DNA and non-radioactive allele specific oligonucleotide probes. New England Journal of Medicine 319:537–541.
13. Kawasaki E, Saiki R, Erlich H 1993 Genetic analysis using polymerase chain reaction-amplified DNA and immobilised oligonucleotide probes: reverse dot-blot typing. Methods in Enzymology 218:369–381.
14. Old J 1996 Haemoglobinopathies. Prenatal Diagnosis 16:1181–1186.
15. Clark BE, Thein SL 2004 Molecular diagnosis of haemoglobin disorders. Clinical and Laboratory Haematology 26:159–176.
16. Liu YT, Old JM, Miles K, et al 2000 Rapid detection of alpha-thalassaemia deletions and alpha-globin triplication by multiplex polymerase chain reactions. British Journal of Haematology 108:295–299.
17. Bain BJ, Chapman C 1998 A survey of current United Kingdom practice for antenatal screening for inherited disorders of globin chain synthesis. UK Forum for Haemoglobin Disorders. Journal of Clinical Pathology 51:382–389.
18. Cumming AM, Shiach CR 1999 The investigation and management of inherited thrombophilia. Clinical and Laboratory Haematology 21:77–92.
19. Poort SR, Rosendaal FR, Reitsma PH, et al 1996 A common genetic variation in the 3′-untranslated region of the prothrombin gene is associated with elevated plasma prothrombin levels and an increase in venous thrombosis. Blood 88:3698–3703.

20. Bertina RM, Koeleman BP, Koster T, et al 1994 Mutation in blood coagulation factor V associated with resistance to activated protein C. Nature 369:64–67.

21. Greaves M, Baglin T 2000 Laboratory testing for heritable thrombophilia: impact on clinical management of thrombotic disease annotation. British Journal of Haematology 109:699–703.

22. Vidal F, Farssac E, Altisent C, et al 2001 Rapid hemophilia A molecular diagnosis by a simple DNA sequencing procedure: identification of 14 novel mutations. Thrombosis and Haemostasis 85:580–583.

23. Lakich D, Kazazian HH Jr, Antonarakis SE, et al 1993 Inversions disrupting the factor VIII gene are a common cause of severe haemophilia A. Nature Genetics 5:236–241.

24. Wion KL, Tuddenham EGD, Lawn R 1986 A new polymorphism in the factor VIII gene for prenatal diagnosis of haemophilia A. Nucleic Acids Research 14:4535–4542.

25. Liu Q, Nozari G, Sommer SS 1998 Single-tube polymerase chain reaction for rapid diagnosis of the inversion hotspot of mutation in hemophilia A. Blood 92:1458–1459.

26. Secker-Walker LM, Craig JM, Hawkins JM, et al 1991 Philadelphia-positive acute lymphoblastic leukaemia in adults: age distribution. BCR-breakpoint and prognostic significance. Leukaemia 5:196–199.

27. Macintyre EA, Delabesse E 1999 Molecular approaches to the diagnosis and evaluation of lymphoid malignancies. Seminars in Hematology 36:373–389.

28. Biondi A, Rambaldi A, Pandolfi PP, et al 1992 Molecular monitoring of the myl/retinoic acid receptor-α fusion gene in acute promyelocytic leukaemia by polymerase chain reaction. Blood 80:492–497.

29. Delabesse E, Asnafi V, Macintyre E 2003 Application of molecular biology techniques to malignant haematology. Transfusion Clinique et Biologique 10:335–352.

30. Cross NCP, Melo JV, Lin F, et al 1994 An optimised multiplex polymerase chain reaction for detection of BCR–ABL fusion mRNAs in haematological disorders. Leukaemia 8:186–189.

31. Lin F, Goldman JM, Cross NCP 1994 A comparison of the sensitivity of blood and bone marrow for the detection of minimal residual disease in chronic myeloid leukaemia. British Journal of Haematology 86:683–685.

32. Cross NCP, Lin F, Chase A et al 1993. Competitive polymerase chain reaction to estimate the number of BCR–ABL transcripts in chronic myeloid leukaemia after bone marrow transplantation. Blood 82:1929–1936.

33. Gabert J, Beillard E, van der Velden et al 2003. Standardization and quality control studies of "real-time" quantitative reverse transcriptase polymerase chain reaction of fusion gene transcripts for residual disease detection in leukemia—a Europe Against Cancer program. Leukaemia 17:2318–2357.

34. Menisk E, van de Locht A. Schattenberg A 1998 Quantification of minimal residual disease in Philadelphia chromosome positive chronic myeloid leukaemia patients using real-time quantitative RT-PCR. British Journal of Haematology 102:768–774.

35. Holland PM, Abramson RD, Watson R, et al 1991 Detection of specific polymerase chain reaction product by utilising the 5′-3′ exonuclease activity of Thermus aquaticus DNA polymerase. Proceedings of the National Academy of Science 88:7276–7280.

36. Livak KJ, Flood SJ, Marmaro J, et al 1995 Oligonucleotides with fluorescent dyes at opposite ends provide a quenched probe system useful for detecting PCR product and nucleic acid hybridization. PCR Methods Application 4:357–362.

37. Kaeda J, Chase A, Goldman JM 2002 Cytogenetic and molecular monitoring of residual disease in chronic myeloid leukaemia. Acta Haematologica 107:64–75.

38. Hochhaus A, Lin F, Reiter A, et al 1996 Quantification of residual disease in chronic myeloid leukaemia on interferon—alpha therapy by competitive polymerase chain reaction. Blood 87:1549–1555.

39. Hughes T, Kaeda J, Branford S et al 2003 For the International Randomised Study of Interferon Versus STI571 (IRIS) Study Group. Frequency of Major Molecular Responses to Imatinib or Interferon Alfa plus Cytarabine in Newly Diagnosed Chronic Myeloid Leukaemia. New England Journal of Medicine 349:1397–1431.

40. van Dongen JJ, Langerak AW, Bruggemann M, et al 2003 Design and standardization of PCR primers and protocols for detection of clonal immunoglobulin and T-cell receptor gene recombinations in suspect lymphoproliferations: report of the BIOMED-2 Concerted Action BMH4-CT98-3936. Leukaemia 17:2257–2317.

41. Deane M, Norton JD 1990 Detection of immunoglobulin gene rearrangement in B lymphoid malignancies by polymerase chain

reaction gene amplification. British Journal of Haematology 74:251–256.

42. Cave H, van der Werff ten Bosch J, Suciu S, et al 1998 Clinical significance of minimal residual disease in childhood acute lymphoblastic leukemia. New England Journal of Medicine 339:591–598.

43. van der Velden VH, Hochhaus A, Cazzaniga G et al 2003 Detection of minimal residual disease in hematologic malignancies by real-time quantitative PCR: principles, approaches, and laboratory aspects. Leukemia 17:1013–1034.

44. Bassam BJ, Caetano-Anolles G, Gresshoff PM 1991 Fast and sensitive silver staining of DNA in polyacrylamide gels. Annals of Biochemistry 196:80–83.

45. Van Deerlin VM, Leonard DG 2000 Bone marrow engraftment analysis after allogeneic bone marrow transplantation. Clinical and Laboratory Medicine 20:197–225.

46. Mann K, Fox SP, Abbs SJ et al 2001 Development and implementation of a new rapid aneuploidy diagnostic service within the UK National Health Service and implications for the future of prenatal diagnosis. Lancet 358:1057–1061

47. Beutler E, Vulliamy TJ 2002 Hematologically important mutations: glucose-6-phosphate dehydrogenase. Blood Cells Molecules and Disease 28:93–103.

48. Harris S, Jones DB 1997 Optimisation of the polymerase chain reaction. British Journal of Biomedical Science 54:166–173.

49. Chomczynski P, Sacchi N 1987 Single step method of RNA isolation by acid guanidinium thiocyanate–phenol–chloroform extraction. Annals of Biochemistry 162:156–159.

22 Miscellaneous tests

S. Mitchell Lewis

TESTS FOR THE ACUTE-PHASE RESPONSE

Inflammatory response to tissue injury (the acute-phase response) includes alteration in serum protein concentration, especially increases in fibrinogen, haptoglobin, caeruloplasmin, immunoglobulins (Ig), and C-reactive protein (CRP), and decrease in albumin. The changes occur in acute infection, during active phases of chronic inflammation, with malignancy, in acute tissue damage (e.g., following acute myocardial infarction), or with physical injury.

Measurement of the acute-phase response is a helpful indicator of the presence and extent of inflammation or tissue damage and response to treatment. The usual tests are estimation of CRP and measurement of the erythrocyte sedimentation rate (ESR); some studies have suggested that plasma viscosity is also a useful indicator, but there is debate on the relative value of these tests.[1,2]

Kits that are sensitive and precise are available for CRP assay; small increases in serum levels of CRP can often be detected before any clinical features become apparent, whereas as a tissue-damaging process resolves, the serum level rapidly decreases toward zero, or at least within the normal range (less than 5 mg/l). The ESR is slower to respond to acute disease activity and it is insensitive to small

changes in the disease activity. It is less specific than CRP because it is also influenced by immunoglobulins (which are not acute-phase reactants) and by anaemia. Moreover, because the rate of change of ESR is slower than that of CRP, it rarely reflects the current disease activity and clinical state of the patient as closely as does CRP. However, the ESR is a useful screening test, and the conventional manual ESR method is simple, cheap, and not dependent on power supply, thus making it suitable for point-of-care (near patient) testing.

Because CRP assay is a biochemical test usually performed in the clinical chemistry laboratory, it will not be further discussed here.

Erythrocyte Sedimentation Rate

The method for measuring the ESR recommended by the International Council for Standardization in Haematology (ICSH)[3] and also by various national authorities[4] is based on that of Westergren, who developed the test in 1921 for studying patients with pulmonary tuberculosis.

Essentially it is the measurement after 1 hour of the sedimentation of red cells in diluted blood in an open-ended glass tube of 30 cm length mounted vertically on a stand.

Conventional Westergren Method

The recommended tube is a straight glass or rigid transparent plastic tube 30 cm in length and not less than 2.55 mm in diameter. The bore must be uniform to within 5% throughout. A scale graduated in mm extends over the lower 20 cm. The tube must be clean and dry and kept free from dust.

If reusable, before being reused it should be thoroughly washed in tap water, then rinsed with deionised or distilled water and allowed to dry. Specially made racks with adjustable levelling screws are available for holding the sedimentation tubes firmly in an exactly vertical position. The rack must be constructed so that there will be no leakage of the blood from the tube. It is conventional to set up sedimentation-rate tests at room temperature (18–25°C). Sedimentation is normally accelerated as the temperature increases, and if the test is to be carried out at a higher ambient temperature, a normal range should be established for that temperature. Exceptionally, when high thermal amplitude cold agglutinins are present, sedimentation becomes noticeably less rapid as the temperature is increased toward 37°C.

For the diluent prepare a solution of 109 mmol/l trisodium citrate (32 g/l $Na_3Ca_6H_5O_7.2H_2O$). Filter through a micropore filter (0.22 mm) into a sterile bottle. It can be stored for several months at 4°C but must be discarded if it becomes turbid through the growth of moulds.

Method

Either collect venous blood in ethylenediaminetetra-acetic acid (EDTA) and dilute a sample accurately in the proportion of 1 volume of citrate to 4 volumes of blood, or collect the blood directly into the citrate solution. The test should then be carried out on the diluted sample within 4 h of collecting the blood, although a delay of up to 6 h is permissible provided that the blood is kept at 4°C. EDTA blood can be used within 24 h if the specimen is kept at 4°C, provided that 1 volume of 109 mmol/l (32 g/l) trisodium citrate is added to 4 volumes of blood immediately before the test is performed.

Mix the blood sample thoroughly and then draw it up into the Westergren tube to the 200 mm mark by means of a teat or a mechanical device; mouth suction should never be used. Place the tube exactly vertical and leave undisturbed for exactly 60 min, free from vibrations and draughts and not exposed to direct sunlight. Then read to the nearest 1 mm the height of the clear plasma above the upper limit of the column of sedimenting cells. The result is expressed as ESR = X mm in 1 h. A poor delineation of the upper layer of red cells may sometimes occur, especially when there is a high reticulocyte count.

Range in Health

The mean values and the upper limit for 95% of normal adults are given in Table 22.1. There is a progressive increase with age, but older than 70 years it is difficult to define a strictly healthy population for determining normal values.

In the newborn, the ESR is usually low. In childhood and adolescence, it is the same as for normal men with no differences between boys and girls. It is increased in pregnancy, especially so in the later stages, and independent of anaemia.[5]

Table 22.1 Erythrocyte sedimentation rate ranges in health	
Age (years)	95% Upper limit (mm in 1h)
Men	
17–50	10
51–60	12
61–70	14
>70	about 30
Women	
17–50	12
51–60	19
61–70	20
>70	about 35
Pregnancy	
First half	48 (62 if anaemic)
Second half	70 (95 if anaemic)

Modified Methods

Length of Tube

The overall length of the tube is not a critical dimension for the test provided that it fits firmly in an appropriate holding device. The tube must, however, be long enough to ensure that packing of the cells does not start before the test has been completed.

Plastic Glass Tubes

A number of plastic materials (e.g., polypropylene and polycarbonate) are recommended as substitutes for glass in Westergren tubes. Nevertheless, not all plastics have similar properties, and it must be demonstrated that the ESR with the chosen tubes is reproducible and not affected by the plastic.

Disposable Glass Tubes

Disposable glass tubes should be supplied clean and dry and ready for use. It is necessary to show that neither the tube material nor the manufacturer's cleaning process affect the ESR.

Capillary Method

Short tubes of narrower bore than in the standard tube are available mainly for tests on infants. These are, however, no longer in general use, and it is necessary to establish normal ranges or a correction factor to convert results to an approximation of ESR by the Westergren method.

Time

Sedimentation is measured after aggregation has occurred and before the cells start to pack (see p. 598), usually at 18–24 min. From the rate during this time period the sedimentation that would have occurred at 60 min is derived and converted to the conventional ESR equivalent by an algorithm.[6]

Sloping Tube

Red cells sediment more quickly when streaming down the wall of a sloped tube. This phenomenon has been incorporated into automated systems in which the end-point is read after 20 min with the tube held at an angle of 18 degrees from the vertical. This has been shown to give results comparable to the conventional method.[7]

Anticoagulant

EDTA blood can be used without citrate dilution, at least if packed cell volume (PCV) is below 0.36 (haemoglobin < 110 g/l); less precise results are obtained when the PCV is higher. The readings from undiluted samples must then be adjusted as for the standardised method (see below).

Because of the biohazard risk of blood contamination inherent in using open-ended tubes, it is now recommended that, where possible, a closed system be used in routine practice. Manual methods are available that avoid transfer of the blood into the sedimentation tube. Automated closed systems use either blood collected in special evacuated tubes containing citrate or EDTA blood. A sample is taken up through a pierceable cap and then automatically diluted in the system if this is required. Some systems use sloping tubes at an angle of 18 degrees to obtain results rapidly, and one model of the *Vesmatic (Diesse)* also incorporates centrifugation.

Whenever a different method or tube is planned, a preliminary test should be carried out to check precision and to compare results with those obtained by the standardised method described in the following section.

ICSH Standardised Method

The ICSH standardised method is intended to provide a reference method for verifying the reliability of any modification of the test. It is carried out on EDTA blood not diluted in citrate, using Westergren tubes as described earlier and applying an experimentally derived formula for correction.[3]

Select 10 blood samples with PCV 0.30–0.36 and, if possible, with ESRs in a wide range between 15 and 105 mm; if necessary, adjust the PCV to within the required range by centrifuging the specimens, removing an appropriate amount of plasma or red cells, and then resuspending the cells by thorough mixing.

Immediately before filling the ESR tube, mix the specimen by at least eight complete inversions. Measure the ESR on each specimen (undiluted) by the standardized Westergren method.

Adjust the reading for lack of dilution as follows:

Corrected ESR (mm in 1 hour) =
$$(\text{undiluted ESR} \times 0.86) - 12.$$

At the same time, carry out the ESR by the method that is to be verified on samples from the same specimens or on blood collected separately from the same subjects in accordance with specified requirements (e.g., directly into tubes containing citrate).

Any new method may be considered to be satisfactory if 95% of results are within the limits given in Table 22.2. However, because the ESR may be affected by several uncontrolled variables, the reference method cannot be used to adjust the measurements that are obtained. Thus, if the new method

Table 22.2 Erythrocyte sedimentation rate values (mm) for verification of comparability of working (routine) method with the international council for standardisation in haematology standardised method[3]

Standardised method*	Working method limits[†]	Standardised method*	Working method limits[†]	Standardised method*	Working method limits[†]
15	3–13	45	18–37	75	40–68
16	4–14	46	18–38	76	40–69
17	4–15	47	19–38	77	41–70
18	4–15	48	20–39	78	42–71
19	5–16	49	20–40	79	43–72
20	5–17	50	21–41	80	44–73
21	6–17	51	22–42	81	45–74
22	6–18	52	22–43	82	45–76
23	6–19	53	23–44	83	46–77
24	7–19	54	24–45	84	47–78
25	7–20	55	24–46	85	48–79
26	8–21	56	25–47	86	49–80
27	8–21	57	26–48	87	50–82
28	9–22	58	26 –49	88	51–83
29	9–23	59	27–50	89	52–84
30	10–24	60	28–51	90	53–85
31	10–25	61	29–52	91	53–86
32	11–25	62	29–53	92	54–88
33	11–26	63	30–54	93	55–89
34	12–27	64	31–56	94	56–90
35	12–28	65	32–57	95	57–91
36	13–29	66	32–58	96	58–93
37	13–30	67	33–59	97	59–94
38	14–30	68	34–60	98	60–95
39	14–31	69	35–61	99	61–96
40	15–32	70	35–62	100	62–98
41	15–33	71	36–63	101	63–99
42	16–34	72	37–64	102	64–100
43	17–35	73	38–65	103	65–101
44	17–36	74	39–66	104	66–103
					67–104

*Standardized method: Ethylenediaminetetra-acetic acid (EDTA) anticoagulated but undiluted whole blood of haematocrit of 0.35 or less.
[†]Working method: 4 volumes EDTA blood plus 1 volume citrate diluent or EDTA blood without diluent. Proposed working method is valid if 95% of results are within indicated limits. Reproduced with permission from Journal of Clinical Pathology.

gives disparate readings, it will be necessary to establish a normal range specifically for the method.

Quality Control

The standardised method can also be used as a quality-control procedure for the routine tests. Select one blood sample with a PCV between 0.30 and 0.36 and perform the ESR by the routine method and by the standardized method as described earlier. Apply the formula to obtain the corrected ESR for the undiluted sample.

The test is satisfactorily controlled if the results by the routine method do not differ from those obtained by the ICSH standardised method by more than the limits shown in Table 22.2.

This procedure may be too laborious for routine use; instead, stabilised whole blood preparations are now available that are suitable as a daily control for use with different automated systems (e.g., *ESR-Chex [Streck]*).[8] Three or four specimens of EDTA blood kept at 4°C will also serve as a control on the following day.[9]

Another control procedure is to calculate the daily cumulative mean, which is relatively stable when at least 100 specimens are tested each day in a consistent clinical setting (see p. 665). A co-efficient of variation of less than 15% between daily sets appears to be a satisfactory index for monitoring instrument performance.[9]

Semiquantitative Slide Method

A method has been suggested to demonstrate enhanced red cell adhesion/aggregation by allowing a drop of citrated blood to dry on a slide. Estimate of the amount of cell aggregation on the film by image analysis provides a semiquantitative measure of the acute-phase response that appears to correlate with the ESR.[10]

Mechanism of Erythrocyte Sedimentation

The rate of fall of the red cells is influenced by a number of interreacting factors.[1] Basically, it depends on the difference in specific gravity between red cells and plasma, but it is influenced very greatly by the extent to which the red cells form rouleaux, which sediment more rapidly than single cells. Other factors that affect sedimentation include the ratio of red cells to plasma, (i.e., the PCV), the plasma viscosity, the verticality or otherwise of the sedi-

mentation tube, the bore of the tube, and the dilution (if any) of the blood.

The all-important rouleaux formation and red cell clumping that are associated with increased ESR are mainly controlled by the concentrations of fibrinogen and other acute-phase proteins (e.g., haptoglobin, ceruloplasmin, $\alpha_1$acid-glycoprotein, $\alpha_1$antitrypsin, and CRP). Rouleaux formation is also enhanced by the immunoglobulins. It is retarded by albumin. Defibrinated blood normally sediments extremely slowly—not more than 1 mm in 1 hour—unless the serum-globulin concentration is increased or there is an unusually high globulin:albumin ratio.

Anaemia, by altering the ratio of red cells to plasma, encourages rouleaux formation and accelerates sedimentation. In anaemia, too, cellular factors may affect sedimentation. Thus, in iron deficiency anaemia, a reduction in the intrinsic ability of the red cells to sediment may compensate for the accelerating effect of an increased proportion of plasma.

Sedimentation can be observed to take place in three stages: a preliminary stage of at least a few minutes during which time rouleaux occur and aggregates form; then a period in which the sinking of the aggregates takes place at approximately a constant speed; and, finally, a phase during which the rate of sedimentation slows as the aggregated cells pack at the bottom of the tube. It is obvious that the longer the tube used, the longer the second period can last and the greater the sedimentation rate may appear to be.

Clinical Significance of the Measurement of the Erythrocyte Sedimentation Rate

Overall, ESR is useful as a screening test in the routine examination of any patient. Although it is a nonspecific phenomenon, its measurement is clinically useful in disorders associated with an increased production of acute-phase proteins. In rheumatoid arthritis or tuberculosis it provides an index of progress of the disease, and it is of considerable value in diagnosis of temporal arteritis and poly-myalgia rheumatica. It is often used if multiple myeloma is suspected, but when the myeloma is nonsecretory or light chain, a normal ESR does not exclude this diagnosis.

An elevated ESR occurs as an early feature in myocardial infarction.[11] Although a normal ESR cannot be taken to exclude the presence of organic disease, the fact remains that the vast majority of acute or chronic infections and most neoplastic and degenerative diseases are associated with changes in the plasma proteins that lead to an acceleration of sedimentation. An increased ESR in subjects who are HIV seropositive seems to be an early predictive marker of progression toward acquired immune deficiency syndrome (AIDS).[12] The ESR is less helpful in countries where chronic diseases are rife; however, one study has shown that very high ESRs (higher than 100 mm/h have a specificity of 0.99 and a positive predictive value of 0.9 for an acute or chronic infection.[13] The ESR is higher in women than in men and correlates with sex differences in fibrinogen levels.[14] An increase in fibrinogen occurs in normal pregnancy, resulting in increased red cell aggregation and elevated sedimentation.[5,15] The ESR is influenced by age, stage of the menstrual cycle, and medications taken (e.g., corticosteroids, contraceptive pills); it is especially low (0-1 mm) in polycythaemia, hypofibrinogenaemia, and congestive cardiac failure and when there are abnormalities of the red cells such as poikilocytosis, spherocytosis, or sickle cells.

Plasma Viscosity

The ESR and plasma viscosity in general increase in parallel with each other.[1] Plasma viscosity is, however, primarily dependent on the concentration of plasma proteins, especially fibrinogen, and it is not affected by anaemia. Changes in the ESR may lag behind changes in plasma viscosity by 24-48 hours, and viscosity seems to reflect the clinical severity of disease more closely than does the ESR.[16]

There are several types of viscometers, including rotational and capillary types, that are suitable for routine use.[1] However, it has fallen out of fashion with the advent of automated and closed-tube ESR methods, and perhaps its main use is in investigation of suspected hyperviscosity. The actual test should be carried out as described in the instruction manual for the particular instrument used.

Reference Values

Each laboratory should establish its own reference values. As a general guide, ICSH has recorded that with the Harkness capillary viscometer normal plasma has a viscosity of 1.16-1.33 mPa/s* at 37°C and 1.50-1.72 mPa/s at 25°C.[17] Plasma viscosity is lower in the newborn (0.98-1.25 mPa/s at 37°C), increasing to adult values by the third year; it is slightly higher in old age. There are no significant differences in plasma viscosity between men and women or in pregnancy. It is remarkably constant in health, with little or no diurnal variation, and it is not affected by exercise. A change of only 0.03-0.05 mPa/s is thus likely to be clinically significant.

Whole Blood Viscosity

The viscosity of whole blood reflects its rheological properties; it is influenced by PCV, plasma viscosity, red cell aggregation, and red cell deformability. It is especially sensitive to PCV, with which it is closely correlated. The clinical interpretation of its measurement must also take into account the interaction of the red cells with blood vessels, which greatly influences blood flow *in vivo*.

Guidelines for measuring blood viscosity and red cell deformability by standardised methods have been published.[18] Rotational and capillary viscometers are suitable for measuring blood viscosity; deformability can be measured by recording the rate at which red cells in suspension pass through a filter with pores 3-5 mm in diameter.

HETEROPHILE ANTIBODIES IN SERUM: DIAGNOSIS OF INFECTIOUS MONONUCLEOSIS

Infectious mononucleosis (IM) is caused by Epstein-Barr virus.[19] Every infected cell contains viral capsid antigens, which give rise to specific heterophile antibodies. Before this identity was known, Paul and Bunnell[20] demonstrated them as agglutinins directed against sheep red cells; they are, in fact, not specific for sheep red cells but also react with horse and ox, but not human, red cells. They are IgM globulins, which are immunologically related to, but distinct from, antibodies that occur in response to the Forssman antigens. The latter are widely spread in animal tissue; they occur at low titre in healthy

---

*If expressed in poise (P), 1 cP = 1 mPa/s.

individuals and at high titre in serum sickness and in some leukaemias and lymphomas.[21,22] In these non-IM conditions, the antibody can be absorbed out by guinea pig cells. Thus, for the diagnosis of IM, it is necessary to demonstrate that the antibody present has the characters of the Paul–Bunnell antibody (i.e., it is absorbed by ox red cells but not by guinea pig kidney). This is the basis of the absorption tests for IM. Immunofluorescent antibody tests have been developed (e.g., *Launce Diagnostics Product 487003*) that distinguish the IgM antibody, which occurs at high titre in the early phase of IM and diminishes during convalescence, from the IgG antibody, which persists at high titre for years after infection[23,24] and which also occurs in the non-IM infections.[19,25]

Screening Tests for Infectious Mononucleosis

The quantitative Paul–Bunnell test described in previous editions is laborious and no longer in common use, having been replaced by rapid screening tests. There are a large number of commercial kits (see later), but the reagents can also be prepared in the individual laboratory.[26]

Reagents

Sera. Patient's serum (fresh or inactivated by heating at 56°C for 30 min) and positive and negative control sera.

Red cell suspension. 20% suspension of horse blood in 109 mmol/l (32 g/l) trisodium citrate. Before use, the suspension must be well mixed by repeated inversion. For the screening test, it is unnecessary to wash the cells.

Guinea pig kidney emulsion. See p. 693.

Ox red cell suspension. See p. 693.

Method

Place 1 large drop (c 30 μl) of guinea pig kidney emulsion and 1 large drop of ox-cell suspension on two adjacent squares on an opal glass tile. Add 1 drop of patient or control serum adjacent to each. Deliver 10 μl of horse-blood suspension to the corner of each square by means of a disposable plastic micropipette, avoiding contact with the drops in the squares. With a wooden applicator stick, mix the reagents (guinea pig kidney emulsion or ox-cell suspension, serum and horse-blood suspension) and then examine with the naked eye for agglutination, using oblique light at an angle over a dark background. Negative and positive serum controls should always be set up at the same time. The appearances are shown in Figure 22.1.

Interpretation

Positive.
Agglutination is stronger in the square containing guinea pig kidney emulsion than in the square containing ox-cell suspension.

Negative.
Agglutination is absent in both squares.

The reagents for this screening method are available commercially in diagnostic kits from several manufacturers. Other kits are based on agglutination of stabilised horse red cells or antigen-coated latex particles to which IM antibody binds. An extensive evaluation of 14 slide tests for the UK Medical Devices Agency (MDA), showed them to have a

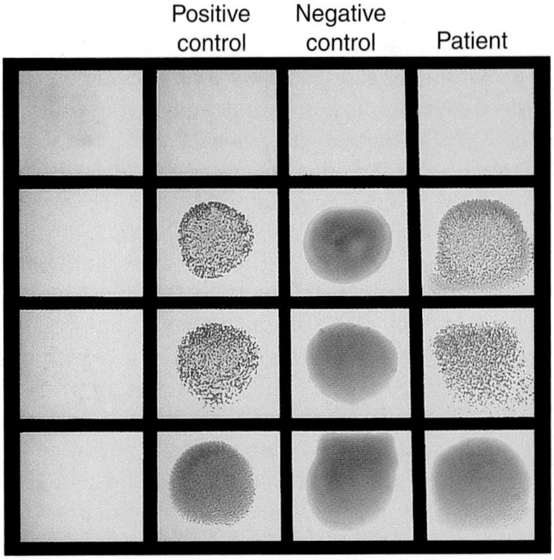

Figure 22.1   Slide screening test for infectious mononucleosis. **Top row:** guinea pig kidney. **Middle row:** ox-cell suspension. **Bottom row:** saline.

sensitivity between 0.87 and 1.00 and specificity of 0.97 to 1.00, with an overall accuracy (positive and negative) in the order of 91–100%.[27] False-positive reactions have been reported in malaria, toxoplasmosis, and cytomegaloid virus infection; autoimmune diseases; and even occasionally without any apparent underlying disease.[28,29] False-negative reactions occur if the test is carried out before the level of heterophile antibody has increased or conversely when it has decreased. False-negative reactions may also occur in the very young and the very old. In the UK MDA study the best performance was obtained with the Clearview test *(Unipath)*, which uses latex-labelled bovine erythrocyte glycoprotein; IM heterophile antibody binds to this to form a complex that presents as a band in the result window (Fig. 22.2). The test can be performed with diluted whole blood as well as with plasma or serum.

Screening tests are also available based on enzyme-linked immunosorbent assay (ELISA) and immunochromatographic assay. These tests are more elaborate than the slide screening test described earlier, but they are less likely to give a false result.

Clinical Value

Tests for the heterophile antibody are useful for diagnosis. Antibodies are often present as early as the 4th to 6th day of the disease and are almost always found by the 21st day. They disappear as a rule within 4–5 months. There is no unanimity as to how frequently negative reactions are found in "true" IM. Occasionally, the characteristic antibodies develop very late in the course of the disease, perhaps weeks or even months after the patient becomes ill, and it is also known that a positive reaction may be transient and that the antibodies may be present at such low titres that they may be missed or may produce anomalous agglutination reactions when associated with the naturally occurring antibody at similar titres. For all of these reasons, it is difficult to state categorically that any particular patient has not or will not produce antibodies. Antibodies specific for Epstein-Barr virus have been demonstrated in the serum of 86% of patients with clinical and/or haematological features of IM.[30]

As far as false-positive reactions are concerned, there is no substantial evidence that sera containing agglutinins in high concentration giving the typical reactions of IM are ever found in other diseases uncomplicated by IM. In particular, the heterophile-antibody titres in the lymphomas are similar to those found in unselected patients not suffering from IM.[31]

Demonstration of Lupus Erythematosus Cells

Antinuclear antibodies, or antinuclear factors (ANF), occur in the serum in a wide range of autoimmune disorders, including systemic lupus erythematosus (SLE). They can be detected and measured quantitatively by sensitive and specific immunological methods; simple qualitative screen test kits are also available from a number of suppliers. They have superseded the LE cell test; this is based on reaction between the patient's autoantibodies and nuclear antigens, with subsequent phagocytosis by neutrophils, which can be demonstrated morphologically. For many years, this was the standard criterion for diagnosing SLE[32] and was described in the eighth and earlier editions of this book. It has been superseded by the immunological tests, but it may be useful if these are not available

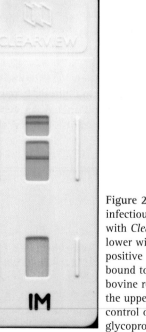

Figure 22.2 Screening for infectious mononucleosis with *Clearview* slide test. The lower window shows a positive result with antibody bound to latex-labelled bovine red cell glycoprotein; the upper window is a control of unbound glycoprotein.

ERYTHROPOIETIN

Erythropoietin regulates red cell production. It is a heat-stable glycoprotein with a molecular weight of about 34 kDa. It is produced mainly in the kidney. Only a small quantity is demonstrable in normal plasma or urine.

A pure form of human erythropoietin from recombinant DNA (r-HuEpo) is available for diagnostic assay methods by ELISA, enzyme immunoassay, and radioimmune assay. Commercial kits are available that are reliable and sensitive,[33] although there is some intermethod variability.[34] However, it is impractical to undertake the assay in laboratories where the test is required only occasionally; it is preferable to send the serum sample to a laboratory where the test is performed regularly or to a designated reference centre. In the United Kingdom, there is a *supraregional assay service** where analysis is carried out by ELISA.

Results are expressed in international units by reference to an international (WHO) standard. This was originally a urinary extract, and a preparation is available with a potency of 10 iu per ampoule.[35] The present standard has been established for r-HuEpo with a potency of 86 iu per ampoule.[36]

Reference Range

The normal reference range in plasma or serum varies considerably according to the method of assay.[33] For the ELISA method used by the UK supraregional service, the normal range is 9.1–30.8 iu/l. With test kits, in the steady state without anaemia, it is usually given as 5–25 iu/l or slightly higher. In normal children, the levels are the same as in adults, except for infants younger than 2 months when the level is low.[37]

There is a diurnal variation, with the highest values at night.[38] In pregnancy, erythropoietin concentration increases with gestation.[39]

Significance

Increased levels of erythropoietin are found in the plasma (or serum) in various anaemias,[40] and there is normally an inverse relationship between haemoglobin and erythropoietin. In thalassaemia, it is lower than in iron deficiency with the same degree of anaemia, but there is a close inverse correlation with the red cell count.[41] In renal disease, there is a progressive decline in the erythropoietin response to anaemia, and in end-stage renal failure the concentration is normal or even lower than normal despite increasing anaemia. Some impairment of production of erythropoietin may also occur in the anaemia of neoplasies and in association with chronic inflammatory diseases. Increased concentrations of erythropoietin occur in secondary polycythaemia owing to respiratory and cardiac disease; in the presence of abnormal haemoglobins with high oxygen affinity; and in association with carcinoma of the kidney and other erythropoietin-secreting tumours such as hepatoma, uterine fibroma, and ovarian carcinoma.[40]

In primary proliferative polycythaemia ("polycythaemia vera"), the plasma erythropoietin level is usually lower than normal even when the haemoglobin has been reduced by venesection.[42,43] In secondary polycythaemia, the level of erythropoietin is never below normal. Assay is particularly useful in patients with erythrocytosis of undetermined cause; low erythropoietin has a specificity of 0.92 with moderate sensitivity for diagnosing primary polycythaemia.[42] However, in such cases there may be an intermittent increase in erythropoietin secretion. Thus, determining its level in a single sample of plasma may be misleading. Low levels have been found in one third of cases of primary (essential) thrombocythaemia, especially when haemoglobin is at a high normal level.[42]

Measurement of plasma erythropoietin is useful in predicting if anaemia in a patient with a myelodysplastic syndrome is likely to respond to erythropoietin therapy.

Autonomous *in Vitro* Erythropoiesis

When bone marrow of mononuclear cells from blood are cultured, erythroid colonies (CFU-E) will normally develop only when erythropoietin is present in the culture medium. However, growth will occur in erythropoietin-free medium in primary polycythaemia. This provides a method for distinguishing primary from secondary polycythaemia.[44–46]

Mononuclear cells are collected from a blood sample by density separation (see p. 68 and p. 514) and added to an appropriate serum-free liquid culture

---

*See www.sas_centre.org/centres/hormones/london_Kings.html

medium[45,46] or collagen gel medium,[47] which is then divided into two portions. To one portion is added 1 iu/ml of Epo. Both portions are plated and incubated for 7 days at 37°C. They are then stained with benzidene and examined directly under an inverted microscope or after spreading onto slides. The numbers of benzidene-positive cell clusters in the erythropoietin-free and erythropoietin-containing samples are counted and compared. A diagnosis of primary polycythaemia is indicated if there is an approximately equal growth in both samples. A method has been described in which flow cytometry with immunofluorescence is used to detect growth of the erythroid cells after only 2–5 days of culture.[48]

Thrombopoietin

Thrombopoietin regulates megakaryocyte development and platelet production. It is a protein produced by the liver and has been purified from serum.[49] It is considerably larger than erythropoietin, with a molecular weight of about 335 kDa. A recombinant human thrombopoietin (rhTPO) has been produced and used to prepare a monoclonal antibody and develop a sensitive and specific ELISA test. This has been used to measure thrombopoietin in normal serum and serum from patients with various blood disorders.[50] The normal range (mean and 2 SD) was 0.79 ± 0.35 fmol/ml for men and 0.70 ± 0.26 fmol/ml for women. It was increased in thrombocytopenias, especially high at 18.5 ± 12.4 fmol/ml in aplastic anaemia with severe thrombocytopenia. In essential thrombocythaemia, it was in the range of 1.01–4.82 fmol/ml.[51]

SUPPLEMENTARY TESTS FOR MALARIA

In addition to morphological examination by microscopy, as described in Chapter 4, there are other methods for screening for the presence of malaria.[50]

Immunological Methods

Simple "dipstick" or slide screening tests for *Plasmodium falciparum* are based on binding of monoclonal antibody to histidine rich protein 2 (HRP-2), which occurs specifically in *P. falciparum*. The methods include the following:

ELISA (e.g., *ParaSight F [BD]*), which has a sensitivity of 0.95 but is less sensitive in low levels of parasitaemia.[50,52] It is negative when only gametocytes are present and is unhelpful in the immediate posttreatment follow-up because it remains positive for 1–2 weeks after clinical cure and disappearance of parasites from the blood, thus making it difficult to monitor response to therapy.[50]

Immunochromatography (e.g., *ICT Malaria Pf [Binax]*), which is reported to have a sensitivity of 100% and specificity of 96.2%.[53] A cheap version of this method, *Falciparum Malaria IC Strip*, is manufactured by the Program for Appropriate Technology for Health (PATH) especially as a diagnostic tool in malaria-endemic areas.[54]

There are also kits capable of demonstrating *P. vivax* infection by combining the *P. falciparum*-specific HRP-2 antibody with antibody against parasite glycolytic enzyme lactic dehydrogenase, which occurs in other types of plasmodium.[50] These include *ICT Malaria Pf/Pv (Binax)* and *OptiMAL (Diamed)*. The latter has a sensitivity of more than 0.95 for both *P. falciparum* and *P. vivax*, and it has the advantage that it correlates with parasite viability, so that the test is negative when treatment is effective.[55,56] It is less sensitive for *P. ovale* and *P. malariae*, and occasionally there is a false-positive reading as a result of cross-reaction with heterophile antibodies in the plasma.[56]

With any of the screening tests, it must be borne in mind that it is always necessary to confirm a positive result by microscopy. Moreover, for clinical management of patients with *P. falciparum* infection, it is essential to examine a blood film to obtain an estimate of the percentage of red cells that are infected, both when making the diagnosis and for monitoring response to treatment. However, immunological screening tests can be useful outside routine laboratory hours if on-call staff are not very experienced in morphological diagnosis.

Polymerase Chain Reaction

Polymerase chain reaction provides highly sensitive and specific results for diagnosis of *P. falciparum* and *P. vivax*. It is especially useful for epidemiological studies, but it is impractical as a routine diagnostic tool when rapid results are required.[57,58]

REFERENCES

1. International Committee for Standardization in Haematology 1988 Guidelines on the selection of laboratory tests for monitoring the acute-phase response. Journal of Clinical Pathology 41:1203–1212.
2. Lowe GDO 1994 Annotation: Should plasma viscosity replace the ESR? British Journal of Haematology 86:6–11.
3. International Council for Standardization in Haematology 1993 ICSH recommendations for measurement of erythrocyte sedimentation rate. Journal of Clinical Pathology 46:198–203.
4. National Committee for Clinical Laboratory Standards 2000 Reference and selected procedures for the erythrocyte sedimentation rate (ESR) test (H2-A4). NCCLS, Wayne, PA.
5. van den Broek NR, Letsky EA 2001 Pregnancy and the erythrocyte sedimentation rate. British Journal of Obstetrics and Gynaecology 108:1164–1167.
6. Kallner A, Engervall P, Björkholm M 1994 Kinetic measurement of the erythrocyte sedimentation rate. Upsala Journal of Medical Science 99:179–186.
7. Happe MR, Buttafarono DF, Dooley DP, et al 2002 Validation of the Diesse Mini-Ves erythrocyte sedimentation rate (ESR) analyzer using the Westergren method in patients with systemic inflammatory conditions. American Journal of Clinical Pathology 118:14–17.
8. Garvey BJ, Mahon A, Parker-Williams J, et al 1999 An evaluation of ESR-Chex control material for erythrocyte sedimentation rate determination (MDA 99/28). Medical Devices Agency, Stationery Office, Norwich NR3 IPD.
9. Plebani M, Piva E 2002 Erythrocyte sedimentation rate: use of fresh blood for quality control. American Journal of Clinical Pathology 117:621–626.
10. Rotstein R, Fusman R, Berliner S, et al 2001 The feasibility of estimating the erythrocyte sedimentation rate within a few minutes by using a simple slide test. Clinical and Laboratory Haematology 23:21–25.
11. Froom P, Margaliot S, Caine Y, et al 1984 Significance of erythrocyte sedimentation rate in young adults. American Journal of Clinical Pathology 82:198–200.
12. Lefrère JJ, Salmon D, Doinel C, et al 1988 Sedimentation rate as a predictive marker in HIV infection. AIDS 2:63–64.
13. Fincher RF, Page MI 1986 Clinical significance of extreme elevation of the erythrocyte sedimentation rate. Archives of Internal Medicine 146:1581–1583.
14. Bain BJ 1983 Some influences on the ESR and the fibrinogen level in healthy subjects. Clinical and Laboratory Haematology 5:45–54.
15. Huisman A, Aarnoudse JG, Krans M, et al 1988 Red cell aggregation during normal pregnancy. British Journal of Haematology 68:121–124.
16. Harkness J 1971 The viscosity of human plasma: its measurement in health and disease. Biorheology 8:171–193.
17. International Committee for Standardization in Haematology 1984 Recommendation for selected method for the measurement of plasma viscosity. Journal of Clinical Pathology 37:1147–1152.
18. International Committee for Standardization in Haematology 1986 Guidelines for measurement of blood viscosity and erythrocyte deformability. Clinical Hemorheology 6:439–453.
19. Henle W, Henle GE, Horwitz CA 1974 Epstein-Barr virus specific diagnostic tests in infectious mononucleosis. Human Pathology 5:551–565.
20. Paul JR, Bunnell WW 1932 The presence of heterophile antibodies in infectious mononucleosis. American Journal of Medical Science 183:90.
21. Huh J, Cho K, Heo DS, et al 1999 Detection of Epstein-Barr virus in Korean peripheral T-cell lymphoma. American Journal of Haematology 60:205–214.
22. Klein G 1994 Epstein-Barr virus strategy in normal and neoplastic B cells. Cell 77:791–793.
23. Strand BC, Schuster TC, Hopkins RF, et al 1981 Identification of an Epstein-Barr virus nuclear antigen by fluoro-immuno-electrophoresis and radioimmuno-electrophoresis. Journal of Virology 38:996–1004.
24. Edwards JMB, McSwiggen DA 1974 Studies on the diagnostic value of an immunofluorescence test for EB virus-specific IgM. Journal of Clinical Pathology 27:647–651.
25. Rea TD, Ashley RL, Russo JE, et al 2002 A systematic study of Epstein-Barr virus serological assays following acute infection. American Journal of Clinical Pathology 117:156–161.
26. Lee CL, Davidsohn I, Panczyszyn O 1968 Horse agglutinins in infectious mononucleosis. II The spot test. American Journal of Clinical Pathology 49:12–18.
27. Garvey BJ, Mahon A, Parker-Williams J, et al 1998 Evaluation report: fourteen commercial IM screening kits (MDA 98/63). Medical Devices Agency, Stationery Office, Norwich NR3 1PD.

28. Reed RE 1974 False-positive monospot tests in malaria. American Journal of Clinical Pathology 61:173–174.

29. Horwitz CA, Henle W, Henle G, et al 1979 Persistent falsely positive rapid tests for infectious mononucleosis. Report of five cases with four-six year follow-up data. American Journal of Clinical Pathology 72:807–811.

30. Evans AS, Niederman JC 1982 EBV-IgA and new heterophile antibody tests in diagnosis of infectious mononucleosis. American Journal of Clinical Pathology 77:555–560.

31. Goldman R, Fishkin BG, Peterson E 1950 The value of the heterophile antibody reaction in the lymphomatous diseases. Journal of Laboratory and Clinical Medicine 35:681–687.

32. Zinkham WH, Conley CL 1956 Some factors influencing the formation of L. E. cells. A method for enhancing L. E. cell production. Bulletin of the Johns Hopkins Hospital 98:102–119.

33. Marsden JT, Sherwood RA, Peters TJ 1995 Evaluation of six erythropoietin kits. (MDA 95/57) Medical Devices Agency, Stationery Office, Norwich NR3 1PD.

34. Bechensteen AG, Lappin TRJ, Marsden J, et al 1993 Unreliability in immunoassays of erythropoietin: anomalous estimates with an assay kit. British Journal of Haematology 83:663–664.

35. Annable L, Cotes PM, Mussett MV 1972 The second international preparation of erythropoietin, human, urinary, for bioassay. Bulletin of the World Health Organization 47:99.

36. Storring PL, Gaines Das RE 1992 The international standard for recombinant DNA-derived erythropoietin: collaborative study of four recombinant DNA-derived erythropoietins and two highly purified human erythropoietins. Journal of Endocrinology 134:459–484.

37. Hellebostad M, Haga P, Cotes MP 1988 Serum immunoreactive erythropoietin in healthy normal children. British Journal of Haematology 70:247–250.

38. Wide L, Bengtsson C, Birgegard G 1988 Circadian rhythm of erythropoietin in human serum. British Journal of Haematology 72:85–90.

39. Cotes PM, Canning CE, Lind T 1983 Changes in serum immunoreactive erythropoietin during the menstrual cycle and normal pregnancy. British Journal of Obstetrics and Gynaecology 90:304–311.

40. Kendall RG 2001 Erythropoietin. Clinical and Laboratory Haematology 23:71–80.

41. Tassiopoulos T, Konstantopoulos K, Tassiopoulos S, et al 1997 Erythropoietin levels and microcytosis in heterozygous beta-thalassaemia. Acta Haematologica 98:147–149.

42. Messinezy M, Westwood NB, El-Hemaidi I, et al 2002 Serum erythropoietin values in erythrocytoses and in primary thrombocythaemia. British Journal of Haematology 117:47–53.

43. Carneskog J, Safai-Kutti S, Wadenvik H, et al 1999 The red cell mass, plasma erythropoietin and spleen size in apparent polycythaemia. European Journal of Haematology 62:43–48.

44. Weinberg RS 1997 In vitro erythropoiesis in polycythemia vera and other myeloproliferative disorders. Seminars in Hematology 34:64–69.

45. Lemoine F, Najman A, Baillou C, et al 1986 A prospective study of the value of bone marrow erythroid progenitor cultures in polycythemia. Blood 68:996–1002.

46. Beckman BS, Anderson WF, Beltran GS, et al 1983 Diagnostic use of CFU-E formation from peripheral blood in polycythemia vera. American Journal of Clinical Pathology 79:496–499.

47. Dobo I, Mossuz P, Campos L, et al 2001 Comparison of four serum-free, cytokine-free media for analysis of endogenous erythroid colony growth in polycythemia vera and essential thrombocythemia. Hematology Journal 2:396–403.

48. Manor D, Rachmilewitz EA, Fibach E 1997 Improved method for diagnosis of polycythemia vera based on flow cytometric analysis of autonomous growth of erythroid precursors in liquid culture. American Journal of Hematology 54:47–52.

49. Kaushansky K 1995 Thrombopoietin: the primary regulator of platelet production. Blood 86:419–431.

50. Hänscheid T 1999 Diagnosis of malaria: a review of alternatives to conventional microscopy. Clinical and Laboratory Haematology 21:235–245.

51. Tahara T, Usuki K, Sato H, et al 1996 A sensitive sandwich ELISA for measuring thrombopoietin in human serum: serum thrombopoietin levels in healthy volunteers and in patients with haemopoietic disorders. British Journal of Haematology 93:783–788.

52. Chiodini PL, Cooke AH, Moody AH, et al 1996 MDA evaluation of the Becton Dickinson ParaSight F test for the diagnosis of Plasmodium falciparum. (MDA 96/33). Medical Devices Agency, Stationery Office, Norwich NR3 1PD.

53. Garcia M, Kirimoama S, Marlborough D, et al 1996 Immunochromatographic test for malaria diagnosis. Lancet 347:1549.

54. Mills CD, Burgess DCH, Taylor HJ, et al 1999 Evaluation of a rapid and inexpensive dipstick

assay for the diagnosis of Plasmodium falciparum malaria. Bulletin of the World Health Organization 77:553–558.

55. Moody A, Hunt-Cooke A, Gabbett E, et al 2000 Performance of the OptiMAL malaria antigen capture dipstick for malaria diagnosis and treatment monitoring at the Hospital for Tropical Diseases, London. British Journal of Haematology 109:891–894.

56. Moody AH, Chiodini PL 2002 Non-microscopic method for malaria diagnosis using OptiMAL IT, a second generation dipstick for malaria pLDH antigen detection. British Journal of Biomedical Science 59:228–231.

57. Seesod N, Nopparat P, Hedrum A, et al 1997 An integrated system using immunomagnetic separation polymerase-chain-reaction and colorimetric detection for diagnosis of Plasmodium falciparum. American Journal of Tropical Medicine and Hygiene 56:322–328.

58. Hang VT, Be TV, Thanh CT, et al 1995 Screening donor blood for malaria by polymerase chain reaction. Transactions of the Royal Society of Tropical Medicine and Hygiene 89:44–47.

Approach to the diagnosis and classification of blood diseases

Imelda Bates and Barbara J. Bain

COMMON PRESENTATIONS OF HAEMATOLOGICAL DISEASES

An abnormal blood count or blood cell morphology does not necessarily indicate a primary haematology problem because it may reflect an underlying non-haematological condition or may be the result of therapeutic interventions. Anaemia occurs in many conditions, but a primary blood disease should be considered when a patient has splenomegaly; lymphadenopathy; a bleeding tendency or thrombosis; and/or non-specific symptoms (malaise, sweats, or weight loss).

As with any clinical problem, the first steps in determining the diagnosis include obtaining a careful clinical and drug history and thorough physical examination. The result of these, in combination with the patient's age, sex, ethnic origin, social and family history, and knowledge of the locally prevalent diseases, will determine subsequent laboratory investigations.

INITIAL SCREENING TESTS

Although the range of haematological tests available to support clinical and public health services is broad, it is often the simplest investigations that are most useful in indicating the diagnosis. Even poorly resourced laboratories are usually able to provide an initial panel of tests such as haemoglobin concentration (Hb), white blood cell count (WBC) and platelet count (Chapter 27), and examination of a peripheral blood smear for a differential leucocyte count (Chapter 3) and cellular morphology (Chapter 5). These screening tests will often enable the underlying pathological processes to be suspected promptly and point to a few key diagnostic tests.

The investigation of specific haematological problems is covered in detail in Chapters 7 (iron deficiency anaemia), 8 (megaloblastic anaemia), 9, 10, and 11 (haemolytic anaemias), 12 (haemoglobinopathies), and 16 and 17 (coagulation disorders).

Interpretation of Screening Tests

Results of laboratory screening tests should always be interpreted with an understanding of the limitations of the tests and the physiological variations that occur with sex, age, and conditions such as pregnancy and exercise. Physiological variations in cell counts are detailed in Chapter 2. Abnormalities of red cells, white cells, or platelets may be quantitative (increased or reduced numbers) or qualitative (abnormal appearance and/or function).

Quantitative Abnormalities of Blood Cells

Increased Numbers of Cells

Increases Affecting More Than One Cell Line

A simultaneous increase in the cells of more than one cell line suggests that the overproduction of cells originates in an early precursor cell. This occurs in myeloproliferative disorders in which one cell type may predominate, e.g., platelets in essential thrombocythaemia and red cells in polycythaemia vera (primary proliferative polycythaemia), but there are often increases in other cell lines. The diagnosis will depend on which cell line expansion is dominant.

Erythrocytosis

Increases in red cells may be one of the following:

- "Relative" (pseudopolycythaemia) owing to reduced plasma volume
- "Primary" (polycythaemia vera) as part of the spectrum of myeloproliferative disorders
- "Secondary" to chronic hypoxia (e.g., chronic lung disease, congenital heart disease, high-affinity haemoglobins) or aberrant erythropoietin production

Secondary polycythaemia can generally be excluded by the clinical history and examination, assessment of serum erythropoietin concentration and arterial oxygen saturation, haemoglobin electrophoresis, and abdominal ultrasound. The presence of splenomegaly is suggestive of polycythaemia vera, and this diagnosis can be confirmed by demonstrating an absolute increase in total red cell volume and excluding other causes of erythrocytosis. Measurement of red cell and/or plasma volume (Chapter 15) will identify pseudopolycythaemia.

Leucocytosis

Neutrophilia

Neutrophils are commonly increased in number during pregnancy and in acute infections, inflammation, intoxication, corticosteroid therapy, and acute blood loss or destruction. Neutrophilia with the neutrophils showing heavy cytoplasmic granulation ("toxic" granulation) is a common finding in severe bacterial infections. In the absence of any underlying cause, a high neutrophil count with immature myeloid cells suggests chronic granulocytic leukaemia; cytogenetic and molecular studies to look for t(9;22) and the *BCR–ABL* fusion gene are indicated (Chapter 21).

Lymphocytosis

Lymphocytosis is a feature of certain infections, particularly infections in children. It may be especially marked in pertussis, infectious mononucleosis, cytomegalovirus infection, infectious hepatitis, tuberculosis, and brucellosis. Lymphocytosis is also a common transient reaction to severe physical stress. Elderly patients with lymphoproliferative disorders, including chronic lymphocytic leukaemia and lymphomas, often present with lymphadenopathy and a lymphocytosis. Morphology and immunophenotyping of the cells combined with histological examination of a bone marrow trephine biopsy are used to classify these disorders and to give an indication of management and prognosis. It is occasionally difficult to differentiate between a reactive and a neoplastic lymphocytosis. In this situation, immunophenotyping, immunophenotypic evidence of light chain restriction, and polymerase chain reaction for immunoglobulin or T-cell receptor gene rearrangements may indicate the presence of a monoclonal population of lymphocytes, thereby supporting a diagnosis of neoplastic, rather than reactive, lymphoproliferation. If lymph nodes are enlarged, a fine needle aspirate for cytology and immunocytochemistry or a lymph node biopsy for histology and immunohistochemistry may be helpful in diagnosis.

Monocytosis

A slight to moderate monocytosis may be associated with some protozoal, rickettsial, and bacterial infections including malaria, typhus, and tuberculosis. High levels of monocytes (monocyte count $>1 \times 10^9/l$) in an elderly patient suggest chronic myelomonocytic leukaemia or, sometimes, atypical chronic myeloid leukaemia. Because these conditions fall into the myeloproliferative/myelodysplastic group of disorders, the diagnosis would be supported by finding splenomegaly, quantitative and qualitative abnormalities in other cell lines, and a clonal cytogenetic abnormality.

Eosinophilia

Eosinophilia is typically associated with allergic disorders including drug sensitivity, skin diseases, and parasitic infections. In most cases, the cause is indicated from the clinical history, which should include details of all medications and foreign travel, and by examination of the stool and urine for parasites and ova. A diagnosis of chronic eosinophilic leukaemia is made if there is an increase in blast cells in the blood or marrow or if there is cytogenetic or molecular evidence of an abnormal myeloid clone. Idiopathic hypereosinophilic syndrome is an unusual cause of eosinophilia in which release of the contents of eosinophil granules results in damage to the heart, lungs, and other tissues. This is a diagnosis of exclusion, made only when detailed investigations exclude all known causes. It is necessary to specifically exclude eosinophilic leukaemia and cytokine-induced eosinophilia resulting from the presence of a neoplastic clone of T cells before diagnosing a condition as the idiopathic hypereosinophilic syndrome.

Basophilia

Basophilia as an isolated finding is unusual. However, it is a common feature of myeloproliferative disorders and basophils may be particularly prominent in chronic granulocytic leukaemia. In this condition, an increasing basophil count may be the first indication of transformation to a more aggressive course.

Thrombocytosis

Thrombocytosis is often associated with infectious and inflammatory conditions such as osteomyelitis and rheumatoid arthritis. Haematological causes of thrombocytosis include chronic blood loss, red cell destruction, splenectomy, and rebound following recovery from marrow suppression. Under these circumstances, a moderately increased platelet count (e.g., $400-800 \times 10^9/l$) does not usually have any pathological consequences. Primary (essential) thrombocythaemia belongs to the spectrum of myeloproliferative diseases and is characterized by a persistently high platelet count (often arbitrarily defined as greater than $600 \times 10^9/l$) and thrombotic or haemorrhagic complications. Further investigations to confirm primary thrombocythaemia include bone marrow examination for increased and abnormal megakaryocytes and cytogenetic analysis.

Reduced Numbers of Cells

Reductions in More Than One Cell Line

A reduction in cell numbers occurs because of increased destruction, reduced production, or increased pooling in the spleen or other organ. Reduced production of cells may be the result of aplastic anaemia, a lack of haematinics such as folate or vitamin B_{12}, or interference with normal haemopoiesis by infiltration (e.g., leukaemia, lymphoma, multiple myeloma, metastatic carcinoma − often with secondary myelofibrosis), infection (e.g., human immunodeficiency virus [HIV] infection, tuberculosis, leishmaniasis), or exposure to toxins (e.g., alcohol) or myelosuppressive drugs (e.g., hydroxycarbamide* or busulphan). Certain myeloid neoplasms (e.g., "idiopathic" myelofibrosis) and the myelodysplastic syndromes (MDS) are characterised by cytopenias, and this is also sometimes a feature of acute myeloid leukaemia (AML). A relatively common cause of a global reduction in circulating cells is pooling of the cells in a grossly enlarged spleen (hypersplenism), which may be secondary to conditions such as myelofibrosis and portal hypertension. Examination of a bone marrow aspirate and trephine biopsy specimen is often helpful in

---

*Previously known as hydroxyurea.

determining the cause of bicytopenia or pancytopenia for which no obvious cause can be found.

Anaemia

There are many causes of anaemia, and a logical classification would be according to mechanism:

Decreased production
Reduced lifespan of red cells
Blood loss
Splenic pooling

In practice, if the cause is not readily apparent from the clinical circumstances and an automated blood count is available, classification according to cell size is more practicable. The choice of further investigations is then guided by the mean cell volume (MCV) and red cell morphology in addition to clinical features. Anaemia is thus broadly divided into three types:

Microcytic (low MCV)
Macrocytic (high MCV)
Normocytic (normal MCV)

Low MCV may be associated with low mean cell haemoglobin (MCH). A low mean cell haemoglobin concentration (MCHC) is less common and correlates with hypochromia.

Figures 23.1–23.3 are flow charts that provide an orderly sequence of investigations for the different types of anaemia on the basis of these indices. Examination of a blood film will usually suggest the quickest route to the diagnosis; confirmation may require the more specific tests, which are given in the text. The presence of basophilic stippling in a patient with microcytic red cells suggests thalassaemia trait or lead poisoning. A dimorphic blood film is typical of congenital sideroblastic anaemia but is more often the result of iron deficiency responding to treatment. Pappenheimer bodies suggest that a microcytic anaemia is the result of sideroblastic erythropoiesis.

Microcytic Anaemia (See Fig. 23.1)

The most common cause of anaemia worldwide is iron deficiency (Fig. 23.1). It can be suspected from a low MCV and the presence of hypochromic, microcytic red cells. Laboratory confirmation of iron deficiency may include measurements of serum ferritin, serum iron plus either total iron-binding capacity or transferrin assay, red cell protoporphyrin, and staining of bone marrow aspirates for iron (see Chapter 4). A diagnosis of iron deficiency requires a search for the cause. This should include specific questions relating to blood loss and dietary insufficiency and may require stool examination for parasites and occult blood, endoscopic examination

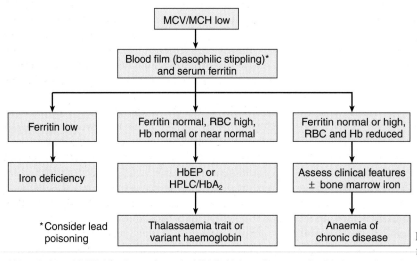

Figure 23.1 Investigation of a microcytic hypochromic anaemia.

Abbreviations: HbEP, Hb electrophoresis; HPLC, high performance liquid chromatography

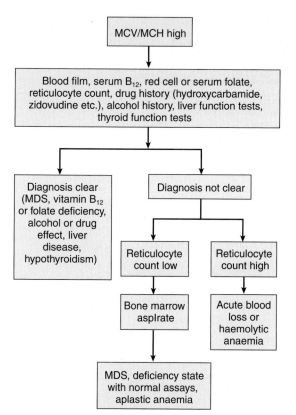

Figure 23.2   Investigation of a macrocytic anaemia. MDS, myelodysplastic syndrome.

of the gastrointestinal tract to exclude occult malignancy, and serological or other tests for coeliac disease. The differential diagnosis of iron deficiency anaemia includes anaemia of chronic disease. Clinical and laboratory features of inflammation may suggest this diagnosis, which is confirmed by demonstration of normal or high serum ferritin, low serum iron, and low transferrin and iron binding capacity.

The thalassaemias also cause microcytosis, but both α and β thalassaemia are usually associated with an increased red blood cell count and a normal or near-normal Hb despite a considerable reduction of the MCV and MCH, whereas in iron deficiency the MCV and MCH do not fall until the Hb is significantly reduced. Further investigations, such as haemoglobin electrophoresis, high-performance liquid chromatography (HPLC), or measurement of HbA$_2$ and HbF usually confirm the diagnosis of β thalassaemia trait. The diagnosis of α thalassaemia trait is more

difficult; detection of infrequent HbH inclusions is usually possible in α^0 thalassaemia trait, but definitive diagnosis requires DNA analysis. The diagnosis of α^+ thalssaemia trait is of less clinical importance; HbH inclusions may not be detected, so DNA analysis is needed.

Macrocytic Anaemia (See Fig. 23.2)

A high MCV with oval macrocytes and hypersegmented neutrophils suggests folate or vitamin B$_{12}$ deficiency and is an indication for assays of these vitamins (see Chapter 8); subsequent investigations could include malabsorption studies, serological test for coeliac disease, and either tests for intrinsic factor antibodies or a Schilling test to detect pernicious anaemia (p. 180). If intrinsic factor antibodies are detected, a Schilling test is not necessary. A high MCV may also be associated with alcohol excess and liver disease or drugs such as hydroxycarbamide or zidovudine. Macrocytosis resulting from chronic haemolysis is associated with increased numbers of immature red cells, which appear slightly larger and more blue than normal red cells on a Romanowsky-stained peripheral blood film. Supravital staining of blood films (p. 40) or an automated reticulocyte count can be used to confirm reticulocytosis. Untreated anaemia associated with polychromasia is likely to indicate blood loss or haemolysis. The combination of red cell fragments, thrombocytopenia, and polychromasia indicates microangiopathic haemolytic anaemia and should trigger further tests such as a platelet count, coagulation studies, assessment of renal function, and a search for infection or neoplastic disease. This further assessment is urgent because these may be features of thrombotic thrombocytopenic purpura, which requires speedy treatment by plasma exchange.

Normocytic Anaemia (See Fig. 23.3)

Normochromic, normocytic anaemia is frequently the result of an underlying chronic, non-haematological disease. Investigations should include screening for renal insufficiency, subclinical infections, autoimmune diseases, and neoplasia. In the presence of anaemia, a lack of polychromasia, confirmed by reticulocytopenia, points toward a primary failure of erythropoiesis or blood loss or haemolysis without compensatory red cell production. Examination of the bone marrow may be help-

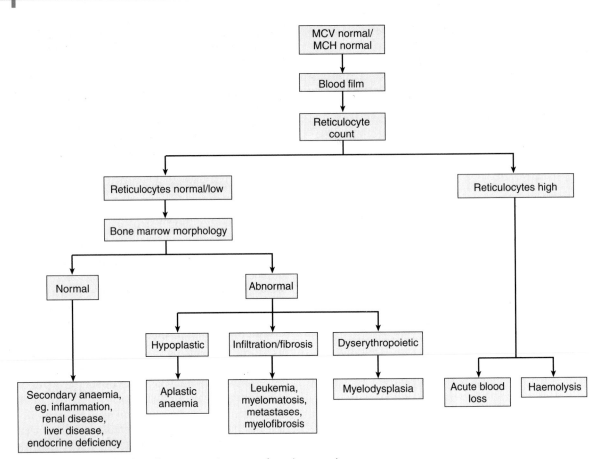

Figure 23.3   Investigation of a normocytic, normochromic anaemia.

ful in demonstrating haematological causes for the normochromic, normocytic anaemia such as aplastic anaemia or early myelodysplastic syndrome. Staining for iron may also show that there is a block in iron metabolism suggestive of anaemia associated with chronic inflammatory disease.

Leucopenia

Neutropenia

Once physiological variation, ethnicity, and familial or cyclic neutropenia have been excluded (p. 20), the non-haematological causes of isolated neutropenia to be considered include overwhelming infection, autoimmune disorders such as systemic lupus erythematosus, irradiation, drugs (particularly anticancer agents), and large granular lymphocyte leukaemia. Bone marrow examination may assist in

determining whether the problem is the result of peripheral destruction (increased marrow myeloid precursors) or stem cell failure (lack of narrow myeloid precursors). Typical marrow appearances occur in drug-induced neutropenia, in which there is a relative paucity of mature neutrophils and in Kostmann's syndrome (infant genetic agranulocytosis) where there is maturation arrest at the promyelocytic stage.

Reduced Numbers of Lymphocytes, Monocytes, Eosinophils, and Basophils

Lymphocytes, eosinophils, and basophils may all be reduced by stress such as surgery, trauma, and infection. Lymphopenia with neutrophilia is a common combination of haematological abnormalities in severe acute respiratory syndrome. Lymphopenia, especially affecting the CD4 cells, may occur in HIV infection and renal failure. Monocytopenia (<0.2 × 10^9/l) is typically found in hairy cell leukaemia, which is also associated with pancytopenia, typical bone marrow histology, and lymphocytes with a characteristic cytology and immunophenotype.

Thrombocytopenia

Thrombocytopenia is a common isolated finding, and it is important to ensure that the laboratory result reflects a true reduction in platelet count before embarking on further diagnostic tests. Frequent causes of spurious thrombocytopenia include blood clots in the sample, platelet aggregation, and platelet satellitism. Platelet aggregation, which can be seen on the blood film, may occur in *vitro* as the result of a temperature-dependent or anticoagulant-dependent autoantibody. Small platelet aggregates are also seen in slides that have been made directly from a fingerprick sample. True thrombocytopenia is most frequently the result of anticancer chemotherapy, HIV infection, autoantibodies ("idiopathic" autoimmune thrombocytopenic purpura), other drugs (such as thiazide diuretics), alcohol excess, hypersplenism, and MDS (in the elderly). The clinical circumstances, together with bone marrow examination and relevant serological tests, should enable these conditions to be differentiated. Thrombocytopenia associated with other complications, such as thromboses, disturbed renal or hepatic function, and haemolytic anaemia, should prompt investigations for other diseases such as thrombotic thrombocytopenic purpura or the HELLP (Haemolysis + Elevated Liver enzymes + Low Platelet count) syndrome. A bone marrow examination is often carried out early in the investigation of thrombocytopenia because it is helpful in excluding conditions such as acute leukaemia, which occasionally present with isolated thrombocytopenia.

Pancytopenia

Pancytopenia (reduction in the white cell count, Hb, and platelet count) is most often the result of anticancer chemotherapy, HIV infection, hypersplenism, and bone marrow infiltration or failure. Careful examination of a blood film is important if the reason for the pancytopenia is not apparent from the clinical history. If this does not reveal the cause, bone marrow aspiration and trephine biopsy may be needed.

Qualitative Abnormalities of Blood Cells

In health, only the most mature forms of cells appear in the peripheral blood. Earlier, less mature cells, such as nucleated red blood cells, polychromatic red cells, myelocytes, and metamyelocytes, may be released from the bone marrow in conditions where the bone marrow is overactive (e.g., acute haemolytic states or recovery after suppression) or functionally abnormal. Their presence in the peripheral blood indicates that active haemopoiesis is taking place.

Abnormalities of All Cell Lines

The combination of anisopoikilocytosis, mild macrocytosis, hypogranular neutrophils with abnormal nuclear morphology, and platelet anisocytosis, often with quantitative abnormalities, is virtually pathognomonic of a myelodysplastic syndrome. These features are reflected in the bone marrow with disturbance of the normal developmental pathway and nuclear:cytoplasmic asynchrony. Cytogenetic studies can confirm the diagnosis when cytological abnormalities are minor and also can assist in determining the prognosis.

Abnormalities of Individual Cell Lines
Red Cells
Congenital abnormalities of the red cell affecting the structure (e.g., spherocytosis, elliptocytosis) and content (e.g., haemoglobinopathies, enzymopathies) often produce typical morphological changes (see Chapter 5). The type of changes will guide further investigations toward analysis of structural proteins, haemoglobin electrophoresis, or HPLC and enzyme assays. Acquired red cell abnormalities may also help to indicate underlying pathology. For example, target cells may prompt investigation of liver function, whereas rouleaux may indicate the need for investigations for multiple myeloma or inflammatory conditions such as rheumatoid arthritis.

White Cells
Congenital abnormalities of neutrophils are unusual, but similar morphological abnormalities (e.g., Pelger–Huët cells) may be seen in acquired conditions such as myelodysplastic syndrome. Reactive

changes in lymphocytes including basophilic, faceted cytoplasm, are typically seen in infectious mononucleosis, which can be diagnosed using an appropriate screening test (p. 601) or, if this is negative, by demonstration of immunoglobulin M (IgM) antibodies to the Epstein–Barr virus. These atypical lymphocytes can sometimes be difficult to differentiate from circulating lymphoma cells. Bone marrow histology, combined with immunophenotyping studies and determination of lymphocyte clonality by demonstration of light chain restriction or by gene rearrangement studies, may be needed to reach a firm conclusion.

Platelets

Platelets that function poorly may not necessarily appear morphologically abnormal, although sometimes they are hypogranular or larger than normal. A normal platelet count with a prolonged bleeding time is characteristic of a disorder of platelet function, but some patients with abnormal platelet function are also thrombocytopenic. Hereditary disorders of platelet function are uncommon and usually present as a bleeding diathesis. When a qualitative disorder of platelets is suspected, platelets should be examined to assess size and to detect the cytological features of the grey platelet syndrome. They can broadly be divided into two categories: abnormalities of the platelet membrane (e.g., Bernard–Soulier syndrome, Glanzmann's thrombasthenia) and of platelet secretory function (e.g., storage pool diseases). In comparison, acquired disorders of platelet function are common. Haematological conditions associated with platelet dysfunction include myeloproliferative and myelodysplastic disorders and dysproteinaemias. Many widely prescribed drugs can interfere with platelet function, including aspirin and non-steroidal anti-inflammatory agents, whereas systemic conditions, particularly chronic renal failure and cardiopulmonary bypass, are associated with a bleeding tendency as a result of qualitative platelet defects. Most of these acquired functional defects are not associated with any abnormality in platelet appearance but in the myelodysplastic and, to a lesser extent, in the myeloproliferative disorders there may be hypogranular and giant platelets.

SPECIFIC TESTS FOR COMMON HAEMATOLOGICAL DISORDERS

Common haematological disorders are outlined in the following sections with suggestions for investigations that may be helpful in confirming the diagnosis. The lists are not intended to be exhaustive because the range of tests provided locally will depend on the availability of expertise and technology. The investigations discussed are those that are likely to be available within a general haematology department.

Red Cell Disorders

Microcytic Hypochromic Anaemias

For more information, see Chapters 7 and 12.

- Measurement of serum ferritin or iron plus either total iron-binding capacity or transferrin assay, red cell protoporphyrin
- Bone marrow aspirate with staining for iron
- Stool examination for occult blood; blood loss studies with ^{51}Cr-labelled red cells
- Tests for malabsorption
- Serological tests for coeliac disease
- Endoscopic examination with biopsy
- Serum lead (if lead poisoning is suspected)

If thalassaemia is suspected:
- Haemoglobin electrophoresis plus Hb A$_2$ and Hb F measurements or HPLC
- Haemoglobin H preparation
- Family studies
- DNA analysis

Macrocytic Anaemias

Where macrocytic, megaloblastic erythroid maturation is demonstrated, further investigations should be undertaken as described in Chapter 8. If the blood film is typical of megaloblastic anaemia, relevant assays and further investigations are often performed without a bone marrow aspirate being done. Macrocytosis may also be secondary to common conditions such as alcohol excess, liver disease, myelodysplastic syndrome, hydroxycarbamide administration, and hypothyroidism. Reticulocytosis from any cause can also increase the MCV.

Aplastic Anaemia

- Bone marrow aspirate and trephine biopsy
- Acidified serum (Ham's) test for paroxysmal nocturnal haemoglobinuria (urine examination for haemosiderin and neutrophil alkaline phosphatase if Ham's test is positive)
- Vitamin B_{12} and folate assays
- Viral studies, particularly for Epstein–Barr and hepatitis viruses.

If Fanconi's anaemia is suspected:
- Studies of sensitivity of chromosomes to breakage by DNA crosslinking agent
- Radiology of hands and forearms

Haemolytic Anaemias

A haemolytic process may be suspected by the presence of a falling haemoglobin, a reticulocytosis, and jaundice with an increase in unconjugated bilirubin level (see Chapters 9, 10, and 11).

White Cell Disorders

The blood may appear entirely normal in some patients with white cell disorders (e.g., lymphoma, myelomatosis, immune deficiency, neutrophil dysfunction). Changes in white cell numbers or morphology may occur rapidly in response to local or systemic disorders. The investigation of white cell disorders is more likely to require marrow examination than investigation of red cell disorders, especially when a primary marrow disorder is suspected. In chronic leukaemias, bone marrow examination may add little to the diagnosis, but the pattern of infiltration may have prognostic significance, e.g., in chronic lymphocytic leukaemia. The distribution of white cells is better appreciated in trephine biopsies, which are particularly important in lymphomas.

Acute Leukaemia

- Bone marrow aspirate
- Bone marrow trephine biopsy if an adequate bone marrow aspirate is not obtained
- Cytochemical stains
- Blood or marrow immunophenotyping, unless obviously myeloid
- Cytogenetic analysis
- Molecular studies (e.g., fluorescence *in situ* hybridization) for rearrangements of specific oncogenes

Neutropenia

- Serial neutrophil counts for cyclical neutropenia
- Tests for antineutrophil antibodies
- Bone marrow aspirate and trephine biopsy
- Autoantibody screen and investigations for systemic lupus erythematosus
- Vitamin B_{12} and folate assays
- Acidified serum (Ham's) test

Chronic Granulocytic Leukaemia

- Bone marrow aspirate
- Cytogenetic analysis
- Molecular studies (e.g., fluorescence *in situ* hybridization) for *BCR–ABL* rearrangement
- Neutrophil alkaline phosphatase score, if cytogenetic and molecular genetic analysis are not available

Chronic Lymphoproliferative Disorders/ Lymphadenopathy

- Serological screening for infectious mononucleosis, cytomegalovirus infection, HIV infection, and toxoplasmosis (if infectious cause suspected)
- Bone marrow aspirate and trephine biopsy (for detection of the presence and distribution of abnormal lymphocytes)
- Immunophenotyping
- Serum protein electrophoresis and immunoglobulin concentrations
- Serum urate, calcium, and lactate dehydrogenase (LDH)
- Lymph node biopsy (aspiration or surgical)
- Cytogenetic or molecular genetic analysis including investigation for immunoglobulin heavy chain or T-cell receptor gene rearrangement if the diagnosis of lymphoma is in doubt
- Radiological studies (X-ray, ultrasonography, computed tomography scan, magnetic resonance imaging)

Myelomatosis

- Bone marrow aspirate
- Bone marrow trephine biopsy if a cellular aspirate is not obtained
- Serum protein electrophoresis and immunoglobulin concentrations

- Serum albumin and calcium measurements
- β_2-microglobulin
- Urine (random and 24 hours) for Bence–Jones protein detection and quantitation
- Tests of renal function
- Radiological skeletal survey
- Serum free light chain quantification and ratio

Other Disorders

Myeloproliferative Disorders

- Blood volume, red cell mass, and plasma volume (for polycythaemia) measurements
- Bone marrow aspirate and trephine biopsy
- Arterial oxygen saturation and carboxyhaemoglobin level
- Abdominal ultrasound examination
- Neutrophil alkaline phosphatase
- Vitamin B_{12} (or B_{12}-binding capacity)
- Serum urate
- JAK2 analysis

Myelodysplasia

- Bone marrow aspirate and trephine biopsy
- Cytogenetic analysis

"Idiopathic" Myelofibrosis

- Bone marrow trephine biopsy
- Red cell folate assay
- Urate

If splenectomy is contemplated:
- Ferrokinetic and red cell survival studies
- Spleen scan and red cell pool measurement.

Pancytopenia with Splenomegaly
- Bone marrow aspirate and trephine biopsy
- Bacterial culture of marrow for tuberculosis
- Marrow examination for amastigotes of *Leishmania donovani*
- Biopsy of palpable lymph nodes (aspiration or surgical)
- Vitamin B_{12} and folate assays
- Liver biopsy
- Splenic aspirate
- Acidified serum (Ham's) test
- Serum rheumatoid factor and autoantibody screen
- Laparotomy and splenectomy.

The rationale behind these tests, and details of investigations outside general haematology practice, can be found in comprehensive haematology textbooks, in electronic databases, and on Web sites.

CLASSIFICATION OF HAEMATOLOGICAL NEOPLASMS

Since the late 1970s, acute leukaemia and the MDS have usually been defined and further classified according to the proposals of the French–American–British (FAB) group. These classifications are now being supplanted by the World Health Organization (WHO) classifications, published in definitive form in 2001. The WHO classifications are much broader in their aims and include myeloproliferative and chronic lymphoproliferative disorders.[1,2]

Application of the WHO criteria requires the results of immunophenotyping and cytogenetic analysis. The FAB classifications therefore continue to have a place (a) when these techniques are not available and (b) in making a provisional morphological diagnosis while awaiting the results of further tests. It may be necessary to issue a provisonal report, so that treatment can commence, with a supplementary report following when all diagnostic procedures have been completed. It is important that, whichever classification is used, the criteria are strictly observed so that there is consistency between different centres and countries. To avoid any possibility of confusion, FAB terminology (e.g., M1, M2) should not be applied if the WHO classsification is being used.

Classification of Acute Myeloid Leukaemia

The FAB criteria for a diagnosis of AML (Table 23.1) are as follows:

1. Blast cells must constitute at least 30% of all bone marrow cells **or**
2. When erythroid cells are at least 50% of bone marrow cells and blasts cells must be at least 30% of non-erythroid cells (lymphocytes, plasma cells, macrophages, and mast cells also being exluded from the count) **or**

Table 23.1	The French–American–British (FAB) classification of acute myeloid leukaemia
Category	Criteria
M0	<3% of blasts MPO or SBB positive Lymphoid markers negative Immunological or ultrastructural features of myeloid differentiation
M1	Blasts ≥90% of bone marrow NEC ≥3% of blasts MPO or SBB positive Maturing monocytic component in bone marrow ≤10% Maturing granulocytic component in bone marrow ≤10%
M2	Blasts 30–89% of BM NEC Maturing granulocytic component >10% NEC BM monocytic component <20% of NEC and other criteria of M4 not met
M3	Characteristic morphology
M4	Blasts ≥30% of BM NEC Granulocytic component ≥20% of BM NEC Monocytic component ≥20% of BM NEC and either PB monocytes ≥5 × 10^9/l or BM like M2 but PB monocytes ≥5 × 10^9/l and cytochemical proof of monocytic differentiation
M5a	Blasts ≥30% of NEC BM monocytic component ≥80% of NEC Monoblasts ≥80% of BM monocytic component
M5b	Blasts ≥30% of NEC BM monocytic component ≥80% of NEC Monoblasts <80% of BM monocytic component
M6	Erythroid cells ≥50% of BM cells BM blasts ≥30% of NEC
M7	Blasts shown to be predominantly megakaryoblasts

MPO, myeloperoxidase; SBB, Sudan black B; BM, bone marrow; NEC, non-erythroid cells; PB, peripheral blood.

3. The characteristic cytological features of acute hypergranular promyelocytic leukaemia or its variant form are present **and**
4. Blast cells are shown to be myeloid by either there being at least 3% of blast cells positive for Sudan black B, myeloperoxidase, or nonspecific esterase or by demonstration of myeloid antigens on immunophenotyping.

The WHO classification categorises cases as AML if the following criteria are met:

1. There are at least 20% of blast cells of myeloid lineage in the blood or bone marrow **or**
2. If the erythroid cells are at least 50% of bone marrow cells, blast cells are at least 20% of nonerythroid cells, **or**
3. Primitive erythroid cells constitute at least 80% of bone marrow cells **or**
4. There is a myeloid sarcoma (granulocytic sarcoma) **or**
5. One of a number of specified chromosomal rearrangements is present (Table 23.2).

In the FAB classification, AML is further classified as shown in Table 23.1. In the WHO classification, AML is further categorised as shown in Table 23.2. It should be noted that the WHO classification is hierachical. If appropriate, cases are first assigned to the category of therapy-related leukaemia. Next, cases are assigned, if appropriate, to the category of AML with recurrent genetic abnormalities. Cases continue to be assigned to successive categories in the order shown in Table 23.2 with remaining cases finally being categorised as "AML not otherwise categorized." This final group is further subdivided into categories resembling those of the FAB classification (but defined in quite a different manner). The "not-otherwise-categorized" group includes several entities that are either newly defined (acute panmyelosis with myelofibrosis and pure erythroid leukaemia) or were not specifically mentioned in the FAB classification (acute basophilic leukaemia and myeloid sarcoma, either granulocytic or monocytic).

Table 23.2   The World Health Organization classification of acute myeloid leukaemia (AML)

Therapy-related AML and myelodysplastic syndrome*
  Alkylating agent related
  Topo-isomerase II inhibitor related
  Other types
AML with recurrent genetic abnormalities*
  AML with t(8;21)(q22;q22)/*AML1-ETO* fusion
  AML with abnormal bone marrow eosinophils and inv(16)(p13q22) or t(16;16)(p13;q22)/*CBFB-MYH11* fusion
  Acute promyelocytic leukaemia with t(15;17)(q22;q12)/*PML-RARA* fusion, and variants
  AML with 11q23 rearrangement and *MLL* abnormality
AML with multilineage dysplasia†
  Following a myelodysplastic syndrome or a myelodysplastic/myeloproliferative syndrome
  Without antecedent myelodysplastic syndrome
AML not otherwise categorized
  AML, minimally differentiated (resembles FAB M0)
  AML without maturation (resembles FAB M1)
  AML with maturation (resembles FAB M2)
  Acute myelomonocytic leukaemia (resembles FAB M4)
  Acute monoblastic and acute monocytic leukaemia (resembles FAB M5a, M5b)
  Acute erythroid leukaemia
    Erythroleukaemia (resembles FAB M6)
    Pure erythroid leukaemia
  Acute megakaryoblastic leukaemia (resembles FAB M7)
  Acute basophilic leukaemia
  Acute panmyelosis with myelofibrosis
  Myeloid sarcoma (granulocytic or monocytic)

*If therapy-related cases have recurrent cytogenetic abnormalities, this is noted.
†Defined as having at least 50% of cells dysplastic in at least 2 lineages

Classification of the Myelodysplastic Syndromes

The FAB criteria for a diagnosis of MDS are that there is evidence for a myeloid neoplasm with ineffective haemopoiesis but the criteria for AML are not met. Blast cells must be less than 30% in the bone marrow. In the WHO classification, there must be evidence for a myeloid neoplasm with ineffective haemopoiesis and blasts must be less than 20% in both blood and bone marrow. In additon, the specific cytogenetic abnormalities shown in Table 23.2 must be absent (or the case is categorized as AML, regardless of the blast count). There is a further major difference between the two classifications, specifically that chronic myelomonocytic leukaemia is classified as MDS in the FAB classification, whereas in the WHO classification it is assigned to a new category of disorder designated myelodysplastic/myeloproliferative diseases. The details of the FAB classification of MDS are shown in Table 23.3 and of the WHO classification in Table 23.4. It will be noted that cytogenetic analysis is essential for the application of the WHO classification because cases of the 5q- syndrome cannot otherwise be recognized. Like the WHO classification of AML, this is a hierachical classification. Therapy-related MDS is categorized with therapy-related AML. Remaining cases are then assessed as to whether they meet the criteria for the 5q- syndrome. If they do not, they are assigned to the remaining categories, depending on the number of lineages showing dyplasia, the percentage of ring sideroblasts, the presence or absence of Auer rods, and the percentage of blast cells in the blood and marrow. The details of the WHO classification of the myelodysplastic/myeloproliferative diseases are shown in Table 23.5.

Table 23.3   The French–American–British classification of the myelodysplastic syndromes

Category	Peripheral blood criteria	Bone marrow criteria
Refractory anaemia (RA) or refractory cytopenia*	Anaemia,* blasts ≤1%, monocytes ≤1 × 10⁹/l	Blasts <5%, ringed sideroblasts ≤15% of erythroblasts
Refractory anaemia with ringed sideroblasts (RARS)	Anaemia, blasts ≤1%, monocytes ≤1 × 10⁹/l	Blasts <5%, ringed sideroblasts >15% of erythroblasts
Refractory anaemia with excess of blasts (RAEB)	Anaemia, blasts >1% <5%, monocytes ≤1 × 10⁹/l [or] blasts <5% and	[and] Blasts ≥5% <20% [but] blasts <20%
Refractory anaemia with excess of blasts in transformation (RAEB-T)	Anaemia, blasts ≥5% [or]	Auer rods in blood or marrow [or] Blasts ≥20% but blasts <30%
Chronic myelomonocytic leukaemia (CMML)	Monocytes >1 × 10⁹/l, granulocytes often increased, blasts <5%	Blasts <20%, promonocytes often increased

*Or in the case of refractory cytopenia, either neutropenia or thrombocytopenia.

Classification of Acute Lymphoblastic Leukaemia

Both the FAB and WHO classifications require that an acute leukaemia be positively shown to be lymphoid before it is categorized as acute lymphoblastic leukaemia (ALL) so as to avoid inadvertently categorising FAB M0 and M7 AML as ALL. The WHO classification groups together ALL and lymphoblastic lymphoma, using the designations precursor B lymphoblastic leukaemia/lymphoblastic lymphoma and precursor T lymphoblastic leukaemia/lymphoblastic lymphoma. These designations are clearly too cumbersome to use in clinical practice, and undoubtedly haematologists will continue to refer to "acute lymphoblastic leukaemia." The FAB group classified ALL into three morphological categories, designated L1, L2, and L3 ALL. It is of little significance whether a case falls into the L1 or L2 category, and this distinction can be dropped. However, L3 morphology—the presence of "blast cells" with basophilic cytoplasm and vacuolation—is of considerable clinical significance. In most, but not all, of these cases the cells are immunologically mature, expressing surface membrane immuno-globulin, and the condition represents a leukaemic presentation of Burkitt's lymphoma. The WHO classification categorizes such cases as Burkitt's lymphoma. This is more appropriate than their being categorized as ALL because the treatment of these cases differs very considerably from the treatment of ALL.

Classification of Myeloproliferative Disorders

The WHO classification of the myeloproliferative disorders is summarized in Table 23.6. Most of these conditions are defined in accordance with established haematological practice. However, the method of distinguishing between essential thrombocythaemia and idiopathic myelofibrosis differs from previous practice with many cases that would previously have been categorized as essential thrombocythaemia now being classified as the cellular phase of myelofibrosis; whether this classsification will be widely accepted remains to be seen. The WHO classification of myeloproliferative disorders takes little account of cytogenetic or molecular genetic analysis, only Ph-positive chronic myeloid leukaemia being defined

Text continued on p. 624.

Table 23.4 Summary of World Health Organization classification of the myelodysplastic syndromes (MDS)

Disease	Peripheral blood findings	Bone marrow findings
MDS associated with isolated del(5q)	Anaemia, platelet count usually normal or elevated, <5% blasts	Megakaryocytes normal or increased but with hypolobated nuclei, <5% blasts, no Auer rods
Refractory anaemia (RA)	Anaemia, no or rare blasts	Dysplasia confined to erythroid lineage, <5% blasts, <15% ringed sideroblasts
Refractory anaemia with ringed sideroblasts (RARS)	Anaemia, no blasts	Dysplasia confined to erythroid lineage, <5% blasts, ≥15% ringed sideroblasts
Refractory cytopenia with multilineage dysplasia (RCMD)	Cytopenias (bicytopenia or pancytopenia), no or rare blasts, no Auer rods, $< 1 \times 10^9$/l monocytes	Dysplasia in ≥10% of the cells of two or more myeloid cell lineages, <5% blasts, <15% ringed sideroblasts, no Auer rods
Refractory cytopenia with multilineage dysplasia and ringed sideroblasts (RCMD-RS)	Cytopenias (bicytopenia or pancytopenia), no or rare blasts, no Auer rods, $< 1 \times 10^9$/l monocytes	Dysplasia in ≥10% of the cells of two or more myeloid cell lineages, <5% blasts, ≥15% ringed sideroblasts, no Auer rods
Refractory anaemia with excess blasts-1 (RAEB-1)	Cytopenias, <5% blasts, no Auer rods, $<1 \times 10^9$/l monocytes	Unilineage or multilineage dysplasia, 5–9% blasts, no Auer rods
Refractory anaemia with excess blasts-2 (RAEB-2)	Cytopenias, 5–19% blasts, Auer rods sometimes present, $<1 \times 10^9$/l monocytes	Unilineage or multilineage dysplasia, 10–19% blasts, Auer rods sometimes present
Myelodysplastic syndrome-unclassifiable (MDS-U)	Cytopenias, no or rare blasts, no Auer rods	Unilineage dysplasia (megakaryocytic or granulocytic), <5% blasts, no Auer rods

Table 23.5   Summary of the World Health Organization categories of myelodysplastic/myeloproliferative diseases

Category	Criteria
Chronic myelomonocytic leukaemia (CMML)	A Ph-negative, BCR–ABL-negative disorder with monocyte count > 1 × 10^9/l Fewer than 20% blasts plus promonocytes in peripheral blood (PB) or bone marrow (BM) Either dysplasia of one or more myeloid lineages or alternative criteria met (acquired clonal cytogenetic abnormality or monocytosis persisting for at least 3 months and alternative causes of monocytosis excluded)
Atypical chronic myeloid leukaemia (aCML)	A Ph-negative, BCR–ABL-negative disorder with leucocytosis resulting from an increase in neutrophils and their precursors, the precursors (promyelocyte to metamyelocytes) constituting a least 10% of PB white cells Basophils less than 2% of white cells Monocytes less than 10% of white cells Hypercellular BM with granulocytic hyperplasia and dysplasia, with or without dysplasia of other lineages Fewer than 20% blasts plus promonocytes in peripheral blood or bone marrow

Juvenile myelomonocytic leukaemia (JMML)	A Ph-negative, BCR–ABL-negative disorder with monocyte count > 1 × 10^9/l
	 Fewer than 20% blasts plus promonocytes in peripheral blood or bone marrow
	 Plus two or more of the following
	     Haemoglobin F increased for age
	     Immature granulocytes in the PB
	     WBC greater than 10 × 10^9/l
	     Clonal chromosomal abnormality (monosomy 7 not excluded)
	     GM-CSF hypersensitivity of myeloid precursors *in vitro*

Myelodysplastic/myeloproliferative disease, unclassifiable	A myelodysplastic/myeloproliferative disorder in which the criteria of one of the myelodysplastic syndromes are met There are prominent proliferative features (e.g., a platelet count of greater than 600 × 10^9/l or a white cell count of greater than 13 × 10^9/l) The condition has developed *de novo* The criteria for other MDS/MPD (CMML, aCML, and JMML) are not met There is no Philadelphia chromosome, BCR–ABL fusion gene, 5q–, inv(3)(q21q26) or t(3;3)(q21;q26)

Table 23.6   Summary of World Health Organization classification of the myeloproliferative disorders

Chronic myelogenous leukaemia, Philadelphia chromosome positive (t(9;22)(q34;q11), *BCR–ABL* fusion)

Chronic neutrophilic leukaemia

Chronic eosinophilic leukaemia/hypereosinophilic syndrome*

Chronic idiopathic myelofibrosis

Polycythaemia vera

Essential thrombocythaemia

Myeloproliferative disorders, unclassifiable

*Cases of hypereosinophilic syndrome are categorized as eosinophilic leukaemia if there are more than 2% blast cells in the blood or more than 5% (but less than 20%) blast cells in the bone marrow or if the myeloid cells have a clonal cytogenetic abnormality or other evidence of clonality; other examples of the hypereosinophilic syndrome continue to be classified as idiopathic and are not regarded as myeloproliferative disorders.

on this basis. It should be noted that the WHO classification defines a case with hypereosinophilia as eosinophilic leukaemia, rather than as the idiopathic hypereosinophilic syndrome, when there is evidence of clonality. The 4q12 syndrome, resulting from a cryptic deletion at 4q12 with formation of a *FIP1L1-PDGFRA* fusion gene, is therefore categorized as eosinophilic leukaemia.

REFERENCES

1. Jaffe ES, Harris NL, Stein H, et al 2001 WHO classification of tumours: pathology and genetics of tumours of haematological and lymphoid tissues. IARC Press, Lyon, France.
2. Vardiman JW, Harris NL, Brunning RD 2002 The World Health Organization (WHO) classification of the myeloid neoplasms. Blood 100:2292–2302.

24 Laboratory organization and management

S. Mitchell Lewis and Anne Bradshaw

The essential function of a haematology laboratory is to obtain reliable and reproducible data for health screening and epidemiological studies and to provide clinicians with timely, unambiguous, and meaningful reports to assist in diagnosing disease and monitoring its response to treatment. Advancing technology and increasing health care legislation have added to the complexity of modern laboratory practice, whose area of responsibility should include the preanalytic stage (i.e., test ordering, blood collection, specimen transport) and the postanalytic stage (i.e., maintaining a data file, preparing reports, transmission of results). Laboratory organization and management are essential for good laboratory practice. The principles outlined in this chapter apply to small as well as to large departments, although the latter requires more complex management arrangements.

MANAGEMENT STRUCTURE AND FUNCTION

The management structure of a haematology laboratory should indicate a clear line of accountability of each member of staff to the head of department. In turn, the head of department may be managerially accountable to a clinical director (of laboratories) and then to a hospital or health authority executive committee. The head of department is responsible for departmental leadership, for ensuring that the laboratory has authoritative representation within the hospital, and for ensuring that managerial and administrative tasks are performed efficiently. Management requires an integrated team effort with individual members of staff contributing managerial skills to specified aspects. All medical and senior technical staff should receive some training in laboratory management. Where the head of department delegates managerial tasks to others, these responsibilities must be clearly defined and stated.

Management of a department requires an executive committee, and under this executive, answerable to the head of department, there should be a number of designated individuals responsible for implementing the functions of the department (Table 24.1). Clearly the activities of the various members of staff overlap, and there must be adequate effective communication between them. There should be regular briefings at meetings of technical heads with their section staff. The only way to avoid unauthorized leakage of information from policy-making committees is to ensure that all members of staff are kept fully informed of any plans that might have bearing on their careers, working practices, and well-being.

Because of the requirements established by regulatory agencies for accreditation of laboratories and audit of their performance (see p. 639), documents on laboratory management and practice from standards-setting authorities, and the plethora of guidelines from national and international professional bodies, there may be need for a special subcommittee of the executive committee whose duty is to keep abreast of these matters and to interrelate with the different sections in the same way as the safety officer.

Staff Appraisal

All members of staff should receive training to enhance their skills and to develop their careers. This requires setting goals and conducting regular appraisals of progress for both management and technical ability. The appraisal process should cascade down from the head of department, and appropriate training must be given to those who undertake appraisals at successive levels. The appraiser should provide a short list of topics to the person to be interviewed who should be encouraged to add to the list so that each understands the topics to be covered. These must not include considerations of pay. An appraisal interview should be open-ended and should be a constructive dialogue of the present state of development and the progress made to date. Ideally, the staff members should leave the interviews with the knowledge that their personal development and future progress are of importance to the department, that priorities have been identified, that an action plan with milestones and a timescale has been agreed, and that progress will be monitored. Formal appraisal interviews (annually for senior staff and more often for others) should be complemented by less formal follow-up discussions to monitor progress. Documentation of formal interviews can be limited to a short list of agreed objectives.

Performance appraisal can have lasting value in the personal development of individuals, but the process can easily be mishandled and should not be started without training in how to hold an appraisal interview.[1]

Continuing Professional Development

Continuing professional development, linked with continuing medical education, is a process of systematic learning that enables health workers to be constantly brought up to date on developments in their profession and thus ensure their competence to practice throughout their entire career. Policies and programmes have already been established in a number of countries and, in some, participation is a

Table 24.1   Suggested components of a management structure

Executive committee
    Head of department
    Business manager
    Consultant haematologists
    Principal Scientific Officer

Safety officer
Quality-control officer
Computer and data processing supervisor

Sectional technical heads
    Cytometry
    Blood film morphology
    Immunohaematology
    Haemostasis
    Blood transfusion
    Special investigations
       (haemolytic anaemias, haemoglobinopathies,
       cytochemistry, etc.)
    Molecular techniques

Clerical supervisor

mandatory requirement for the right to practice. Schemes for continuing professional development are run by national professional bodies that are responsible for the practice standards of their members. In the United Kingdom, a scheme relevant to clinical haematologists is administered by the Royal College of Pathologists.[2,3] The Institute for Biomedical Science undertakes a scheme for scientists/technologists working in the laboratory, which is mandatory for laboratory accreditation by Clinical Pathology Accreditation (p. 641); details of the Institute's scheme are available on their Web site (www.ibms.org). The continuing professional development process is based on obtaining "credits" for various qualifying activities, such as attendance at specified lectures, workshops, and conferences; giving lectures; writing books or journal articles, using computer- or journal-based programmes; and taking part in peer review discussions. The credit points accumulate toward an annual required score.

Strategic and Business Planning

The head of department is responsible for determining the long-term (usually up to 5 years) strategic direction of the department. Strategic planning requires awareness of any national and local legislation that may affect the laboratory and of changes in local clinical practice that may alter workload. It is conventional to perform an analysis of the internal Strengths and Weaknesses of the laboratory and its ability to respond to external Opportunities and Threats ("SWOT" analysis). Expansion of a major clinical service, such as organ transplantation, or the opportunity to compete for the laboratory service of other hospitals and clinics may pose both an external opportunity and threat to the laboratory depending on its ability to respond to the consequential increase in workload. Internal strengths may include technical or scientific expertise, whereas a heavy workload that precludes any additional developmental work would be a weakness.

Increasingly, laboratories must meet financial challenges and the need for greater cost-effectiveness. This may require rationalisation by eliminating unused laboratory capacity, avoiding unnecessary tests, and ensuring more efficient use of skilled staff and expensive equipment. This may require centralisation of multiple laboratory sites, or conversely there may be advantages in establishing satellite centres for the benefit of patients and clinicians if these can be shown to be cost-effective.

A business plan is primarily concerned with determining short-term objectives that will allow the strategy to be implemented over the next financial year or so. It requires prediction of future work level and expansion. Planning of these objectives should involve all staff because this will heighten awareness of the issues and will develop "ownership" of the strategy. In all but the smallest laboratory, a business manager is required to coordinate such planning and to liase with the equivalent business managers in other clinical and laboratory areas. Business planning also requires a sophisticated laboratory accounting process with an up-to-date record of workload and costs so that the realistic price of tests can be established.

Workload Assessment and Costing of Tests

Laboratories should maintain accurate records of workload and costs in order to apportion resources to each section. Computerization of laboratories has greatly facilitated this process. In assessing workload, account must be taken of the entire cycle from test receipt to issue of a report, whether the test is by manual or semi-automated method or by high-volume multiple-analyte automated analyzers, the roles of biomedical scientists/senior technologists and junior technicians, supervised laboratory assistants, clerical staff, and medical personnel responsible for reviewing the report. Out of hours service requires a different calculation of costs.

Methods for determining the workload of individual laboratory sections, adjusted for test complexity, are described in "Guidelines of the Canadian Health Service Organizations."[4] Similar workload scoring systems have been published by the College of American Pathologists[5] and the Welcan system in the United Kingdom.[6] In most areas, however, these have been largely replaced by benchmarking (see p. 642).

Financial Control

Full costing of tests includes all aspects of laboratory function (Table 24.2). The amount allocated for staff salaries should include the cost of training and should take into account absences for annual leave or sickness. It needs also to take into account

Table 24.2 Factors contributing to cost of laboratory tests
Direct costs
Staff salaries
Laboratory equipment purchases
Reagents and other consumables
Equipment maintenance
Quality control
Specific technical training on equipment
Indirect costs
Capital costs and mortgage factor
Depreciation
Building repairs and routine maintenance
Lighting, heating, and waste disposal
Personnel services
Cleaning services
Transport and portering
Laundry services
Computers
Telephone and fax
Postage

E = Annual equipment cost based on initial cost divided by expected life of the item*
M = Annual maintenance and servicing of equipment
0 = Laboratory overheads (see Table 24.2)
S = Supervision
T = Transport and communication
A = Laboratory administration, including salaries of clerical and other nontechnical staff.

Efficient budgeting requires regular monitoring, at least monthly. Computer spreadsheets are a useful means to obtain an easily comprehended view of the financial state and the likely outcome.

In general, staff cost is by far the largest component of the total costs of running a laboratory. Furthermore, most of the other costs are obligations outside the direct control of the laboratory. If financial savings become necessary, they can be achieved in a variety of ways, but large savings usually necessitate a reduction in staff because employment costs can account for three-fourths of total expenditure. Possible initiatives include the following:

Rationalization of service with other local hospitals to eliminate duplication
Restructuring within a hospital laboratory for cross-discipline working (e.g., between haematology and clinical chemistry)
Subcontracting of labour-intensive tests to a specialist laboratory
Employment of part-time contract staff (e.g., for overnight and weekend emergency service or for the phlebotomy service) and sharing of emergency service between local hospitals
Review of price setting on the basis of workload and calculated cost per test

Increasing use of automated systems will allow for staff reduction,[7] although an estimate of savings must take account of capital and running costs of the equipment, especially the high cost of some reagents, and whether the system can be used to high capacity and throughout a 24-hour service.

Purchasing expensive equipment outright adds to the capital assets of the laboratory, with the con-

the extent to which staff of various levels, as described earlier, are involved. Indirect costs may be apportioned to different sections of a department who share common overhead costs.

Calculation of Test Costs

When preparing a budget, the following formula provides a reasonably reliable estimate of the total annual costs:

$$[L \times N] + [C \times N] + E + M + 0 + S + T + A, \text{ where}$$

L = Labour costs for each test from estimate of time taken and the salary rate of the staff member(s) performing the tests
N = Number of tests in the year
C = Cost of consumables per test (including controls)

---

*Either a proportion of the original cost or the annual cost of hire, as discussed later.

sequential cost of depreciation (usually 8–10% per annum). Leasing equipment can be a better alternative, and, in some countries, most equipment is obtained in this way. Careful calculation of the lease cost is required because this can be up to 20% higher than outright purchase. An advantage of leasing is flexibility to upgrade equipment should workload increase or technology change. If maintenance and consumable costs are included in the agreement, it is important to neither underestimate nor overestimate the annual requirements that will be included in the contract.

When automation is coupled with centralization of the service to another site, care must be taken to maintain service quality. Failure to do so will encourage clinicians to establish independent satellite laboratories. Loss of contact between clinical users and laboratory staff may compromise the preanalytic phase of the test process and may lead to inappropriate requests, excessive requests, and test samples that are of inadequate volume or are poorly identified. When services are centralized, attention must be paid to all phases (preanalytic, analytic, and postanalytic) of the test process, including the need for packaging the specimens and the cost of their transport to the laboratory.

Table 24.3   Systematic errors in analyses
Analyzer calibration uncertain (no reference standard available)
Bias in instrument, equipment, or glassware
Faulty dilution
Faults in the measuring steps (e.g., reagents, spectrometry, calculations)
Sampling not representative of specimen
Specimens not representative of *in vivo* status
Incomplete definition of analyte or lack of critical resolution of analyzer
Approximations and arbitrary assumptions inherent in analyzer's function
Environmental effects on analyzer
Preanalytic deterioration of specimens

TEST RELIABILITY

The reliability of a quantitative test is defined in terms of the *uncertainty of measurement* of the analyte (sometimes referred to in documents as "measurand"). This is based on its accuracy and precision.[8]

Accuracy is the closeness of agreement between the measurement that is obtained and the true value; the extent of discrepancy is the *systematic error,* or *bias.* The most important causes of systematic error are listed in Table 24.3. The error can be eliminated or at least greatly reduced by using a reference standard with the test, together with internal quality control and regular checking by external quality assessment (see p. 667).

Precision is the closeness of agreement when a test is repeated a number of times. Imprecision is the result of random errors; it is expressed as standard deviation (SD) and coefficient of variance (CV%).

When the data are spread normally (Gaussian distribution), for clinical purposes there is a 95% probability that results that fall within a range of +2 SD to −2 SD of the target value are correct.

Some of the other factors listed in Table 24.3 can be quantified to calculate the combined uncertainty of measurement. Thus, for example, when a calibration preparation is used, its uncertainty is usually stated on the label or accompanying certificate. The standard uncertainty is then calculated as follows:

$$\sqrt{(SD_1)^2 + (SD_2)^2}$$

Expanded uncertainty of measurement takes account of nonquantifiable items by multiplying the previous amount by a "coverage factor" (k), which is usually taken to be ×2 for 95% level of confidence.[8,9]

It may be necessary to decide by statistical analysis whether two sets of data differ significantly. The t-test is used to assess the likelihood of significant difference at various levels of probability by comparing the means or individually paired results. The F-ratio is useful to assess the influence of random errors in two sets of test results.

TEST SELECTION

To evaluate the diagnostic reliability and predictive value of an individual laboratory test, it is necessary to calculate test sensitivity and specificity.[10] *Sensitivity* is the fraction of true positive results when a test is applied to patients known to have the relevant disease or when results have been obtained by a reference method. *Specificity* is the fraction of true negative results when the test is applied to normals.

Diagnostic sensitivity = TP ÷ (TP + FN)
Diagnostic specificity = TP ÷ (TP + FN)
Positive predictive value = TP ÷ (TP + FP)
Negative predictive value = TN ÷ (TN + FN)

where TP = true positive; TN = true negative; FP = false positive; FN = false negative

Overall reliability can be calculated as

$$\frac{TP + TN}{Total\ number\ of\ tests} \times 100\%.$$

Sensitivity and specificity should be near 1.0 (100%) if the test is unique for a particular diagnosis. A lower level of sensitivity or specificity may still be acceptable if the results are interpreted in conjunction with other tests as part of an overall pattern. It is not usually possible to have both 100% sensitivity and 100% specificity. Whether sensitivity or specificity is more important depends on the particular purpose of the test. Thus, for example, if haemoglobinometry is required in a clinic for identifying patients with anaemia, sensitivity is important, whereas in blood donor selection, for selecting individuals who are not anaemic, specificity is more important.

Likelihood Ratio

The ratio of positive results in disease to the frequency of false-positive results in normals gives a statistical measure of the discrimination by the test between disease and normality. It can be calculated as follows:

Sensitivity / 1 – Specificity.[11]

The higher the ratio, the greater is the probability of disease, whereas a ratio <1 makes the possibility of the disease being correctly diagnosed by the test much less likely. Conversely, the likelihood of normality can be calculated as (1-sensitivity)/specificity.

An alternative method is that of Youden, which is obtained by calculating Specificity/(1– Sensitivity).[12] Values range between –1 and +1. With a positive ratio rising above zero toward +1 there is an increasing probability that the test will discriminate the presence of the specified disease, and there is decreasing likelihood that the test is valid when the ratio falls from 0 to –1.

Receiver–Operator Characteristic Analysis

The relative usefulness of different methods for the same test or of a new method against a reference method can also be assessed by the receiver–operator characteristic (ROC).[11] This is demonstrated graphically by plotting *sensitivity* on the vertical axis against *1-specificity* on the horizontal axis at a series of cut-off points for the different methods being compared. A result at the top left of the graph indicates high sensitivity and specificity, and a plot lying above and to the left of another plot shows greater reliability of that method.

Test Utility

To ensure cost-effectiveness of the laboratory service, tests with no proven value should be eliminated, and new tests for which there is independent evidence of effectiveness should be introduced. There is still unresolved debate on the economics of providing an automated total screening programme in contrast to specifically selected tests. Undoubtedly, few clinicians are familiar with all 11 (or possibly more) blood count parameters, which are reported routinely by some automated analyzers. One study, for example, indicated that the differential leucocyte count is overused and only occasionally clinically useful.[13]

For assessing cost-effectiveness of a test, account must be taken of (a) cost per test as compared with other tests that provide similar clinical information; (b) diagnostic reliability; and (c) clinical usefulness as assessed by the extent with which the test is relied on in clinical decisions, whether the results are likely to change the physician's diagnostic opinion and the clinical management of the patient, taking account of disease prevalence and a specified clinical or public health situation.[14] This requires audit by an independent assessor to judge what proportion of the requests for a particular test are actually used intelligently and what percentage are unnecessary or wasted tests[14,15] (see p. 677). Information on the utility of various tests can also be obtained from published guidelines and benchmarking (see p. 642).

The realistic cost-effectiveness of any test

may be assessed by $\dfrac{A}{B \times C}$

where A = cost/test as described on p. 628
B = diagnostic reliability as described on p. 630
C = clinical usefulness as described earlier.

INSTRUMENTATION

Equipment Evaluation

Evaluation of equipment to match the nature and volume of laboratory workload is a very important exercise. Protocols for evaluating blood cell analyzers and other haematology instruments have been published by the International Council for Standardization in Haematology.[16] The following are usually included in such evaluations:

1. Verification of instrument requirements for space and services
2. Extent of technical training required to operate the instrument
3. Clarity and usefulness of instruction manual
4. Assessment of safety (mechanical, electrical, microbiological, and chemical)
5. Determination of the following:
   a. linearity
   b. precision/imprecision
   c. carryover
   d. extent of inaccuracy by comparison with measurement by definitive or reference methods
   e. comparability with an established method used in the laboratory
   f. sensitivity (i.e., determination of the smallest change in analyte concentration that gives a measured result)
   g. specificity (i.e., extent of errors caused by interfering substances
6. Throughput time and number of specimens that can be processed within a normal working day

7. Cost per test
8. Reliability of the instrument when in routine use and adequacy of service and maintenance provided
9. Staff acceptability, impact on laboratory organization, and level of technical expertise required to operate the instrument.

As a rule, this type of evaluation is carried out by a reference laboratory on behalf of a national consumer organization or government health agency such as the Medical Devices Agency* of the Department of Health, London, who list a large number of such reports in their catalogue (see www.medical-devices.gov.uk). A CE mark on a device indicates that it conforms to defined specifications of the *in-vitro* diagnostic medical devices directive (see p. 649).

After an instrument has been purchased and installed, a less extensive check of performance with regard to precision, linearity, carryover, and comparability is often useful:

Precision

Carry out appropriate measurements 10 times consecutively on three or more specimens selected in the pathological range so as to include a low, a high, and a normal concentration of the analyte. Calculate the replicate SD and CV as shown on p. 698.

Table 24.4   Test precision for different purposes

Purpose of test	Expected CV% (automated counters)		
	Hb	RBC	WBC
Scientific standard	<1	1	1–2
State of art:			
best performance	1.5	2	3
routine laboratories	2–3	3	5–6
Clinical needs	5–10	5	10–15

CV, coefficient of variance; Hb, haemoglobin concentration; RBC, red blood cell count; WBC, white blood cell count.

*Medicines and Healthcare products Regulatory Agency (MHRA)

The degree of precision that is acceptable depends on the purpose of the test (Table 24.4). To check between-batch precision, measure three samples in several successive batches of routine tests; calculate the SD and CV in the same way.

Linearity

Linearity demonstrates the effects of dilution. Prepare a specimen with a high concentration of the analyte to be tested and, as accurately as possible, make a series of dilutions in plasma so as to obtain 10 samples with evenly spaced concentration levels between 10% and 100%. Measure each sample three times and calculate the means. Plot results on arithmetic graph paper. Ideally, all points should fall on a straight line that passes through the zero of the horizontal and vertical axes. In practice, the results should lie within 2SD limits of the means calculated from the CVs, which have been obtained from analysis of precision (see earlier). Inspection of the graph will show whether there is linearity throughout the range or whether it is limited to part of the range.

Carryover

Carryover indicates the extent to which measurement of an analyte in a specimen is likely to be affected by the preceding specimen. Measure a specimen with a high concentration in triplicate, immediately followed by a specimen with a low concentration of the analyte.

$$\text{Carryover (\%)} = \frac{l_1 - l_3}{h_3 - l_3} \times 100, \text{ where } l_1 \text{ and } l_3$$

are the results of the first and third measurements of the samples with a low concentration and h_3 is the third measurement of the sample with a high concentration.

Accuracy and Comparability

Accuracy and comparability test whether the new instrument (or method) gives results that agree satisfactorily with those obtained with an established procedure and with a reference method. Test specimens should be measured alternately, or in batches, by the two procedures. If results by the two methods are analysed by correlation coefficient (r), a high correlation does not mean that the two methods agree. Correlation coefficient is a measure of relation and not agreement. It is better to use the limits of agreement method.[17] For this, plot the differences

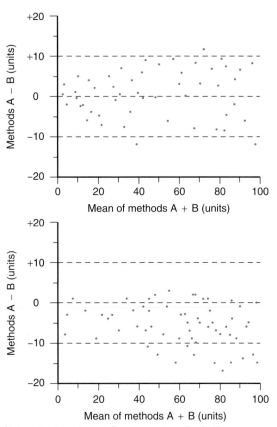

Figure 24.1   Limits of agreement method. Shows mean values for paired results by two methods A plus B (*horizontal axis*) plotted against the differences (*A minus B*) between the paired results (*vertical axis*). Horizontal lines represent equality with range of ±10 units (mean ±SD). Upper figure shows no bias between methods A and B, whereas lower figure shows false high results (negative values) for method B.

between paired results on the vertical axis of linear graph paper against the means of the pairs on the horizontal axis (Fig. 24.1); differences between the methods are then readily apparent over the range from low to high values. If the scatter of differences increases at high values, logarithmic transformed data should be plotted.

It is also useful to check for bias by including the instrument or method under test in the laboratory's participation in an external quality-assessment scheme (p. 667). Bias is expressed by $\dfrac{R - M}{M} \times 100$, where R = measurement by the device/method being tested and M = target EQAS result.

An alternative method to check for bias is the variance index.[18] This uses a *chosen coefficient of variance (CCV)*, which is based on an optimal CV for a reliable method, and the variance index (VI%) is calculated by $\frac{R - M}{M} \times \frac{100}{CCV} \times 100$.

Maintenance Logs

All laboratory equipment should be inspected regularly, and specific maintenance procedures should be carried out. Each item of laboratory equipment should have a maintenance log to document what maintenance is required, the desired frequency, and when it was last carried out. The log includes servicing and repairs by the manufacturer. Equipment used to test biological specimens must be cleaned thoroughly before a maintenance procedure is carried out to reduce the biohazard. The procedure for such cleaning must be documented (as a standard operating procedure) together with the name of the responsible worker and the date.

DATA PROCESSING

It is essential that accurate records of laboratory results are kept for whatever period is stipulated by national legislation. Computer-assisted data handling is essential for all but the smallest laboratory. For long-term storage of data, possibilities include a printed (hard) copy, a floppy disk, compact disk, or Zip disk, or a local server should be used. Laboratory results are usually issued as numeric data with abnormal results highlighted for the clinician. Report

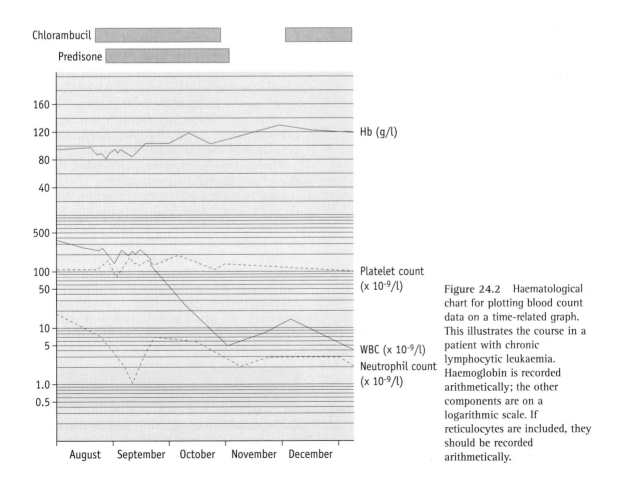

Figure 24.2   Haematological chart for plotting blood count data on a time-related graph. This illustrates the course in a patient with chronic lymphocytic leukaemia. Haemoglobin is recorded arithmetically; the other components are on a logarithmic scale. If reticulocytes are included, they should be recorded arithmetically.

forms should be reader friendly. Serial data are particularly useful to illustrate any trend with time and may be in the form of a cumulative tabulation or a graph. For the latter an arithmetic scale should be used for haemoglobin, red cell count, and reticulocytes, whereas platelet and leucocyte counts are best displayed on a logarithmic scale (Fig. 24.2). A graph is particularly useful for displaying results in relation to target intervals because this facilitates adjustment of dosage of drugs that are likely to affect the blood. Furthermore, this method of archiving reduces the number of pages of laboratory reports in the patient's file.[19,20]

Laboratory Computers

Developments in computer technology have made available powerful microcomputers and sophisti-

Table 24.5 Some uses of laboratory personal computers
Statistics
Graphics
Word processing
Creating lecture slides
Desktop publishing
Database files
Spreadsheets
Workload recording
Test costing and invoicing
Managing budgets
Stock control
Quality-control procedures
Audit systems
Internet information
Electronic mail
Teaching/training materials, including morphology
Expert systems—clinical decision support

cated computer software at moderate prices. Such computers may be an integral part of an analytic instrument or interfaced to it by cable. A modem is required to link the computer to the telephone or broadband for access to the Internet and electronic mail, and also to interconnect within a local area network, so as to provide for data interchange and to enable multiple workers to use a common database.

Computers are developing at such a rate that it is essential to seek expert advice to ensure that the instrument being purchased has an adequate *random access memory* (RAM) capacity and other specifications to run the planned programs (Table 24.5).

Helpful advice on the use of personal computers is provided in *ABC of Medical Computing* by Lee and Millman,[21] and there are also monographs dealing specifically with applications of the Internet for health professions.[22]

The Internet provides access to a vast amount of information. Medline and a number of other libraries provide citations and abstracts of articles in almost every medical journal in the world; some journals provide full articles, which can be read directly on the computer or printed out as a pdf file. This usually requires a subscription fee, but by an agreement between the World Health Organization (WHO) and the world's leading publishers this access is available free of charge or at greatly reduced prices in more than 100 low-income countries.

Some search engines give an automatic translation of non-English language articles.

Many individual experts have their own Web sites for presenting dissertations and comments in their specialities, whereas manufacturers provide up-to-date information on their products. It is impractical to provide a comprehensive index of all relevant Web sites; however, Table 24.6 lists some that are of particular interest to the haematology laboratory. In any event, entering a key word or phrase is likely to provide access to a vast amount of information on virtually any topic as well as links to related items.

PREANALYTIC AND POSTANALYTIC STAGES OF TESTING

The haematology laboratory should be involved in the preanalytic stage (test requesting, blood sample

Table 24.6 Selected internet sites of haematological interest

scholar.google.com>ICSH	Access to an extensive bibliography on scientific and medical topics; ICSH link lists publications from International Council for Standardization in Haematology
www.who.int/entity/en/	Home page of the World Health Organization; *Essential health technology:* guidelines on laboratory practice; *Blood transfusion safety:* information on blood transfusion devices and safety. Lists WHO publications for downloading
www.ish–world.org	International Council for Standardization in Haematology, with a listing of all its publications
www.ish–world.org	Home page of International Society of Haematology
www.ifbls.org	International Federation of Biomedical Laboratory Science; arranges international congresses and educational resources
www.isth.org	International Society of Thrombosis and Haemostasis; includes bibliography and full reports of official communications from their scientific and standardization committees
www.isbt-web.org	Home page of International Society of Blood Transfusion
http://www.rcpath.org.uk	General information from Royal College of Pathologists
www.ibms.org	General information from Institute of Biomedical Science, including various aspects of CPD
www.ukneqas.org.uk	Home page of UK NEQAS; click onto Haematology for information on the various tests included in their surveys
www.cpa-uk.co.uk	Clinical Pathology Accreditation, with details of its functions and the procedures for a laboratory applying for accreditation
www.ncbi.nlm.nih.gov/entrez/	National Library of Medicine with access to MEDLINE
www.haem.net	Electronic journal published from the Department of Haematology of Hammersmith Hospital; it includes information on laboratory management.
www.bloodmed.org/home (a subscription publication from Blackwell Publishing)	Electronic journal of haematological research, practice, and education, including review papers, guidelines, and news of regulatory affairs
www.mhra.gov.uk	MDA reports of instrument and kits evaluations
www.bcshguidelines.com	Home page of the British Committee for Standards in Haematology, providing the full text of all current and past guidelines, whether published in book or journal format
www.transfusionguidelines.org.uk/uk_guidelines/	UK blood transfusion and tissue transplant guideline documents
www.rph.wa.gov.au/labs/haem/malaria/index.html	Malaria training programme from Royal Perth Hospital, Australia
www.westgard.com	J.O. Westgard's "Lesson of the Month" and other tutorials on quality assurance

collection, and transport to the laboratory) as well as the postanalytic stage (return of results to the clinician). Both stages have a significant impact on test reliability, laboratory performance, and client satisfaction.[23]

Test Requesting

There is considerable variation between clinicians in their test ordering patterns, and laboratory staff have historically exerted little influence on test request patterns, although sustained educational programmes have sometimes achieved more selective testing.[24] Unnecessary requests often result from inappropriate request forms, such as those that permit clinicians to tick from a list instead of requesting specific tests. Innovations in modifying requesting patterns have included use of problem-orientated request forms[25] and computer-assisted ordering of tests according to protocols written by specialist clinical teams.[26]

Sample Collection and Delivery

It is important to have positive identification of patient and sample. Failure to do so is a serious cause of error, especially in blood transfusion (see p. 483) but also in routine diagnostic tests, where patient-sample and intersample identification must be checked at all times. Methods have been developed* for electronic ordering of tests using the hospital's patient identification bar code for checking the patient's identity at the time of phlebotomy, printing the bar code onto the specimen containers, and checking this by means of a handheld scanner at all stages in the laboratory until the report is issued.[27]

After the blood has been collected every effort must be made to ensure its delivery to the laboratory without delay. If this is not coordinated, samples may remain in clinical areas awaiting collection by porters who then follow a fixed circuit of other hospital areas before eventually reaching the laboratory. However, if responsibility for blood collection and transport is held by the laboratory, these separate activities can be coordinated. Alternative and faster means of specimen delivery to laboratories include rail track or pneumatic tube conveyor systems.[28]

---

*For example, BD Dx system.

Preanalytic Phase

The time of receipt should be registered, and specimens must be checked to ensure that they are appropriate for the tests that are requested and that there has been no contamination by leakage on the outside of the tubes and/or the request forms. Requests should be registered and the specimens should be separated into "routine" and "urgent," the latter being handed directly to the appropriate staff member.

Postanalytic Phase

After the tests have been carried out, the following procedures are required to ensure proficiency in the postanalytic phase:

1. Processing of results for transcription on to report forms.
2. Immediate scrutiny of urgent results with issue of provisional report and its delivery to the requesting clinician.
3. Assessment of the significance of results in the context of established reference values and decision for further tests.
4. Transmission of final report without unreasonable delay to the location indicated on the request form. Computer-assisted reporting of results to linked monitors and printers located in clinical areas is very helpful, but in some countries most hospitals rely on manual transport of result sheets and this can significantly prolong request completion times. Pneumatic tube and rail track conveyor systems used for the preanalytic stage can also be used for rapid return of results to wards and clinics. Return of results is, of course, no guarantee that ward or clinic staff will react in a timely way to change a patient's treatment or even file report forms in the patient's medical record.

   It is the responsibility of the clinician to ensure that the reports of tests requested by them are received, noted, and acted on. However, good laboratory practice includes speedy notification to the responsible clinical staff of a result that shows an apparently **unexpected** serious abnormality.
5. As an audit of utility of the laboratory there should be regular contact with users to ensure that the reports arrive in due time for optimal use

during clinical management and that the clinicians are satisfied that results are presented in a clear and unambiguous form; there should also be discussions on test selection, taking account of the clinical relevance of the tests that are undertaken, the introduction of new tests, and evaluation of benefit versus cost, as discussed earlier.

Test Turnaround Time

There is increasing pressure from clinicians for rapid reports of results. Improving test turnaround time (TAT) is a complex task involving work scheduling, education, and selection of equipment.[29-31] TAT is most easily measured as the time lapse between arrival of a blood specimen in the laboratory and issue of the validated result. This can be undertaken manually, albeit tediously, in a small unit. In a computerized laboratory, however, it is relatively easy to record these times and then to analyze the data to calculate the median time and the 95th percentile for completing each test; the percentage of tests completed within a preselected time is also of value.[32] Computer-assisted graphic presentation of the frequency distribution of completed tests is a useful way of displaying turnaround times for individual tests (Fig. 24.3).

Turnabout time, as defined earlier, refers to the analytic stage of testing and excludes the time delay of the preanalytic and postanalytic stages of testing. When the laboratory has responsibility for all three stages, it becomes possible to extend the measurement of analytic turnaround time to the more meaningful parameter of request completion time (total time from initiation of the request to delivery of the result to a clinician). The speed with which modern systems perform reduces the need for interrupting the routine specimens for urgent tests, but they still require an effective way to convey the urgent results to the clinician.[33]

Point-of-Care Testing

Point-of-care testing (POCT), also known as *near-patient testing*, functions at two levels, either within a hospital as an adjunct to the laboratory or for primary health care outside the hospital.

Specialist clinical areas within hospitals have an increasing need for a customized laboratory service to meet their particular requirements. When rapid results are especially important, laboratory testing within the clinical area may be the best arrangement. Intensive care units have a long established need for near-patient monitoring of blood gases, but other clinicians use laboratory tests for monitoring ill patients and for making rapid decisions on treatment (e.g., in oncology outpatient clinics), and this has increased demand for a rapid results service. POCT may also be necessary when a test is performed on nonanticoagulated capillary blood.

Diagnostic laboratories are often located in areas of the hospital that are remote from critical care and outpatient areas. Rapid transit systems, including pneumatic tubes (see earlier), may be the preferred

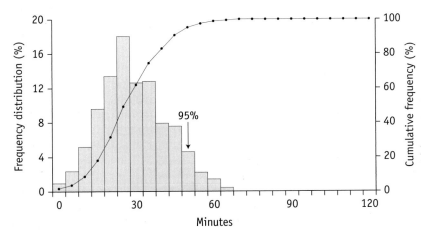

Figure 24.3 Frequency histogram, cumulative percentage (•-•-•), and 95th percentile (*arrow*) showing analytical completion time for nonurgent prothrombin times.

alternative to multiple satellite testing areas, particularly when the main laboratory already offers a rapid results service. Knowledge of test turnaround time (Fig. 24.3) is required to make an informed decision on the need for near-patient testing in satellite areas. When POCT equipment is the preferred option, the running of the satellite laboratory and maintenance of its equipment should be the responsibility of the appropriate pathology discipline. This is essential for quality control, safety, and accreditation, whether the satellite is staffed by laboratory staff, as in busy locations, or used by medical staff or nurses as a marginal activity. A designated member of laboratory staff should supervise this service, visiting each test location daily and ensuring that all results and quality-control data are integrated into the main laboratory computer system. Some instruments designed for POCT will store quality-control data on a computer floppy disk, which can be removed and taken to the main laboratory. Guidelines on the organization of a POCT service have been published by the British Committee for Standards in Haematology,[34] the Joint Working Group on Quality Assurance,[35] and the UK Medical Devices Agency*.[36] There is also an international standard (ISO 22870).

Point-of-Care Testing Beyond the Laboratory

POCT beyond the laboratory is increasingly popular in some countries, and it is particularly useful when patients live a distance away from a hospital laboratory. Instrument manufacturers are now producing tabletop or handheld devices that are simple to use, autocalibrated, and require minimum maintenance. The haematology tests that are usually undertaken include haemoglobin concentration, blood cell counting by simple analyzers, erythrocyte sedimentation rate, and prothrombin time for oral anticoagulation control.[37–40]

Although this use of POCT is independent, the local hospital laboratory should encourage the doctors and clinics to seek advice and help with selection of appropriate instruments; their standardization/calibration; and quality control, including a link into the external quality-assessment scheme in which the laboratory participates. Harmonization of reports

with laboratory records is helpful when a patient is referred to the hospital. Studies on the management of anticoagulation control have shown that with appropriate training and cooperation from the laboratory, pharmacists are able to provide as reliable a service as the hospital-based one and with more convenience for the patient.[41]

A major source of error in POCT outside the hospital is faulty specimen collection, whether for venous or finger-prick samples. Clinic staff who undertake this procedure should be given supervised training (see Chapter 1).

Patient Self-Testing

There is an increasing trend toward self-testing by patients, and glucose checks for self-management of diabetes are now routine practice. Simple portable precalibrated coagulometers, which use capillary blood to measure prothrombin time and International Normalized Ratio, are now available.[38] It has been shown that patients are able to use these instruments correctly, and once their treatment has been established, the individual patients can be relied on to maintain their anticoagulation within the therapeutic range[41] (see also p. 470). There are International Organization for Standardization (ISO) and European standards to ensure that such instruments are reliable and that the instructions for their use are clear, unambiguous and written for the users (see p. 631).

Laboratory Services for General Practitioners

The customers of a haematology laboratory include not only hospital clinicians but also general practitioners/family doctors who have different priorities from hospital practitioners. Close attention to the general practitioner's needs is an important demonstration of the quality of the laboratory, and this will encourage continued referral of patients after the initial use of laboratory services. Appropriate customized service is outlined in the following sections.

Quality Assurance

General practitioners are not specialists in laboratory medicine and require evidence that a hae-

---

*UK Medicines and Healthcare-products Regulatory Agency.

matology laboratory provides a service of high quality. This may be based on accreditation of the laboratory, its participation in external quality control schemes, a good local reputation among other laboratory users, and a willingness to collaborate with general practitioners in a mutually beneficial audit programme, including participation in POCT.

Preanalytic Service

Education of the general practitioner is important. This may include a users' handbook or wall chart (to show the correct specimen container and volume of blood required), reference ranges, requirements for patient preparation (e.g., fasting), the timing of any medication that may affect the test result, and the turnaround time for each test. The latter is important so that patients can be given a follow-up appointment to be told the result. Handbooks should be of loose-leaf format to facilitate updating. An occasional laboratory news sheet may also be of value, particularly when a new test or service is introduced. Education should also cover safety aspects, such as how to deal with blood spillage or a needle-stick injury.

Efficient specimen collection and transport are also of high priority. A general practitioner may require health centre staff to be trained and accredited for collecting blood samples. A specimen transport system at an agreed time of day is particularly important so that patients can be given a suitable appointment for blood collection. Request forms should, as far as possible, be standardized, with one request form for all pathology requests.

Postanalytic Service

The general practitioner needs a fast report service for abnormal test results to a direct telephone number or fax at the health centre. To facilitate contact with the laboratory there should be a direct dial helpline to the haematologist of the day. With transmission of results by telefax or e-mail, confidentiality must be ensured by secure identification of the recipient. In some countries Web-enabled access with secure password entry is being developed. When there is no electronic link to the laboratory, it may prove economical to use the specimen transport service to return test results to general practitioners.

Standard Operating Procedures

Standard operating procedures (SOPS) are written instructions that are intended to maintain optimal consistent quality of performance in the laboratory. They should cover all aspects of work, with some relating to test procedures and others relating to specimen collection, laboratory safety, handling of urgent requests, data storage, telephone reporting policy, and so on. They may be based on standard textbook descriptions or an instrument manufacturer's instruction manual, but they should reflect daily practice, and each laboratory must prepare its own individual set of SOPs. They should be reviewed once a year, and any revisions must be highlighted with the date. Older versions must be destroyed, and numbered copies of the new version must be distributed to authorized locations. A suggested format for an SOP is given in Table 24.7.

LABORATORY AUDIT AND ACCREDITATION

Audit

Laboratory audit is the systematic and critical analysis of the quality of the laboratory service. The essence of audit is that it should be continuous and designed to achieve incremental improvement in quality of the day-to-day service. It should encompass the preanalytic, analytic, and postanalytic stages of laboratory practice; some examples are given in Table 24.8.

The first stage of audit is to define the standard to be achieved; this may be in the form of a standard operating procedure for an analytic procedure, a protocol for test ordering, presurgery blood transfusion order schedule, or a target turnaround time. These standards will have been agreed within the laboratory and, whenever possible, in conjunction with relevant users of the laboratory. Clinical input is invaluable in relation to the clinical significance of analyzer-generated results, test utility (see p. 630), appropriate laboratory utilization,[15] and the advantages and disadvantages of point-of-care tests.[42-43] To monitor performance against agreed-on standards, each laboratory section should form its own audit group, or, if there is an audit group for the whole department, it should be open to all grades of

Table 24.7   Format for a standard operating procedure (SOP)

Cover page
Title, reference number, date of preparation, name of composer, name of authorizer

Scope
Purpose of the SOP; principles of procedure or test; grade(s) of staff permitted to undertake the task(s)

Specimen requirements
Type and amount; delivery arrangements; storage conditions, and any time or temperature restrictions

Specimen reception
Registration and check of request form; criteria for rejecting a specimen

Safety precautions
Obligatory protection requirements

Handling "high-risk" samples

Equipment and reagents
Lists of equipment, apparatus, reagents, controls, calibrators, forms, and other stationery

Test procedure
Step-by-step details of method, calculation of results, quality-control checks

Reporting
Procedure for reporting results for routine and urgent requests

Clinical significance
An understanding of the clinical reason for the test and significance of abnormal results

Reference range for healthy subjects and confidence limits

Test limitations
How to recognize errors and steps to avoid or correct them

Maintenance of equipment
List of schedule for routine in-house maintenance (daily, weekly), and servicing

Specimen storage posttest
Period of retention and conditions for storage: instructions for disposal of specimens and diluted subsamples

List of relevant literature

Date when SOP is due to be reviewed

staff to allow peer review and to take advantage of the educational value of audit. Laboratory staff should lead the audit process rather than having it imposed on them. It is good practice to make a short report of each audit meeting, recording attendance, the items identified for improvement, and an action list.

In the United Kingdom a national steering group has been set up by the relevant professional organizations to monitor serious hazards of transfusion ("SHOT"). A large proportion of the incidents that

have occurred have been the result of incorrect identification of patient–specimen link, with the wrong blood being collected from the hospital blood bank or satellite refrigerator, or with there being failure in bedside checking procedures.[44] (see also p. 523).

The audit process improves quality simply by examining and questioning established standards and guidelines. The ever-increasing need for cost-effectiveness is likely to forge closer working relation-

Table 24.8 Examples of laboratory audit
Education of laboratory users
Appropriateness of test requests
Test menu in response to clinical needs
Appropriateness of blood samples (e.g., adequate volume)
Interpretation of abnormal results
Timeliness of reports
Internal quality-control results
External quality-assessment scheme performance
Cost-effectiveness of specialist tests
Reporting of abnormal results
Compliance with safety policies
Use of blood and blood products
Frequency and cause of transfusion reactions
Turnaround time for emergency requests
Satisfaction of outpatients undergoing venepuncture
Satisfaction of laboratory users

ships between the different pathology disciplines, as well as between laboratories within the same discipline. This changing laboratory environment highlights the need for continuous training of haematology staff in good laboratory management and in the importance of audit.

Accreditation

The purpose of laboratory accreditation schemes is to allow external audit of a laboratory's organization, management, quality-assurance programme, and level of user satisfaction. The advantage to the accredited laboratory is that this indicates to clinical users that it has a defined standard of practice that has been independently confirmed by external peer review. Such review should include assessment of basic functional structure (laboratory facilities such as staff and equipment), processes (test analyses),

outcome (quality of test results including timeliness and interpretation), interaction with clinical users and optimal use of resources.

In some countries certification for accreditation is undertaken by government-authorized bodies. In the United Kingdom this function is the responsibility of the UK Accreditation Service (UKAS) and the National Measurement Accreditation Service (NAMAS),[45] which does not accredit laboratories in general terms but validates specified tests that are undertaken by a laboratory, certifying that these tests are up-to-date, recognized as standard practice, and comply with ISO standards (see p. 642). In the United States control is similarly undertaken by the regulations of the Clinical Laboratories Improvement Amendments (CLIA 1988) policy.[46,47] In Australia control is maintained by a government authority, National Pathology Accreditation Advisory Council (NPAAC), which sets the standards for accreditation of laboratories. By contrast, in the United Kingdom the majority of clinical laboratories are accredited by UK Clinical Pathology Accreditation Ltd (CPA);[48,49] this is a nongovernment professional body but with a link to UKAS. It is less restrictive on the range of tests that a particular laboratory is permitted to carry out, but it checks the ability of a laboratory to provide a satisfactory standard, as demonstrated by adequate quality control; participation in an external quality-assessment scheme; and on-site inspection of its facilities, staffing, and direction.

Some national schemes have established formal links with each other, such as the European Co-operation for Accreditation of Laboratories (EAL) and the Western European Laboratory Accreditation Co-operation (WELAC).

Descriptions of the requirements for national accreditation programmes are available for the United States,[47] United Kingdom,[49] and Australia.[50] Updated versions of these documents are available on their Web sites. An important component of all accreditation programmes is participation in proficiency testing/external quality-assessment schemes. These schemes are expected to conform to standards that are specified in ISO/IEC Guide 43 and by the International Laboratory Accreditation Co-operative (ILAC) in the ILAC Guidance document G13/2000 (*Requirements for the competence of providers of proficiency testing schemes*).

INTERNATIONAL STANDARDS OF PRACTICE

The International Standards Organization (ISO) has established guidelines for laboratory practice. Of special importance are ISO 15189: *"Medical laboratories—particular requirements for quality and competence,"* which sets out the rules for laboratory management; ISO 9000 series: *"Quality management and quality systems";* and Guide 25: *"General requirements for the technical competence of testing laboratories."* Other relevant standards from ISO and the European authority CEN are listed in Table 24.9.

BENCHMARKING

The objective of benchmarking[51] is to provide a reference point for laboratories to assess their performance by comparison with their peers and the leaders in the field. Departments are divided into several categories on the basis of their size, whether academic or nonteaching and whether responsible for special activities. Their responses to a lengthy annual questionnaire permit evaluation of various aspects of laboratory practice. By standardizing definitions of tests and requests it is possible to establish an agreed method for estimating workload

Table 24.9	ISO and European (EN) standards relating to medical laboratory practice
ISO9000	A series of standards and guidelines on selection and use of quality-management systems and quality assurance (complementary aspects are specified in ISO 9001-9004)
ISO15189	Medical laboratories: particular requirements for quality and competence.
ISO22869	Guidance document on implementation of ISO 15189 (formerly ISO Guide 25)
ISO22870	Appendix to ISO 15189 relating to quality management for point-of-care testing
ISO15194	*In vitro* diagnostic medical devices: measurement of quantities in samples of biological origin: description of reference materials
EN12286	*In vitro* diagnostic medical devices: presentation of reference measurement procedures
EN13612	Performance evaluation of *in vitro* diagnostic medical devices
ISO15198	Validation of manufacturers' recommendations for user quality control
EN375	Information supplied by manufacturers with *in vitro* diagnostic reagents
EN591	Instructions for use of *in vitro* diagnostic instruments
EN592	Instructions for use of *in vitro* diagnostic instruments for self-testing
EN13532	General requirements for *in vitro* diagnostic medical devices for self-testing
ISO17593	Requirements for *in vitro* monitoring systems for self-testing of oral anticoagulation therapy
EN14136	Use of external quality-assessment schemes in assessment of performance of *in vitro* diagnostic procedures
ISO6710	Single-use containers for venous blood specimen collection
ISO15190	Safety management for medical laboratories
ISO, International Organization for Standardization; EN, Comité Européen de Normalisation.	

in a standard way and to provide the optimal criteria for staffing levels, skill-mix, productivity, and cost-effectiveness, taking account of clinical needs and local patient population ("case-mix"). Thus, benchmarking judges the quality of service of a laboratory by assessing whether it can be run more efficiently with improved cost-effectiveness and clinical effectiveness. It provides an assessment of the adequacy of staffing with realistic measure of workload parameters, how test throughput and reporting time might be improved, taking account of how variation in clinical practice might affect the laboratory service, and whether cost-effectiveness and clinical benefit might be improved by decentralising some components or conversely by eliminated satellite units. This has become an essential method for achieving continuous sustainable improvement based on evidence rather than intuition.

In the United States a scheme known as *Q-probe* was established in 1989 by the College of American Pathologists Laboratory Improvement Program to facilitate implementation of CLIA '88 requirements by providing laboratories with continuing peer review and education with periodic on-site audit. Reports of various Q-probe studies are published regularly in the *Archives of Pathology and Laboratory Medicine*. In the United Kingdom a similar scheme has been developed in keeping with the requirements of the Commission for Health Improvement (CHI). It is undertaken by the Clinical Benchmarking Company, which is a partnership established by the Clinical Management Unit of the Centre for Health Planning at Keele University with Newchurch Limited, an informatics service company. For haematology and other laboratory-based disciplines, this scheme operates with a team of advisers appointed by the Royal College of Pathologists. Assessment of performance of an individual laboratory is based on comparison with best performance in a comparable peer cluster. The Web site is www.newchurch.co.uk/consulting, and their contact e-mail address is benchmarking@newchurch.co.uk. Another Web site that describes appropriate programs is www.4sdawn.com/benchmarking.

REFERENCES

1. Stuart J, Hicks JM 1991 Good laboratory management: an Anglo-American perspective. Journal of Clinical Pathology 44:793–797.
2. Royal College of Pathologists 2002 Background information on the continuing professional development (CPD) scheme. Royal College of Pathologists, London.
3. Du Boulay C 1999 Continuing professional development: some new perspectives. Journal of Clinical Pathology 52:162–164.
4. Canadian Institute for Health Information 2002 Management information systems guidelines: clinical laboratory workload measurement system. CIHI, Ottawa K1N 9N8.
5. College of American Pathologists Workload and personnel management committee 1992 Workload Recording Method and Personnel Management Manual. College of American Pathologists, Northfield, IL.
6. Bennett CHN 1991 Welcan UK: its development and future. Journal of Clinical Pathology 44:617–620.
7. Macdonald AJ, Bradshaw AE, Holmes WA, et al 1996 The impact of an integrated haematology screening system on laboratory practice. Clinical and Laboratory Haematology 18:271–276.
8. International Organization for Standardization 1994 Accuracy (trueness and precision) of measurement, methods and results. ISO 5725 Parts 1–4. ISO, Geneva.
9. Ellison SLR, Rosslein M, Williams A 2000 Eurachem-CITAC Guide: Quantifying uncertainty in analytic measurement, 2nd ed. Eurachem Secretariat, eurochem@fc.ul.pt.
10. Galen RS, Gambino S 1975 Beyond normality: the predictive value and efficiency of medical diagnoses. Wiley, New York.
11. Griner PF, Nayawski RJ, Mushlin AI, et al 1981 Selection and interpretation of diagnostic tests and procedures: principles and applications. Annals of Internal Medicine 94:553–592.
12. Youden WJ 1950 Index for rating diagnostic tests. Cancer 3:32–35.
13. Shapiro MF, Hatch RL, Greenfield S 1984 Cost containment and labor-intensive tests: the case of the leukocyte differential count. Journal of the American Medical Association 252:231–234.

14. Hernandez JS 2003 Cost-effectiveness of laboratory testing. Archives of Pathology and Laboratory Medicine 127:440–445.

15. van Walraven C, Naylor CD 1998 Do we know what inappropriate laboratory utilization is? A systematic review of laboratory clinical audits. Journal of the American Medical Association 280:550–558.

16. International Council for Standardization in Haematology1994 Guidelines for the evaluation of blood cell analysers including those used for differential leucocyte and reticulocyte counting and cell marker applications. Clinical and Laboratory Haematology 16:157–174.

17. Bland JM, Altman D G 1986 Statistical methods for assessing agreement between two methods of clinical measurement. Lancet i:307–310.

18. Bullock DG, Wilde CE 1985 External quality assessment of urinary pregnancy oestrogen assay: further experience in the United Kingdom. Annals of Clinical Biochemistry 22:273–282.

19. Henry JB, Kelly KC 2003 Comprehensive graphic-based display of clinical laboratory data. American Journal of Clinical Pathology 119:330–336.

20. Powsner SM, Tufte ER 1999 Graphical summary of patient status. Lancet 344:386–389.

21. Lee N, Millman A 1996 ABC of Medical Computing. BMA Publishing, London.

22. Kiley R 1999 Medical information on the internet: a guide for health professionals. Churchill Livingstone, Edinburgh.

23. Narayanan S 2000 The preanalytic phase: an important component of laboratory medicine. American Journal of Clinical Pathology 113:429–452.

24. Bareford D, Hayling A 1990 Inappropriate use of laboratory services: long term combined approach to modify request patterns. British Medical Journal 301:1307.

25. Fraser CG, Woodford FP 1987 Strategies to modify the test-requesting patterns of clinicians. Annals of Clinical Biochemistry 24:223–231.

26. Mutimer D, McCauley B, Nightingale P, et al 1992 Computerised protocols for laboratory investigation and their effect on use of medical time and resources. Journal of Clinical Pathology 45:572–574.

27. Bologna LJ, Lind C, Riggs RC 2002 Reducing major identification errors within a deployed phlebotomy process. Clinical Leadership and Management Review 16:22–26.

28. Keshgegian AA, Bull GE 1992 Evaluation of a soft-handling computerized pneumatic tube specimen delivery system. Effects on analytical results and turnaround time. American Journal of Clinical Pathology 97:535–540.

29. Howanitz JH, Howanitz PJ 2000 Laboratory results: timeliness as a quality attribute and strategy. American Journal of Clinical Pathology 116:311–315.

30. Hilbourne LH, Oye RK, McArdle JE, et al 1989 Use of specimen turnaround time as a component of clinician expectations with laboratory performance. American Journal of Clinical Pathology 92:613–618.

31. Winkelman JW, Tansijevic MJ, Wynbenga DR, et al 1997 How fast is fast enough for clinical laboratory turnabout time: Measurement of the interval between result entry and inquiries for reports. American Journal of Clinical Pathology 108:400–405.

32. Valenstein PN 1996 Laboratory turnaround time. American Journal of Clinical Pathology 105:676–688.

33. Hillbourne L, Lee H, Cathcart P 1996 STAT testing? a guideline for meeting clinician turnaround time requirements. American Journal of Clinical Pathology 105:671–675.

34. England JM, Hyde K, Lewis SM, et al 1995 Guidelines for near patient testing: haematology. Clinical and Laboratory Haematology 17:301–310.

35. Joint Working Group on Quality Assurance 1999 Guidelines: Near to patient or point of care testing. Clinical and Laboratory Haematology 21(Supplement, Advancing Laboratory Haematology):31–34.

36. Medical Devices Agency 2002 Management and use of IVD Point of care test devices. MDA, UK Department of Health, London.

37. Baer DM, Belsey RE 1995 Physician's office testing. In: Lewis S M, Koepke JA (eds) Haematology laboratory management and practice. Butterworth Heinemann, Oxford, Ch. 5.

38. Machin SJ, Mackie IJ, Chitolie A, et al 1996 Near patient testing (NPT) in haemostasis—a synoptic review. Clinical and Laboratory Haematology 18:69–74.

39. Cachia PG, McGregor E, Adlakha S, et al 1998 Accuracy and precision of the TAS analyzer for near-patient INR testing by non-pathology staff in the community. Journal of Clinical Pathology 51:68–72.

40. Rose PE, Fitzmaurice D 1998 New approaches to the delivery of anticoagulant services. Blood Reviews 12:84–90.

41. Ansell JE, Patel N, Ostrovsky D, et al 1995 Long term patient self-management of oral anticoagulation. Archives of Internal Medicine 155:2185–2189.

42. Gray TA, Freedman DB, Burnett D, et al 1996 Evidence based practice: clinicians' use and attitudes to near patient testing. Journal of Clinical Pathology 49:903–908.

43. Klee GG, Spackman KA, Habermann TM 1995 Targeting the usage and reporting of hematological laboratory tests to help streamline patient care. In: Lewis S M, Koepke JA (eds) Hematology laboratory management and practice. Butterworth Heinemann, Oxford, Ch. 17

44. Asher D, Atterbury CLJ, Chapman C et al 2002 6th Annual report: Serious hazards of transfusion. This and all previous reports are available on the SHOT website.

45. UK Accreditation Service (UKAS) 2000 The conduct of UKAS laboratory assessments. UKAS Publications, Feltham TW13 4UN, UK.

46. Bachner P, Hamlin WB 1995 Regulatory and professional standards affecting clinical laboratories. In: Lewis S M, Koepke JA (eds) Hematology laboratory management and practice. Butterworth Heinemann, Oxford, Ch. 20.

47. College of American Pathologists 1998 Standards for laboratory accreditation. College of American Pathologists, Northfield, IL.

48. CPA (UK) Ltd 2000 Standards for the medical laboratory. CPA(UK)Ltd, Sheffield S10 2PB.

49. CPA (UK) Ltd 2000 Accreditation Handbook. CPA(UK)Ltd, Sheffield S10 2PB.

50. Hynes AF, Lea AR, Hailey DM 1989 Pathology laboratory accreditation in Australia. Australian Journal of Medical Laboratory Science 10:12.

51. Galloway M, Nadin L 2001 Benchmarking and the laboratory. Journal of Clinical Pathology 54:590–559.

25 Laboratory safety

S. Mitchell Lewis

Every laboratory worker should be aware of the potential hazards in their workplace, including sites where point-of-care tests are carried out, reagent stores, and satellite storage refrigerators that hold blood and blood products. It is important for them to ensure safety in their practice from specimen collection to waste disposal. The head of the department should develop a strategy to protect the health and well-being of all members of the staff and legitimate visitors. The procedures to be followed must take account of mandatory rules and regulations as well as local practices.

There should be a designated safety officer of sufficient seniority with authority to implement departmental safety policy in all sections of the laboratory. The safety officer should be responsible for daily management of safety issues and should be directly accountable to the head of department. There must be an established protocol for handling needlestick injury to a member of staff, with immediate referral to the appropriate hospital department of occupational health, which should provide a 24-hour advisory service. All incidents must be recorded, safety protocol must be reviewed, and measures must be taken to prevent recurrence.

The safety officer must have the training and time to do the job well and provide training for other staff who must not be allowed to handle potentially hazardous materials until they have completed training in accordance with the safety requirements.

The safety officer should represent the laboratory on relevant safety committees and work closely with hospital occupational health, control of infection, and radiation protection officers. Within the department, a safety committee should be established as a useful forum for safety audit.

Departmental safety policy should be documented as "standard operating procedures" (SOPs) that are readily accessible in each section of the laboratory. It must provide a comprehensive account of departmental safety policy (Table 25.1). Attention must be drawn to known and potential hazards in relation to infection, toxic substances, fire, radiation, and mechanical injury. Where a hazard cannot be eliminated, the risk should be reduced so far as is reasonably practicable (e.g., by reducing the frequency and period of exposure). The safety booklet should refer to relevant local, national, and international safety legislation.

In addition to the documentation that sets out laboratory safety policy, SOPs should also include information on handling reagents that are classified by relevant authorities as *hazardous to health*, together with relevant safety and decontamination protocols as described in this chapter.

A standard for safety management in medical laboratories has been established by the International Organization for Standardization (ISO 15190).[1] This provides rules for a safe working environment in the laboratory and includes a

Table 25.1   Items to be included in laboratory safety policy document

Blood collection
Labelling, transport, and reception of specimens
Handling of specimens and containment of high-risk specimens
Location of protective equipment
Managing and reporting of needlestick injury
Management of eyesplash
Disposal of used needles, syringes, and lancets
Procedure for blood spillage
Hazard risk assessment for all substances in the laboratory
Safety in near-patient testing
Protective clothing
Health records of staff, including immunization
Laboratory security, out-of hours working, and visitors to the department
Waste disposal
Electrical equipment testing
Recording of accidents
Safety cabinet monitoring
Laboratory cleaning policies
Policy for receiving and sending postal specimens
Radiation protection
Fire precautions
Staff training programmes
Safety inspections
Schedule for safety committee meeting

comprehensive list of items to be checked when auditing safety practice. A similar document on safety of electrical equipment used in the laboratories has been established by the International Electrotechnical Commission (IEC).[2]

The World Health Organization (WHO) has also published comprehensive manuals on safety in health care laboratories,[3,4] and there is a WHO Web site linked to the Safe Injection Global Network (www.who.int/injection_safety), which describes strategies for safe handling of blood. This includes (a) selection of blood donors, testing of blood units, appropriate clinical use of blood, and (when applicable) viral inactivation of human material for therapeutic use; (b) safe and appropriate use of injections, sharps waste management, and prevention of cross infection; and (c) procedures conducted according to universal precautions. Global activities on this topic are reported regularly by e-mail on application to sign@who.int.

In many countries there are mandatory requirements for safety at work at a national level; these include hospitals and clinical laboratories. In the United Kingdom the authority for this is the Health and Safety Executive, which has established procedures for prevention of infections in clinical laboratories.[5] Other essential sets of regulations for the laboratory are *Ionizing Radiation Regulations* (2000),[6] *Control of Substances Hazardous to Health (COSHH) Regulations* (2002),[7] and *Genetically Modified Organisms Regulations* (2000).[8] The toxicity of all chemical reagents, including those incorporated into kits, should be categorised and certified by COSHH with regard to degree of physical and biological hazard, safety measure for use, handling of spillage, and waste disposal. The management of these regulations and methods for investigation of accidents are described by Holt.[9]

The specific safety requirements to be considered in laboratory practice are described in the following sections. They include design of premises, electrical and radiation safety, fire hazard, toxic and carcinogenic reagents, handling of biohazardous material, and waste disposal.

DESIGN OF PREMISES

The area where work is carried out should be sufficiently large to easily accommodate items of equipment, all of which should be installed on fixed surfaces or stable trolleys. If possible, equipment that makes excessive noise should be kept separate from the general working area. Optimal lighting should be ensured, and there should be adequate ventilation with protection from dust. There should be appropriate storage facilities for chemicals (see later). Fire extinguishers and first-aid cabinets should be placed in easily accessible sites. The laboratory working area must meet design standards for "level 2 containment"; there should be restricted access that should be enforced where possible.

Electrical and Radiation Safety

All electrical equipment used should be certified by its manufacturer to comply with the national or international safety standards. Electrical equipment should not interfere electrically with *in vivo* medical devices (e.g., pacemakers) unless clearly marked with an appropriate caution. Before installation, all electrical devices should be inspected by someone trained in portable appliance testing, who must ensure that all plugs, fuses, and electrical cables are appropriate and functional and that the plugs and cables are not adjacent to water taps. There should be a planned programme of preventive maintenance for each item of electrical equipment. All equipment should be decontaminated before inspection or repair.

Protection when handling radioactive material and using equipment for measuring radioactivity is described on p. 359.

Fire Hazard

Most fires result from accidents with flammable substances such as alcohol and solvents. All manipulations of such substances must be carried out away from naked flames. Bulk stocks should be kept in flame-protected bins in a storage area separated from the laboratory and clearly marked as **FIRE RISK**. Not more than 400 ml should be kept on an open bench or shelf. Gas burners must never be left unattended, and pilot lights must never be left on overnight. The burners should be as close as possible to the gas source, and lengthy connecting tubes must be avoided.

Fire extinguishers, especially those suitable for dealing with electrical and chemical fires, and fire blankets should be placed near to doors of rooms and at strategic points in corridors. They should be inspected regularly.

Chemical Safety

Dangerous chemicals such as strong acids and alkalis must be stored at floor level. Chemicals that are likely to react with each other must be stored well apart; poisons should be stored in locked cabinets. Manufacturers' product safety data sheets must be checked for advice on safe handling of any potentially toxic or carcinogenic substances. Such reagents must be stored in a secure place with restricted access; they should be handled only by experienced staff wearing protective clothing, and weighing should be carried out in an air-flow cabinet at face velocity of around 0.8 m/s.

Eyewash Facilities

An eyewash station should be conveniently located where hazardous chemicals or biological materials are handled. This should consist of a spray device attached to the water supply by a flexible hose. If access to plumbing is not available, the alternative is an ample supply of easy-open containers of sterile water or isotonic saline.

BIOHAZARDOUS SPECIMENS

When handling blood the most commonly encountered pathogens are human immunodeficiency virus (HIV) and hepatitis viruses.

All specimens of human origin should be regarded as potentially infectious and must be handled appropriately by means of *universal precautions* to minimise exposure of skin and mucous membranes to the hazard. Special precautions are necessary with highly infectious specimens (see below).

Universal Precautions

1. Personal hygiene precautions to be adopted in areas where blood is collected, specimens are handled, and analytic work is carried out:
    Eating, drinking, and application of cosmetics are absolutely forbidden.

Staff should not wear jewelry, and ideally watches and rings should be removed.

Disposable latex rubber or plastic gloves should be worn during sample handling and analytic work.*

Personal clothing should not be allowed to protrude beyond the sleeves of protective clothing.

Any exposed cuts or abrasions must be kept covered with waterproof dressings.

Hands must be washed when leaving analytical areas.

2. Venepuncture should be performed wearing disposable thin plastic or rubber latex gloves. Care must be taken to prevent injuries when handling syringes and disposing of the needles. Do not recap used needles by hand; do not detach the needle from the syringe or break, bend, or otherwise manipulate used needles by hand. Used disposable syringes and needles, lancets, and other sharp items such as glass slides must be placed in a puncture-resistant plastic "sharps" container for disposal. Care must be taken to avoid blood contamination of tourniquets as a potential cause of cross-infection. If necessary, they should be washed with soap and water.

3. As far as possible, only disposable syringes, needles, and lancets should be used. Disposable syringes and lancets must never be reused on a different person.

4. Specimens should be sent to the laboratory in individual closed plastic bags, separated from the request forms to prevent their contamination should there be any leakage from the specimens. Ideally, the plastic bag should be placed inside another container. Tubes that minimise the risk of leakage are described on p. 3.

5. Mouth pipetting is absolutely prohibited.

6. Centrifugation must be performed in sealed centrifuge buckets.

7. Blood and bone marrow slides must be handled in the same way as blood samples until they are fixed in methanol, stained, and covered with a cover glass.

8. Used material must be placed in designated biohazard plastic bags awaiting disposal (see below).

9. Protective laboratory clothing (e.g., white coats) must never be worn outside the laboratory.

10. Additional precautions with highly infectious material include the following:

   a. Only experienced staff should perform procedures.

   b. Specimens should be handled in a microbiological safety cabinet (if the procedure involves generation of an aerosol) or in a clearly segregated and designated area of the laboratory.

   c. Specimens should be handled using protective clothing (close-fitting disposable gloves, disposable plastic apron, glasses or goggles, face mask).

   d. Disposable plastic should be used instead of glassware, and sharp-pointed instruments (e.g., scissors) should not be used.

   e. There should be special arrangements for waste disposal (see p. 653).

Chemical Disinfectants

There are several types of chemicals that can be used as germicides, including aldehydes, phenols, halogens, alcohols, and hypochlorites. However, there is no single disinfectant effective against all pathogens, and their effectiveness depends on the nature of the organism (Table 25.2).[4,10]

Sodium Hypochlorite (Chlorine)

Sodium hypochlorite (chlorine) is the most commonly used disinfectant in the laboratory because it is very active against all micro-organisms, although less effective for fungi. Its disadvantage is that it is corrosive to metal. Because hypochlorite solutions gradually lose their strength, fresh dilutions must be made daily. For general use a concentration of 1 g/l (1000 ppm) as available chlorine is required; a

---

*Irritant reactions to latex rubber or plastic gloves may result from mechanical friction of the skin from poor fitting, prolonged use without changing the gloves, perspiration, or a specific allergy. Hand washing with a mild antiseptic soap and application of an anti-inflammatory hand cream may be helpful. It may also be helpful to wear powder-free gloves and to wear a larger-sized glove to increase air circulation until the hands heal. In the event of a specific allergy to the chemical ingredients within the gloves, it may be worthwhile trying a different type or brand of glove.

Table 25.2   Properties of common disinfectants

Reagent	Concentration (%)*	Active against					
		Fungi	Bacteria	Mycobacteria	Spores	Lipid–coated viruses	Nonlipid–coated viruses
A: Hypochlorites	1–10	+	+++	++	++	+	+
B: Phenolic compounds	1–5	+++	+++	++	0	+	(±)
C: Formaldehyde	2–8	+++	+++	+++	+++	+	+
D: Glutaraldehyde	2	+++	+++	+++	+++	+	+
E: Ethyl alcohol	70–80	0	+++	+++	0	+	(±)
F: Isopropyl alcohol	70	0	+++	+++	0	+	(±)
G: Iodoform	0.1–2	+++	+++	+++	+	+	+

*See text.
+, ++, and +++, Extent of effectiveness; (±), variable, dependent on virus; 0, not effective.

Reagent	Inactivated by organic matter	Corrosive*	Skin irritant*	Eye irritant*	Respiratory irritant*
A: Hypochlorites	+++	+	+	+	+
B: Phenolic compounds		+	+	+	
C: Formaldehyde			+	+	+
D: Glutaraldehyde		+	+	+	
E: Ethyl alcohol				+	
F: Isopropyl alcohol				+	
G: Iodoform	+++	+	+	+	

*Apart from these specific hazards, all disinfectants are toxic substances.

stronger solution containing 5 g/l (5000 ppm) is necessary for dealing with blood spillage.

Household bleaches usually contain 50 g/l as available chlorine and should thus be diluted 1:50 for general use and 1:10 for blood contamination. Other chlorine-containing compounds that can be used are prepared as follows:

Calcium hypochlorite (70% available chlorine): 1.4 g/l; 7 g/l for blood contamination.
Sodium dichloroisocyanurate (NaDCC) (60% available chlorine): 1.7 g/l; 20 g/l for blood contamination.

Chloramine (25% available chlorine): 20 g/l in all conditions.

Formaldehyde

Formaldehyde is active against all organisms, but it is less effective at temperatures below 20°C. A solution of 5% formalin in water is recommended for use against viruses.

Gluteraldehyde

Gluteraldehyde is active against all microorganisms at a concentration of 20 g/l (2%). It is especially useful for decontaminating equipment with metal components. Before use, the solution must be activated by addition of bicarbonate to make it alkaline, and it must be used within 2 weeks. It must be handled with caution, avoiding contact with skin, eyes, and respiratory tract.

Phenolic Compounds

Several common disinfectants are based on phenolic compounds. They are active against fungi and all vegetative bacteria but not against spores, and they vary in their activity against viruses.

Alcohols

Ethanol and isopropyl alcohol have similar disinfectant properties at a concentration of 70–80% in water; higher or lower concentrations reduce their germicidal effectiveness. They are active against vegetative bacteria and lipid viruses but not against spores or fungi. Their effect on nonlipid viruses is variable. Alcohol is especially effective when mixed with other agents for example, 80% alcohol with 100 g/l of formaldehyde or with 2 g/l of sodium hypochlorite (2000 ppm available chlorine.)

Applications of Disinfectants

Routine

On completion of the day's work the working area should be wiped with a freshly prepared 1% w/v sodium hypochlorite solution (chlorine bleach). Reusable pipettes should be soaked in a 2.5% solution for 30 min or longer. A 10% solution must be used for cleaning up blood spillage. The diluted sodium hypochlorite solution should be freshly made each day. It is helpful to add detergent to the solution because disinfectants are most active on clean surfaces.

A stabilised blend of peroxide with surfactant and organic acids in a buffer system is available as a commercial product ("Virkon," Antec-DuPont). It appears to be effective as a general disinfectant for all hard surfaces, plastic and stainless steel laboratory equipment, medical instruments, and laundry; it also absorbs spilled blood or other body fluids.

Automated Equipment

Some automated equipment can be disinfected by flushing several times with 10% w/v sodium hypochlorite, or with 2% w/v glutaraldehyde, followed by several flushes with water. Only glutaraldehyde should be used on instruments with a metal surface because hypochlorite causes corrosion. Other instruments have special requirements for decontamination; always refer to the manufacturer's instructions.

Centrifuges

Laboratory centrifuges require particular attention. Any spillage of blood should be dealt with immediately, and the bowl, head, and buckets (including rubber pads) should be disinfected regularly with 2% w/v glutaraldehyde solution. Centrifuges should never be cleaned using hypochlorite solution or other metal corrosives. Special care is required when a glass or plastic tube breaks in a centrifuge (Table 25.3).

Syringes and Needles

Although single-use disposable syringes and needles are strongly recommended, circumstances may require reusables. These must be washed thoroughly in running water to remove all traces of

Table 25.3   Procedure for decontaminating a centrifuge after breakage of a tube
1. Switch off centrifuge motor and do not open lid for 30 min. Inform the safety officer.
2. When breakage involves a high-risk specimen, gloves, goggles, and a protective apron must be worn and the bucket must be opened in a safety cabinet.
3. Strong gloves must be worn and forceps must be used when removing broken tubes and any solid debris. These together with buckets, trunnions, and rotor should be placed in 2% w/v glutaraldehyde solution for 24 hours.
4. The centrifuge bowl should be washed with 2% w/v glutaraldehyde solution, left to dry, and washed again.
5. All contaminated disposable material must be placed in appropriate containers for autoclaving.

blood. Syringes are then soaked for at least 30 min in 10% hypochlorite bleach and needles are soaked overnight in freshly diluted 2% glutaraldehyde. They are then rinsed under running tap water and soaked in two changes of distilled or deionised water. Finally, before reuse they must be sterilised by heating in an oven at 120°C for 30 min.

Gloves

Disposable gloves must not be reused because they may retain contaminated material and may deteriorate when cleaned. Rubber household gloves may be washed and decontaminated by soaking in 1% hypochlorite solution for 30 min, but they must be discarded if they have punctures or tears or if they show signs of deterioration such as beginning to peel or crack.

Laundry

Soiled laundry must be placed in leak-proof labelled bags for transport to the laundry where the items should be washed in hot water (>70°C) with detergent for 25–30 min before being rinsed, or alternatively this can be soaked in 1% w/v sodium hypochlorite solution (see p. 650) before being washed by hand.

WASTE DISPOSAL

The safe disposal of laboratory waste is of prime importance. Laboratory waste and contaminated materials present a health hazard both to laboratory workers and to the community. The careless dumping of solid, liquid, chemical, and biological waste is also a threat to the environment. WHO has a useful Web site (www.healthcarewaste.org) that provides up-to-date information on various aspects of waste management, including country-specific and region-specific problems and legal requirements.

Laboratory waste is classified under the following headings:

Infectious materials
Pathological materials
Radioactive materials
Genotoxic substances
Sharps
Chemicals, including analyser effluents
Pharmaceuticals
Heavy metals, including batteries and broken thermometers
Pressurized containers
General, nonclinical waste

A practical document on health care waste management has been published by WHO Euro Regional office[11]; this manual can be downloaded from www.healthcarewaste.org. See also www.noharm.org >medicalwaste.

Blood and other potentially infected body fluids can safely be poured down a drain only if it is connected to a sanitary sewer. The drain should then be immediately flushed with water, followed by 250 ml of 10% hypochlorite, and finally again flushed with water. If there is not a sewer system the material should be ducted into holding tanks for steam heating or chemical treatment before final discharge to the public sewers. Specimen containers, used syringes, swabs, and tissues, should be collected in special colour-coded bags for subsequent incineration or autoclaving before being disposed of in a rubbish dump. "Sharps" containers should be incinerated without opening.

Highly infectious specimens require special management, as follows[11]:

Segregate from other potentially infectious waste and place immediately in a leakproof bag or container.
If possible, disinfect immediately by autoclaving or chemical treatment; the waste can then be handled alongside other clinical waste.
If not immediately disinfected, place in identifiable (e.g., yellow) bags with biohazard symbol marked "HIGHLY INFECTIOUS WASTE." These must be taken immediately to a central storage point for disposal.

Information about the disposal of specific chemicals is usually given in the manufacturer's safety data sheet, and a waste control strategy should be established, taking account of toxic and carcinogenic materials, corrosive substances, flammable substances, and reactive chemicals with risk of explosion. Analyser effluents that do not contain chemicals that potentially react with metal waste piping can be discharged directly into a main sewer.

Pressurised containers must not be punctured or incinerated. They should be carefully discharged in the open air away from people and then discarded in nonhazardous waste containers.

General waste includes domestic, packaging, and other substances not hazardous to human health. This may either be incinerated or disposed of according to local facilities.

SPECIMEN TRANSPORT

There are strict national and international regulations about packaging and shipment of patients' specimens and other biological material by post or air transport, and they also apply to courier services.[12-14] The International Air Transport Association (IATA) requires that specimens must be packaged in accordance with *IATA Packing Instructions 650,* which are described on their Web site.

The following is a summary of the requirements:

A primary sealed, leakproof container for the specimen.

Absorbent material surrounding the primary container; if several primary containers are packed together they must be individually wrapped to prevent contact with each other and to ensure a tight packing.

Secondary protecting container (e.g., rigid plastic tube, corrugated fibre-board, or polystyrene box). If being sent by air this container must be capable of withstanding a 95 kPa pressure differential without leakage.

Outer packaging such as a secure rigid cardboard or fibre-board box or a bubble-wrap mailing envelope.

The outer package must be clearly labelled "BIOHAZARD" together with the universal biohazard symbol. It is also advisable to add a warning that the parcel must only be opened by an authorised person, preferably in the laboratory. If sent by air the label must state "Packed in compliance with IATA Packing Instruction 650."

When plasma or serum must be maintained in a frozen state, the packed specimen should be placed in an insulated container surrounded by dry ice. Conversely, care must be taken to prevent freezing of whole blood specimens. The container must also permit release of CO_2 gas to prevent build-up of pressure. Specific airline regulations should be checked to ensure that dry ice is not deemed a hazardous material.

REFERENCES

1. International Organization for Standardization 2003 Medical laboratories—requirements for safety: ISO 15190. ISO, Geneva.
2. International Electrotechnical Commission 2001 Safety requirements for electrical equipment for measurement, control and laboratory use: Part 1: General requirements IEC/ISO/EN 61010. ISO, Geneva. **Other sections of this standard relate to particular requirements (e.g., Part 020: laboratory centrifuges; Part 081: semi-automated analyzers; Part 101 in-vitro diagnostic (IVD) medical equipment.)**
3. World Health Organization 1997 Safety in health-care laboratories—Document LAB/97.1. WHO, Geneva.
4. World Health Organization 1993 Laboratory Biosafety Manual, 2nd ed. WHO, Geneva.
5. United Kingdom Health and Safety Executive 1991 Safe working and the prevention of infections in clinical laboratories. HSE Books, Sudbury, Suffolk CO10 2WA.*
6. National Radiological Protection Board 2002 The ionizing radiation (Medical exposure) regulations 2000. NRPB, Didcot, Oxon OX11 0RQ.
7. United Kingdom Health and Safety Executive 2002 Control of substances hazardous to health (COSHH) regulations. HSE Books, Sudbury, Suffolk CO10 2WA.
8. United Kingdom Health and Safety Executive 2000 Genetically modified organisms (GMOs) including genetically modified micro-organisms (GMMs) regulation. HSE Books, Sudbury, Suffolk CO10 2WA.
9. Holt AStJ 2000 Principles of health and safety at work, 5th ed. reprint. Institute of Occupational Safety and Health, Wigston LE18 1NN.
10. Gardner JF, Peel MM 1998 Sterilization, disinfection and infection control 3rd ed. Churchill Livingstone, London.
11. Rushbrook P, Chandra C, Gayton S 2000 Starting health care waste management in medical institutions: a practical approach.

*A full list of publications from HSE can be found at www.HSEbooks.com.

WHO/EURO/00/502187. WHO Regional Office for Europe, Copenhagen.

12. National Committee for Clinical Laboratory Standards 1994 Procedures for handling and transport of diagnostic specimens and etiological agents H5-A3. NCCLS, Wayne, PA.

13. United Nations 1993 Recommendations on the transport of dangerous goods, 8th ed. United Nations, New York.

14. European Committee for Standardization 1996 Transport packages for medical and biological specimens—requirements, tests EN 829. CEN, Brussels.

26 Quality assurance

S. Mitchell Lewis and Barbara De la Salle

Quality assurance in the haematology laboratory is intended to ensure reliable test results with the necessary degree of precision and accuracy, as described on p. 629. *Accuracy* refers to the closeness of the estimated value to that considered to be true. *Precision* refers to the reproducibility of a result, but a test can be precise without being accurate. Inaccuracy, imprecision, or both occur as a result of using unreliable standards or reagents, incorrect instrument calibration, or poor technique (e.g., consistently faulty dilution or the use of a method that gives a reaction that is incomplete or not specific for the substance to be measured).

Precision can be controlled by replicate tests and by repeated tests on previously measured specimens. Accuracy can, as a rule, be checked only by the use of reference materials that have been assayed by reference methods.

A quality-assurance programme includes internal quality control, external quality assessment, and standardisation. It must also ensure adequate control of the preanalytic and postanalytic stages from specimen collection (see Chapter 1) to the timely dispatch of an informative report (see p. 636).

Internal quality control is based on monitoring the haematology test procedures that are performed in the laboratory. It includes measurements on specially prepared materials and repeated measurements on routine specimens, as well as daily statistical analysis of data obtained from the tests that have been routinely carried out. This should ensure continual evaluation of the reliability of the work of the laboratory with validation of tests before reports are released.

External quality assessment (EQA) is evaluation by an outside agency of the performance by numerous laboratories on specially supplied samples. Analysis of performance is retrospective. The objective is to achieve between-laboratory and between-method comparability, but this does not necessarily guarantee accuracy unless the specimens have been assayed by a reference laboratory alongside a reference preparation of known value. Schemes are usually organised nationally or regionally. National schemes are frequently known by the acronym NEQAS (National External Quality Assessment Scheme). There is an international EQA scheme organized by WHO, and a regional scheme has been established by the *Asian Network of Clinical Laboratory Standardization and Harmonization* as Asian Quality Assurance Surveys (contact: Kaplee @korea.ac.kr). "Proficiency testing" describes the procedures by which an EQA scheme functions.

Standardisation encompasses both materials and methods. *Material standard* or *reference preparations* are used to calibrate analytic instruments and to assign quantitative values to calibrators. Where possible they must be traceable to defined physical or chemical measurement based on the metrological units of length (metre), mass (kilogram), amount of substance (mole), and time (seconds).

A *reference method* is an exactly defined technique that is used in association with a reference preparation, when available, to provide sufficiently precise and accurate data for scientific purposes and for assessing the validity of other methods.

A *selected method* is one that is directly comparable with and traceable to the international reference method; it serves as an alternative to the reference method when an international reference material is not available; it should be used for evaluation and validation of a proposed routine (working) method.

A *working* (or *recommended*) *method* is intended for use in routine practice, taking account of economy of labour and materials and ease of performance and having been shown by a validation study with a reference method to be sufficiently reliable for its intended purpose.

The main international authority concerned with material standards (reference preparations) for laboratory medicine is the World Health Organization. Most of these are held by the WHO International Laboratory at the UK National Institute for Biological Standards and Control (NIBSC). In the European Union, the Institute for Reference Materials and Measurements (IRMM) has established numerous standards termed "certified reference materials" for haematology and clinical chemistry (see p. 694). International standards are not intended for routine use but serve as stable standards for assigning values to commercial (or laboratory-produced) "secondary standards" or *calibrators.*

Controls are preparations that are used for either internal quality control or external quality assessment. Some control preparations have assigned values (see later), but they should not be used as standards because the assigned values are usually only approximations, and they are often stable for a limited time only.

Standardisation of methods and devices used in haematology are the concern of the International Council for Standardization in Haematology (ICSH), whose recommendations are published in haematology journals. The International Organization of Standardization (ISO) and the Comité Européen de Normalisation (CEN) have also established standards for medical laboratory practice and for the use of *in vitro* diagnostic medical devices (see below). In the United Kingdom, the British Committee for Standards in Haematology (BCSH) publishes guidelines in books or as journal articles. In the United States, a wide range of practice guidelines have been published by the Clinical and Laboratory Standards Institute (CLSI) (formerly the National Committee for Clinical Laboratory Standards, NCCLS).

Lists of published documents and catalogues from these various organizations can be found on their Web sites. Some may be confused with other bodies with the same initials if the full title is not stated:

WHO: Home page > Biologicals > International reference preparations > Catalogue

NIBSC: Home page >Catalogues > Catalogue of biological standards > Blood products

IRMM: Home page > Reference material sales > Catalogue > Clinical chemistry

ISO: Home page > Products & services > ISO catalogue > 11. Health care technology > ISO catalogue 11.100 > Laboratory medicine (or identify a particular standard

CEN: Home page > TC140

ICSH: Home page > Publications

BCSH: Home page > Guidelines

NCCLS: Home page > Shop > Hematology

In Europe *in vitro* diagnostic medical devices (IVDMD) used in the laboratory, including instruments and equipment, reagents, calibrators, and test materials, are now controlled by a European Parliament and Council directive. This requires that manufacturers use the CE mark on their products to certify that they conform to their performance claims.[1] Details of the directive are available on the MDA website (see Table 24.6). A number of firms also provide useful information, e.g.,

www.ce-marking.org. This process is supervised nationally by appropriate authorities (e.g., in the United Kingdom, by the Medicines and Healthcare Products Regulatory Agency [MHRA], formerly the Medical Devices Agency). External quality-assessment schemes have a role in identifying unsatisfactory performance by the devices.

The following ISO (and CEN) standards are concerned with laboratory practice and the requirements of the IVDMD directive; conformity to them may also be mandatory in countries outside Europe.

ISO 9000 and 10000 series: A set of standards that specify various aspects of quality-management systems for any organization

EN ISO 15189: Medical laboratories—particular requirements for quality and competence. This takes into account the requirements of the ISO 9000 series where they are relevant to medical laboratory practice; it also includes a supplementary document on point-of-care testing (ISO 22870)

ISO 22869: Guidance on laboratory implementation of ISO 15189

EN ISO 17511: IVDMD—metrological traceability of values assigned to calibrators and control materials

ISO 15198: IVDMD—validation of user quality-control procedures by the manufacturer

EN 14136: Use of external quality-assessment schemes in the assessment of the performance of *in vitro* diagnostic examination procedures

ISO Guide 43: Proficiency testing by interlaboratory comparisons

  Part 1: Development and operation of proficiency testing schemes

  Part 2: Selection and use of proficiency testing schemes by laboratory accreditation bodies

The use of reference preparations and the principles of quality assurance are described in this chapter. The blood count is used as an illustrative model. Standards available for other tests are referred to in the sections of this book where these are described.

REFERENCE PREPARATIONS

Haemoglobin

The availability of an international reference preparation of haemiglobincyanide (HiCN) has contributed to improved accuracy of haemoglobin measurement.[2] In some countries, preparations that conform to the international standard are certified by the appropriate national authorities. A limited quantity of the international standard can be obtained from WHO, and a comparable certified reference material is available from IRMM (see p. 695). An important feature of this material is that it is stable for at least several years. Where the use of cyanide reagent for routine haemoglobinometry is prohibited, the haemiglobincyanide standard can still be used to assign a haemoglobin value to a lysate or a whole blood preparation (p. 661), which is then used as the local secondary standard after appropriate dilution. Undiluted lysate is usually stable for up to 6 months, and whole blood is stable for about 3 weeks, but after dilution for only a few days.

Both whole blood and lysates are useful for quality assurance of haemoglobinometry; whole blood reference samples should be introduced into batches of blood samples, and all the samples should be assayed together. This is applicable to both automated and manual methods.

Blood Cells

Standard preparations are essential for the calibration of electronic particle counters, especially automated systems that can be adjusted arbitrarily. This means that to obtain a true result the machine has to be calibrated using a reference preparation with assigned values of known accuracy.

Natural blood, collected into ethylenediaminetetraacetic acid (EDTA), is of no value as a reference preparation because of its short life in the laboratory. Various methods have been tried to preserve blood without affecting the components of the blood count,[3,4] and commercial products using preserved blood are available, but they may be instrument specific. Blood keeps for a few weeks at 4°C if acid–citrate–dextrose (ACD) or citrate–phosphate–dextrose (CPD) has been added to it. Even so, the mean cell volume (MCV) slowly increases and some of the red cells lyse, with the result that the blood cannot be regarded as a reference material, although it can be used as a control preparation to check the precision and reliable functioning of a cell counting system over relatively short periods.[3]

Attempts have been made to provide suitably sized particles in stable suspension as substitutes for normal blood cells. These include fixed red cells and spherical latex particles.[5] The cells can be permanently stabilized by fixation (e.g., in glutaraldehyde solution). The glutaraldehyde causes red cells to shrink in size immediately, and the shrinking process continues for 3–4 days. Thereafter, the cells remain constant in size and shape, and the results of cell counts and cell size distribution remain the same for months or even years. Thus these fixed cells can be used to check the consistency of an instrument's function, but because they are inflexible, biconcave discs with flow properties that differ from those of fresh blood in analytic systems, they cannot be used to calibrate an instrument for natural blood measurements.[6,7]

For total leucocyte counts, two types of material have been used successfully as standard reference materials, at least with simple analysers, but these fixed preparations may not be suitable for use with some modern systems.

1. Leucocytes concentrated from human blood and fixed in the following solution[8]: glacial acetic acid, 42 mg; sodium sulphate, 7 g; sodium chloride, 7 g; and water, to 1 litre.
2. Glutaraldehyde-fixed erythrocytes suspended in leucocyte-free mammalian whole blood.[9] Turkey or chicken blood,* in which the red cells are nucleated, is suitable for the total leucocyte count. Different animal species can provide cells of sizes comparable to those of the differential leucocytes count; however, other physical properties of the different types of leucocyte are not paralleled in the reference materials, so that such preparations are unsuitable as direct standards for automated differential counts based on identifying cells by their various physical properties.

Assigning Values

Methods used for assigning values to reference materials must be as accurate and precise as is practical. Standardised reference methods have been described for haemoglobin concentration (Hb), red blood cell count (RBC), white blood cell count (WBC), and packed cell volume (PCV) (Chapter 3).

---

*Available commercially (e.g., TCS Biosciences Ltd, Buckingham MK18 2LR, UK).

QUALITY-CONTROL MATERIALS

Commercial products are available, and control materials can also be made locally, although there may be technical difficulties in preparing such "homemade" materials. For example, stored plasma may become turbid, chemical or serological analysis may be affected by instability of enzymes, and immunological reactions may be interfered with by added preservatives. With the blood count, there are especially difficult problems because of the need to ensure homogeneity in aliquot samples and the instability of blood cells, whereas procedures that enhance the stability of blood samples distort the behaviour of the cells, so that control material is not strictly analogous to fresh blood. Nonetheless, provided attention is paid to these difficulties, preserved or stabilised blood provides suitable material for internal quality-control procedures for haemoglobin, red cell counts, and leucocyte counts. Blood collected into ACD or CPD (see p. 689) and passed through a blood-infusion set to remove any clots is suitable. For lysates, blood in EDTA or heparin is also suitable. Care should be taken at all stages to avoid contamination. Where possible, sterile glassware and reagents should be used and aseptic handling procedures should be adopted. To help maintain sterility, broad-spectrum antibiotics should be added to the product (e.g., 1 mg of penicillin together with 5 mg of gentamycin per 100 ml).

When human blood is used, it should be handled in the same way as a patient's sample, and if possible, it should first be checked to ensure that it is negative for hepatitis B and C and human immunodeficiency virus (HIV).

Preparation of Preserved Blood

Preparing preserved blood involves the following steps[9,10]:

1. Collect blood into a sterile container (e.g., a blood transfusion donor bag) with ACD or CPD anticoagulant (p. 689). Leave for 2–3 days at 4°C.
2. Centrifuge the blood for 20 min at approximately 2000 g. Separate (and keep) the supernatant plasma but discard the buffy coat. Transfer the red cell concentrate into 500 ml bottles.

3. Mix 3 volumes of the red cells with 1.5 volumes of 9 g/l NaCl, centrifuge for 20 min at approximately 2000 g and remove the supernatant and upper layer of the red cells by suction.
4. Repeat step 3.
5. Dilute 5 volumes of the plasma with 2 volumes of 9 g/l NaCl and add antibiotic.
6. Add the diluted plasma from step 5 to the red cell concentrate at an appropriate ratio to obtain a preparation suitable for use as a red cell count control.
7. Mix well and, with continuous mixing, dispense in aliquot volumes into clean sterile vials,* and cap tightly. Store at 4°C.

Assign values for Hb, RBC, and PCV by at least 5 replicate measurements, using the counter on which the subsequent tests will be performed. Before analysis, mix the sample on a roller mixer or continuously by hand for 5 min before opening. The between-test coefficient of variation (CV) should not exceed 2%. Check between-sample homogeneity of dispensing by repeated counts on 5 randomly selected vials. Unopened vials of human blood should keep in good condition for about 3 weeks at 4°C and equine blood should keep for up to 2 months.[10] Equine blood has an added advantage that it can be used to simulate microcytic human blood because horse red cells have an MCV of approximately 50 fl.

Preparation of Lysate

1. Collect blood as described earlier (e.g., into a blood transfusion donor bag). Out-of-date donor blood can be used provided that it is not lysed. Centrifuge at approximately 2000 g for 20 min and discard the plasma and buffy coat.
2. Add an equal volume of 9 g/l NaCl, mix well, transfer to a sterile centrifuge bottle, and recentrifuge; discard the supernatant. Repeat the

saline wash 3 times to ensure complete removal of the plasma, leucocytes, and platelets.
3. To each 10 ml volumes of the washed cells, add 6 volumes of water and 4 volumes of toluene, cap, and shake vigorously on a mechanical shaker or vibrator for 1 h. Then keep overnight at 4°C to allow the lipid/cell debris to form a semisolid surface between the toluene and lysate.
4. On the following day, centrifuge at approximately 2000 g for 20 min, remove the lysate layers, and pool them in a clean bottle.
5. Using gentle vacuum suction (e.g., by water pump), filter the lysate through coarse filter paper (e.g., Whatman No. 1) in a Buchner funnel. Repeat filtration using 0.22 μm micropore filter or fine filter paper (e.g., Whatman No. 42), changing the paper whenever the filtration slows down. It is important not to overload the funnel with lysate.
6. To each 70 ml of lysate, add 30 ml of glycerol and broad-spectrum antibiotic (see p. 660). If a lower Hb is required, add 30% glycerol in saline. Mix well, dispense into sterile containers, and cap tightly.

Assign a value for Hb by the spectrophotometric method (p. 30); carry out 10 replicate tests, taking samples at random from several vials of the batch. The CV should be less than 2%. Stored at 4°C, the product should retain its assigned value for at least several months or for 1–2 years if kept at –20°C.

Preparation of Stabilised Whole Blood Control[12]

Reagent

Formaldehyde 37–40%	6.75 ml
Glutaraldehyde 50%	0.75 ml
Trisodium citrate	26 g
Water	to 100 ml

Method

1. Obtain whole blood in CPD or ACD. This should be as fresh as possible and never more than 3 days old. Filter through a 40 μm blood filter into a series of plastic bottles.
2. If an increased red cell count is required, centrifuge the blood and remove part of the

---

*A mixing-dispensing unit as described by Ward and colleagues[11] is recommended for large-scale dispensing (e.g., for NEQAS samples; see p. 667). It can be constructed using standard glassware and so on, except for the specially manufactured flask head. Information on this is available from the Department of Medical Engineering, Imperial College Hammersmith Campus, London W12 0NN.

plasma; if a lower red cell count is required, dilute the blood with an appropriate amount of that plasma. If paired bottles are gently centrifuged (approximately 1500 g) for 15 min to produce buffy coats, these can then be manipulated in a similar way to provide different levels of leucocyte and platelet counts. Add broad-spectrum antibiotic (see p. 660) to each sample.

3. Mix well and add 1 volume of reagent to 50 volumes of the cell suspension. Mix on a mechanical mixer for 1 h at room temperature and leave for 24 h at 4°C.
4. With continuous mixing, dispense into sterile containers; cap tightly and seal with plastic tape. Refrigerate at 4°C until needed. Unopened vials should keep in good condition for several months at 4°C.

For analysis, samples should be gently mixed on a roller mixer or by hand before opening. Assign values for Hb and cell counts by at least 5 replicate tests and check between-sample homogeneity by repeated counts on 5 randomly selected vials. CV should not exceed 2%. Note, however, that the PCV by centrifugation will be approximately 10% higher than the haematocrit obtained by automated counters.

Simple Method for Blood Count Quality-Control Preparations

The method described in the following provides a suitable preparation for control of total red cell, leucocyte, and platelet counting by some semi-automated blood cell counters, but it is not suitable for some automated systems. It should be stable for approximately 3 weeks if kept at 4°C.

Method

1. Collect a unit of human blood into CPD anticoagulant (p. 689). Carry out the subsequent procedure within 1 day after collection.
2. Filter the blood through a blood transfusion recipient set into a 500 ml glass bottle.
3. Add 1 ml of fresh 40% formaldehyde. Mix well by inverting and then leave on a roller mixer for 1 hour.
4. Leave at 4°C for 7 days, mixing by inverting a few times each day. At the end of this period of storage, mix well on a roller mixer for 20 min and then, with constant mixing by hand, dispense in 2 ml volumes into sterile containers.

Preparation of Surrogate Leucocytes

Chicken and turkey red blood cells are nucleated, and when fixed their size is within the human leucocyte range as recognised on electronic cell counters. They are thus suitable to serve as surrogate leucocytes.[13] However, such material may not be suitable for counting systems that are based on technologies other than impedance cell sizing.

For use as a white blood cell control, 25 ml of blood collected into any anticoagulant should suffice; after processing, an appropriate amount is added to preserved whole blood. Sterility must be maintained throughout the procedure.

Method

1. Centrifuge blood at approximately 2000 g for 20 min and remove the plasma aseptically.
2. Add an equal volume of 0.15 mol/l phosphate buffer, pH 7.4 (p. 691); mix and transfer to a sterile centrifuge bottle; recentrifuge and discard the supernatant and buffy coat.
3. Repeat the wash and centrifugation twice. To the washed cells, add 10 times their volume of glutaraldehyde fixative (0.25% in 0.15 mol/l phosphate buffer, pH 7.4). Leave overnight at 4°C.
4. On the next day, shake vigorously to ensure complete resuspension. Mix on a mechanical mixer for 1 h. To check that fixation has been complete, centrifuge 2–3 ml of the suspension, discard the supernatant, and add water to the deposit. If lysis occurs, the stock glutaraldehyde requires replacement.
5. When fixation is complete (i.e., after 18 hours of exposure), centrifuge the suspension at approximately 2000 g for 10 min and discard the supernatant. Add an equal volume of water to the fixed cell deposit, resuspend, and mix by stirring and shaking; recentrifuge at approximately 2000 g for 10 min and discard the supernatant; repeat twice.
6. Resuspend the fixed cells to approximately 30% concentration in 9 g/l NaCl. Mix well with vigorous shaking. Add antibiotic (see p. 660), cap tightly, seal with a plastic seal, and store at 4°C.

Before use, stand vial at room temperature for 10–20 min; then resuspend by vigorous shaking by hand or on a vortex mixer until no clumps remain at the base of the container, and then mix on a rotary mixer for at least 20 min before opening the vial.

For use as a WBC surrogate, after resuspension as described earlier, transfer an appropriate amount to a volume of preserved blood from which the leucocytes have been depleted by passing through a leucocyte filter. Establish the count by 5–10 replicate measurements on 3 vials and check intersample homogeneity by counts on 3 random vials from the batch. The CV should be not more than 5%.

An occasional batch may be found to be unsatisfactory and should be discarded.

Quality-Control Preparation for Platelet Counts[9]

Reagents

Alsever's solution. (A) Trisodium citrate, 16 g; NaCl, 8.2 g to 1 litre with water; (B) dextrose, 41 g to 1 litre with water. Store at 4°C. Immediately before use, mix equal volumes of A and B; filter through 0.2 μm micropore filter.

EDTA solution. 100 g/l of K_2 EDTA in the Alsever's solution; stable for 6 months at 4°C.

Method

1. Collect a unit of blood into ACD or CPD anticoagulant. Centrifuge for 10 min at 200 g and collect the platelet suspension into a plastic container.
2. Add 1 ml of EDTA solution. Mix well and leave at 37°C for 2 h to allow the platelets to disaggregate.
3. Add 200 ml of glutaraldehyde fixative (0.25% in 0.15 mol/l phosphate buffer, pH 7.4). Shake vigorously by hand to ensure complete platelet distribution, and leave for 48 h at room temperature with occasional shaking.
4. Centrifuge for 30 min at 3500 g. Wash the deposit twice in Alsever's solution and finally resuspend in 15–20 ml of Alsever's solution.
5. Carry out a rough platelet count to determine the approximate concentration, and add an appropriate amount of the suspension to preserved blood

(p. 660). Mix well for 20 min and, with continuous mixing, dispense into sterile containers. Cap and seal. At 4°C, the preparation should have a shelf life of 3–4 months. Before use, resuspend by thorough shaking by hand, followed by mechanical mixing for approximately 15 min.

A simpler method for preserving platelets by adding prostaglandin E_1 to blood in ACD has been reported to provide a control preparation with stability of about 14 days.[14]

ANALYSIS OF DATA

Standard Deviation of Controls

Control material may be prepared by the individual laboratory as described earlier or obtained from commercial sources. To ensure homogeneity, the stock should be dispensed into vials with continuous mixing; this is conveniently undertaken by means of a rotating flask. A mixing unit that is suitable has been designed specifically for this (see footnote, p. 661). Intertube homogeneity should then be checked by measuring the relevant analytes in at least 3 (preferably 10) vials taken at random from the batch. Their results should be within 2 standard deviations (SD) of 5–10 replicate measurements on 1 sample from the batch. The SD is calculated as shown on p. 698. Calculating the CV provides an alternative way of expressing the dispersion of results. The advantage of CV is that it describes the significance of SD irrespective of the measured value.

Control Charts

The use of control charts was first applied in clinical chemistry by Levey and Jennings.[15] They are now widely used in haematology for both automated and manual procedures.

Samples of the control specimen are included in every batch of patients' specimens, and the results are checked on a control chart. To check precision, it is not necessary to know the exact value of the control specimen. If, however, its value has been determined reliably by a reference method, the same material can also be used to check accuracy or to calibrate an instrument. If possible, controls with high, low, and normal values should be used. It is advisable to use at least one control sample per batch even if the batch is very small. Because the controls are intended to simulate random sampling, they must be treated exactly like the patients' specimens. The results obtained with the control samples can be plotted on a chart as described later.

The mean value and SD of the control specimen should first be established, as described earlier, in the laboratory where the tests on specimens are performed. Using arithmetic graph paper, a horizontal line is drawn to represent the mean (as a base), and on an appropriate scale of quantity and unit, lines representing +2 SD and –2 SD are drawn above and below the mean. The results of successive control sample measurements are plotted. If the test is satisfactory, sequential results oscillate about the mean value and less than 5% of the results fall outside 2 SD. Figure 26.1 illustrates a control chart from an automated system; a similar principle can be used for simple methods in which the data are plotted manually (Fig. 26.2).

The following indicate a fault in technique or in the instrument or reagent:

One widely deviant result outside 3 SD = a gross error or "blunder"
One or two results on or beyond the +2 SD or –2 SD limits = random error

Several consecutive similar results on one side of the mean = calibration fault causing a consistent bias
Consecutive fluctuating values, rising and falling by 2 SD = imprecision

The fault may be in the reagents or the laboratory ware, or it may be caused by incorrect adjustment/calibration of the instrument, technical error, or even clerical error in transcribing the results. Before an intensive investigation, the test should be repeated with another sample, and the possibility must also be considered that the inconsistency may be the result of deterioration or infection of the batch of material. This control process is unlikely to detect an error in an individual specimen, which can only be detected by correlation checks (described later). For haemoglobinometry, it may be useful to use both whole blood and lysate in a quality-control check because differences in results obtained with these two preparations help to identify errors resulting from incorrect dilution, inadequate mixing, or failure of a reagent to bring about complete lysis.

If the control specimen is included with each batch of tests during the course of a day, their measurements should not differ by more than the established CV. A trend of sequentially increasing or decreasing values with the repeated measurements is indicative of drift.

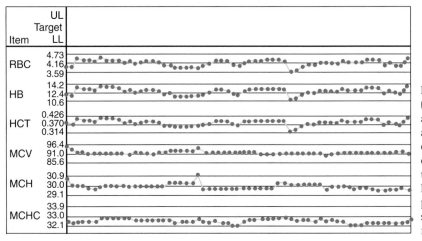

Figure 26.1 Control chart (Levey–Jennings chart) with automated blood count analyser. The mean value for each component of the blood count is shown on the right together with the upper and lower limits for satisfactory performance, which have been set at +2 SD and –2 SD, respectively.

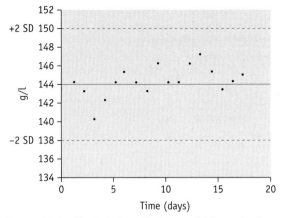

Figure 26.2   Control chart for haemoglobinometry by manual method. The limits for satisfactory performance have been set at ± 2 SD

Duplicate Tests on Patients' Specimens

Duplicate tests on patients' specimens[16] provide another way of checking the precision of routine work. To start the process, test 10 consecutive specimens in duplicate under careful conditions. Calculate the differences between the pairs of results, and derive the SD (p. 698). Subsequent duplicate measurements on any specimen in the same batch of tests should not differ from each other by more than 2 SD. This method detects random errors, but it does not detect incorrect calibration. It is also not sensitive to gradual drift, which, however, may be detected if the duplicate measurement is carried out in a later batch, provided that the specimen has not altered on standing. If the test is always badly done or has an inherent fault, the SD is wide.

These procedures are suitable for both manual and automated methods; they are impractical for routine blood counts in a busy laboratory, where three or four specimens in a batch should be tested in duplicate from time to time as a rough check of consistency.

"Delta" Check

The blood count on any patient should not differ from their counts that have been obtained during the previous 2–3 weeks by more than an amount that takes into account both test CV and physiological variation, provided that the patient's clinical con-

dition has not altered significantly. With automated counters, the differences should generally be not more than 10% for haemoglobin and RBC, 20% for WBC, and 50% for the platelet count. This procedure detects any deterioration of apparatus and reagents that may have developed between tests.

The test can also be carried out on the blood of healthy individuals whose blood count remains virtually constant day by day, subject only to the physiological changes (see p. 17).

Use of Patient Data for Quality Control

In hospitals with at least 100 test requests each day, there should be no significant daily variability in the means of their red cell indices obtained by an automated blood counter provided that the population of patients remains stable and that samples from a particular clinical source are not processed all in the same set, thus disproportionately influencing the mean. Assuming that the sample population is stable, any significant change in the means of the red cell indices indicates a change in instrument calibration or a drift owing to a fault in its function.

The procedure was developed by Bull[17,18] using a computerised algorithm to estimate the daily patient means of red cell indices (mean cell volume [MCV], mean cell haemoglobin [MCH], and mean cell haemoglobin concentration [MCHC]). To start this program, it is first necessary to assay samples from at least 300–500 patients in an automated blood counter over several days and to establish the means of MCV, MCH, and MCHC. Then, using the algorithm, it is possible to analyse the means in successive batches of 20 specimens. By plotting these on a graph, any drift of the three indices can be readily recognised and used to identify instrument faults; an increased SD signifies loss of precision. To ensure that each batch is representative, the samples should be randomised before analysis and, if possible, within any batch of 20, no more than 7 should come from one clinical source or have the same clinical condition.

The method is now incorporated in many automated blood counters (Fig. 26.3). In laboratories using manual methods, a simple adaptation of the same principle can be applied, confined to MCHC and excluding results from any special clinic that

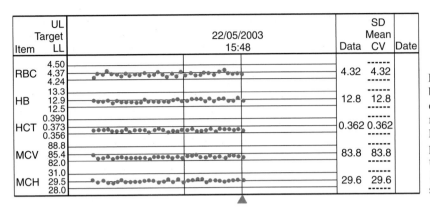

Item	UL Target LL	22/05/2003 15:48			SD Mean Data CV		Date
RBC	4.50 4.37 4.24				4.32	4.32 ------	
HB	13.3 12.9 12.5				12.8	12.8 ------	
HCT	0.390 0.373 0.356				0.362	0.362 ------	
MCV	88.8 85.4 82.0				83.8	83.8 ------	
MCH	31.0 29.5 28.0				29.6	29.6 ------	

Figure 26.3 Quality control based on patients' data. Control of automated blood counts by mean results for red cell indices MCV, MCH, and MCHC. The predetermined means are shown together with the upper limits (UL) and lower limits (LL) for satisfactory control.

are likely to be specifically biased. From the daily means for all measurements on 10 consecutive working days, an overall daily mean and SD are established. The mean MCHC is then calculated at the end of each day. If the test does not vary by more than 2 SD, it is considered satisfactory but may be misleading if there is an error in the same direction in both haemoglobin and PCV. The results may be displayed graphically, as illustrated in Figure 26.4. It is useful in validating successive batches of calibrators.

A similar instrument-specific procedure is used by some manufacturers who gather the data submitted through network links by users of their instruments. This enables them to maintain a constant check of performance of these instruments overall and to detect any that require recalibration or investigation of faults.

Correlation Check

Correlation check implies that any unexpected result of a test must be checked to see whether it can be explained on clinical grounds or whether it correlates with other tests. Thus, for example, un-expectedly higher or lower haemoglobin might be explained by a blood transfusion or a haemorrhage, respectively. A low MCHC should be confirmed by demonstrating hypochromic red cells on a Romanowsky-stained blood film; a high MCV must correlate with macrocytosis. Similarly, the blood films should be examined to confirm marked leucocytosis or leucopenia or thrombocytosis or thrombocytopenia, to distinguish between platelets and red cell fragments or conversely between giant

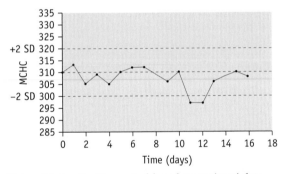

Figure 26.4 Quality control based on patients' data. Control of manual blood counts using the mean cell haemoglobin concentration (MCHC) as an indicator.

platelets and normal-sized red cells (e.g., Fig. 5.95), or to check an erroneously high leucocyte count as a result of incompletely lysed red cells in haemoglobinopathies or liver disease—but be careful because the blood film itself may be misleading if not correctly made and stained.

Recording blood count data on cumulative report forms or charts is good clinical practice and provides an inbuilt quality-control system by making it easy to detect an aberrant result when compared with a previously determined baseline. This is especially useful in detecting the occasional wild errors caused by incorrect labelling of the specimen, inadequate suspension of the blood before sampling, partial clotting of a blood sample, or deterioration on storage. A discrepant result without apparent clinical reason must be suspect until confirmed by a repeat test on a fresh specimen. The occurrence of a similar discrepancy in two different specimens on the same day would suggest that two specimens have been mixed up.

EXTERNAL QUALITY ASSESSMENT

An external quality assessment scheme (EQAS)[10,19-21] is an important complement to internal control. Even when all precautions are taken to achieve accuracy and precision in the laboratory, errors arise that are only detectable by objective external assessment. The principle is that the same material is sent from a national or regional centre to numerous participating laboratories, at least 20. Results that are returned to the EQAS centre are analysed, a target value and an acceptable range around the target are established, and the performance of the individual participants is judged. It is important that surveys should be performed at regular intervals, although their frequency may vary, depending on the diagnostic importance of the particular test, how frequently they are requested, and their technical reliability. Thus, for example, in the UK national scheme (NEQAS) for haematology, specimens are distributed at 4-weekly intervals for blood counts and every 3 months for most other tests.*

The main purposes of EQAS are to ensure reliable performance by individual laboratories and to achieve harmonisation or concordance between laboratories. However, some analysers handle preserved blood differently from routine specimens and, even if correctly calibrated, different types of counter may differ in their responses to EQA samples.[22,23] It may thus be necessary to analyse results separately for different groups of instruments. When there are unexplained differences in counts on EQA samples with different instruments in the same laboratory, counts should be made on fresh EDTA blood samples with the different instruments to ascertain their true comparability, and, if necessary, recalibration of one should be undertaken to achieve concordance.

EQAS also has other complementary functions:

Collecting information on the reliability of particular methods, materials, and equipment

Identifying problems with any *in vitro* diagnostic medical device (IVDMD) that requires reaction from the manufacturer and/or reporting to the responsible national authority as described in EN 14136 (p. 659).

Providing information on performance required for the purpose of licensing or accreditation

Identifying laboratories whose performance provides a benchmarking standard

Recommending state-of-the-art procedures for various analytic tests, organizing workshops for education and training of laboratory staff, and advising on best-practice guidelines

Analysis of EQA Data

Deviation Index

From the results returned by the participants the median or mean and SD are calculated. An individual laboratory can then compare its performance in the survey with that of other laboratories and with its own previous performance from the deviation index (DI) (or z-score, as it is sometimes called). This is calculated as the difference between the individual laboratory's result and the median or mean relative to the SD. Thus,

$$DI = \frac{[\text{Actual results for test} - \text{Adjusted mean or median}]}{\text{Trimmed SD}}$$

When results have a Gaussian distribution the mean and SD are adjusted in a preliminary calculation by excluding all results in the highest and lowest 5%.

When distribution of results is non-Gaussian, median should be used rather than mean. In this case SD is calculated as follows:

$$\text{Central 50\% spread} \div 1.349$$

Instead of using a trimmed SD as described earlier, the SD may be calculated from a constant CV, which takes account of technical variance of the method, clinical utility of the test, and the critical range of measurement for diagnostic discrimination.

In this method, a DI (score) of less than 0.5 denotes excellent performance, a score between 0.5 and 1.0 is satisfactory, and a score between 1.0 and 2.0 is still acceptable. A score higher than 2.0 suggests that the analyser calibration should be

---

*Information on UK NEQAS is available on the Web site www.ukneqas.org.uk or by e-mail to haem@ukneqas.org.uk.

checked, whereas a DI >3.0 indicates a serious defect requiring attention.

Consecutive Monitoring

It is essential to monitor EQA results in consecutive surveys, noting any fluctuations in the DI. A convenient way for quantifying this is to add 6 recent DI scores (e.g., from the 2 samples in the last 3 surveys); any values >3.5 are rounded down to 3.5 to avoid an isolated very high value having an excessive effect on the calculation. The total is then multiplied by 6. Failure to submit results in a survey suffers a penalty of 50.

A score of 100 or more indicates persistent unsatisfactory performance. It is, however, to be hoped that participants have corrected any problems before this stage is reached.

Outwith Consensus Method

The "Outwith consensus" method, which is a refinement of the non-Gaussian procedure described earlier, is used in the UK NEQAS for blood coagulation. The median is calculated and all the participant results are then ranked in five grades as follows:

Group A: 25% of all results that are immediately adjacent to and above the median and 25% that are immediately adjacent to and below the median

Group B: The next 10% on each side of A

Group C: The next 5% on each side of B

Group D: The next 5% on each side of C

Group E: The final 5% on each side of D (and also nonparticipation)

Performance in any particular test is assessed from the grades obtained in two consecutive exercises. Unsatisfactory performance is designated when the combination is D-D, E-C, E-D, or E-E.

Target Values and Bias

The true value for a test can usually be assumed to be the result obtained by best performance of selected participants in the survey or by experts using reference methods or total participant consensus after trimming, as described earlier. This is the target value (TV) to be aimed for by all the participants. The percent bias by an individual participant's result (R) can then be calculated as follows:

$$[(R-TV) \div TV] \times 100$$

The pattern of bias in successive surveys indicates whether there is a constant calibration error or a progressive fault or whether the original defect has been corrected.

Youden (xy) Plot

The Youden plot is a useful method for relating measurements on two samples in a survey to provide a graphic display and, when a participant's results are unsatisfactory, for distinguishing between a consistent bias and random error. Results for the two samples are plotted on the horizontal (x) and the vertical (y) axis, respectively, and the standard deviations (2 SD or 3 SD) for the two sets are drawn, as shown in outline in Fig. 26.5.

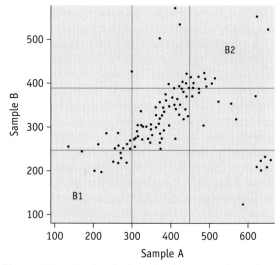

Figure 26.5   Youden (xy) graph. The range of standard deviations (SDs) calculated from the overall results with sample x and sample y, respectively, are drawn on the x axis and the y axis; the individual paired results are then plotted on the graph. Results in the central square are satisfactory; those in B demonstrate a consistent bias with measurements that are too low (B1) or too high (B2), whereas results in other areas indicate random errors.

Results that fall in the central block are satisfactory; those in blocks B indicate a consistent bias that may be positive (to right) or negative (to left), whereas results in other areas indicate random errors (inconsistency) in the two samples.

Methodology Check

It is sometimes useful to check separate components of a method. Thus, appropriate samples can be used to check adequacy of mixing to ensure sample homogeneity, the reliability of the dilution procedure, and how an instrument is used. As an example, a survey might include a pair of identical whole blood samples and lysates from the same specimen for measuring haemoglobin, together with a prediluted haemoglobin solution.

Clinical Significance

In assessing performance, using limits based on the SD in some cases is too rigid and in other cases it is too lenient. To ensure that results are clinically reliable, they should be within a certain percentage of the assigned value. This must take account of unavoidable imprecision of the method and normal diurnal variations. The following limits are adequate to meet these requirements in practice:

Hb and RBC (by cell counter)	3–4%
PCV, MCV, MCH, MCHC	4–5%
Leucocyte count	8–10%
Platelet count	10–15%
Vitamin B_{12}, folate, iron, ferritin	20%
HbA_2 and HbF quantitation	5%

Semiquantitative Tests

Reactions such as lysis, agglutination, or colour change are recorded as 0, 1+, 2+, 3+, or 4+. Assessment of performance should be based on extent of divergence from the target value, which might be a consensus of participant results or a referee's results. Account must be taken of the diagnostic and clinical significance of an incorrect or confusing result.

Qualitative Tests

In assessing qualitative or interpretative tests (e.g., blood film morphology), participant results are compared with the consensus obtained from a panel of referees or by concordance of 75% or more of the participants. The features reported are graded on

their clinical significance, taking account of the specific medical condition, as follows:

Essential for diagnosis: 5 points
Likely to influence diagnostic decision: 2–3 points
Could be helpful in reaching a diagnosis, but only
   as a secondary consideration: 1 point
Provides no useful information: 0 points.

All correct observations are given a positive score, and false-positive observations are subtracted in accordance with the grading. The result is expressed as percentage of total possible score established by the referees.

QUALITY-ASSURANCE PROTOCOL FOR DIAGNOSTIC LABORATORIES

The procedures that should be included in a quality-assurance programme vary with the tests undertaken; the instruments used; and (especially if these include a fully automatic counting system) the size of the laboratory and the numbers of specimens handled, the computer facilities available, and the amount of time that can be devoted to the programme. At least some form of internal quality control must be undertaken, and there must be participation in an external quality-assessment scheme where one is available. Some control procedures should be performed daily, and other performance checks should be done at appropriate intervals. The latter is particularly important when there is a change in staff and after a maintenance service or repair has been carried out on equipment. The comprehensive protocol is summarised in Table 26.1.

All laboratory staff require training in these various aspects of quality assurance. A useful training manual from WHO* describes the principles and methods together with practical exercises to illustrate these.[9] Another good teaching source is J.O. Westgard's Web site (www.westgard.com); this includes a "Lesson of the Month" and other current topics that are regularly updated.

---

*Available on request to the Department of Essential Health Technology, WHO, 1211 Geneva 27, Switzerland.

Table 26.1 Quality-assurance procedures

Calibration with reference standards

Instruments: At 6-month intervals, if control chart or EQA indicates bias or fluctuation in results, and after any repair/service
Diluting systems: Initially and at 1- to 2-week intervals

Control cart with control material: daily or more frequently with each batch of specimens

Delta check on selected patients' samples: daily

Duplicate tests on two or three patients' samples: if control chart or delta check shows discrepancies

Analysis of patients' results: constancy of mean MCV, MCH, MCHC: daily

Correlation assessment of test reports

Cumulative results: following previous tests
Blood film: if unusual test results and/or counter flags appear
Clinical state

EQAS performance

REFERENCES

1. European Parliament and Council 1998 Directive 98/79 on *in vitro* diagnostic medical devices. Official Journal of the European Communities 331/1–331/37.
2. International Council for Standardization in Haematology 1996 Recommendations for reference methods of haemoglobinometry in human blood (ICSH Standard 1995) and specifications for international haemiglobincyanide standard, 4th ed. Journal of Clinical Pathology 49:271–274.
3. International Council for Standardization in Haematology 1988 The assignment of values to fresh blood used for calibrating automated blood cell counters. Clinical and Laboratory Haematology 10:203–212.
4. Springer W, Prohaska W, Neukammer J, et al 1999 Evaluation of a new reagent for preserving fresh blood samples and its potential usefulness for internal quality controls of multichannel haematology analyzers. American Journal of Clinical Pathology 111:387–396.
5. Lewis SM, England JM, Rowan RM 1991 Current concerns in haematology 3: blood count calibration. Journal of Clinical Pathology 44:881–884.
6. Richardson Jones A 1982 Counting and sizing of blood cells using aperture-impedance systems. In: van Assendelft OW, England JM (eds) Advances in hematological methods: the blood count. CRC Press, Boca Raton, FL, Ch 5.
7. Thom R 1972 Hemocytometry: method and results by improved electronic blood-cell sizing. In: Izak G, Lewis SM (eds) Modern concepts in hematology. Academic Press, New York, p. 191–200.
8. Torlontano G, Tata A 1972 Stable standard suspension of white blood cells suitable for calibration and control of electronic counters. In: Izak G, Lewis SM (eds) Modern concepts in hematology. Academic Press, New York, p. 230–234.
9. Lewis SM 1998 Quality assurance in haematology: document LAB/98.4. World Health Organization, Geneva.
10. Deom A, El Aouad R, Heuck CC, et al 2000 Requirements and guidance for external quality assurance programmes for health laboratories: document LAB/2000. World Health Organization, Geneva.
11. Ward PG, Chappel DA, Fox JGC, et al 1975 Mixing and bottling unit for preparing biological fluids used in quality control. Laboratory Practice 24:577–583.
12. Reardon DM, Mack D, Warner B, et al 1991 A whole blood control for blood count analysers, and source material for an external quality assessment scheme. Medical Laboratory Sciences 48:19–26.
13. International Council for Standardization in Haematology 1994 Reference method for the

enumeration of erythrocytes and leucocytes. Clinical and Laboratory Haematology 16:131–138.

14. Zhang Z, Tatsumi N, Tsuda I, et al 1999 Long-term preservation of platelet count in blood for external quality control surveillance using prostaglandin E_1. Clinical and Laboratory Haematology 21:71.

15. Levey S, Jennings ER 1950 The use of control charts in the clinical laboratory. American Journal of Clinical Pathology 20:1059–1066.

16. Cembrowski GS, Lunetsky ES, Patrick CC, et al 1988 An optimized quality control procedure for hematology analyzers with the use of retained patient specimens. American Journal of Clinical Pathology 89:203–210.

17. Korpman RA, Bull BS 1976 The implementation of a robust estimator of the mean for quality control on a programmable calculator or a laboratory computer. American Journal of Clinical Pathology 65:252–253.

18. Smith FA, Kroft SH 1996 Exponentially adjusted moving mean procedure for quality control: an optimized patient sample control procedure. American Journal of Clinical Pathology 105:44–51.

19. Lewis SM 1995 External quality assessment. In: Lewis SM, Koepke JA (eds) Haematology laboratory management and practice. Butterworth Heinemann, Oxford, Ch 19.

20. International Council for Standardization in Haematology 1998 Guidelines for organization and management of external quality assessment using proficiency testing. International Journal of Haematology 68:45–52.

21. International Organization for Standardization 1997 Guide 43–1 Proficiency testing by interlaboratory comparisons. I Development and operation of proficiency testing schemes. ISO, Geneva.

22. Wardle J, Ward PG, Lewis SM 1985 Response of various blood counting systems to CPD-A1 preserved whole blood. Clinical and Laboratory Haematology 7:245–250.

23. Leyssen MHJ, DeBruyere MJG, van Druppen et al 1985 Problems related to CPD preserved blood used for NEQAS trials in haematology. Clinical and Laboratory Haematology 7:239–243.

27 Haematology in under-resourced laboratories

Imelda Bates and Barry Mendelow

INTRODUCTION: TYPES OF LABORATORIES

In most countries, there are likely to be some laboratories with limited resources, but in under-resourced countries, there are few laboratories with highly trained technologists and sophisticated equipment; in these countries it is not unusual for laboratory tests to be carried out by nurses and orderlies in outpatient consulting rooms, corridors, and in rural health centres. Understaffing, poor morale, inadequate equipment, and erratic supplies of reagents are chronic problems in laboratories in poorer countries, and these factors have a major impact on the range and quality of services that can be offered. Many smaller laboratories are multifunctional, performing haematology, parasitology, clinical chemistry, and microbiology tests. A blood transfusion service is usually available at the larger institutions and, unless there is a national blood service, laboratory staff will be responsible for donor selection, blood collection, and issuing of blood. If there is no organisation of public health laboratories, routine laboratories will be required to provide high-quality health surveillance data for epidemiological and public health monitoring.

In a number of under-resourced countries the difficulties are compounded by the fact that health services are becoming overwhelmed by expanding epidemics of HIV/AIDS (human immunodeficiency virus/acquired immune deficiency syndrome), tuberculosis, and malaria. Diagnosis and monitoring of these diseases require a robust and reliable laboratory service. Thus, malaria diagnosis must be confirmed by a laboratory test because other disorders can masquerade clinically as malaria.[1] The diagnosis of tuberculosis may require bone marrow aspiration and culture and trephine biopsy examination, especially in patients who are also HIV positive because in these cases sputum tests for acid-fast organisms are frequently negative.[2] Monitoring of HIV progression to AIDS and the effectiveness of antiretroviral therapy requires haemoglobin estimations, CD4-positive lymphocyte counts, and plasma viral load determinations.[3-5]

The purpose of this chapter is to point toward an effective haematology service that can be provided despite serious limitations. In planning such a service, it is necessary to identify what facilities are needed and to plan a network for referral when a clinical problem requires investigations beyond the facilities and expertise that are available locally. Thus, for example, successful management of haematological malignancies in countries with limited resources might involve enthusiastic local haematologists forming partnerships with institutions in developed countries with consequent adaptation of standard protocols and improvement of local supportive care facilities.[6]

ORGANIZATION OF CLINICAL LABORATORY SERVICES

In under-resourced countries clinical laboratory services may be considered at three levels according to their size, staffing, and the work they undertake. These are (A) subdistrict facilities including health centres; (B) district hospitals; and (C) central, regional, and teaching hospitals (Fig. 27.1).

Level A. Subdistrict Facilities Including Health Centres

The level A "laboratory" generally provides the means for helping to determine whether a patient should be referred to the local hospital. It may be simply an estimation of haemoglobin concentration (Hb) during the clinical consultation (i.e., point-of-care testing) or it may be a side room where basic laboratory tests are often carried out by nurses, assistants, or orderlies with no technical qualifications. The haematology equipment available may include a simple method for estimating Hb and a microscope for examination of slides for tuberculosis or malaria. However, maintenance of microscopes in the rural areas is often poor and this can significantly compromise the quality of results (see p. 707).

Level of Laboratory	Haematology Services Performed
Health Centres	Simple haemoglobin estimation
	Screening for malaria
	HIV testing
District Hospitals	Haemoglobin measurement
	Examination of blood films (morphology and differential white cell count)
	Total platelet and white cell counts
	Screening for sickle haemoglobin (when appropriate)
	Malaria rapid test
	CD4 count
Central/Regional Hospitals	Automated blood count
	G6PD screen
	Haemoglobin electrophoresis
	Immunophenotyping
	HIV viral load estimation
	Basic clotting tests
	Oral anticoagulant control
	Processing of bone marrow aspirates
	Cross-matching and antibody screening
	Basic blood components production
National Reference Centre	All relevant tests

Figure 27.1   Network of laboratories.

Level B. District Hospitals

District hospital laboratories are usually multipurpose, performing microbiological and biochemical as well as haematological tests. Laboratory staff consist of one or two qualified technicians supported by assistants who often have little or no training. The minimum equipment available for haematology is a microscope and centrifuge and possibly a simple colorimeter for measurement of haemoglobin concentration.

Level C. Central and Teaching Hospitals

At this level the laboratory staff receive multidisciplinary training and each laboratory generally has a specialist technical head, whereas many of the more senior staff will have received postgraduate training in their chosen discipline. Equipment generally includes centrifuges, colorimeters, microscopes, haemoglobin electrophoresis equipment, and possibly blood bank centrifuges for the separation of blood components. Automated haematology analysers may be found in such laboratories. In many cases, these have been supplied by donor agencies, but long-term funding to support maintenance and training for using these systems is often lacking and consequently they may be unreliable or not used at all owing to a shortage of appropriate reagents and inadequate maintenance and staff training.

AVAILABILITY OF TESTS AT EACH LEVEL

In under-resourced countries the haematology tests that are available at the different levels of health care services are very variable and depend on local clinical needs, the equipment available, the number of laboratory staff, and their technical skill. The following is a general description of the tests that are likely to be required, but all may not necessarily be available at the specified levels.

Level A

Haemoglobin estimation by simple method (p. 678)
Malaria screen on peripheral blood thin and thick films (p. 71)

HIV serology tests supported by voluntary counselling and testing

Level B

Haemoglobin measurement (p. 26)
Peripheral blood morphology, especially to identify the cause of anaemia (Chapter 5)*
Platelet and total white blood cell counts (p. 680)
Differential white cell count (p. 35)
CD4 lymphocyte count (p. 684; see also p. 337)
Malaria screening by thick and thin peripheral blood smears (p. 71) or rapid immunological test for *Plasmodium falciparum* and possibly other species (p. 604)
Screening test for sickle haemoglobin in areas where this is relevant (p. 294).

Level C

In addition to tests carried out at level B, the haematology services offered by level C might include the following:

Automated Hb, MCV, MCH, MCHC, platelet counts, white blood cell total, and differential counts (p. 36).
Haemoglobin electrophoresis or high-performance liquid chromatography (Chapter 12)
Haemoglobin A_2 and haemoglobin F measurements (pp. 298 and 302)
Glucose-6-phosphate dehydrogenase screen (by fluorescent spot or methaemoglobin reduction method) (p. 217)
Flow cytometry immunophenotyping (Chapter 14)
Polymerase chain reaction (PCR) or other method for diagnosis of mutations associated with haematological malignancies (Chapter 21)
HIV plasma viral load estimations
Staining of bone marrow smears for morphological assessment (p. 119) and estimation of iron status (p. 311)
Bone marrow trephine examination (p. 124)
Blood grouping and crossmatching (Chapter 20)
Identification of blood group antibodies (Chapter 19)
Basic clotting screen (prothrombin time, thrombin

---

*A bench-aid on morphology is available from the World Health Organization (WHO).[7]

time, and activated partial thromboplastin time) (p. 398)

Oral anticoagulant control (p. 466)

Separation of whole blood into packed cells, plasma, and, occasionally, platelets (p. 661).

Microscopes

The microscope is the most important piece of equipment in laboratories in under-resourced countries. It is essential for the diagnosis of anaemia, tuberculosis, malaria, and other blood parasitic infections and for performing absolute and differential cell counts. Reliable assessment of these morphological features requires that the microscope is clean and correctly set up with aligned lenses and inbuilt or reflected light to ensure clear images at high magnification. Failure to maintain the quality of microscopes to a high standard by routine maintenance and regular professional servicing can lead to inaccurate diagnoses and inefficient use of technician time.[8,9] Routine maintenance of the microscope is described on p. 707.

"ESSENTIAL" HAEMATOLOGY TESTS

Despite the relatively high cost of running a laboratory service and the low per capita health care budget in under-resourced countries, there are very few data available on which to base rational decisions about "essential" laboratory tests.[10,11] In many of these countries, decisions for the laboratories are made at central level by health care planners whose interests are wider that those of the laboratory manager, but it is important to ensure that the viewpoint of the laboratory manager is respected. In deciding which tests are "essential," it is important to have reliable information concerning the clinical and public health needs of the local community and to collaborate with health planners in projecting the medium- and long-term trends. The need for such information is especially urgent in countries where an overwhelming burden has been placed on the health services by the HIV/AIDS epidemic.

To ensure cost-effectiveness of the laboratory service, tests with no proven value should be eliminated, and new tests for which there is inde-

pendent evidence of effectiveness should be introduced, as described in Chapter 24 p. 627. For laboratories without access to computerised data systems, an index of realistic cost-effectiveness can be obtained from the following formula, which takes account of various factors[3]:

$$\frac{A \times 100}{C} \times \frac{100}{B} \text{ where}$$

A = cost per test, B = its diagnostic reliability, and C = its clinical usefulness.

However, in laboratories with limited facilities these factors must be interpreted with caution because it is not possible to draw up a list of such tests that will be applicable to all countries or even to different regions within a country. The following aspects should be taken into account.

Cost Per Test

Often the cost of a test is calculated from the price of reagents divided by the number of tests performed. However, this oversimplifies the situation and is not accurate enough to form the basis for national policy decisions and budget allocation. The factors that need to be taken into account when calculating the total annual costs for a laboratory, including a formula for the calculation, are given on p. 628. As an example of the effect of various factors on costs, in a typical district hospital laboratory in Africa, malaria and tuberculosis microscopy comprised 22% and 46% respectively of the total number of tests performed, but when these factors are taken into account, tuberculosis smears actually accounted for 43% and malaria microscopy for 9% of the overall laboratory budget.[11]

Diagnostic Reliability

The quality of all tests carried out by a laboratory should be regularly monitored; systems for doing this are well-established (see Chapter 24). The quality of the test will influence its utility. For example, if the result of a test in routine practice is only correct 80% of the time, then 1 in 5 tests will be wasted, reducing the effectiveness of the test by 20%. Furthermore, the inaccurate test may result in a patient receiving inappropriate treatment. It is also important to know the sensitivity and specificity of the test and its predictive value, as calculated on p. 627. However, in many under-resourced countries, it is difficult to establish these figures because the "gold standard" diagnostic services needed to determine "true positive" and "true negative" data are lacking.

Clinical Usefulness

An assessment of the clinical usefulness of a test should be carried out by an independent clinician who is familiar with local diseases and the diagnostic support services that are available. This assessor needs to compare actual clinical practice with locally agreed "best practice" or, if available, local guidelines. From observation of a range of clinical interactions, the percentage of times that ideal practice is followed can be calculated. For example, transfusion guidelines may recommend that transfusions are given routinely to children with an Hb of less than 5 g/dl. The assessor can record how many children with Hb below this level failed to receive a transfusion and how many transfusions were given without waiting for the Hb result or at an inappropriate Hb concentration. For each test, the assessor needs to judge whether it has been appropriately requested and is used to influence patient management or public health decisions. The percentage of tests that are not used to guide clinical decisions will provide a figure for "clinical wastage" of the test that can be entered into the formula (p. 676).

MAINTAINING QUALITY AND RELIABILITY OF TESTS

Paradoxically, it is in under-resourced laboratories, where equipment and supplies are limited and training and supervision may be minimal, that the level of skills and motivation required to maintain quality of service need to be highest. Even the most basic of laboratories should ensure that procedures are in place to monitor quality (see Chapter 26). In addition to monitoring the technical quality of each test, the quality of the whole service must be ensured both within the laboratory (internal control) and between laboratories (external control). Standard operating procedures (p. 639) should be drafted for every method. In addition to providing standardised techniques, these are excellent teaching resources, and adherence to these procedures will minimise errors. They need to be regularly reviewed and updated to keep pace with technical developments and changes in local circumstances (e.g., nonavailability of reagents, technical limitations).

Quality Control of a Test Method (Technical Quality)

Methods for the control for various haematology tests are described in Chapter 26, but some may need to be adapted to specific local circumstances in resource-poor countries. For example, each batch of sickle screening tests should include known positive and negative samples; for monitoring constancy of haemoglobin estimations, a high and a low value sample can be remeasured several times during the day.

Internal Quality Control

Internal quality control is a system within an individual laboratory for ensuring that the whole test process, rather than just one technical element, is of acceptable quality. Monitoring of quality by the use of controls that are put through the whole process, and plotting a control chart (p. 663), will highlight problems with the system. For example, an inaccurate white cell differential count may point toward problems with sample collection and handling, slide preparation, fixing and staining, morphological interpretation, and microscope quality as well as inadequate microscopy technique. Measures such as the introduction of standard operating procedures, in-service training, and equipment maintenance schedules are designed to improve performance and prevent problems.

External Quality Assessment

The principles of external quality assessment (EQA) are described on p. 667. Poor communications and transport facilities make it difficult to establish EQA in under-resourced laboratories. Although participation in an international or a national or even local regional external quality assessment system may be beyond the capabilities of a small rural laboratory, it should be possible for them to link with neighbouring facilities. Rural laboratories can take advantage of programmes with established communications between the districts, to exchange materials and results between different laboratories. Such programmes might include district medical officer supervisory visits or national vertical programmes such as tuberculosis monitoring or health education visits. A rural laboratory that detects a problem with its results needs to have a clearly defined reporting system to a higher level facility, which is in turn responsible for addressing the problem. Accreditation schemes (p. 639), either national or local, can be set up to formally recognise laboratories that are performing well and to assist those that are not.

BASIC HAEMATOLOGY TESTS

Haemoglobinometry

Various methods for the measurement of haemo-globin concentration are given in Chapter 3. The most accurate method that may be available in under-resourced laboratories is the haemiglobin-cyanide (cyanmethaemoglobin) method. However, this requires a power source and considerable technical expertise to carry out accurate dilutions and to prepare the standard curve.

Methods for measuring the Hb that are robust, accurate, and can be used by unskilled health workers are described below.

Direct Reading Haemoglobinometers

HemoCue Blood Hemoglobin System*
HemoCue Blood Hemoglobin System (see p. 30) is a battery- or mains-operated portable, direct read-out machine that uses disposable dry-chemistry cuvettes. It is precise and accurate (provided that only the specified cuvettes are used) and, unlike most other systems, it does not require predilution of the sample. Although the use of the unique disposable cuvettes makes this method relatively expensive, it is very simple to use so that the cost may be offset by savings on training and supervision.

---

*Available from HemoCue AB, Box 1204, SE-262 23, Angelholm, Sweden. Tel: +46 431 45 82 00.

DHT Haemoglobinometer[†]

DHT Haemoglobinometer (see p. 30) is a portable, battery- or mains-operated, direct read-out machine. It has been specifically designed for use in poorer tropical countries. It uses a stable, inexpensive diluting fluid and has low power consumption. It is simple to use because the diluted sample is placed in a cuvette that is inserted into the machine. This automatically initiates the reading and display of the haemoglobin value.

Haemoglobin Colour Scale[‡]

Many colour comparison methods have been developed in the past, but these have become obsolete because the colours were not sufficiently comparable to blood or were not durable. The World Health Organization (WHO) has now developed a low-cost haemoglobin colour scale for anaemia screening where there is no laboratory.[12,13] It consists of a set of printed colour shades representing haemoglobin levels between 4 and 14 g/dl. The colour of a drop of blood collected onto a specific type of matrix is compared to that on the chart (Fig. 27.2). It is intended for detecting the presence of anaemia and estimating its severity in 2 g/dl (20 g/l) increments. The utility of the scale in clinical practice has been demonstrated by field trials in rural antenatal clinics and peripheral health centres.[14,15] However, care must be taken to follow the instructions exactly because poor lighting, allowing the blood spot to dry out, and using the incorrect type of matrix for the test strips can have detrimental effects on the results.[§]

Packed Cell Volume

Although the packed cell volume can be used as a simple screen for anaemia and as a rough guide to the accuracy of haemoglobin measurements, it is not a substitute for a well-performed haemoglobin

---

[†]Available from Developing Health Technology, Bridge House, Worlington Road, Barton Mills, IP28 7DX, U.K. Tel: + 44 1603 416058.
[‡]Available from Copack GmbH, AmKrick 9, 22113 Oststeinbek, Germany, e-mail:into@copackservice.de
[§]Information on the Hb Colour Scale can be obtained from: Department of Essential Health Technology, WHO, 1211 Geneva 27; Fax: +41 22 791 4836. See also Table 24.6, p. 635.

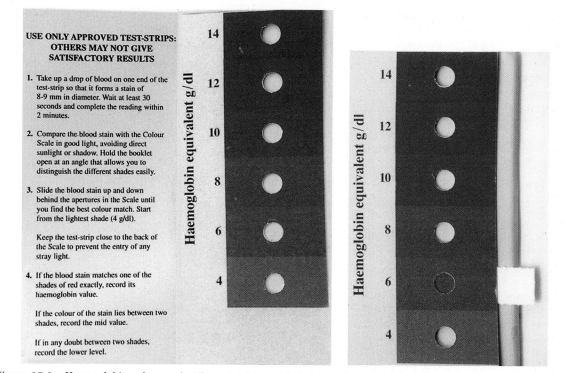

USE ONLY APPROVED TEST-STRIPS: OTHERS MAY NOT GIVE SATISFACTORY RESULTS

1. Take up a drop of blood on one end of the test-strip so that it forms a stain of 8-9 mm in diameter. Wait at least 30 seconds and complete the reading within 2 minutes.

2. Compare the blood stain with the Colour Scale in good light, avoiding direct sunlight or shadow. Hold the booklet open at an angle that allows you to distinguish the different shades easily.

3. Slide the blood stain up and down behind the apertures in the Scale until you find the best colour match. Start from the lightest shade (4 g/dl).

   Keep the test-strip close to the back of the Scale to prevent the entry of any stray light.

4. If the blood stain matches one of the shades of red exactly, record its haemoglobin value.

   If the colour of the stain lies between two shades, record the mid value.

   If in any doubt between two shades, record the lower level.

Figure 27.2   Haemoglobin colour scale. The stained test-strip being read on the right indicates a severe anaemia with a haemoglobin value of about 6 g/dl.

measurement. In addition to the technical problems outlined on p. 30 there are particular problems with this method in resource-poor settings that may lead to errors in estimating the packed cell volume. The lack of a mechanical mixing device means that specimens may not be adequately mixed. A lack of high-quality sealant for the microhaematocrit tubes means that they often leak during centrifugation. Because the microhaematocrit tubes are difficult to label, samples may get mixed up in the centrifuge, especially when pressure of work is high and there is a lack of supervision. Erratic power supplies, lack of devices for measuring g forces, and poor equipment maintenance result in inadequate centrifugation with incomplete packing of the red cells.

Manual Cell Counts Using Counting Chambers

Visual counting of blood cells is an acceptable alternative to electronic counting for white cell and platelet counts. It is not recommended for routine red cell counts because the number of cells that can be counted within a reasonable time in the routine laboratory (e.g., about 400) will be too few to ensure a sufficiently precise result (see below).

Counting Chambers

The visibility of the rulings in the counting chamber[16] is as important as the accuracy of calibration, so that chambers with a "metallised" surface and Neubauer or Improved Neubauer rulings are recommended. These have nine 1 mm × 1 mm ruled areas, which, when covered correctly with the special thick coverglass, each contain a volume of 0.1 µl of diluted blood (Figs. 27.3 and 27.4). Coverslips designed for mounting of microscopy preparations must not be used with counting chambers. The sample is introduced between the chamber and the coverglass using a pipette or capillary tube, and the preparation is viewed using a ×40 objective and ×6 or ×10 eyepieces. With

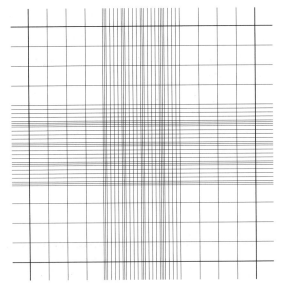

Figure 27.3   Neubauer counting chamber. The total ruled area is 3 mm × 3 mm; the central ruled area is 1 mm × 1 mm. In the central area, 16 groups of 16 small squares are separated by triple rulings.

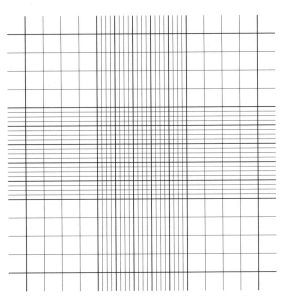

Figure 27.4   Improved Neubauer counting chamber. The central area consists of 25 groups of 16 small squares separated by closely ruled triple lines (which appear as thick black lines in the photograph).

Neubauer and Improved Neubauer chambers, count the cells in 4 or 8 horizontal rectangles of 1 mm × 0.05 mm (80 or 160 small squares) or in 5 or 10 groups of 16 small squares, including the cells that touch the bottom and left-hand margins of the small squares.

Total White Blood Cell Count

To make the counting of white cells easier, diluted whole blood is mixed with a fluid to lyse the red cells and stain the white cell nuclei deep violet-black.

Diluent

The diluent is 2% (20 ml/l) acetic acid coloured pale violet with gentian violet.

Method

Make a 1 in 20 dilution of blood by adding 0.1 ml of *well-mixed* blood (lack of adequate mixing is a major source of error) to 1.9 ml of diluent* in a 75 × 10 mm plastic (or glass) tube. After sealing the

---

*Or a proportionately smaller volume: 20 μl of blood in 0.38 ml of lysing fluid.

tube with a lid or tightly fitting bung, mix the diluted blood in a mechanical mixer or by hand for at least 2 min by tilting the tube to an angle of about 120 degrees combined with rotation, thus allowing the air bubble to mix the suspension. Fill a clean dry counting chamber, with its coverglass already in position, without delay. This is simply accomplished with the aid of a plastic Pasteur pipette or a length of stout capillary glass tubing that has been allowed to take up the suspension by capillarity. Take care that the counting chamber is filled in one action and that no fluid flows into the surrounding moat.

Leave the chamber undisturbed on a bench for at least 2 min for the cells to settle, but not much longer, because drying at the edges of the preparation initiates currents that cause movement of the cells after they have settled. The bench must be free of vibrations, and the chamber must not be exposed to draughts or to direct sunlight or other sources of heat. It is important that the coverglass should be of a special thick glass and perfectly flat, so that when laid on the counting chamber, diffraction rings are seen. The coverglass should be of such a size that when placed correctly on the counting chamber the central ruled areas lie in the centre of the rectangle to be filled with the cell suspension.

If any of the following filling defects occur, the preparation must be discarded and the filling procedure must be repeated using another clean dry chamber:

Overflow into moat
Chamber area incompletely filled
Air bubbles anywhere in chamber area
Any debris in chamber area

To obtain a coefficient of variation of 5%, it is necessary to count about 400 cells (Table 27.1); in practice, it is reasonable to count 100 white cells. To minimise distribution errors, count the cells in the entire ruled area (i.e., $9 \times 0.1\ \mu l$ areas in an Improved Neubauer counting chamber).

Calculation
White blood cell count per litre (WBC/l)

$$= \frac{\text{No of cells counted} \times \text{dilution} \times 10^6}{\text{Volume counted } (\mu l)}$$

Thus, if N cells are counted in $0.1\ \mu l$, then the WBC/l is as follows:

$$\frac{N \times 20 \times 10^6}{0.1} = N \times 200 \times 10^6$$

(e.g., if 115 cells are counted, the WBC is $115 \times 200 \times 10^6/l = 23 \times 10^9/l$)

Range of White Blood Cell Count in Health
See pp. 14 to 17.

Platelet Count

Manual counts are used routinely in under-resourced laboratories, and they are still needed even in well-equipped laboratories for blood samples with a significant proportion of giant platelets. However, for all other samples, automated

No. of areas	Total no. of cells counted	√	σ	Uncertainty of total count	Range per 1 mm² area	Calculated count/μl
1	50	7	14	36–64	36–64	7.2–12.8
2	100	10	20	80–120	40–60	8.0–12.0
4	200	14	28	172–228	43–57	8.6–11.4
6	300	17	34	266–334	44–56	8.9–11.1
8	400	20	40	360–440	45–55	9.0–11.0
10	500	22	44	456–544	46–54	9.2–10.8
16	800	28	56	744–856	47–53	9.4–10.6
20	1000	32	64	936–1064	47–53	9.4–10.6
30	1500	39	78	1422–1578	47–52	9.4–10.4
200	10000	100	200	9800–10,200	49–51	9.8–10.2

Table 27.1   Variance of haemocytometry count

The inherent error of a cell count results from the random way in which the cells are distributed in the counting chamber. This is known as the count variance (σ); it is calculated as $\sqrt{n} \div n$, where n = number of cells actually counted and variance is expressed as a percentage. The uncertainty of the count is in the range $n \pm \sigma$.
In this theoretical example the final (calculated) count is based on the number of cells in a 1 mm² area at a dilution of 1:20. There were approximately 50 cells in each 1 mm² area. For convenience, results have been rounded to the nearest whole number.
Counting in only one or two fields results in a wide variance that is reduced as more cells are counted. However, high precision is achieved only when thousands of cells are counted, which is only possible with automated cell counters.

full blood counters produce platelet counts with a precision that is much superior to that of manual platelet counts. Platelet counts are best performed on ethylenediaminetetra-acetic acid (EDTA)-anticoagulated blood that has been obtained by clean venipuncture. They can also be carried out on blood obtained by skin prick, but the results are less satisfactory than those on venous blood. Skin-prick platelet counts are significantly lower than counts on venous blood and less constant[17]; a variable number of platelets are probably lost at the site of the skin puncture. Manual platelet counts are performed by visual examination of diluted, lysed whole blood using a Neubauer or Improved Neubauer counting chamber as for total white cell counts.[18,19]

Method

The diluent consists of 1% aqueous ammonium oxalate in which the red cells are lysed. This method is recommended in preference to that using formal-citrate as diluent, which leaves the red cells intact and is more likely to give incorrect results, when the platelet count is low.

Before diluting the blood sample, examine it carefully for the presence of blood clots. If these are present, a fresh specimen should be requested because clots will cause the platelet count to be artificially low. Make a 1 in 20 dilution of well-mixed blood in the diluent by adding 0.1 ml of blood to 1.9 ml of ammonium oxalate diluent (10 g/l). Not more than 500 ml of diluent should be made at a time, using scrupulously clean glassware and fresh glass-distilled or deionised water. If possible, the solution should be filtered through a micropore filter (0.22 µm) and kept at 4°C. For use, a small part of the stock is refiltered and dispensed in 1.9 ml volumes in 75 × 12 mm tubes.

Mix the suspension on a mechanical mixer for 10–15 min. Fill a Neubauer counting chamber with the suspension, using a stout glass capillary or Pasteur pipette. Place the counting chamber in a moist Petri dish and leave untouched for at least 20 min to give time for the platelets to settle.

Examine the preparation with the ×40 objective and ×6 or ×10 eyepieces. The platelets appear under ordinary illumination as small (but not minute) highly refractile particles if viewed with the condenser racked down; they are usually well-separated, and clumps are rare if the blood sample

has been skillfully collected. To avoid introducing into the chamber dirt particles, which might be mistaken for platelets, all equipment must be scrupulously clean. Platelets are more easily seen with the phase-contrast microscope. A special, thin-bottomed (1 µm) counting chamber is best for optimal phase-contrast effect. The number of platelets in one or more areas of 1 mm² should be counted. The total number of platelets counted should always exceed 200 to ensure a coefficient of variation of 8–10%.

Calculation

$$\text{Platelet count per litre} =$$

$$\frac{\text{No. of cells counted} \times \text{Dilution} \times 10^6}{\text{Volume counted (µl)}}$$

Thus, if N is the number of platelets counted in an area of 1 mm² (0.1 µl in volume), the number of platelets per litre of blood is:

$$N \times 10 \times 20 \text{ (dilution)} \times 10^6 = N \times 200 \times 10^6$$

Range of Platelet Counts in Health

See pp. 14 to 17.

Errors in Manual Cell Counts

The errors associated with manual cell counts are *technical* and *inherent*.

Technical errors can be minimised by avoiding the following:

Poor technique in obtaining the blood specimen
Insufficient mixing of the blood specimen
Inaccurate pipetting and the use of badly calibrated pipettes or counting chambers
Inadequate mixing of the cell suspension
Faulty filling of the counting chamber
Careless counting of cells within the chamber

Standardised Counting Chambers

To reduce errors, it is important to have a good-quality counting chamber. The exact chamber depth depends also on the coverglass, which should be free from bowing and sufficiently thick so as not to bend when pressed on the chamber. It must be free from scratches, and even the smallest particle of dust may cause unevenness in its lie on the chamber. The specifications described by WHO[16] outline a tolerance of dimensions for counting chambers that provides reasonable accuracy.

Accurate Dilutions

Bulb-diluting pipettes are not recommended; they are difficult to calibrate and easily broken. The volumes of blood used are unnecessarily small, and it is difficult to fill the counting chamber so that the exact amount of fluid is delivered. Pipettes of 0.1 ml and 0.02 ml (20 µl) are relatively inexpensive and easy to calibrate. With a 2 ml volume in a glass or plastic tube provided with a tightly fitting rubber or plastic bung, a suspension is obtained that is easy to label and handle, and with a little practice, perfect filling of the counting chamber can regularly be accomplished with the aid of a fine plastic Pasteur pipette or stout glass capillary tube. Automatic diluter units are useful. These consist of a dual metering system that enables a volume of diluent and the appropriate volume of blood to be dispensed consecutively into a tube (see p. 705). A variety of automatic diluting systems are now available that have good accuracy and precision. Handheld semiautomatic microsamplers with a detachable tip are designed to operate as "to deliver" pipettes, but a regular supply of the disposable tips may be too expensive and difficult to maintain for poorer laboratories. Pipetting errors apply to all tests that involve dilution of the blood sample, and they also occur with autodiluters that are prone to error with viscid fluids and when the delivery volume of the unit is not correctly adjusted.

Microscopy Artifacts

Dirt or clumped red cell debris may be mistaken for white cells or platelets. Clumping of white cells occurs particularly in heparinised blood, especially when the concentration of heparin exceeds 25 iu/ml of blood. The clumps are most frequently seen in blood that has been allowed to stand for several hours before undertaking the count.

Inherent errors result from uneven distribution of cells in the counting chamber, and no amount of mixing will minimise this inherent variation in numbers between areas. Inherent error can only be reduced by counting more cells in a preparation. In theory, the count varies in proportion to the square root of the number of cells counted (i.e., if four times the number of cells are counted, the variation

is halved [Table 27.1]). For example, when performing a manual white cell count, 95% of the observed counts on a sample of true value 5.0×10^9 cells per litre would lie within the range 4.0–6.0. In practice, the difference between 5.0 and 6.0×10^9 cells per litre for a white cell count is of little clinical significance.

It is also important for the observer not to bias the count by foreknowledge of what result might be expected or by selecting certain areas in the chamber for counting.[20]

Peripheral Blood Morphology

Examination of the peripheral blood film is of utmost importance. In addition to providing information about quantitative changes in blood cells, careful analysis of the qualitative changes may help in elucidating the underlying reasons for clinical problems. These observations may identify the cause of anaemia or undiagnosed fever or the presence of a haemoglobinopathy (see Chapter 5). Problems that might occur when preparing blood films relate to the slides themselves and to the quality of fixing the films and the staining reagents. When glass slides are in short supply, laboratories sometimes find it necessary to wash and reuse slides (see p. 695). Traces of detergent can result in misleading appearances of the red cells (Fig. 27.5), as can residual stain and scratches on the slide. In humid conditions, particularly during the rainy season, water may be absorbed by the methanol used for fixing slides and this can cause gross artefactual changes in red cell appearance (Fig. 4.2, p. 65). To avoid this problem, stock bottles of methanol should be kept tightly closed after use; small amounts should be aliquoted into a bottle with a tightly fitting cap for daily use and replaced regularly from the stock bottle.

Modified (One-Tube) Osmotic Fragility Test

This simple and inexpensive test for screening for β thalassaemia trait is useful when quantification of haemoglobin A_2 is not possible and standardised automated analysers are not available for accurate measurement of MCV and MCH.[21]

A variety of concentrations of buffered saline have been used. A concentration of 0.36% in

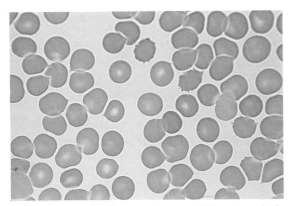

Figure 27.5   Red cell appearances on detergent washed slide.

buffered saline (see p. 691 for preparation) is recommended to ensure a high sensitivity with an acceptable specificity.[22,23] Because the false-positive rate is around 10%, confirmation of a positive result requires referral of a sample to a laboratory able to quantitate haemoglobin A$_2$. The test can also be used to screen for α^0 thalassaemia trait, with positive samples being referred to a reference centre for DNA analysis. About 50% of samples containing haemoglobin E also give a positive result; this is an advantage rather than a disadvantage because detection of haemoglobin E is important in predicting the possibility of thalassaemia major or intermedia in compound heterozygotes with β-thalassemia.

Haemoglobin E Screening Test

Ideally, the diagnosis of haemoglobin E heterozygosity or homozygosity should be by haemoglobin electrophoresis at alkaline pH or high-performance liquid chromatography with a second method being used to confirm the provisional identification (see Chapter 12). When these facilities are not available, a screening test using the blue dye, 2,6-dichlorophenolindophenol (DCIP),* can be used. Samples containing haemoglobin E become faintly turbid when incubated with DCIP.[24,25]

---

*A suitable kit for this test is available from PCL Holding Co. Ltd., Sirinthorn Road, Bangplad, Bangkok (Fax: 662 881 0989).

LABORATORY SUPPORT FOR MANAGEMENT OF HIV/AIDS: CD4-POSITIVE T-CELL COUNTS

Facilities for CD4-positive counts are essential in countries with a high incidence of HIV/AIDS, both for diagnosis and for identifying and monitoring patients who would benefit from antiretroviral drugs.

A method using a simple low-cost single platform flow cytometer is now available and suitable for district hospital laboratories.[26] (See www.guava technologies.com.) However, it may still be too complex to maintain and too expensive for peripheral facilities in some under-resourced countries. A "field friendly" enzyme-linked immunosorbent assay (ELISA) technique for quantifying CD4-positive cells on dried blood spots has been described.[27] However, it is not yet confirmed whether this method is effective for samples with low CD4+ counts. Other methods including dipstick systems are being developed, and still require field trials.

LABORATORY MANAGEMENT

Interlaboratory Communication

A well-planned logistical service is necessary to facilitate flow of communication between remote clinics and central laboratories and clinical consultants. This enables reports on specimens received from the periphery and relevant advice on diagnosis and patient management to be sent without delay from the central laboratory to the periphery. The major delay in test turnaround time (see p. 637) is the result of slow delivery of reports after the test has been performed. TeleFax and e-mail facilities have helped to eliminate this delay, but they are dependent on fixed line communications and electrical supplies, both of which are frequently absent at remote rural clinics.

A potential solution is the use of a digital wireless data communications system such as the Global System of Mobile (GSM) network for laboratory reporting.[28] In some under-resourced countries rural populations have access to wireless communications that are relatively well-maintained. The data volume required for text-based laboratory reports is extremely modest and their transmission is low cost. Newer enhanced and multimedia message services also allow for two-way data communications and remote database interrogation. Result reporting can either be incorporated into the mainstream laboratory information system or by individual handsets for smaller independent laboratories.

Specimen Transport

The need to ensure appropriate conditions for keeping specimens after they have been collected and other aspects of specimen transport to the laboratory are described in Chapter 1. The special problem of transporting specimens from remote clinics to laboratories and reference centres requires further consideration. Relatively well-resourced peripheral laboratories can assist in rural development initiatives by creating employment opportunities for bicycle riders, motorcyclists, taxi operators, formal and informal courier companies, and even helicopter service providers. The location of clinics is helped if Global Positioning System (GPS) coordinates are available for each clinic.[29] By making use of the digital wireless data communication systems currently available* laboratory services in under-resourced countries can be models for the health service as a whole.

Staff Training

In poorer countries, there is often no system for regular supervision of an individual's performance in the laboratory, and many staff do not receive continuing professional development (see p. 626). Monitoring standards of practice should continue for the whole professional life of laboratory staff to ensure high-quality results. For under-resourced countries, training may be provided in association with vertical health programmes such as HIV or tuberculosis control, but the need for training in basic haematological techniques is often overlooked because tests such as haemoglobin estimation and white cell counts are usually not linked to specific diseases and are therefore not amenable to incorporation in a vertical programme. However, because anaemia is the most prevalent disorder worldwide and is often the first sign of underlying disease, the importance of reliable haemoglobin measurements cannot be overemphasised. Thus, continuing education should include the whole range of tests offered by the laboratory and not only tests that are used to support the diagnosis of specific diseases.

Individuals need to keep their own training record, perhaps in the form of a log book, and to have their training achievements and plans regularly reviewed by their line managers. Central records of all training should also be maintained for monitoring purposes and to ensure equitable and appropriate distribution of training between different levels of staff. Regular monitoring of the quality of results from individual laboratories will enable specific problems to be identified, and issues such as equipment failures, discontinuity of supplies, and communication breakdowns should be brought to the attention of regional management teams. In addition, this quality monitoring will allow discrete training needs to be identified, enabling limited teaching resources to be specifically targeted.

Many medical and technical journals now publish their articles in full on the Internet; by an arrangement between the main international publishers and WHO they can be accessed free of charge or at significantly discounted cost in most under-resourced countries.[†]

Clinical Staff Interaction

Appropriate clinical use of the laboratory has a direct impact on the cost-effectiveness of the service (p. 676). Laboratory tests may be initiated by nurses, health field workers, and public health officers as well as doctors. Many of these persons have little or no training in how to request appropriate tests, how to provide timely and suitable samples, and how to use the results for maximal benefit to the patients. Training for laboratory users needs to be incorporated into laboratory training programmes and closely monitored. In poorer countries, there is often a dearth of clinicians with both clinical and laboratory experience who are qualified to provide such training. Under these circumstances, the relationship between the laboratory and clinical

---

*MTN (www.mtn.co.za); Vodacom (www.vodacom.co.za/default.aspx); Exactmobile (www.exactmobile.com).

†www.who.int/hinari/en

staff can be enhanced, and use of the laboratory can be optimised, by using a clinician/technologist team to provide joint training in both disciplines.

Health Management Teams

Local health management teams are often responsible for ensuring that their laboratories are provided with the necessary tools to deliver high-quality service. As a rule, these teams do not include members of the laboratory profession who are only represented by other allied professionals such as pharmacists. Staff in under-resourced laboratories are therefore not always responsible for purchasing supplies and equipment for the laboratory, and this results in wastage through the purchase of inappropriate or poor-quality equipment and reagents. In addition to encouraging adequate representation of laboratory professionals at management level, it is important to ensure that nonlaboratory personnel responsible for making decisions about under-resourced laboratories are educated about the needs of their laboratory service.

Health and Safety

Details of laboratory safety issues are described in Chapter 25. Awareness of these issues should be constantly promoted within all laboratories, and the working environment needs to be made as safe as possible. A "Code of Safe Laboratory Practice" should be prepared that is affordable and relevant to the local circumstances. It should include the following:

Risk assessment—identification of the potential workplace hazards and the risk they pose to individuals working or visiting the laboratory
Education on safe working practices
Monitoring of adherence to health and safety regulations
Prompt reporting and investigation of laboratory accidents

Disposable syringes (p. 2) are intended for single-use only. They cannot withstand sterilisation and should never be reused. Similarly, disposable lancets for skin puncture must never be reused. The practice of using a single lancet on several patients consecutively, and cleaning it with alcohol between use, is unacceptable.

REFERENCES

1. Faiz MA, Yunus EB, Rahman MR, et al 2002 Failure of national guidelines to diagnose uncomplicated malaria in Bangladesh. American Journal of Tropical Medicine and Hygiene 67:396–399.
2. Akpek G, Lee SM, Gagnon DR, et al 2001 Bone marrow aspiration, biopsy, and culture in the evaluation of HIV-infected patients for invasive mycobacteria and histoplasma infections. American Journal of Hematology 67:100–106.
3. Sherman GG, Galpin JS, Patel JM, et al 1999 CD4+ T cell enumeration in HIV infection with limited resources. Journal of Immunological Methods 222:209–217.
4. Glencross D, Scott LE, Jani IV, et al 2002 CD45-assisted PanLeucogating for accurate, cost-effective dual-platform CD4+ T-cell enumeration. Cytometry 50:69–77.
5. Glencross DK, Mendelow BV, Stevens WS 2003 Laboratory monitoring of HIV/AIDS in a resource-poor setting. South African Medical Journal 93:262–263.
6. Eden T 2002 Translation of cure for acute lymphoblastic leukaemia to all children. British Journal of Haematology 118:945–951.
7. Lewis SM, Bain BJ, Swirsky DM 2000 Bench-aid for morphological diagnosis of anaemia. WHO, Geneva.
8. Mundy C, Ngwira M, Kadawele G, et al 2000 Evaluation of microscope condition in Malawi. Transactions of the Royal Society of Medicine and Hygiene 94:583–584.
9. Opoku-Okrah C, Rumble R, Bedu-Addo G, et al 2000 Improving microscope quality is a good investment for under-resourced laboratories. Transactions of the Royal Society of Medicine and Hygiene 94:582.
10. World Health Organization 1998 Laboratory services for primary heath care: requirements for essential clinical laboratory tests. Document: LAB/98.1. WHO, Geneva.
11. Mundy CJF, Bates I et al 2003. The operation, quality and costs of a district hospital laboratory service Malawi. Transactions of the Royal Society of Tropical Medicine and Hygiene 97:403–408.
12. Lewis SM, Stott GJ, Wynn KJ 1998 An inexpensive and reliable new haemoglobin colour scale for assessing anaemia. Journal of Clinical Pathology 51:21–24.
13. Timan IS, Tatsumi N, Aulia D, Wangsasaputra E 2004 Comparison of haemoglobinometry by WHO haemoglobin colour scale and copper sulphate

against haemiglobincyanide reference method. Clinical and Laboratory Haematology 26:253–258.

14. Van den Broek NR, Ntonya C, Mhanga E, et al 1999 Diagnosing anaemia in pregnancy in rural clinics: assessing the potential of the haemoglobin colour scale. Bulletin of the World Health Organization 77:15–21.

15. Montresor A, Ramsan M, Khalfan N, et al 2003. Performance of the Haemoglobin Colour Scale in diagnosing severe and very severe anaemia. Tropical Medicine International Health 8:1–6.

16. World Health Organization 2000 Recommended methods for the visual determination of white blood cell count and platelet count. Document WHO/DIL/00.3. WHO, Geneva.

17. Brecher G, Schneiderman M, Cronkite EP 1953 The reproducibility and constancy of the platelet count. American Journal of Clinical Pathology 23:15–26.

18. Brecher G, Cronkite EP 1950 Morphology and enumeration of human blood platelets. Journal of Applied Physiology 3:365–377.

19. Lewis SM, Wardle J, Cousins S, et al 1979 Platelet counting–development of a reference method and a reference preparation. Clinical and Laboratory Haematology 1:227–237.

20. Sanders C, Skerry DW 1961 The distribution of blood cells on haemocytometer counting chambers with special reference to the amended British Standards Specification 748 (1958). Journal of Clinical Pathology 48:298–304.

21. Thomas S, Srivastava A, Jeyaseelan L, et al. 1996 Nestroft as a screening test for the detection of thalassaemia and common haemoglobinopathies– an evaluation against a high performance liquid chromatographic method. Indian Journal of Medical Research. 104:194–197.

22. Kattamis C, Efremov G, Pootrakul S 1981 Effectiveness of one tube osmotic fragility screening in detecting β-thalassaemia trait. Journal of Medical Genetics 18:266–270.

23. Chow J, Phelan L, Bain BJ 2005 The role of a single-tube osmotic fragility for thalassemia screening in under-resourced laboratories. American Journal of Hematology 79:198–201.

24. Fucharoen G, Sanchaisuriya K, Sae-ung N, et al 2004 A simplified screening strategy for thalassaemia and haemoglobin E in rural communities in south-east Asia. Bulletin of the World Health Organization 82:364–372.

25. Chapple L, Harris A, Phelan L, et al 2005 Reassessment of a simple chemical method using DCIP for screening for haemoglobin E. Journal of Clinical Pathology 59:74–76.

26. Scott LE, Lawrie D, Harvey J, et al 2004 A comparison of the Guava Personal Cell Analyser (PCA) with PLG CD4 T cell enumeration: a pilot evaluation. 11th Conference on Retroviruses and Opportunistic Infections, San Francisco, Feb. 8–11, 2004.

27. Mwaba P, Cassol S, Pilon R, et al 2003 Use of dried whole blood spots to measure CD4+ lymphocyte counts in HIV-1-infected patients. Lancet 362:1459–1460.

28. Wright B. Rural Doctors Advance Care with Wireless: www.hst.org.za/news/20011026.

29. Medical Research Council of South Africa 2001 Geographic Information Systems in health www.mrc.ac.za/mrcnews/june2001/geoinformation. htm.

Uuseful Publications not Specifically Referred to in the Text

Laboratory Organization and Management

World Health Organization 1990 Primary health care– towards the year 2000. WHO/SHS/901. WHO, Geneva.

Houng L, El-Nageh MM 1993 Principles of management of health laboratories. WHO Regional Publications, Eastern Mediterranean Series No. 3.

World Health Organization 1993 Laboratory equipment preventative maintenance programme. In: Principles of management of health laboratories. WHO Regional Publications, Eastern Mediterranean Series No 3.

World Health Organization 1994 Health laboratory facilities in emergency and disaster situations. WHO Regional Publications, Eastern Mediterranean Series No. 6.

World Health Organization 1999 Health laboratory services in support of primary health care in South East Asia. WHO South East Asia Regional Office (SEARO), Publication No. 24 (2nd ed.).

Practical Methods

World Health Organization 1986 Methods recommended for essential clinical chemical and haematological tests for intermediate hospital laboratories. WHO/LAB/86.3. WHO, Geneva.

Carter JY, Lema OE 1994 Practical laboratory manual for health centres in Eastern Africa. African Medical and Research Foundation, PO Box 31025, Nairobi, Kenya.

World Health Organization 1995 Production of basic diagnostic laboratory reagents. WHO Regional Publications, Eastern Mediterranean Series No. 2.

World Health Organization 2000 Manual of basic techniques (revised 2nd ed.). WHO Distribution and Sales, Geneva.

Quality Assurance

World Health Organization 1992 Basics of quality assurance for intermediate and peripheral laboratories. WHO Regional Publications, Eastern Mediterranean Series No. 2.

World Health Organization 1993 Quality assurance related to health laboratory technology. WHO, Geneva.

World Health Organization 1995 Quality systems for medical laboratories: Guidelines for implementation and monitoring. WHO Regional Publications, Eastern Mediterranean Series No. 14.

Lewis SM 1998 Quality Assurance in Haematology WHO Document: LAB/98.4. WHO, Geveva.

Preventive Maintenance of Equipment

World Health Organization 1992 Calibration and maintenance of semi-automated haematology equipment: Document: LBS/92.8. WHO, Geneva.

World Health Organization 1994 Maintenance and repair of laboratory, diagnostic imaging, and hospital equipment. WHO Distribution and Sales, Geneva.

Training for Laboratories

Abbott FR 1992 Teaching for better learning: a guide for teachers of primary health care staff. WHO, Geneva.

World Health Organization 1992 Technical training requirements: report of meeting on development of appropriate technology to support primary health care. WHO, Geneva.

The WHO documents on this list are generally available, without charge, from the Department of Essential Health Technologies, WHO, 1211 Geneva 27 (Fax: +41 22 791 4836) or from the Internet sites (see Table 24.6, p. 635). Documents are also available from the regional offices:

Eastern Mediterranean: PO Box 1517, Alexandria 21511, Egypt.

Southeast Asia: World Health House, Indraprastha Estate, New Delhi, 110002, India.

Other publications from WHO Distribution and Sales are available at reduced prices in developing countries.

Sources of Teaching Material and Equipment for Under-resourced Laboratories

Echo Joint Mission Hospital Equipment Board
Ullswater Crescent, Coulsdon, Surrey, CR3 2HR, UK
Tel: +44 (0) 208 660 2220; Fax: +44 (0) 208 668 0751; e-mail: cs@echohealth.org.uk

Developing Health Technology
Bridge House, Worlington Road, Barton Mills, IP28 7DX, UK
Tel: +44 (0) 1603 416058; Fax: +44 (0) 1603 416066; e-mail: dht@gordon-keeble.co.uk
www.dht-online.co.uk

Tropical Health Technology
PO Box 50, Fakenham, Norfolk, NR21 8XB
Tel: +44 (0) 1328 855805; Fax: +44 (0) 1328 853799; e-mail: thtbooks@tht.ndirect.co.uk

Teaching Aids At Low Cost (TALC)
PO Box 49, St Albans, Herts. AL1 5TX, UK
Tel: +44 (0) 1727 853869; Fax: +44 (0) 1727 846852; e-mail: Info@talcuk.org
www.talcuk.org

TALC Library/Resource Centre
Institute of Child Health, 30 Guilford Street, London, WC1N 1EH, UK
Tel: +44 (0) 207 242 9789, ext. 2424

28 Appendices

S. Mitchell Lewis

PREPARATION OF COMMONLY USED REAGENTS, ANTICOAGULANTS, AND PRESERVATIVE SOLUTIONS

Water

For most purposes, still-prepared distilled water or deionized water is equally suitable. Throughout this text, this is implied when "water" is referred to. When doubly distilled or glass-distilled water is required, this has been specially indicated, and when tap water is satisfactory or indicated, this, too, has been stated.

Acid–Citrate–Dextrose (ACD) Solution–NIH-A

Trisodium citrate, dihydrate (75 mmol/l)	22 g
Citric acid, monohydrate (42 mmol/l)	8 g
Dextrose (139 mmol/l)	25 g
Water to 1 litre	

Sterilize the solution by autoclaving at 121°C for 15 min. Its pH is 5.4. For use, add 10 volumes of blood to 1.5 volumes of solution. For use in red cell survival studies, see p. 369.

Acid–Citrate–Dextrose (Alsever's) Solution

Dextrose (114 mmol/l)	20.5 g
Trisodium citrate, dihydrate (27 mmol/l)	8.0 g
Sodium chloride (72 mmol/l)	4.2 g
Water to 1 litre	

Adjust the pH to 6.1 with citric acid (c 0.5g) and then sterilize the solution by micropore filtration (0.22 μm) or by autoclaving at 121°C for 15 min. For use, add 4 volumes of blood to 1 volume of solution.

Citrate–Phosphate–Dextrose (CPD) Solution, pH 6.9

Trisodium citrate, dihydrate (102 mmol/l)	30 g
Sodium dihydrogen phosphate, monohydrate (1.08 mmol/l)	0.15 g
Dextrose (11 mmol/l)	2 g
Water to 1 litre	

Sterilize the solution by autoclaving at 121°C for 15 min. After cooling to c 20°C, it should have a brown tinge and its pH should be 6.9.

Citrate–Phosphate–Dextrose (CPD) Solution, pH 5.6–5.8

Trisodium citrate, dihydrate (89 mmol/l)	26.30 g
Citric acid, monohydrate (17 mmol/l)	3.27 g
Sodium dihydrogen phosphate monohydrate (16 mmol/l)	2.22 g
Dextrose (142 mmol/l)	25.50 g
Water to 1 litre	

Sterilize the solution by autoclaving at 121°C for 15 min. For use as an anticoagulant preservative, add 7 volumes of blood to 1 volume of solution.

Citrate–Phosphate–Dextrose–Adenine (CPD-A) Solution, pH 5.6–5.8

Trisodium citrate, dihydrate (89 mmol/l)	26.30 g
Citric acid, monohydrate (17 mmol/l)	3.27 g
Sodium dihydrogen phosphate, monohydrate (16 mmol/l)	2.22 g
Dextrose (177 mmol/l)	31.8 g
Adenine (2.04 mmol/l)	0.275 g
Water to 1 litre	

Sterilize the solution by autoclaving at 121°C for 15 min. For use as an anticoagulant preservative, add 7 volumes of blood to 1 volume of solution.

Low Ionic Strength Solution (LISS)[1]

Sodium chloride (NaCl) (30.8 mmol/l)	1.8 g
Disodium hydrogen phosphate (Na_2HPO_4) (1.5 mmol/l)	0.21 g
Sodium dihydrogen phosphate (NaH_2PO_4) (1.5 mmol/l)	0.18 g
Glycine (NH_2CH_2COOH) (240 mmol/l)	18.0 g
Water to 1 litre	

Dissolve the sodium chloride and the two phosphate salts in c 400 ml of water; dissolve the glycine separately in c 400 ml of water; adjust the pH of each solution to 6.7 with 1 mol/l NaOH. Add the 2 solutions together and make up to 1 litre. Sterilize by Seitz filtration or autoclaving. The pH should be within the range of 6.65–6.85, the osmolality 270–285 mmol, and conductivity 3.5–3.8 mS/cm at 23°C.

EDTA

Ethylenediamine tetra-acetic acid (EDTA), dipotassium salt	100 g
Water to 1 litre	

Allow appropriate volumes to dry in bottles at c 20°C so as to give a concentration of 1.5 ± 0.25 mg/ml of blood.

Neutral EDTA, pH 7.0, 110 mmol/l

EDTA, dipotassium salt	44.5 g
or disodium salt	41.0 g
1 mmol/l NaOH	75 ml
Water to 1 litre	

Neutral buffered EDTA, pH 7.0

EDTA, disodium salt (9 mmol/l)	3.35 g
Disodium hydrogen phosphate (Na_2HPO_4) 26.4 mmol/l)	3.75 g
Sodium chloride (NaCl) (140 mmol/l)	8.18 g
Water to 1 litre	

Saline

Sodium chloride (NaCl) (154 mmol/l)	9.0 g
Water to 1 litre	

Trisodium Citrate ($Na_3C_6H_5O7.2H2O$), 109 mmol/l

Dissolve 32 g* in 1 litre of water. Distribute convenient volumes (e.g., 10 ml) into small bottles and sterilise by autoclaving at 121°C for 15 min.

Heparin

Powdered heparin (lithium salt) is available with an activity of c 160 iu/mg. Dissolve it in water at a concentration of 4 mg/ml. Sodium heparin is available in 5 ml ampoules with an activity of 1000 iu/ml. Add appropriate volumes of either solution to a series of containers and allow to dry at c 20°C so as to give a concentration not exceeding 15–20 iu/ml of blood.

BUFFERS

Barbitone Buffer, pH 7.4

Sodium diethyl barbiturate ($C_8H_{11}O_3N_2Na$) (57 mmol/l)	11.74 g
Hydrochloric acid (HCl) (100 mmol/l)	430 ml

Barbitone buffered saline, pH 7.4

NaCl	5.67 g
Barbitone buffer, pH 7.4	1 litre

*Or 38 g of $2Na_3C_6H_5O_7$. 11 H_2O.

Before use, dilute with an equal volume of 9 g/l NaCl.

Barbitone Buffered Saline, pH 9.5

Sodium diethyl barbiturate ($C_8H_{11}O_3N_2Na$) (98 mmol/l)	20.2g
Hydrochloric acid (HCl) (100 mmol/l)	20 ml
NaCl	5.67 g

Before use, dilute the buffer with an equal volume of 9 g/l NaCl.

Barbitone–Bovine Serum Albumin Buffer, pH 9.8

Sodium diethyl barbiturate ($C_8H_{11}O_3N_2Na$) (54 mmol/l)	10.3 g
NaCl (102 mmol/l)	6.0 g
Sodium azide (31 mmol/l)	2.0 g
Bovine serum albumin (BSA)	5.0 g
Water to 1 litre	

Dissolve the reagents in c 900 ml of water. Adjust the pH to 9.8 with 5 mol/l HCl. Make up the volume to 1 litre with water. Store at 4°C.

Citrate–Saline Buffer

Trisodium-citrate ($Na_3C_6HO_7 \cdot 2H_2O$) (5 mmol/l)	1.5 g
NaCl (96 mmol/l)	5.6 g
Barbitone buffer, pH 7.4	200 ml
Water	800 ml

Glycine Buffer, pH 3.0

Glycine (NH_2CH_2COOH) (82 mmol/l)	6.15 g
NaCl (82 mmol/l)	4.80 g
Water	820 ml
0.1 mol/l HCl	180 ml

HEPES Buffer, pH 6.6

N-2-hydroxyethylpiperazine-N′-2-ethanesulfonic acid (100 mmol/l)	23.83 g

Dissolve in c 100 ml of water. Add a sufficient volume of 1 mol/l NaOH (c 1 ml) to adjust the pH to 6.6. If the buffer is intended for use with Romanowsky staining (p. 62), then add 25 ml of dimethyl sulphoxide (DMSO). Make up the volume to 1 litre with water.

HEPES–Saline Buffer, pH 7.6

HEPES (20 mmol/l)	4.76 g
NaCl	8.0 g

Dissolve in c 100 ml of water. Add a sufficient volume of 1 mol/l NaOH to adjust the pH to 7.6. Make up volume to 1 litre with water.

Imidazole Buffered Saline, pH 7.4

Imidazole (50 mmol/l)	3.4 g
NaCl (100 mmol/l)	5.85 g

Dissolve in c 500 ml of water. Add 18.6 ml of 1 mol/l HCl and make up the volume to 1 litre with water. Store at room temperature (18–25°C).

Phosphate Buffer, Iso-osmotic

(A) $NaH_2PO_4 \cdot 2H_2O$ (150 mmol/l)	23.4 g/l
(B) NaH_2PO_4 (150 mmol/l)	21.3 g/l

pH	Solution A	Solution B
5.8	87 ml	13 ml
6.0	83 ml	17 ml
6.2	75 ml	25 ml
6.4	66 ml	34 ml
6.6	56 ml	44 ml
6.8	46 ml	54 ml
7.0	32 ml	68 ml
7.2	24 ml	76 ml
7.4	18 ml	82 ml
7.6	13 ml	87 ml
7.7	9.5 ml	90.5 ml

Normal human serum has an osmolality of 289 ± 4 mmol. Hendry[2] recommended slightly different concentrations of the stock solution, namely, 25.05 g/l NaH_2PO_4 $2H_2O$ and 17.92 g/l Na_2HPO_4 for an iso-osmotic buffer.

Phosphate Buffered Saline

Equal volumes of iso-osmotic phosphate buffer and 9 g/l NaCl.

Phosphate Buffer, Sörensen's

Stock solutions:

	66 mmol/l	100 mmol/l	150 mmol/l
(A) KH_2PO_4	9.1 g/l	13.8 g/l	20.7 g/l
(B) Na_2HPO_4	9.5 g/l	14.4 g/l	21.6 g/l
or $Na_2HPO_4 \cdot 2H_2O$	11.9 g/l	18.0 g/l	27.1 g/l

To obtain a solution of the required pH, add A and B in the indicated proportions:

pH	A	B
5.4	97.0	3.0
5.6	95.0	5.0
5.8	92.2	7.8
6.0	88.0	12.0
6.2	81.0	19.0
6.4	73.0	27.0
6.6	63.0	37.0
6.8	50.8	49.2
7.0	38.9	61.1
7.2	28.0	72.0
7.4	19.2	80.8
7.6	13.0	87.0
7.8	8.5	91.5
8.0	5.5	94.5

This buffer is not iso-osmotic with normal plasma (see earlier).

Tris–HCl Buffer (200 mmol/l)

Tris (hydroxymethyl) aminomethane (24.23 g/l)	250 ml

To obtain a solution of the required pH, add the appropriate volume of 1 mol/l HCl and then make up the volume to 1 litre with water.

pH	Volume
7.2	44.5 ml
7.4	42.0 ml
7.6	39.0 ml
7.8	33.5 ml
8.0	28.0 ml
8.2	23.0 ml
8.4	17.5 ml
8.6	13.0 ml
8.8	9.0 ml
9.0	5.0 ml

100 mmol/l, 150 mmol/l, 300 mmol/l, and 750 mmol/l stock solutions may be similarly prepared with an appropriate weight of Tris and volume of acid.

Tris–HCl Bovine Serum Albumin (BSA) Buffer, pH 7.6, 20 mmol/l

Tris (hydroxymethyl) aminomethane (20 mmol/l)	2.42 g
EDTA, disodium salt (10 mmol/l)	3.72 g
NaCl (100 mmol/l)	5.85 g
Sodium azide (3 mmol/l)	0.2 g

Dissolve the reagents in c 800 ml of water. Adjust the pH to 7.6 with 10 mol/l HCl. Add 10 g of BSA and make up to 1 litre with water.

Buffered Formal Acetone

Dissolve 20 mg Na_2HPO_2 and 100 mg KH_2PO_4 in 30 ml distilled water. Add 45 ml acetone and 25 ml of 40% formalin. Mix well and store at 4°C. Use cold. Make up new fixative every 4 weeks.

REAGENTS

Rabbit Brain Thromboplastin

Freeze-dried rabbit brain thromboplastins are now widely available commercially with a shelf life of 2–5 years or longer. Usually, they are calibrated against the World Health Organization (WHO) International Reference Preparation of thromboplastin and are supplied with an International Sensitivity Index (ISI) and a table converting prothrombin times to International Normalized Ratios (INR).

If a commercial preparation is not available, it is possible to prepare a homemade substitute using rabbit brain that does not require freeze drying and that is relatively stable.

Acetone-Dried Brain Powder

Strip the membrane off freshly collected rabbit brain, wash free from blood, and place in about 3 times its volume of cold acetone. Macerate for 2–3 min and then filter through absorbent lint (BP or USP grade) on a Büchner funnel. Repeat the extraction 7 times; after 2 extractions increase the time of exposure to acetone to *c* 20 min for each subsequent extraction. The material should become "gritty" by the fourth or fifth extraction. After the last extraction, spread the acetone-dried brain on a piece of paper and allow to dry in air for 30 min. Rub through a 1 mm mesh nylon sieve to produce a coarse powder. Dispense into a batch of screw-capped bottles and dry over phosphorus pentoxide in a vacuum desiccator. After drying, screw down the caps tightly and store at 4°C or –20°C. At –20°C, the material should be stable for at least 5 years. One hundred g of whole brain yield *c* 15 g of dried powder.

Preparation of Liquid Suspension

Dissolve 0.9 g of NaCl and 0.9 g of phenol in 100 ml of water. Suspend 3.6 g of the acetone-dried brain in 100 ml of the phenol–saline solution at 15–20°C and allow to stand at this temperature for 4–5 h, mixing at 30-min intervals. Transfer to a 4°C refrigerator for 24 h, and occasionally mix it. Thereafter, leave undisturbed at 4°C for 3 h and then decant the supernatant carefully through fine muslin or similar material. The ISI should be not more than 1.4 (see p. 466), and the mean normal prothrombin time should be 12–13 s. Store the suspension at 4°C. At this temperature, it will be stable for at least 6 months; at room temperature it will be stable for at least 7 days. It must not be allowed to freeze because freezing results in flocculation of the smooth suspension with deterioration of thromboplastic activity.

APTT Phospholipid Reagent

Acetone-dried rabbit brain is suitable for preparing an APTT (activated partial thromboplastin time) reagent. Bovine brain may also be used.

Prepare acetone-dried brain powder as described above. Suspend 5 g of the powder in 20 ml of chloroform (analytic grade) in a covered beaker for 1–2 hours. Filter through filter paper to obtain a clear filtrate. Wash the brain deposit on the filter paper with 20 ml of chloroform and pool the clear filtrate with the previous filtrate. Evaporate the filtrate to dryness in a beaker of known weight in a waterbath at 60–70°C and weigh the residual deposit: 5 g of dried brain should yield *c* 1.5 g of phospholipid deposit. Emulsify in saline to give a 5% emulsion; 1.5 g of deposit should provide 30 ml of emulsion. Distribute the emulsion in small volumes in stoppered tubes. At –20°C it should be stable for at least 1 year.

For use, dilute 1 in 100 in saline and mix with an equal volume of 2.5 mg/ml kaolin suspension in imidazole buffer.

Guinea Pig Kidney Suspension

Strip the capsules and perirenal fat from at least 2 pairs of kidneys. Then wash them well in running water. Homogenise the tissue in 9 g/l NaCl (saline) in a blender for 2 min, sterilise it at 121°C (by autoclaving at 15 lb pressure for 20 min), and blend it again so as to obtain a fine suspension. Then centrifuge the suspension in saline and wash the deposit in 2 changes of saline. Finally, add to the deposit about 4 times its volume of 5 g/l phenol in saline. After resuspension, centrifuge the sample in a haematocrit tube to estimate its concentration. Then add sufficient phenol–saline to the remainder to produce a 1 in 6 suspension. Use it without further dilution. Its absorbing power must be tested with known positive and negative sera. The reagent will remain potent for at least 1 year if stored at 4°C.

Ox Red Cell Suspension

Wash ox cells in several changes of 9 g/l NaCl (saline) and make a 30% suspension. Then sterilise it at 121°C (by autoclaving at 15 lb pressure for 20 min). When cool, adjust the packed cell volume to 0.20 with saline and add an equal volume of 10 g/l phenol–saline to give a 10% suspension.

The ability of the suspension to absorb the infectious mononucleosis antibody must be tested with known positive sera. It should remain potent for several years if stored at 4°C.

REFERENCE STANDARDS AND REAGENTS

A wide range of international reference materials has been established by WHO, and these are held at designated institutions. The majority of the materials of haematological interest listed below are held at the National Institute for Biological Standards and Control (NIBSC). Those indicated by an asterisk are held at the WHO International Laboratory for Biological Standards, Central Laboratory of the Netherlands Red Cross Blood Transfusion Service (CLB). A comprehensive catalogue is available on the WHO website (www.who.int/bloodproducts/catalogue/en/index.html), and details can also be found on the NIBSC website (www.nibsc.ac.uk/products/catalogue.html).

General Haematology

Erythropoietin, human, urinary
Erythropoietin, recombinant DNA-derived
Ferritin, human, recombinant
Haemiglobincyanide
HbA$_2$
HbF
Folate, whole blood
C-reactive protein (CRP)
Human serum protein for immunoassay: includes transferrin*

Immunohaematology

Anti-A blood-typing serum*
Anti-B blood-typing serum*
Anti-D (anti-Rh^0) incomplete blood-typing serum*
Anti-D (anti-Rh^0) complete blood-typing serum*
Anti-E complete blood-typing serum*

Immunology

Human serum immunoglobulins immunoglobulin G (IgG), IgA, and IgM
Human serum immunoglobulin IgE
Antinuclear factor, homogeneous*
Horseradish peroxidase-conjugated sheep anti-human IgG*
Human serum complement components C1q, C4, C5, factor B, and functional CH$_{50}$*

Coagulation

Ancrod
Antithrombin, plasma
Antithrombin concentrate
Factors II, VII, IX, X (combined as concentrates)
Factor VIII and von Willebrand factor, plasma
Factor VIII concentrate
Factor IXa concentrate
Heparin, low molecular weight
Plasma fibrinogen
Plasmin
Plasminogen activator inhibitor
Tissue plasminogen activator, recombinant
Streptokinase
α-Thrombin
β-Thromboglobulin
Antihuman platelet antigen-1a
Platelet factor 4
Protein S, plasma
Protein C, plasma
Protamine
Urokinase, high molecular weight
Thromboplastin, bovine, combined*
Thromboplastin, human, recombinant*
Thromboplastin, rabbit, plain*
Von Willebrand factor, concentrate
Von Willebrand factor: Ag (antigen); RCO (ristocetin cofactor activity); CB (collagen binding activity)

The following Certified Reference Materials have been established by the European Union (BCR):
Haemiglobincyanide
Monosized latex particles:
CRM165: 2.2 mm (5.7 fl); CRM166: 4.8 mm (60.0 fl); CRM167: 9.5 mm diameter
Thromboplastin, bovine (CRM148)
Thromboplastin, rabbit, plain (CRM149)
Human serum proteins (CRM470), including haptoglobin

Contact Addresses

National Institute for Biological Standards and Control (NIBSC)
Blanche Lane, South Mimms, Herts EN6 3QH, England
Tel: 44 1707 646399
Fax: 44 1707 646977
Email: standards@nibsc.ac.uk
Central Laboratory of Netherlands Red Cross Blood Transfusion Service (CLB)
125 Plesmanlaan, 1066 AD Amsterdam Netherlands

Tel: 31 20 512 9222
Fax: 31 20 512 3252
European Union (BCR)
Institute for Reference Materials and Measure-ments (IRMM)
Retieseweg B2440, Geel, Belgium
Fax: 32 14 590 406
Email: bcr.sales@irmm.jrc.be

PREPARATION OF GLASSWARE

Siliconised Glassware

Use c 2% solution of silicone (dimethyldichloro-silane) in solvent. Immerse the clean glassware or syringes to be coated in the fluid and allow to drain dry. (Rubber gloves should be worn and the procedure should be performed in a fume cupboard provided with an exhaust fan.) Then rinse the coated glassware thoroughly in water, and allow to dry in an oven at 100°C for 10 min or overnight in an incubator.

Cleaning Slides

New Slides

Boxes of clean, grease-free slides are available commercially. If these are not available, the following procedure should be carried out. Leave the slides overnight in a detergent solution. Then wash well in running tap water, rinse in distilled or deionised water, and store in 95% ethanol or methanol until used. Dry with a clean linen cloth and carefully wipe free from dust before they are used.

Dirty Slides

When discarded, place in a detergent solution; heat at 60°C for 20 min; and then wash in hot, running tap water. Finally, rinse in water before being dried with a clean linen cloth.

Cleaning Glassware

Wash in running tap water. Then boil in a detergent solution; rinse in acid; and wash in hot, running tap water, as described above. Alternatively, the apparatus can be soaked in 3 mol/l HCl.

For the removal of deposits of protein and other organic matter, "biodegradable" detergents are recommended. Decon 90 (*Decon Laboratories Ltd*, Hove BN3 3LY, UK) is suitable, but a number of similar preparations are also available.

Iron-Free Glassware

Wash in a detergent solution, then soak in 3 mol/l HCl for 24 hours; finally, rinse in deionised, double-distilled water.

SIZES OF TUBES

The sizes of tubes recommended in the text have been chosen as being appropriate for the tests described. The dimensions given are the length and external diameter (in mm). The equivalent in inches, as given in some catalogues, and certain corresponding internal diameters, are as follows:

75×10 mm
   (internal diameter 8 mm) = $3 \times {}^3/_8$ inch
75×12 mm
   (internal diameter 10 mm) = $3 \times {}^1/_2$ inch
65×10 mm = $2{}^1/_2 \times {}^3/_8$ inch
38×6.4 mm = $1{}^1/_2 \times {}^1/_4$ inch ("precipitin tubes")
100×12 mm = $4 \times {}^1/_2$ inch
150×16 mm = $6 \times {}^5/_8$ inch
150×19 mm = $6 \times {}^3/_4$ inch

SPEED OF CENTRIFUGING

Throughout the book, the unit given is the relative centrifugal force (g). Conversion of this figure to rpm (rev/min) depends on the radius of the centrifuge; it can be calculated by reference to the nomogram illustrated in Figure 28.1 or from the formula for relative centrifugal force (RCF):

$$RCF = 118 \times 10^{-7} \times r \times N^{-2}$$

where r = radius (cm) and N = speed of rotation (rpm).
The following centrifugal forces are recommended:

"Low-spun" platelet-rich plasma: 150–200 g (for 10–15 min)
"High-spun" plasma   1200–1500 g (for 15 min)
Packing of red cells   2000–2300 g (for 30 min)

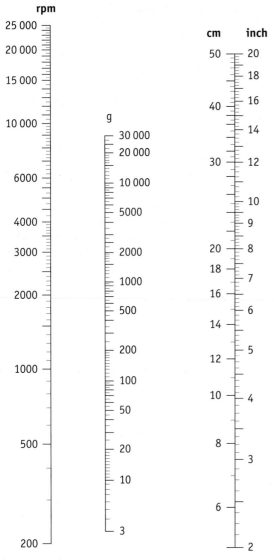

rpm

Figure 28.1 Nomogram for computing relative centrifugal forces.

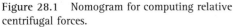

UNITS OF WEIGHT AND MEASUREMENT IN COMMON USE IN HAEMATOLOGY

Throughout the book, measurements have been expressed in SI units, in accordance with international recommendations.[3] These units are derived from the metric system. The base units are shown in the following, and the abbreviated forms are indicated alongside.

Weight – unit: gram (g)

$\times 10^3$ = kilogram (kg)
$\times 10^{-3}$ = milligram (mg)
$\times 10^{-6}$ = microgram (µg)
$\times 10^{-9}$ = nanogram (ng)
$\times 10^{-12}$ = picogram (pg)
$\times 10^{-15}$ = femtogram (fg)

Length – unit: metre (m)

$\times 10^{-1}$ = decimetre (dm)
$\times 10^{-2}$ = centimetre (cm)
$\times 10^{-3}$ = millimetre (mm)
$\times 10^{-6}$ = micrometre (µm)
$\times 10^{-9}$ = nanometre (nm)

Volume – unit: litre (l or L) = dm³

$\times 10^{-1}$ = decilitre (dl) (formerly 100 ml)
$\times 10^{-3}$ = millilitre (ml) = cm³ (formerly cc)
$\times 10^{-6}$ microlitre (µl) = mm³
$\times 10^{-9}$ = nanolitre (nl)
$\times 10^{-12}$ = picolitre (pl)
$\times 10^{-15}$ femtolitre (fl)

Amount of substance – unit: mole (mol)

$\times 10^{-3}$ = millimole (mmol)
$\times 10^{-6}$ = micromole (µmol)

Substance concentration – unit: moles per litre (mol/l) (formerly M)

$\times 10^{-3}$ = millimole per litre (mmol/l)
$\times 10^{-6}$ = micromole per litre (µmol/l)

Mass concentration – unit: gram per litre (g/l)

$\times 10^{-3}$ = milligram per litre (mg/l)
$\times 10^{-6}$ = microgram per litre (µg/l)

When preparing a small amount of a reagent, it is more appropriate to express its concentration per ml or dl.

To convert a measurement from mass concentration to molar concentration, divide by the molecular mass. Thus, for example, the molecular mass of human Hb (as 4Fe tetramer) is 64,458 (see p. 27) or 16,114 as the Fe monomer. Then, when Hb is 160 g/l, this is equivalent to 160 ÷ 16 114 mol/l (i.e., 9.9 mmol/l).

ATOMIC WEIGHTS AND MOLECULAR CONCENTRATIONS

The concentration of a substance in solution can be expressed either in g/l or in mol/l. The latter is also indicated by M (e.g., 0.1 M HCl = 0.1 mol/l). A mole (mol) is the molecular weight or relative molecular mass (RMM) of the substance (including water of crystallization if present). Thus, for example:

$$\text{RMM of NaCl} = 58.5; \text{ then } 1 \text{ mol/l}$$
$$= 58.5 \text{ g/l and } 9 \text{ g/l} = 9 \div 58.5 = 0.154 \text{ mol/l}$$
$$= 154 \text{ mmol/l}.$$

The atomic weights of some chemicals commonly used in preparation of reagents are as follows:

Calcium	40
Carbon	12
Chlorine	35
Chromium	52
Hydrogen	1
Iron	56
Magnesium	24
Nitrogen	14
Oxygen	16
Phosphorus	31
Potassium	39
Sodium	23
Sulphur	32

RADIATION DOSES

When using radionuclides, account must be taken of their potential risk for the recipient and for the laboratory workers. The extent of radiation hazard in relation to the small amount of radionuclide used in diagnostic work depends on a number of factors, namely, the energy and range of the radiations; whether the radionuclide is widely distributed in the body or becomes localised in specific organs, the physical half-life of the radionuclide, and its biological half-time in the body.

Formerly, radioactivity was expressed in curies (Ci); 10^{-3} Ci = 1 mCi and 10^{-6} = 1 μCi. The preferred SI unit of radioactivity is the Bequerel (Bq). 1 Bq corresponds to one disintegration per second, so that 1 Ci = 3.7×10^{10} Bq, 1 millicurie (mCi) = 3.7 × 10^7 Bq or 37 megabequerels (MBq), and 1 microcurie (μCi) = 3.7×10^4 Bq or 0.037 MBq; 10^3 MBq = 1 gigabequerel (GBq).

The effect of radiation on the body depends, essentially, on the amount of energy deposited. This is expressed in grays (Gy); 1 Gy is the dose of radiation that deposits 1 joule of energy per kg of tissue. In the past, this has been expressed in rads (1 Gy = 100 rad). The reaction of the body to the radiation is also affected by the type of the particular ionizing ray. The biological effect of the radiation is calculated from the amount of Gy (or rad) multiplied by an ionization quality factor; this factor varies with the type of ray, and it is 20 times more for α-rays than for β- and γ-rays. The unit for describing biological effect of radiation (i.e., the unit of "effective dose") is the Sievert (Sv). The annual dose limit for the whole body for somebody working with radionuclides is 50 mSv, with a larger amount for individual organs. Lower dose limits, of 5 mSv, apply to members of the public.

STATISTICAL PROCEDURES

Mean ($\bar{x}$) is the sum of all the measurements (Σ) divided by the number of measurements (n).

Median (m) is the point on the scale that has an equal number of observations above and below.

Mode is the most frequently occurring result.

Gaussian distribution describes events or data that occur symmetrically about the mean (see Fig. 2.1, p. 12); with this type of distribution, mean, median, and mode will be approximately equal. The extent of spread of measurements about the mean is expressed as the standard deviation (SD). Its calculation is described below. This means that 68% of the measurement will be within the ±1 SD range, 95% will be within ± 2 SD, and 99% will be within ±3 SD.

Confidence intervals indicate the upper and lower limits between which a specified proportion of results (e.g., 95%) on a particular population may be expected to occur.

Log normal distribution describes events that are asymmetrical (skewed) with a larger number of observations toward the end. The mean will thus be nearer that end; the mean, median, and mode may differ from each other. To calculate geometric mean and SD, the data are first converted to their logarithms, and after calculating the mean and SD of the logarithms, the results are reconverted to the antilog.

Poisson distribution describes events that are random in their occurrence. This will be the case, for example, when blood cells are counted in a diluted suspension. The number of cells that are counted in a given volume will vary on each occasion; this count variation (σ) is $0.92 \sqrt{\lambda}$, where λ = the total number of cells counted (see p. 682). It is an estimate of the standard deviation of the entire population, whereas SD denotes the standard deviation of the items that were actually measured.

Coefficient of variation (CV) is another way of indicating standard deviation, related to the actual measurement, so that variation at different levels can be compared. It is expressed as a percentage.

Standard error of mean (SEM) is a measure of dispersion of the mean of a set of measurements. It is used to compare means of two sets of data.

Calculations

Variance (s^2)

$$\frac{\Sigma(x - \bar{x})^2}{n-1}$$

Standard deviation (SD)

$$\sqrt{s^2}$$

Coefficient of variation (CV) as percentage

$$\frac{SD \times 100\%}{\bar{x}}$$

Standard error mean (SEM)

$$\frac{SD}{\sqrt{n}}$$

Standard deviation of paired results

$$\sqrt{\frac{\Sigma d^2}{2n}}$$

where d = differences between paired measurements and n = number of paired measurements

Standard deviation of median

$$\frac{\text{Central } 50\%}{1.35} \text{ (between 25\% and 75\%)}$$

Confidence interval

Decide on required confidence interval (e.g., 95% or 99%).

From t-test Table (see p. 699) find number at n–1 degrees of freedom.

Calculate SD and SEM as above.

Then confidence interval will be between $\bar{x} - (t \times SEM)$ and $\bar{x} + (t \times SEM)$

When the original data are non-Gaussian, convert to their logs, use these figures throughout the calculation, and convert the final results to their antilogs.

Analysis of Differences by t-Test

Analysis of differences by t-test is a method for comparing two sets of data (e.g., to assess the accuracy of a new method against a reference method).

Calculation

Determine the difference in each pair of tests (d) and the mean difference ($\bar{d}$)

Variance is obtained from $\dfrac{(d - \bar{d})^2}{n-1}$; $t = \bar{d} \div \dfrac{s^2}{n}$

From the t-test chart (Table 28.1) read the value of t for the appropriate degree of freedom (i.e., n – 1). Express results as the level of probability (p) that there is *no* significant difference between the sets of data that are being compared.

Analysis of Variation by F-Ratio

Analysis of variation by F-ratio is a method to assess the relative precision of two sets of measurements.

Calculation

Determine variance (s^2) as described above for each set. Because the ratio must not be less than 1, use the higher variance as the numerator. Then, from the chart (Table 28.2), read the value at either 95% or 99% probability (i.e., p = 0.05 or p = 0.01) for the appropriate degrees of freedom (i.e., n – 1) for the two sets of data.

Interpretation

There is a significant difference in variation between the two sets when the calculated ratio is greater than the value read from the chart.

Table 28.1 Critical values of t–test

df	50 (0.5)	40 (0.4)	30 (0.3)	20 (0.2)	10 (0.1)	5 (0.05)	1 (0.01)
				% Probability level			
1	1.000	1.376	1.963	3.078	6.314	12.706	63.657
2	0.816	1.061	1.386	1.886	2.920	4.303	9.925
3	0.765	0.978	1.250	1.638	2.353	3.182	5.841
4	0.741	0.941	1.190	1.533	2.132	2.776	4.604
5	0.727	0.920	1.156	1.476	2.015	2.571	4.032
6	0.718	0.906	1.134	1.440	1.943	2.447	3.707
7	0.711	0.896	1.119	1.415	1.895	2.365	3.499
8	0.706	0.889	1.108	1.397	1.860	2.306	3.355
9	0.703	0.883	1.100	1.383	1.833	2.262	3.250
10	0.700	0.879	1.093	1.372	1.812	2.228	3.169
11	0.697	0.876	1.088	1.363	1.796	2.201	3.106
12	0.695	0.873	1.083	1.356	1.782	2.179	3.055
13	0.694	0.870	1.079	1.350	1.771	2.160	3.012
14	0.692	0.868	1.076	1.345	1.761	2.145	2.977
15	0.691	0.866	1.074	1.341	1.753	2.131	2.947
16	0.690	0.865	1.071	1.337	1.746	2.120	2.921
17	0.689	0.863	1.069	1.333	1.740	2.110	2.989
18	0.688	0.862	1.067	1.330	1.734	2.101	2.878
19	0.688	0.861	1.066	1.328	1.729	2.093	2.861
20	0.687	0.860	1.064	1.325	1.725	2.086	2.845
21	0.686	0.859	1.063	1.323	1.721	2.080	2.831
22	0.686	0.858	1.061	1.321	1.717	2.074	2.819
23	0.685	0.858	1.061	1.321	1.717	2.074	2.819
24	0.685	0.857	1.059	1.318	1.711	2.064	2.797
25	0.684	0.856	1.058	1.316	1.708	2.060	2.787
26	0.684	0.856	1.058	1.315	1.706	2.056	2.779
27	0.684	0.855	1.057	1.314	1.703	2.052	2.771
28	0.683	0.855	1.056	1.313	1.701	2.048	2.763
29	0.683	0.854	1.055	1.311	1.699	2.045	2.756
30	0.683	0.854	1.055	1.310	1.697	2.042	2.750

Table 28.1   Critical values of t-test (Cont'd)

df	50 (0.5)	40 (0.4)	30 (0.3)	20 (0.2)	10 (0.1)	5 (0.05)	1 (0.01)
				% Probability level			
40	0.681	0.851	1.050	1.303	1.684	2.021	2.704
50	0.680	0.849	1.048	1.299	1.676	2.008	2.678
60	0.679	0.848	1.046	1.296	1.671	2.000	2.660
120	0.677	0.845	1.041	1.289	1.658	1.980	2.617
∞	0.674	0.842	1.036	1.282	1.645	1.960	2.576

ANOVA

ANOVA is another method for sum of squares analysis of variation when comparing two sets of data (e.g., two different methods for doing a test or results from two individuals, A and B, doing the same test).

	Set A	Set B
Number of measurements	n	n
Add all results from each of the two sets	Σ A	Σ B
Square each sum	$(Σ A)^2$	$(Σ B)^2$

Combine the sets and divide by number of

$$\text{measurements:} \quad \frac{(Σ A)^2 + (Σ B)^2}{n}$$

Subtract correction factor:
$(Σ A + Σ B)^2 \div (\text{Total n of A} + B)$

Compare this measurement with the values given in the F-distribution table at 95% or 99% for the appropriate degree of freedom. If the calculated sum is greater than the table reading, it can be concluded that there is a 95% (or 99%) probability that the differences between the sets are significant and are not the result of chance alone.

AUTOMATED (MECHANICAL) PIPETTES

Accurate pipetting is an essential requirement for all quantitative tests. A variety of automated handheld pipettes are available, many of which incorporate a disposable tip with an ejector mechanism, which allows the user to remove it without hand contact. Some pipettes have a fixed capacity; in others a range of volumes can be obtained by means of an adjusting screw, and the delivery volume is displayed on a digital readout.

Because the designs are varied, the specific manufacturer's instructions must be carefully followed. The following important points are common to all:

1. Always use the specified tip.
2. Never wash and reuse tips.
3. Ensure that the tip is fitted firmly to the pipette.
4. Keep the pipette clean of dirt and grease.
5. Always pipette in a vertical position.
6. Never leave the pipette on its side with liquid in the tip.
7. Return the pipette to its stand after use.
8. Operate by a slow, smooth, consistent procedure, avoiding bubbles or foaming.
9. Use "reverse pipetting" for plasma, high-viscosity fluids, and/or very small volumes. With the plunger pressed all the way down (2nd stop), dip the tip well below the surface of the fluid and release the plunger knob slowly. Remove the pipette; wipe the outside of the tip carefully with a tissue; and then, with the tip against the inside wall of the receiving container, deliver its contents by depressing the plunger knob to the 1st stop. Then discard the tip with its residual contents.
10. For blood dilution, fill and empty the tip with the blood 2–3 times, then depress the plunger to

Table 28.2 F distribution tables (a) 99% probability (p = 0.01)

df Numerator	df Numerator 1	2	3	4	5	6	7	8	9	10	12	15	20	24	30	40	60	120	∞
1	4052	4999.5	5403	5625	5764	5859	5928	5981	6022	6056	6106	6157	6209	6235	6261	6287	6313	6339	6366
2	98.50	99.00	99.17	99.25	99.30	99.33	99.36	99.37	99.39	99.40	99.42	99.43	99.45	99.46	99.47	99.47	99.48	99.49	99.50
3	34.12	30.82	29.46	28.71	28.24	27.91	27.67	27.49	27.35	27.23	27.05	26.87	26.69	26.60	26.50	26.41	26.32	26.22	26.13
4	21.20	18.00	16.69	15.98	15.52	15.21	14.98	14.80	14.66	14.55	14.37	14.20	14.02	13.93	13.84	13.75	13.65	13.56	13.46
5	16.26	13.27	12.06	11.39	10.97	10.67	10.46	10.29	10.16	10.05	9.89	9.72	9.55	9.47	9.38	9.29	9.20	9.11	9.02
6	13.75	10.92	9.78	9.15	8.75	8.47	8.26	8.10	7.98	7.87	7.72	7.56	7.40	7.31	7.23	7.14	7.06	6.97	6.88
7	12.25	9.55	8.45	7.85	7.46	7.19	6.99	6.84	6.72	6.62	6.47	6.31	6.16	6.07	5.99	5.91	5.82	5.74	5.65
8	11.26	8.65	7.59	7.01	6.63	6.37	6.18	6.03	5.91	5.81	5.67	5.52	5.36	5.28	5.20	5.12	5.03	4.95	4.86
9	10.56	8.02	6.99	6.42	6.06	5.80	5.61	5.47	5.35	5.26	5.11	4.96	4.81	4.73	4.65	4.57	4.48	4.40	4.31
10	10.04	7.56	6.55	5.99	5.64	5.39	5.20	5.06	4.94	4.85	4.71	4.56	4.41	4.33	4.25	4.17	4.08	4.00	3.91
11	9.65	7.21	6.22	5.67	5.32	5.07	4.89	4.74	4.63	4.54	4.40	4.25	4.10	4.02	3.94	3.86	3.78	3.69	3.60
12	9.33	6.93	5.95	5.41	5.06	4.82	4.64	4.50	4.39	4.30	4.16	4.01	3.86	3.78	3.70	3.62	3.54	3.45	3.36
13	9.07	6.70	5.74	5.21	4.86	4.62	4.44	4.30	4.19	4.10	3.96	3.82	3.66	3.59	3.51	3.43	3.34	3.25	3.17
14	8.86	6.51	5.56	5.04	4.69	4.46	4.28	4.14	4.03	3.94	3.80	3.66	3.51	3.43	3.35	3.27	3.18	3.09	3.00
15	8.68	6.36	5.42	4.89	4.56	4.32	4.14	4.00	3.89	3.80	3.67	3.52	3.37	3.29	3.21	3.13	3.05	2.96	2.87
16	8.53	6.23	5.29	4.77	4.44	4.20	4.03	3.89	3.78	3.69	3.55	3.41	3.26	3.18	3.10	3.02	2.93	2.84	2.75
17	8.40	6.11	5.18	4.67	4.34	4.10	3.93	3.79	3.68	3.59	3.46	3.31	3.16	3.08	3.00	2.92	2.83	2.75	2.65
18	8.29	6.01	5.09	4.58	4.25	4.01	3.84	3.71	3.60	3.51	3.37	3.23	3.08	3.00	2.92	2.84	2.75	2.66	2.57
19	8.18	5.93	5.01	4.50	4.17	3.94	3.77	3.63	3.52	3.43	3.30	3.15	3.00	2.92	2.84	2.76	2.67	2.58	2.49
20	8.10	5.85	4.94	4.43	4.10	3.87	3.70	3.56	3.46	3.37	3.23	3.09	2.94	2.86	2.78	2.69	2.61	2.52	2.42
21	8.02	5.78	4.87	4.37	4.04	3.81	3.64	3.51	3.40	3.31	3.17	3.03	2.88	2.80	2.72	2.64	2.55	2.46	2.36
22	7.95	5.72	4.82	4.31	3.99	3.76	3.59	3.45	3.35	3.26	3.12	2.98	2.83	2.75	2.67	2.58	2.50	2.40	2.31
23	7.88	5.66	4.76	4.26	3.94	3.71	3.54	3.41	3.30	3.21	3.07	2.93	2.78	2.70	2.62	2.54	2.45	2.35	2.26

Table 28.2 F distribution tables (a) 99% probability (p = 0.01)—cont'd

df Numerator	1	2	3	4	5	6	7	8	9	10	12	15	20	24	30	40	60	120	∞
24	7.82	5.61	4.72	4.22	3.90	3.67	3.50	3.36	3.26	3.17	3.03	2.89	2.74	2.66	2.58	2.49	2.40	2.31	2.21
25	7.77	5.57	4.68	4.18	3.85	3.63	3.46	3.32	3.22	3.13	2.99	2.85	2.70	2.62	2.54	2.45	2.36	2.27	2.17
26	7.72	5.53	4.64	4.14	3.82	3.59	3.42	3.29	3.18	3.09	2.96	2.81	2.66	2.58	2.50	2.42	2.33	2.23	2.13
27	7.68	5.49	4.60	4.11	3.78	3.56	3.39	3.26	3.15	3.06	2.93	2.78	2.63	2.55	2.47	2.38	2.29	2.20	2.10
28	7.64	5.15	4.57	4.07	3.75	3.53	3.36	3.23	3.12	3.03	2.90	2.75	2.60	2.52	2.44	2.35	2.26	2.17	2.06
29	7.60	5.42	4.54	4.04	3.73	3.50	3.33	3.20	3.09	3.00	2.87	2.73	2.57	2.49	2.41	2.33	2.23	2.14	2.03
30	7.56	5.39	4.51	4.02	3.70	3.47	3.30	3.17	3.07	2.98	2.84	2.70	2.55	2.47	2.39	2.30	2.21	2.11	2.01
40	7.31	5.18	4.31	3.83	3.51	3.29	3.12	2.99	2.80	2.80	2.66	2.52	2.37	2.29	2.20	2.11	2.02	1.92	1.80
60	7.08	4.98	4.13	3.65	3.34	3.12	2.95	2.82	2.72	2.63	2.50	2.35	2.20	2.12	2.03	1.94			
120	6.85	4.79	3.95	3.48	3.17	2.96	2.79	2.66	2.56	2.47	2.34	2.19	2.03	1.95	1.86	1.76	1.66	1.53	1.38
∞	6.63	4.61	3.78	3.32	3.02	2.80	2.64	2.51	2.41	2.32	2.18	2.04	1.88	1.79	1.70	1.59	1.47	1.32	1.00

Table 28.2 F distribution tables (cont'd.) 95% probability (p = 0.05)

df Numerator	1	2	3	4	5	6	7	8	9	10	12	15	20	24	30	40	60	120	∞
1	161.4	199.5	215.7	224.6	230.2	234.0	236.8	238.9	240.5	241.9	243.9	245.9	248.0	249.1	250.1	251.1	252.2	253.3	254.3
2	18.51	19.00	19.16	19.25	19.30	19.33	19.35	19.37	19.38	19.40	19.41	19.43	19.45	19.45	19.46	19.47	19.48	19.49	19.50
3	10.13	9.55	9.28	9.12	9.01	8.94	8.89	8.85	8.81	8.79	8.74	8.70	8.66	8.64	8.62	8.59	8.57	8.55	8.53
4	7.71	6.94	6.59	6.39	6.26	6.16	6.09	6.04	6.00	5.96	5.91	5.86	5.80	5.77	5.75	5.72	5.69	5.66	5.63
5	6.61	5.79	5.41	5.19	5.05	4.95	4.88	4.82	4.77	4.74	4.68	4.62	4.56	4.53	4.50	4.46	4.43	4.40	4.36
6	5.99	5.14	4.76	4.53	4.39	4.28	4.21	4.15	4.10	4.06	4.00	3.94	3.87	3.84	3.81	3.77	3.74	3.70	3.67
7	5.59	4.74	4.35	4.12	3.97	3.87	3.79	3.73	3.68	3.64	3.57	3.51	3.44	3.41	3.38	3.34	3.30	3.27	3.23
8	5.32	4.46	4.07	3.84	3.69	3.58	3.50	3.44	3.39	3.35	3.28	3.22	3.15	3.12	3.08	3.04	3.01	2.97	2.93
9	5.12	4.26	3.86	3.63	3.48	3.37	3.29	3.23	3.18	3.14	3.07	3.01	2.94	2.90	2.86	2.83	2.79	2.75	2.71

Table 28.2 F distribution tables (cont'd.) 95% probability (p = 0.05)—cont'd

df Numerator							df Numerator											
1	2	3	4	5	6	7	8	9	10	12	15	20	24	30	40	60	120	∞
161.4	199.5	215.7	224.6	230.2	234.0	236.8	238.9	240.5	241.9	243.9	245.9	248.0	249.1	250.1	251.1	252.2	253.3	254.3
18.51	19.00	19.16	19.25	19.30	19.33	19.35	19.37	19.38	19.40	19.41	19.43	19.45	19.45	19.46	19.47	19.48	19.49	19.50
10.13	9.55	9.28	9.12	9.01	8.94	8.89	8.85	8.81	8.79	8.74	8.70	8.66	8.64	8.62	8.59	8.57	8.55	8.53
7.71	6.94	6.59	6.39	6.26	6.16	6.09	6.04	6.00	5.96	5.91	5.86	5.80	5.77	5.75	5.72	5.69	5.66	5.63
6.61	5.79	5.41	5.19	5.05	4.95	4.88	4.82	4.77	4.74	4.68	4.62	4.56	4.53	4.50	4.46	4.43	4.40	4.36
5.99	5.14	4.76	4.53	4.39	4.28	4.21	4.15	4.10	4.06	4.00	3.94	3.87	3.84	3.81	3.77	3.74	3.70	3.67
5.59	4.74	4.35	4.12	3.97	3.87	3.79	3.73	3.68	3.64	3.57	3.51	3.44	3.41	3.38	3.34	3.30	3.27	3.23
5.32	4.46	4.07	3.84	3.69	3.58	3.50	3.44	3.39	3.35	3.28	3.22	3.15	3.12	3.08	3.04	3.01	2.97	2.93
5.12	4.26	3.86	3.63	3.48	3.37	3.29	3.23	3.18	3.14	3.07	3.01	2.94	2.90	2.86	2.83	2.79	2.75	2.71
4.96	4.10	3.71	3.48	3.33	3.22	3.14	3.07	3.02	2.98	2.91	2.85	2.77	2.74	2.70	2.66	2.62	2.58	2.54
4.84	3.98	3.59	3.36	3.20	3.09	3.01	2.95	2.90	2.85	2.79	2.72	2.65	2.61	2.57	2.53	2.49	2.45	2.40
4.75	3.89	3.49	3.26	3.11	3.00	2.91	2.85	2.80	2.75	2.69	2.62	2.54	2.51	2.47	2.43	2.38	2.34	2.30
4.67	3.81	3.41	3.18	3.03	2.92	2.83	2.77	2.71	2.67	2.60	2.53	2.46	2.42	2.38	2.34	2.30	2.25	2.21
4.60	3.74	3.34	3.11	2.96	2.85	2.76	2.70	2.65	2.60	2.53	2.46	2.39	2.35	2.31	2.27	2.22	2.18	2.13
4.54	3.68	3.29	3.06	2.90	2.79	2.71	2.64	2.59	2.54	2.48	2.40	2.33	2.29	2.25	2.20	2.16	2.11	2.07
4.49	3.63	3.24	3.01	2.85	2.74	2.66	2.59	2.54	2.49	2.42	2.35	2.28	2.24	2.19	2.15	2.11	2.06	2.01
4.45	3.59	3.20	2.96	2.81	2.70	2.61	2.55	2.49	2.45	2.38	2.31	2.23	2.19	2.15	2.10	2.06	2.01	1.96
4.41	3.55	3.16	2.93	2.77	2.66	2.58	2.51	2.46	2.41	2.34	2.27	2.19	2.15	2.11	2.06	2.02	1.97	1.92
4.38	3.52	3.13	2.90	2.74	2.63	2.54	2.48	2.42	2.38	2.31	2.23	2.16	2.11	2.07	2.03	1.98	1.93	1.88
4.35	3.49	3.10	2.87	2.71	2.60	2.51	2.45	2.39	2.35	2.28	2.20	2.12	2.08	2.04	1.99	1.95	1.90	1.84
4.32	3.47	3.07	2.84	2.68	2.57	2.49	2.42	2.37	2.32	2.25	2.18	2.10	2.05	2.01	1.96	1.92	1.87	1.81
4.30	3.44	3.05	2.82	2.66	2.55	2.46	2.40	2.34	2.30	2.23	2.15	2.07	2.03	1.98	1.94	1.89	1.84	1.78

df Numerator (row labels): 1, 2, 3, 4, 5, 6, 7, 8, 9, 10, 11, 12, 13, 14, 15, 16, 17, 18, 19, 20, 21, 22

Table 28.2 F distribution tables (cont'd.) 95% probability (p = 0.05)—cont'd

df Numerator	1	2	3	4	5	6	7	8	9	10	12	15	20	24	30	40	60	120	∞
23	4.28	3.42	3.03	2.80	2.64	2.53	2.44	2.37	2.32	2.27	2.20	2.13	2.05	2.01	1.96	1.91	1.86	1.81	1.76
24	4.26	3.40	3.01	2.78	2.62	2.51	2.42	2.36	2.30	2.25	2.18	2.11	2.03	1.98	1.94	1.89	1.84	1.79	1.73
25	4.24	3.39	2.99	2.76	2.60	2.49	2.40	2.34	2.28	2.24	2.16	2.09	2.01	1.96	1.92	1.87	1.82	1.77	1.71
26	4.23	3.37	2.98	2.74	2.59	2.47	2.39	2.32	2.27	2.22	2.15	2.07	1.99	1.95	1.90	1.85	1.80	1.75	1.69
27	4.21	3.35	2.96	2.73	2.57	2.46	2.37	2.31	2.25	2.20	2.13	2.06	1.97	1.93	1.88	1.84	1.79	1.73	1.67
28	4.20	3.34	2.95	2.71	2.56	2.45	2.36	2.29	2.24	2.19	2.12	2.04	1.96	1.91	1.87	1.82	1.77	1.71	1.65
29	4.18	3.33	2.93	2.70	2.55	2.43	2.35	2.28	2.22	2.18	2.10	2.03	1.94	1.90	1.85	1.81	1.75	1.70	1.64
30	4.17	3.32	2.92	2.69	2.53	2.42	2.33	2.27	2.21	2.16	2.09	2.01	1.93	1.89	1.84	1.79	1.74	1.68	1.62
40	4.08	3.23	2.84	2.61	2.45	2.34	2.25	2.18	2.12	2.08	2.00	1.92	1.84	1.79	1.74	1.69	1.64	1.58	1.51
60	4.00	3.15	2.76	2.53	2.37	2.25	2.17	2.10	2.04	1.99	1.92	1.84	1.75	1.70	1.65	1.59	1.53	1.47	1.39
120	3.92	3.07	2.68	2.45	2.29	2.17	2.09	2.02	1.96	1.91	1.83	1.75	1.66	1.61	1.55	1.50	1.43	1.35	1.25
∞	3.84	3.00	2.60	2.37	2.21	2.10	2.01	1.94	1.88	1.83	1.75	1.67	1.57	1.52	1.45	1.39	1.32	1.22	1.00

the 1st stop. With the tip well below the surface of the specimen, release the plunger to fill the tip with blood. Withdraw the pipette from the specimen, wipe the outside of the tip carefully with a tissue, dip the tip into the diluent well below the surface, and press the plunger knob repeatedly to fill and empty the tip until the interior wall is clear. Then depress the plunger to the 2nd stop to empty the tip completely.

11. At intervals, monitor the reliability of the pipette by checking its accuracy and precision.

Quality control of pipette reliability involves the following:

1. Ensure that all the items to be used are at ambient room temperature.
2. Record the weight of a weighing beaker using a precision balance sensitive to 0.1 mg.
3. Record the temperature of a tube of distilled water, fill the pipette with the water, wipe the outside of the tip, and dispense the water into the weighing beaker with the tip touching the side of the beaker.
4. Record the weight of the beaker plus water and calculate the weight of the water.
5. Calculate the volume (in μl) from the weight (in mg) ÷ the ambient temperature factor (Table 28.3).
6. Repeat the procedure ten times, changing the tip each time.
7. Calculate the mean, SD, and CV of the dispensed volume. From the mean, calculate the percentage deviation from the expected volume by the formula:

$$\frac{\text{Expected volume} - \text{Delivered volume}}{\text{Expected volume}} \times 100.$$

For routine purposes, this should not differ by more than 1.5%. The CV should be <1%.

AUTODILUTERS

Autodiluter systems provide a constant dilution of blood in reagent by a single process. To check their accuracy, a calibrated 0.2 ml pipette and 50 ml volumetric flask are required. Equipment certified as conforming to these measurements in accordance with national standards is available commercially, or their accuracy can be checked by the procedure described above.

Mix well a 2–3 ml specimen of fresh whole blood and lyse (see p. 281). Then dilute manually 1:251 in haemiglobincyanide reagent (see p. 27) using the calibrated pipette and volumetric flask. At the same time, dilute a sample of the blood in haemiglobincyanide solution, in duplicate, by means of the autodiluter. Read the absorbance of each solution at 540 nm in a spectrophotometer. The dilution by the autodiluter is obtained from the formula:

$$A_1 \times \frac{\text{dilution (i.e., 1:251)}}{A_2}$$

where A_1 = absorbance at 540 nm of manual dilution and A_2 = absorbance at 540 nm of autodiluted sample.

If indicated, an appropriate adjustment should be made to the autodiluter in accordance with the manufacturer's instructions or a correction factor should be applied whenever the autodiluter is used.

Table 28.3 Ambient temperature factor for correction of weight:volume ratio

Temp (°C)	Volume factor
18	0.9986
19	0.9984
20	0.9982
21	0.9980
22	0.9978
23	0.9976
24	0.9973
25	0.9971
26	0.9968
27	0.9965
28	0.9963
29	0.9960
30	0.9957

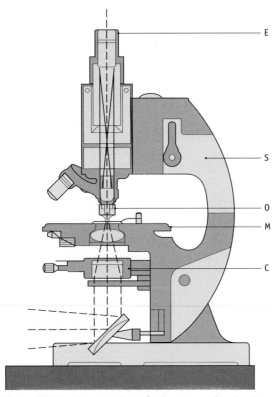

Figure 28.2 Cross-section of microscope, showing its components. E, eyepiece; S, stand; O, objective; M, mechanical stage; C, condenser. The broken lines indicate the light path. Note that this shows an external light source being directed into the microscope. In most modern microscopes there is an built-in lamp in the base.

MICROSCOPY

Microscope Components

The main components of most routine microscopes are illustrated in Figure 28.2. The objectives are usually marked with their magnifying power, but older lenses may be marked by their focal length instead. The approximate equivalents are as follows:

Focal length (mm)	Magnification
2	×100
4	×40
16	×10
40	×4

The working distance of the objective is the distance between the objective and the object to be visualised. The greater the magnifying power of the objective, the smaller the working distance:

Objective	Working distance
×10	5–6 mm
×40	0.5–1.5 mm
×100	0.15–0.20 mm

These specifications mean that when a coverglass is used, if it is too thick it will not be possible to focus at high magnification. Thus, the coverglass should be no more than 0.15 mm thick for examination of covered preparations by the ×100 oil-immersion. Furthermore, if the glass slide is too thick, this may prevent correct focus of the light path through the condenser to the object, as described later.

Setting Up the Microscope Illumination

1. If the microscope requires an external light source, using the mirror at the base direct the light into the condenser. If the illumination is built in, make sure that the lamp voltage is turned down before switching on the microscope; then turn up the lamp until it is c 70% of maximum power.
2. Place a slide of a blood film with a coverglass on the stage.
3. Lower the condenser, open the iris diaphragm fully, and bring the preparation on the slide into focus with the ×10 objective.
4. Check that the eyepieces are adjusted to the operator's interpupillary width and that the specimen is in focus for each eye by rotating the focusing mechanism on the adjustable eyepiece.
5. Close the diaphragm and raise the condenser slowly until the edge of the circle of light comes into sharp focus.
6. Using the condenser centering screws, adjust its position so that the circle of light is in the centre of the field.
7. Open the diaphragm completely so that light fills the whole field of view.
8. Remove the eyepieces, so that the upper lens of the objective is seen to be filled with a circle of

light. Close the diaphragm slowly until the circle of light occupies about two-thirds of the surface.

9. Replace the eyepieces, refocus the specimen, and if necessary readjust the condenser aperture and lamp brightness to obtain the sharpest possible image.

Examination of Slides

Low power (×10). Start with the objective just above the slide preparation. Then raise the objective with the coarse adjustment screw until a clear image is seen in the eyepiece. If there is insufficient illumination, rack up the condenser slightly.

High power (×40). Rack the condenser halfway down; lower the objective until it is just above the slide preparation. Use the coarse adjustment to raise the objective very slowly until a blurred image appears. Then bring into focus using the fine adjustment. If necessary, raise the condenser to obtain sufficient illumination.

Oil immersion (×100). Place a small drop of immersion oil on the part to be examined. Rack up the condenser as far as it will go. Lower the objective until it is in contact with the oil. Bring it as close as possible to the slide, but avoid pressing on the preparation. Look through the eyepiece and turn the fine adjustment very slowly until the image is in focus.

After using the oil-immersion objective, to avoid scratching the lens or coating the ×40 lens with oil, first swing the ×10 objective (or an empty lens space on the nosepiece) into place before removing the slide. As far as possible, use oil only when essential (e.g., for determining malaria species), and examine blood films for morphology or differential leucocyte count with the ×40 lens without oil.

ROUTINE MAINTENANCE OF MICROSCOPE

The microscope is a delicate instrument that must be handled gently. It must be installed in a clean environment away from chemicals, direct sunlight, heating source, or moisture. If the stage is contaminated with saline, it must be cleaned immediately to avoid corrosion. Even in a temperate climate humidity and high temperatures cause growth of fungus, which can damage optical surfaces. Because storage in a closed compartment encourages fungal growth, do not store it in its wooden box, but keep it standing on the bench protected by a light plastic cover.

After use of optics, wipe the immersion objective with lens tissue, absorbent paper, soft cloth, or medical cotton wool. If other lenses are smeared with oil, wipe them with a little toluene or a solution of 40% petroleum ether, 40% ethanol, and 20% ether.

Lenses must never be soaked in alcohol because this may dissolve the cement.

Clean nonoptical parts with mild detergent and remove grease or oil with petroleum ether, followed by 45% ethanol in water. Remove dust from the inside and outside of the eyepieces with a blower or soft camel-hair brush.

Clean the condenser in the same way as the lenses with a soft cloth or tissue moistened with toluene, and clean the mirror (if present) with a soft cloth moistened with 5% alcohol. The iris diaphragm is very delicate, and if damaged or badly corroded it is usually beyond repair.

Never force the controls. If movement of the focusing screws or mechanical stage becomes difficult, lubricate them with a small drop of machine oil. All accessible moving parts should be cleaned occasionally and given a touch of oil to protect against corrosion. Do not use vegetable oils because they become dry and hard. Always keep the surface of the fixed stage dry because moving wet slides requires increased force, which may damage the mechanical stage.

Hot, Humid Climates

In hot, humid climates, if no precautions are taken, fungus may develop on the microscope—particularly on the surface of the lenses, in the grooves of the screws, and under the paint—and the instrument will soon be useless. This can be prevented as follows.

Every evening fit the microscope into an airtight dust cover together with silica gel. When necessary, dry the silica out and reuse it. An alternative method is to place the microscope in a warm cupboard. This is a cupboard with a tight-fitting door, heated by a 40-watt light bulb. Check that the temperature inside the cupboard is at least 5°C warmer than that of the laboratory, but take care that it does not overheat.

Hot, Dry Climates

In hot, dry climates, the main problem is dust. Fine particles work their way into the threads of the screws and under the lenses. This can be avoided as follows:

1. Always keep the microscope under a dustproof plastic cover when not in use.
2. At the end of the day's work, clean the microscope thoroughly by blowing air on it from a rubber bulb.
3. Finish cleaning the lenses with a lens brush or fine paintbrush. If dust particles remain on the surface of the objectives, remove with clean paper.

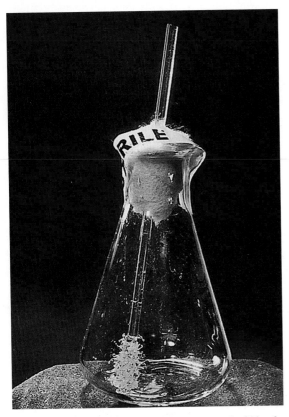

Figure 28.3   Flask for defibrinating 10–50 ml of blood. The glass rod has had some small pieces of drawn-out glass capillary fused to its lower end.

DEFIBRINATING BLOOD

To obtain unclotted red cells without adding an anticoagulant (e.g., for the investigation of certain types of haemolytic anaemia) the sample can be defibrinated. This can be performed by placing the blood in a receiver such as a conical flask containing a central glass rod on to which small pieces of glass capillary have been fused (Fig. 28.3). The blood is whisked around the central rod by moderately rapid rotation of the flask. Coagulation is usually complete within 5 min, with most of the fibrin collecting on the central rod. When fibrin formation seems complete, the glass rod should be removed from the flask. The morphology of the red cells (and also the leucocytes) is well-preserved. If serum is also required, the defibrinated blood may be centrifuged and the serum can be obtained quickly and in relatively large volumes.

REFERENCES

1. Moore HC, Mollison PL 1976 Use of a low-ionic-strength medium in manual tests for antibody detection. Transfusion 16:291.
2. Hendry EB 1961 Osmolarity of human serum and of chemical solutions of biological importance. Clinical Chemistry 7:156.
3. World Health Organization 1977 The SI for the health professions. WHO, Geneva.

Index

Note: Italic page numbers refer to illustrations.